Neurosurgical Aspects of Craniosynostosis

Federico Di Rocco • John Kestle
Editors

Neurosurgical Aspects of Craniosynostosis

Springer

Editors
Federico Di Rocco
Pediatric Neurosurgery Department
Hôpital Femme Mère Enfant, French
Referral Center for Craniosynostosis
INSERM 1033
Lyon, France

John Kestle
Department of Neurosurgery
University of Utah
Salt Lake City, UT, USA

ISBN 978-3-031-69388-5 ISBN 978-3-031-69386-1 (eBook)
https://doi.org/10.1007/978-3-031-69386-1

This Springer imprint is published by the registered company Springer Nature Switzerland AG
The registered company address is: Gewerbestrasse 11, 6330 Cham, Switzerland

Preface

Cranial artificial deformation has accompanied the human race for thousands of years. The history of the surgical correction of congenital or acquired cranial deformities is considerably shorter, extending for little more than a century. Though commonly associated with the Andean civilisation, the practice of artificial cranial deformation may be encountered in the history of various populations in all continents. The aim of such practice has been extensively discussed by historians and anthropologists. For what concerns the Andean people, the common belief is that the artificial alteration of the cranial shape was utilised to distinguish ethnic differences among groups and in the same group to individuate castes, social classes and professions. The main goal of the surgical correction of craniosynostosis is just the opposite: to 'normalise' the altered cranial shape and prevent the affected subjects from suffering from the social stigma brought about by the physical deformity. We don't know much about the possible cognitive defects that the artificially restricted growth of the skull could have generated, but we are aware of the possible cerebral damage following an abnormally increased intracranial pressure, due to a decreased cranial volume, or distorted vectors of cerebral growth. The correction of such possible causes of cerebral damage is the main aim of the surgical management besides the normalisation of the head shape and the prevention of possible secondary morphologic and functional anomalies and justifies the current attention to provide the appropriate surgical correction carried out already in the first few months of life.

To operate a newborn requires several conditions to be met. First of all, the knowledge of the disease on the part of the family physician and the family itself. Then, the contribution of the paediatrician and the radiologist for a timely recognition. The neurosurgeon has also a role in the diagnosis, but they are called to have the necessary skills to operate the infant or the young child, or to be able to provide the best cranial reconstruction in case of delayed diagnosis.

Even though to a superficial analysis the surgical treatment of craniosynostosis seems to have come back from complex reconstruction with bone displacement and replacement which characterised the operative procedures in the end of the last century to the original linear craniectomies, a more thorough, deeper evaluation shows the great advances made in the management of craniosynostosis; advances made possible, as this book wants to demonstrate, thanks to the newly introduced diagnostic tools, refinements in anaesthesiological intraoperative care, extended and appropriate postoperative follow-ups as well as the acquisition of craniofacial surgical techniques.

Indeed, during recent years the knowledge of the pathophysiologic mechanisms leading to the early fusion of cranial sutures has substantially improved thanks to the genetic studies and the utilisation of animal models.

While different surgical techniques have blossomed, the risks associated with surgical and anaesthesiological manoeuvres have been reduced. New surgical tools have been developed allowing less-invasive procedures, especially in very young subjects. The long follow-up of a large series of patients has allowed clinicians to better appreciate the results and long-term outcomes and at the same time to recognize the still existing limits of the surgical treatment in terms of late recurrences or incomplete corrections leading to the necessity of redo-surgeries. Also some functional difficulties in operating on patients which burden the life of patients and their families have been identified and addressed.

Nevertheless, in spite of these relevant progresses in the understanding of craniosynostosis, most of the recent papers have been focusing on aesthetical results of the surgical management rather than the functional neurological issues. The neurosurgical aspects of the conditions have been little by little put aside with the studies focusing either on the length of the hospital stay and the costs of surgery or the cosmetic outcomes.

Because managing a craniosynostosis is more than correcting a cranial index, we wanted, with this book, to focus on the role of the neurosurgeon, and in the same time to raise the interest of all the specialists that form the team involved in the management of craniosynostosis on neurosurgical issues with the ultimate goal of enhancing its effectiveness for the best cure of our patients.

Lyon, France — Federico Di Rocco
Salt Lake City, UT, USA — John Kestle

Acknowledgement

We would like to acknowledge the contributions of Prof. David F. Jimenez MD, FACS, who passed away before his contributions to this book were published. Thanks to his work, "strip and helmet" has become a big part of the current management of craniosynostosis.

Contents

Part IV The Multidisciplinary Team and the Neurosurgeon

Part V Technical Aspects

Part I

Introduction

1 Historical Perspective on the Evolution of the Techniques and Controversies

Federico Di Rocco, Carmine Mottolese, and Ashwaq Al Nadabi

1.1 Introduction

The beginning of the history of the surgical management of craniosynostosis resembles a fairytale: *Once upon a time a mother noticed that her child's head did not grow as expected and asked a doctor to "unlock" its skull...* This event happened in real life when the French neurosurgeon accepted a mother's request and performed the first operation to release the skull of a child with sagittal craniosynostosis by carrying out two linear strip craniectomies in the parietal bone parallel to an early fused sagittal suture in 1890 [1] (Fig. 1.1).

The operation was successful and stimulated further surgical attempts to manage craniosynostosis surgically. Two years later, in San Francisco L C Lane responded again to a mother's desire: *Early in the month of August, 1888, I received a letter from a lady residing in the interior of California, stating that she desired to consult me concerning her infant, then nearly 9 months of age, which presented signs of mental imbecility. At the time appointed for the consultation, the lady presented herself with her infant. The child, otherwise in good health and well nourished, was decidedly microcephalic. The cranium was symmetrical, and only deviated from normal type in the smallness of its volume. The mother stated that at birth the anterior fontanelle was wholly closed, and the posterior one nearly so. The mother was especially solicitous to learn whether the child's brain was otherwise healthy; and on being assured that there was no evidence to the contrary, she asked if an operation were not possible whereby the brain could enlarge* [2]. Once

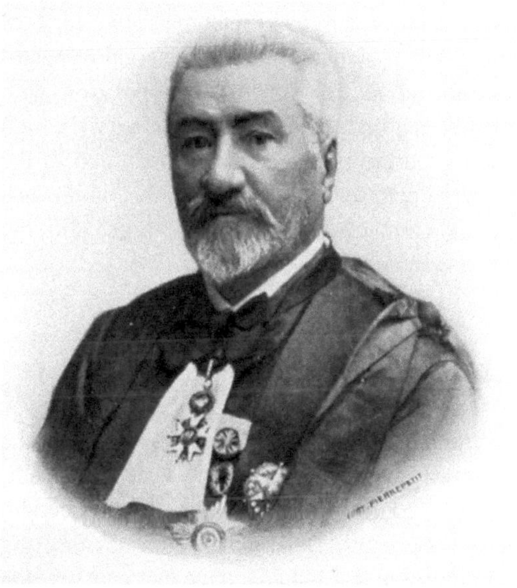

Fig. 1.1 Prof Odilon Lannelongue, 1840–1911

F. Di Rocco (✉) · C. Mottolese · A. Al Nadabi
Department of Pediatric Neurosurgery, French Referral Center for Craniosynostosis of Lyon, INSERM 1033, Université de Lyon, Hospices Civils de Lyon, Lyon, France
e-mail: federico.dirocco@chu-lyon.fr; carmine.mottolese@chu-lyon.fr; Ashwaq.Alnadabi@chu-lyon.fr

F. Di Rocco, J. Kestle (eds.), *Neurosurgical Aspects of Craniosynostosis*,
https://doi.org/10.1007/978-3-031-69386-1_1

more on a sagittal craniosynostosis Lane performed an operation similar to that of Lannelongue, that is strip parietal craniectomies, with, however, the removal of the fused sagittal suture. Consequently, the surgical management of craniosynostosis has been marked by technical controversy since its beginning! It is worth noting how the title of Lane's report translated an unappropriated enthusiasm as his operation was proposed "for relief of mental imbecility due to *the premature sutural closure and microcephalus*", thus likely contributing to possible operations on microcephalic children. The wrong surgical indication to treat microcephaly and the unsatisfactory surgical outcomes, the lack of improvement in patients with true craniosynostosis too old at the time of the operation with already established neurological deficits, the high rate of morbidity and mortality recorded in the pioneer operations arose deep doubts on the surgical attempt of "unlocking" the brain utilizing linear craniectomies.

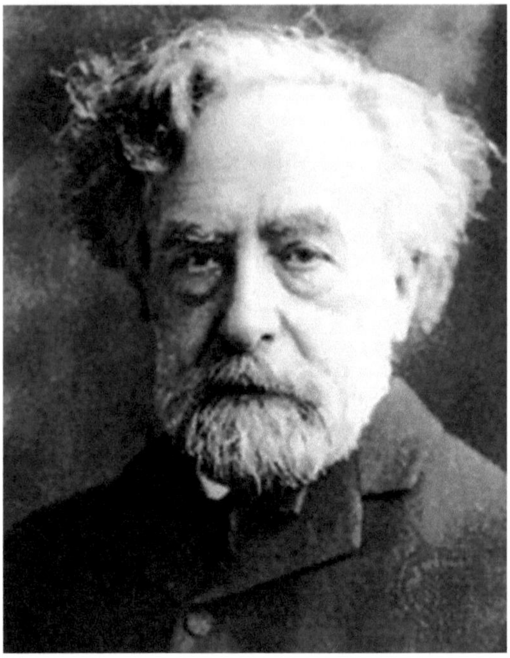

Fig. 1.2 Abraham Jacobi, 1830–1919

1.2 Non Nocere

Such doubts found their severe interpreter in the person of the founder of modern American paediatrics Abraham Jacobi who blamed the procedure at an American Academy of Pediatrics meeting held in Rome in 1894 and in a paper entitled *Non nocere* [3] (Fig. 1.2).

On the grounds of the analysis of a series of 33 children who had undergone linear craniectomies, 15 of them have died because of the operation, he criticized these early attempts to release the skull with vehement words: "The relative impunity of operative interference accomplished by modern asepsis and antisepsis has developed an undue tendency to, and rashness in, handling the knife. The hands take too frequently the place of brains…Is it sufficient glory to don a white apron and swing a carbonized knife, and is therein a sufficient indication to let daylight into a deformed cranium and on top of the hopelessly defective brain, and to proclaim a success because the victim consented not to die of the assault? Such rash feats of indiscriminate surgery…are stains on your hands and sins on your soul. No ocean of soap and water will clean those hands, no power of corrosive sublimate will disinfect the souls". Even though an atlas describing the various linear craniectomies was published in 1895 [4], the surgical treatment of craniosynostosis was practically abandoned for nearly three decades because of great Jacobi's influence Also some eminent neurosurgeons, like Cushing, contributed to the neurosurgeons' disinterest of treating craniosynostosis surgically at the beginning of the twntieth century, though, however, he operated on craniosynostosis children later on [5].

The paper by Faber and Towne on five children who responded favourably to the surgical "release" of the skull sutures when the correction was done early in infancy re-established the due attention of the effects of the premature fusion of the cranial sutures on the brain development so contributing to the return of linear craniectomy in the neurosurgical armamentarium [6].

The first surgical attempts to treat craniosynostosis by "releasing" the skull were based on pathogenetic interpretations of the role of the cranial sutures and the consequences of their early fusion on the cranial growth already propounded at the beginning of the nineteenth century when the German physician, anatomist, anthropologist and inventor Samuel Thomas von Soemmering had published important studies indicating the role of the cranial sutures in the active growth of the skull and had pointed out the effect of their premature fusion on skull growth and shape [7] (Fig. 1.3).

Another German scientist Rudolph Virchow is associated with the surgical management of craniosynostosis because of the so-called *law or rule of Virchow* which states that skull growth is arrested in the direction perpendicular to a fused suture while expanding at the sites of unaffected sutures, in a direction parallel to the fused suture leading to characteristic skull deformations on which the various types of craniosynostosis are still named (Fig. 1.4).

Craniosynostosis was considered by Virchow in a complex frame of malformed skull shapes in a quite influential paper *Über den Cretinismus, namentlich in Franken, und über pathologische Schädelformen* [8]. It is quite interesting reading about the great debate about the cause of mental retardation that took place in the second half of the nineteenth century in the absence of a clear disease definition, as described by Schlich in his paper *Changing disease identities: cretinism, politics and surgery (1844–1892)* [9].

The reinstatement of linear craniectomies and suturectomies for treating craniosynostosis and their diffusion in the 1930s and 1940s were mainly based on the assumption that an early release of the constricted skull, possibly carried out during the first 2 months of life, could prevent secondary damage of the developing brain and also decreasing the risk of re-ossification because of the expansive forces of the growing brain. Indeed, re-ossification of the linear craniectomies was observed to occur more frequently in older children. In the 50s, several methods were suggested in the attempts to prevent this type of failure from the mechanical obstacle created by enwrapping the cut bone edges with tantalum foils [10] or polyethylene films [11] and to the application of chemical agents, such as Zenker's solution, on the dura underlying the linear craniectomies to impair the osteoblastic activity of the outer layer of the dura mater [12]. Failures to pre-

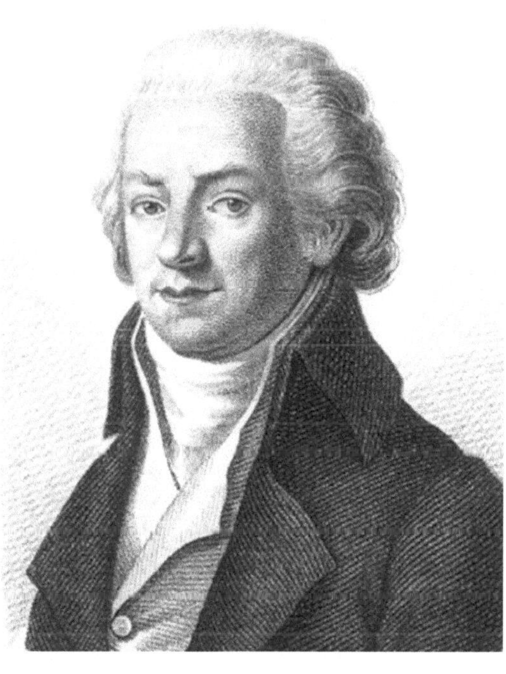

Fig. 1.3 Samuel Thomas Soemmering, 1755–1830

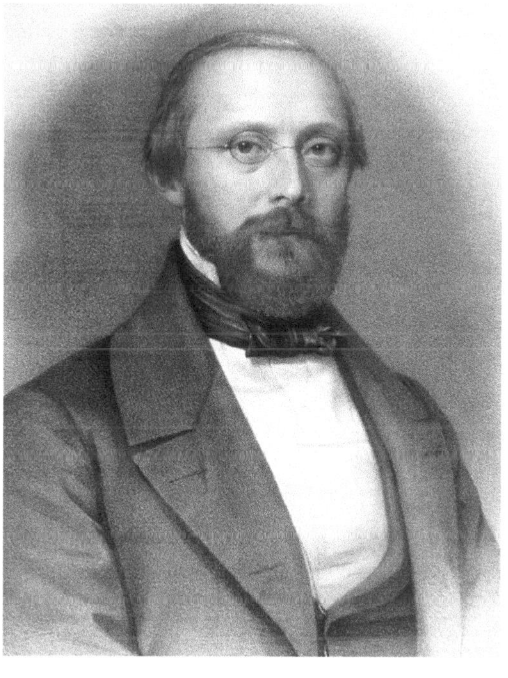

Fig. 1.4 Rudolph Virchow, 1821–1902

vent re-ossification and infective complications related to the foreign material led to the progressive abandonment of the attempts to block bone formation at the borders of the craniectomies. Also, the use of Zenker's solution, a tissue fixative containing mercuric chloride, potassium bichromate, sodium sulphate and glacial acetic acid, was suspended in the late 1970s and early 1980s after clinical reports of postoperative seizures in operated children and the experimental demonstration of the immediate breakdown of the blood–brain barrier and inflammatory response in the underlying brain with thickening of the arachnoid membrane, associated with the procedure, likely being the cause of the postoperative seizures [13–15].

In the second half of the twentieth century, linear craniectomies and suturectomies were widely performed on the grounds of clinical reports describing good results in large series of patients with low morbidity and mortality rate such as, for example, that by Shillito and Matson who recorded three deaths out of 519 operated on infants [16]. Linear craniectomies evolved in more complex surgical procedures aimed at correcting some specific deformations of the head associated with the craniosynostosis already at the time of the operation while assuring a better prevention of the secondary re-ossification. Most of the surgical variants concerned the management of sagittal synostosis such as a major widening of suturectomy, the enlargement of the restricted transverse diameters by out-fracturing the parietal bone after having performed additional suturectomy along the coronal and the lambdoid sutures, decreasing the resistance of the parietal bone with additional bone vertical cuttings or bone morcellation, maintaining the fractured parietal bones in the newly expanded position by interposing bone fragments at the level of the sagittal suturectomy, as well as addressing the frontal and occipital bossing [17–27]. All the newly introduced surgical techniques corresponded to the understanding that removing the fused suture was not sufficient and that it was necessary to manage also the abnormal compensatory calvarial growth that occurred at the level of the normal cranial sutures. In other words, it became clear that surgical management should not be limited to the "release" of the skull in the first months of life, necessary to correct the increased intracranial pressure and its possible effect on cognition, by profiting from the forces of the developing brain to normalize the cranial shape but that the operation also should have aimed at improving the child's cosmetic aspect. The improvement of the cosmetic aspects should have prevented the psychological consequences eventually related to self-estimation and acceptance by the social environment. The cosmetic indication was then accepted as a further criterion for the surgical indication justifying the more extended surgical corrections that had become possible for the concomitant improvement in anaesthesiology intraoperative assistance and in post-operative care.

1.3 The Functional Matrix

In the same years, a great debate was going on among orthodontists on the reciprocal influences of developmental anomalies of the face, skull base and cranial vault stimulated by the paper published in 1962 by Melvin Moss [28], and his numerous publications in the subsequent three decades [29–35] thatpropounded the so-called *functional matrix theory* [28] (Fig. 1.5).

The theory criticized the classic osteology the various bones of the skull and facies classically distinguished as specific entities with a pre-established pattern of growth suggesting that they had to be considered a series of segments related to a specific function and responding to specific functional demands during their development. Grossly, the theory could be simplified in the concept that bones do not grow but are grown in response to the growth and function of soft tissue matrices. The functional matrix, that is the soft tissue mass enclosed by bones to form a functional unit, elicits secondary growth responses by its corresponding skeletal unit. Functional matrices were individualized into two main types: periosteal matrices serving as the functional muscle/tendon attachments to skeletal units and capsular matrices enclosing a mass or volume within

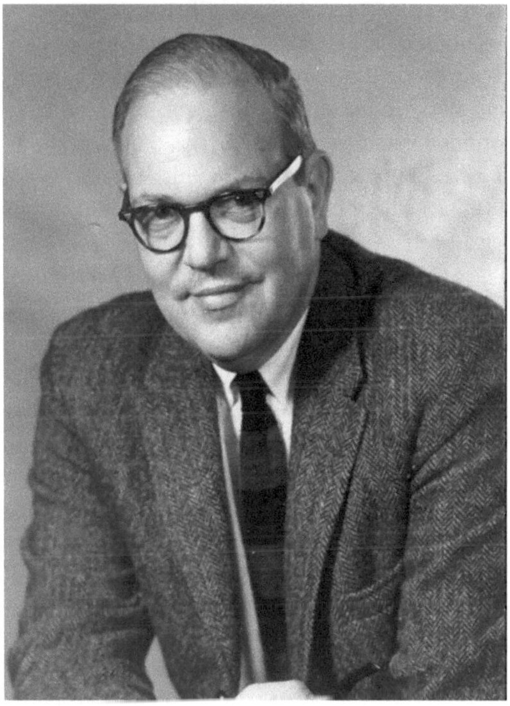

Fig. 1.5 Melvin Lionel Moss (1923–2006) (published under CC BY-SA 3.0)

a functional space. Anomalies of functional matrices, according to the theory, were responsible for abnormal bone growth, for example, the cranial alterations secondary to defects in neural mass [34]. The actual role of cranial sutures as an independent centre of bone formation, similar to the epiphyseal growth plates, was challenged on the grounds of several experimental observations, such as the possibility of halting their function by extrinsic mechanical strains or the lack of bone formation in subcutaneously transplanted sutures. Furthermore, clinical and experimental evidence proved that the growth of the cranial and facial bones could be determined by extrinsic factors as demonstrated by the vertical growth of the facies and the skull in children with respiratory problems or the unilateral hypo development of the maxillar and mandibular bone induced by the homolateral muscle palsy obtained by the unilateral sectioning of the facial nerve in perinatal rabbits [36–38].

To summarize: (1) The neurocranial capsular matrix, which is an enclosure having contents that exert pressure, is the basic component of cranial growth which in turn stimulates compensatory growth of its skeletal unit. (2) Neuronal function and peripheral innervation appear crucial for normal craniofacial development. (3) In ontogenesis, genomic (intrinsic, prior) and epigenetic (extrinsic, proximate) factors are each a necessary cause, but neither alone is sufficient as only the interaction of both provides both the necessary and sufficient causes of morphogenesis.

Though still debated, the concepts originated by Moss's theory influenced the neurosurgeon to develop new strategies beyond the mere opening of the cranial sutures and eventually to elaborate pluri-stage surgical methodologies to face the more complex forms of craniofacial stenosis, considered as inoperable for a long time. Multi-stage operations offered the possibility to offer the infant with complex craniosynostosis an early protection of the developing brain with a reasonable surgical risk, controlling the intracranial pressure and assuring space for the growth of the brain prior to taking care of the cosmetic problem at a later age.

1.4 The Modern Craniofacial Era

In the late 60s and 70s, Paul Tessier, and his colleague neurosurgeon Gerard Guiot marked a significant step in the treatment of craniofacial malformation introducing new surgical procedures for craniofacial reconstruction that influenced the plastic and maxillofacial surgeons and impacted on the neurosurgeons as well (Fig. 1.6).

Tessier's innovative techniques led to the creation of a new subspecialty, namely craniofacial surgery. Patients with complex facio-craniosynostoses, once considered inoperable, could finally be treated with new surgical procedures with rewarding results [39]. Autologous bone grafts and bone substitutes became increasingly utilized and new instruments to bend and shape the bone grafts were progressively introduced [40–42].

As an effect of Tessier's contribution craniofacial surgeons were increasingly participating in

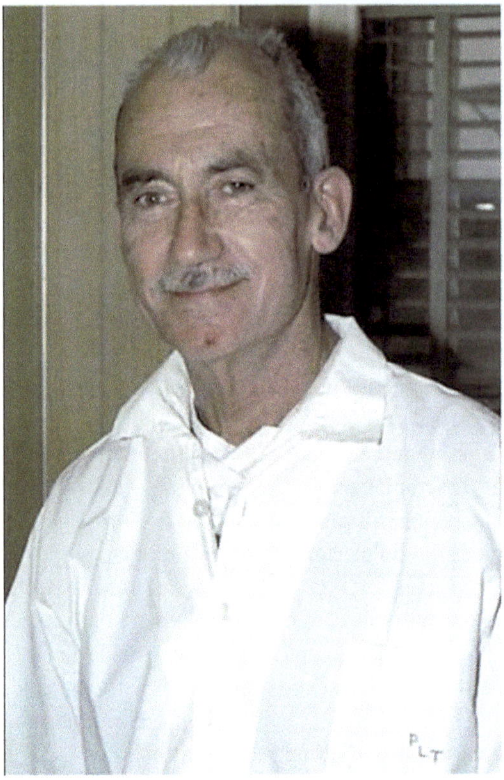

Fig. 1.6 Paul Tessier (1917–2008)

surgical teams involved in the treatment of the most severe forms of craniosynostosis though neurosurgeons remained the essential components dealing with the calvarial reconstruction, the safety of the underlying meninges and the management of the neurological disturbances associated to craniosynostosis, namely hydrocephalus and Chiari type 1 anomaly. On the other hand, the neurosurgeon became acquainted with techniques that utilize autologous calvarial bone grafts or bone substitutes and the manipulation/dislocation/repositioning of the calvarial bones for both increasing the intracranial volume and correcting the cranial dysmorphia. In this direction, several techniques have been proposed since the 70s, especially for the immediate reconstruction of the frontal region and the orbit in simple craniosynostoses. The lateral canthal advancement of the supraorbital margin in unilateral coronal synostosis was introduced by Hoffman and Mohr with an explicit reference to Tessier's technique "The facility with which the supraorbital margin could be mobilized in Tessier's method of craniofacial repair suggested to us that we could easily modify our approach to coronal synostosis and advance the supraorbital margin, creating an artificial suture at the base of the skull and allowing for proper correction of this disorder" [43, 44] and widely utilized. Technical modifications have been proposed in the subsequent years such as, for example, the fronto-orbital advancement using an en bloc frontal bone craniectomy [45] or the reconstruction of the frontal region using reverse frontal bone graft without the use of an orbital bar [46]. Fronto-orbital advancement has been also widely utilized to correct the metopic synostosis associating the creation and correction of a fronto-orbital bar, prepared according to Tessier's and Marchac's principles [47] and repositioned in a more anterior position with advancement, remodelling and rotation of the frontal bone, in one or two pieces [48]. Also, for the correction of metopic craniosynostosis several technical variants have been proposed [49–51]. At the end of the twentieth century, the fronto-orbital and facial monobloc advancement started to utilize the osteogenic property of the external dura mater with temporary or internal distractors device which allowed higher degrees of anterior dislocation of the cranial vault [52].

Posterior cranial vault expansion was introduced to increase the skull volume available for cerebral growth, decrease intracranial pressure, counteract the evolution towards turricephaly and prevent or at least diminish the impact of secondary cerebellar tonsils descent in syndromic and non-syndromic coronal or bi-lambdoid synostosis [53–57]. Nowadays, the procedure is frequently adopted as the initial treatment of syndromic complex craniosynostosis in order to postpone the fronto-orbital advancement. Also, for the posterior cranial vault, the introduction of osteogenic distraction resulted in more favourable and long-lasting outcomes. The introduction of resorbable distractors contributed to the current wide use of this type of procedure avoiding the necessity of a second operation to remove the distraction devices [58]. One of the major limits of the just described techniques was the morbidity associated with the external manipulation of the distraction devices, besides the child's discomfort and the possibility of infective complications.

All the above-described techniques are gratified by results that were not possible in the previous years. However, they are weighted by the major surgical risk of mortality and morbidity. It is not surprising that the introduction of the device that did not need external manipulation such as the internal springs devised by Claes Lauritzen [59] with the goal of assuring a dynamic force acting on the margins of the osteotomies is able to maintain the anatomical correction of the malformed skull beyond the operation matching with the natural growth of the child [60]. The obvious limit of the technique is again the necessity of a second operation for the removal of the spring-mediated distractors.

Cranial reconstruction with calvarial remodelling, fronto-orbital advancement and prolonged osteogenic distraction has certainly met the expectancy of families and patients for excellent functional and cosmetic outcomes, nevertheless, they are relatively severe surgical procedures with associated mortality and morbidity that seem to be not justified in simple craniosynostosis. Hence, the return to linear craniectomies currently carried out in very young infants with minimal scalp incisions [61, 62], the aid of endoscopy and postoperative moulding helmet mostly in sagittal synostosis but also anterior plagiocephaly and trigonocephaly [63–68]. The effective advantages of this minimal approach in terms of late outcome are currently under evaluation [69–71].

To conclude, at first sight the surgical evolution of craniosynostosis surgery from the early strip craniectomies to the complete calvarial remodelling and now minimally invasive surgical interventions seems to have come full circle. However, during such a journey a deep understanding of the disease has been reached with the possibility to select the most appropriate surgical procedure. The technical instrumentation has been enriched considerably and the intraoperative and postoperative care greatly improved. In this evolution, the neurosurgeon has not been alone but accompanied by ever-enlarging teams involving several surgical and medical specialists: anaesthesiologists, maxilla-facial surgeons, plastic surgeons, radiologists, ophthalmologists, otolaryngologists, paediatricians, geneticists, neurologists, dentists, psychologists, speech therapists, social workers…and families.

References

1. Lannelongue M. De la craniectomie dans la microcéphalie. Compt Rend Seances Acad Sci. 1890;50:1382–5.
2. Lane LC. Pioneer craniectomy for relief of mental imbecility due to premature sutural closure and microcephalus. JAMA. 1892;18:49–50.
3. Jacobi A. Non nocere. Med Rec. 1894;45:609–18.
4. Dennis FS, editor. System of surgery, vol. 1. Philadelphia: Lea Brothers; 1895.
5. Maher CO, Buchman SR, O'Hara E, Cohen-Gadol AA. Harvey Cushing's experience with cranial deformity. Neurosurg Focus. 2010;29(6):E6. https://doi.org/10.3171/2010.9.FOCUS10191.
6. Faber HK, Towne EB. Early craniectomy as a preventive measure in oxycephaly and allied conditions with special reference to the prevention of blindness. Am J Med Sci. 1927;173:701–11.
7. Von Soemmerring ST. Vom Bau des menschlichen Körpers (Frankfurt am Main 1791–96, 6 Bde.; 2. Aufl. 1800; neue Aufl. von Bischoff, Henle u. a., Leipzig 1839–45, 8 Bde.
8. Virchow R. Über den Cretinismus, namentlich in Franken, und über pathologische Schädelformen. Verh Phys Med Gesell Wurzburg. 1851;2:230–71.
9. Schlich T. Changing disease identities: cretinism, politics and surgery (1844-1892). Med Hist. 1994;38(4):421–43. https://doi.org/10.1017/s0025727300036929.
10. Simmons DR, Peyton WT. Premature closure of the cranial sutures. J Pediatr. 1947;31:528–47.
11. Ingraham FD, Alexander E Jr, Matson DD. Clinical studies in craniosynostosis analysis of 50 cases and description of a method of surgical treatment. Surgery. 1948;24:518–41.
12. Anderson FM, Johnson FL. Craniosynostosis; a modification in surgical treatment. Surgery. 1956;40:961–70.
13. Sugar O, Pawl RP. Dural application of Zenker's solution. Neurosurgery. 1980;6(6):729. https://doi.org/10.1097/00006123-198006000-00020.
14. Marlin AE, Brown WE Jr, Huntington HW, Epstein F. Effect of the dural application of Zenker's solution on the feline brain. Neurosurgery. 1980;6:45–8.
15. McComb JG, Withers GJ, Davis RL. Cortical damage from Zenker's solution applied to the dura mater. Neurosurgery. 1981;8(1):68–71. https://doi.org/10.1227/00006123-198101000-00013.

16. Shillito J Jr, Matso DD. Craniosynostosis: a review of 519 surgical patients. Pediatrics. 1968;41(4):829–53.
17. Venes JL, Sayers MP. Sagittal synostectomy. Technical note. J Neurosurg. 1976;44:390–2.
18. Stein SC, Schut L. Management of scaphocephaly. Surg Neurol. 1977;7:153–5.
19. Jane JA, Edgerton MT, Futrell JW, Park TS. Immediate correction of sagittal synostosis. J Neurosurg. 1978;49:705–10.
20. Epstein N, Epstein F, Newman G. Total vertex craniectomy for the treatment of scaphocephaly. Childs Brain. 1982;9:309–16.
21. Vollmer DG, Jane JA, Park TS, Persing JA. Variants of sagittal synostosis: strategies for surgical correction. J Neurosurg. 1984;61:557–62.
22. Persing JA, Nichter LS, Jane JA, Edgerton MT Jr. External cranial vault molding after craniofacial surgery. Ann Plast Surg. 1986;17:274–83.
23. Greene CS Jr, Winston KR. Treatment of scaphocephaly with sagittal craniectomy and biparietal morcellation. Neurosurgery. 1988;23:196–202.
24. Delashaw JB, Persing JA, Broaddus WC, Jane JA. Cranial vault growth in craniosynostosis. J Neurosurg. 1989;70:159–65.
25. Goodrich JT. Craniofacial reconstruction for craniosynostosis. In: Goodrich JT, Post KD, Argamaso RV, editors. Plastic techniques in neurosurgery. New York: Thieme; 1991. p. 75–108.
26. Di Rocco C. Surgical management of craniosynostosis and craniofacial deformities. In: Schmidek HH, Sweet WH, editors. Operative neurosurgical techniques: indications, methods, and results, vol. 2. 3rd ed. Philadelphia: Saunders; 1995. p. 135–48.
27. Mehta VA, Bettegowda C, Jallo GI, Ahn ES. The evolution of surgical management for craniosynostosis. Neurosurg Focus. 2010;29(6):E5.
28. Moss ML. The functional matrix. In: Kraus BS, Riedel R, editors. Vistas in orthodontics. Philadelphia: Lea & Febiger; 1962. p. 85–98.
29. Moss ML, Greenberg SN. Functional cranial analysis of the human maxillary bone: I, basal bone. Angle Orthod. 1967;37:151–61.
30. Moss ML, Rankow RM. The role of the functional matrix in mandibular growth. Angle Orthod. 1968;38:95–103.
31. Moss ML, Salentijn L. The primary role of functional matrices in facial growth. Am J Orthod. 1969;55:566–5.
32. Moss ML, Salentijn L. The capsular matrix. Am J Orthod. 1969;56:474–90.
33. Moss ML. Twenty years of functional cranial analysis. Am J Orthod. 1972;61:479–85.
34. Moss ML. Experimental alteration of basisynchondrosal cartilage growth in rat and mouse. In: Bosma JF, editor. Development of the basicranium. Bethesda: U.S. Department of Health, Education, and Welfare; 1976. p. 541–75.
35. Moss-Salentijn L, Melvin L. Moss and the functional matrix. J Dent Res. 1997;76:1814–7.
36. Pawłowska-Seredyńska K, Umławska W, Resler K, Morawska-Kochman M, Pazdro-Zastawny K, Kręcicki T. Craniofacial proportions in children with adenoid or adenotonsillar hypertrophy are related to disease duration and nasopharyngeal obstruction. Int J Pediatr Otorhinolaryngol. 2020;132:109911.
37. Chambi-Rocha A, Cabrera-Domínguez ME, Domínguez-Reyes A. Breathing mode influence on craniofacial development and head posture. J Pediatr. 2018;94(2):123–30.
38. Calvo-Henríquez C, Martins-Neves S, Faraldo-García A, Ruano-Ravina A, Rocha S, Mayo-Yáñez M, Martinez-Capoccioni G. Are pediatricians and otolaryngologists well prepared to identify early signs of vertical facial growth. Int J Pediatr Otorhinolaryngol. 2019;119:161–5.
39. Tessier P. The definitive plastic surgical treatment of the severe facial deformities of craniofacial dysostosis. Crouzon's and Apert's diseases. Plast Reconstr Surg. 1971;48:419–42.
40. Tessier P, Kawamoto H, Matthews D, Posnick J, Raulo Y, Tulasne JF, et al. Autogenous bone grafts and bone substitutes—tools and techniques: I. A 20,000-case experience in maxillofacial and craniofacial surgery. Plast Reconstr Surg. 2005;116(5 Suppl):6S–24S.
41. Tessier P. Relationship of craniostenoses to craniofacial dysostoses, and to faciostenoses: a study with therapeutic implications. Plast Reconstr Surg. 1971;48:224–37.
42. Tessier P. [Treatment of facial dysmorphias in craniofacial dysostosis, Crouzon's and Apert's diseases]. Total osteotomy and sagittal displacement of the facial massive. Faciostenosis, sequelae of Lefort 3 fracture. Dtsch Zahn Mund Kieferheilkd Zentralbl Gesamte. 1971;57:302–320.
43. Hoffman HJ, Mohr G. Lateral canthal advancement of the supraorbital margin. A new corrective technique in the treatment of coronal synostosis. J Neurosurg. 1976;45(4):376–81. https://doi.org/10.3171/jns.1976.45.4.0376.
44. Hoffman HJ. Procedure of lateral canthal advancement for the treatment of coronal synostosis. Childs Nerv Syst. 1996;12:678–82.
45. Guzman R, Looby J, Schendel S, Edwards M. Fronto-orbital advancement using an en bloc frontal bone craniectomy. Oper Neurosurg. 2011;68:ons68–74. https://doi.org/10.1227/NEU.0b013e31820780cd.
46. Robins JMW, Sheikh AJ, Shastin D, Schramm MWJ, Carter P, Russell JL, Liddington M, Chumas PD. Fronto-orbital advancement and reconstruction using reverse frontal bone graft without the use of orbital bar: a technical note. Childs Nerv Syst. 2020;36:1295–9.
47. Marchac D. Radical forehead remodeling for craniostenosis. Plast Reconstr Surg. 1978;61(6):823–35.
48. Wojcicki P, Prudel B. Trigonocephaly: long-term results after surgical correction of metopic suture synostosis. Adv Clin Exp Med. 2019;28(5):625–35.
49. Di Rocco C, Velardi F, Ferrario A, Marchese E. Metopic synostosis: in favour of a "simplified" surgical treat-

ment. Childs Nerv Syst. 1996;12(11):654–63. https://doi.org/10.1007/BF00366147. PMID: 9118127.
50. Di Rocco C, Frassanito P, Tamburrini G. The shell technique: bilateral fronto-orbital reshaping in trigonocephaly. Childs Nerv Syst. 2013;29(12):2189–94. https://doi.org/10.1007/s00381-012-1766-0. Epub 2012 Aug 23. PMID: 22914920.
51. Messi M, Consorti G, Lupi E, Girotto R, Valassina D, Balercia P. A new operative open-wings technique to correct the frontoforehead unit in metopic synostosis. J Craniofac Surg. 2015;26(3):902–5.
52. Cohen SR, Boydston W, Hudgins R, Burstein FD. Monobloc and facial bipartition distraction with internal devices. J Craniofac Surg. 1999;10:244–51.
53. Renier D, Lajeunie E, Arnaud E, Marchac D. Management of craniosynostoses. Childs Nerv Syst. 2000;16:645–58.
54. Levitt MR, Niazi TN, Hopper RA, Ellenbogen RG, Ojemann JG. Resolution of syndromic craniosynostosis-associated Chiari malformation type I without suboccipital decompression after posterior cranial vault release. J Neurosurg Pediatr. 2012;9:111–5.
55. Nowinski D, Saiepour D, Leikola J, Messo E, Nilsson P, Enblad P. Posterior cranial vault expansion performed with rapid distraction and time-reduced consolidation in infants with syndromic craniosynostosis. Childs Nerv Syst. 2011;27:1999–2003.
56. Nowinski D, Di Rocco F, Renier D, SainteRose C, Leikola J, Arnaud E. Posterior cranial vault expansion in the treatment of craniosynostosis. Comparison of current techniques. Childs Nerv Syst. 2012;28:1537–44.
57. Di Rocco F, Usami K, Protzenko T, Collet C, Giraudat K, Arnaud E. Results and limits of posterior cranial vault expansion by osteotomy and internal distractors. Surg Neurol Int. 2018,9.217. Published online 2018 Oct 30. https://doi.org/10.4103/sni.sni_465_17.
58. Burstein FD, Williams JK, Hudgins R, Graham L, Teague G, Paschal M, et al. Single stage craniofacial distraction using resorbable devices. J Craniofac Surg. 2002;13:776–82.
59. Lauritzen CG, Davis C, Ivarsson A, et al. The evolving role of springs in craniofacial surgery: the first 100 clinical cases. Plast Reconstr Surg. 2008;121(2):545–54.
60. Shakir S, Humphries LS, Lanni MA, Kalmar CL, Vu G, Heuer G, Lang SS, Bartlett SP, Taylor JA, Swanson JW. What is the role of force in correcting scaphocephaly through spring-mediated cranial vault expansion for sagittal craniosynostosis? J Craniofac Surg. 2021;32(8):2615–20. https://doi.org/10.1097/SCS.0000000000007780.
61. Di Rocco C. How to decrease the impact of surgical scar in the correction of sagittal synostosis. Childs Nerv Syst. 2003;19:42–5.
62. Massimi L, Di Rocco C. Mini-invasive surgical technique for sagittal craniosynostosis. Childs Nerv Syst. 2012;28(9):1341–5. https://doi.org/10.1007/s00381-012-1799-4. Epub 2012 Aug 8.
63. Jimenez DF, Barone CM. Endoscopic craniectomy for early surgical correction of sagittal craniosynostosis. J Neurosurg. 1998;88:77–81.
64. Barone CM, Jimenez DF. Endoscopic craniectomy for early correction of craniosynostosis. Plast Reconstr Surg. 1999;104:1965–73.
65. Johnson JO, Jimenez DF, Barone CM. Blood loss after endoscopic strip craniectomy for craniosynostosis. J Neurosurg Anesthesiol. 2000;12:60.
66. Barone C, Jimenez DF. Endoscopic approach to coronal craniosynostosis. Clin Plast Surg. 2004;31:415–22.
67. Berry-Candelario J, Ridgway EB, Grondin RT, Rogers GF, Proctor MR. Endoscope-assisted strip craniectomy and postoperative helmet therapy for treatment of craniosynostosis. Neurosurg Focus. 2011;31(2):E5.
68. Hinojosa J. Endoscopic-assisted treatment of trigonocephaly. Childs Nerv Syst. 2012;9:1381–7.
69. Goyal A, Lu VM, Yolcu YU, Elminawy M, Daniels DJ. Endoscopic versus open approach in craniosynostosis repair: a systematic review and meta-analysis of perioperative outcomes. Childs Nerv Syst. 2018;34:1627–37.
70. Marupudi NI, Reisen B, Rozzelle A, Sood S. Endoscopy in craniosynostosis surgery: evolution and current trends. J Pediatr Neurosci. 2022;17(Suppl 1):S44–53. https://doi.org/10.4103/jpn.JPN_47_22. Epub 2022 Sep 19.
71. Valetopoulou A, Constantinides M, Eccles S, Ong J, Hayward R, Dunaway D, Jeelani NUO, James G, Silva AHD. Endoscopic strip craniectomy with molding helmet therapy versus spring-assisted cranioplasty for nonsyndromic single-suture sagittal craniosynostosis: a systematic review. J Neurosurg Pediatr. 2022;30:455–62. https://doi.org/10.3171/2022.7.PEDS2232. Epub ahead of print.

2 Embryology and Skull Growth: What Is Important for the Neurosurgeon?

Yann Heuzé

2.1 Foreword

As a biological anthropologist, I was trained in Anatomy and Evolution. During my postdoc in the Richtsmeier lab in the Department of Anthropology at the Pennsylvania State University, I had the opportunity to study developmental biology and birth defects such as craniosynostosis which then became central to my research. The purpose of this chapter is to present the embryology and growth of the skull from an evolutionary and developmental perspective (evo-devo). As such, the goal of this chapter is not to provide an up-to-date highly detailed description of skull embryology and early skull growth in humans. Those data have been previously published by other authors and should be consulted for a thorough treatment of these important topics. Many helpful reviews and original research exist in the current literature. For my chapter, I have leaned heavily on "Larsen's human embryology" by Gary Schoenwolff et al. [1], "Craniofacial embryogenetics and development" by Geoffrey H. Sperber and Steven M. Sperber [2], and "Bones and cartilage" by Brian K. Hall [3].

Y. Heuzé (✉)
Univ. Bordeaux, CNRS, Ministère de la Culture, Pessac, France
e-mail: yann.heuze@u-bordeaux.fr

2.2 From Fertilization to Gastrula: Fundamental Processes

Though the initial 2 days of human embryo formation are under the control of factors expressed only by the oocyte, subsequent differentiation of cells is governed by the genetic material inherited from both parents. Three days after the fertilization of the ovum by the spermatozoon that results in the formation of the totipotential zygote, the first mitotic cycles have produced 16 smaller pluripotential cells achieving the morula stage. In addition to the expression of genetic material within the cell, interactions between cells and their environment are essential for differentiation. These interactions between newly differentiated cells happen by induction. Induction can occur by direct cellular contact, diffused agents, or agents embedded in vesicles targeting mechanisms such as gene activation or inactivation, protein translation, modification of cell membrane selectivities, intercellular adhesion or repulsion, and cell migration. Timing is an additional dimension that is crucial to normal development. Alteration or disruption of this complex symphony referred to as morphogenesis can lead to abnormal development.

At the end of the first week after fertilization (preimplantation period), the embryonic period starts with the implantation of the blastocyst (around 100 cells at the time) into the decidual

F. Di Rocco, J. Kestle (eds.), *Neurosurgical Aspects of Craniosynostosis*,
https://doi.org/10.1007/978-3-031-69386-1_2

layer of the uterine wall. The embryonic period comprises 7 weeks of embryogenesis. The polarized blastocyst consists of an outer layer (trophoblast) and an inner cell mass adherent to the trophoblast, filling only one part of the newly formed blastocyst cavity. Eventually, the inner cell blast will give rise to the definitive structures of the fetus, while the trophoblast will form the extra-embryonic tissues.

At day 10, newly formed structures called fetal membranes are visible: the chorion deriving from the trophoblast and delimiting the embryo; the amnion, a membrane delimiting the future amniotic sac filled with amniotic fluid; the yolk sac, providing nutrition and gas exchange before the forming placenta becomes functional; and the allantois, a transient sac allowing gas exchange and liquid waste handling. With the establishment of the two layers, the dorsoventral axis is defined. The two-layer germ disk is connected dorsally to the amnion through the epiblast and ventrally to the yolk sac through the hypoblast. The germ disk, amnion, and yolk sac derive from the inner cell blast.

Between days 14 and 17, a process called gastrulation initiates and will reorganize the two-layer blastocyst into a three-layer embryo (gastrula) consisting of ectoderm, mesoderm, and endoderm. Signaling pathways such as Hedgehog (HH), fibroblast growth factor (FGF), wingless (Wnt), bone morphogenetic protein (BMP), and Notch are active and regulate the activity of Nodal (a transforming growth factor beta, TGF-β) that is essential to the formation of mesoderm and the establishment of left–right asymmetry of visceral organs. At the caudal end of the two-layer germ disk, nodal signaling causes epiblast cells to proliferate, differentiate, and migrate toward the midline of the germ disk. This accumulation of cells produces a bulge and ultimately forms a linear band of cells called the primitive streak. The primitive streak elongates cranially in the midline and the progression stops when the streak is about halfway across the embryonic disk. While the lengthening stops, epiblast cells are still migrating toward the rostral end of the primitive streak creating the primitive node and thereby establishing the cranial-caudal axis. The primitive node is a major signaling center and will subsequently induce the formation of the neural plate and notochord rostrally (see below). Epiblast cells continue to migrate toward the primitive streak and primitive node and eventually pass through the primitive groove and primitive pit, respectively, via a process known as ingression. Ingression is made possible by the epithelial–mesenchymal transition (EMT, see for a review [4]) in which epiblast cells lose their polarity and adhesive properties and migrate ventrally to form a layer between the epiblast and hypoblast. Through EMT, these cells proliferate and form the intraembryonic mesoderm. As the ingression process continues, the hypoblast and epiblast form the endoderm and ectoderm, respectively. The embryonic disk is now trilaminar and the three primary germ layers, ectoderm, endoderm, and mesoderm, will give rise to all structures and organs of the body.

The role of the primitive node is essential during gastrulation. At day 16, epiblast cells migrating through the primitive node differentiate to form the notochord which develops cranially and stops caudally to the prechordal plate. The notochord, surrounded ventrally by the endoderm, dorsally by the ectoderm, and laterally by the mesoderm (now called paraxial mesoderm), is achieved around day 20.

2.3 Neurulation: A Focus on Cranial Neural Crest Cells

One of the main evolutionary innovations of vertebrates is the appearance of an embryonic stem-cell population from the neuroectoderm called the neural crest. With the "new head hypothesis," Gans and Northcutt [5] proposed that many elements of the vertebrate head represent an addition rather than a modified portion of the protochordates' trunk. More precisely, anterior structures such as sensory, integrative, and motor systems, as well as the associated supportive skeletal structures derive from the neural crest and epidermal placodes [5]. These structures are pivotal in functions such as the detection and capture of prey as well as the exchange and distribution of respiratory gases [5].

The specification of neural tissues creates the neural plate which is an ectodermal structure that forms cranially to the primitive node and dorsally to the forming notochord (i.e., notochordal process). The neural plate results from a process called neural induction when signaling (downregulation of *BMP* by *FGF*) causes the apicobasal thickening of epiblast cells. The neural plate then elongates cranially along the midline. The neural plate is composed of neural ectoderm and is separated from the nonneural ectoderm by the neural plate border that will give rise to a population of stem cells called the neural crest and to placodes during the process of neurulation. Neurulation, the transformation of the neural plate into a neural tube, is induced and regulated by *TGF-beta* signaling molecules such as Chordin and Noggin that downregulate BMP signaling [6], as well as FGFs [7], Wnt signals [8] and a Dlx gradient [9]. At day 19, a neural groove appears in the neural ectoderm. The neural groove is bordered laterally by the neural folds formed through the ingression of the neural plate. The folding process and the fusion of the neural folds allow the formation and closure (dorsally) of the neural tube at day 21. The neural crest cells also undergo ingression through EMT and pass momentarily between the ectoderm (dorsally) and the neural tube (ventrally) [10] as they begin their migration process. The closure of the cranial and caudal openings of the neural tube (neuropores) takes place on days 24 and 26–28, respectively.

The neural crest cells are multi-potent stem cells unique to vertebrates that arise on the dorsal aspect of the embryo and stretch from the cranial to the caudal tip. Neural crest cells migrate, proliferate, and differentiate into various tissues (connective, muscle, nervous, and endocrine) and pigment cells (melanocytes). Martik's et al. [11] work on lamprey (jawless fish; agnatha) led them to propose that the neural crest of early vertebrates formed a single and uniform cell population similar to neural crest cells of the amniote trunk, and that during early vertebrate evolution, a new subpopulation of neural crest cells appeared; the cranial neural crest. These authors propose that Hox genes and other regulatory modifications are sufficient to account for the small transcriptional differences observed between the cranial and trunk neural crest subpopulations. Co-option of distinct genes into a cranial neural crest-specific module likely allowed the cranial neural crest gene regulatory network to progressively give rise to morphological novelties such as the lower jaw [11]. After induction, cranial neural crest cells migrate to the frontonasal process and the first four pharyngeal arches [12–14]. Throughout interactions with neighboring structures such as surface ectoderm, neuroectoderm, and endoderm, neural crest cells contribute to the development of many cranial structures and are critical to normal development of the craniofacial region [15]. The cranial neural crest gives rise to the frontal bone, most bones of the facial skeleton, and most facial connective tissues.

The dorsal closure of the neural tube (day 21) ends the presomite period and initiates the somite period marked by the appearance of 42–44 bilaterally paired blocks of paraxial mesoderm along the rostro-caudal axis of the embryo that are characteristic of segmented animals: the somites. Intermediate and lateral plate mesoderm are situated lateral to the paraxial mesoderm. Somitogenesis starts rostrally with paraxial mesoderm condensations forming incompletely segmented structures called somitomeres. Cranial somitomeric mesoderm migrates ventrally to contribute to the future pharyngeal arches. Caudal to the somitomeres, a craniocaudal sequence characterizes the formation of the somites establishing the segmented nature of the body with 4 occipital, 8 cervical, 12 thoracic, 5 lumbar, 5 sacral, and 8–10 coccygeal somites. The segmentation of the somites is driven by a number of "clock" genes. Periodical activation of these clock "genes" generates a signaling wave propagating in the rostral direction involving *Notch*, *Wnt*, and *FGF*. Boundaries between somites are formed through EMT. The somites subsequently differentiate into three parts: the sclerotome (ventromedial aspect), dermatome (lateral aspect), and myotome (intermediate portion). The sclerotome contributes to the vertebral column except in the occipital region where it fuses to form the occipital bone. The dermatome gives rise to the dermis of the skin. The myotome differentiates into muscles. By the end of the somite period, the cardiovascular, digestive, respiratory, nervous, urinary, and reproductive systems are established. The optic and otic placodes, which will give rise to the eyes and internal ears, respectively, are formed. It is also the time when the embryo folds ventrally. At day 31, the head of the embryo is composed of a prominent brain ventrally associated with the pharyngeal arches prefiguring the face and neck, altogether flexed over the developing heart due to this folding. At this time the nasal placode and limb buds are also visible. The postsomite period initiates at day 32. Head development occurs at the center of the postsomite period when eyes, ears, and nose acquire a human characteristic morphology. At the end of the postsomite period (day 56, end of the eighth week), the embryo is termed a fetus.

2.4 Role of Neural Crest Cells in Head Development: The Example of the Frontonasal Ectodermal Zone (FEZ)

At the end of the fourth week (day 28), while the neural tube is closed, the cranial section of the embryo experiences major expansion, bending, folding, and constriction. The neural tube then forms three primitive brain regions: the prosencephalon or forebrain, the mesencephalon or midbrain, and the rhombencephalon or hindbrain. The segmentation process goes on and at the end of the seventh week (day 49), the secondary brain regions are visible. The prosencephalon gives rise to the telencephalon and diencephalon, and the rhombencephalon to the metencephalon and myelencephalon. Later, the telencephalon will differentiate into the cerebral cortex, hippocampus, basal ganglia, basal forebrain nuclei, and olfactory bulbs. The diencephalon will differentiate into the thalamus, hypothalamus, and neural portion of the eye. The metencephalon will differentiate into the cerebellum and pons, and the myelencephalon into the medulla (for a review on brain patterning and associated signaling pathways, see [16]).

During the fourth week of development (at the time the neural tube is closing), seven prominences prefiguring the face and organized around the stomodeum (future mouth) are visible: the midline frontonasal prominence and three paired lateral structures, the lateral nasal (sometimes considered part of the frontonasal prominence), maxillary, and mandibular prominences. The maxillary and mandibular prominences derive from the first pharyngeal arch. Craniofacial development results from interactions between neural crest cells and the surrounding epithelia such as the neural ectoderm of the forebrain, the facial ectoderm of the frontonasal prominence, and pharyngeal arches, as well as the endoderm of the inner surface of the pharyngeal arches. Pioneering experiments on chick and quail by Le Douarin and lab members showed that the fate of neural crest cells is restricted by *Hox* genes such as *Hoxa2* (reviewed in [17]). However, the neural crest is not pivotal in the formation and patterning of the pharyngeal arches. The pharyngeal endoderm is involved in the patterning of the pharyngeal arch skeleton [18].

Many transcription factors contribute to craniofacial development. Brugman et al. (2008), for example, provide a review that highlights the role of FGF8 in normal craniofacial development. Fgf8 signaling from the neuroectoderm promotes the development of the jaws in birds, while the expression of *Fgf8* in the first branchial arch ectoderm is dependent on signaling from the neural crest [19]. This illustrates how interactions between epithelia and mesenchyme are pivotal to craniofacial morphogenesis. Another key signaling pathway in craniofacial development is associated to *sonic hedgehog* (*Shh*) from the Hedgehog family. *Shh* expression takes place in the prosencephalon, and then in the ventral part of the telencephalon [20]. Shh signaling is pivotal for the proper morphogenesis of the frontonasal prominence. Fgf and Shh signaling emanating from the forebrain neuroectoderm are essential for the patterning and differentiation of the frontonasal neural crest [21]. Of particular importance to facial development is the frontonasal ectodermal zone (FEZ). The FEZ was defined by Hu et al. [22] as a key signaling center for the morphogenesis of the face located in the surface cephalic ectoderm in mammals and avians. The FEZ is formed by the boundary between *Shh* and *Fgf8* expressing cells located within the frontonasal prominence ectoderm [22]. While the FEZ is a single site of expression, in mice the FEZ is divided into paired regions associated with the median nasal prominence [23]. *Shh* expression in the FEZ starts with the arrival of NC cells into the frontonasal prominence and is probably induced and maintained by Bmps [24]. Several ectopic transplantation experiments demonstrated that the FEZ induces skeletogenesis and determines the dorsoventral polarity of the upper jaw as well as its morphogenesis through patterning of the underlying mesenchymal cells [22, 23]. However, when the FEZ was transplanted into regions expressing homeobox genes such as the second pharyngeal arch, no effects on the mesenchymal cells were observed [23]. FEZ positively regulates Bmp expression in NC mesenchyme of the upper jaw in birds [23] and as such participates in craniofacial phenotypic variation. For example, Young et al. [25] showed that downregulation of *Shh* in the brain caused a continuous narrowing of the frontonasal prominence, hypotelorism, and medial maxillary rotation, while upregulation of *Shh* causes the opposite phenotype. Besides physical interactions between the developing brain and face (see [26] on the role of brain growth on the positioning of the facial prominences and eyes), FEZ is an example of a molecular signaling center active in craniofacial morphogenesis.

2.5 Different Units of the Skull in Evolutionary and Developmental Biology

The skull is a complex skeletal system whose primary function is to protect the brain and the major sense organs (olfactory, optic, and auditory) as they carry out their functions. Multiple and sometimes conflicting definitions of the different elements of the skull exist depending on the authors' area of study; e.g., human anatomy, comparative anatomy, embryology, evolution, or developmental biology. The skull is often compartmentalized into divisions on the basis of varying criteria and/or based on certain developmental derivatives. Examples of these divisions include regions or modules labeled as facial skeleton, braincase, cranial base, cranial vault, chondrocranium, splanchnocranium, dermatocranium, pharyngeal skeleton, and viscerocranium. Most researchers and clinicians have a fairly clear idea of what each division comprises, though these definitions are rarely made explicit. To more clearly define aspects of the craniofacial skeleton, Kawasaki and Richtsmeier [27] proposed to follow the nomenclature used in evolutionary and developmental biology that defines the skull into the cranial endoskeleton (composed of the chondrocranium and pharyngeal skeleton) and the cranial dermal skeleton (dermatocranium). The pharyngeal skeleton, composed primarily of cartilage, arose as simple gill supports in stem jawless vertebrates and became specialized into the more complex lower jaw that includes the ear ossicles. The chondrocranium, composed of cartilage and cartilage bone arose to support the brain. The dermatocranium composed primarily of dermal bone, enamel, and enameloid was the last to evolve [28]. Bone forming from the endoskeletal precursors (cartilage bone) and from the dermal or exoskeleton (dermal bone and membrane bone) is distinct ontogenetically and/or phylogenetically [3, 29]. The dermal bone of the exoskeleton forms in contact with the epithelial ectoderm through intramembranous ossification, whereas the endoskeleton forms mainly through endochondral ossification but not in contact with the epithelial ectoderm.

The two principal skeletal tissues are bone and cartilage (the other two being enamel and dentin). Cranial cartilage and bone that form endochondrally and intramembranously can derive from either the mesoderm or neural crest. Endochondral ossification is a process in which cartilaginous models are replaced by bone. Intramembranous ossification occurs when aggregated mesenchymal cells directly differentiate into osteoblasts and form bone. In both types of ossification, bone consists of cells distributed on a collagen matrix that is mineralized into a vascularized skeletal tissue. Ossification per se starts with the condensation of mesenchymal cells and upregulation of tissue-specific genes. Condensation consists of successive stages; initiation, formation of boundaries, cell adhesion, proliferation, growth, and end of growth [3].

Osteoblasts manufacture the extracellular matrix called osteoid and also mineralize that matrix trapping them within the mineralized tissue where they differentiate into osteocytes and function in bone homeostasis. The bone grows by apposition and mineralization of new osteoid perichondrially (outer surface of cartilage), periosteally (outer surface of bone), or endosteally (inner surface of bone).

Cartilage consists of cells and extracellular matrix that may or may not mineralize and is avascular. Cartilage is formed by chondroblasts and chondrocytes and resorbed by chondroclasts. The extracellular matrix is rich in water, glycosaminoglycans, and type II collagen. Cartilage grows by apposition, but unlike the bone, it can also grow interstitially and is therefore capable of changing its shape rather quickly during development.

Though the two modes of ossification are active in craniofacial development, the relationship between the chondrocranium and dermatocranium during intrauterine development remains elusive. This is in part related to the transient nature of the chondrocranium. However, a recent study by Motch et al. [30] provides experimental data on a mouse model for Crouzon syndrome (*Fgfr2c*$^{C342Y/+}$) supporting the existence of a developmental relationship between cartilaginous elements of the chondrocranium and bones of the dermatocranium. Together with the data published earlier by Kawasaki and Richtsmeier [27] and Pitirri et al. [28], these studies lead the members of this group to hypothesize that the chondrocranium is pivotal in establishing the initial formation and spatial distribution of the dermal bones during embryogenesis. These authors propose that the chondrocranial elements serve as a scaffold guiding and influencing the location and morphology of developing dermal bones. If these results were to be confirmed in future studies, they would advocate for a reassessment of the classic definition of intramembranous ossification which is not supposed to involve cartilage elements.

2.6 Neural Crest Vs. Mesoderm-Derived Tissues and Premature Suture Fusion

Bones forming the craniofacial skeleton are either derived from the cranial neural crest or paraxial mesoderm. The facial skeleton, anterior parts of the braincase floor, the squamous temporal, and frontal bones are derived from the cranial neural crest. The mesoderm gives rise to the occipital bones, parietal bones, and the nonsquamous part of the temporal bone [31–33]. Many of these bones articulate at cranial sutures (and synchondroses) which form major bone growth sites as long as the mesenchyme forming the suture remains undifferentiated [34]. As a consequence, the coronal suture forms a boundary between the neural crest and mesoderm-derived bones of the skull.

When a craniosynostosis-associated mutation is present in a human patient, that mutation is present in all cells of the body—including all bone cells whether derived from neural crest or from mesoderm. Laboratory animals and recent developments in Cre-mediated DNA recombination provide an established method for the conditional control of gene expression in animal models. There exist Cre-LoxP systems that allow spatial and/or temporal control over the recombination of the target gene. For example, it is possible to create an Apert mouse model bearing a Cre-inducible mutation on fibroblast growth factor receptor 2 (*Fgfr2*^{S252W}). When using mesoderm-specific Cre driver (i.e., *Mesp1Cre*) and neural crest-specific Cre driver (i.e., *Wnt1Cre*) and such Cre-inducible Apert mouse model, it then becomes possible to express the

Apert mutation only in mesoderm- or neural crest-derived tissues [35].

Premature fusion of the coronal suture (i.e., coronal craniosynostosis) can be caused by the expression of the *Fgfr2*^{S252W} Apert syndrome mutation in the mesoderm-derived mesenchyme of the coronal suture in mouse. In the conditional expression mouse model for Apert syndrome, the expression of this mutation is responsible for abnormal osteogenesis though it does not alter the lineage border integrity between mesoderm and neural crest [35]. A subsequent study on the same mouse models showed that the conditional expression of the *Fgfr2*^{S252W} mutation in the suture mesenchyme of other craniofacial sutures was not sufficient to induce its premature fusion and that suture-specific variation in the timing of fusion might also play a significant role [36]. Though mice expressing the *Fgfr2*^{S252W} mutation only in the neural crest-derived tissues possess a patent coronal suture at birth, these mice displayed a more severe phenotype than the mice expressing this same mutation only in the mesoderm-derived tissues (and possessing a fused coronal suture) [36]. This can be explained by the fact that the majority of the craniofacial bones are neural crest-derived and that mice expressing the *Fgfr2*^{S252W} mutation only in the neural crest-derived tissues displayed a premature fusion of several facial sutures such as the premaxillary–maxillary, maxillary–palatine, and maxillary–zygomatic sutures.

Paralleling the dual nature of brain influence on craniofacial development (physical and molecular) besides the primary effect on craniofacial phenotype of the expression of a specific mutation, secondary effects related to physical interactions between the neural-crest derived and mesoderm-derived tissues exist as well. Indeed, both mouse models conditionally expressing the FGFR2 S252W mutation either in the neural crest- or mesoderm-derived tissues also displayed dysmorphologies in bones not expressing the mutation. The authors proposed that these secondary changes could be caused by four potential sources: (1) disrupted morphogenesis of the bone not expressing the mutation caused by a neighboring prematurely fused suture; (2) displacement of the bone not expressing the mutation caused by neighboring dysmorphic mutant bones; (3) abnormal physical constraints of soft tissues expressing the mutation; and (4) abnormal signaling or soluble factors produced by mutant cells that alter the development of the neighboring nonmutant cells [36].

2.7 Conclusion: What Is Important for the Neurosurgeon?

This chapter is an attempt to deliver a solid, not-too-detailed summary of the early development of the whole embryo and then of the bones of the head which, I hope, will be of interest to neurosurgeons. Throughout this chapter, the complex developmental stages and associated mechanisms were described from an evolutionary and developmental perspective. After the first 3 weeks of development and the establishment of the three primary germ layers, I focused on the activities of cranial neural crest cells during neurulation with some insights on their evolutionary origin. A focus was then provided with the interesting example of the frontonasal ectodermal zone illustrating the pivotal role of interactions between epithelia and mesenchyme in craniofacial morphogenesis. The FEZ also allowed illustrating the integrative nature of craniofacial development with the complex interactions between the growing brain and skull either through physical interactions or molecular signaling centers. Subsequently, osteogenesis of the skull was described providing an evolutionary and developmental perspective on the cranial endoskeleton formed by the chondrocranium and pharyngeal skeleton, and the cranial dermal skeleton or dermatocranium. The work from the Richtsmeier group was used to illustrate how the chondrocranial elements might serve as a scaffold guiding and influencing the location and morphology of developing dermal bones. Finally, through the example of the conditional expression of the *Fgfr2*^{S252W} Apert syndrome mutation in mouse models, the role of sutures in craniofacial morphogenesis was described as well as the nature of the interactions between the mesoderm- and neural crest-derived craniofacial bones.

Surgical techniques to operate on patients with craniosynostosis, either syndromic or nonsyndromic, sometimes focus on the rearrangement of bones that make up the facial skeleton and cranial vault. However, we need to remember that these causative mutations (for a review, see [37]) affect all cells and all tissues (soft and hard) and that understanding how different tissues impact the growth pattern of others is critical to the proper correction of craniofacial anomalies.

Acknowledgments I thank Federico Di Rocco for the kind invitation to write this chapter. I am grateful to Joan T. Richtsmeier for her inspiring influence on my research and for helpful comments on previous versions of this manuscript. This research benefited from the scientific framework of the University of Bordeaux's IdEx "Investments for the Future" program/GPR "Human Past."

References

1. Schoenwolf GC, Bleyl SB, Brauer PR, Francis-West PH. Larsen's human embryology. 6th ed. Philadelphia: Elsevier—Health Sciences Division; 2021.
2. Sperber GH, Sperber SM. Craniofacial embryogenetics and development. 3th ed. Raleigh: PMPH-USA Limited; 2018.
3. Hall BK. Bones and cartilage: developmental and evolutionary skeletal biology. 2nd ed. Elsevier/AP, Academic Press is an imprint of Elsevier: Amsterdam; 2015.
4. Kalluri R, Weinberg RA. The basics of epithelial-mesenchymal transition. J Clin Invest. 2009;119:1420–8.
5. Gans C, Northcutt RG. Neural crest and the origin of vertebrates: a new head. Science. 1983;220:268–73.
6. Anderson RM, Stottmann RW, Choi M, Klingensmith J. Endogenous bone morphogenetic protein antagonists regulate mammalian neural crest generation and survival. Dev Dyn. 2006;235:2507–20.
7. Mayor R, Guerrero N, Martínez C. Role of FGF and noggin in neural crest induction. Dev Biol. 1997;189:1–12.
8. García-Castro MI, Marcelle C, Bronner-Fraser M. Ectodermal Wnt function as a neural crest inducer. Science. 2002;297:848–51.
9. McLarren KW, Litsiou A, Streit A. DLX5 positions the neural crest and preplacode region at the border of the neural plate. Dev Biol. 2003;259:34–47.
10. Noden DM, Trainor PA. Relations and interactions between cranial mesoderm and neural crest populations. J Anat. 2005;207:575–601.
11. Martik ML, Gandhi S, Uy BR, Gillis JA, Green SA, Simoes-Costa M, Bronner ME. Evolution of the new head by gradual acquisition of neural crest regulatory circuits. Nature. 2019;574:675–8.
12. Hunt P, Gulisano M, Cook M, Sham MH, Faiella A, Wilkinson D, Boncinelli E, Krumlauf R. A distinct Hox code for the branchial region of the vertebrate head. Nature. 1991;353:861–4.
13. Le Lièvre CS, Le Douarin NM. Mesenchymal derivatives of the neural crest: analysis of chimaeric quail and chick embryos. J Embryol Exp Morphol. 1975;34:125–54.
14. Lumsden A, Sprawson N, Graham A. Segmental origin and migration of neural crest cells in the hindbrain region of the chick embryo. Development. 1991;113:1281–91.
15. Creuzet S, Couly G, Le Douarin NM. Patterning the neural crest derivatives during development of the vertebrate head: insights from avian studies. J Anat. 2005;207:447–59.
16. Altmann CR, Brivanlou AH. Neural patterning in the vertebrate embryo. Int Rev Cytol. 2001;203:447–82.
17. Le Douarin NM, Creuzet S, Couly G, Dupin E. Neural crest cell plasticity and its limits. Development. 2004;131:4637–50.
18. Couly G, Creuzet S, Bennaceur S, Vincent C, Le Douarin NM. Interactions between Hox-negative cephalic neural crest cells and the foregut endoderm in patterning the facial skeleton in the vertebrate head. Development. 2002;129:1061–73.
19. Creuzet S, Schuler B, Couly G, Le Douarin NM. Reciprocal relationships between Fgf8 and neural crest cells in facial and forebrain development. Proc Natl Acad Sci U S A. 2004;101:4843–7.
20. Cordero D, Marcucio R, Hu D, Gaffield W, Tapadia M, Helms JA. Temporal perturbations in sonic hedgehog signaling elicit the spectrum of holoprosencephaly phenotypes. J Clin Invest. 2004;114:485–94.
21. Brugmann SA, Tapadia MD, Helms JA. The molecular origins of species-specific facial pattern. Curr Top Dev Biol. 2006;73:1–42.
22. Hu D, Marcucio RS, Helms JA. A zone of frontonasal ectoderm regulates patterning and growth in the face. Development. 2003;130:1749–58.
23. Hu D, Marcucio RS. Unique organization of the frontonasal ectodermal zone in birds and mammals. Dev Biol. 2009;325:200–10.
24. Marcucio RS, Young NM, Hu D, Hallgrimsson B. Mechanisms that underlie co-variation of the brain and face. Genesis. 2011;49:177–89.
25. Young NM, Chong HJ, Hu D, Hallgrímsson B, Marcucio RS. Quantitative analyses link modulation of sonic hedgehog signaling to continuous variation in facial growth and shape. Development. 2010;137:3405–9.
26. Diewert VM, Lozanoff S, Choy V. Computer reconstructions of human embryonic craniofacial morphology showing changes in relations between the face and brain during primary palate formation. J Craniofac Genet Dev Biol. 1993;13:193–201.

27. Kawasaki K, Richtsmeier JT. Association of the chondrocranium and dermatocranium in early skull development. In: Percival C, Richtsmeier JT, editors. Building bones: early bone development informing anthropological inquiry. Cambridge: Cambridge University Press; 2017. p. 52–78.
28. Pitirri MK, Kawasaki K, Richtsmeier JT. It takes two: building the vertebrate skull from chondrocranium and dermatocranium. Vertebr Zool. 2020;70:587–600.
29. Hall BK. Endoskeleton/Exo (dermal) skeleton—mesoderm/neural crest: two pair of problems and a shifting paradigm. J Appl Ichthyol. 2014;30:608–15.
30. Motch Perrine SM, Pitirri MK, Durham EL, Kawasaki M, Zheng H, Chen DZ, Kawasaki K, Richtsmeier JT. A dysmorphic mouse model reveals developmental interactions of chondrocranium and dermatocranium. Elife. 2022;11:e76653.
31. Jiang X, Iseki S, Maxson RE, Sucov HM, Morriss-Kay GM. Tissue origins and interactions in the mammalian skull vault. Dev Biol. 2002;241:106–16.
32. McBratney-Owen B, Iseki S, Bamforth SD, Olsen BR, Morriss-Kay GM. Development and tissue origins of the mammalian cranial base. Dev Biol. 2008;322:121–32.
33. Yoshida T, Vivatbutsiri P, Morriss-Kay G, Saga Y, Iseki S. Cell lineage in mammalian craniofacial mesenchyme. Mech Dev. 2008;125:797–808.
34. Opperman LA. Cranial sutures as intramembranous bone growth sites. Dev Dyn. 2000;219:472–85.
35. Holmes G, Basilico C. Mesodermal expression of Fgfr2S252W is necessary and sufficient to induce craniosynostosis in a mouse model of Apert syndrome. Dev Biol. 2012;368:283–93.
36. Heuzé Y, Singh N, Basilico C, Jabs EW, Holmes G, Richtsmeier JT. Morphological comparison of the craniofacial phenotypes of mouse models expressing the Apert FGFR2 S252W mutation in neural crest- or mesoderm-derived tissues. Bone. 2014;63:101–9.
37. Heuzé Y, Holmes G, Peter I, Richtsmeier JT, Jabs EW. Closing the gap: genetic and genomic continuum from syndromic to nonsyndromic craniosynostoses. Curr Genet Med Rep. 2014;2:135–45.

Genetics of Craniosynostoses: What Is Important for the Neurosurgeon?

3

Federica Tiberio and Wanda Lattanzi

3.1 Introduction

Craniosynostosis (CS) represents a highly clinically and genetically heterogeneous group of congenital craniofacial malformations due to the premature ossification of cranial sutures. Cranial sutures are fibrous joints interposed between skull flat bones that play a key role during craniofacial development, enabling the physiological synchronous growth of the skull and the brain [1, 2]. The premature suture fusion occurring in CS leads to a skull growth constraint perpendicularly to the closed suture, with a compensatory growth in the direction of lower resistance (perpendicularly to the patent sutures) according to "Virchow's law" [3].

CS occurs overall in 1 of 2000–2500 live births, being the second most prevalent craniofacial defect [4, 5]. Indeed, the number of children diagnosed with CS worldwide has been recently estimated to be nearly 85,000 in a year [6].

F. Tiberio
Department of Life Science and Public Health, Università Cattolica del Sacro Cuore, Rome, Italy
e-mail: federica.tiberio@unicatt.it

W. Lattanzi (✉)
Department of Life Science and Public Health, Università Cattolica del Sacro Cuore, Rome, Italy

Fondazione Policlinico Universitario A. Gemelli IRCCS, Rome, Italy
e-mail: wanda.lattanzi@unicatt.it

CS treatment is predominantly surgical, representing a major indication of decompressive craniectomy and cranioplasty procedures in newborns and infants (see dedicated chapters in this volume). Therefore, not only CS contributes significantly to infant morbidity and disability, but represents a major economic burden, with millions of dollars spent annually, considering the costs for genetic diagnosis, imaging, neurodevelopmental, and standard surgical treatments, which may vary in types and number of procedures and for associated care.

Despite CS being ethologically heterogeneous as in most cases it results from a combination of environmental and genetic factors, genetic testing is an essential part of the diagnostic workup of patients.

This chapter aims to provide a detailed and comprehensive update on the genetic causes and risk factors for CS, integrating the consolidated knowledge of genetic pathophysiology with recent scientific findings achieved during the last decades. With a dedicated focus on the relevance of genetic knowledge for neurosurgical planning, and on the implications for prognosis, it may serve as a useful guide for pediatric neurosurgeons in the management and treatment of these conditions.

F. Di Rocco, J. Kestle (eds.), *Neurosurgical Aspects of Craniosynostosis*,
https://doi.org/10.1007/978-3-031-69386-1_3

3.2 CS Types and Classification

CS is classified according to different alternative criteria. Firstly, based on the number of fused sutures, simple CS refers to single-suture ossification, whereas complex CS is used to describe a multi-suture ossification pattern [7].

Based on the underlying pathophysiological mechanism, CS is defined as primary when the skull developmental abnormality is caused directly by a genetic mutation, acting alone or in combination with environmental factors, and secondary when it results from other conditions that indirectly affect cranial suture biology during the perinatal stage (e.g., maternal hyperthyroidism, hypercalcemia, or rickets, and/or neurodevelopmental abnormalities of the fetus, such as microcephaly) [5, 8, 9].

More commonly, CS is classified based on the clinical manifestation as nonsyndromic craniosynostosis (NCS), when it occurs as an isolated phenotypic trait, or syndromic (SCS) when it represents a feature of a complex syndrome with associated extracranial defects [5].

NCS represents around 70% of all CS cases and usually occurs as a primary simple CS [10, 11]. They are classified according to the affected suture site (sagittal, metopic, uni- or bi-coronal, and uni- or bi-lambdoid CS) and to the resulting skull dysmorphism (scaphocephaly or dolichocephaly, trigonocephaly, and anterior or posterior plagiocephaly/brachycephaly) [10].

NCS etiology is yet to be entirely clarified. They can be due to genetic background (more commonly single gene mutations and/or polymorphisms) with the concurrence of environmental factors (e.g., intrauterine fetal head constraint due to multiple pregnancies, primiparity, abnormal fetal position, oligohydramnios, and prenatal exposures to teratogens) that delineate a multifactorial etiology [11, 12]. Large cohort studies revealed that a genetic cause is detectable more frequently in NCS cases affecting coronal and/or multiple sutures [13], despite novel causative and/or risk-associated genes being very recently identified also in CS affecting midline sutures [14–16].

In syndromic forms, which comprise 25–30% of all CS cases, the premature fusion of sutures is associated with additional variable inborn defects, and/or developmental delay, defining the phenotypes of more than 150 Mendelian disorders annotated in the OMIM database (www.omim.org) [17]. Currently, a genetic etiology—single gene mutations or chromosomal structural abnormalities—can be confirmed in about 80% of syndromic cases [5]. In the last two decades, significant progress has been made in understanding the genetic basis of CS as a whole, with diverse large cohort studies that enabled identifying causative gene mutations and/or risk-associated polymorphisms also in NCS [5, 13, 18, 19]. These studies have strongly contributed to defining the influence of specific gene mutations on the surgical outcome and on the overall clinical prognosis for most CS patients [5, 13, 19, 20].

3.3 Molecular Genetics of Craniosynostosis

The etiology of CS is extremely heterogeneous and an identifiable genetic basis is estimated to be found in up to 45% of CS cases nowadays [5, 13, 19]. Among all genetic diagnoses, 86% of cases represent single-gene mutations, while the remainder are chromosomal structural aberrations [4]. As a rule, syndromic CS is most frequently associated with a genetic defect (75–80% of cases); instead, nonsyndromic CS results from multifactorial etiopathogenesis involving strong genetic and epigenetic influences usually combined with environmental factors, which contribute to the onset to this congenital defect [4, 19].

During the last decades, genetic studies focused on the molecular mechanisms of craniosynostosis have greatly improved enabling the discovery of new disease genes and disease-causing mutations in previously identified genes associated with the syndromic phenotype [5, 13, 18, 19]. In addition, recent genomic discoveries have extensively elucidated the genetic basis for nonsyndromic cases, implicating the newly identified genes in signaling pathways previously found in syndromic cases [21, 22]. In this regard, both CS forms will be considered altogether in this paragraph as parts of a unique nosological continuum.

Currently, the OMIM (online Mendelian inheritance in Men database (www.omim.org, accessed on January 5, 2022) reports 150 conditions that feature CS either as a hallmark (CS syndrome properly said) or as a frequent clinical feature (other syndromes) (Table 3.1). Currently, these conditions can be associated with mutations in 125 different genes, corroborating the wide genetic and allelic heterogeneity of CS.

Interestingly, the best characterized CS-associated genes (highlighted in Table 3.1) are part of functionally interconnected signaling cascades mainly involved in skeletal and craniofacial development [5, 12, 23]. In approximately 75–80% of all syndromic cases, the phenotype is caused by monogenic mutations in either of a short list of 7 genes encoding for developmental and bone-related signaling molecules, namely, Fibroblast Growth Factor Receptor 1–3 (*FGFR-1, -2,* and *-3*), TWIST family bHLH transcription factor 1 (*TWIST1*), Muscle Segment Homeobox 2 (*MSX2*), Ephrin B1 (*EFNB1*), and Transcription Factor 12 (*TCF12*) [4, 5, 19].

The most frequently diagnosed CS syndromes include Muenke syndrome (1/10,000–1/30,000, 4% of all CS), Saethre-Chotzen syndrome (1/25,000–1/50,000), Crouzon syndrome (1/25,000–1/61,000, 4.8% of all CS), Apert syndrome (1/65,000–1/100,000, 3% of all CS), Pfeiffer syndrome (1/100,000, 1–2% of all CS), and craniofrontonasal syndrome (1/120,000, 0.8% of all cases) [5, 24]. These tend to share an autosomal dominant pattern of inheritance, due to either gain-of-function (e.g., *FGFR2–3* and *MSX2* mutations), loss-of-function, or dominant negative mutations (e.g., *TWIST1*, *EFNB1*, and *TCF12* mutations). Indeed, the genetic pathophysiology of CS mostly results from gain-of-function and haploinsufficiency, whereas rarely consists in a complete loss-of-function as these genes play key roles during embryonic development and thus, their complete loss is lethal in utero [12, 23]. Nonetheless, other alternative patterns of inheritance are described for additional rare syndromes encompassing the CS spectrum (e.g., Carpenter syndrome, autosomal recessive; Craniofrontonasal dysplasia, and X-linked dominant, among others; see Table 3.1).

The best-characterized disease-associated genes along with recently identified pathogenic and risk-related gene variants are systematically described.

3.3.1 Fibroblast Growth Factor Receptors (FGFRs)

FGFRs are single-pass transmembrane proteins that serve as high-affinity tyrosine kinase receptors for fibroblast growth factors (FGFs). FGFs binding to the extracellular IgII-IgIII domains of FGFR induces receptor activation triggering the intracellular downstream signaling that culminates in the phosphorylation of target proteins [25–27].

FGFRs are expressed in a spatial-dependent manner by controlling the proliferation and differentiation of mesenchymal and neuroectodermal cells during skeletal development [27]. Specifically, in cranial sutures, FGFR2 is predominantly expressed in osteoprogenitor cells, FGFR1 is located in more differentiated osteoblasts, whereas FGFR3 has lower expression in the periosteum and in sutural osteogenic fronts at the late stage of suture niche development [28].

Gain-of-function missense mutations affecting hot spot domains in *FGFR* -1, -2, and -3 have been extensively associated with syndromic CS [5, 29, 30]. The clinical spectrum of these conditions varies from complex multi-suture CS syndromes (including Apert syndrome, Beare-Stevenson cutis gyrata syndrome, Bent bone dysplasia, Crouzon syndrome, Crouzon syndrome with acanthosis nigricans, Jackson-Weiss syndrome, Muenke syndrome, and Pfeiffer syndrome) to isolated monosutural CS [30].

Specifically, the majority of FGFR-related CS syndromes have been associated with autosomal dominant mutations located within exons 8 and 10 of the *FGFR2* gene (encoding IgIIIa and IgIIIc domains, respectively) or in the intron sequence

Table 3.1 Craniosynostosis-associated genes and corresponding syndromes

Cytogenetic location	Gene	Phenotype	MIM number	Inheritance
1p36.33	GNB1	Intellectual developmental disorder, autosomal dominant 42	616973	Autosomal dominant
1p36.33-p36.32	SKI	Shprintzen-Goldberg syndrome	182212	Autosomal dominant
1p36.31	CHD5	Parenti-Mignot neurodevelopmental syndrome	619873	Autosomal dominant
1p36.12	ALPL	Hypophosphatasia, infantile	241500	Autosomal recessive
1p36.11-p35.3	AHDC1	Xia-Gibbs syndrome	615829	Autosomal dominant
1p34.3	SNIP1	Neurodevelopmental disorder with hypotonia, craniofacial abnormalities, and seizures	614501	Autosomal recessive
1p32.3	ORC1	Meier-Gorlin syndrome 1	224690	Autosomal recessive
1p31.3	NFIA	Brain malformations with or without urinary tract defects	613735	Autosomal dominant
1p13.3	SLC25A24	Fontaine progeroid syndrome	612289	Autosomal dominant
1p13.3	ALX3	Frontonasal dysplasia 1	136760	Autosomal recessive
1q21.3	EFNA4	–	–	–
1q24.1	TMCO1	Craniofacial dysmorphism, skeletal anomalies, and impaired intellectual development 1	213980	Autosomal recessive
1q42.12	H3-3A	Bryant-Li-Bhoj neurodevelopmental syndrome 1	619720	Autosomal dominant
2p25.3	COLEC11	3MC syndrome 2	265050	Autosomal recessive
2p24.1	WDR35	Cranioectodermal dysplasia 2	613610	Autosomal recessive
		Short-rib thoracic dysplasia 7 with or without polydactyly	614091	Autosomal recessive
2p23.2	PPP1CB	Noonan syndrome-like disorder with loose anagen hair 2	617506	Autosomal dominant
2p22.3	LTBP1	Cutis laxa, autosomal recessive, type IIE	619451	Autosomal recessive
2p13.2	CYP26B1	Craniosynostosis with radiohumeral fusions and other skeletal and craniofacial anomalies	614416	–
2q34-q36	IHH	Syndactyly, type 1, with or without craniosynostosis	185900	Autosomal dominant
2q34	PTH2R	–	–	–
2q35	NHEJ1	Severe combined immunodeficiency with microcephaly, growth retardation, and sensitivity to ionizing radiation	611291	–
3p24.1	TGFBR2	Loeys-Dietz syndrome 2	610168	Autosomal dominant
3p22.3	CRTAP	Osteogenesis imperfecta, type VII	610682	Autosomal recessive
3p21.31	SETD2	Rabin-Pappas syndrome	620155	Autosomal dominant

(continued)

Table 3.1 (continued)

Cytogenetic location	Gene	Phenotype	MIM number	Inheritance
3q21.3-q22.1	IFT122	Cranioectodermal dysplasia 1	218330	Autosomal recessive
3q24	ZIC1	Craniosynostosis 6	616602	Autosomal dominant
		Structural brain anomalies with impaired intellectual development and craniosynostosis	618736	Autosomal dominant
3q26.31	FNDC3B	–	–	–
3q27.3	MASP1	3MC syndrome 1	257920	Autosomal recessive
4p16	–	Craniosynostosis, Adelaide type	600593	?Autosomal dominant
4p16.3	**FGFR3**	Crouzon syndrome with Acanthosis nigricans	612247	Autosomal dominant
		Muenke syndrome	602849	Autosomal dominant
		Thanatophoric dysplasia, type I	187600	Autosomal dominant
		Thanatophoric dysplasia, type II	187601	Autosomal dominant
4p16.3	SH3BP2	Cherubism	118400	Autosomal dominant
4p14	WDR19	Cranioectodermal dysplasia 4	614378	Autosomal recessive
		Short-rib thoracic dysplasia 5 with or without polydactyly	614376	Autosomal recessive
4q24	PPP3CA	Arthrogryposis, cleft palate, craniosynostosis, and impaired intellectual development	618265	Autosomal dominant
4q24	SLC39A8	Congenital disorder of glycosylation, type IIn	616721	Autosomal recessive
4q26	SEC24D	Cole-Carpenter syndrome 2	616294	Autosomal recessive
4q28.1	SPRY1	–		
4q33	NEK1	Short-rib thoracic dysplasia 6 with or without polydactyly	263520	Autosomal recessive; Digenic recessive
5p13	–	Chromosome 5p13 duplication syndrome	613174	Isolated cases
5p13.2	NIPBL	Cornelia de Lange syndrome 1	122470	Autosomal dominant
5p12	FGF10	LADD syndrome	149730	Autosomal dominant
5q11.2	IL6ST	Hyper-IgE recurrent infection syndrome 4B, autosomal recessive	618523	Autosomal recessive
5q12.1	ZSWIM6	Acromelic frontonasal dysostosis	603671	Autosomal dominant
5q12.3	CWC27	Retinitis pigmentosa with or without skeletal anomalies	250410	Autosomal recessive
5q23.2	CEP120	Joubert syndrome 31	617761	Autosomal recessive
		Short-rib thoracic dysplasia 13 with or without polydactyly	616300	Autosomal recessive

(continued)

Table 3.1 (continued)

Cytogenetic location	Gene	Phenotype	MIM number	Inheritance
5q31.3	PCDHGC4	Neurodevelopmental disorder with poor growth and skeletal anomalies	619880	Autosomal recessive
5q31.3	SPRY4	Hypogonadotropic hypogonadism 17 with or without anosmia	615266	Autosomal dominant
5q32-q33.1	TCOF1	Treacher Collins syndrome 1	154500	Autosomal dominant
5q35.2	**MSX2**	Craniosynostosis 2	604757	Autosomal dominant
6p22.1	H4C9	Tessadori-van Haaften neurodevelopmental syndrome 4	619951	Autosomal dominant
6p12.3	TFAP2B	Char syndrome	169100	Autosomal dominant
6p12.1-p11.2	RAB23	Carpenter syndrome	201000	Autosomal recessive
6q21	OSTM1	Osteopetrosis, autosomal recessive 5	259720	Autosomal recessive
7p21.1	**TWIST1**	Craniosynostosis 1	123100	Autosomal dominant
		Robinow-Sorauf syndrome	180750	Autosomal dominant
		Saethre-Chotzen syndrome with or without eyelid anomalies	101400	Autosomal dominant
		Sweeney-Cox syndrome	617746	Autosomal dominant
7p21.1	POLR1F	–	–	–
7p14.1	GLI3	Greig cephalopolysyndactyly syndrome	175700	Autosomal dominant
7q11.23	–	Chromosome 7q11.23 deletion syndrome, distal, 1.2 Mb	613729	
7q11.23	–	Williams-Beuren syndrome	194050	Autosomal dominant
7q11.23	POR	Antley-Bixler syndrome with genital anomalies and disordered steroidogenesis	201750	Autosomal recessive
7q32.1	SMO	Curry-Jones syndrome, somatic mosaic	601707	–
8p23.1	MCPH1	Microcephaly 1, primary, autosomal recessive	251200	Autosomal recessive
8p21.1	ESCO2	Roberts-SC phocomelia syndrome	268300	Autosomal recessive
8p21.1	EXTL3	Immunoskeletal dysplasia with neurodevelopmental abnormalities	617425	Autosomal recessive
8p12	GTF2E2	Trichothiodystrophy 6, nonphotosensitive	616943	Autosomal recessive

(continued)

Table 3.1 (continued)

Cytogenetic location	Gene	Phenotype	MIM number	Inheritance
8p11.23	**FGFR1**	Hartsfield syndrome	615465	Autosomal dominant
		Jackson-Weiss syndrome	123150	Autosomal dominant
		Osteoglophonic dysplasia	166250	Autosomal dominant
		Pfeiffer syndrome	101600	Autosomal dominant
		Trigonocephaly 1	190440	Autosomal dominant
8p11.21	KAT6A	Arboleda-Tham syndrome	616268	Autosomal dominant
8q12.1	BPNT2	Chondrodysplasia with joint dislocations, GPAPP type	614078	Autosomal recessive
8q12.2-q21.2	–	Hydrocephalus, autosomal dominant	123155	Autosomal dominant
8q22.1	–	Nablus mask-like facial syndrome	608156	Autosomal dominant
8q24.12	COLEC10	3MC syndrome 3	248340	Autosomal recessive
8q24.3	RECQL4	Baller-Gerold syndrome	218600	Autosomal recessive
9p	–	Chromosome 9p deletion syndrome	158170	Autosomal dominant
9p24.2	GLIS3	Diabetes mellitus, neonatal, with congenital hypothyroidism	610199	Autosomal recessive
9p22.3	FREM1	Trigonocephaly 2	614485	Autosomal dominant
9p13.3	IL11RA	Craniosynostosis and dental anomalies	614188	Autosomal recessive
9q21.2	PSAT1	Phosphoserine aminotransferase deficiency	610992	Autosomal recessive
9q21.32	HNRNPK	Au-Kline syndrome	616580	Autosomal dominant
9q21.33	NTRK2	Obesity, hyperphagia, and developmental delay	613886	Autosomal dominant
9q22.33	TGFBR1	Loeys-Dietz syndrome 1	609192	Autosomal dominant
9q31.2	ZNF462	Weiss-Kruszka syndrome	618619	Autosomal dominant
10p12.1	WAC	Desanto-Shinawi syndrome	616708	Autosomal dominant
10q22.1	KIFBP	Goldberg-Shprintzen megacolon syndrome	609460	Autosomal recessive
10q26	–	Chromosome 10q26 deletion syndrome	609625	Autosomal dominant

(continued)

Table 3.1 (continued)

Cytogenetic location	Gene	Phenotype	MIM number	Inheritance
10q26.13	**FGFR2**	Scaphocephaly, maxillary retrusion, and impaired intellectual development	609579	–
		Antley-Bixler syndrome without genital anomalies or disordered steroidogenesis	207410	Autosomal dominant
		Apert syndrome	101200	Autosomal dominant
		Beare-Stevenson cutis gyrata syndrome	123790	Autosomal dominant
		Bent bone dysplasia syndrome	614592	Autosomal dominant
		Craniofacial-skeletal-dermatologic dysplasia	101600	Autosomal dominant
		Craniosynostosis, nonspecific		
		Crouzon syndrome	123500	Autosomal dominant
		Jackson-Weiss syndrome	123150	Autosomal dominant
		Pfeiffer syndrome	101600	Autosomal dominant
		Saethre-Chotzen syndrome	101400	Autosomal dominant
		Scaphocephaly and Axenfeld-Rieger anomaly		
		Saethre-Chotzen syndrome	101400	Autosomal dominant
		Scaphocephaly and Axenfeld-Rieger anomaly	–	–
11p15.4	CDKN1C	Beckwith-Wiedemann syndrome	130650	Autosomal dominant
		IMAGE syndrome	614732	Autosomal dominant
11p15.2	SOX6	Tolchin-Le Caignec syndrome	618971	Autosomal dominant
11p11.2	ALX4	Frontonasal dysplasia 2	613451	Autosomal recessive
		{Craniosynostosis 5, susceptibility to}	615529	Autosomal dominant
11q12.1	FAM111A	Gracile bone dysplasia	602361	Autosomal dominant
11q12.2	TMEM216	Joubert syndrome 2	608091	Autosomal recessive
11q13.1	DPF2	Coffin-Siris syndrome 7	618027	Autosomal dominant
11q21	CEP57	Mosaic variegated aneuploidy syndrome 2	614114	Autosomal recessive
12p12.1	KRAS	Noonan syndrome 3	609942	Autosomal dominant
12q13.3	PRIM1	Primordial dwarfism-immunodeficiency-lipodystrophy syndrome	620005	Autosomal recessive
13q12.11	FGF9	Multiple synostoses syndrome 3	612961	Autosomal dominant
13q33-q34	–	Chromosome 13q33-q34 deletion syndrome	619148	Autosomal dominant

(continued)

Table 3.1 (continued)

Cytogenetic location	Gene	Phenotype	MIM number	Inheritance
14q22.2	BMP4	Microphthalmia, syndromic 6	607932	Autosomal dominant
14q24.3	IFT43	Cranioectodermal dysplasia 3	614099	Autosomal recessive
14q32.12	LYSET	Dysostosis multiplex, Ain-Naz type	619345	Autosomal recessive
14q32.2	YY1	Gabriele-de Vries syndrome	617557	Autosomal dominant
15q21.1	FBN1	Marfan lipodystrophy syndrome	616914	Autosomal dominant
15q21.3	**TCF12**	Craniosynostosis 3	615314	Autosomal dominant
15q22.31	SMAD6	{Craniosynostosis 7, susceptibility to}	617439	Autosomal dominant
15q26-qter	–	Levy-Shanske syndrome	614846	
16p13.3	IFT140	Short-rib thoracic dysplasia 9 with or without polydactyly	266920	Autosomal recessive
16q12.2	IRX5	Hamamy syndrome	611174	Autosomal recessive
16q13	RSPRY1	Spondyloepimetaphyseal dysplasia, Faden-Alkuraya type	616723	Autosomal recessive
17p13.3	DPH1	Developmental delay with short stature, dysmorphic facial features, and sparse hair	616901	Autosomal recessive
17p13.1	MYH3	Contractures, pterygia, and spondylocarpostarsal fusion syndrome 1A	178110	Autosomal dominant
17q21.2	STAT3	Hyper-IgE recurrent infection syndrome	147060	Autosomal dominant
17q23.2	TLK2	Intellectual developmental disorder, autosomal dominant 57	618050	Autosomal dominant
17q25.3	P4HB	Cole-Carpenter syndrome 1	112240	Autosomal dominant
18q21.32	CCBE1	Hennekam lymphangiectasia-lymphedema syndrome 1	235510	Autosomal recessive
18q22.2	RTTN	Microcephaly, short stature, and polymicrogyria with seizures	614833	Autosomal recessive
19p13.13	–	Chromosome 19p13.13 deletion syndrome	613638	
19p13.13	–	Chromosome 19p13.13 duplication syndrome	613638	
19q13.2	EXOSC5	Cerebellar ataxia, brain abnormalities, and cardiac conduction defects	619576	Autosomal recessive
19q13.2	ERF	Craniosynostosis 4	600775	Autosomal dominant
19q13.2	MEGF8	Carpenter syndrome 2	614976	Autosomal recessive
19q13.32	KPTN	Intellectual developmental disorder, autosomal recessive 41	615637	Autosomal recessive
20p12.2	JAG1	Alagille syndrome 1	118450	Autosomal dominant
20q11.22	GDF5	Brachydactyly, type C	113100	Autosomal dominant
20q13.13	SNAI1	–	–	–

(continued)

Table 3.1 (continued)

Cytogenetic location	Gene	Phenotype	MIM number	Inheritance
21q22.11	SON	ZTTK syndrome	617140	Autosomal dominant
21q22.11	DONSON	Microcephaly-micromelia syndrome	251230	Autosomal recessive
22q11.21	CDC45	Meier-Gorlin syndrome 7	617063	Autosomal recessive
22q11.21	SCARF2	Van den Ende-Gupta syndrome	600920	Autosomal recessive
22q11.23	SPECC1L	Teebi hypertelorism syndrome 1	145420	Autosomal dominant
22q12-q13	–	CDAGS syndrome	603116	Autosomal recessive
22q12.1	MN1	CEBALID syndrome	618774	Autosomal dominant
22q13.2	TCF20	Developmental delay with variable intellectual impairment and behavioral abnormalities	618430	Autosomal dominant
Xp11.23	OTUD5	Multiple congenital anomalies-neurodevelopmental syndrome, X-linked	301056	X-linked recessive
Xp11.22	HUWE1	Intellectual developmental disorder, X-linked syndromic, Turner type	309590	X-linked
Xq13.1	**EFNB1**	Craniofrontonasal dysplasia	304110	X-linked dominant
Xq13.1	MED12	Opitz-Kaveggia syndrome	305450	X-linked recessive
Xq28	CCNQ	STAR syndrome	300707	X-linked dominant
Xq28	NAA10	Microphthalmia, syndromic 1	309800	X-linked

flanking exon 10 (IIIa/exon 8 and IIIc/exon 10) [29, 31]. Additional mutations have been described in the IgI–IgII domains and in the tyrosine-kinase domains of this receptor [31–33].

Interestingly, identical *FGFR2* mutations (i.e., C278F, G298P, and C342T) have been found in patients with Crouzon, Pfeiffer, and Jackson-Weiss syndromes, suggesting that unknown genetic modifiers could contribute to the wide phenotypic heterogeneity observed in patients carrying the same FGFR2 mutation [34].

Furthermore, mutations in *FGFR2* (c.1576A>G; p.Lys526Glu, and c.1032G>A; p. Ala344Ala) have been found in familial cases of sagittal synostosis [20, 35].

A mutation affecting the *FGFR1* gene (p. Pro252Arg) has been found in 5% of individuals with Pfeiffer syndrome 1 (the less severe phenotype) and in a patient with Jackson-Weiss syndrome [36, 37]. *FGFR1* variants have also been associated with NCS cases. In particular, a heterozygous missense mutation (c.899T>C, p. Ile300Thr) and a frameshift mutation (due to a c.730_731insG insertion) in *FGFR1* were found in two nonsyndromic cases presenting metopic and sagittal synostosis, respectively [11, 38].

Furthermore, heterozygous mutations in *FGFR3* have been specifically associated with Crouzon syndrome with acanthosis nigricans (p. Ala391Glu) and with Muenke syndrome (p. Pro250Arg) as well as with nonsyndromic cases [39–42]. Specifically, the latter is one of the most common alterations in the human genome with a mutation rate of 8×10^{-6} [43].

FGFR-related syndromes usually display an overall decreased reproductive fitness, with probands carrying, in most cases, de novo mutations [5, 29, 30]. Nonetheless, due to the extremely variable phenotypic expression, familial forms, with wide intrafamilial heterogeneity, have been described. The widely variable expression and penetrance of FGFR missense mutations also explain the rare occurrence of milder phenotypes that may be sometimes disguised.

Mutations in *FGFR* genes represent a significant surgical prognostic factor, being associated with a worse clinical course, including the frequent need for re-intervention to treat relapses (i.e., re-synostosis; [44]). In this regard, it has been suggested that patients operated on below 6 months of age have a three-fold greater risk of developing re-synostosis compared with children treated between 6 months and 2 years old [45]. However, it is not clear whether the high risk of developing postoperative reossification results from the progressive nature of these conditions, the age at the time of surgery, or the presence of germline mutations in these patients [44, 46, 47].

Overall, it is reasonable to consider *FGFR* -1, -2, and -3 genetic testing in complex nonsyndromic and syndromic cases, especially in the presence of additional clinical features and developmental delay (Fig. 3.1) [4, 48].

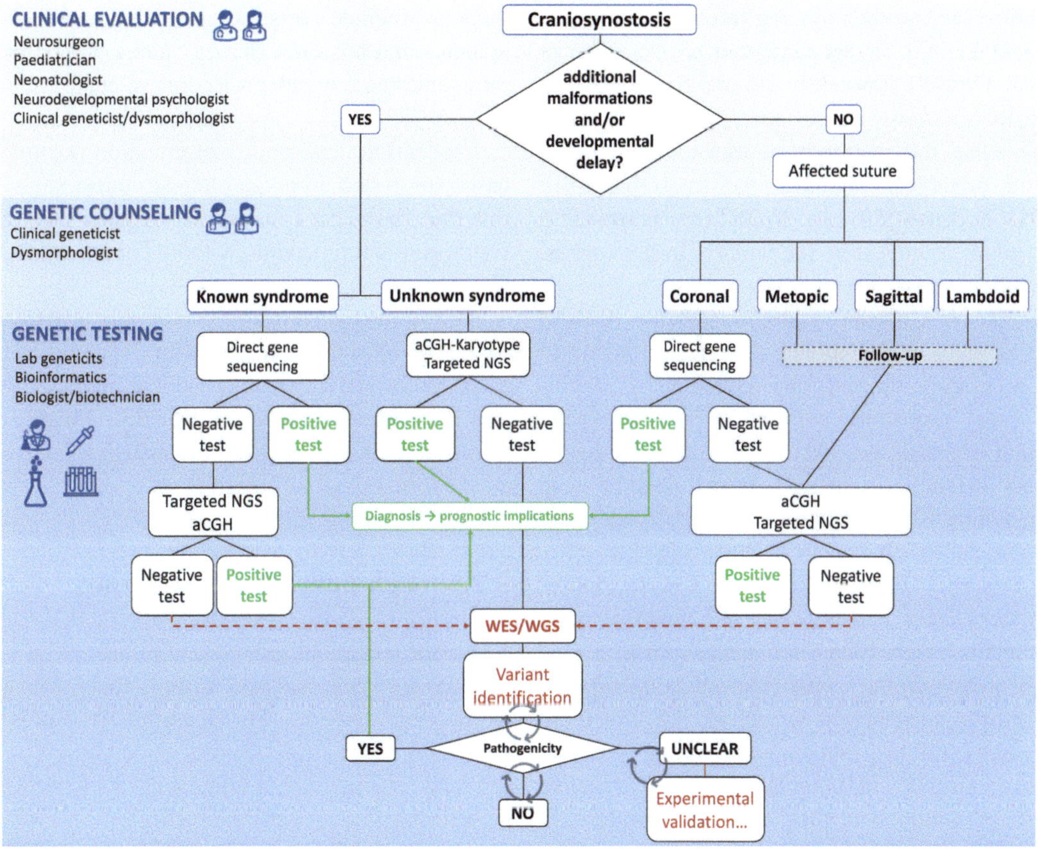

Fig. 3.1 Tentative flowchart for genetic diagnosis. The path toward a complete and correct diagnosis of a CS case starts with the clinical evaluation, which should be based on the shared effort of a multidisciplinary team of specialized medical and surgical professionals. To achieve the correct categorization of the specific CS subtype, the neurosurgeon must first establish the site and number of affected suture(s). Experienced clinical geneticists/dysmorphologists should physically examine the patient to assess the presence of additional malformations and anomalies throughout the body and analyze the pedigree for intrafamilial recurrence. Pediatric neuropsychologists/psychiatrists will assess the psychomotor performance of patients. Genetic counseling will then serve to complete the differential diagnosis and plan the correct testing, which largely varies based on CS type. If genetic testing is mandatory for syndromic and/or unclear complex CS forms, a more temporizing strategy, with careful follow-up may be exploited in the management of nonsyndromic CS, which may disguise genetic forms, especially in the case of coronal involvement, of familial recurrence, or in the presence of subtle and often neglected associated cognitive or somatic anomalies. See the chapter text for additional details

3.3.2 TWIST Family bHLH Transcription Factor 1 (TWIST1) and Related Genes

The basic helix-loop-helix transcription factor (bHLH) TWIST1 is a key regulator of skeletal development. Specifically, during calvarial development, TWIST1 controls the specification and the differentiation of cells within the cranial suture mesenchyme and osteogenic fronts by first homo- or heterodimerizing with other bHLH molecules and then binding to conserved motifs on DNA [49]. In this context, it has been shown that TWIST1 transiently inhibits the expression of RUNX family transcription factor 2 (*RUNX2*), encoding the master bone transcription factor, and negatively regulates the transcription of *FGFR* genes [50–52]. TWIST1 is believed to regulate osteogenesis particularly in the coronal suture domain [53].

Saethre-Chotzen syndrome (OMIM 101400) is an autosomal dominant disorder belonging to CS syndromes and characterized by uni/bicoronal synostosis with additional facial and limb abnormalities [54]. The disorder is due to loss-of-function mutations in the *TWIST1* gene including SNPs, deletions, insertions, duplications, and complex rearrangements [13].

Also for *TWIST1* mutations, a wide clinical heterogeneity can be described. Indeed, point mutations were found in patients with an apparent nonsyndromic phenotype, affecting sagittal, metopic, and coronal sutures [5, 38]. For these reasons, *TWIST1* mutational screening is widely recommended in complex CS with negative *FGFR* mutation results, and in coronal NCS, even in the absence of clear syndromic traits (Fig. 3.1) [4, 48].

Also, *TWIST1* mutations are associated with a worse surgical course due to increased risk of developing intracranial hypertension, thus requiring more invasive surgery and/or multiple procedures [44, 54].

The transcription factor 12 gene (*TCF12*) encodes another member of the bHLH transcription factor family, which is involved in the maintenance of coronal suture patency by forming heterodimers with TWIST1 and thus inhibiting osteogenic differentiation acting on RUNX2 and FGFR signaling pathways [55]. TCF12-related CS (OMIM 615314) caused by heterozygous mutations in *TCF12* was identified in syndromic multi-suture CS associated with additional abnormalities closely resembling the Saethre-Chotzen phenotype. Also, *TCF12* mutations have been found in apparently nonsyndromic patients with unilateral/bilateral coronal synostosis, though in most cases a mild to moderate cognitive impairment was observed in patients [5, 55, 56]. *TCF12* variants include small frameshift, nonsense, splicing, and missense changes, along with large intragenic rearrangements leading to haploinsufficiency [55, 57].

Epidemiological studies of mutation-positive cases suggested a benign clinical course showing that these patients usually require only a single surgical procedure without complications [57, 58].

TCF12 molecular testing is currently included in first level tests in patients with unilateral and bilateral coronal CS (with or without syndactyly) and is recommended in all *FGFR3*-, *TWIST1*-negative patients, and aCGH-negative multi-suture forms (Fig. 3.1) [23, 58].

3.3.3 Eph-Ephrin Pathway Genes

Eph-ephrin is another important family of tyrosine kinase receptors and ligands that control skull development [5]. Specifically, EphB/EphrinB1 interaction controls skeletal patterning and craniofacial morphogenesis, whereas Ephrin A4 is a downstream effector of Twist regulating coronal suture formation and patency [12, 59, 60]. In this regard, loss-of-function mutations in *EFNA4* and *EFNB1* encoding Ephrin A4 and Ephrin B1 ligands have been found in nonsyndromic coronal CS and in X-linked craniofrontonasal syndrome (featuring coronal CS), respectively [5]. Mutations in *EFNB1* are also described in unclear syndromic phenotypes, including both coronal and multi-suture CS, and should be considered for second-level genetic testing in these cases (Fig. 3.1) [23, 44].

3.3.4 ETS2 Repressor Factor (ERF)

The ETS2 repressor factor gene (*ERF*) encodes a repressor transcription factor expressed by neural crest cells that antagonizes RUNX2-induced osteogenic signaling [61, 62]. *ERF* loss-of-function mutations have been found in 2% of syndromic CS cases and in 0.7% of clinically nonsyndromic patients. ERF haploinsufficiency causes the loss of RUNX2 inhibition enhancing osteoprogenitors' differentiation within the cranial sutures niche [62]. *ERF* mutations are typically associated with sagittal and uni-/bi-lateral lambdoid synostoses or less frequently a multi-suture involvement up to pansynostosis [13, 61, 62].

Regarding the clinical management of ERF-related craniosynostosis, it is extremely important to consider that these patients develop a progressive ossification of sutures, presenting an asymptomatic course until the appearance of multi-suture synostoses and raised ICP during early infancy [61]. For these reasons, *ERF* mutation screening could be considered in suspect nonsyndromic CS and in complex CS cases involving at least sagittal or lambdoid suture (Fig. 3.1) [61].

3.3.5 Msh Homeobox 2 (MSX2) and Homeotic Transcription Factors

The Msh homeobox 2 (*MSX2*) encodes a homeodomain transcription factor mainly expressed by the neural crest cells and strongly contributes to craniofacial development [5].

MSX2 gain-of-function was the first genetic abnormality described in a CS phenotype, later named Boston-type CS [63]. This is a rare condition, with full penetrance and variable expressivity, involving either sagittal, coronal, or multi-suture CS [5]. *MSX2* copy number variations have also been associated with CS, confirming that correct cranial suture development requires an appropriate MSX2 dosage [64].

Similarly, gain-of-function mutations in the homeobox gene named aristaless-like homeobox 4 (*ALX4*) have been associated with both syndromic multi-suture CS involving at least sagittal suture (i.e., frontonasal dysplasia) and nonsyndromic sagittal, coronal, or metopic phenotype [65, 66]. Similar to MSX2, a high dosage of ALX4 causes CS, while loss-of-function mutations lead to defective ossification of the skull (i.e., parietal foramina 2) [5, 66].

Whole exome and genome sequencing (WES/WGS) in unsolved CS cases allowed the identification of heterozygous variants in the SIX homeobox 1 (*SIX1*) gene, which encodes a homeodomain-containing transcription factor of the sine oculis class [15]. The patients presented sagittal and/or bi-lambdoid sutures' fusion associated with additional features that are typically found in SIX1-related syndromes (branchio-otic syndrome, MIM 608389; nonsyndromic, MIM 605192; and branchio-oto-renal syndrome) [15].

Finally, the SIX homeobox 2 (*SIX2*), another member of the aristaless family, was found mutated in patients with syndromic complex CS or single-sagittal suture synostosis, resembling frontonasal phenotype [67]. *SIX2* encodes a transcription factor that controls neural crest cells' proliferation and migration during early skull development [67].

Given the low prevalence and the poor reproducibility of associated phenotypes, mutation analyses of homeotic genes are not currently suggested as a first-line test, although *MSX2* testing is advised in the presence of Boston-type CS (Fig. 3.1) [68]. Based on the available pieces of evidence, it should be also considered in nonsyndromic sagittal and/or unicoronal synostosis with familial recurrence and/or history of syndactyly (Fig. 3.1) [68].

3.3.6 Ciliary Genes

Primary cilium (CP) is a nonmotile cellular organelle that protrudes from the apical surface of almost all human cells, receiving and transducing physical and biochemical extracellular stimuli into intracellular cascades (i.e., Hedgehog (HH) and Wnt family member (WNT)) to regulate tissue development and homeostasis [69].

Ciliopathies are a group of Mendelian conditions due to mutations in primary cilium-related genes and are characterized by several anomalies (i.e., retinal degeneration, renal disease, and cerebral anomalies) including skeletal defects [70]. Among these, craniosynostosis has been recurrently reported in ciliopathies caused by mutations in over 18 CP-related genes, becoming a clinically relevant phenotype [69].

Specifically, genes encoding the intraflagellar transport (IFT) components involved in protein traffickings along CP such as *IFT122*, *IFT43*, and *IFT140* have been implicated in the etiopathogenesis of cranio-ectodermal dysplasia 1 and 3 (CED, also named Sensenbrenner syndrome) and of short-rib thoracic dysplasia 9 (SRTD 9), respectively [69, 71]. These conditions are characterized by limb and facial abnormalities and sagittal or metopic CS [69].

Furthermore, biallelic mutations in the Centrosomal protein 120 (*CEP120*) and in NIMA-related kinase 1 (*NEK1*) genes, both involved in centrosome organization, centriole biogenesis, and cell cycle progression control, have been associated with different forms of STRD characterized by uni- and bicoronal synostosis, respectively [69].

In addition, the dysregulation of the HH pathway, one of the most important cilia-related signaling, has been found in ciliopathies characterized by complex clinical defects including sagittal synostosis. Of these, Joubert syndrome 2 is caused by a homozygous mutation in the transmembrane protein 216 (*TMEM216*) gene, encoding for a ciliary base protein that regulates the HH pathway and ciliary membrane composition [69]. In addition, microduplications of the *IHH* (Indian hedgehog signaling molecule) gene have been found in the Syndactyly type 1 featuring syndactyly and sagittal CS [72].

A recurrent somatic mosaic mutation in the gene encoding the ciliary membrane receptor Smoothened, frizzled class receptor (*SMO*) causes Curry–Jones syndrome, a multisystem disorder characterized by patchy skin lesions, polysyndactyly, cerebral malformations, and unicoronal craniosynostosis [73].

Besides, HH signaling is mediated by the GLI family zinc finger proteins, including GLI3 which is involved in the intramembranous ossification process of skull bones [74]. Heterozygous loss-of-function mutations in the *GLI3* gene are indeed associated with Greig cephalopolysyndactyly syndrome, characterized by craniofacial anomalies, including sagittal and metopic CS, along with hand/foot abnormalities, and cognitive impairment [75].

Finally, loss-of-function mutations in the RAB23, member RAS oncogene family (*RAB23*) gene, acting as a negative regulator of HH and ERK1/2 signaling, cause Carpenter Syndrome 1, a rare pleiotropic disorder featuring either single (sagittal) or multi-suture (sagittal and metopic; cloverleaf skull) synostosis as a hallmark [76]. These patients also present multisystem developmental impairment, with variable severities, affecting the brain, genitourinary system, heart, and appendicular skeleton [69].

Genome-wide association study (GWAS) identified susceptibility loci for sagittal nonsyndromic craniosynostosis near Bone Morphogenetic Protein 2 (*BMP2*) and within the Bardet-Biedl syndrome gene 9 (*BBS9*) gene, which encodes a protein of the multimeric complex "BBSome" required for ciliogenesis [77]. In this regard, Barba et al. [78] observed specific upregulated splice variants of BBS9 in nonsyndromic patients with sagittal or metopic synostosis.

Recently, a WGS study detected a novel variant of the CP-related fuzzy planar cell polarity protein gene (*FUZ*) (c.851 G>C, p.(Arg284Pro)) in monozygotic twins exhibiting metopic craniosynostosis [79]. In this study, the authors highlighted that the FUZ protein is a planar cell polarity (PCP) effector, which is essential for normal ciliogenesis, although it also acts as a negative regulator of osteogenesis [79].

In this context, to date, it has become important to consider genetic screening of CP-related genes in patients featuring single- or multi-suture synostosis and core phenotypic manifestations of ciliopathy (Fig. 3.1).

3.3.7 Recently Identified Genes

Next-generation sequencing has greatly enhanced the discovery of new disease-associated genes expanding the genetic spectrum of CS disorders at an unprecedented pace [5, 13, 19].

Homozygous missense and nonsense mutations along with a duplication in the gene encoding the IL11 receptor alpha (***IL11RA***) have been reported in patients showing a Crouzon-like phenotype with multi-suture synostosis and dental anomalies [80–84]. *IL11RA* testing is hence recommended in familial pansynostosis CS, specifically in complex form associated with teeth anomalies [4] (Fig. 3.1).

The ZIC family member 1 (***ZIC1***) gene encodes another regulator of embryo development that drives the membranous ossification by regulating FGF signaling and Sonic hedgehog signaling molecule (SHH) within calvarial suture mesenchyme [85]. Heterozygous gain-of-function mutations in *ZIC1* have been found in patients with severe bicoronal and complex CS phenotypes, including learning disability [85]. The diagnosis of a *ZIC1* mutation has significant implications for prognosis; hence, ZIC1 testing is advisable for FGFRs/TWIST1/TCF12-negative coronal synostosis and complex CS forms [85] (Fig. 3.1).

A unique homozygous mutation in the beta-1,3-glucuronyltransferase 3 (***B3GAT3***) gene, known to be involved in linkeropathy syndrome, was found in 6 patients exhibiting a severe clinical spectrum consisting in craniosynostosis, midface hypoplasia, skeletal defects involving limbs and extremities, bone fragility, and cardiovascular abnormalities [86].

De novo variants of ***CD96***, a member of the immunoglobulin superfamily, were identified in two cases with C syndrome/Opitz trigonocephaly (OMIM 211750) exhibiting trigonocephaly, facial deformities, wide alveolar ridges, multiple buccal frenula, limb defects, visceral anomalies, redundant skin, psychomotor retardation, and hypotonia resembling Bohring-Opitz syndrome (caused by mutations in *ASXL1*) [87, 88]. It has been supposed that mutations in *CD96* affect cell adhesion and cell growth [88].

Homozygous mutations in the diphthamide biosynthesis 1 (***DPH1***) gene have also been associated with a phenotype characterized by unusual skull shape due to sagittal/coronal synostosis, developmental delay, central nervous system malformations, cardiac defect, short stature, and early lethality [13, 89, 90].

Heterozygous missense mutations in ***FGF9*** were identified in 2 families with multiple synostoses syndromes, 3 exhibiting multiple synostoses including the premature fusion of sagittal suture [91, 92]. It has been suggested that these mutations led to dysregulation of FGFR3 signaling by impairing the homodimerization of FGF9 and its binding to the receptor FGFR3 [92].

Craniosynostosis involving metopic suture has been reported in few patients with severe polymalformative syndrome associated with homozygous missense mutations in the FTO alpha-ketoglutarate dependent dioxygenase (***FTO***) gene [13, 93]. FTO belongs to the AlkB-related dioxygenase family, playing a role in genome integrity only partially known [94].

Skeletal abnormalities, including sagittal synostosis, have been associated also with heterogeneous nuclear ribonucleoprotein K (***HNRNPK***) haploinsufficiency resulting in Au-Kline syndrome (OMIM 616580) [13, 95]. Affected individuals also showed intellectual disability, unique craniofacial phenotype, and brain and connective tissue anomalies [95].

Two male patients with sagittal suture synostosis and a clinical spectrum extending from Lin-Gettig syndrome to genitopatellar (GPS) and Say Barber Biesecker Young Simpson (SBBYS) syndromes have been associated with de novo frameshift mutations in the lysine acetyltransferase 6B (***KAT6B***) gene [96]. The affected individuals also showed hypoplastic male genitalia, agenesis of the corpus callosum, thyroid abnormalities, and dysmorphic features such as short palpebral fissures and retrognathia [96].

Mutations in genes encoding proteins of the lectin complement pathway such as MBL-associated serine protease 1 (***MASP1***) and collectin subfamily member 11 (***COLEC11***) have been reported in 3MC syndromes (Carnevale, Mingarelli, Malpuech, and Michels syndromes) associated with a clinical spectrum comprising craniosynostosis [13, 97, 98].

A heterozygous missense mutation and a deletion in the prolyl 4-hydroxylase subunit beta (***P4HB***) gene have been associated with Cole-Carpenter syndrome (OMIM 112240), which consists of frequent fractures, coronal and metopic synostosis, ocular proptosis, hydrocephalus, and distinctive facial features [99, 100].

Compound heterozygous mutations in the sodium voltage-gated channel alpha subunit 4 (***SCN4A***) gene have been reported in two siblings featuring lower facial weakness, highly arched palate, synostosis of the sagittal and metopic sutures, axial hypotonia, proximal muscle weakness, and mild scoliosis [101]. Nevertheless, Gonorazky et al. [101] revealed that these mutations caused full and partial loss of function of the Nav1.4 channel leading to a reduction of muscle contraction. These data did not correlate with the premature fusion of cranial sutures suggesting that craniosynostosis could be an incidental finding in these two patients [101].

De novo missense mutations in the SLC25A24 pseudogene 2 (***SLC25A24***) gene, which encodes for the calcium-binding mitochondrial carrier protein (SCaMC-1, also known as SLC25A24) have been described in complex syndromes including Gorlin-Chaudhry-Moss syndrome (GCMS; OMIM 233500) and Fontaine syndrome cases both including coronal craniosynostosis, among their clinical spectrum [102, 103]. In addition, a potential influence between TWIST signaling and SLC25A24 function has emerged due to the overlapping clinical features between disorders caused by TWIST2 (i.e., Barber-Say syndrome and Ablepharon-Macrostomia syndrome) and GCMS [102].

Moreover, recent data reported craniosynostosis as a novel phenotype of RASopathies that are caused by gene mutations in the RAS-MAPK (mitogen-activated protein kinase) signal cascade [104]. Specifically, alterations in the KRAS proto-oncogene, GTPase (***KRAS***), protein tyrosine phosphatase nonreceptor type 11 (***PTPN11***), SHOC2 leucine-rich repeat scaffold protein (***SHOC2***), B-Raf proto-oncogene, and serine/threonine kinase (***BRAF***) genes have been described in patients with sagittal and/or lambdoid synostosis and additional features like-Noonan syndrome or like-cardio-facio-cutaneous syndrome (CFC) syndrome [104–107]. In this context, it has been postulated that the insurgence of craniosynostosis in these patients could be due to downstream signaling interaction between FGFR and the RAS/MAPK pathways [105, 107].

Whole-exome sequencing studies of a large nonsyndromic craniosynostosis cohort (sagittal and/or metopic; sagittal and coronal) revealed that SMAD family member 6 (***SMAD6***) damaging variants comprise about 5% of all midline NCS (including ~8% of all metopic, 2% of all sagittal, and 30% of cases with both sagittal and metopic) [14, 42]. Specifically, these variants were mostly transmitted by apparently unaffected parents and resulted in the loss of SMAD6 inhibitory effects, thus promoting BMP signaling and the premature fusion of cranial sutures [42, 108]. Concerning this, it is still debated if the presence of *BMP2* polymorphism, detected in some SMAD6-positive patients, can predict their phenotype [14, 42].

In addition, these patients presented worse clinical outcomes due to an increased risk of developing raised ICP after surgical procedures, highlighting that *SMAD6* genetic testing is recommended in unsolved CS patients [14] (Fig. 3.1). Moreover, echocardiographic screening is suggested in asymptomatic SMAD6-positive cases since it has been reported that patients with cardiovascular disorders ((i.e., bicuspid aortic valve (BAV) and ascending thoracic aortic aneurysm (TAA)) were enriched for *SMAD6* variants [14].

In addition, damaging de novo mutations in other inhibitors of WNT, BMP, and RAS/ERK signaling pathways have been documented in a wide cohort of patients with nonsyndromic midline craniosynostosis [20, 42, 109]. These included mutations in negative regulators of WNT signaling as axin 1 (***AXIN1***), mesoderm posterior bHLH transcription factor 1 (MESP1), nephrocystin 4 (***NPHP4***), proteasome 26S subunit, ATPase -2 and -5 (***PSMC2*** and ***PSMC5***), and Dishevelled segment polarity protein 3

(***DVL3***) as well as inhibitors of Ras/ERK signaling including sprouty RTK signaling antagonist 1 and 4 (***SPRY1*** and ***SPRY4***), RAS protein activator like 2 (***RASAL2***), and ArfGAP with RhoGAP domain, ankyrin repeat, and PH domain 3 (***ARAP3***) [42].

Miller et al. [109] described a boy showing sagittal synostosis, blue sclerae, micrognathia, ligamentous laxity, bilateral recurrent inguinal herniae, tall stature, and mildly abnormal aortic contour on echocardiography caused by two rare heterozygous variants in the fibrillin 1 (***FBN1***) gene.

In addition, a heterozygous mutation in the SH2 domain encoded by the signal transducer and activator of transcription 3 (***STAT3***), which was previously reported in a case of hyper-IgE/Jobs syndrome, was also found in a patient with midfacial hypoplasia, progressive airway distress, and pansynostosis [109].

Heterozygous nonsense mutation in the neurotrophic receptor tyrosine kinase 2 (***NTRK2***) gene has been associated with a female proband exhibiting an asymmetric face, left coronal synostosis, and later developmen [109].

Loss-of-function variants in the zinc finger protein 462 (***ZNF462***) have been described in nine individuals with multiple congenital syndromes including metopic ridging/craniosynostosis [40, 110].

Biallelic variants in cell division cycle 45 (***CDC45***), which encode a member of the pre-initiation complex in DNA replication, have been reported in Meier-Gorlin syndrome (MGS) associated with craniosynostosis [111, 112]. Clinical presentation of these patients varied from uni- and bicoronal synostosis and mild short stature, to a severe phenotype of MGS associated with multi-suture synostosis [111, 112].

Furthermore, a novel homozygous missense variant in the GINS complex subunit 2 (***GINS2***) gene was identified in a patient with MGS associated with bilateral coronal synostosis, phenotypically overlapping with the CDC45-related MGS [113]. The authors supposed that missense change disrupted the effective interaction between the GINS complex and CDC45, which is necessary for the correct function of the CMG helicase complex (Cdc45/MCM2–7/GINS) [113].

Pathogenic variants in the BCL11 transcription factor B (***BCL11B***), which play a key role in the maintenance of cranial suture patency, have been associated with about 20 cases featuring immunodeficiency, neurological disorders, dermal defects, congenital diaphragmatic hernia, and craniosynostosis [13, 114]. In this context, Zhao et al. [114] have recently described a novel frameshift variant in the *BCL11B* gene in a 25-month-old Chinese boy with severe multi-suture craniosynostosis and global developmental delay.

Furthermore, recent studies described craniosynostosis as an unseen clinical feature in chromatinopathies, which are genetically and clinically heterogeneous Mendelian disorders caused by genetic alterations of various components of the epigenetic machinery [115–117]. These conditions are characterized by a distinctive phenotype comprising intellectual disabilities, limb malformations, immune dysfunction, growth impairment, and skeletal anomalies [117]. In this regard, the craniosynostosis phenotype observed in a few cases could reflect the alteration of molecular pathways acting downstream of the mutated genes [116, 117].

Indeed, CS has been rarely associated with ***KANSL1*** (KAT8 regulatory NSL complex subunit 1) haploinsufficiency in Koolen-de Vries and Mowat-Wilson syndromes, with **KAT6B** (lysine acetyltransferase 6B)-related disorders and with pathogenic variants of ***KMT2D*** (lysine-specific methyltransferase 2D) in Kabuki syndrome [117].

In addition, Bukowska-Olech et al. [118] described six patients carrying pathogenic alterations in epigenetic regulators such as **ARID1A** (AT-rich interaction domain 1A), **KMT2A** (lysine methyltransferase 2A), and **NSD1** (nuclear receptor binding SET domain protein 1) resulting in Coffin-Siris syndrome type 2, Wiedemann-Steiner syndrome, and Sotos syndrome type 1, respectively. They were all characterized by intellectual disability, immune deficiencies, or skeletal anomalies including CS as a rare observation [118].

Metopic CS (trigonocephaly) has been recurrently described in Bohring-Opitz syndrome resulting from mutations of the chromatin modifier ASXL transcriptional regulator 1 (***ASXL1***) gene [117].

Based on such evidence, cranial sutures' evaluation and genetic testing should be considered in intellectual disabilities, to allow an accurate diagnosis and to improve the clinical outcomes of the patients (Fig. 3.1).

3.3.8 Chromosomal Structural Rearrangements

Despite CS being frequently regarded as a monogenic disorder, structural chromosomal aberrations can be identified in up to 15% of cases, mostly syndromic [5, 44]. These alterations are usually assessed by integrating standard karyotyping with array comparative genomic hybridization (aCGH) [5].

Chromosomal alterations are poorly reproducible across patients, as the involved loci are extremely heterogeneous; nevertheless, some recurrent mutation hotspots can be identified and may allow identifying additional putative candidate genes [5, 11].

In this regard, Gajecka et al. [119] proposed a list of candidate genes regulating cranial suture closure based on the analysis of subjects with duplication/triplication or the deletion of 1p chromosome presenting or not anomalies in suture ossification. Indeed, chromosome **1p36 duplication and triplication** have been reported in complex conditions including metopic or coronal craniosynostosis [119–121]. Conversely, monosomy 1p36, the most commonly observed terminal deletion, has been associated with late-closing anterior fontanelle, mental retardation along with other signs [119].

Among genes identified, the authors supposed that the matrix metalloproteinase-23A and -23B genes (*MMP23A* and *MMP*23B), which map to 1p36 and are responsible for extracellular matrix remodeling also during osteogenesis, could be involved in the suture phenotype in these patients [119].

In addition, two different intragenic microdelections in the *NFIA* gene (Chromosome **1p31.1 deletion**) have been reported in four patients with developmental delay, macrocephaly, hypoplastic corpus callosum, metopic/sagittal or lambdoid synostosis, and hematuria [122, 123]. Subsequently, Serra et al. [124] described a female with **1p31.3p22.2 deletion** exhibiting craniosynostosis, facial dysmorphisms, and a severe global developmental and growth delay. The deleted region of the proband contains about 90 genes including interleukin 23 receptor (*IL23R*), *RPE65* (retinoid isomerohydrolase RPE65), *LRRC7* (leucine rich re-peat containing 7), *SRSF11* (serine and arginine rich splicing factor 11), *ANKRD13C* (ankyrin repeat domain 13C), *CTH* (cystathionine gamma-lyase), *NEGR1* (neuronal growth regulator 1), *TNNI3K* (TNNI3 interacting kinase), *LHX8* (LIM homeobox 8), *ACADM* (acyl-CoA dehydrogenase medium chain), *PIGK* (phosphatidylinositol glycan anchor biosynthesis class K), *ZZZ3* (zinc finger ZZ-type containing 3), *USP33* (ubiquitin specific peptidase 33), *NEXN* (nexilin F-actin binding protein), *FUBP1* (far upstream element binding protein 1), *ADGRL2* (adhesion G protein-coupled receptor L2), *LPAR3* (lysophosphatidic acid receptor 3), *BCL10* (BCL10 immune signaling adaptor), *CCN1* (cellular communication network factor 1), *CLCA3P* (chloride channel accessory 3, pseudogene), and *SH3GLB1* (SH3 domain containing GRB2 like, endophilin B1) [124]. Of these, *IL23R* may have a potential association with craniosynostosis since it was already described in a patient with atypical CS [125].

Sowińska-Seidler et al. [126] identified a previously unreported de novo 1.26 Mb **duplication at chromosome 1q22–q23.1** in a male proband affected by complex CS, including metopic and lambdoid synostosis, muscular hypotonia, psychomotor retardation, and facial dysmorphism. The chromosome region described encompasses two genes involved in osteoblast differentiation: bone gamma-carboxyglutamate protein (*BGLAP*), encoding osteocalcin protein, and lamin A/C (LMNA), encoding lamin A/C [126].

In addition, a **duplication of the *RUNX2* locus on 6p21.1** was associated with metopic CS as well as **partial trisomy 6p12.3–p21.1** and ***RUNX2* locus quadruplication** was found in patients with more complex syndromic phenotypes, including combined coronal and sagittal synostosis or pan-craniosynostosis, respectively [127, 128]. These data suggest a dosage effect of RUNX2 alterations, with midline (metopic and sagittal) sutures appearing to be the primary target sites of the dysmorphic insult [127–129]. *RUNX2* encodes a transcription factor critical for skull development, considered as the bone master gene as its function is key to initiate skeletal formation during early prenatal stages [130]. Interestingly, a recent study in a sagittal NCS cohort reported the presence of gain-of-function nonsynonymous variants in the *RUNX2* locus [129].

Interstitial **deletions of chromosome 7p** have been found in patients with complex Saethre-Chotzen-like phenotypes [5, 131]. The *TWIST1* gene along with *HOXA* (homeobox A cluster) genes, mapping to this locus, could be involved in the pathogenesis of these patients [5, 131].

Karyotyping by both G-bind staining and array-based DNA hybridization allowed the identification of novel **microduplications on chromosomes 8p11.22 q12.1 and 16q11.2 q21** in a 2-year-old boy with dolichocephaly craniosynostosis [132]. The authors hypothesized that being 8p11.22 q12.1 merely 1 Mb downstream of *FGFR1*, duplication of this region might regulate the expression of *FGFR1*, thereby causing the development of craniosynostosis [132]. In addition, *BBS2* (Bardet-Biedl syndrome 2, Ch-Band: 16q21), *SALL1* (spalt-like transcription factor 1, Ch-Band: 16q12.1), and *CDH8* (cadherin 8, Ch-Band: 16q22.1) genes are plausible candidates of patients' phenotype [132].

The **9p deletion** syndrome (MIM 158170) is a multiple congenital disorder characterized by dysmorphic facial features, trigonocephaly, multiple congenital anomalies, and mental delay [133]. In the majority of cases, the 9p22.3 deletion position is a specific hotspot for metopic CS, causing over 15% of syndromic trigonocephaly [134, 135]. The FRAS1-related extracellular matrix 1 (*FREM1*) gene, mapping to this locus, is considered a putative candidate for the CS phenotype since it usually acts as an inhibitor of FGF signaling within the suture mesenchyme [136]. Further studies have identified additional genes that could be responsible for the 9p deletion syndrome phenotype, such as Cerberus 1 DAN family BMP antagonist (*CER1*), tyrosinase-related protein 1 (*TYRP1*), and protein tyrosine phosphatase receptor type D (*PTPRD*) [133, 137].

Duplications at chromosome 11q locus (**11q11-q13.3 duplications**), including *FGF3* and *FGF4* genes, have been also rarely found in patients with complex syndromic CS involving coronal/multi suture synostosis, congenital heart defect, and developmental delay [138, 139].

Microdeletion at 9p22–p24 and 11q23–q24 has also been associated with syndromic metopic craniosynostosis [134].

In addition, a de novo **balanced translocation t(9;11)(q33;p15)** was observed in a patient, who exhibited synostoses of both the lambdoid and the distal part of the sagittal sutures with a gaping anterior fontanelle and midfacial dysmorphisms [140]. The breakpoint disrupts the SRY-box transcription factor 6 (*SOX6*) gene locus on chromosome 11p15, known to be involved in skeletal growth and differentiation processes and a region on chromosome 9 with a large number of highly conserved nongenic sequences [140]. In addition, heterozygous missense mutations in the *SOX6* gene and a partial gene deletion encompassing exons 5–7 have been found in four patients with mild/moderate sagittal, coronal, and/or sutures synostosis and additional clinical features [140, 141].

Metopic synostosis has been reported also in a few cases of **partial and complete trisomy 13** (Patau syndrome) as well as in less severe **trisomy 13 mosaicism** characterized by a triad of the cleft lip and palate, postaxial polydactyly, and microcephaly [142, 143].

Cases of **partial distal trisomy (or tetrasomy) of chromosome 15q25qter**, housing the insulin-like growth factor 1 receptor (*IGF1R*) gene, have been reported in patients featuring craniosynostosis [144 150]. In addition, Cunningham et al. [151] identified five variants in *IGF1R* in patients with isolated sagittal or coronal suture synostosis, corroborating the idea that these genes could be associated with premature fusion suture. IGF1R is a tyrosine kinase growth factor receptor expressed in the developing cranial sutures, where it regulates osteoblasts' differentiation in response to tensile force [151].

1-bp duplication in the ring finger and the SPRY domain containing 1 (***RSPRY1***) **on chromosome 16q13** leading to a frameshift and premature truncation of this protein have been found in a Saudi family presenting premature ossification of the right coronal suture and progressive skeletal dysplasia phenotype [152].

Variable degrees of CS, ranging from simple metopic or bicoronal synostosis to severe multisuture CS, have been also observed in a rare **22q11 deletion** syndrome, although the molecular basis of this defect is still unknown [153–155].

3.4 From Genetics to Clinical Management of Craniosynostosis

3.4.1 Relevance of Genetics in CS Diagnosis

The clinical management of patients with craniosynostosis is complex and requires a multidisciplinary team of specialists including neurosurgeons, clinical geneticists, pediatricians, maxillofacial, and plastic surgeons, depending on the case complexity [24, 156–158].

Craniosynostosis is usually diagnosed at birth or shortly after, through clinical evaluation, physical assessment, and genetic testing [157–159]. As far as genetic diagnosis is concerned, the improved knowledge of the genetic causes along with the rapid progress of genome sequencing technologies and data analysis pipelines have been recently showing an even wider etiological heterogeneity and complexity than originally thought. This scenario offers unprecedented opportunities for patient-tailored management of each single CS case, improving genetic counseling and testing, risk assessment, reproductive advice, prognostic guidance, treatment planning, and, last but not least, favoring the study of disease mechanisms and the development of advanced therapies.

Nonetheless, the management of a correct molecular genetic diagnosis of CS and its clinical interpretation is extremely challenging and debated due to the complex and heterogeneous genetic background previously described.

Tentative diagnostic flowcharts [4, 48] have been proposed based on more recent discoveries to drive tailored patients' management but need to be constantly updated. Figure 3.1 displays a tentative and extremely simplified flowchart for CS genetic diagnosis, which does not take into account a number of country- and institution-specific issues that may cause significant variation in the overall management of patients.

The updated guidelines for the care and treatment of craniosynostosis recommend genetic counseling and testing for patients with proven disease (following clinical and physical evaluations) [156, 157]. Indeed, a genetic cause, represented by either a mutation in a single gene or a structural chromosomal aberration, is increasingly detected in CS cases and can dramatically affect the surgical outcome and the overall clinical prognosis [4, 5, 156, 157].

Specifically, the direct sequencing of one or a few specific target genes is advised for children with proven and clearly recognizable Mendelian syndromes with reduced genetic heterogeneity and a defined set of disease-associated genes, in order to have faster results with fewer costs (Fig. 3.1) [156, 157].

Since NGS allows scalable high-throughput analysis of large portions of the genome, wide panels of multiple target genes can be sequenced altogether, after a clinical-driven hypothesis. The cost for NGS technologies is slowly but progressively decreasing, enabling their implementation in the diagnostic routine of many developed countries.

Indeed, extended diagnostic CS gene panels tested through Next Generation Sequencing (NGS), along with karyotyping plus aCGH, are currently often proposed for patients presenting craniosynostosis and additional birth defects and/or developmental disorders, which overall refer to Mendelian disorders or complex syndromic phenotypes with inherent genetic heterogeneity, or for patients with proven craniosynostosis without a recognizable phenotype, as they grant the highest chance of identifying rare genetic causes [156, 157].

Targeted sequencing of selected genes can be not suitable whenever the scarcity of genetic data or the poor definition of the phenotype impedes the correct selection and completion of the target gene list. In this case, whole exome sequencing (WES) could be exploited to detect new mutations in unpredicted sites of the coding portion of the DNA. Furthermore, whole genome sequencing (WGS) could be finally considered to also analyze noncoding (putatively regulatory) regions of the DNA.

It is worth noting that NGS technologies cannot be considered yet a manageable tool without the correct interpretation of the wide data sets that they yield. While increasing the chance to find new variants, WES and WGS also increase dramatically the volume of yielded data and the complexity of their interpretation, hence the possibility of translating NGS data into a relevant diagnostic outcome. The vast majority of sequencing results, especially when obtained through WGS, are represented by "variants of unknown significance" (VUS). These remain in the limbo of experimental data, requiring a long and detailed path of research to validate and confirm their clinical significance, before translating them into a diagnostic outcome to be transferred to patient families.

3.4.2 Relevance of Genetics in CS Prognosis

Patients with proven single gene mutations require more frequent multiple surgical procedures and develop peri- and post-operative complications [44]. These include hyperthermia, severe blood loss (transfusion-related adverse events), wound infection, meningitis, subgaleal and subcutaneous hematoma, rupture of the dura mater, cerebrospinal fluid (CSF) leakage, intracranial empyema, venous air embolism, and seizures [160–162]. In addition, up to 40% of complex syndromic cases develop delayed complications such as basal encephalocele and resynostosis [46, 162, 163].

Conversely, chromosomal abnormalities seem not to significantly affect the surgical course in these patients [44]. Current guidelines recommend standard karyotyping and aCGH in complex patterns of suture fusion CS or isolated metopic synostosis cases mostly associated with developmental delay and cannot be clearly classified as a known monogenic disorder (see the previous section).

The updated guideline recommends skull remodeling within the first year of life in nonsyndromic craniosynostosis [157]. Specifically, surgery is indicated for sagittal, unilateral coronal, unilateral lambdoid, and moderate metopic synostosis since no spontaneous improvement of the abnormal skull shape is expected [157].

In addition, the indications suggest performing minimally invasive surgery on NCS patients from the ages of 3–6 months to prevent peri- and post-operative risks and to avoid an increased ossified skull area [157]. Conversely, open cranial vault remodeling is counseled in NCS cases older than 6 months to reduce the risk of growth limitation of the skull [157].

Literature data reported that surgical treatment is indicated as soon as there are signs of increased ICP in syndromic CS and multi-suture cases [157]. In this context, occipital cranial expansion with distraction performed within the first year, especially between the age of 6 and 9 months, results in greater clinical outcomes in patients with Apert and Crouzon syndrome or with multi-suture synostosis involving at least both lambdoid sutures [157]. Skull remodeling through fronto-supraorbital expansion is strongly encouraged for Saethre-Chotzen and Muenke syndrome [157].

Finally, surgical procedures should be chosen based on cranial deformity for other types of syndromic craniosynostosis [157].

References

1. Opperman LA. Cranial sutures as intramembranous bone growth sites. Dev Dyn. 2000;219(4):472–85.
2. Yilmaz E, Mihci E, Nur B, Alper OM. Coronal craniosynostosis due to TCF12 mutations in patients from Turkey. Am J Med Genet A. 2019a;179(11):2241–5.
3. Persing JA, Jane JA, Shaffrey M. Virchow and the pathogenesis of craniosynostosis: a translation of his original work. Plast Reconstr Surg. 1989;83:738–42.
4. Johnson D, Wilkie AO. Craniosynostosis. Eur J Hum Genet. 2011;19(4):369–76.
5. Lattanzi W, Barba M, Di Pietro L, et al. Genetic advances in craniosynostosis. Am J Med Genet A. 2017;173(5):1406–29.
6. Shlobin NA, Baticulon RE, Ortega CA, et al. Global epidemiology of craniosynostosis: a systematic review and meta-analysis. World Neurosurg. 2022;164:413–423.e3.
7. Slater BJ, Lenton KA, Kwan MD, et al. Cranial sutures: a brief review. Plast Reconstr Surg. 2008;121(4):170e–8e.
8. Cohen MM. Perspectives on craniosynostosis. West J Med. 1980;132(6):507–13.
9. Flaherty K, Singh N, Richtsmeier JT. Understanding craniosynostosis as a growth disorder. Wiley Interdiscip Rev Dev Biol. 2016;5(4):429–59.
10. Garza RM, Khosla RK. Nonsyndromic craniosynostosis. Semin Plast Surg. 2012;26(2): 53–63.
11. Lattanzi W, Bukvic N, Barba M, et al. Genetic basis of single-suture synostoses: genes, chromosomes and clinical implications. Childs Nerv Syst. 2012;28(9):1301–10.
12. Stanton E, Urata M, Chen JF, et al. The clinical manifestations, molecular mechanisms and treatment of craniosynostosis. Dis Model Mech. 2022;15(4):dmm049390.
13. Goos JAC, Mathijssen IMJ. Genetic causes of craniosynostosis: an update. Mol Syndromol. 2019;10(1–2):6–23.
14. Calpena E, Cuellar A, Bala K et al.; Genomics England Research Consortium. SMAD6 variants in craniosynostosis: genotype and phenotype evaluation. Genet Med. 2020;22(9):1498–1506.
15. Calpena E, Wurmser M, McGowan SJ, et al. Unexpected role of SIX1 variants in craniosynostosis: expanding the phenotype of SIX1-related disorders. J Med Genet. 2022;59(2):165–9.
16. Justice CM, Musolf AM, Cuellar A, et al. Targeted sequencing of candidate regions associated with sagittal and metopic nonsyndromic craniosynostosis. Genes (Basel). 2022;13(5):816.
17. Sawh-Martinez R, Steinbacher DM. Syndromic Craniosynostosis. Clin Plast Surg. 2019;46(2):141–55.
18. Armand T, Schaefer E, Di Rocco F, et al. Genetic bases of craniosynostoses: an update. Neurochirurgie. 2019;65(5):196–201.
19. Wilkie AOM, Johnson D, Wall SA. Clinical genetics of craniosynostosis. Curr Opin Pediatr. 2017;29(6):622–8.
20. Roscioli T, Elakis G, Cox TC, et al. Genotype and clinical care correlations in craniosynostosis: findings from a cohort of 630 Australian and New Zealand patients. Am J Med Genet C Semin Med Genet. 2013;163C(4):259–70.
21. Clarke CM, Fok VT, Gustafson JA, et al. Single suture craniosynostosis: identification of rare variants in genes associated with syndromic forms. Am J Med Genet A. 2018;176:290–300.
22. Timberlake AT, Persing JA. Genetics of nonsyndromic craniosynostosis. Plast Reconstr Surg. 2018;141(6):1508–16.
23. Twigg SR, Wilkie AO. A genetic-pathophysiological framework for craniosynostosis. Am J Hum Genet. 2015;97(3):359–77.
24. O'Hara J, Ruggiero F, Wilson L, et al. Syndromic craniosynostosis: complexities of clinical care. Mol Syndromol. 2019;10(1–2):83–97.
25. Park OJ, Kim HJ, Woo KM, et al. FGF2-activated ERK mitogen-activated protein kinase enhances Runx2 acetylation and stabilization. J Biol Chem. 2010;285(6):3568–74.
26. Pfaff MJ, Xue K, Li L, et al. FGFR2c-mediated ERK-MAPK activity regulates coronal suture development. Dev Biol. 2016;415(2):242–50.
27. Su N, Jin M, Chen L. Role of FGF/FGFR signalling in skeletal development and homeostasis: learning from mouse models. Bone Res. 2014;2: 14003.
28. Xie Y, Su N, Yang J, et al. FGF/FGFR signalling in health and disease. Signal Transduct Target Ther. 2020;5(1):181.
29. Azoury SC, Reddy S, Shukla V, et al. Fibroblast growth factor receptor 2 (FGFR2) mutation related syndromic craniosynostosis. Int J Biol Sci. 2017;13(12):1479–88.
30. Wenger T, Miller D, Evans K. FGFR craniosynostosis syndromes overview. In: Adam MP, Everman DB, Mirzaa GM, Pagon RA, Wallace SE, Bean LJH, et al., editors. GeneReviews®. Seattle: University of Washington; 1998.
31. Kan SH, Elanko N, Johnson D, et al. Genomic screening of fibroblast growth-factor receptor 2 reveals a wide spectrum of mutations in patients with syndromic craniosynostosis. Am J Hum Genet. 2002;70(2):472–86.
32. Sharma VP, Wall SA, Lord H, et al. Atypical Crouzon syndrome with a novel Cys62Arg mutation in FGFR2 presenting with sagittal synostosis. Cleft Palate Craniofac J. 2012;49(3):373–7.
33. Suh YJ, Bae HS, Choi JY, et al. A novel FGFR2 mutation in tyrosine kinase II domain, L617F, in Crouzon syndrome. J Cell Biochem. 2014;115(1): 102–10.
34. Tartaglia M, Di Rocco C, Lajeunie E, et al. Jackson-Weiss syndrome: identification of two novel FGFR2 missense mutations shared with Crouzon and

Pfeiffer craniosynostotic disorders. Hum Genet. 1997;101:47–50.
35. Lo Vecchio F, Tabolacci E, Nobile V, et al. Mother and daughter carrying of the same pathogenic variant in FGFR2 with discordant phenotype. Genes (Basel). 2022;13(7):1161.
36. Rai R, Iwanaga J, Dupont G, et al. Pfeiffer type 2 syndrome: review with updates on its genetics and molecular biology. Childs Nerv Syst. 2019;35:1451–5.
37. Roscioli T, Flanagan S, Kumar P, et al. Clinical findings in a patient with FGFR1 P252R mutation and comparison with the literature. Am J Med Genet. 2000;93:22–8.
38. Ye X, Guilmatre A, Reva B, et al. Mutation screening of candidate genes in patients with nonsyndromic sagittal craniosynostosis. Plast Reconstr Surg. 2016;137(3):952–61.
39. Doherty ES, Lacbawan F, Hadley DW, et al. Muenke syndrome (FGFR3-related craniosynostosis): expansion of the phenotype and review of the literature. Am J Med Genet A. 2007;143A(24):3204–15.
40. Kruszka P, Hu T, Hong S, et al. Phenotype delinea tion of ZNF462 related syndrome. Am J Med Genet A. 2019;179(10):2075–82.
41. Rymer K, Shiang R, Hsiung A, et al. Expanding the phenotype for the recurrent p.Ala391Glu variant in FGFR3: beyond Crouzon syndrome and acanthosis nigricans. Mol Genet Genomic Med. 2019;7(6):e656.
42. Timberlake AT, Furey CG, Choi J, et al. De novo mutations in inhibitors of Wnt, BMP, and Ras/ERK signalling pathways in nonsyndromic midline craniosynostosis. Proc Natl Acad Sci U S A. 2017;114(35):E7341–7.
43. Moloney DM, Wall SA, Ashworth GJ, et al. Lancet. 1997;349(9058):1059–62.
44. Wilkie AO, Byren JC, Hurst JA, et al. Prevalence and complications of single-gene and chromosomal disorders in craniosynostosis. Pediatrics. 2010;126(2):e391–400.
45. Panchal J, Uttchin V (2003) Management of craniosynostosis. Plast Reconstr Surg 111(6):2032–2048.
46. Hermann CD, Hyzy SL, Olivares-Navarrete R, et al. Craniosynostosis and resynostosis: models, imaging, and dental implications. J Dent Res. 2016;95(8):846–52.
47. Wilkie AO, Bochukova EG, Hansen RM, et al. Clinical dividends from the molecular genetic diagnosis of craniosynostosis. Am J Med Genet A. 2007;143A(16):1941–9.
48. Agochukwu NB, Solomon BD, Muenke M. Impact of genetics on the diagnosis and clinical management of syndromic craniosynostoses. Childs Nerv Syst. 2012;28(9):1447–63.
49. Quarto N, Senarath-Yapa K, Renda A, et al. TWIST1 silencing enhances in vitro and in vivo osteogenic differentiation of human adipose-derived stem cells by triggering activation of BMP-ERK/FGF signalling and TAZ upregulation. Stem Cells. 2015;33(3):833–47.
50. Bialek P, Kern B, Yang X, et al. A twist code determines the onset of osteoblast differentiation. Dev Cell. 2004;6:423–35.
51. Rice DP, Aberg T, Chan Y, et al. Integration of FGF and TWIST in calvarial bone and suture development. Development. 2000;127:1845–55.
52. Yang DC, Tsai CC, Liao YF, et al. Twist controls skeletal development and dorsoventral patterning by regulating runx2 in zebrafish. PLoS One. 2011;6:e27324.
53. Zhou Y, Koelling N, Fenwick AL, et al. Disruption of TWIST1 translation by 5′ UTR variants in Saethre-Chotzen syndrome. Hum Mutat. 2018;39(10):1360–5.
54. Woods RH, Ul-Haq E, Wilkie AOM, et al. Reoperation for intracranial hypertension in TWIST1-confirmed Saethre-Chotzen syndrome: a 15-year review. Plast Reconstr Surg. 2009;123(6):1801–10.
55. Goumenos A, Tsoutsou E, Traeger-Synodinos J, et al. Two novel variants in the *TCF12* gene identified in cases with craniosynostosis. Appl Clin Genet. 2019;12:19–25.
56. Yilmaz E, Mihci E, Nur B, et al. Recent advances in craniosynostosis. Pediatr Neurol. 2019b;99:7–15.
57. Sharma RK. Craniosynostosis. Indian J Plast Surg. 2013;46(1):18–27.
58. Di Rocco F, Baujat G, Arnaud E, et al. Clinical spectrum and outcomes in families with coronal synostosis and TCF12 mutations. Eur J Hum Genet. 2014;22(12):1413–6.
59. Bush JO, Soriano P. Ephrin-B1 forward signalling regulates craniofacial morphogenesis by controlling cell proliferation across Eph-ephrin boundaries. Genes Dev. 2010;24(18):2068–80.
60. Ting MC, Wu NL, Roybal PG, et al. EphA4 as an effector of Twist1 in the guidance of osteogenic precursor cells during calvarial bone growth and in craniosynostosis. Development. 2009;136(5):855–64.
61. Glass GE, O'Hara J, Canham N, et al. ERF-related craniosynostosis: the phenotypic and developmental profile of a new craniosynostosis syndrome. Am J Med Genet A. 2019;179(4):615–27.
62. Twigg SR, Vorgia E, McGowan SJ, et al. Reduced dosage of ERF causes complex craniosynostosis in humans and mice and links ERK1/2 signalling to regulation of osteogenesis. Nat Genet. 2013;45(3):308–13.
63. Jabs EW, Müller U, Li X, et al. A mutation in the homeodomain of the human MSX2 gene in a family affected with autosomal dominant craniosynostosis. Cell. 1993;75(3):443–50.
64. Pelegrino Kde O, Sugayama S, Lezirovitz K, et al. MSX2 copy number increase and craniosynostosis: copy number variation detected by array comparative genomic hybridization. Clinics (Sao Paulo). 2012;67(8):981–5.

65. Fonteles CS, Finnell RH, Lei Y, et al. De novo ALX4 variant detected in child with nonsyndromic craniosynostosis. Braz Med Biol Res. 2021;54(11):e11396.
66. Yagnik G, Ghuman A, Kim S, et al. ALX4 gain-of-function mutations in nonsyndromic craniosynostosis. Hum Mutat. 2012;33(12):1626–9.
67. Hufnagel RB, Zimmerman SL, Krueger LA, et al. A new frontonasal dysplasia syndrome associated with deletion of the SIX2 gene. Am J Med Genet A. 2016;170A(2):487–91.
68. Janssen A, Hosen MJ, Jeannin P, et al. Second family with the Boston-type craniosynostosis syndrome: novel mutation and expansion of the clinical spectrum. Am J Med Genet A. 2013;161A(9):2352–7.
69. Tiberio F, Parolini O, Lattanzi W. Ciliary signalling and mechanotransduction in the pathophysiology of craniosynostosis. Genes (Basel). 2021;12(7):1073.
70. Focșa IO, Budișteanu M, Bălgrădean M. Clinical and genetic heterogeneity of primary ciliopathies (Review). Int J Mol Med. 2021;48(3):176.
71. Schock EN, Brugmann SA. Discovery, diagnosis, and etiology of craniofacial ciliopathies. Cold Spring Harb Perspect Biol. 2017;9(9):a028258.
72. Klopocki E, Lohan S, Brancati F, et al. Copy-number variations involving the IHH locus are associated with syndactyly and craniosynostosis. Am J Hum Genet. 2011;88(1):70–5. https://doi.org/10.1016/j.ajhg.2010.11.006. Epub 2010 Dec 17. PMID: 21167467; PMCID: PMC3014361.
73. Twigg SRF, Hufnagel RB, Miller KA, et al. A recurrent mosaic mutation in SMO, encoding the hedgehog signal transducer smoothened, is the major cause of Curry-Jones syndrome. Am J Hum Genet. 2016;98(6):1256–65.
74. Yang J, Andre P, Ye L, et al. The hedgehog signalling pathway in bone formation. Int J Oral Sci. 2015;7:73–9.
75. Vortkamp A, Gessler M, Grzeschik KH. GLI3 zinc-finger gene interrupted by translocations in Greig syndrome families. Nature. 1991;352:539–40.
76. Hasan MR, Takatalo M, Ma H, et al. RAB23 coordinates early osteogenesis by repressing FGF10-pERK1/2 and GLI1. Elife. 2020;9:e55829.
77. Justice CM, Yagnik G, Kim Y, et al. A genome-wide association study identifies susceptibility loci for nonsyndromic sagittal craniosynostosis near BMP2 and within BBS9. Nat Genet. 2012;44(12):1360–4.
78. Barba M, Di Pietro L, Massimi L, et al. BBS9 gene in nonsyndromic craniosynostosis: role of the primary cilium in the aberrant ossification of the suture osteogenic niche. Bone. 2019;112:58–70.
79. Barrell WB, Adel Al-Lami H, Goos JAC, et al. Identification of a novel variant of the ciliopathic gene FUZZY associated with craniosynostosis. Eur J Hum Genet. 2022;30(3):282–90.
80. Brischoux-Boucher E, Trimouille A, Baujat G, et al. IL11RA-related Crouzon-like autosomal recessive craniosynostosis in 10 new patients: resemblances and differences. Clin Genet. 2018;94(3–4):373–80.
81. Keupp K, Li Y, Vargel I, et al. Mutations in the interleukin receptor IL11RA cause autosomal recessive Crouzon-like craniosynostosis. Mol Genet Genomic Med. 2013;1(4):223–37.
82. Korakavi N, Prokop JW, Seaver LH. Evolution of the phenotype of craniosynostosis with dental anomalies syndrome and report of IL11RA variant population frequencies in a Crouzon-like autosomal recessive syndrome. Am J Med Genet A. 2019;179(4):668–73.
83. Nieminen P, Morgan NV, Fenwick AL, et al. Inactivation of IL11 signalling causes craniosynostosis, delayed tooth eruption, and supernumerary teeth. Am J Hum Genet. 2011;89(1):67–81.
84. Topa A, Rohlin A, Andersson MK, et al. The outcome of targeted NGS screening in patients with syndromic forms of sagittal and pansynostosis—IL11RA is an emerging core-gene for pansynostosis. Eur J Med Genet. 2022;65(5):104476.
85. Twigg SR, Forecki J, Goos JA, et al. Gain-of-function mutations in ZIC1 are associated with coronal craniosynostosis and learning disability. Am J Hum Genet. 2015;97(3):378–88.
86. Yauy K, Tran Mau-Them F, Willems M, et al. B3GAT3-related disorder with craniosynostosis and bone fragility due to a unique mutation. Genet Med. 2018;20(2):269–74.
87. Chinen Y, Kaname T, Yanagi K, et al. Opitz trigonocephaly C syndrome in a boy with a de novo balanced reciprocal translocation t(3;18)(q13.13;q12.1). Am J Med Genet A. 2006;140(15):1655–7.
88. Kaname T, Yanagi K, Chinen Y, et al. Mutations in CD96, a member of the immunoglobulin superfamily, cause a form of the C (Opitz trigonocephaly) syndrome. Am J Hum Genet. 2007;81(4):835–41.
89. Loucks CM, Parboosingh JS, Shaheen R, et al. Matching two independent cohorts validates DPH1 as a gene responsible for autosomal recessive intellectual disability with short stature, craniofacial, and ectodermal anomalies. Hum Mutat. 2015;36(10):1015–9.
90. Urreizti R, Mayer K, Evrony GD, et al. Correction: DPH1 syndrome: two novel variants and structural and functional analyses of seven missense variants identified in syndromic patients. Eur J Hum Genet. 2020;28(1):138.
91. Dobson SM, Kiss C, Borschneck D, et al. Novel FGF9 variant contributes to multiple synostoses syndrome 3. Am J Med Genet A. 2022;188(7):2162–7.
92. Rodriguez-Zabala M, Aza-Carmona M, Rivera-Pedroza CI, et al. FGF9 mutation causes craniosynostosis along with multiple synostoses. Hum Mutat. 2017;38(11):1471–6.
93. Rohena L, Lawson M, Guzman E, et al. FTO variant associated with malformation syndrome. Am J Med Genet A. 2015;170A(4):1023–8.
94. Gerken T, Girard CA, Tung YC, et al. The obesity-associated FTO gene encodes a 2-oxoglutarate-dependent nucleic acid demethylase. Science. 2007;318:1469–72.

95. Au PYB, Innes AM, Kline AD. Au-Kline syndrome. In: Adam MP, Everman DB, Mirzaa GM, et al., editors. GeneReviews®. Seattle: University of Washington; 2019. https://www.ncbi.nlm.nih.gov/books/NBK540283/.
96. Bashir RA, Dixit A, Goedhart C, Parboosingh JS, Innes AM, Care for Rare Canada Consortium, Ferreira P, Hasan SU, Au PB. Lin-Gettig syndrome: craniosynostosis expands the spectrum of the KAT6B related disorders. Am J Med Genet A. 2017;173(10):2596–604.
97. Atik T, Koparir A, Bademci G, et al. Novel MASP1 mutations are associated with an expanded phenotype in 3MC1 syndrome. Orphanet J Rare Dis. 2015;10:128.
98. Rooryck C, Diaz-Font A, Osborn DP, et al. Mutations in lectin complement pathway genes COLEC11 and MASP1 cause 3MC syndrome. Nat Genet. 2011;43(3):197–203.
99. Balasubramanian M, Padidela R, Pollitt RC, et al. P4HB recurrent missense mutation causing Cole-Carpenter syndrome. J Med Genet. 2018;55(3):158–65.
100. Rauch F, Fahiminiya S, Majewski J, et al. Cole-Carpenter syndrome is caused by a heterozygous missense mutation in P4HB. Am J Hum Genet. 2015;96(3):425–31.
101. Gonorazky HD, Marshall CR, Al-Murshed M, et al. Congenital myopathy with "corona" fibres, selective muscle atrophy, and craniosynostosis associated with novel recessive mutations in SCN4A. Neuromuscul Disord. 2017;27(6):574–80.
102. Ehmke N, Graul-Neumann L, Smorag L, et al. De novo mutations in SLC25A24 cause a craniosynostosis syndrome with hypertrichosis, progeroid appearance, and mitochondrial dysfunction. Am J Hum Genet. 2017;101(5):833–43.
103. Writzl K, Maver A, Kovačič L, et al. De novo mutations in SLC25A24 cause a disorder characterized by early aging, bone dysplasia, characteristic face, and early demise. Am J Hum Genet. 2017;101(5):844–55.
104. Ueda K, Yaoita M, Niihori T, et al. Craniosynostosis in patients with RASopathies: accumulating clinical evidence for expanding the phenotype. Am J Med Genet A. 2017;173(9):2346–52.
105. Addissie YA, Kotecha U, Hart RA, et al. Craniosynostosis and Noonan syndrome with KRAS mutations: expanding the phenotype with a case report and review of the literature. Am J Med Genet A. 2015;167A(11):2657–63.
106. McDonald BS, Pigors M, Kelsell DP, et al. Noonan syndrome with multiple lentigines and associated craniosynostosis. Clin Exp Dermatol. 2018;43(3):357–9.
107. Takenouchi T, Sakamoto Y, Miwa T, et al. Severe craniosynostosis with Noonan syndrome phenotype associated with SHOC2 mutation: clinical evidence of crosslink between FGFR and RAS signalling pathways. Am J Med Genet A. 2014;164A(11):2869–72.
108. Timberlake AT, Choi J, Zaidi S, et al. Two locus inheritance of nonsyndromic midline craniosynostosis via rare SMAD6 and common BMP2 alleles. Elife. 2016;5:e20125.
109. Miller KA, Twigg SR, McGowan SJ, et al. Diagnostic value of exome and whole genome sequencing in craniosynostosis. J Med Genet. 2017;54(4):260–8.
110. Weiss K, Wigby K, Fannemel M, et al. Haploinsufficiency of ZNF462 is associated with craniofacial anomalies, corpus callosum dysgenesis, ptosis, and developmental delay. Eur J Hum Genet. 2017;25(8):946–51.
111. Fenwick AL, Kliszczak M, Cooper F, et al. Mutations in CDC45, encoding an essential component of the pre-initiation complex, cause Meier-Gorlin syndrome and craniosynostosis. Am J Hum Genet. 2016;99(1):125–38.
112. Knapp KM, Fellows B, Aggarwal S, et al. A synonymous variant in a non-canonical exon of CDC45 disrupts splicing in two affected sibs with Meier-Gorlin syndrome with craniosynostosis. Eur J Med Genet. 2021;64(4):104182.
113. Nabais Sá MJ, Miller KA, McQuaid M, et al. Biallelic GINS2 variant p.(Arg114Leu) causes Meier-Gorlin syndrome with craniosynostosis. J Med Genet. 2022;59(8):776–80.
114. Zhao X, Wu B, Chen H, et al. Case report: a novel truncating variant of BCL11B associated with rare feature of craniosynostosis and global developmental delay. Front Pediatr. 2022;10:982361.
115. Di Fede E, Grazioli P, Lettieri A, et al. Epigenetic disorders: lessons from the animals-animal models in chromatinopathies. Front Cell Dev Biol. 2022;10:979512.
116. Poot M. Structural genome variations related to craniosynostosis. Mol Syndromol. 2019;10(1–2):24–39.
117. Zollino M, Lattante S, Orteschi D, et al. Syndromic craniosynostosis can define new candidate genes for suture development or result from the non-specific effects of pleiotropic genes: rasopathies and chromatinopathies as examples. Front Neurosci. 2017;11:587.
118. Bukowska-Olech E, Sowińska-Seidler A, Larysz D, et al. Results from genetic studies in patients affected with craniosynostosis: clinical and molecular aspects. Front Mol Biosci. 2022;9:865494.
119. Gajecka M, Yu W, Ballif B, et al. Delineation of mechanisms and regions of dosage imbalance in complex rearrangements of 1p36 leads to a putative gene for regulation of cranial suture closure. Eur J Hum Genet. 2015;13:139–49.
120. Garcia-Heras J, Corley N, Garcia MF, et al. De novo partial duplications 1p: report of two new cases and review. Am J Med Genet. 1999;82(3):261–4.
121. Heilstedt HA, Shapira SK, Gregg AR, et al. Molecular and clinical characterization of a patient with duplication of 1p36.3 and metopic synostosis. Clin Genet. 1999;56(2):123–8.

122. Nyboe D, Kreiborg S, Kirchhoff M, et al. Familial craniosynostosis associated with a microdeletion involving the NFIA gene. Clin Dysmorphol. 2015;24(3):109–12.
123. Rao A, O'Donnell S, Bain N, et al. An intragenic deletion of the NFIA gene in a patient with a hypoplastic corpus callosum, craniofacial abnormalities and urinary tract defects. Eur J Med Genet. 2014;57(2–3):65–70.
124. Serra G, Antona V, Giuffrè M, et al. Interstitial deletions of chromosome 1p: novel 1p31.3p22.2 microdeletion in a newborn with craniosynostosis, coloboma and cleft palate, and review of the genomic and phenotypic profiles. Ital J Pediatr. 2022;48(1):38.
125. Rivera-Pedroza CI, Barraza-García J, Paumard-Hernández B, et al. Chromosome 1p31.1p31.3 deletion in a patient with craniosynostosis, central nervous system and renal malformation: case report and review of the literature. Mol Syndromol. 2017;8(1):30–5.
126. Sowińska-Seidler A, Olech EM, Socha M, et al. Novel 1q22-q23.1 duplication in a patient with lambdoid and metopic craniosynostosis, muscular hypotonia, and psychomotor retardation. J Appl Genet. 2018;59(3):281–9.
127. Greives MR, Odessey EA, Waggoner DJ, et al. RUNX2 quadruplication: additional evidence toward a new form of syndromic craniosynostosis. J Craniofac Surg. 2013;24(1):126–9.
128. Varvagiannis K, Stefanidou A, Gyftodimou Y, et al. Pure de novo partial trisomy 6p in a girl with craniosynostosis. Am J Med Genet A. 2013;161A(2):343–51.
129. Cuellar A, Bala K, Di Pietro L, et al. Gain-of-function variants and overexpression of RUNX2 in patients with nonsyndromic midline craniosynostosis. Bone. 2020;137:115395.
130. Komori T. Runx2, a multifunctional transcription factor in skeletal development. J Cell Biochem. 2002;87(1):1–8.
131. Fryssira H, Makrythanasis P, Kattamis A, et al. Severe developmental delay in a patient with 7p21.1-p14.3 microdeletion spanning the TWIST gene and the HOXA gene cluster. Mol Syndromol. 2011;2(1):45–9.
132. Yu D, Li S, Liu Q, Zhang K. Novel chromosomal microduplications associated with dolichocephaly craniosynostosis: a case report. Medicine (Baltimore). 2017;96(49):e8729.
133. Mohamed AM, Kamel AK, Eid MM, et al. Chromosome 9p terminal deletion in nine Egyptian patients and narrowing of the critical region for trigonocephaly. Mol Genet Genomic Med. 2021;9(11):e1829.
134. Jehee FS, Johnson D, Alonso LG, et al. Molecular screening for microdeletions at 9p22-p24 and 11q23-q24 in a large cohort of patients with trigonocephaly. Clin Genet. 2005;67(6):503–10.
135. Spazzapan P, Arnaud E, Baujat G, et al. Clinical and neuroradiological features of the 9p deletion syndrome. Childs Nerv Syst. 2016;32(2):327–35.
136. Vissers LE, Cox TC, Maga AM, et al. Heterozygous mutations of FREM1 are associated with an increased risk of isolated metopic craniosynostosis in humans and mice. PLoS Genet. 2011;7:e1002278.
137. Choucair N, Mignon-Ravix C, Cacciagli P, et al. Evidence that homozygous PTPRD gene microdeletion causes trigonocephaly, hearing loss, and intellectual disability. Mol Cytogenet. 2015;8:39.
138. Grillo L, Greco D, Pettinato R, et al. Increased FGF3 and FGF4 gene dosage is a risk factor for craniosynostosis. Gene. 2014;534(2):435–9.
139. Jehee FS, Bertola DR, Yelavarthi KK, et al. An 11q11-q13.3 duplication, including FGF3 and FGF4 genes, in a patient with syndromic multiple craniosynostoses. Am J Med Genet A. 2007;143A(16):1912–8.
140. Tagariello A, Heller R, Greven A, et al. Balanced translocation in a patient with craniosynostosis disrupts the SOX6 gene and an evolutionarily conserved non-transcribed region. J Med Genet. 2016;43(6):534–40.
141. Tolchin D, Yeager JP, Prasad P, et al. De novo SOX6 variants cause a neurodevelopmental syndrome associated with ADHD, craniosynostosis, and osteochondromas. Am J Hum Genet. 2020;106(6):830–45.
142. Aypar E, Yildirim MS, Sert A, et al. A girl with metopic synostosis and trisomy 13 mosaicism: case report and review of the literature. Am J Med Genet A. 2011;155A(3):638–41.
143. Karabel M, Yolbaş I, Kelekçi S, et al. A newborn with trisomy 13 who had tetralogy of Fallot and metopic synostosis: case report. Hippokratia. 2013;17(3):268–70.
144. Hu J, McPherson E, Surti U, et al. Tetrasomy 15q25.3 --> qter resulting from an analphoid supernumerary marker chromosome in a patient with multiple anomalies and bilateral Wilms tumors. Am J Med Genet. 2002;113(1):82–8.
145. Kant SG, Kriek M, Walenkamp MJ, et al. Tall stature and duplication of the insulin-like growth factor I receptor gene. Eur J Med Genet. 2007;50(1):1–10.
146. Nagai T, Shimokawa O, Harada N, et al. Postnatal overgrowth by 15q-trisomy and intrauterine growth retardation by 15q-monosomy due to familial translocation t(13;15): dosage effect of IGF1R? Am J Med Genet. 2002;113(2):173–7.
147. Pedersen C. Letter: partial trisomy 15 as a result of an unbalanced 12/15 translocation in a patient with a cloverleaf skull anomaly. Clin Genet. 1976;9(3):378–80.
148. Van Allen MI, Siegel-Bartelt J, Feigenbaum A, et al. Craniosynostosis associated with partial duplication of 15q and deletion of 2q. Am J Med Genet. 1992;43(4):688–92.
149. Van den Enden A, Verschraegen-Spae MR, Van Roy N, et al. Mosaic tetrasomy 15q25-->qter in a newborn infant with multiple anomalies. Am J Med Genet. 1996;63(3):482–5.

150. Zollino M, Tiziano F, Di Stefano C, et al. Partial duplication of the long arm of chromosome 15: confirmation of a causative role in craniosynostosis and definition of a 15q25-qter trisomy syndrome. Am J Med Genet. 1999;87(5):391–4.
151. Cunningham ML, Horst JA, Rieder MJ, et al. IGF1R variants associated with isolated single suture craniosynostosis. Am J Med Genet A. 2011;155A(1):91–7.
152. Faden M, AlZahrani F, Mendoza-Londono R, et al. Identification of a recognizable progressive skeletal dysplasia caused by RSPRY1 mutations. Am J Hum Genet. 2015;97:608–15.
153. Al-Hertani W, Hastings VA, McGowan-Jordan J, et al. Severe craniosynostosis in an infant with deletion 22q11.2 syndrome. Am J Med Genet A. 2013;161A(1):153–7.
154. McDonald-McGinn DM, Gripp KW, Kirschner RE, et al. Craniosynostosis: another feature of the 22q11.2 deletion syndrome. Am J Med Genet A. 2005;136A(4):358–62.
155. Rojnueangnit K, Robin NH. Craniosynostosis and radial ray defect: a rare presentation of 22q11.2 deletion syndrome. Am J Med Genet A. 2013;161A(8):2024–6.
156. Mathijssen IMJ. Guideline for care of patients with the diagnoses of craniosynostosis: working group on craniosynostosis. J Craniofac Surg. 2015;26:1735–807.
157. Mathijssen IMJ, Working Group Guideline Craniosynostosis. Updated guideline on treatment and management of craniosynostosis. J Craniofac Surg. 2021;32(1):371–450.
158. Xue AS, Buchanan EP, Hollier LH Jr. Update in management of craniosynostosis. Plast Reconstr Surg. 2022;149(6):1209e–23e.
159. Kajdic N, Spazzapan P, Velnar T. Craniosynostosis—Recognition, clinical characteristics, and treatment. Bosn J Basic Med Sci. 2018;18(2):110–6.
160. Esparza J, Hinojosa J. Complications in the surgical treatment of craniosynostosis and craniofacial syndromes: apropos of 306 transcranial procedures. Childs Nerv Syst. 2008;24(12):1421–30.
161. Melville H, Wang Y, Taub PJ, et al. Genetic basis of potential therapeutic strategies for craniosynostosis. Am J Med Genet A. 2010;152A(12):3007–15.
162. Wu SH, Liu TJ, Fan SS, et al. Severe chemosis and treatment following fronto-orbital advancement surgery for Crouzon syndrome: a case report. Medicine (Baltimore). 2021;100(7):e24693.
163. Caplan J, Angel M, Parent A. Encephalocele as a late complication of cranial vault reconstruction in a patient with Crouzon's syndrome. J Craniofac Surg. 2002;13(4):501–4.

4 Craniofacial Anomalies and Neurocognitive Aspects in *Fgfrs*-Craniosynostoses Mouse Models

Anne Morice, Federico Di Rocco, and Laurence Legeai-Mallet

4.1 Introduction

Craniosynostoses—reported in 1:2000 to 1:3000 live births, comprising at least 20% of syndromic cases [1]—are defined by the premature fusion of one or more cranial and facial sutures, leading to various craniofacial anomalies, among which: skull vault deformation, potentially causing increased intracranial pressure, shallow orbits leading to exorbitism and midfacial retrusion that can be associated with obstructive sleep apnoea syndrome [2–4].

To better understand the physiopathology of these anomalies several mouse models have been generated in the past decades, based on the underlying mutations found in syndromic craniosynostoses.

Indeed, various mutations have been reported in patients with syndromic craniosynostoses, and several key signalling pathways involved in craniofacial development are affected by these variants. Mutations in FGFR (fibroblast growth factor receptor) genes are reported in almost 75% of syndromic craniosynostoses [5]. Such FGFR-related conditions are caused by specific heterozygous activating mutations in FGFR1 (Pfeiffer syndrome type 1) [1], FGFR2 (Apert, Crouzon, Pfeiffer type 2 and 3 syndromes, Antley-Bixler, Beare-Stevenson cutis gyrata syndromes, Bent Bone Dysplasia and Saethre-Chotzen like syndrome) [5–9] and FGFR3 (Muenke syndrome and Crouzonodermoskeletal syndrome). Muenke syndrome is the most frequent FGFR-related syndromic craniosynostosis [10]. Crouzonodermoskeletal syndrome is an exceedingly rare syndrome sharing similarities with Crouzon syndrome and including skin lesions (*acanthosis nigricans*) [11]. Most of these FGFR variants are gain of function mutations, inducing high receptor activity in the presence or in the absence of its FGF ligands, which disrupts bone formation. Today, the impact of FGFRs activat-

A. Morice
Unité de Paris Cité, Laboratory of Molecular and Physiopathological Bases of Osteochondrodysplasia, Imagine Institute, INSERM UMR 1163, Paris, France

Service de Chirurgie Maxillo-faciale et plastique, Centre de Compétence CRANIOST et MAFACE, CHRU de Tours, Tours, France
e-mail: a.morice@chu-tours.fr

F. Di Rocco
Hôpital Femme Mère Enfant, Hospices Civils de Lyon, Université Claude Bernard Lyon, Lyon, France

Centre de Référence Maladies Rares Craniosténose Lyon, INSERM 1033, Lyon, France
e-mail: federico.dirocco@chu-lyon.fr

L. Legeai-Mallet (✉)
Unité de Paris Cité, Laboratory of Molecular and Physiopathological Bases of Osteochondrodysplasia, Imagine Institute, INSERM UMR 1163, Paris, France
e-mail: laurence.legeai-mallet@inserm.fr

F. Di Rocco, J. Kestle (eds.), *Neurosurgical Aspects of Craniosynostosis*,
https://doi.org/10.1007/978-3-031-69386-1_4

ing mutations on skull formation is well understood, however neurocognitive development remains to be elucidated.

Here, we describe mouse models carrying *Fgfrs*-activating mutations generated in the past decades allowing a better understanding of the impact of these mutations during craniofacial and suture formation. In addition, we describe the impact of an Fgfr variant on the brain and in particular on behaviour.

4.2 *Fgfrs*-Craniosynostosis Mice Models

Several mice models carrying *Fgfr1*, *Fgfr2* and *Fgfr3* activating mutations known to be involved in human FGFRs-related craniosynostoses have been reported.

4.2.1 Mouse Model Mimicking Pfeiffer Syndrome (*Fgfr1*$^{P250R/+}$)

The *Fgfr1*$^{P250R/+}$ mouse model has been generated by Zhou et al., by inserting the P250R mutation in the *Fgfr1* gene by homologous recombination [12], corresponding to the human Pro252Arg mutation, leading to the mild form of Pfeiffer syndrome. Heterozygous mice (*Fgfr1*$^{P250R/+}$) developed an abnormal craniofacial phenotype from postnatal day 3 with premature fusion of coronal, frontal and sagittal sutures, without skull base anomalies. Although heterozygous mice showed decreased body size, analyses of the growth plates did not reveal any anomalies, highlighting that *Fgfr1*$^{P250R/+}$ mutation preferentially impacts membranous ossification but not endochondral ones [12, 13].

4.2.2 Mice Models Mimicking Apert Syndrome (*Fgfr2*$^{S252W/+}$, *Fgfr2*$^{P253R/+}$)

The first mouse model for Apert syndrome to be reported is the *Fgfr2*$^{S252W/+}$ mouse model, generated by the ubiquitous expression of the Ser252Trp mutation in the *Fgfr2* gene, corresponding to the most frequent mutation observed in human pathology. Mutant mice showed early premature fusion of coronal sutures, from embryonic stage E18.5, with thinner calvaria bones, and reduced presphenoid bone length, leading to significant craniofacial anomalies (dome-shaped skull, midface hypoplasia, wide-spaced eyes and malocclusion). Mutant mice presented reduced naso-anal length, without significant anomalies of the growth plates [14].

The second mouse model for Apert syndrome to be described is the *Fgfr2*$^{P253R/+}$ mouse model, generated by the insertion of the Pro253Arg mutation in the *Fgfr2* gene, reported to be of concern in one-third of Apert patients. Mutant mice presented brachycephaly, with dome-shaped skull, wide-spaced eyes, midface hypoplasia and malocclusion, and a shortened skull base. Syndactyly was also observed. As for the *Fgfr2*$^{S252W/+}$ mouse model, *Fgfr2*$^{P253R/+}$ mice presented reduced size, but contrary to the first mouse model, growth plate anomalies were observed, highlighting the impact of the *Fgfr2*$^{P253R/+}$ mutation in the process of endochondral ossification [15].

4.2.3 Mice Models Mimicking Crouzon Syndrome (*Fgfr2*$^{C342Y/+}$, *Fgfr2*$^{W290R/+}$)

The first mouse model mimicking Crouzon syndrome has been generated by Eswarakumar et al. [16]. This model has been established by the insertion of the Cys342Tyr mutation, frequently associated with Crouzon/Pfeiffer syndromes, into the *Fgfr2* gene by a Cre recombinase under the control of the PKG promoter. The Cys342Tyr mutation affects exon 9 of the gene and only affects the *Fgfr2IIIc* isoform. *Fgfr2*$^{C342Y/+}$ mutant mice present a dome-shaped skull, shortened face, exophthalmia, shortened skull base and malocclusion. Frontal and parietal bones overlapped from embryonic stage E16.5, and premature closure of coronal and lambdoid sutures occurred postnatally [16].

The second Crouzon model reported is the *Fgfr2*$^{W290R/+}$ mouse model, generated by the N-ethyl-N-nitrosourea (ENU) mutagenesis screen. The mutation affects both the b (epithelial) and c (mesenchymal) isoforms of the *Fgfr2* gene. *Fgfr2*$^{W290R/+}$ mutant mice presented premature fusion of coronal and lambdoid sutures, with a dome-shaped skull, short snout and malocclusion of the incisors. The presence of skull base anomalies, thickened nasal septum cartilage and abnormal sternum cartilage highlight the impact of this mutation on endochondral ossification processes [17].

4.2.4 Mouse Model Mimicking Beare-Stevenson Syndrome (*Fgfr2*$^{Y394C/+}$)

This mouse model has been generated by the ubiquitous insertion of the Tyr394Cys mutation into the *Fgfr2* gene. Heterozygous mice presented reduced growth and premature death at 2 weeks of age. Premature fusion of coronal, zygomatic and squamosal sutures occurred with subsequent brachycephalic skull and midface hypoplasia. In addition to the skeletal anomalies, mutant mice present cutaneous anomalies, including cutis gyrata, epidermal acanthosis and papillomatosis [18].

4.2.5 Mouse Model Mimicking Muenke Syndrome (*Fgfr3*$^{P244R/+}$)

To generate this mouse model, the *Fgfr3*$^{P244R/+}$ mutation located in exon 7 of the *Fgfr3* gene was inserted using a Cre-LoxP system. The craniofacial phenotype was mostly mild and variable, and premature fusion of coronal sutures did not frequently affect mutant animals. Fusion of zygomatic bone and synostosis of the premaxillary suture were observed. Premature closure of the intersphenoidal and spheno-occipital synchondroses frequently affected mutant mice, highlighting the impact of the mutation during endochondral ossification. In addition, delayed development of the mandibular condylar head was observed with condylar cartilage anomalies, harvesting arthritic features. Sensorineural hearing loss was also detected in mutants, in accordance with otologic impairments observed in patients with Muenke syndrome [19, 20].

4.2.6 Mouse Model Mimicking Crouzon Syndrome with *Acanthosis Nigricans* (CAN) (*Fgfr3*$^{A385E/+}$)

This mouse model has been generated by inserting the A385E mutation, located in exon 9 of the *Fgfr3* gene, using a Cre-LoxP system, under the control of a Prm1 promoter [21]. No significant craniofacial morphological changes have been observed in mutant mice, without abnormal premature fusion of cranial sutures. Abnormal transient morphological changes of the mandible have been reported, as observed in human pathology [21, 22]. No obvious cutaneous anomalies were observed in mutant mice, unlike in patients.

The absence of significant craniofacial phenotype in the CAN *Fgfr3*$^{A385E/+}$ mouse model, *Fgfr3*$^{P244R/+}$ Muenke mouse model and *Fgfr3*$^{-/-}$ knock-out mice [23–25] emphasises that the Fgfr3 receptor is less involved during craniofacial formation and intramembranous suture formation in mice than in human or in zebrafish [13, 26].

4.3 Neurocognitive Aspects in Human FGFR-Related Craniosynostoses and New Insights Using Fgfr3$^{A385E/+}$ Crouzon with Acanthosis nigricans Mouse Model

Cognitive impairment, including mental retardation, learning disabilities and behaviour/psychopathology, has been reported in up to 24% of the patients with single-suture craniosynostosis [27]. In syndromic multiple-suture craniosynostoses, the exact incidence of cognitive impairments is difficult to determine, depending on the clinical assessment performed, with the lack of standardised protocols. In addition, the highly heterogeneous cerebral conditions of these patients, depending on the intrinsic brain anomalies and those linked to intracranial pressure, increase the lack of objective data concerning cognitive impairments in syndromic craniosynostosis.

Among *FGFR*-craniosynostoses, Pfeiffer syndromes type II and type III, linked to activating *FGFR2* mutations, are generally associated with severe neurological impairments and severe developmental delay [28–30]. In Crouzon syndrome, craniofacial phenotype and the impact of neurocognitive functions are highly heterogeneous, linked to the numerous distinct mutations described in this spectrum [31–33]. In Apert syndrome, although normal cognitive development has been reported, mild to severe mental retardation is often described [34, 35]. In other rare FGFR2-related craniosynostosis syndromes, including Jackson-Weiss syndrome and Beare Stevenson syndrome, there is a lack of reported data on cognitive impairment, especially in Beare Stevenson syndrome leading to frequent premature death [36, 37].

In *FGFR3*-related craniosynostoses, severe neurocognitive disorders have been reported, including anxiety, learning impairments, as well as memory, attention and emotional control disturbances [13, 38–40].

Cognitive impairment in syndromic patients is multifactorial, resulting from a combination of the raised intracranial pressure due to the synostosis, alterations in cerebrospinal fluid dynamics and anomalies in venous outflow. The possibility of a direct impact of the underlying mutation on the brain function has also been hypothesised [41].

To study the potential direct impact of the FGFR3 mutation, *Fgfr3*$^{A385E/+}$ knock-in mice without a craniofacial phenotype are particularly interesting [21].

Indeed, neuro behavioural experiments performed in the mouse model for Crouzon with *acanthosis nigricans* (CAN) *Fgfr3*$^{A385E/+}$ for the first time give new insights into the impact of FGFR3 activating mutations on neurocognitive functions. *Fgfr3*$^{A385E/+}$ mutant mice presented severe memory and learning impairments, a structurally abnormal hippocampus, low activity-dependent synaptic plasticity and overactivation of MAPK/ERK and Akt signalling pathways in the hippocampus. Pharmacological inhibition by infigratinib (BGJ398), a tyrosine kinase inhibitor, rescued memory impairments in *Fgfr3*$^{A385E/+}$ mutant mice [13], Fig. 4.1. These results demonstrate for the first time the impact of activating *Fgfr3* mutation on brain development and neurocognitive functions, independently of craniofacial anomalies and premature closure of cranial sutures and skull base synchondroses. Overall, this study provides a better understanding of the role of *Fgfr3* on brain development and neurocognitive functions and gives new therapeutic perspectives in neurocognitive disorders with the potential use of tyrosine kinase inhibitors.

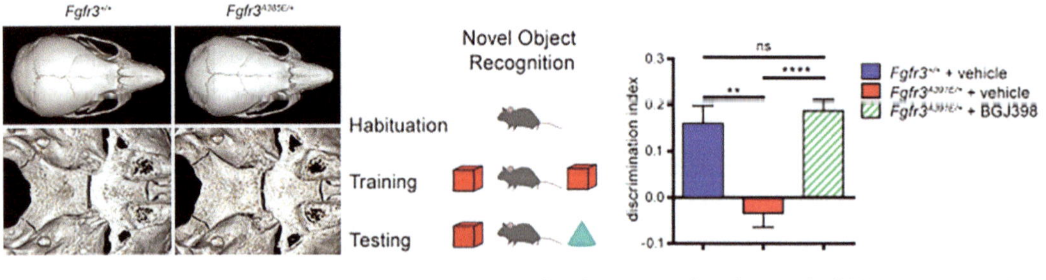

Fig. 4.1 MicroCT of Crouzon with *acanthosis nigricans* (CAN) *Fgfr3*$^{A385E/+}$ and controls mice showing a normal craniofacial phenotype without skull vault and base anomalies in CAN mutant mice. Behavioural studies showing memory impairments in CAN mutant mice when compared with controls, 7 days of subcutaneous injections of a tyrosine kinase inhibitor (BGJ398) in 4-month-old mice rescued memory impairment [13]

4.4 Therapeutic Approaches in FGFR-Related Growth Anomalies

Current therapeutic approaches are many and varied and include targeting the FGFR3 receptor, inhibiting the tyrosine kinase activity of FGFR3 and antagonisation of *FGFR3* downstream signalling pathways. Several preclinical studies have demonstrated the positive effects of FGFR3 antagonists on bone growth in mouse models of achondroplasia carrying an *Fgfr3*-activating mutation, including tyrosine kinase inhibitor (Infigratinib) [42–44], CNP analogs (vosoritide) [45, 46] and more recently (−)-Epicatechin [47] (Fig. 4.2). The treatments rescued the bone phenotype of an *Fgfr3*-related mouse model of achondroplasia bearing a $Fgfr3^{Y367C/+}$ gain-of-function mutation [42, 45, 47].

Interestingly, taking advantage of the Fgfr3-related Crouzon mouse model which has no craniosynostosis, Cornille et al. confirmed that memory impairments in FGFR3-related Crouzon mice were due to the increased activation of the Fgfr3 in the central nervous system. This concept is also in line with a hypothesis raised several years ago, in which certain cognitive impairments found in patients with FGFR-related synostosis are caused by abnormal FGFR expression in the brain—rather than through an effect of the skull size or the associated hydrocephalus [41]. Daily intraperitoneal and intracerebroventricular administration of the Fgfr3 inhibitor BGJ398 (Infigratinib) to adult mice rescued the learning and memory impairments observed in the FGFR3-related Crouzon mice suggesting that the modulation of FGFR3 signalling might be of value for treating the neurological disorders associated with craniosynostosis (Fig. 4.1) [21].

These findings suggest that in the future patients might benefit from a combination of medical and surgical treatments aiming to correct the different aspects of craniosynostosis-related impairments. The different surgical approaches that have been developed in the last years allow the correction of the suture synostosis and more in general of the associated skull deformation but also to reduce effectively a raised intracranial pressure (ICP) or decompress a too small foramen magnum and thus indirectly improve the functional outcome of the patients. Pharmacological treatments seem to directly improve the functional outcome. But these treatments because they improve bone growth metabolism will probably also reduce the risk of developing a raised ICP or a significant descent of cerebellar tonsils (Table 4.1).

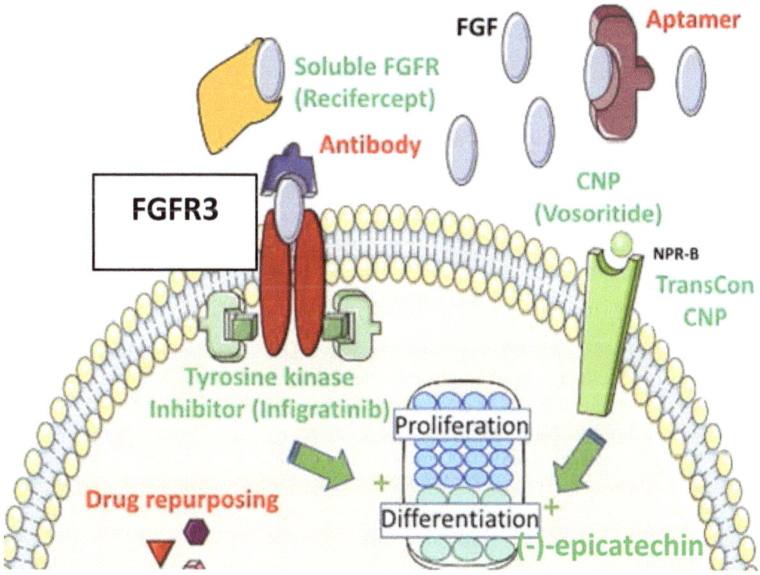

Fig. 4.2 Pharmacological approaches using FGFR3 antagonists to rescue the defective endochondral ossification process in mouse models of achondroplasia (adapted from [48])

Table 4.1 Correction of morphological and functional consequences of craniosynostosis: comparison between pharmacological and surgical approaches

	Pharmacological approach	Surgical approach
Craniosynostosis	?	Immediate correction
Bone growth	Improved[a]	?
Raised intracranial pressure	?	Immediate reduction
Cerebellar tonsil's descent	?	Immediate correction
Functional outcome	Improved[b]	Indirect effect

[a] Increase in bone size and increase in the size of the foramen magnum [42, 45]
[b] Learning and memory impairments improvement [21]

In conclusion, thanks to the promising results observed in mouse models we can expect pharmacological approaches to play a role in the management of patients with craniosynostosis in the near future.

References

1. Johnson D, Wilkie AO. Craniosynostosis. Eur J Hum Genet. 2011;19(4):369–76. https://doi.org/10.1038/ejhg.2010.235. Epub 2011 Jan 19.
2. Heuzé Y, Holmes G, Peter I, Richtsmeier JT, Jabs EW. Closing the gap: genetic and genomic continuum from syndromic to nonsyndromic craniosynostoses. Curr Genet Med Rep. 2014a;2(3):135–45.
3. Heuzé Y, Martinez-Abadias N, Stella JM, Arnaud E, Collet C, Fructuoso GG, Alamar M, Lo LJ, Boyadjiev SA, Di Rocco F, et al. Quantification of facial skeletal shape variation in fibroblast growth factor receptor-related craniosynostosis syndromes. Birth Defects Res A Clin Mol Teratol. 2014b;100:250–9.
4. Flaherty K, Singh N, Richtsmeier JT. Understanding craniosynostosis as a growth disorder. Wiley Interdiscip Rev Dev Biol. 2016;5(4):429–59. https://doi.org/10.1002/wdev.227.
5. Lattanzi W, Barba M, Di Pietro L, Boyadjiev SA. Genetic advances in craniosynostosis. Am J Med Genet A. 2017;173(5):1406–29.
6. Armand T, Schaefer E, Di Rocco F, Edery P, Collet C, Rossi M. Genetic bases of craniosynostoses: an update. Neurochirurgie. 2019;65(5):196–201. https://doi.org/10.1016/j.neuchi.2019.10.003. Epub 2019 Oct 9.
7. Wilkie AO, Slaney SF, Oldridge M, Poole MD, Ashworth GJ, Hockley AD, Hayward RD, David DJ, Pulleyn LJ, Rutland P, et al. Apert syndrome results from localized mutations of FGFR2 and is allelic with Crouzon syndrome. Nat Genet. 1995;9(2):165–72.
8. Azoury SC, Reddy S, Shukla V, Deng CX. Fibroblast growth factor receptor 2 (FGFR2) mutation related syndromic craniosynostosis. Int J Biol Sci. 2017;13(12):1479–88. https://doi.org/10.7150/ijbs.22373.
9. Rutland P, Pulleyn LJ, Reardon W, Baraitser M, Hayward R, Jones B, Malcolm S, Winter RM, Oldridge M, Slaney SF, et al. Identical mutations in the FGFR2 gene cause both Pfeiffer and Crouzon syndrome phenotypes. Nat Genet. 1995;9(2):173–6.
10. Muenke M, Gripp KW, McDonald-McGinn DM, Gaudenz K, Whitaker LA, Bartlett SP, et al. A unique point mutation in the fibroblast growth factor receptor 3 gene (FGFR3) defines a new craniosynostosis syndrome. Am J Hum Genet. 1997;60(3):555–64.
11. Meyers GA, Orlow SJ, Munro IR, Przylepa KA, Jabs EW. Fibroblast growth factor receptor 3 (FGFR3) transmembrane mutation in Crouzon syndrome with acanthosis nigricans. Nat Genet. 1995;11(4):462–4.
12. Zhou YX, Xu X, Chen L, Li C, Brodie SG, Deng CX. A Pro250Arg substitution in mouse Fgfr1 causes increased expression of Cbfa1 and premature fusion of calvarial sutures. Hum Mol Genet. 2000;9(13):2001–8. https://doi.org/10.1093/hmg/9.13.2001. PMID: 10942429.
13. Cornille M, Dambroise E, Komla-Ebri D, Kaci N, Biosse-Duplan M, Di Rocco F, Legeai-Mallet L. Animal models of craniosynostosis. Neurochirurgie. 2019;65(5):202–9. https://doi.org/10.1016/j.neuchi.2019.09.010. Epub 2019 Sep 26. PMID: 31563616.
14. Chen L, Li D, Li C, Engel A, Deng CX. A Ser252Trp [corrected] substitution in mouse fibroblast growth factor receptor 2 (Fgfr2) results in craniosynostosis. Bone. 2003;33(2):169–78. https://doi.org/10.1016/s8756-3282(03)00222-9. Erratum in: Bone. 2005 Dec;37(6):876. PMID: 14499350.
15. Yin L, Du X, Li C, Xu X, Chen Z, Su N, Zhao L, Qi H, Li F, Xue J, Yang J, Jin M, Deng C, Chen L. A Pro253Arg mutation in fibroblast growth factor receptor 2 (Fgfr2) causes skeleton malformation mimicking human Apert syndrome by affecting both chondrogenesis and osteogenesis. Bone. 2008;42(4):631–43. https://doi.org/10.1016/j.bone.2007.11.019. Epub 2008 Jan 31. PMID: 18242159.
16. Eswarakumar VP, Horowitz MC, Locklin R, Morriss-Kay GM, Lonai P. A gain-of-function mutation of Fgfr2c demonstrates the roles of this receptor variant in osteogenesis. Proc Natl Acad Sci U S A. 2004;101(34):12555–60. https://doi.org/10.1073/pnas.0405031101. Epub 2004 Aug 17. PMID: 15316116; PMCID: PMC515096.

17. Mai S, Wei K, Flenniken A, Adamson SL, Rossant J, Aubin JE, Gong SG. The missense mutation W290R in Fgfr2 causes developmental defects from aberrant IIIb and IIIc signaling. Dev Dyn. 2010;239(6):1888–900. https://doi.org/10.1002/dvdy.22314. PMID: 20503384.
18. Wang Y, Zhou X, Oberoi K, Phelps R, Couwenhoven R, Sun M, Rezza A, Holmes G, Percival CJ, Friedenthal J, Krejci P, Richtsmeier JT, Huso DL, Rendl M, Jabs EW. p38 Inhibition ameliorates skin and skull abnormalities in Fgfr2 Beare-Stevenson mice. J Clin Invest. 2012;122(6):2153–64. https://doi.org/10.1172/JCI62644. Epub 2012 May 15. PMID: 22585574; PMCID: PMC3366414.
19. Laurita J, Koyama E, Chin B, Taylor JA, Lakin GE, Hankenson KD, Bartlett SP, Nah HD. The Muenke syndrome mutation (FgfR3P244R) causes cranial base shortening associated with growth plate dysfunction and premature perichondrial ossification in murine basicranial synchondroses. Dev Dyn. 2011;240(11):2584–96. https://doi.org/10.1002/dvdy.22752. PMID: 22016144.
20. Twigg SR, Healy C, Babbs C, Sharpe JA, Wood WG, Sharpe PT, Morriss-Kay GM, Wilkie AO. Skeletal analysis of the Fgfr3(P244R) mouse, a genetic model for the Muenke craniosynostosis syndrome. Dev Dyn. 2009;238(2):331–42. https://doi.org/10.1002/dvdy.21790. PMID: 19086028.
21. Cornille M, Moriceau S, Khonsari RH, Heuzé Y, Loisay L, Boitez V, Morice A, Arnaud E, Collet C, Bensidhoum M, Kaci N, Boddaert N, Paternoster G, Rauschendorfer T, Werner S, Mansour SL, Di Rocco F, Oury F, Legeai-Mallet L. FGFR3 overactivation in the brain is responsible for memory impairments in Crouzon syndrome mouse model. J Exp Med. 2022;219(4):e20201879. https://doi.org/10.1084/jem.20201879. Epub 2022 Mar 7. PMID: 35254402; PMCID: PMC8906494.
22. Morice A, Cornette R, Giudice A, Collet C, Paternoster G, Arnaud É, Galliani E, Picard A, Legeai-Mallet L, Khonsari RH. Early mandibular morphological differences in patients with FGFR2 and FGFR3-related syndromic craniosynostoses: a 3D comparative study. Bone. 2020;141:115600. https://doi.org/10.1016/j.bone.2020.115600. Epub 2020 Aug 18. PMID: 32822871.
23. Colvin JS, Bohne BA, Harding GW, McEwen DG, Ornitz DM. Skeletal overgrowth and deafness in mice lacking fibroblast growth factor receptor 3. Nat Genet. 1996;12(4):390–7. https://doi.org/10.1038/ng0496-390. PMID: 8630492.
24. Deng C, Wynshaw-Boris A, Zhou F, Kuo A, Leder P. Fibroblast growth factor receptor 3 is a negative regulator of bone growth. Cell. 1996;84(6):911-21. https://doi.org/10.1016/s0092-8674(00)81069-7. PMID: 8601314.
25. Su N, Xu X, Li C, He Q, Zhao L, Li C, Chen S, Luo F, Yi L, Du X, Huang H, Deng C, Chen L. Generation of Fgfr3 conditional knockout mice. Int J Biol Sci. 2010;6(4):327–32. https://doi.org/10.7150/ijbs.6.327. PMID: 20582225; PMCID: PMC2892296.
26. Dambroise E, Ktorza I, Brombin A, Abdessalem G, Edouard J, Luka M, Fiedler I, Binder O, Pelle O, Patton EE, Busse B, Menager M, Sohm F, Legeai-Mallet L. Fgfr3 is a positive regulator of osteoblast expansion and differentiation during zebrafish skull vault development. J Bone Miner Res. 2020;35(9):1782–97. https://doi.org/10.1002/jbmr.4042. Epub 2020 May 26. PMID: 32379366.
27. Lekovic GP, Bristol RE, Rekate HL. Cognitive impact of craniosynostosis. Semin Pediatr Neurol. 2004;11(4):305–10. https://doi.org/10.1016/j.spen.2004.12.001. PMID: 15828715.
28. Cohen MM Jr. Pfeiffer syndrome update, clinical subtypes, and guidelines for differential diagnosis. Am J Med Genet. 1993;45(3):300–7.
29. Vogels A, Fryns JP. Pfeiffer syndrome. Orphanet J Rare Dis. 2006;1(1):1–3.
30. Ko JM. Genetic syndromes associated with craniosynostosis. J Korean Neurosurg Soc. 2016;59(3):187–91.
31. Shiller JG. Craniofacial dysostosis of Crouzon: a case report and pedigree with emphasis on heredity. Pediatrics. 1959;23(1):107–12.
32. Schmetz A, Amiel J, Wieczorek D. Genetics of craniofacial malformations. Semin Fetal Neonatal Med. 2021;26(6):101290. WB Saunders.
33. Passos-Bueno MR, Sertié AL, Jehee FS, Fanganiello R, Yeh E. Genetics of craniosynostosis: genes, syndromes, mutations and genotype-phenotype correlations. Front Oral Biol. 2008;12:107–43.
34. Kreiborg S, Cohen MM Jr. Characteristics of the infant Apert skull and its subsequent development. J Craniofac Genet Dev Biol. 1990;10(4):399–410.
35. Wenger, T. L., Hing, A. V., & Evans, K. N. (2019). Apert syndrome. In M. P. Adam (Eds.) et al, GeneReviews®. University of Washington, Seattle.
36. Jackson CE, Weiss L, Reynolds WA, Forman TF, Peterson JA. Craniosynostosis midface hypoplasia, and foot abnormalities: an autosomal dominant phenotype in a large Amish kindred. J Pediatr. 1976;88(6):963–8.
37. Przylepa KA, Paznekas W, Zhang M, Golabi M, Bias W, Bamshad MJ, et al. Fibroblast growth factor receptor 2 mutations in Beare–Stevenson cutis gyrata syndrome. Nat Genet. 1996;13(4):492–4.
38. Maliepaard M, Mathijssen IM, Oosterlaan J, Okkerse JM. Intellectual, behavioral, and emotional functioning in children with syndromic craniosynostosis. Pediatrics. 2014;133(6):e1608–15. https://doi.org/10.1542/peds.2013-3077. PMID: 24864183.
39. Yarnell CM, Addissie YA, Hadley DW, Guillen Sacoto MJ, Agochukwu NB, Hart RA, Wiggs EA, Platte P, Paelecke Y, Collmann H, Schweitzer T, Kruszka P, Muenke M. Executive function and adaptive behavior in Muenke syndrome. J Pediatr. 2015;167(2):428–34. https://doi.org/10.1016/j.jpeds.2015.04.080. Epub 2015 May 28. PMID: 26028288; PMCID: PMC4516644.
40. Kruszka P, Addissie YA, Agochukwu NB, Doherty ES, Muenke M. Muenke syndrome. In: Adam MP, Ardinger HH, Pagon RA, Wallace SE, Bean LJ, Stephens K, Amemiya A, editors. GeneReviews®. Seattle: University of Washington, Seattle; 1993.

41. Raybaud C, Di Rocco C. Brain malformation in syndromic craniosynostoses, a primary disorder of white matter: a review. Childs Nerv Syst. 2007;23(12):1379–88. https://doi.org/10.1007/s00381-007-0474-7. Epub 2007 Sep 20. PMID: 17882438.
42. Komla-Ebri D, Dambroise E, Kramer I, et al. Tyrosine kinase inhibitor NVP-BGJ398 functionally improves FGFR3-related dwarfism in mouse model. J Clin Invest. 2016;126(5):1871–84. https://doi.org/10.1172/JCI83926.
43. Di Rocco F, Biosse Duplan M, Heuzé Y, Kaci N, Komla-Ebri D, Munnich A, Mugniery E, Benoist-Lasselin C, Legeai-Mallet L. FGFR3 mutation causes abnormal membranous ossification in achondroplasia. Hum Mol Genet. 2014;23(11):2914–25. https://doi.org/10.1093/hmg/ddu004. Epub 2014 Jan 12. PMID: 24419316.
44. Biosse Duplan M, Komla-Ebri D, Heuzé Y, Estibals V, Gaudas E, Kaci N, Benoist-Lasselin C, Zerah M, Kramer I, Kneissel M, Porta DG, Di Rocco F, Legeai-Mallet L. Meckel's and condylar cartilages anomalies in achondroplasia result in defective development and growth of the mandible. Hum Mol Genet. 2016;25(14):2997–3010. https://doi.org/10.1093/hmg/ddw153. Epub 2016 Jun 3. PMID: 27260401; PMCID: PMC5181594.
45. Lorget F, Kaci N, Peng J, et al. Evaluation of the therapeutic potential of a CNP analog in a Fgfr3 mouse model recapitulating achondroplasia. Am J Hum Genet. 2012;91(6):1108–14. https://doi.org/10.1016/j.ajhg.2012.10.014.
46. Wendt DJ, Dvorak-Ewell M, Bullens S, Lorget F, Bell SM, Peng J, et al. Neutral endopeptidase-resistant C-type natriuretic peptide variant represents a new therapeutic approach for treatment of fibroblast growth factor receptor 3–related dwarfism. J Pharmacol Exp Ther. 2015;353(1):132–49.
47. Martin L, Kaci N, Benoist-Lasselin C, et al. Theobroma cacao improves bone growth by modulating defective ciliogenesis in a mouse model of achondroplasia. Bone Res. 2022;10(1):8. Published 2022 Jan 25. https://doi.org/10.1038/s41413-021-00177-7.
48. Legeai-Mallet L, Savarirayan R. Novel therapeutic approaches for the treatment of achondroplasia. Bone. 2020;141:115579. https://doi.org/10.1016/j.bone.2020.115579. Epub 2020 Aug 11. PMID: 32795681.

5 Neurocranial Growth in Craniosynostosis

Maarten te Dorsthorst and Hans Delye

Within the broad array of neurosurgical procedures, craniosynostosis surgery is somewhat of an outsider, as the final result can only be evaluated many years later. Even when all short-term surgical goals are reached, it could be that in time mid-term and long-term results are not reached at all, due to the continuing growth of the brain and skull. Therefore, taking into account the physiological growth of the cranial vault and the underlying brain is of paramount importance during the consideration of all viable surgical options and the corresponding timing of the surgery as part of the optimal treatment plan.

5.1 Underlying Principles and Mechanisms

Understanding the physiological growth of the cranial vault is fundamental to understanding the pathophysiology involved in craniosynostosis. It is clear that a detailed description of the complex processes giving rise to the development and growth of the craniofacial skeleton is far beyond the scope of this chapter and the interested reader is referred to textbooks focussing only on this subject [1]. But still, it is good to have a notion of the main processes at play.

The physiological growth and development of the neurocranium start with osteogenesis, both as intramembranous ossification and enchondral ossification. Intramembranous ossification begins with the differentiation of mesenchymal cells into groups of osteoblasts in ossification centres. In these centres, the connective membrane is turned into bone, with the remainder of this membrane giving rise to the endosteum, periosteum and sutures. In this way, most of the cranial vault is formed from the intramembranous bone of paraxial mesodermal origin: the frontal and parietal bones and parts of the occipital and temporal bones. Endochondral ossification occurs on a segment of hyaline cartilage. The chondrocytes grow, the cartilaginous matrix mineralizes and decreases, and the chondrocytes are replaced by capillaries and adjacent connective tissue cells, which differentiate into osteoblasts. The cranial base is formed in this way from the endochondral bone of neural crest origin [1].

These mechanisms of osteogenesis are well studied and agreed upon in histology literature. However, on a larger scale, the subsequent processes regulating the (mainly postnatal) further growth and development of the neurocranium are far more complex and less understood. Historically, the role of the sutures and growth centres in bone formation and the regulation of the mechanisms at play have been extensively

M. te Dorsthorst · H. Delye (✉)
Department of Neurosurgery, Radboud University Medical Centre, Nijmegen, Netherlands
e-mail: Maarten.teDorsthorst@Radboudumc.nl

F. Di Rocco, J. Kestle (eds.), *Neurosurgical Aspects of Craniosynostosis*,
https://doi.org/10.1007/978-3-031-69386-1_5

debated. Basically, two main theories have been postulated. The genetic theory in which the phenotypic expression is determined by genetic transcription: the growth and development of the neurocranium are to a high degree independent from environmental influences and interaction with surrounding tissues. This is opposed by the theory stating that growth and development are a major result of complex interaction with environmental factors and surrounding tissues and are only basically defined by the genetic constitution. Both theories have been used to try to offer an understanding of mechanisms involved in pathology, such as craniosynostosis [2].

We will shortly discuss some historical milestones, but the interested reader is referred to the recent publications giving a concise overview of the history of craniofacial studies and evolving theories [2, 3].

The first reports on craniofacial growth date back to 1791, when Sömmering described cranial deformity resulting from cranial suture pathology. Otto described microcephaly or premature sutural closure resulting in craniosynostosis 40 years later. In 1851, Virchow put forth the hypothesis that cranial growth perpendicular to the fused suture was limited and growth in the plane parallel to the fused suture was enhanced [4].

In the early twentieth century, with the advent of X-ray, cephalometric studies were undertaken. At first, these were merely descriptive and focussed on the description of the craniofacial growth pattern with little interest in the relation between growth and function of parts of the craniofacial skeleton. Growth of the craniofacial skeleton was considered to be intrinsic and following growth of the rest of the body, more or less equal in all mankind, not influenced by interaction with surrounding tissues nor a resultant of function. It was believed that growth and development were genetically determined. However, in time, it became apparent that craniofacial growth showed more variation than what could be explained by genetic patterns only. Now, more and more studies have shifted towards the relationship between function and anatomy and it became clear that, to some extent, growth and variation could be considered an adaptation to changing functional demands.

In the 1960s, Moss and co-workers put forward the functional matrix hypothesis. In this hypothesis (which did apply to the whole body and not only to the head), they stated that the head served different functions, and every function was carried out by a 'functional cranial component'. Each cranial component consisted of a 'functional matrix' carrying out the function and a 'skeletal unit' designed to protect and support its functional matrix. They hypothesized that any change in size, shape, spatial position and maintenance in all skeletal units were always secondary to primary changes in their specific functional matrices. On a larger level, all the functional cranial components were organized in the form of 'cranial capsules', mainly the neurocranial capsule and the orofacial capsule. A 'capsule' was defined as an envelope that contains a series of functional cranial components which are sandwiched in between two covering layers. For the neurocranial capsule, this was the skin and the dura mater. Each capsule surrounds and protects a 'capsular' functional matrix. For the neurocranial capsule, this is the 'neural mass', consisting of the brain, leptomeninges and cerebrospinal fluid. Capsular matrices, as the neural mass, are defined and act as a volume. With this neurocranial functional matrix hypothesis, Moss and co-workers posed that the cranium is in large formed due to secondary passive growth at the sutures, in response to the active growth of the cerebral mass, where the sutural location, morphology and patency give direction to this growth [5]. This hypothesis shifted the presumed role of the sutures from being active growth centres creating the cranial vault in the genetically predetermined form and dimensions towards passive, compensatory growth centres that only reacted to the changes of the neural mass. In this hypothesis, the structural growth and shape of the cranial vault bones are not genetically predetermined, but reactive in nature to the functional matrix-neural mass. Although the functional matrix hypothesis has been criticized (mainly on the notion of the intrinsic growth propensities of the cephalic cartilage at the skull base), the concept of skull growth being the result of driving intracranial forces being limited by diminishing growth potential of sutures and growth centres has been widely observed and accepted. So what about the undeniable role of genes in regulating the growth of the neurocranium and what about their role in the occurrence of craniosynostosis? Richtsmeier and Flaherty built an argument that the brain and skull phenotypes take shape resulting from communication between cells and tissues by regulating gene expression affecting morphogenesis [6]. Twigg and Wilkie described clearly the way bone formation processes at the sutures are influenced/regulated by genetic transcription in response to internal/external stimuli, see also Fig. 5.1 [7]. Disruption of this equilibrium could then result in early, pathological, closure and the occurrence of craniosynostosis [7].

To summarize, the current understanding is that the origin of neurocranial growth is genetically predefined up to the point that the calvarial growth at the sutures is becoming the resultant of intracranial driving forces, regulated by a complex interplay of different genes that control the

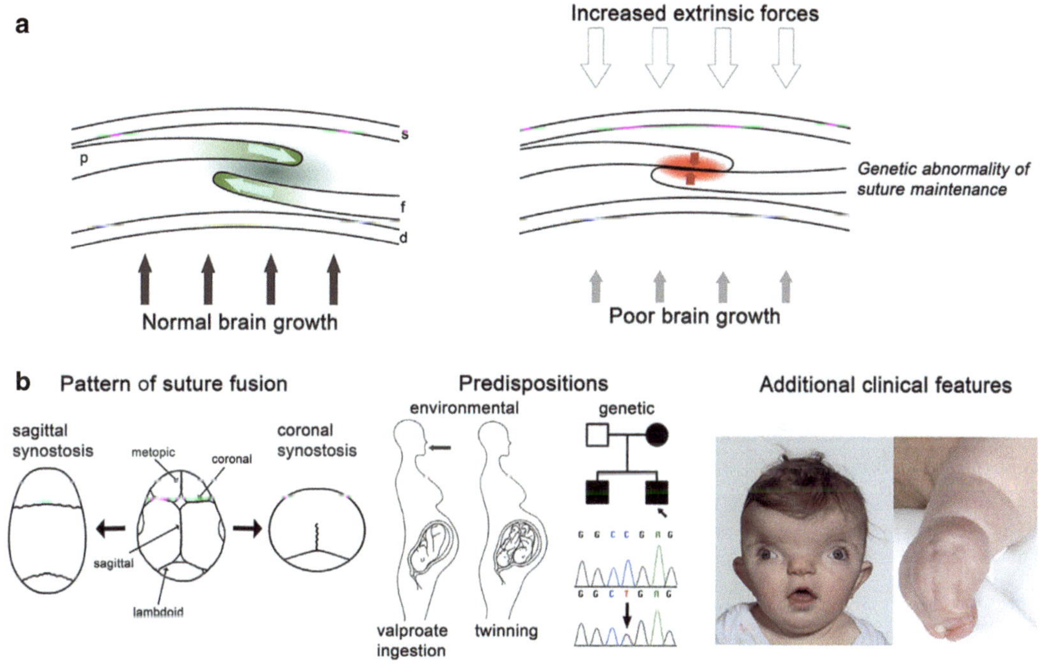

Fig. 5.1 Overview of clinical causes and classification of craniosynostosis. (**a**) Cross-section of coronal suture showing the developing parietal bone (p) overlying the frontal bone (f). Internally, the dura mater (d) separates the calvaria from the brain; skin (s) is external. Left, normal growth of the skull vault is regulated by a delicate balance of proliferation and differentiation occurring within the suture (green shading) co-ordinated with the enlargement of the underlying brain (black arrows). Right, in craniosynostosis this balance has been disturbed by excessive external force on the skull, usually during pregnancy (unfilled arrows), inefficient transduction of stretch from the growing brain (grey arrows), or intrinsic abnormality of signalling within the suture itself (red shading). (**b**) Approaches to clinical classification. Left: view of the skull from above (front at top). Normal skull with major vault sutures identified is central. To either side, the examples show skull shapes resulting from sagittal synostosis (left) and bilateral coronal synostosis (right). Note the metopic suture closes physiologically at the age of 3–9 months. Centre: the clinical history can reveal possible environmental predispositions such as teratogen exposure (most commonly maternal treatment with the anticonvulsant sodium valproate) or twinning (intrauterine constraint); affected relatives with craniosynostosis (filled symbols in pedigree) suggest a likely genetic cause, which can be confirmed by diagnostic genetic testing. Right: clinical examination can reveal facial dysmorphic features such as hypertelorism (wide spaced eyes) and grooved nasal tip, suggesting craniofrontonasal syndrome (left), or other physical features such as syndactyly characteristic of Apert syndrome (right). (Clinical photographs reproduced, with permission, from Johnson and Wilkie and Twigg et al. Reproduced with permission from Elsevier [7])

proliferation-differentiation balance of a population of undifferentiated stem cells in the midsutural mesenchyme.

5.2 Neurocranial Growth Patterns

How does this give rise to normal growth patterns? And how do these differ from what is seen in craniosynostosis? Although many cephalometric studies have been done in the twentieth century [8], the timing and amplitude of regional growth of different calvarial skull bones and resultant skull shape are not totally elucidated yet. The same holds true for the regional growth patterns of the developing brain. Research investigating the growth of the cranial vault and the cerebrum in the first stages after birth has always been difficult because of limitations with regard to data collection. Computed tomography (CT) has been used only in the case of suspected abnormalities, due to its use of ionizing x-rays. Magnetic resonance (MR) imaging may not use harmful radiation, but MR images are often degraded due to the neonates' motion [9]. Additionally, unmyelinated white matter can be difficult to differentiate from grey matter [10] and myelination of white matter may cause changes in contrast and brightness inhomogeneities on MR imaging [11]. Recent advances in using non-ionizing 3D-stereophotogrammetry have provided the first limited data sets on normal growth patterns of the head. However, this technique only covers the outer surface of the head and cannot distinguish the skull from the intracranial mass [12].

5.2.1 Brain Growth Patterns

The increase in the cerebral volume results from progressive phenomena, such as cell proliferation, arborization and myelination [13]. The traditional quantification of neonate cranial growth is based on the head circumference, where the head circumference shows a natural logarithmic growth pattern, as displayed in Fig. 5.2 [12]. Although the direct measurement of the head circumference is still widely used as a parameter, this metric has shown low reliability and high inter-and intra-observer variability [14]. Pfefferbaum and colleagues were the first to publish the overall brain, white and grey matter volume of infants, children and adolescents based on MR imaging, though the number of infants in the subject group was very limited [13]. Matsuzawa showed that MR image analyses showed that volumetric growth of the cerebrum followed a

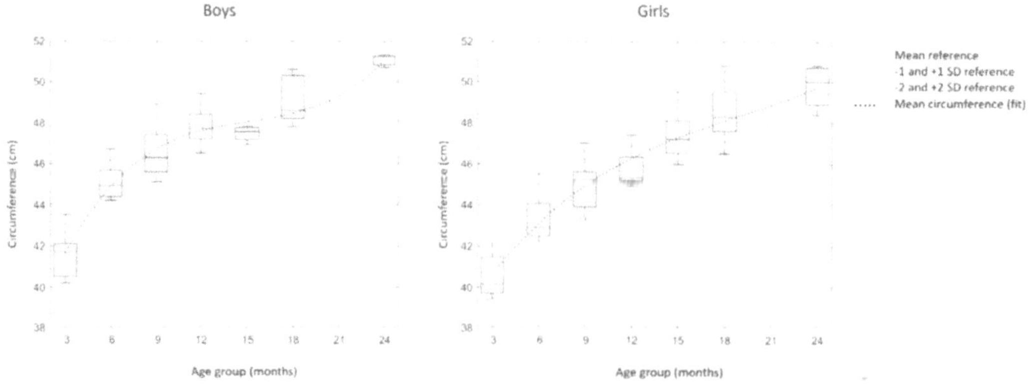

Fig. 5.2 Boxplots of circumference measured on 3D photographs for boys (left) and girls (right). Circumference reference values based on the Dutch cross-sectional growth study are plotted in the background. (Reproduced with permission from Elsevier [12])

natural logarithmic curve, similar to the curve of the head circumference [15].

The total brain volume increase is the largest in the first year of life (from ~36% of adult volume at 4 weeks of age to ~72% of adult volume at 1 year), and then starts to slow down (with total brain volume reaching ~83% of adult volume at 2 years of age) and reaching an approximation of its final volume at around 5 years of age [11, 15]. Knickmeyer found that the cerebellum showed disproportionate enlargement when compared to the cerebral hemispheres in the first 2 years of life. Within the cerebral hemispheres, volume enlargement was larger in grey matter than white matter, with a doubling of the cortical grey matter volume during the first year of life. However, they did not report on volumetric changes of the separate lobes or regions of the brain, with an exception for the cerebellum, see Table 5.1 [11].

The early fast growth rate of the cerebellum was confirmed by Holland et al., who defined regional growth rates and left-right asymmetries in the first 3 months of infant brain development. They found a volume increase of the cerebellum of 108% at 90 days postnatally, in contrast to a total brain volume increase of only 64%. They did not study the grey and white matter and did not look at the volume increase of separate lobes or regions of the brain [9].

Matsuzawa and colleagues were the first to compartmentalize the cerebrum partly based on anatomical boundaries and analysed (relative) volumetric data on the compartments. However, the volumetric evolution of these cerebral compartments over time was not publicized [15].

With the development of new MRI techniques, brain development in neonates and infants is gaining more attention and regional differences

Table 5.1 Age-related changes in brain volume (Reproduced from [11])

	Neonate	1 year	2 year	Percentage change: 95% CI (neonate to 1 year)		Percentage change: 95% CI (1 year–2 years)	
Region				ANOVA	ANCOVA (adjusted for TBV)	ANOVA	ANCOVA (adjusted for TBV)
TBV	425,387 (4806)	855,540 (12,492)	983,866 (15,393)	95–107%[a]	N/A	11–19%[a]	N/A
Cerebral hemispheres	370,685 (4185)	699,378 (10,199)	801,501 (12,577)	83–94%[a]	−6 to −5%[a]	11–19%[a]	−1 to 1%
Cerebellum	26,985 (371)	91,962 (1712)	105,154 (2084)	228–253%[a]	71–83%[a]	10–19%[a]	−1 to 9%[b]
Subcortical + brainstem	27,679 (453)	64,214 (868)	73,227 (1140)	126–138%[a]	18–22%[a]	11–18%[a]	−2 to 5%
Hemispheric gray	206,480 (2396)	514,048 (6679)	588,441 (9100)	143–155%[a]	25–29%[a]	11–18%[a]	2–4%
Hemispheric white	164,133 (1901)	183,280 (4122)	217,883 (5142)	6–16%[a]	−60 to −56%[a]	13–24%[a]	−24 to −4%[b]
Lateral ventricles	2109 (149)	8069 (723)	7406 (786)	213–352%[a]	−73 to −22%	−28 to 11%	−160 to −17%[a]
Right caudate	N/A	3221 (69)	3778 (83)	N/A	N/A	12–23%[a]	1–11%[c]
Left caudate	N/A	3012 (68)	3607 (91)	N/A	N/A	14–26%[a]	3–15%[c]
Right hippocampus	N/A	2113 (39)	2377 (65)	N/A	N/A	6–19%[c]	−4 to 7%
Left hippocampus	N/A	2075 (43)	2367 (68)	N/A	N/A	7–21%[b]	−6 to 6%

All volumes are mean (SD) in mm^3

N/A Not applicable

[a] $p < 0.0001$

[b] $p < 0.001$

[c] $p \leq 0.05$

are being studied and slowly clarified. Lyall et al. looked at the development of the regional cortical thickness and cortical surface area. They found that cortical thickness and cortical surface area have distinct and regionally heterogeneous growth patterns. In the first 2 years of life, primary and secondary sensory cortices displayed a slower increase in thickness when compared to cortices of regions involved with speech and language as well as the insula and cingulate cortex. In general, cortical thickness approaches 97% of adult values in the first 2 years of life. However, the cortical thickness did not show a clear relationship to the total cortical volume, whereas the cortical surface area had a strong and direct relationship to the total cortical volume [16].

During the first 2 years of life, the cortical surface area showed an average increase of 115%, three-quarters of which occurred during the first year. Almost all regions of the brain show a large increase in surface area in the first year of life, but the most expanding regions include lateral frontal lobes, lateral parietal lobes and occipital lobes, as well as left Heschl's and left inferior temporal gyri, as is displayed in Fig. 5.3 [16]. This includes typical sensory-specific association cortices, such as superior occipital gyrus (visual association), superior and middle temporal gyrus (auditory association) and superior parietal gyrus (sensory/tactile association and spatial correspondence). The rapid increase in the surface area of these cortices could be related to the rapid expansion of the topographic maps that each of these area's harbour early in childhood. These maps are highly plastic and refined with increased experience. However, they noted that many of these regions did not show a large amount of cortical thickness growth, suggesting that topographic map plasticity could be regulated primarily by surface area expansion [16, 17].

Although Lyall has given us insight into the development of cortical thickness and cortical surface area in the first 2 years of life in relation to possible functional developmental stages, their data did not provide data on the regional differences in volume gain on the level of separate lobes or regions of the brain, including white matter [16].

With regard to the timeframe in which most craniosynostosis treatments are performed, we can summarize the growth as follows: it is shown that the total volume of the brain, the volume of the cerebral hemispheres and the volume of the cerebellum increase dramatically during the first year of life, with an increase of 101%, 88% and an extraordinary 240%, respectively. The volume increase of the cerebral hemispheres is mainly the result of the volume increase of the grey mat-

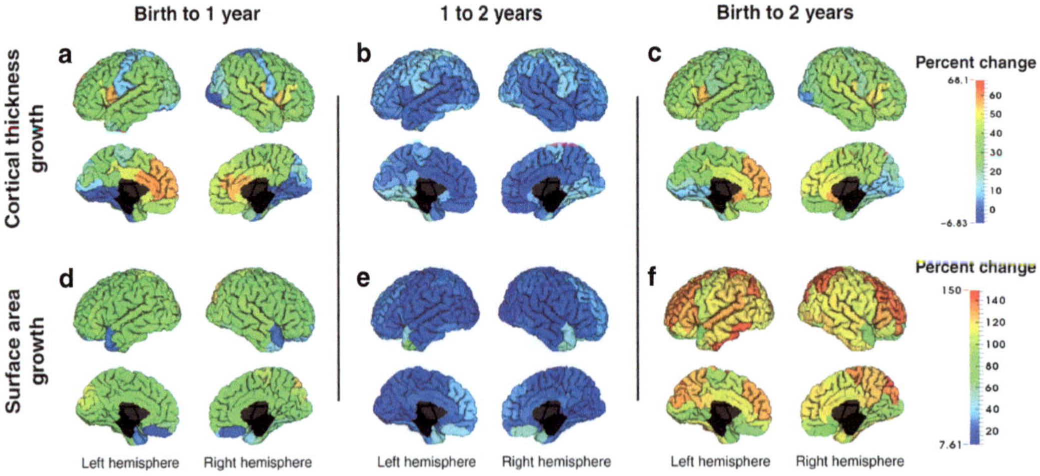

Fig. 5.3 Early cortical surface measures development from birth to 2 years. Regional percent change for CT. (**a–c**) and SA (**d–f**) from birth to 1 year (**a, d**), 1–2 years (**b, e**), and birth to 2 years (**c, f**). Warmer colours indicate larger per cent changes than cooler colours. (Reproduced with permission of Oxford University Press [16])

ter. In turn, the volume increase of the cortical grey matter has a strong relationship with the cortical surface area and less with the cortical thickness. The increase of the cortical surface area is large for almost all regions of the brain in the first year of life, but the most expanding regions include lateral frontal lobes, lateral parietal lobes and occipital lobes, as well as left Heschl's and left inferior temporal gyri.

Currently, there are no data available on the specific timing of the volume increase of separate regions of the hemispheres during the first year of life, it is nonetheless becoming increasingly clear that the brain development in early childhood is very complex and regionally and temporally diverse. This has not been properly clarified in the literature to date, one can assume that this heterogenous development would result in non-uniform volume gain of the brain during the first year of life. If so, bearing in mind the functional matrix hypothesis, this would mean that skull growth is not uniform either in the first year of life.

5.2.2 Skull Growth Patterns

Despite the long history of two-dimensional cephalometric studies, the interest in the 3D skull growth patterns in infants has gained new interest in only recent years. Even though some studies still report using radiation techniques [18, 19] the renewed interest is mainly due to the development of radiation-free evaluation methods, such as stereophotogrammetry, allowing for a prospective and longitudinal study on the skull growth patterns in infants [12, 20, 21]. We strongly believe that this knowledge is crucial to understanding deviations of what is considered 'normal growth' and to evaluating both pathology and treatment results of growth deviations, such as craniosynostosis. The use of radiation-free stereophotogrammetry allows for repetitive, longitudinal and prospective measurements in large groups of individuals without the concerns of radiation on the developing brain. This is a huge benefit over traditional radiation-based techniques, still, a critical note needs to be addressed: this technique only captures the surface and is therefore prone to measurement errors induced by increasingly larger amounts of hair. This means that this study method is feasible and reliable on a group level up to the age of 18–24 months and can allow for individual follow-up and comparison in selected individuals up to the age of 4–5 years [12]. Another important feature to remember is that stereophotogrammetry techniques always include soft tissue and the measurements and growth patterns derived from it are strongly correlated with the measurements and growth patterns of the skull, but are not the same. In general, stereophotogrammetry-based measurements tend to be larger, depending on the age of the subject and type of measurement.

Using prospectively collected stereophotogrammetry data, comparing them to retrospectively collected CT data, Meulstee et al. documented the very fast growth of the cranium in the first 2 years in infants, showing the fastest expansion during the first 6 months and generally slower rate of growth after 12 months. They looked at more regionally detailed growth patterns and found that, between age 3 months and 6 months, the largest growth occurred in the frontal and parietal regions and, between age 6 months and 12 months, most growth was anteriorly located, resulting in an elongation of the head shape. In the following period of 12–18 months, the posterior part of the skull developed more rapidly. Because of the overall slowing of the growth after 12 months, they looked at a larger time interval of up to 24 months. This showed that most growth was located at the frontal and posterior parts of the skull. This focus on posterior growth from 12 to 24 months corresponds to the time when toddlers start developing walking skills, increasing balance and muscle coordination, and suggests a relationship with the continuing volume increase of the cerebellum at that time. See also Fig. 5.4 [12].

Meyer-Marcotty et al. looked at the growth patterns of infants' heads with stereophotogrammetry techniques from age 4 until 10 months. Unfortunately, they did not produce growth maps but presented 2D measurements such as length, width, cephalic index and vertex height. Even so,

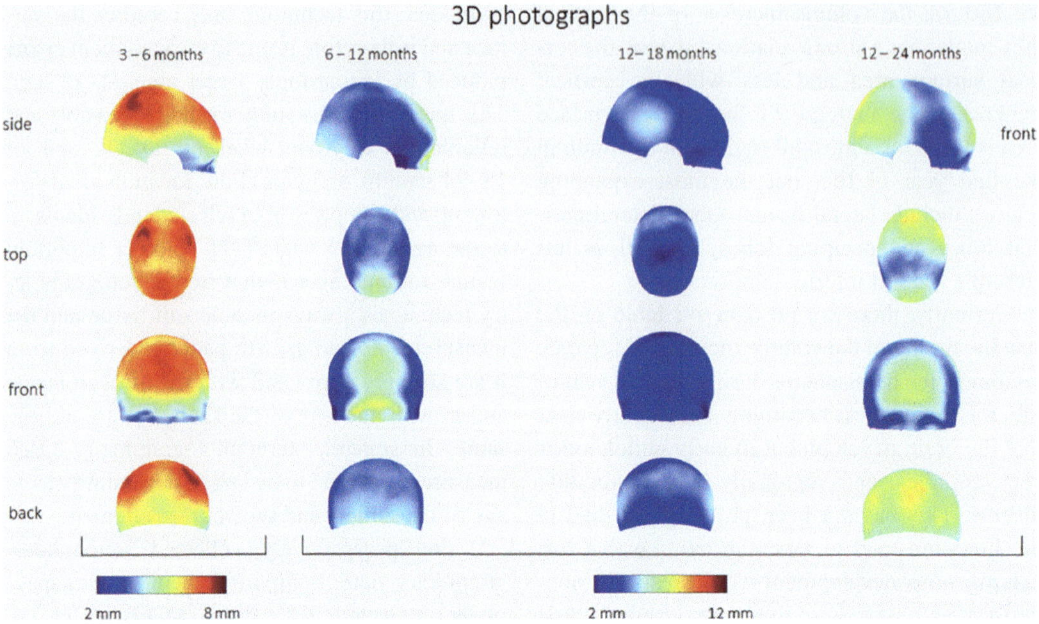

Fig. 5.4 Growth maps of 3D photographs, illustrating the focus of growth between the different time intervals. (Reproduced with permission from Elsevier [12])

they confirmed the fast growth in the first year of life, showing that the fastest growth was seen between age 4 and 6 months, with a total head volume increase of 13%. In the time span of 6–8 months, this dropped to 8.6% increase and was only 5.6% between 8 and 10 months. Of importance, they found that the initial relative increase in head length and head width was equal from 4 to 6 months, but thereafter the increase in head width was less than head length, showing a decrease in the cephalic index after 6 months of age. This was even more pronounced in the timespan of 8–10 months, with a relative increase of head width of 1% and head length of 2.4% [21]. In an earlier study of the same group, they looked at the time interval of 6–12 months and found a relative decrease of CI of 2.5% [22].

This finding was also documented by Kuwahara et al. who recently produced skull growth patterns of Japanese infants based on CT scan data. They created 6 'average' skull models of infants ranging from age 1 to 17 months producing 2D measurements and detailed 3D growth patterns, see Figs. 5.5 and 5.6 [19].

In their study, they found the same fast growth up to the age of 5 months as described by Meyer-Marcotty et al. and Meulstee et al. [12, 19, 21] The detailed growth patterns showed a more homogeneous growth during the early phases (up to the age of 5 months), with the exception of the occipital region. In the time span from 4–5 to 6–8 months, they found frontal and occipital growth, leading to a higher increase in length and elongation of the head with a cephalic index decrease of 5%. The following period from 6–8 to 9–11 months showed a higher relative increase of width, with most growth occurring at the posterior temporal and lower parietal sites. After this short period of increase in the cephalic index (2.2%), they found for the last period from 9–11 to 12–17 months again a decrease of the cephalic index of 2%, with growth now focusing on the occipital region [19].

It would be interesting to compare the growth patterns found by Meulstee et al. and Kuwahara et al. Unfortunately, this is rather difficult because of the different grouping according to age in both studies. Being the result of a mathematical difference in the position of vertices of created average skull/head models for a certain age group, the presented heat maps of both studies are highly influenced by the grouping of the original CT

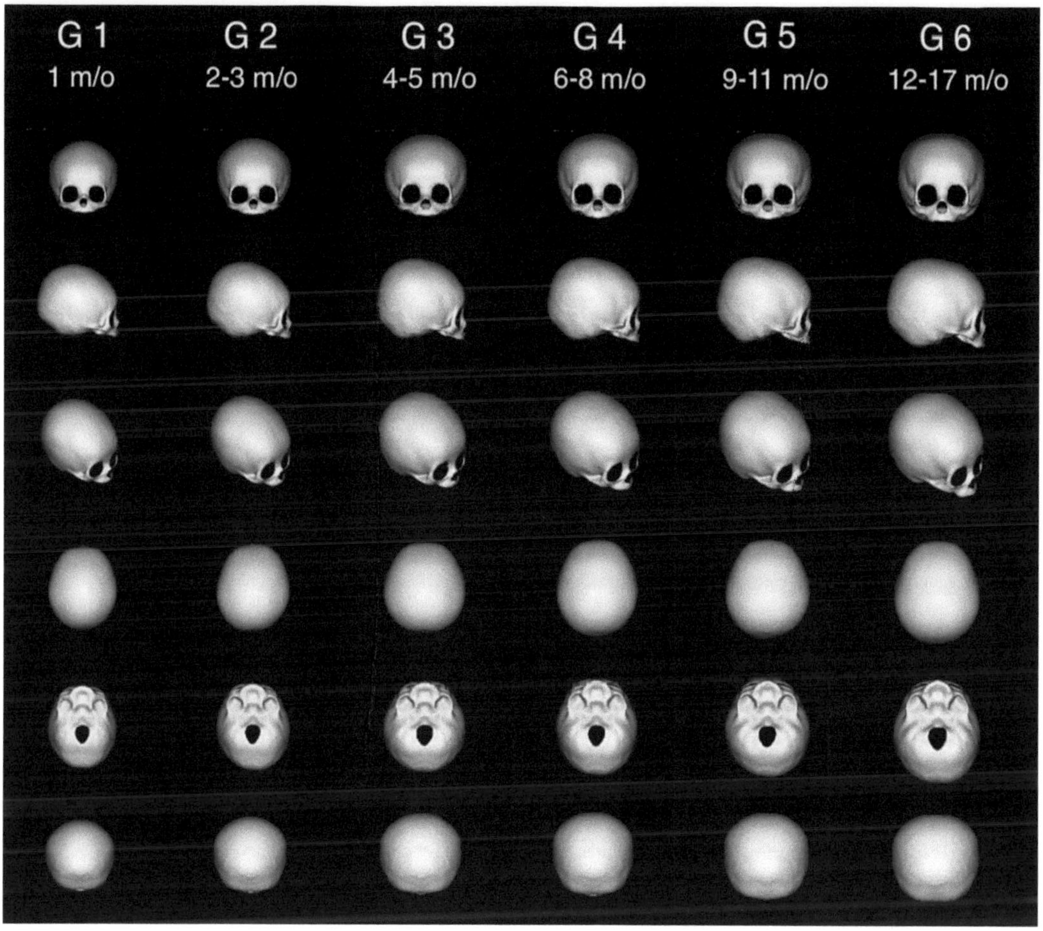

Fig. 5.5 The average cranial models of six different age groups, viewed in six directions. (Reproduced with permission of author [19])

scans/stereophotogrammetry data. However, it looks like the general trend reported by Meulstee et al. is also reported by Kuwhara et al.: at first a more evenly distributed growth, followed by a clear growth of frontal and then posterior parts. Interestingly, when comparing the 2D data of Meulstee et al., Meyer-Marcotty et al. and Kuwahara et al., the same trend of increase in length of the head/skull is seen after 6 months, even when considering that the study population of Kuwahara et al. displayed a more brachycephalic head shape overall [12, 19, 22].

To summarize, we can state that skull growth shows a very fast expansion in the first year of life, with a peculiar fast rate during the first 6 months of life accommodating the exceptional volumetric increase of the developing brain. Although studies on skull/head growth patterns differ in timing and methodology, in general, we can state that skull growth is more evenly distributed in the first 5–6 months of life. Thereafter, an elongation of the head occurs, with first a period of frontal growth up to the age of 8–12 months, followed by a period of increased posterior and occipital growth up to the age of 17–18 months (or longer), which is then again followed by frontally located growth. We hope that more studies with uniform methods regarding age grouping and larger study groups will elucidate these growth patterns further in the future.

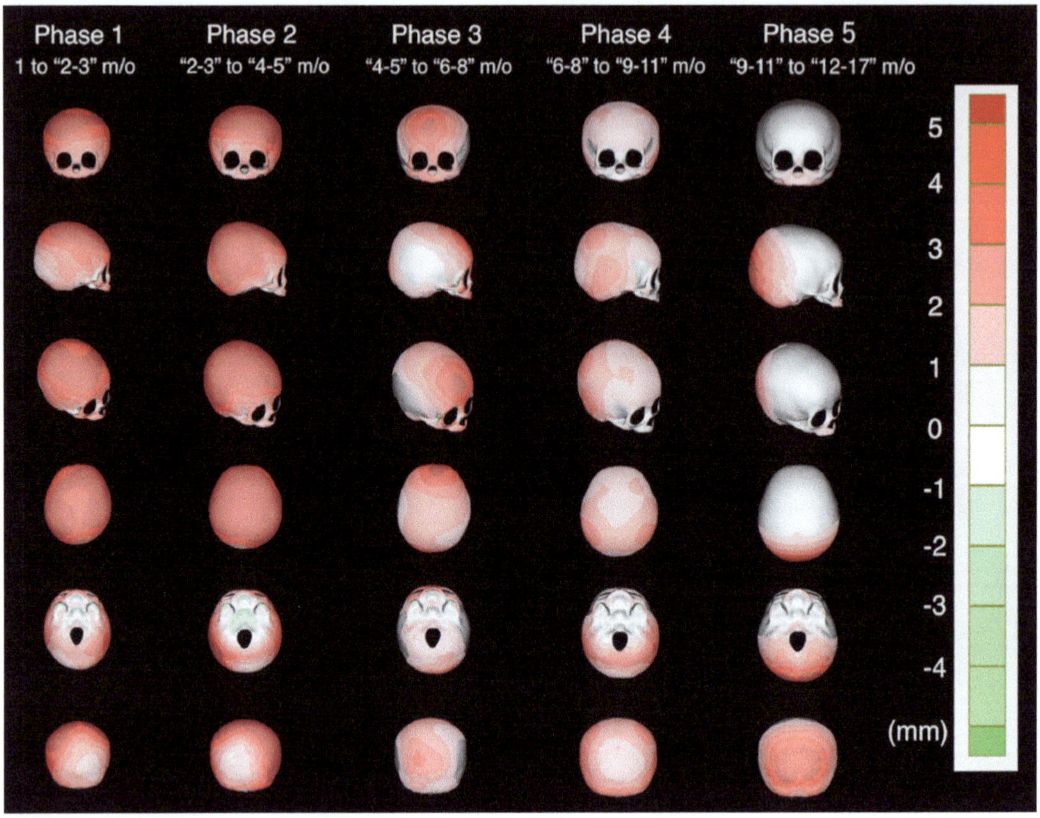

Fig. 5.6 Heat map showing the shortest interplanar distance in the perpendicular direction between two average models of adjacent age groups. The larger the increase related to growth, the more reddish the colour will be. (Reproduced with permission of author [19])

5.3 Implications for Craniosynostosis Treatment

Notwithstanding the fast-increasing knowledge about the different genes that control the proliferation-differentiation balance of the mid-sutural mesenchyme, there are no medical/genetic therapies yet that can prevent or cure the premature fusion of sutures in craniosynostosis. As soon as a suture closes too early, the normal growth pattern of the skull is disrupted. Because of the lack of growth potential at the fused suture, the intracranial driving forces (i.e. the fast-expanding brain) will induce increased growth at the remaining non-fused sutures and will continue to do so as long as the fused suture is not treated. Both lack of growth and compensatory growth will in turn give rise to the well-known deviant head shapes.

It is clear that the uniform growth of the cranial vault is the fastest during the first 6 months of life. Already half of the total volumetric growth of the neurocranium has been completed at 6 months after birth [1]. The cranial vault reaches approximately 86% of its adult size by 1 year of age and 94% of adult size by 5 years of age [8].

By extension, the influence of a prematurely closed suture on normal growth and shape development, including the occurrence of possible compensatory growth, is the greatest in the first

6 months of life but will continue and slowly diminish after 1 year.

Bearing in mind the functional matrix hypothesis, in which the expanding intracranial mass is designated the motor for the calvarial growth by stimulating and inducing growth at the sutures, we strongly advocate an early re-opening of a prematurely closed suture in order to restore as fast as possible the normal growth potential of the skull and limit both the duration of growth restriction and the increasing amount of compensatory growth.

This argument for very early surgical treatment of craniosynostosis should, of course, be balanced by the risks and morbidity of the proposed type of surgery.

The surgical treatment of craniosynostosis can generally be divided into two main modalities: open cranial vault reconstruction surgery (OCVRS) and minimally invasive surgery, such as endoscopically assisted craniosynostosis surgery (EACS) [23]. A detailed description and comparison of both open and minimally invasive techniques would exceed the scope of this chapter.

To be brief, OCVRS has been considered the 'golden standard' in the treatment of craniosynostosis for a long time. As it entails large craniectomies and thorough remodelling of the skull, it is considered a major surgery and is typically performed at the age of 10–12 months in order to allow some general body growth to balance the surgical risks. This means that growth restriction and subsequent compensatory growth continue upto 10–12 months, possibly leading to disturbing secondary changes that are not routinely dealt with during primary surgery (e.g. biparietal widening in trigonocephaly that is not corrected with a fronto-orbital advancement).

More and more treatment centres, however, are shifting towards the use of minimally invasive techniques such as EACS. Because of the much better safety profile, these techniques can be performed in very young infants and are typically performed around the age of 3–5 months [24].

In endoscopically assisted suturectomy followed by helmet therapy, the goal is to shorten the time between sutural closure and re-opening, reducing the development of progressive cranial deformity. The helmet moulding therapy then guides the multidirectional driving force of the expanding cranial mass, without being constrictive, towards the region that was previously restricted in order to compensate for the inability to surgically reconstruct the already existing deformity at the time of surgery.

When comparing our postoperative stereophotogrammetry data of trigonocephaly patients treated with endoscopically assisted suturectomy followed by helmet therapy to the normative data of Meulstee et al., we see a remarkable shift towards a normal growth pattern, as depicted in Fig. 5.7 [12, 25].

Directly after surgery, the growth pattern between 0 and 6 months is quite distinct from the early growth pattern in normal infants (3–6 months), but the growth pattern at 6–12 months post-surgery is very similar to the normal growth pattern of infants age 6–9 months! [25].

To summarize, the fast-expanding brain is the motor of the fast-growing skull, especially in the first 6 months of life. If this normal growth is limited by the premature closure of a suture, we believe it is paramount to lift this growth restriction as soon as possible to restore the normal growth potential and avoid progressive deformation of the skull. Treatment before the age of 6 months should be the goal and is only possible if there are no diagnostic delays. Therefore, it is crucial that every patient in which the diagnosis of craniosynostosis is suspected is instantly referred to a craniofacial unit for further diagnosis and treatment.

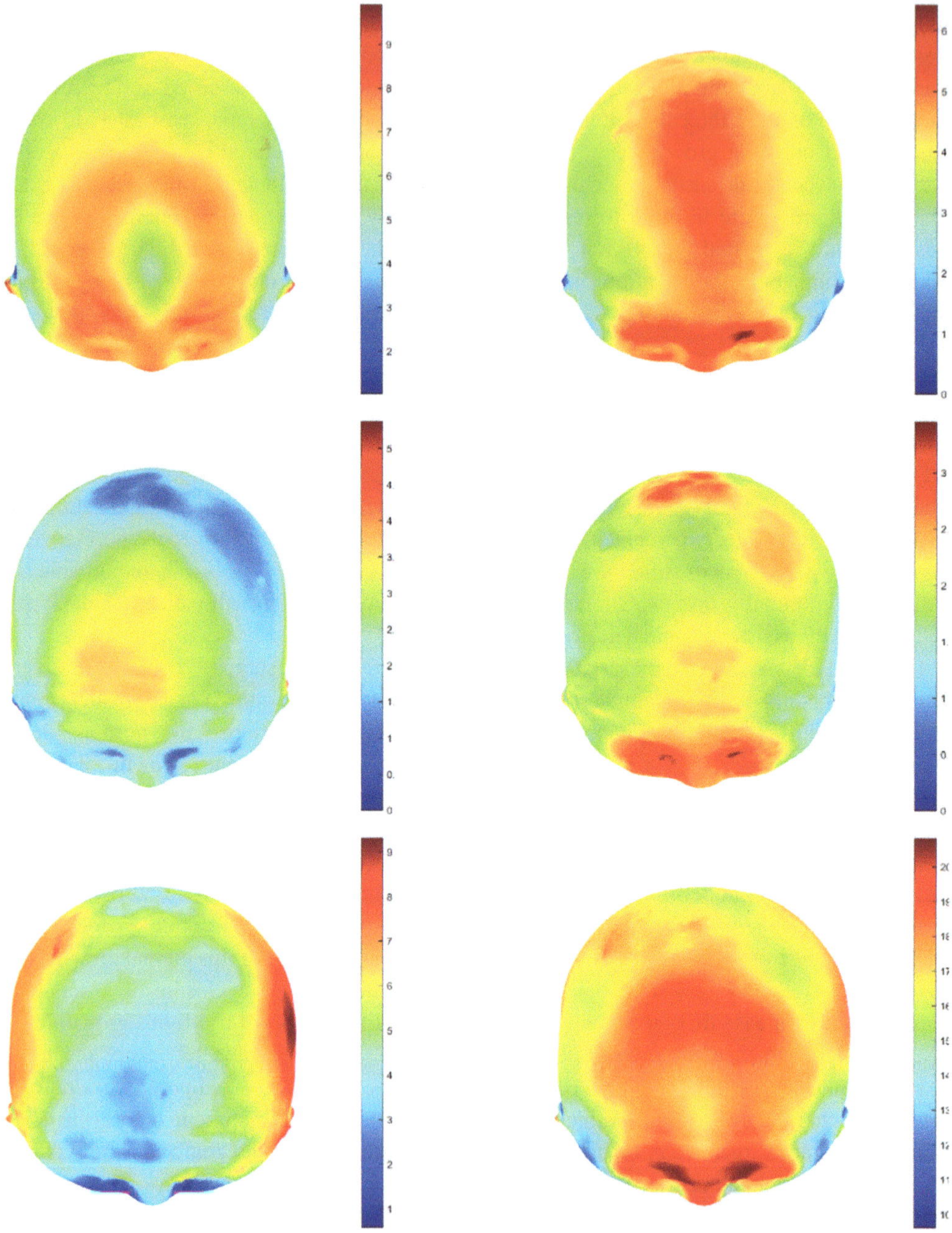

Fig. 5.7 Mean head shapes with heatmaps of the absolute head growth in mm for the trigonocephaly group (please note the different colour scales). Top-left: Pre-surgery to 6 months post-surgery. Top-right: 6–12 months post-surgery. Middle-left: 12–18 months post-surgery. Middle-right: 18–24 months post-surgery. Bottom-left: 24 months post-surgery to 36–48 moths post-surgery. Bottom-right: Pre-surgery to 36–48 months post-surgery. (Reproduced with permission of Elsevier [25])

References

1. Sperber GH, Sperber SM. Craniofacial embryogenetics and development, third edition. Br Dent J. 2019;227(9):773.
2. Dos Santos Silva A, Cardim VLN. Craniofacial developmental concepts in dynamic osteotomies and the nautilus technique: a procedure created in Brazil for the treatment of craniosynostosis. Anat Rec (Hoboken). 2021;304:1202.
3. Manlove AE, Romeo G, Venugopalan SR. Craniofacial growth: current theories and influence on management. Oral Maxillofac Surg Clin North Am. 2020;32(2):167–75.
4. Delashaw JB, Persing JA, Broaddus WC, Jane JA. Cranial vault growth in craniosynostosis. J Neurosurg. 1989;70(2):159–65.
5. Moss ML, Young RW. A functional approach to craniology. Am J Phys Anthropol. 1960;18(4):281–92.
6. Richtsmeier JT, Flaherty K. Hand in glove: brain and skull in development and dysmorphogenesis. Acta Neuropathol. 2013;125(4):469–89.
7. Twigg SR, Wilkie AO. A genetic-pathophysiological framework for craniosynostosis. Am J Hum Genet. 2015;97(3):359–77.
8. Farkas LG, Posnick JC, Hreczko TM. Anthropometric growth study of the head. Cleft Palate Craniofac J. 1992;29(4):303–8.
9. Holland D, Chang L, Ernst TM, Curran M, Buchthal SD, Alicata D, et al. Structural growth trajectories and rates of change in the first 3 months of infant brain development. JAMA Neurol. 2014;71(10):1266–74.
10. Hüppi PS, Warfield S, Kikinis R, Barnes PD, Zientara GP, Jolesz FA, et al. Quantitative magnetic resonance imaging of brain development in premature and mature newborns. Ann Neurol. 1998;43(2):224–35.
11. Knickmeyer RC, Gouttard S, Kang C, Evans D, Wilber K, Smith JK, et al. A structural MRI study of human brain development from birth to 2 years. J Neurosci. 2008;28(47):12176–82.
12. Meulstee JW, de Jong GA, Borstlap WA, Koerts G, Maal TJ, Delye H. The normal evolution of the cranium in three dimensions. Int J Oral Maxillofac Surg. 2020;49(6):739–49.
13. Pfefferbaum A, Mathalon DH, Sullivan EV, Rawles JM, Zipursky RB, Lim KO. A quantitative magnetic resonance imaging study of changes in brain morphology from infancy to late adulthood. Arch Neurol. 1994;51(9):874–87.
14. Porras AR, Liyun T, Tsering D, Mantilla E, Oh A, Enquobahrie A, et al. Quantification of head shape from three-dimensional photography for pre-and post-surgical evaluation of craniosynostosis. Plast Reconstr Surg. 2019;144(6):1051e.
15. Matsuzawa J, Matsui M, Konishi T, Noguchi K, Gur RC, Bilker W, et al. Age-related volumetric changes of brain gray and white matter in healthy infants and children. Cereb Cortex. 2001;11(4):335–42.
16. Lyall AE, Shi F, Geng X, Woolson S, Li G, Wang L, et al. Dynamic development of regional cortical thickness and surface area in early childhood. Cereb Cortex. 2015;25(8):2204–12.
17. Gilmore JH, Knickmeyer RC, Gao W. Imaging structural and functional brain development in early childhood. Nat Rev Neurosci. 2018;19(3):123–37.
18. Delye H, Clijmans T, Mommaerts MY, Sloten JV, Goffin J. Creating a normative database of age-specific 3D geometrical data, bone density, and bone thickness of the developing skull: a pilot study. J Neurosurg Pediatr. 2015;16(6):687–702.
19. Kuwahara K, Hikosaka M, Takamatsu A, Miyazaki O, Nosaka S, Ogawa R, et al. Average models and 3-dimensional growth patterns of the healthy infant cranium. Plast Reconstr Surg Glob Open. 2020;8(8):e3032.
20. Marcus JR, Domeshek LF, Loyd AM, Schoenleber JM, Das RR, Nightingale RW, et al. Use of a three-dimensional, normative database of pediatric craniofacial morphology for modern anthropometric analysis. Plast Reconstr Surg. 2009;124(6):2076–84.
21. Meyer-Marcotty P, Kunz F, Schweitzer T, Wachter B, Böhm H, Waßmuth N, et al. Cranial growth in infants—A longitudinal three-dimensional analysis of the first months of life. J Craniofac Surg. 2018;46(6):987–93.
22. Meyer-Marcotty P, Böhm H, Linz C, Kochel J, Stellzig Eisenhauer A, Schweitzer T. Three-dimensional analysis of cranial growth from 6 to 12 months of age. Eur J Orthod. 2014;36(5):489–96.
23. Delye H, Borstlap W, Van Lindert E. Endoscopy-assisted craniosynostosis surgery followed by helmet therapy. Surg Neurol Int. 2018;9:59.
24. Arts S, Delye H, van Lindert EJ. Intraoperative and postoperative complications in the surgical treatment of craniosynostosis: minimally invasive versus open surgical procedures. J Neurosurg Pediatr. 2017;21(2):112–8.
25. de Jong G, Tolhuisen M, Meulstee J, van der Heijden F, van Lindert E, Borstlap W, et al. Radiation-free 3D head shape and volume evaluation after endoscopically assisted strip craniectomy followed by helmet therapy for trigonocephaly. J Craniofac Surg. 2017;45(5):661–71.

Part II

Clinical Aspects and Management Principles

Clinical Diagnosis of Craniosynostosis: What Is Important for the Surgeon

6

Federico Di Rocco, Alexandru Szathmari, Pierre-Aurélien Beuriat, and Matthieu Vinchon

6.1 Introduction

When the neurosurgeon is faced with a cranial deformity, a reliable diagnosis on the ground of the clinical features is possible in the great majority of cases based on the specific morphological features the skull develops in case of premature fusion of one or more sutures. However, the clinician should keep in mind that there are some limitations in the clinical diagnosis as different nosographic entities can share similar abnormal features in early life which then can evolve successively with specific features that characterise distinct syndromes. This is the case for example in Crouzon syndrome due to the asynchronous closure of the sutures starting with the fusion of the sagittal suture that may lead to an early clinical scaphocephaly and progressing later on with the fusion of the remaining sutures resulting in oxycephaly and specific facial phenotype. The diagnosis can also be unclear in some newborns presenting with cranial moulding secondary to a prolonged abnormal position of the foetus in the intrauterine life, or after a difficult delivery where the skull deformation can be induced by instrumental manoeuvres. Patent sutures are mobile at birth and during the first weeks of life, giving the possibility to mobilise calvarial bones manually for differential diagnosis. However, in most cases, this type of mechanical skull deformation tends to resolve spontaneously in the first weeks of life (Fig. 6.1). Finally, the clinical diagnosis can remain doubtful in case of partial fusion of a suture as the resulting deformation might be mild or atypical so requiring further radiological or echographic exploration.

F. Di Rocco (✉) · A. Szathmari · P-A Beuriat · M. Vinchon
Department of Pediatric Neurosurgery, French Referral Center for Craniosynostosis of Lyon ERN Cranio, INSERM 1033, Hôpital Femme Mère Enfant, Université de Lyon, Lyon, France
e-mail: federico.dirocco@chu-lyon.fr; alexandru.szathmari@chu-lyon.fr; pierre-aurelien.beuriat@chu-lyon.fr; matthieu.vinchon@chu-lyon.fr

F. Di Rocco, J. Kestle (eds.), *Neurosurgical Aspects of Craniosynostosis*,
https://doi.org/10.1007/978-3-031-69386-1_6

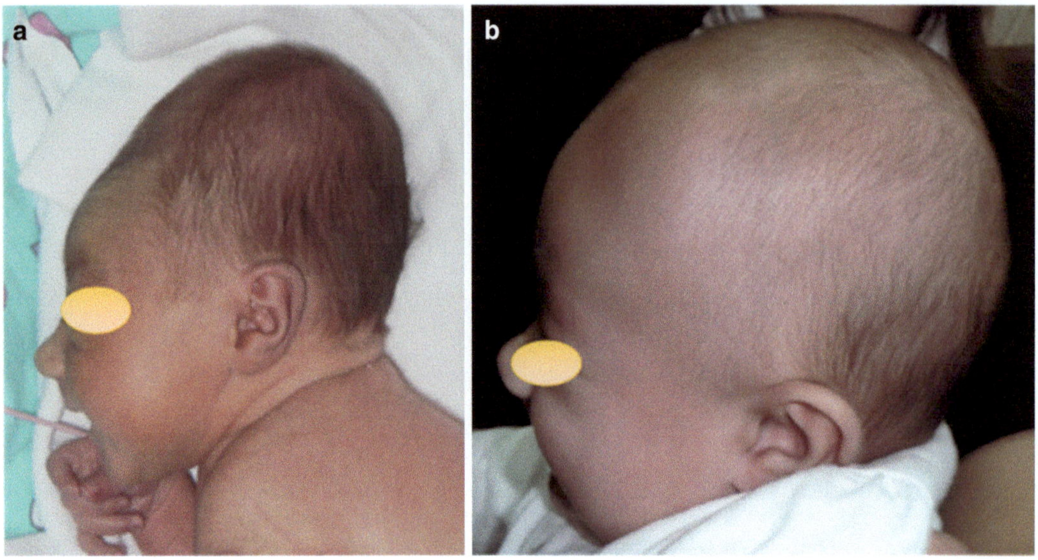

Fig. 6.1 Cranial molding with the head at birth (**a**), when the child was referred for suspicion of scaphocephaly, rapidly dismissed on account of a mobile sagittal suture and the lack of parietal narrowing, frontal bossing, occipital bullet and temporal narrowing. The deformation corrected spontaneously in less than a month (**b**)

6.2 Diagnostic Features

6.2.1 Clinical Diagnosis of the Synostosis

In most of the cases of craniosynostosis, the diagnosis is made at first glance by evaluating the phenotypic appearance of the head and possible associated malformations, for example, finger and toes or external ear. The early fused suture is often seen to bulge under the scalp or the frontal skin.

Firstly, anamnestic information should be collected, namely the family history and family tree (familial cases, pregnancy, delivery modalities, mother's drugs and father's age). In some cases, one of the parents may have a mild form of the same craniosynostosis as their child, and be unaware of it. The neurosurgeon should inquire about the growth pattern of the child's head (rate of increase of its perimeter) and then evaluate its proportions (horizontal, transverse and vertical diameters, symmetry and head circumference) as well as the shape and position of the forehead (bulging, high and flat, retroverted, etc.), the occiput (bossing, flattening and abnormal increased vertical diameter) and the temporal regions (protruding and flattened). Also, the preferred craniocervical posture can provide important information.

The face should also be assessed (symmetry, exorbitism, midface retrusion, mandible malocclusion, etc.).

The different suture-related skull deformities associated with the most common forms of craniosynostosis have been described extensively and are well known to the paediatrician, the neurosurgeon and the craniofacial surgeons. We will review here briefly the key features of the various types of craniosynostosis that are described in dedicated chapters of this book extensively.

6.2.1.1 Scaphocephaly

The premature fusion of the sagittal suture results in an elongation of the skull and its reduction in width. The skull has a boat-shaped deformation with an increase in the antero-posterior diameter and a reduced bi-parietal diameter. The ratio between these two dimensions, the cranial index (CI), is decreased, whereas the head circumference is compensatory increased. The forehead and the posterior aspect of the skull may be very prominent. The parietal prominences are often absent. The vertex of the skull is lowered. A median ridge corresponding to the fused suture can be apparent in the typical scaphocephaly. The anterior and posterior fontanels are reduced in size or even absent. However, the anterior fontanel may remain open in some subjects, or be even larger than normal and tense in cases of an associated intracranial hypertension. This finding as well as incipient ocular bulging are hints of a possible Crouzon's syndrome.

The degree of head deformation is extremely variable and sometimes limited to the parieto-occipital aspect of the skull sparing the forehead. The orbital region is usually within normal limits as are the maxilla and mandible. However, subtle changes might be present when some measurements are taken [1]. The cranial index can sometimes be deceptively normal because of compensatory bulging of the temporal squama, making the CI a poorly accurate criterion in the clinical diagnosis of scaphocephaly (Fig. 6.2).

Incomplete fusion of the sagittal suture may result in limited morphological modifications of the calvaria, which can escape the correct recognition or delay the clinical diagnosis until restricted cranial volume becomes apparent at adolescence, on account of tonsillar herniation or "pseudo-pseudotumour".

6.2.1.2 Trigonocephaly

The presence of a crest of bone along the metopic suture should be differentiated from true metopic craniosynostosis as it does not interfere with the volume of the skull, does not induce malformations of the neighbouring structures and tends to

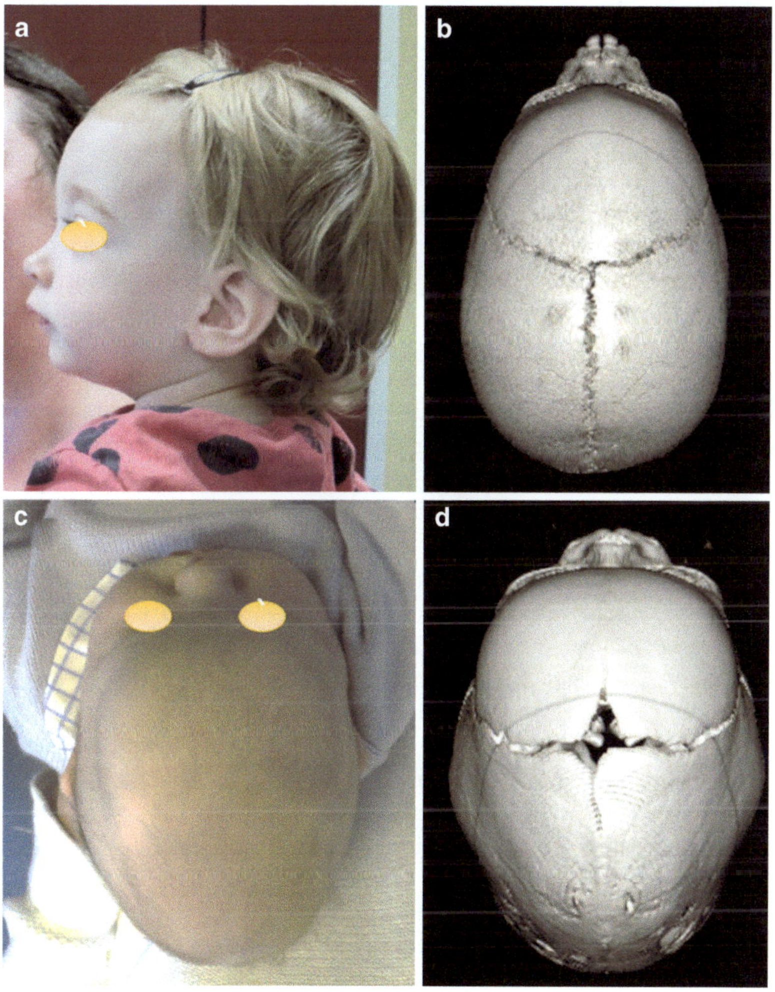

Fig. 6.2 Cranial index (CI) in non-synostotic dolichocephaly (**a, b**) and in authentic sagittal synostosis (**c, d**); the CI is an highly imperfect criterion for the diagnosis

resolve in time spontaneously. The hallmark of true trigonocephaly is the keel-like prominence of the forehead associated with flattened and retruded supraorbital ridges often resulting in exorbitism. Viewed from above, the forehead is small and triangular in shape, whereas in the frontal view hypotelorism is a typical feature. In some infants, the latter is masked by the frequently associated epicanthal fold, which may give a false aspect of hypertelorism. A compensatory widening of the temporal regions may be present too.

6.2.1.3 Frontal Plagiocephaly

Unilateral premature fusion of the coronal suture results in a marked asymmetry of the skull vault and base because of the reduced development of the hemicranium on the side of the fused hemicoronal suture. There is a depression in the supraorbital region on the affected side that may be associated with an actual or only relative protrusion of the contralateral side, which is especially apparent when the metopic suture remains patent. Because of the associated homolateral deviation of the vomer bone, the cranium appears scoliotic when seen from above. The homolateral deviation of the vomer bone shows different degrees of severity from patient to patient from mild to severe and determines the severity of the cranial base asymmetry together with the changes of the sphenoidal wings and the anterior displacement of the nasal bones. Clinically, the changes of the sphenoid account for the increased vertical diameter and flattening of the orbit, which may result in the characteristic "harlequin's eye", with a recessed orbital rim and a relatively bulging globe. The anterior displacement of the pyramidal bone as compared to the contralateral side translates into an anterior displacement of the ear on the side of the affected suture. While the bridge of the nose may be attracted towards the affected suture, the nasal tip is deviated with a variable degree of severity contralaterally. The mandibular bone is also asymmetrical, its branch being shorter on the affected side, while the chin is usually deviated contralaterally, although a significant functional mandibular malocclusion is rare.

Most of the infants and toddlers present with torticollis and a particular type of squint, due to the higher position of the *caruncola*. This torticollis is typically corrected by occlusion of one eye. Older children often develop an obvious cervico-facial scoliosis and torticollis on account of the abnormal posture secondary caused by orbital dystopia and the crossed asymmetry of the cranio-vertebral junction, the occipital *condyle being* smaller and the lateral mass of the first cranial vertebra larger on the affected side.

The rare fronto-shenoidal variant of synostotic anterior plagiocephaly shows typical features, with a lowered orbit on the synostotic side, while the chin is deviated towards the synostotic side, contrary to the classical anterior plagiocephaly caused by unicoronal synostosis (Fig. 6.3).

6.2.1.4 Lambdoid

Similar to hemicoronal synostosis, uni lambdoid synostosis causes an asymmetry of the hemicranium which is hypoplasic on the affected side, especially because of the restricted growth of the posterior cranial vault. The ear on the affected side is drawn backward and downward compared to the contralateral side. Viewed from above the skull has a trapezoid shape, different from the parallelogram resulting from the posterior positional deformation with patent sutures.

In some cases, the deformation of the skull and face can be influenced by the additional closure of other sutures.

6.2.1.5 Brachycephaly

In children with coronal synostosis, the antero-posterior diameter of the head is reduced while the transverse diameter is increased. The forehead is wide, high and flattened in its lower segment with a retrusion of the supraorbital bar, and bulging in its superior aspect with upper frontal bossing. Hypertelorism can also be present. In some cases, the posterior aspect of the skull might be also flattened resulting in a turricephaly (Fig. 6.4).

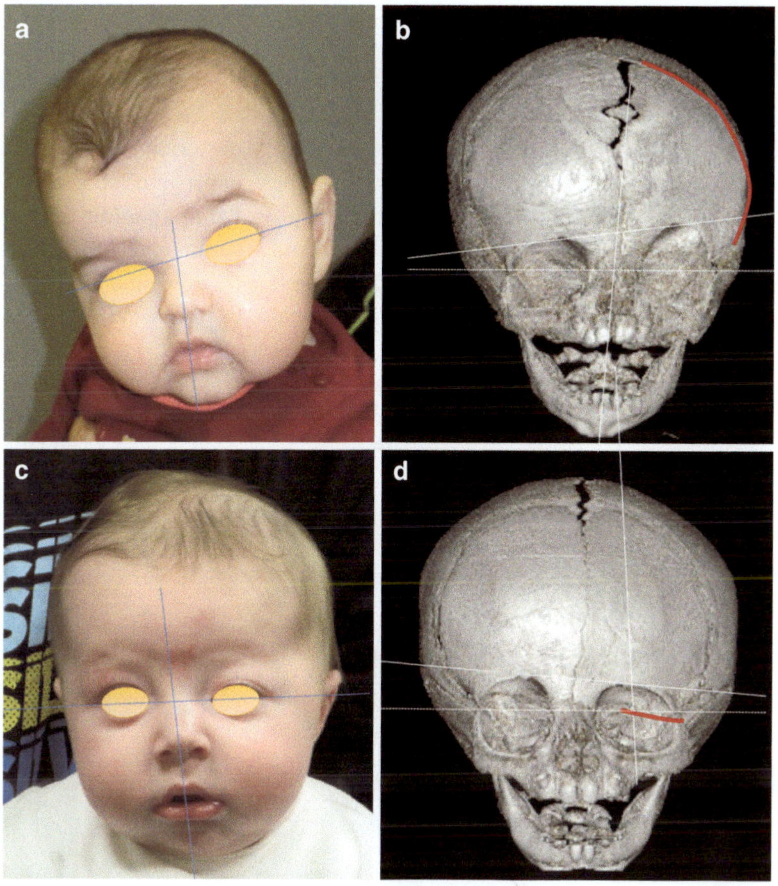

Fig. 6.3 Plagiocephaly: facial features and CT-scanner in typical anterior plagiocephaly caused by unicoronal synostosis (**a**, **b**), and the rare variant fronto-sphenoidal synostosis (**c**, **d**); note the inverted facial features, the orbit being displaced upward (**a**) versus downward (**c**), and the chin deviated toward the non-synostotic side (**a**) versus the synostotic side (**c**)

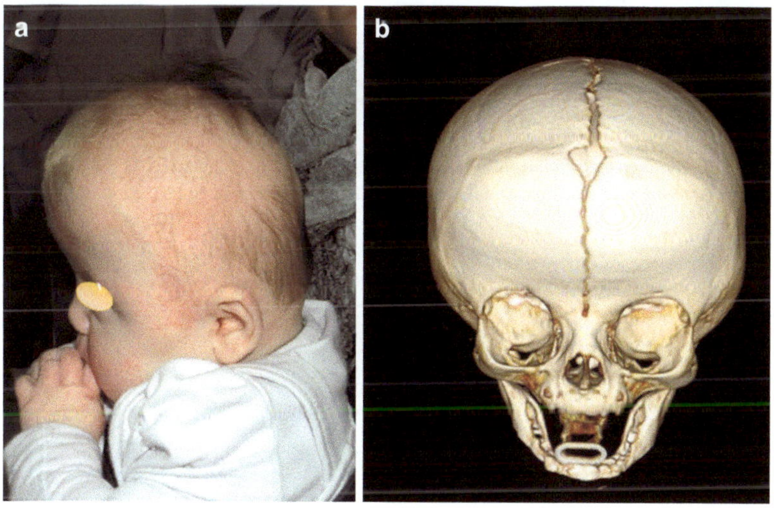

Fig. 6.4 Typical turricephalic appearance of bicoronal synostosis (**a**), with correlated CT scanner showing closed coronal sutures, and persistent metopic suture accounting for the widened and flattened forehead (**b**)

6.2.1.6 Bilambdoid and Sagittal ("Mercedes" type)

In the case of fusion of the sagittal and both lambdoid sutures, the skull is usually short and narrow posteriorly resulting in the so-called "coup de serpe" ("sickle cut"). The skull can be flattened or even introverted in the central occipital region at the confluence of the fused lambdoid and sagittal sutures (Figs. 6.5 and 6.6). The frontal region is usually enlarged and the coronal sutures are displaced posteriorly. It is important to note that in some cases the skull might be dolichocephalic [2].

6.2.1.7 Oxycephaly

In multiple synostoses diagnosed later in infancy and in childhood, the deformation is characterised by a high and steep forehead with a depression above the supraorbital bar. A protrusion of the bregmatic region is often present and gives the head a typical pointed shape. The anteroposterior diameter is reduced. The nasofrontal angle is often extremely obtuse. In some cases, the morphology remains harmonious because all sutures are fused, but the intracranial volume is reduced, and these missed cases can be diagnosed at the time of visual loss caused by optic atrophy.

6.2.1.8 Cloverleaf Skull

Also named Kleeblattschaedel or *crâne en trèfle*, it describes a very early manifestation of multiple-suture synostosis resulting in severe intracranial hypertension. Because all the main sutures are

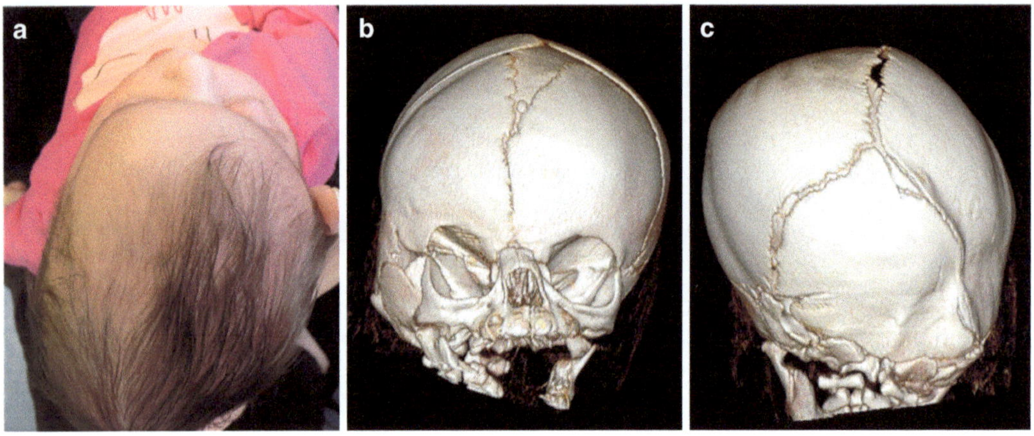

Fig. 6.5 Synostosis of the right coronal and lambdoid sutures cause by FGFR3 P250 familial mutation. (**a**) View from above, note the marked trapezoidal shape, markedly different from positional deformations

Fig. 6.6 Mercedes type synostosis (lambda region synostosis)

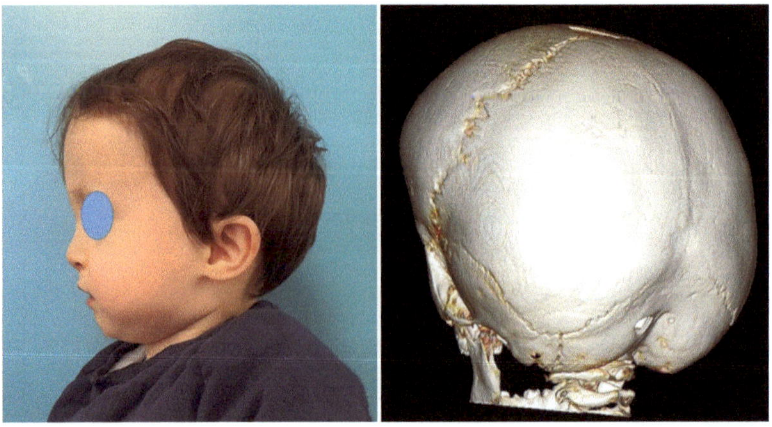

fused, brain growth causes bulging of the bregmatic and pterional fontanels, resulting in the typical three-lobed craniofacial aspect. It is associated with dilated scalp veins, hypotelorism and exorbitism, and a reduced head circumference.

Having made the positive diagnosis of synostosis, the surgeon needs to carefully evaluate the clinical status of the child to search for symptoms and signs related to the restricted skull growth.

The presence of symptoms and signs of raised intracranial pressure (ICP) needs to be taken into account with great attention due to the risk of neurological deterioration. Although clinical signs of significantly increased intracranial pressure may be observed in multiple-suture synostosis already at a very early stage, in most cases they develop later on during the first year of age or even later. Stagnating calvarial growth may precede the clinical evidence of a rise in ICP in multiple-suture synostosis. Parents and children if old enough should be interrogated for chronic headaches. The frequency and time of the episodes of headache should also be noted.

Fundus oculi examination may disclose papilledema and mandate a complete ophthalmological examination.

In the same way, symptoms and signs compatible with a descent of cerebellar tonsils in syndromic synostosis, and more rarely, in sagittal synostosis, as well as breathing difficulties or hearing issues should prompt a specific ENT examination.

6.2.2 Importance of Evaluating the Anomalies of the Middle and Lower Face

After examining the skull, it is essential to examine the face in search of signs of faciostenosis. Indeed, the prognosis will be drastically different in the case of a faciocraniostenosis compared to a non-syndromic single-suture synostosis.

All the different types of craniosynostosis can be associated with a syndrome, where the face might be also affected. Thus, is it essential to examine the face in all types of synostosis. However, the face can also be totally normal in syndromic patients. This is especially the case in bicoronal synostosis, which is rarely non-syndromic.

The essential role of the face shape in establishing the diagnosis is highlighted by the antenatal diagnosis of the synostoses. Ultrasound examination allows the analysis of the forehead, orbits and face permitting a proper diagnosis of faciocranio-synostosis.

The orbits should be carefully examined. Indeed, a proptosis might be present as well as a hypertelorbitism both suggestive of a syndromic craniosynostosis. In case of severe proptosis, the complete ocular occlusion can be impaired, consequently, the integrity of the cornea should be verified. In most severe cases an early tarsorraphy might be needed. Ptosis of the eyelids, in most cases unilateral, more rarely bilateral, is evocative of a TWIST1 or TCF12-related synostosis, and may require specific treatment when the eyelid impinges on the pupil.

Similarly, anomalies of the ear's shape, namely the presence of a crux cymbae, may suggest the just mentioned mutations. In particular, a hammered and thickened aspect of the upper part of the helix is suggestive of TCF12 mutation [3, 4] (Fig. 6.7). Muenke's syndrome, related to the P250 mutation of FGFR3, which affected specifically the coronal sutures, also causes sensorineural and/or conductive hearing loss so that the hearing function should be grossly stimulated during the evaluation.

The aspect of the nose should be assessed. An enlarged bifid nose tip can be seen in craniofrontonasal dysplasias. A beaked nose is associated with syndromic faciosynostosis, such as Crouzon's syndrome. However, in infants, the nose may be apparently normal even in overt syndromic forms. Restricted upper airways can manifest with mouth breathing. The family should be questioned about the nocturnal sleep of their infant, with regard in particular to the occurrence of obstructive sleep apnoeas, poor feeding and recurrent otitis media caused by the constriction of the Eustachian tube.

A maxillary retrusion with an arched palate and an associated malocclusion are highly suggestive of a syndromic form. A palatal cleft can

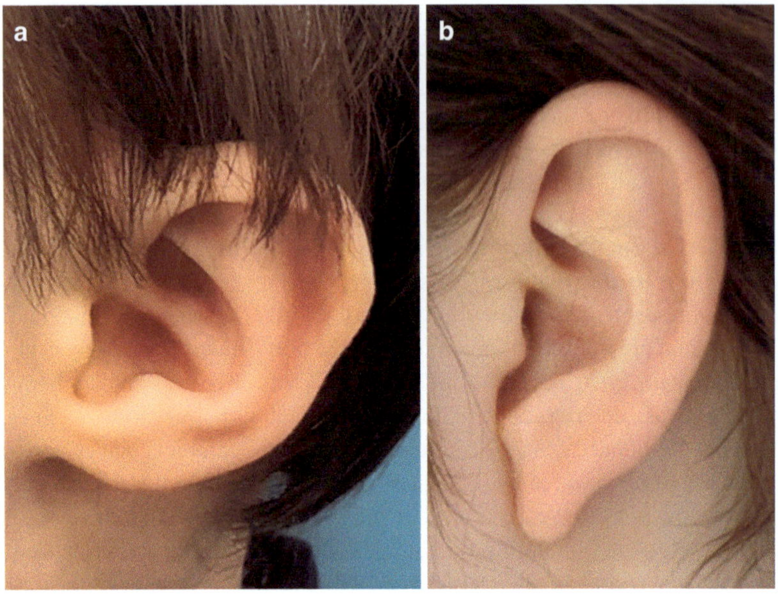

Fig. 6.7 Malformations of the conch; (**a**) typical crux cymbae, characteristic of Twist mutation; (**b**) battered and thickened upper of the upper part of the helix, characteristic of TCF12 mutation

be present and may help compensate for nasal breathing in case of nasopharyngeal constriction. Hypomaxillia can be present at birth, and even be evident on prenatal imaging, but it can also develop later in life, on account of its different growth rate with the calvaria and mandibula.

The mouth shape, the palatal arch and the philtrum length should be checked (a thin mouth and shallow philtrum being features of foetal Valproate syndrome associated with metopic synostosis). The mandible, palate and teeth eruption should also be verified. Delayed dental eruption and dental anomalies, in general, might be an early sign of a bone metabolic anomaly [5]. Buccal hygiene should be checked and encouraged in faciosynostoses because orthodontic treatments, which will be the first step before orthognathic surgery, cannot proceed with poorly maintained teeth.

6.2.3 Importance of Extracranial Features

The examination of the child should not be limited to the head. Indeed, some anomalies in the extremities might be present in children with synostosis and might be an indication of the presence of an underlying syndrome.

Hands and feet should be examined for syndactyly, in the form of paddle-shaped extremities, or a subtle membranous syndactyly. The shape of the fingers and toes should be also carefully assessed for brachydactyly, clinodactyly or abnormal thumbs or big toes. The presence of a palmar crease should also be taken into account as an indicator of possible underlying syndromes.

In case of deformation of the hands and feet in Apert syndrome, the family should be instructed on the necessity of early specific management. Similarly, in some genetic syndromes involving midline craniosynostosis, especially trigonocephaly (smad6-related trigonocephaly for instance), the opportunity of a cardiac evaluation should be suggested because of the possible associated cardiac malformations.

6.3 Limits of the Clinical Diagnosis

The clinical diagnosis of the synostosis is usually based on the phenotypic appearance. However, the improvement of neuroimaging investigations and the availability of echoencephalography as well molecular analyses may overcome the limits of mere clinical observation contributing to the correct diagnosis, especially in doubtful cases. In fact, especially in the neonatal period some syndromes cannot be diagnosed with certainty as their typical phenotypic appearance will develop only later, such as in Crouzon syndrome in which some sutures fuse and the facial anomalies become obvious only in a late phase of the clinical course. Also, the closure of the sagittal synostosis, which characterises some metabolic forms of craniosynostosis [6, 7], occurs in a late phase without affecting significantly the shape of the head. In all these cases, and more broadly whenever the diagnosis remains doubtful, the clinical evaluation should be coupled with laboratory investigations, namely genetic and metabolic tests and neuroimaging studies when necessary.

Ultrasound examination may confirm or rule out the closure of the sagittal suture in the case of a newborn with a dolichocephalic skull without the necessity of irradiating the child. The exam could also detect an associated ventricular enlargement. Ultrasounds, computed tomography scanners (TDM) or magnetic resonance imaging (MRI) is widely used in order to assess abnormally enlarged or compressed cerebrospinal fluid (CSF) spaces, the presence of bony spiculae or craniolacuniae, cerebral abnormalities, namely cerebellar tonsillar herniation, that can be associated in particular with syndromic synostosis but might also be present in single suture synostosis, and also study the cerebral circulation, in particular the venous drainage.

6.4 Importance of Follow-Up

6.4.1 Evolution in Time

The evaluation of a child with craniosynostosis and to a certain extent the diagnosis-making process are somehow a dynamic process as the disease and its clinical features evolve over time. This concept is established for specific syndromes but is not yet fully understood for all forms of craniosynostosis. Typically, the synostosis is progressive in Crouzon syndrome, where the sutures fuse also in a late phase of development, as well as in TWIST1-related synostosis that can also progress and has the potential risk of developing a pansynostosis, affecting sutures that were patent at birth. Metabolic synostoses also have a chronic evolution and develop in children despite a previously normal skull. Consequently, prolonged follow-up is necessary, even in subjects who have been operated on. Such control should not be limited to the evolution of the cranial sutures but should involve other organs of the body and cognitive development.

Delayed teeth eruption might for instance suggest a metabolic disorder that might become overt only after the surgery. Some other features related to bone metabolism need also to be checked during the follow-up of children with craniosynostosis, in particular the possibility of late long bone anomalies. Leg bowing in toddlers are potential sign of abnormal phosphocalcic metabolism as in vitamin-resistant rickets that can be associated with metabolic craniosynostosis and treated prior to the associated bone alterations leading to the correct but delayed recognition of the syndrome.

Melanodermia, a hallmark of FGFR3-related Crouzon syndrome, will become evident with time (Fig. 6.8). The parents and the child should be informed of such an evolution.

Indeed, missing an underlying syndrome bears the potential risk of inappropriate management as well as incomplete understanding by the parents of its consequences [5].

Also, some anomalies of the brain may develop in a late phase of the disease; the most known of these is the progressive descent of the cerebellar tonsils, absent at birth in Crouzon's syndrome or in some metabolic craniosynostoses. The phenomenon is progressive and may remain ignored until causing neurological dysfunction or syringomyelia. Thus, closer follow-up controls, coupling clinical examination and MRI investigations until the end of statural growth are mandatory in most syndromic cases. The early genetic confirmation of an underlying mutation might also allow anticipating the potential evolution: for instance, the risk of future closure of other sutures (high in some syndromic

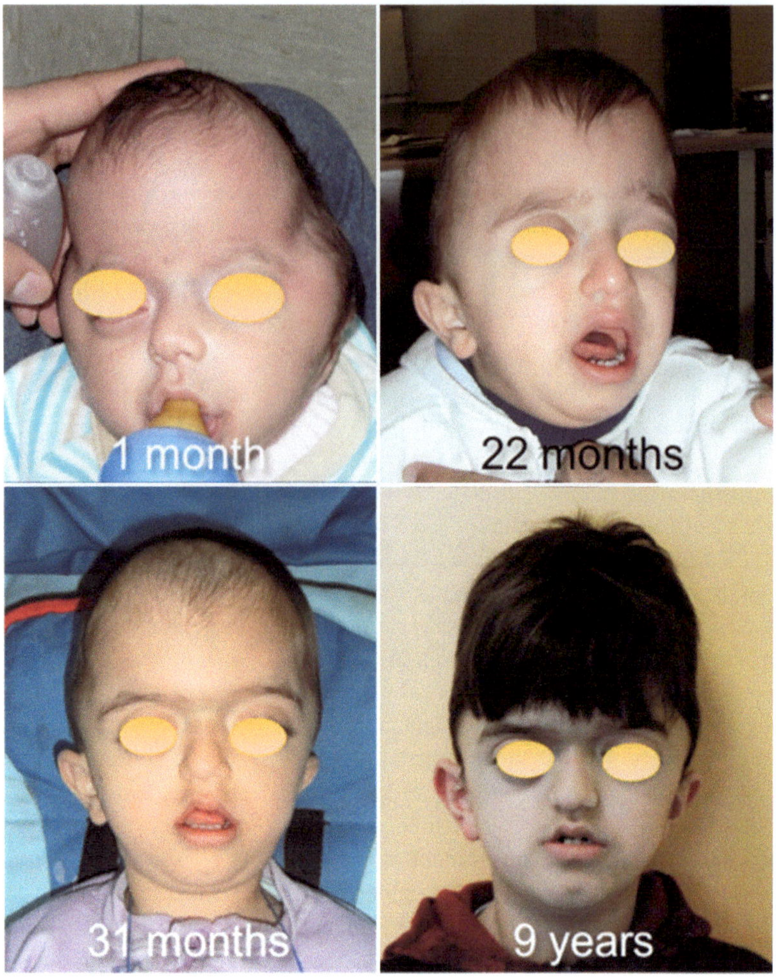

Fig. 6.8 Melanodermia caused by acanthosis nigricans, associated with FGFR3-related Crouzon syndrome

FGFR2-related syndromes) or the risk of postoperative recurrence of the synostosis (high in Twist1 mutation).

Cognitive development might also be hindered either by the synostosis itself or by an associated underlying condition. The incidence of cognitive delay is relatively known for some syndromic synostosis, e.g. Apert's syndrome but it is still unclear for many types of craniosynostoses, the single suture craniosynostoses being included. Cognitive impairment and learning difficulties are often diagnosed when the child enters school. Consequently, specific management (ergotherapy, speech therapy, etc.) and school adaptations are adopted in several cases relatively late, especially if the early post-operative controls do not address cognition appropriately, starting already in the first years of life.

The recognition of neurodevelopmental impairment in an apparently isolated single suture synostosis should prompt a thorough genetic evaluation for an underlying genetic condition. Indeed, some gene mutations are nowadays known to be associated with cognitive impairment and synostosis (e.g. SMAD6).

6.4.2 Interest of Clinical Classification Coupled with Genetic Analysis

As mentioned earlier, the proper diagnosis and classification of the synostosis are of paramount importance for the individual patient, in order to assess and tailor his individual management, and also to analyse clinical series and long-term results. The lack of specific investigations in most of the past series makes them relatively useless for understanding the role of surgical treatment in avoiding the secondary effects of the disease.

Even today different nomenclatures and classifications of craniosynostosis are still based essentially on the type of fused suture and the type of deformation, consequently limiting the meaning of clinical reports in terms of neurological and cognitive development. Indeed, underlying genetic mutations that may participate significantly in the functional outcome independently from the synostotic aspects and their surgical management are investigated in only a minority of cases [8, 9].

The ideal classification should merge the clinical and anatomical description, which is necessary for management purposes, to the potential underlying genetic mutation that may impact the patient's development. Outcome studies of genetically defined cohorts are necessary to help foresee the outcome of operation on children with craniosynostosis and predict their future cognitive development.

Unfortunately, currently, the genetic workup frequently identifies new gene variants of unknown significance or incomplete penetrance [10].

In its present state, this new knowledge does not allow us to establish any reliable prognosis. In the future, a better definition of the associated phenotypes could help to validate the clinical significance of these new variants.

References

1. Nicolini F, Arnaud E, Usami K, Vecchione A, Brunelle F, Di Rocco F. Impact of extra-axial cerebrospinal fluid collection in frontal morphology after surgical treatment of scaphocephaly. Surg Neurol Int. 2018;9:215. https://doi.org/10.4103/sni.sni_13_18. Erratum in: Surg Neurol Int 2019 Feb 13;10:20. Rocco, Federico Di [corrected to Di Rocco, Federico]. PMID: 30505617; PMCID: PMC6219275.
2. Chivoret N, Arnaud E, Giraudat K, O'Brien F, Pamphile L, Meyer P, Renier D, Collet C, Di Rocco F. Bilambdoid and sagittal synostosis: report of 39 cases. Surg Neurol Int. 2018;9:206. https://doi.org/10.4103/sni.sni_454_17. PMID: 30386676; PMCID: PMC6194734.
3. Lacroix G, Karnoub MA, Vinchon M, Wolber A, Martinot V, Guerreschi P. Auricles anomalies in patients with a TCF12 gene mutation. J Craniofac Surg. 2023;34(1):302–5. https://doi.org/10.1097/SCS.0000000000008938. Epub 2022 Aug 22. PMID: 35994750.
4. Di Rocco F, Baujat G, Arnaud E, Rénier D, Laplanche JL, Daire VC, Collet C. Clinical spectrum and outcomes in families with coronal synostosis and TCF12 mutations. Eur J Hum Genet. 2014;22(12):1413–6. https://doi.org/10.1038/ejhg.2014.57. Epub 2014 Apr 16. PMID: 24736737; PMCID: PMC4231413.
5. Quinaux T, Custodi V, Putoux A, Bacchetta J, Rossi M, Di Rocco F. Sensenbrenner syndrome: a further challenge in evaluating sagittal synostosis and a need for a multidisciplinary approach. Childs Nerv Syst. 2021;37(5):1695–701. https://doi.org/10.1007/s00381-021-05075-1. Epub 2021 Feb 19. PMID: 33606107.
6. Di Rocco F, Rothenbuhler A, Cormier Daire V, Bacchetta J, Adamsbaum C, Baujat G, Rossi M, Lingart A. Craniosynostosis and metabolic bone disorder. A review. Neurochirurgie. 2019;65(5):258–63. https://doi.org/10.1016/j.neuchi.2019.09.008. Epub 2019 Sep 25. PMID: 31562881.
7. Rothenbuhler A, Fadel N, Debza Y, Bacchetta J, Diallo MT, Adamsbaum C, Linglart A, Di Rocco F. High incidence of cranial synostosis and chiari I malformation in children with X-linked hypophosphatemic rickets (XLHR). J Bone Miner Res. 2019;34(3):490–6. https://doi.org/10.1002/jbmr.3614. Epub 2018 Nov 20. PMID: 30352126; PMCID: PMC7816089.
8. Cornille M, Moriceau S, Khonsari RH, Heuzé Y, Loisay L, Boitez V, Morice A, Arnaud E, Collet C, Bensidhoum M, Kaci N, Boddaert N, Paternoster G, Rauschendorfer T, Werner S, Mansour SL, Di Rocco F, Oury F, Legeai-Mallet L. FGFR3 overactivation in the brain is responsible for memory impairments in Crouzon syndrome mouse model. J Exp Med. 2022;219(4):e20201879. https://doi.org/10.1084/jem.20201879. Epub 2022 Mar 7. PMID: 35254402; PMCID: PMC8906494.
9. Raybaud C, Di Rocco C. Brain malformation in syndromic craniosynostoses, a primary disorder of white matter: a review. Childs Nerv Syst. 2007;23(12):1379–88. https://doi.org/10.1007/s00381-007-0474-7. Epub 2007 Sep 20. PMID: 17882438.
10. Di Rocco F, Rossi M, Verlut I, Szathmari A, Beuriat PA, Chatron N, Chauvel-Picard J, Mottolese C, Monin P, Vinchon M, Guernouche S, Collet C. Clinical interest of molecular study in cases of isolated midline craniosynostosis. Eur J Hum Genet. 2023;31(6):621–8. https://doi.org/10.1038/s41431-023-01295-y. Epub 2023 Feb 3. PMID: 36732661; PMCID: PMC10250395.

7 Sagittal Suture Synostosis: Key Points for Surgeons and Management Principles (Diagnosis, Surgical Considerations and Timing)

Michael M. McDowell, Ian F. Pollack, Michael R. Bykowski, and Jesse A. Goldstein

7.1 Introduction

Sagittal synostosis (SS) represents 40–60% of all surgically treated craniosynostosis diagnoses and has a prevalence of approximately 1 in 4000–5000 live births [1–5]. Non-syndromic SS affects male patients in approximately 75–80% of cases [6–9]. Sagittal synostosis is widely recognized by the scaphocephalic or synostotic dolichocephalic, cranial morphology, in which the premature closure of the sagittal suture results in the relative elongation of the cranium in the anterior-posterior direction. An underlying genetic syndrome is identified in less than 3% of cases [8]. The causal factor of sporadic cases is frequently unclear but may reflect a combination of genetic predisposition and metabolic and environmental factors.

M. M. McDowell · I. F. Pollack (✉)
Departments of Neurological Surgery, UPMC Children's Hospital of Pittsburgh, University of Pittsburgh School of Medicine, Pittsburgh, PA, USA
e-mail: mcdowellmm2@upmc.edu; ian.pollack@chp.edu

M. R. Bykowski · J. A. Goldstein
Plastic and Reconstructive Surgery, UPMC Children's Hospital of Pittsburgh, University of Pittsburgh School of Medicine, Pittsburgh, PA, USA
e-mail: michael.bykowski@chp.edu; jesse.goldstein@chp.edu

7.1.1 Embryology and Natural History

Craniosynostosis is a dysfunction specific to the membranous type of bone formation, a mechanism most associated with skull and other flat bone development [10]. The common mechanism purported for craniosynostosis is based on an imbalance of osteoblast and osteoclast function, in which excessive osteoblast function is not proportionately compensated for by osteoclastic activity. This results ultimately in premature fusion of one or more sutures. Under normal conditions, the sutures function as the growth centers of each bony plate of the neurocranium which is driven by underlying brain volume and pulsation [6, 11, 12]. Rarely, overdrainage in a neonate with a ventricular shunt may result in premature suture fusion due to a reduction in pressure exerted on the skull from the brain [13, 14]. This phenomenon, in addition to craniosynostosis from other reductions in brain volume or pressure such as peri-natal stroke, is known as secondary craniosynostosis [6]. Sagittal synostosis restricts skull growth along the midline between the fontanelles, resulting in relative overgrowth at other sutures, producing cranial deformity due to excess elongation of the skull relative to its width. Some authors have hypothesized an association between SS and dysfunction of language, speech,

F. Di Rocco, J. Kestle (eds.), *Neurosurgical Aspects of Craniosynostosis*,
https://doi.org/10.1007/978-3-031-69386-1_7

memory, and executive function due to a negative effect on the dorsolateral prefrontal cortex, but data to support this are sparse and typically not specific to SS [3, 15–17]. A direct correlation between intracranial pressure or the timing of surgery and neurocognitive outcomes remains controversial [18–20].

7.2 Diagnosis

The diagnosis of SS is typically made clinically based on the presence of scaphocephaly and often a palpably closed sagittal suture, ridging, or subtle depression between the fontanelles known as a saddle deformity or clinocephaly. During the first year of life, the deformity produced in severe cases is particularly noticeable in part due to the potential for low hair volume combined with the disproportionate size of the head relative to the infant's body [6]. It is our preference to obtain a low-dose volumetric CT scan with 3D post-processing imaging for surgical planning and long-term post-operative comparisons, although some sites will rely on clinical diagnosis alone [21, 22]. CT imaging helps to ensure the appropriate diagnosis of other suture fusions and rule out nonsynostotic scaphocephaly, and is typically of high enough resolution to identify major parenchymal abnormalities such as Chiari malformation which may be associated with craniosynostosis [18, 23]. Other commonly seen associated conditions with SS include extra-axial fluid collections (25%) and copper-beaten skull morphology (3%) [8]. Surgically relevant anatomic characteristics such as sagittal sinus or large emissary vein exposure through atypical bony defects may also be detected.

Despite the classic appearance of single suture synostoses, studies have shown that the presence of additional undiagnosed suture fusions can occur in 2–7% of cases overall [8]. In a study including 235 patients with a clinical diagnosis of SS and a pre-operative CT, Ravinda et al. found that patients with SS were the most likely to have additional suture involvement of all presumed single suture clinical diagnoses, with 8% of patients having one or more additional suture fusion. In addition, six patients with clinical diagnoses of SS were ultimately found to have a syndromic condition [8]. Magnetic resonance imaging is not routinely obtained in the absence of other clinical findings of concern.

7.3 Operative Decision-Making and Timing

Sagittal synostosis is broadly divided into "early presentation" and "late presentation" categories, with the former consisting of children with characteristic scaphocephalic head shapes at or shortly following birth and the latter consisting of children who initially have relatively normal head shapes that either become somewhat scaphocephalic with time or remain relatively normocephalic but are noted on imaging for headaches or after head injuries to have sagittal synostosis. For children who present with obvious scaphocephaly in infancy, the management focuses on deformity correction and in untreated cases, on the detection and treatment of increased intracranial pressure, whereas in those older children with sagittal synostosis in the setting of a relatively normal head shape, intervention centers on identifying and, if needed, treating elevated intracranial pressure.

For children with obvious deformities, early detection and referral of SS are critical to ensure the most versatile opportunity for individualized decision-making in order to take advantage of the doubling of brain volume in the first 6 months of life and again by 2 years of age. There are two main indications for surgical correction of SS: to improve appearance and to prevent or treat intracranial hypertension. Studies have shown a negative cosmetic perception of untreated synostosis from both clinicians and lay-persons [24]. Uncorrected SS may result in significant impairment in self-esteem and socialization. However, a subset of parents elect expectant management, based on their belief that the esthetic issue may stabilize later in life after the completion of head growth, thickening of the scalp, hair growth, and the reduction in head size relative to body size [6]. In such patients, the development of intracranial hypertension provides a more pressing indication for intervention at later time points. At a mean age of 1 year, one cohort of untreated patients with SS who underwent intracranial pressure monitoring were found to have developed intracranial hypertension (15 mmHg or greater) in 13.4% of cases overall; this phenomenon was observed in approximately 25% of patients older than 1 year [25]. Whether 15 mmHg is an appropriate threshold is a matter of some debate, but it is clear that a substantial portion of children do suffer significant intracranial pressure elevations well beyond the normal range that can have adverse visual and cognitive sequelae, making surgical intervention more than simply a cosmetic consideration.

For those children with obvious scaphocephaly, the management options vary depending on the age of the patient and the nature of the deformity. It is imperative that parents are disabused of the notion that one approach is the "right" treatment, since over the years many approaches have been found to yield excellent outcomes with acceptable morbidity. Rather, parents should be counseled that both less-invasive (endoscopic) approaches and open remodeling techniques are valid approaches with different strengths and weaknesses that must be considered in the context of the patient and family in question. For example, if the child has a physical or behavioral issue that might complicate the consistent usage of a molding helmet, open correction at an older age or the use of a spring-mediated cranioplasty may be more optimal.

Although the senior neurosurgeon has done a variety of open approaches over the years in infants younger than 6 months, including open sagittal strip craniectomy with mid-parietal and posterior parietal wedge osteotomies or barrel stave osteotomies [26], and pi and reverse pi techniques [27], and such approaches are well described in the literature, it has been our preference in recent years to perform minimally invasive/endoscopic strip craniectomy with either post-operative helmeting or spring placement in patients between 3–6 months of age. The strategy behind this is well described by previous authors [28–31], and our main innovations (described and illustrated in the spring-mediated cranioplasty chapter), are (1) to accomplish the procedure through a small, well-placed vertex incision, rather than two separate anterior and posterior incisions, to minimize later cosmetic sequelae in patients who may have receding hair lines later in life and (2) to use a diamond burr to achieve bone-thinning and hemostasis over the thick posterior sagittal ridge, simplifying the craniectomy. The general concepts and illustrations in that chapter apply also to craniectomy with helmeting, rather than springs. The preferred timing follows recovery from the transient anemia of infancy that can mark the transition from fetal to adult hemoglobin [32, 33]. One multi-center study found the addition of 33 min of total surgical time for the second-stage spring removal [9], which counterbalances the time commitment and need for compliance with helmet usage that factor into family and surgical decision-making for a given child.

Conceptually, all of the above approaches are considered "early" surgeries and take advantage of the intrinsic growth potential of the brain and pliability of the infant skull to achieve a desirable outcome. The exact consequences of earlier, shorter anesthesia versus later, longer anesthesia in children under the age of 1 year remain under investigation, but the current literature suggests a favorable risk profile in terms of the development of neurocognitive dysfunction and lower IQ due to general anesthesia, provided it is limited in duration. Specifically, good outcomes have been reported in one prospective multicenter study by McCann et al. focused on children in early infancy exposed to approximately an hour of anesthesia and followed until age five [6, 34–37]. Patient families should be counseled that early endoscopic techniques with molding helmets or springs have advantages that include shorter average anesthesia and hospitalization times, lower blood loss, and smaller scars [3, 38, 39]. However, these approaches result in anesthesia exposure at an earlier age compared to open techniques [33, 40]. Families should be counseled on the potential minor dermatological complications such as alopecia from nearly full-time helmet use, and the need for a second short surgery if a spring-mediated approach is used. Additional factors that may inhibit endoscopic intervention with postoperative helmeting in some regions are the availability of insurance to cover the cost of helmeting and easy accessibility to orthotists for helmet adjustments. Because the minor second procedure is required for spring removal if that option is pursued, some families may simply opt for an open strip resection or a deformity-targeted approach with more intraoperative recontouring in slightly older infants, and it is important that the surgeon is comfortable with all the various options, and their pros and cons. From a financial standpoint, however, multiple studies have suggested that the overall cost, including indirect costs such as missed work and travel, tends to strongly favor endoscopic cases, with the cost of the endoscopic surgery alone averaging over $11,000 less than open cases in one study [3, 39, 41, 42].

In contrast to early surgeries, later procedures are typically open operations. Although some surgeons will perform less-extensive surgeries, such as pi or other extended strip approaches in children slightly older than 6 months, the diminishing growth potential with age generally necessitates more extensive surgeries as time goes on, particularly after 9–12 months. In patients who present closer to 1 year of age or develop symptoms of intracranial pressure later in childhood, it is our recommendation to pursue an open cranial remodeling procedure due to the reduced growth potential to drive remodeling from less-invasive operations. These more extensive surgeries typically result in greater blood loss and thus are generally performed at age 6 months or older, although the lower age cutoff varies between centers [3]. The anesthesia time and hospital stay are greater and the scalp incision more extensive. Open approaches typically result in a more immediate cranial expansion, but the clinical and cosmetic consequences of this versus earlier less-invasive interventions are unclear.

A number of studies have suggested that cranial index scores in particular seem to be comparable despite the differences in the operative technique and timing of surgery [24, 39, 40]. However, others have questioned the utility of craniometric metrics in SS beyond a general confirmation of morphological impact. In particular, the outer head circumference may overestimate the inner volume in SS, resulting in overcorrection [43]. More complex metrics such as the Rotterdam scaphocephaly morphology score (RSMS) have been proposed that use a graded rating of specific features such as frontal bossing, temporal pinching, and vertex height, but these are cumbersome and ultimately subjective despite their effectiveness at correlating to correction [43]. One study by Lepard et al. suggested a slight, statistically significant increase in aesthetic outcomes at a median of 20 months post-operatively, perceived both by professionals and laypeople, in favor of endoscopic repair, but the interrater and intrarater reliabilities were low, the mean outcomes for each group favorable, the choice of open procedure varied, and the confounding factor of scar prominence may have affected the perception of cranial deformity [24]. A contrasting study by Millesi et al. reported that at 12 months post-operatively, the cosmetic outcome was rated as good or excellent by 89% of caregivers and 97% of surgeons for open procedures, with 73% of caretakers feeling the head shape was completely normal. Multiple studies have suggested similar cosmetic outcomes and surgical complications, though some have reported a lower rate of revision surgery in endoscopic cases [3, 33, 40, 44]. However, this may reflect substantial differences in patient selection, particularly when factoring in the reduced capacity for further head growth to drive expansion in many open cases.

Also complicating comparison between procedures is that many children who undergo early surgery have unmistakably severe deformity at birth, whereas those undergoing later surgery may have more subtle findings that are initially missed or may present with relatively normal craniometric parameters, but signs of increased intracranial pressure.

7.4 Operative Technique

7.4.1 Endoscopic Surgery

The patient is placed prone with the head secured in a horseshoe and generous local anesthetic with epinephrine injected into the scalp after being scrubbed with a chlorhexidine brush. The head of the bed is rotated 180° away from the anesthesia team. The scalp is the generously sterilized with betadine solution after the incision is marked out. It is our preference to make a 2–3 cm incision just anterior to the midpoint between fontanelles to allow for most of the endoscopic work to be done in a single direction (**Figures and caveats for this are provided in the Spring-Mediated Cranioplasty chapter**). The scalp is incised down to galea sharply and both edges are then elevated with skin hooks. Spot hemostasis is performed as needed and the pericranium is separated bluntly from the galea along the intended craniectomy pathway. Two lines are made off the midline bilaterally with needle electrocautery, marking out the 1 cm bony strip to be removed. A burr hole is drilled at the posterior edge of the incision and off the midline to avoid directly drilling on the sagittal sinus. The dura is dissected off of the adjacent bone with a modified Penfield 4. A Kerrison ronguer is used to extend the burr hole along the demarcated bone anteriorly. It is our preference to always perform the craniectomy first in the dependent direction to prevent additional pooling of blood in the operative field from bony edges in the caudal aspect of the craniectomy. Skin hooks can be used to shift the scalp forward to allow for a greater length of removal with sequential dural dissection. We find that dependent suturectomy is best extended to the fontanelle predominantly with rongeurs via scalp retraction with skin hooks or a lighted retractor. The use of endoscopy in the reverse direction can be disorienting, and in severe cases that require extensive anterior and posterior visualization, we use endoscope monitors at both the head and foot of the patient to allow normal viewing orientation in both directions. However, in most cases, an endoscope monitor is only required at the foot of the patient for the posterior craniectomy.

The lighted endoscope is then inserted by a co-surgeon and additional bites with a small eye rongeur are taken after extending the dural dissection. It is our experience that the utilization of sinus instrumentation greatly reduces the time and difficulty of distal suturectomy. Once the comfortable reach of the rongeur has been exceeded, a straight Blakesley Thru-Cut forcep (Karl Storz, Germany) is utilized to take additional midline bites. Curved Blakesley Ethmoid forceps (Karl Storz, Germany) can be used to add additional lateral width to the suturectomy distally if the Thru-Cut is obstructed. The dura is sequentially dissected as the suturectomy is further extended. It is critical to withdraw the endoscope intermittently to better visualize the course being taken. It is our experience that surgeons typically veer off over time away from the side of their dominant hand without intermittent correction. The sagittal sinus can serve as a good guide to the midline as well, but can become increasingly difficult to visualize during the distal portions of endoscopic work due to the increasingly parallel view of the endoscope relative to the dura. In some cases, the bone thickness may be difficult to address with sinus instruments. By using the endoscope to retract the scalp and a suction tip to retract the dura, this bone can be drilled down to the inner cortex safely under irrigation with a 4 mm coarse diamond round drill bit. A short, angled drill handle (Stryker, Kalamazoo, MI) is more ergonomic and allows for more distal access. This is also helpful in addressing bone bleeding, as the coarse diamond bit provides a cauterizing effect. Depending on the angle, the drill or Thru-Cut can be used to complete the inner cortex craniectomy efficiently until the fontanelle is reached. The parietal bones are palpated through the scalp while being visualized with the endoscope to confirm appropriate mobility. In some cases, the parietal bones are insufficiently mobilized despite extending the suturectomy from fontanelle to fontanelle. In this case, the proximal lambdoid sutures may be dissected off of the dura, and additional suturectomy performed until the mobility is satisfactory. Depending on the operative plan, distractor springs may be inserted at this point of the procedure. It is important if springs are to be applied that the thickness of the bone along the suturectomy be examined. Particularly in young patients the bone may be insufficiently resistant to allow for spring insertion without subsequent erosion and the operative plan may require revision to a helmet-assisted approach, where a slightly wider (2 cm versus 1 cm) craniectomy may be preferable. The dura should also be inspected to ensure a sufficiently wide dissection off of the bone to prevent inadvertent dural injury with the insertion of the spring footplates. The scalp is then closed in a standard fashion with absorbable sutures.

7.4.2 Open Surgery

Since its initial description by Lane in the 1890s, open treatment of craniosynostosis has had numerous variations of fluctuating popularity that can be generally characterized as cranial vault expansion with or without recontouring [45]. Major factors in the determination of operative planning of an open procedure are the timing of surgery, the nature of the deformity, and the presence of increased intracranial pressure. While open surgery is more effective than endoscopic surgery in older patients, some open procedures still make use of remaining skull growth potential, whereas others are better suited to SS that was missed until later in childhood or in cases of late onset SS.

It is our preference to make a zig-zag incision bilaterally starting just anterior and superior to the pinna, ensuring partial exposure of the temporalis muscles, adjusting the curve to best reflect the cranial target. For patients presenting earlier than 9 months in which an open approach is taken, we prefer to perform a modified pi procedure. Burr holes are made lateral to a 3 cm strut of bone covering the sagittal sinus and a linear cut is made parallel to the strut, spanning the distance between each fontanelle. Barrel stave osteotomies are performed every 2–3 cm extending laterally to the extent allowed by the soft tissue exposure or the limits of the cranial vault. Each bony strip is then bent outward using a heavy needle driver or Tessier bone bender.

For patients greater than 9 months of age but still within the skull growth period, a deformity-focused approach is taken. This includes extended frontal-orbital advancement and expansion; posterior vault recontouring with the approach noted in the prior paragraph combined with an occipitotemporal craniotomy and bone remodeling to provide sagittal shortening and coronal widening; biparietal "clam-shell" and barrel-stave expansions; and a frontoparietal/occipitotemporal "switch" cranioplasty approach. These techniques and related variations are discussed in more detail in later chapters. In selected cases with significant deformity of both the frontal and occipital regions, a total calvarial reconstruction [46] or a staged approach may be undertaken. In many cases, families are most concerned about a particular aspect, such as the frontal bossing and biparietal narrowing which can be addressed with an anteriorly or posteriorly focused reconstructive strategy, avoiding the potentially increased morbidity of a total calvarial reconstructive approach.

A special situation relates to those children who present with a relatively normal head shape and size, with increased intracranial pressure associated with presumed late-onset sagittal synostosis. Such children typically present with headaches and have evidence of papilledema or findings of significantly increased intracranial pressure on invasive monitoring. For patients presenting with little or no deformity after the majority of skull growth has been achieved, we focus on achieving a significant expansion without dramatically altering their appearance. In such cases, we have generally proceeded with a "mid-vault" bilateral parietal craniotomy with barrel staves directed toward the frontal, temporal, and parieto-occipital regions for circumferential expansion (Fig. 7.1). Bi-parietal craniotomies are elevated, leaving a midline 3 cm strut of bone covering the sagittal sinus. Barrel stave osteotomies are performed every 2–3 cm circumferentially, except toward the midline, to the extent allowed by the soft tissue exposure or the limits of the cranial vault. Each bony strip is then partially out fractured or bent depending on the rigidity using a large needle driver or Tessier bone

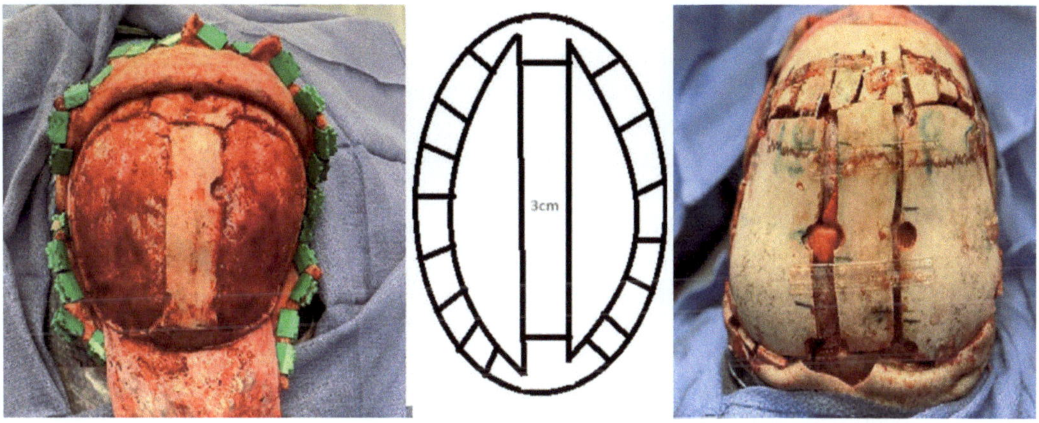

Fig. 7.1 Operative photo of middle vault expansion with bilateral parietal craniotomies and barrel staves (left). Simplified depiction of the cuts made (middle). Post-reconstruction photo (right)

bender. The bone flaps are then secured using resorbable plates and screws to the midline strut and sutures are used laterally to secure the bone flaps to the barrel staves. In some instances where late-onset increased pressure occurs in the context of a metabolic disorder with bone thickening associated with sagittal synostosis, endocranial thinning is used to further expand the intracranial volume [47].

7.5 Complication Avoidance

Synostosis surgeries are by their nature high-risk surgeries, with the potential for life-threatening blood loss as the most serious complication. Avoidance necessitates vigilance in intraoperative monitoring, having adequate intravenous lines for blood infusion, immediate availability of blood in the operating room, and care during the dissection of dura from the bone. Adherence of the sinus to the bone or extension through the bone requires particular attention to dissection. Likewise, a subset of children will have sizeable bridging veins between the dura and bone, which must be identified, coagulated, and divided, regardless of whether the exposure is being done in an open or endoscopic fashion. Venous blood loss can often be controlled with judicious head elevation, but that must be balanced with the risk of air embolism, another potentially life-threatening complication, particularly in the setting of hypovolemia. Treatment requires lowering the head, filling the field with saline, and waxing of the bone edges.

Other complications that can occur include brain injury and dural tears. For the former, it is essential to exercise care in separating the dura from the bone and minimize excessive retraction. This in part applies to the latter as well; particular caution is required when stripping dura that is adherent to a nonclosed suture during extended calvarial expansion techniques. Our preference is to close any visible defect primarily, to avoid the risks of a growing leptomeningeal cyst or late cerebrospinal fluid leakage from the wound. Infection is uncommon with these procedures, but by no means rare, even with the use of careful aseptic technique and perioperative antibiotics. Helpful tactics to avoid this complication are to minimize areas of bone, plate, screw, or spring prominence adjacent to the incision to limit stress on the incision line and the potential for erosion of the skin at nearby pressure points.

Late events that should also be considered are the presence of associated hydrocephalus and the need for further surgical intervention. In children with underlying syndromic or metabolic etiologies for their sagittal synostosis who present primarily with increased intracranial pressure, it is essential to follow them closely for the resolution of papilledema. In some instances, patients with syndromic or metabolic etiologies will also have impaired CSF absorption or cranial venous outflow obstruction, and will have persistent papilledema, with a pseudotumor-like pattern of little or no ventriculomegaly. In such children, secondary shunt insertion may be required. Although postoperative reclosure of the sagittal suture line or other cranial openings is not uncommon after correction, a minority of patients require additional surgery [26, 29, 33]. They nonetheless require ongoing follow-up until approximately 8 years of age, when most cranial growth has been completed. A small percentage of children, ranging from 3 to 5% in most large series, will require a secondary cranial expansion surgery, either for recurrent cosmetic deformity or late onset of increased intracranial pressure or a symptomatic Chiari malformation. A subset of these children will have a mild form of an underlying craniofacial syndrome that only becomes apparent in retrospect, but others will have no discernible genetic etiology. Although this is not a complication that can necessarily be avoided, it is one that can be anticipated and managed expeditiously, before the onset of visual loss or other sequelae. This highlights the importance of conscientious craniofacial follow-up, even for the most straightforward cases of sagittal synostosis.

7.6 Conclusions

The management of sagittal synostosis is aided by multiple operative approaches that allow for satisfactory cosmesis and, where needed, the alleviation of intracranial hypertension. An individualized approach should be taken based on patient's age, deformity, presence or absence of increased intracranial pressure, and family factors and preferences, recognizing that there is no single "right" approach to patient management. The most critical step in management is to ensure early diagnosis and work-up to allow for the greatest flexibility in operative management. In some cases, with late-onset synostosis, this can be challenging, and dependent upon the availability of high-resolution imaging, reliable ophthalmology assessments, and in some cases intracranial pressure monitoring. Pre-operative CT imaging and genetic testing are commonly performed at our site in order to screen for concomitant synostoses and syndromic conditions, which may influence surgical planning.

Acknowledgements None.

Conflicts of InterestNone.

References

1. Kolar JC. An epidemiological study of nonsyndromal craniosynostoses. J Craniofac Surg. 2011;22(1):47–9.
2. Boulet SL, Rasmussen SA, Honein MA. A population-based study of craniosynostosis in metropolitan Atlanta, 1989-2003. Am J Med Genet A. 2008;146A(8):984–91.
3. Yan H, Abel TJ, Alotaibi NM, Anderson M, Niazi TN, Weil AG, et al. A systematic review and meta-analysis of endoscopic versus open treatment of craniosynostosis. Part 1: the sagittal suture. J Neurosurg Pediatr. 2018;22(4):352–60.
4. Di Rocco F, Arnaud E, Renier D. Evolution in the frequency of nonsyndromic craniosynostosis. J Neurosurg Pediatr. 2009;4(1):21–5.
5. Lee HQ, Hutson JM, Wray AC, Lo PA, Chong DK, Holmes AD, et al. Changing epidemiology of nonsyndromic craniosynostosis and revisiting the risk factors. J Craniofac Surg. 2012;23(5):1245–51.
6. Proctor MR, Meara JG. A review of the management of single-suture craniosynostosis, past, present, and future. J Neurosurg Pediatr. 2019;24(6):622–31.
7. Persing JA. MOC-PS(SM) CME article: management considerations in the treatment of craniosynostosis. Plast Reconstr Surg. 2008;121(4 Suppl):1–11.
8. Ravindra VM, Awad AW, Baker CM, Lee A, Anderson RCE, Gociman B, et al. Preoperative imaging patterns and intracranial findings in single-suture craniosynostosis: a study from the synostosis research group. J Neurosurg Pediatr. 2021;28:344–50.
9. Lang SS, Meier PM, Paden WZ, Storm PB, Heuer GG, Bartlett SP, et al. Spring-mediated cranioplasty versus endoscopic strip craniectomy for sagittal craniosynostosis. J Neurosurg Pediatr. 2021;28:1–9.
10. Miura T, Perlyn CA, Kinboshi M, Ogihara N, Kobayashi-Miura M, Morriss-Kay GM, et al. Mechanism of skull suture maintenance and interdigitation. J Anat. 2009;215(6):642–55.
11. Jin SW, Sim KB, Kim SD. Development and growth of the Normal cranial vault : an embryologic review. J Korean Neurosurg Soc. 2016;59(3):192–6.
12. Pattisapu JV, Gegg CA, Olavarria G, Johnson KK, Ruiz RL, Costello BJ. Craniosynostosis: diagnosis and surgical management. Atlas Oral Maxillofac Surg Clin North Am. 2010;18(2):77–91.
13. Davis C, Lauritzen CG. Spring-assisted remodeling for ventricular shunt-induced cranial deformity. J Craniofac Surg. 2008;19(3):588–92.

14. Weinzweig J, Bartlett SP, Chen JC, Losee J, Sutton L, Duhaime AC, et al. Cranial vault expansion in the management of postshunt craniosynostosis and slit ventricle syndrome. Plast Reconstr Surg. 2008;122(4):1171–80.
15. Kapp-Simon KA, Speltz ML, Cunningham ML, Patel PK, Tomita T. Neurodevelopment of children with single suture craniosynostosis: a review. Childs Nerv Syst. 2007;23(3):269–81.
16. Speltz ML, Kapp-Simon KA, Cunningham M, Marsh J, Dawson G. Single-suture craniosynostosis: a review of neurobehavioral research and theory. J Pediatr Psychol. 2004;29(8):651–68.
17. Speltz ML, Kapp-Simon K, Collett B, Keich Y, Gaither R, Cradock MM, et al. Neurodevelopment of infants with single-suture craniosynostosis: presurgery comparisons with case-matched controls. Plast Reconstr Surg. 2007;119(6):1874–81.
18. Thiele-Nygaard AE, Foss-Skiftesvik J, Juhler M. Intracranial pressure, brain morphology and cognitive outcome in children with sagittal craniosynostosis. Childs Nerv Syst. 2020;36(4):689–95.
19. Starr JR, Kapp-Simon KA, Cloonan YK, Collett BR, Cradock MM, Buono L, et al. Presurgical and postsurgical assessment of the neurodevelopment of infants with single-suture craniosynostosis: comparison with controls. J Neurosurg. 2007;107(2 Suppl):103–10.
20. Hashim PW, Patel A, Yang JF, Travieso R, Terner J, Losee JE, et al. The effects of whole-vault cranioplasty versus strip craniectomy on long-term neuropsychological outcomes in sagittal craniosynostosis. Plast Reconstr Surg. 2014;134(3):491–501.
21. Fearon JA, Singh DJ, Beals SP, Yu JC. The diagnosis and treatment of single-sutural synostoses: are computed tomographic scans necessary? Plast Reconstr Surg. 2007;120(5):1327–31.
22. Cerovac S, Neil-Dwyer JG, Rich P, Jones BM, Hayward RD. Are routine preoperative CT scans necessary in the management of single suture craniosynostosis? Br J Neurosurg. 2002;16(4):348–54.
23. Strahle J, Muraszko KM, Buchman SR, Kapurch J, Garton HJ, Maher CO. Chiari malformation associated with craniosynostosis. Neurosurg Focus. 2011;31(3):E2.
24. Lepard J, Akbari SHA, Mooney J, Arynchyna A, Iii SGM, Myers RP, et al. Comparison of aesthetic outcomes between open and endoscopically treated sagittal craniosynostosis. J Neurosurg Pediatr. 2021;28:1–7.
25. Arnaud E, Renier D, Marchac D. Prognosis for mental function in scaphocephaly. J Neurosurg. 1995;83(3):476–9.
26. Adamo MA, Pollack IF. A single-center experience with symptomatic postoperative calvarial growth restriction after extended strip craniectomy for sagittal craniosynostosis. J Neurosurg Pediatr. 2010;5(1):131–5.
27. Lin KY, Gampper TJ, Jane JA. Correction of posterior sagittal craniosynostosis. J Craniofac Surg. 1998;9(1):88–91.
28. Losken HW, Pollack IF, Singhal VK. Vascularized fronto-orbital advancement. J Craniofac Surg. 1996;7(2):107–10.
29. Riordan CP, Zurakowski D, Meier PM, Alexopoulos G, Meara JG, Proctor MR, et al. Minimally invasive endoscopic surgery for infantile craniosynostosis: a longitudinal cohort study. J Pediatr. 2020;216:142–9.e2.
30. Nguyen DC, Farber SJ, Skolnick GB, Naidoo SD, Smyth MD, Kane AA, et al. One hundred consecutive endoscopic repairs of sagittal craniosynostosis: an evolution in care. J Neurosurg Pediatr. 2017;20(5):410–8.
31. Jimenez DF, Barone CM, Cartwright CC, Baker L. Early management of craniosynostosis using endoscopic-assisted strip craniectomies and cranial orthotic molding therapy. Pediatrics. 2002;110(1 Pt 1):97–104.
32. Sankaran VG, Orkin SH. The switch from fetal to adult hemoglobin. Cold Spring Harb Perspect Med. 2013;3(1):a011643.
33. Goyal A, Lu VM, Yolcu YU, Elminawy M, Daniels DJ. Endoscopic versus open approach in craniosynostosis repair: a systematic review and meta-analysis of perioperative outcomes. Childs Nerv Syst. 2018;34(9):1627–37.
34. Davidson AJ, Disma N, de Graaff JC, Withington DE, Dorris L, Bell G, et al. Neurodevelopmental outcome at 2 years of age after general anaesthesia and awake-regional anaesthesia in infancy (GAS): an international multicentre, randomised controlled trial. Lancet. 2016;387(10015):239–50.
35. McCann ME, de Graaff JC, Dorris L, Disma N, Withington D, Bell G, et al. Neurodevelopmental outcome at 5 years of age after general anaesthesia or awake-regional anaesthesia in infancy (GAS): an international, multicentre, randomised, controlled equivalence trial. Lancet. 2019;393(10172):664–77.
36. Davidson AJ, Sun LS. Clinical evidence for any effect of anesthesia on the developing brain. Anesthesiology. 2018;128(4):840–53.
37. Warner DO, Zaccariello MJ, Katusic SK, Schroeder DR, Hanson AC, Schulte PJ, et al. Neuropsychological and behavioral outcomes after exposure of young children to procedures requiring general anesthesia: the mayo anesthesia safety in kids (MASK) study. Anesthesiology. 2018;129(1):89–105.
38. Thompson DR, Zurakowski D, Haberkern CM, Stricker PA, Meier PM, Bannister C, et al. Endoscopic versus open repair for craniosynostosis in infants using propensity score matching to compare outcomes: a multicenter study from the pediatric craniofacial collaborative group. Anesth Analg. 2018;126(3):968–75.
39. Abbott MM, Rogers GF, Proctor MR, Busa K, Meara JG. Cost of treating sagittal synostosis in the first year of life. J Craniofac Surg. 2012;23(1):88–93.
40. Shah MN, Kane AA, Petersen JD, Woo AS, Naidoo SD, Smyth MD. Endoscopically assisted versus open repair of sagittal craniosynostosis: the St. Louis

Children's Hospital experience. J Neurosurg Pediatr. 2011;8(2):165–70.
41. Garber ST, Karsy M, Kestle JRW, Siddiqi F, Spanos SP, Riva-Cambrin J. Comparing outcomes and cost of 3 surgical treatments for sagittal synostosis: a retrospective study including procedure-related cost analysis. Neurosurgery. 2017;81(4):680–7.
42. Vogel TW, Woo AS, Kane AA, Patel KB, Naidoo SD, Smyth MD. A comparison of costs associated with endoscope-assisted craniectomy versus open cranial vault repair for infants with sagittal synostosis. J Neurosurg Pediatr. 2014;13(3):324–31.
43. Vinchon M, Guerreschi P, Karnoub MA, Wolber A. Morphological and surgical results in sagittal synostosis: early craniectomy versus later cranioplasty. Childs Nerv Syst. 2021;37(7):2335–41.
44. Han RH, Nguyen DC, Bruck BS, Skolnick GB, Yarbrough CK, Naidoo SD, et al. Characterization of complications associated with open and endoscopic craniosynostosis surgery at a single institution. J Neurosurg Pediatr. 2016;17(3):361–70.
45. Lane L. Pioneer craniectomy for relief of mental imbecility due to premature sutural closure and microcephalus. JAMA. 1892;18(2):49–50.
46. Pollack IF, Losken HW, Hurwitz DJ. A combined frontoorbital and occipital advancement technique for use in total calvarial reconstruction. J Neurosurg. 1996;84(3):424–9.
47. Herman PI, Marji FP, Anstadt EE, Dvoracek LA, Goldstein JA, Pollack IF, et al. Decompressive cranial vault remodeling in osteosclerotic robinow syndrome. Cleft Palate Craniofac J. 2021;58(1):126–30.

8 Key Points for the Neurosurgeons and Management Principles (Diagnosis, Surgical Principles, Their Rationale, and Timing)

Hannah E. Goldstein, Craig Birgfeld, Amy Lee, Srinivas Susarla, and Scott Boop

Metopic craniosynostosis, premature fusion of the metopic suture, causes the abnormal head shape described as trigonocephaly. It accounts for approximately 5–10% of all single-suture synostoses, with a prevalence of approximately 1 in 15,000 children. Metopic craniosynostosis is sporadic in approximately 75% of cases, though up to 5% of patients have a positive family history, without a known underlying genetic defect; the other 25% are syndromic, associated with Jacobsen/11q23 deletion, chromosome 9p deletion, Opitz C syndromes, and other aneuploidies. Metopic craniosynostosis has also been associated with other congenital malformations, including neuromuscular dysfunction and developmental delay, but without a specific syndromic diagnosis. The metopic suture physiologically closes by 9 months of age, though normal closure can occur as early as 3 months.

8.1 Diagnosis

8.1.1 Clinical Exam

Initial diagnosis of metopic suture synostosis, as with any craniosynostosis, is based on clinical exam findings. From the vertex view, the head is noted to be triangular in shape, with a keel deformity of the forehead, resulting in pseudohypotelorism, anterior displacement of the coronal sutures, posterior displacement of the superolateral orbital rims, temporal narrowing, flattening of the frontal bones, and compensatory bulging of the parieto-occipital region (Fig. 8.1). The anterior fontanelle is also triangular in shape, with a flat edge anteriorly. Because metopic synostosis is a symmetric deformity, more subtle cases may go undiagnosed. It is important to differentiate metopic craniosynostosis from metopic ridging associated with the physiological closure of the suture which occurs in about one-third of people. The former is treated with surgical cranial vault expansion while the latter does not require surgery.

H. E. Goldstein · C. Birgfeld · A. Lee (✉) ·
S. Susarla · S. Boop
Seattle Children's Hospital, University of Washington, Seattle, WA, USA
e-mail: hannah.goldstein@seattlechildrens.org; craig.birgfeld@seattlechildrens.org; amy.lee@seattlechildrens.org; Srinivas.Susarla@seattlechildrens.org; sboop92@uw.edu

F. Di Rocco, J. Kestle (eds.), *Neurosurgical Aspects of Craniosynostosis*,
https://doi.org/10.1007/978-3-031-69386-1_8

8.1.2 Imaging

The imaging modality of choice for workup of any craniosynostosis is a three-dimensional computed tomography (CT) scan. This radiological study is not only diagnostic but can also be used to help guide surgical management and planning. The 3D CT scan provides a detailed look at the fused suture, overall head shape, and facial and skull base deformities (Fig. 8.2).

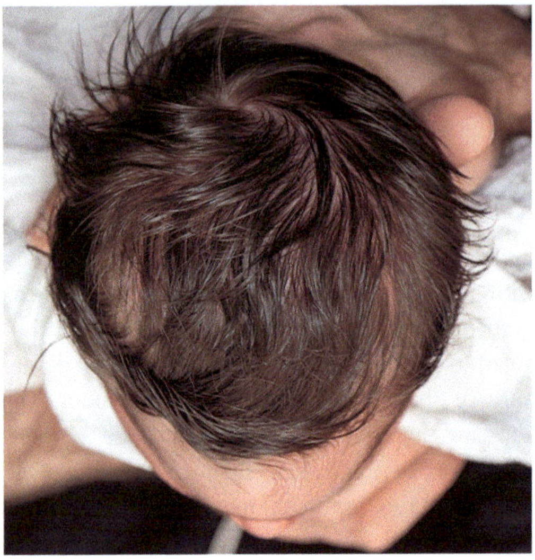

Fig. 8.1 Vertex view of the head. Note the triangular in shape, keel deformity of the forehead, anterior displacement of the coronal sutures, posterior displacement of the superolateral orbital rims, temporal narrowing, flattening of the frontal bones, and compensatory bulging of the parieto-occipital region

8.2 Decision Making

Previous studies have shown that 8–13% of patients with single suture synostosis develop elevated ICP (>15 mmHg); however, to date, there is no way of predicting which patients will fall into this category. Therefore, early surgical intervention is advocated for children with metopic, as well as other forms of craniosynostoses, in order to make adequate room for normal brain growth and development. The surgical intervention also provides the patient with the best esthetic outcome to alleviate the psychosocial impact a skull deformity may cause.

8.3 Surgical Technique

Most craniofacial centers of excellence offer both open cranial vault remodeling (fronto-orbital advancement) and endoscopic techniques. The pros and cons of each are discussed in more detail in the following sections. Often the decision is based on the age of the patient at the time of diagnosis. In cases where the family has the option to proceed with endoscopic treatment or wait until the child is old enough to undergo a fronto-orbital advancement, the decision comes down to the severity of the deformity, surgeon preference, and family preference.

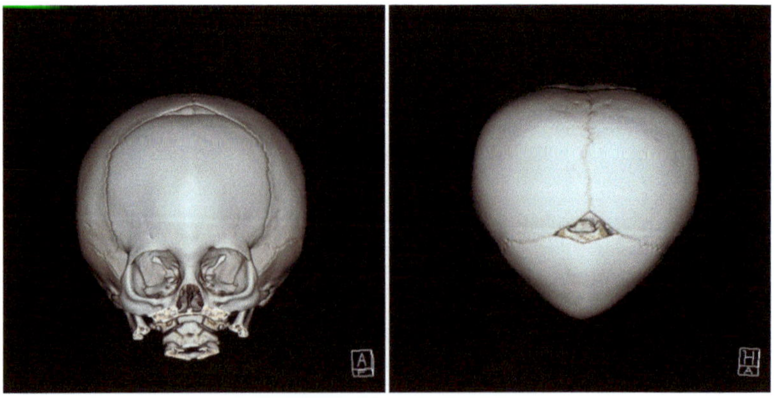

Fig. 8.2 Three3-dimensional computed tomography (CT) scan. The 3D CT scan provides a detailed look at the fused suture, overall head shape, and facial and skull base deformities

8.3.1 Fronto-Orbital Advancement (FOA)

While a detailed discussion of the operative procedure itself is beyond the scope of this chapter, there are important surgical principles to keep in mind. Fronto-orbital advancement is a major operative procedure, with anticipated blood loss, and as such, involves the collaboration of a skilled and experienced pediatric anesthesiology team. The procedure should be done under general anesthesia, with at least two good IVs, an arterial line, a Foley, and precordial Doppler monitoring. All patients should have cross-matched blood available prior to the start of the surgery.

The patient is positioned supine, with the head on a padded horseshoe headrest. Per the preference of the family, either the entire head, or a wide strip is shaved, and a zigzag bicoronal incision is marked out. The zigzag incision results in better cosmesis of scalp alopecia, with the bicoronal approach allowing for access all the way to the nasion. The scalp flaps are elevated in the subperiosteal plane along with the temporalis muscle, anteriorly to the superior orbital rims and laterally to the temporal fossa. If the supraorbital neurovascular bundles are within a true foramen as opposed to a notch, this must be opened with an osteotome in order to release the bundle and protect the nerves bilaterally.

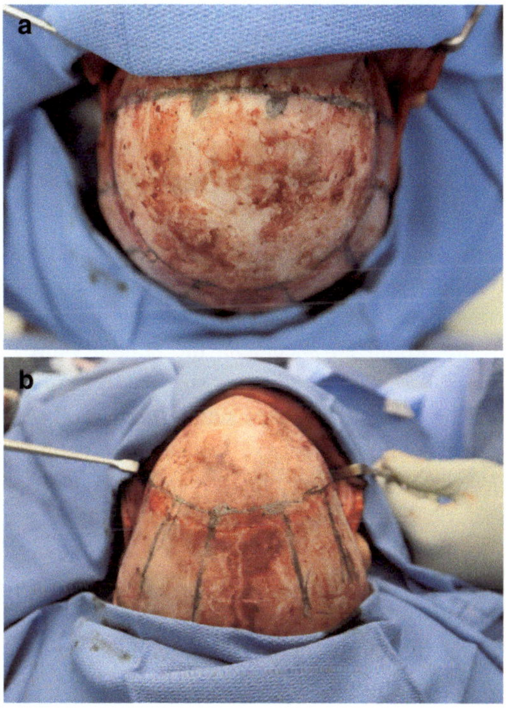

Fig. 8.3 (**a**) Once the exposure is completed, the bifrontal craniotomy is marked using a sterile pencil. Bur holes are drilled and a complete epidural dissection is completed. The craniotomy is completed and the bone flap removed. (**b**) Barrel stave osteotomies are marked out with a sterile pencil. The epidural space is then dissected underneath the parietal bones, and multiple barrel stave osteotomies are made. Out-fracturing of this bone expands the intracranial volume

The planned craniotomy cuts can be drawn out with a bone pencil (Fig. 8.3a). A bifrontal craniotomy is performed, with special care taken when dissecting in the epidural plane along the midline. The epidural space is then dissected underneath the parietal bones, and multiple barrel stave osteotomies are made (Fig. 8.3b). Out-fracturing of this bone expands the intracranial volume. Next, the epidural dissection is carried out on the floor of the anterior and middle fossa, with cotton paddies placed along the interface. Temporal extensions are cut beneath the sphenoid wing on either side, and orbital osteotomies are carried out via cuts along the orbital roof bilaterally and a cut across the nasal glabella medially. The orbital bandeau can then be removed as a single piece. Once the bone is removed, one should carefully inspect the dura to ensure there are no dural tears. If there are any tears in the dura, these can be primarily repaired using 4–0 Nurolon sutures and Tisseal.

The orbital bandeau is split in the middle, with an interpositional bone graft used to both widen and advance the fronto-orbital region. Closing osteotomies are made at the lateral orbit to advance the lateral bandeau. The recontoured bandeau and frontal bones are secured in place with a mix of PDS suture, resorbable plates and screws, and 26-gauge wires. Bone graft is harvested from the inner table of the frontal bone flap. The split calvarial bone graft and bone particulate graft are used to fill in the defects created by the vault expansion. Meticulous hemostasis is achieved, and a #7 Jackson-Pratt drain is left in the subgaleal space. The scalp is reapproximated with absorbable sutures, with antibiotic ointment applied liberally to the incision line.

8.3.2 Endoscopic Suturectomy

Endoscopic suturectomy involves shorter operative time and less blood loss compared to an open cranial vault expansion. However, unlike with a fronto-orbital advancement, the cranial vault is not reshaped at the time of surgery. By cutting out the abnormally fused suture, and then keeping the child in a series of helmets to direct bone growth, endoscopic techniques take advantage of the growing brain and still malleable skull.

The patient is positioned supine, with the head on a padded horseshoe headrest. A small, approximately 1–2 in., zig-zag incision is made just behind the hairline (Fig. 8.4). After the incision is opened, two burr holes are made, one on either side of the fused suture and underlying sagittal sinus. Bone is then removed with a Kerrison rongeur posteriorly to the anterior fontanelle. The epidural space is dissected anteriorly, with the aid of endoscopic visualization. Bone scissors are used to cut out the fused suture as far anteriorly as possible, down to the nasion. After about 4 months of age, the bone becomes too thick to cut in this fashion. Hemostatic agents are used, and the incision is closed with absorbable sutures.

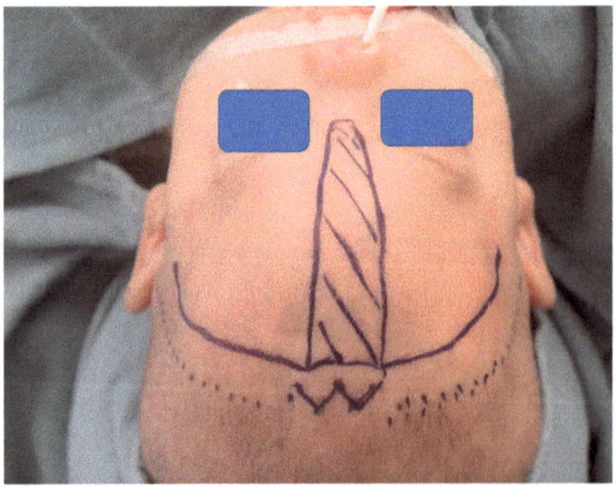

Fig. 8.4 Skin markings for proposed endoscopic suturectomy. A small zig-zag incision is made just behind the hairline. The epidural space is dissected anteriorly, with the aid of endoscopic visualization. Bone scissors are used to cut out the fused suture as far anteriorly as possible, down to the nasion

8.4 Timing of Intervention

It is our practice to offer endoscopic intervention through 4 months of age. As the endoscopic technique relies on the rapidly growing brain to reshape the skull, once the rate of head growth slows, the cosmetic results are arguably not as good. Furthermore, as the child ages and the skull becomes thicker, it becomes technically more challenging to cut through the bone without the use of a drill.

Fronto-orbital advancement is generally performed between 9 and 12 months of age. Though most children will present before this time, the reasons for waiting are twofold: (1) the bone strength increases with age. This allows for a more stable reconstruction and less chance of relapse. Higher revision rates are often seen when an open cranial vault procedure is performed prior to 6 months of age (2). The older child is better able to tolerate the associated blood loss and prolonged anesthetic time associated with the open procedure.

For children who present prior to 4 months of age, families are generally given the option to proceed with endoscopic treatment or wait until the child is old enough to undergo an open fronto-orbital advancement.

8.5 Post-Op Care and Follow-Up

Patients who undergo open fronto-orbital advancement typically spend the first post-operative night in the intensive care unit. Post operative blood counts and electrolytes are checked, and children are transfused as necessary. All patients are started on standing acetaminophen, as well as IV narcotics as needed. Patients are given a total of 24-h of peri-operative antibiotics. Most children transfer to the surgical floor on post-operative day one. Parents should be prepared for the fact that periorbital edema usually peaks on post-operative day two or three, often to the extent that the child cannot open their eyes. Once patients are tolerating a PO diet, pain medications can be transitioned from IV to oral. The Jackson-Pratt drain remains in place until the output decreases. Discharge criteria, once the drain is removed, include pain well controlled with oral pain medications, tolerating a diet, voiding appropriately, and having bowel movements. This usually coincides with at least one of the eyes starting to open. On average, patients are discharged home on post-operative days 3–4. The wound is managed with twice daily application of antibiotic ointment for 7 days.

Patients who undergo endoscopic metopic suturectomy often go directly to the surgical ward post-operatively. Given the shorter anesthesia time, less blood loss, and significantly less post-operative swelling associated with this procedure, many children are able to be discharged home as early as post-operative day 1. They are fitted for their helmet 7–10 days post-operatively once the swelling has subsided and the helmet is delivered 2–3 days later. The helmet is worn 23 h per day, generally until the patient's first birthday. Visits with the orthotist are every 2 weeks for adjustment.

It is our institutional practice for patients to come for a wound check at 2–4 weeks. Then at 1 year and 2 year post op with surface imaging at the 2-year visit. Further visits occur as the patient begins school at age 5 or 6 and finally before graduation at age 16–18.

8.6 Complications and Management

The overall morbidity and mortality rates for craniosynostosis surgery are low, and the surgeries are generally very well tolerated. However, it is important to remember that due to the young age and small size of the patient, their circulating blood volume is relatively small. Given the highly vascular nature of both the scalp and the bone, blood loss, especially during an open cranial vault procedure, can be significant. It is important to maintain euvolemia and transfuse crystalloid, colloid, and blood as necessary. In fact, it is our team's practice not to begin an open cranial vault expansion without cross-matched blood in the room.

During epidural dissection or during bone removal, there can be injury to the venous sinuses. It is of utmost importance to recognize this and treat it expeditiously, to avoid possibly catastrophic complications. Venous sinus injury should be occluded with gelfoam and cotton patties to apply direct pressure, followed by repair with a muscle plug. It is also important to carefully inspect the dura and directly repair any dural tears in order to avoid post-operative CSF leaks and potential infection.

Given the degree of bone work and the head position, which is usually higher than the child's heart, there is a risk of air embolism. It is our practice to pre-operatively place a precordial Doppler on all patients in order to help monitor for air embolism. Significant air embolisms can lead to hemodynamic instability. As soon as there is a concern for an air embolism, the field should be flooded with saline irrigation, the entry site occluded, and the head of the bed lowered below the level of the heart to prevent further air entrapment.

Other complications, though rare, that the family should be counseled preoperatively about injury to the underlying brain parenchyma, transfusion reactions, seizures, and wound infections. Additionally, patients may present years later with post-reconstruction calvarial defects that may require additional surgery to fill the defects.

8.7 Evidence and Outcomes

Generally, outcomes following either open cranial vault expansion or endoscopic strip craniectomy for metopic craniosynostosis are excellent [1–14], both in terms of cosmetic results and long-term neurocognitive development. Short-term, endoscopic strip craniectomy is associated with shorter OR time, less blood loss, lower rates of blood transfusion, and shorter hospital stays. However, long-term, standardized studies are still lacking in comparing the two techniques. It is important to recognize that children even with single-suture craniosynostosis require multidisciplinary care provided by pediatric neurosurgeons, craniofacial plastic surgeons, pediatric anesthesiologists, pediatricians, ophthalmologists, geneticists, and pediatric nurses. Due to the complexity of their care, we recommend treatment at craniofacial centers of excellence that can tailor the approach to each individual child.

References

1. Bennett KG, Hespe GE, Vercler CJ, Buchman SR. Short- and long-term outcomes by procedure type for non-sagittal single-suture craniosynostosis. J Craniofac Surg. 2019;30(2):458–64.
2. Breugem CC, van R Zeeman BJ. Retrospective study of nonsyndromic craniosynostosis treated over a 10-year period. J Craniofac Surg. 1999;10:140–3.
3. Goyal A, Lu VM, Yolcu YU, Elminawy M, Daniels DJ. Endoscopic versus open approach in craniosynostosis repair: a systemic review and meta-analysis of perioperative outcomes. Childs Nerv Syst. 2018;34:1627–37.
4. Jimenez DF, Barone CM, Cartwright CC, Baker L. Early management of craniosynostosis using endoscopic-assisted strip craniectomies and cranial orthotic molding therapy. Pediatrics. 2002;110(1 Pt 1):97–104.
5. JRW K, Lee A, RCE A, Gociman B, Patel KB, Smyth MD, Birgfeld C, Pollack IF, Goldstein JA, Tamber M, Imahiyerobo T, Siddiqi FA, Synostosis Research Group. Variation in the management of isolated craniosynostosis: a survey of the synostosis research group. J Neurosurg Pediatr. 2018;22(6):627–31.
6. Massenburg BB, Nassar AH, Hopper RA. National database reported outcomes following craniosynostosis reconstruction. J Craniofac Surg. 2020;31(1):154–7.
7. Mehta VA, Bettegowda C, Jallo GI, Ahn ES. The evolution of surgical management for craniosynostosis. Neurosurg Focus. 2010;29:E5.
8. Nagaraja S, Anslow P, Winter B. Craniosynostosis. Clin Radiol. 2013;68:284–92.
9. Pattisapu JV, Gegg CA, Olavaria G, Johnson KK, Ruiz RL, Costello BJ. Craniosynostosis: diagnosis and surgical management. Atlas Oral Maxillofac Surg Clin N Am. 2010;18:77–91.
10. Ravindra VM, Awad AW, Baker CM, Lee A, Anderson RCE, Gociman B, Patel KB, Smyth MD, Birgfeld C, Pollack IF, Goldstein JA, Imahiyerobo T, Siddiqi FA, Kestle JRW, Synostosis Research Group (SynRG). Preoperative imaging patterns and intracranial findings in single-suture craniosynostosis: a study from the synostosis research group. J Neurosurg Pediatr. 2021;25:1–7.
11. Renier D, Sainte-Rose C, Marchac D, Hirsch J. Intracranial pressure in craniostenosis. J Neurosurg. 1982;57(3):370–7.
12. Schulz M, Liebe-Puschel L, Seelbach K, Paulikat L, Fehlhaber F, Schwarz K, Blecher C, Thomale U. Quantitative and qualitative comparison of morphometric outcomes after endoscopic and conventional correction of sagittal and metopic craniosynostosis versus control groups. Neurosurg Focus. 2021;50(4):E2.
13. Shillito J, Matson DD. Craniosynostosis: a review of 519 surgical patients. Pediatrics. 1968;41(4):829–53.
14. Warren SM, Proctor MR, Bartlett SP, Blount JP, Buchman SR, Burnett W, Fearon JA, Keating R, Muraszko KM, Rogers GR, Rubin MS, McCarthy JG. Parameters of care for craniosynostosis: craniofacial and neurologic surgery perspectives. Plast Reconstr Surg. 2012;129:731–7.

9 Unilateral Coronal Craniosynostosis: Clinical Presentation and Management Principles

Yosef Dastagirzada, Hammad Khan, Sean Neifert, Henri Kolb, and Richard C. E. Anderson

9.1 Introduction

Unilateral coronal craniosynostosis (UCS, or anterior plagiocephaly) is the second most common type of craniosynostosis, occurring in approximately 1/10,000 births [1]. It accounts for between 20 and 35% of nonsyndromic cases, with a female predominance of 3:2 [2, 3]. Although a number of syndromes, including Apert, Crouzon, and Pfeiffer Syndrome, are associated with coronal craniosynostosis, these account for only 8% of cases overall and are most commonly bilateral [4, 5]. By contrast, sporadic cases account for the vast majority of coronal craniosynostosis and are typically unilateral. Interestingly, authors have identified unilateral craniosynostosis in images of Abraham Lincoln and eight other individuals from his family lineage [6] (Fig. 9.1). This is likely consistent with familial nonsyndromic cases which are shown to have an autosomal dominant pattern of inheritance [7].

Advances in the realm of genomics, specifically next-generation sequencing and molecular classification, have traced the pathology to embryonic gene dysregulation and neural crest migration/proliferation, which are discussed in more detail in Chap. 3 [8, 9]. Although numerous advancements have been made across many disciplines related to craniosynostosis over the last several decades, the clinical management begins with an accurate diagnosis. In this chapter, we will discuss the pathophysiology, clinical presentation (history and physical exam), imaging, and clinical management of unilateral coronal craniosynostosis, including indications and timing of surgery and a brief discussion of surgical techniques.

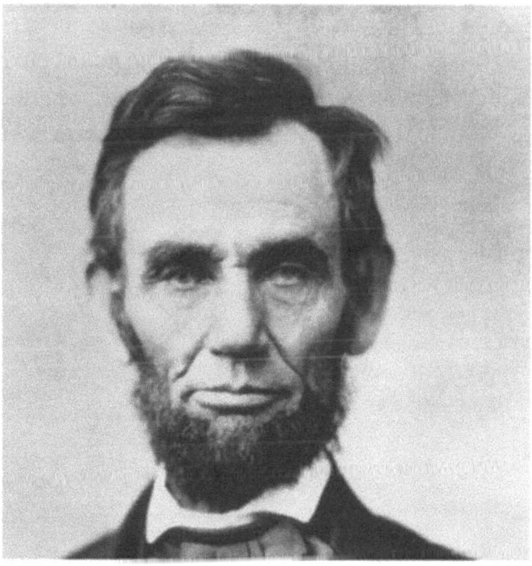

Fig. 9.1 Photo of President Abraham Lincoln demonstrating features of coronal craniosynostosis (elevation and anterior location of left ear, smaller left orbit with elevated ipsilateral eyebrow)

Y. Dastagirzada · H. Khan · S. Neifert · H. Kolb · R. C. E. Anderson (✉)
Department of Neurosurgery, NYU Langone Health, New York, NY, USA
e-mail: randerson@NEUROSURGERYNJ.COM

F. Di Rocco, J. Kestle (eds.), *Neurosurgical Aspects of Craniosynostosis*,
https://doi.org/10.1007/978-3-031-69386-1_9

9.2 Pathophysiology

The cranial vault initially serves as a capsular membrane overlying the developing brain. The process of intramembranous ossification occurs in accordance with the direction of brain growth and leads to the development of the frontal, parietal, occipital, and temporal bones that form the calvarium [10, 11]. Dural attachments strongly adhere to the cranial sutures at the sites of approximation between cranial bones. The dura mater secretes various growth factors that regulate mesenchymal stem cells and largely dictate the growth of the cranial vault. Disruptions in these signaling pathways may lead to premature fusion of the sutures and have been implicated in the pathophysiology of syndromic and nonsyndromic craniosynostosis [12, 13]. These include mutations in three of four fibroblast growth factor receptors (FGFR-1, FGFR-2, and FGFR-3), transforming growth factor-beta (TGF-B), insulin-like growth factors (IGFs), as well as the transcription factors MSX2 and TWIST1 [14–20]. Premature fusion of a suture restricts the growth of the cranial vault perpendicular to the line of the suture, with compensatory growth occurring along nonfused sutures. This phenomenon, known as Virchow's Law, leads to the stereotypical abnormal skull growth and head shape that characterize craniosynostosis, restricting the development of the growing brain [21] (Fig. 9.2).

9.3 Management

9.3.1 Diagnosis

Craniosynostosis typically occurs in utero and is visible at birth. It often becomes more evident to family and providers at one year of age, when the brain and skull growth is most rapid and the architecture of the skull is extremely malleable. In nonsyndromic/unilateral cases, the child is most often neurologically and developmentally normal.

9.3.1.1 Physical Exam Findings

The physical exam is the most important tool in the diagnosis of craniosynostosis, with up to 98% accuracy in cases of nonsyndromic craniosynostosis [22]. Unilateral coronal craniosynostosis presents with anterior plagiocephaly, ridging along the fused suture, retrusion of the lateral superior orbital rim, harlequin eye deformity, nasal root deviation, and other findings. The diagnosis can occasionally be difficult in mild cases, but careful attention to the shape of the craniofacial skeleton (forehead, ear location, orbital shape, and nose) allows for the correct diagnosis in the vast majority of cases. The primary phenotypical findings can be found in (Table 9.1) and a classic appearance of unilateral craniosynostosis from the vertex view is demonstrated in Fig. 9.3.

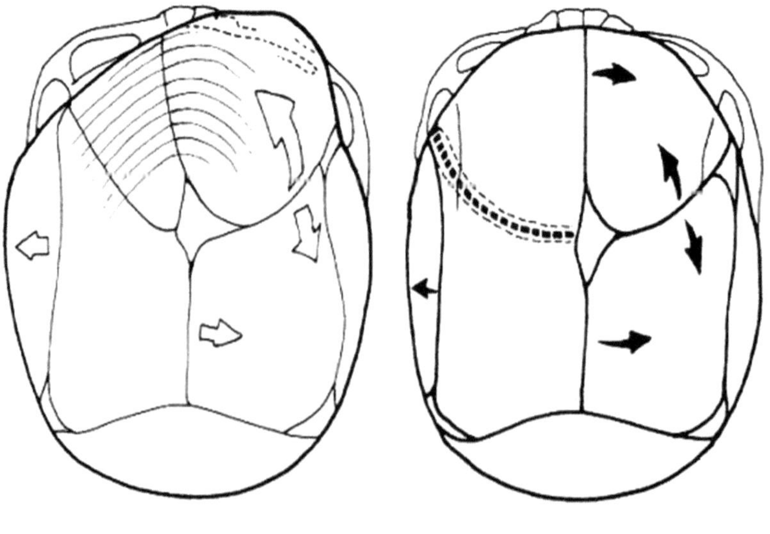

Fig. 9.2 Virchows' law explains the restriction of growth perpendicular to the line of the abnormal suture and compensatory growth along nonfused sutures

Table 9.1 Phenotypical findings of unilateral coronal craniosynostosis

Flattening/retrusion of the *ipsilatera*l forehead and compensatory *contralateral* forehead protrusion or bossing
Ridging along the *ipsilateral* coronal suture
Retrusion of the *ipsilateral* supraorbital rim
Superolateral elevation of the *ipsilateral* sphenoid wing/superior orbital margin (also known as a harlequin eye deformity, a pathognomonic finding)
Elevation of the eye on the *ipsilateral* side (vertical dystopia)
Widening of the *ipsilateral* palpebral fissure
Nasal root deviation to the *ipsilateral* side and nasal tip deviation to the *contralateral* side
Forward displacement of the *ipsilateral* ear
Deviation of the chin to the *contralateral* side

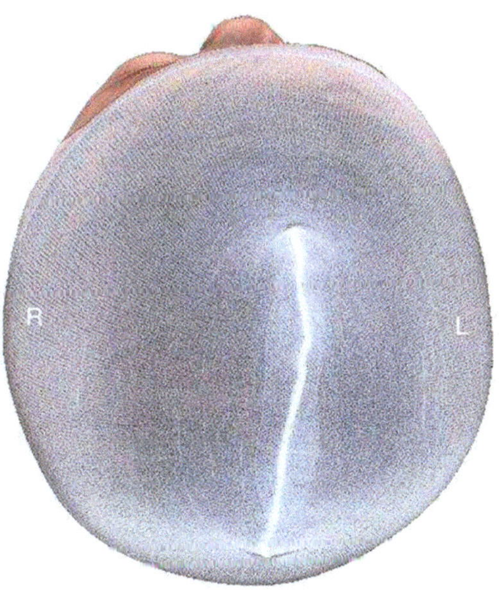

Fig. 9.3 Vertex view of a child with unilateral craniosynostosis demonstrates the classic flattening/retrusion of the ipsilateral forehead (R) with contralateral forehead protrusion (L)

Because of the proximity of the coronal suture to the skull base and its sequelae on the development of the sphenoid wing, ophthalmologic findings including strabismus and amblyopia are also common. It has been postulated that the deformed orbital shape changes the insertion of the orbital muscles and can lead to superior oblique muscle palsy and trochlea displacement [23, 24]. Many patients require ophthalmologic corrective procedures after their primary craniofacial surgery. Papilledema has been noted to be present in up to 10–15% of craniosynostosis cases (more common in syndromic cases) but rare among unilateral craniosynostosis cases [25]. In a study of 84 patients with nonsyndromic unicoronal craniosynostosis, no papilledema was detected in any case preoperatively [26].

9.3.1.2 Imaging

Plain radiographs are not commonly obtained in children with craniosynostosis because the sensitivity and specificity are low. Historic data have reported sensitivities with a range of 57–80% and specificities of 54–100% [27]. However, of all types of nonsyndromic craniosynostosis, plain radiographs are probably the most useful in UCS due to the pathognomonic finding of a harlequin eye deformity (Fig. 9.4).

Computed tomography (CT) scan with three dimensional reconstructions is the gold standard imaging study to diagnose craniosynostosis. However, when the diagnosis of UCS can be made unequivocally from the history and physical exam, CT scans are often bypassed to minimize radiation exposure in young children. There is still equipoise regarding the utility of CT scans, as some studies support its use and others do not. For instance, Ulma et al. reported that preoperative CT for patients with UCS led to changes in management for up to 48% of patients and helped with the avoidance of inadvertent complications (e.g., damage to deviated anterior superior sagittal sinus and anomalous venous drainage) [28]. However, other studies have questioned the need for CT given the high reliability of the physical exam and the low likelihood of altering the surgical plan [22].

There have been some attempts to utilize ultrasound and MRI as radiation-reducing imag-

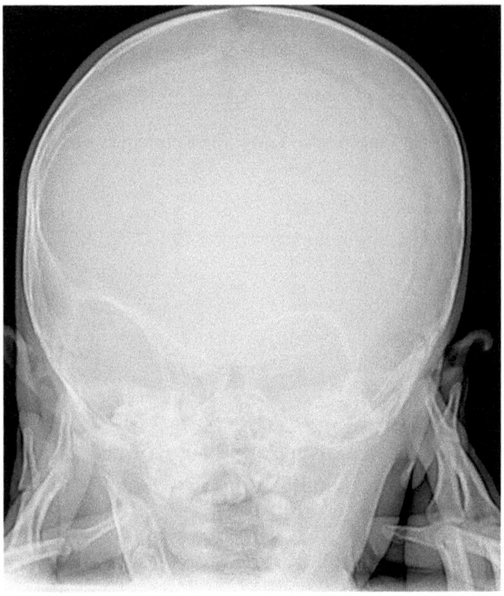

Fig. 9.4 AP radiograph demonstrates the classic Harlequin eye due to the superolateral elevation of the ipsilateral sphenoid wing/superior orbital margin

ing modalities with some promising results, although CT imaging remains the most widely used technique [7].

9.4 Treatment

9.4.1 Indications for Surgery

Surgical techniques have transformed since the first major studies addressing UCS in the 1970s. Historically, orbitofrontal advancement (OFA) has been the primary method of surgical treatment, and it is typically performed between 6 and 12 months of age. The main goals are to immediately expand the intracranial space to preclude intracranial hypertension and restore more symmetric contour to the skull, specifically the frontal/fronto-orbital bar regions [29, 30]. Secondary goals include the potential for preventing psychosocial disadvantages and improving neurological development, although these have not been demonstrated scientifically.

Over the last 20 years, endoscopic-assisted strip craniectomy followed by helmet therapy has become increasingly popular for younger patients. This technique is typically performed between 2 and 6 months of age. In contrast to an OFA, where the skull and orbital bar are removed, recontoured, and replaced, in an endoscopic craniectomy only the fused/abnormal suture is removed, thereby recreating the normal physiology of an open suture. A postoperative orthotic designed to restrict the growth of the contralateral frontal region and facilitate the expansion of the ipsilateral region is then commonly used for 9–12 months postoperatively to facilitate gradual improvement in head shape.

The optimal timing and treatment strategy for UCS remain controversial. Although rare, sequelae that can accompany untreated craniosynostosis include developmental delay, neurologic dysfunction, facial and eye abnormalities, and/or respiratory compromise. The surgical techniques for both approaches will be described in detail in the following chapters and are only briefly reviewed here.

9.4.2 Surgical Principles of Unilateral Craniosynostosis

9.4.2.1 Orbitofrontal Advancement Technique

Patients are typically positioned supine with the head on a Mayfield horseshoe headrest or gel donut. The scalp and upper face are prepped and draped in a fashion that facilitates the exposure of the brows, eyelids, and proximal aspects of the nose. Perioperative antibiotics, decadron, and mannitol are given intravenously. Recent data also support the use of tranexamic acid (TXA) in the perioperative period, with a statistically significant reduction in intraoperative blood loss and transfusion requirements, without adverse outcomes [31, 32].

A bicoronal curvilinear or zig-zag incision behind the hairline is made at the level of the mid-vertex with careful lateral extension to the frontozygomatic sutures. During the incision, the superficial temporal artery and soft tissue at the frontozygomatic suture should be preserved. The anterior flap is reflected to the level of the orbital rims, with care to preserve the supraorbital neurovascular bundle during flap dissection when possible. Exposure typically includes the nasion, supraorbital rims, anterior fontanelle, coronal sutures, and frontozygomatic sutures. Once exposure is complete, the affected and unaffected coronal sutures must be identified. The objective is to fashion and contour the bifrontal bone graft in a manner that achieves bifrontal symmetry; careful measurements of the orbital rim on the unaffected side are taken and used to contour the affected side. Depending on the magnitude of the deformity, a bifrontal craniotomy that extends posteriorly to around the normal coronal suture on the unaffected side and a similar distance on the fused side (typically 1.5–2 cm posterior to the fused suture) is subsequently performed. The orbital rim is transected around 1 cm from the supraorbital ridge to prevent fracture of the bone when the orbital bar is advanced. Several peripheral burr holes or slots are then created, including one across the midline near the anterior fontanelle and one just superior to the orbital rim, to facilitate dissection of the dura from the cranium. The dura is stripped off the bone and the bifrontal bone flap is removed in a single piece.

Removal of the orbital bar is then performed. Cottonoids are placed along the dura to gently retract the frontal lobes as the dura is dissected from the floor of the anterior fossa. The periorbita is dissected from the roof of the orbit. A high-speed drill, ultrasonic bone scalpel, or osteotome is then used to make cuts along the roof of the orbit, medially through the nasion, and laterally through the sphenoid wing to release the orbital bar in a single piece.

At this point, the remodeling and reconstruction are performed, typically together with the plastic surgery team. The orbital bar is contoured and advanced differentially to achieve orbital symmetry and increase the intracranial space, and then it is secured to the nasion and bilateral temporal bones with an absorbable plating system and sutures. The bifrontal bone flap is then divided, trimmed, contoured, replaced, and secured to the orbital bar and surrounding parietal bone. Remaining bone fragments are used to fill in any gaps and the wound is closed in layers after copious irrigation and hemostasis.

9.4.2.2 Endoscopic-Assisted Craniectomy Technique

Patients are typically positioned similarly, supine with the head on a Mayfield horseshoe headrest or gel donut. The abnormal suture is then palpated and an 8–10 mm wide craniectomy extending from the anterior fontanelle to the base of the coronal suture is mapped out and marked on the skin. As the bone thickens inferiorly into the sphenoid bone, the craniectomy is taken posteriorly behind the sphenoid down to the temporal-squamosal suture [33]. A small one-inch incision is marked longitudinally about midway along the fused suture and behind the hairline. The scalp is prepped and draped and perioperative antibiotics and decadron are given intravenously. An incision is made, and an avascular plane is developed between the galea and pericranium from the anterior fontanelle to the temporal squamosal suture using a 0° endoscope and a scalp retractor. A burr hole is then created using a small burr at the level of the incision, and the endoscope is used to dissect and strip the underlying dura from the bone. A strip craniectomy removing the fused suture as described above is then performed using the Kerrison rongeur, Jansen Middleton nasal rongeurs, and other long-handled bone rongeurs. The wound is copiously irrigated, hemostasis is achieved, and the wound is closed with absorbable sutures in the galea and skin.

Approximately 1 week postoperatively, patients are fitted for cranial molding helmets, which are generally worn for 23 hours a day and tolerated very well. Children typically require 2–3 helmets for a total duration of 9–12 months [33].

9.4.2.3 Open Versus Endoscopic Techniques: Rationale and Timing

As previously mentioned, while the optimal timing for surgical correction has not yet been clearly defined, orbitofrontal advancements for coronal craniosynostosis are generally performed between 6 and 12 months of age. This is partially because children have more favorable bone pliability until approximately 1 year of age, and fusion of the nonpathologic sutures occurs around 2 years. Endoscopic-assisted craniectomy, on the other hand, is typically performed only up to 6 months of age [34].

Early data with endoscopic techniques for coronal synostosis demonstrated benefits over open surgery with respect to ophthalmic outcomes (need for strabismus surgery) and correction of variables like vertical dystopia, nasal deviation, and sagittal imbalance [35, 36]. Postoperative cosmetic results also were comparable [37]. Furthermore, reductions in operative time, blood loss, blood transfusions, length of stay, and cost have all been demonstrated with the endoscopic approach compared to orbitofrontal advancement [37, 38]. There is sparse literature surrounding the recurrence rates among cases of unicoronal craniosynostosis treated with endoscopic or open techniques.

Complication rates for both procedures are relatively low, including dural tears, CSF leaks/pseudomeningoceles, and wound infection. Data have demonstrated no significant differences in complication rates among minimally invasive/endoscopic versus open approaches, although a trend towards decreased complication rates in endoscopic treatments has been delineated [39, 40]. The complication rate has been well described to increase in cases with multiple sutures involved [40].

Key Points for the Neurosurgeon

- Unilateral coronal craniosynostosis is the second most common form of craniosynostosis.
- Unilateral cases are almost always sporadic, while bilateral cases are frequently associated with syndromic presentations.
- Stereotypical physical examination findings include ipsilateral plagiocephaly, contralateral frontal bossing, nasal root deviation, ridging along the suture, and a harlequin eye deformity.
- Radiographic confirmation with plain radiographs or CT scans is generally performed when a definitive diagnosis cannot be made based on the physical exam.
- OFA is generally performed between 6 and 12 months of age, while endoscopic-assisted craniectomy is performed up to 5–6 months of age.
- Unlike OFA, endoscopic-assisted surgery typically requires the use of a contoured helmet for 9–12 months after surgery.
- The most common complication of surgical intervention for coronal synostosis is blood loss requiring transfusion. The overall complication rate for these surgical interventions is relatively low.

References

1. Garza RM, Khosla RK. Nonsyndromic craniosynostosis. Semin Plast Surg. 2012;26:53–63.
2. Kalantar-Hormozi H, Abbaszadeh-Kasbi A, Sharifi G, Davai NR, Kalantar-Hormozi A. Incidence of familial craniosynostosis among patients with nonsyndromic craniosynostosis. J Craniofac Surg. 2019;30:e514–7.
3. Persing JA. MOC-PS(SM) CME article: management considerations in the treatment of craniosynostosis. Plast Reconstr Surg. 2008;121(4 Suppl):1–11.
4. Jezela-Stanek A, Krajewska-Walasek M. Genetic causes of syndromic craniosynostoses. Eur J Paediatr Neurol. 2013;17:221–4.
5. Lajeunie E, Crimmins DW, Arnaud E, Renier D. Genetic considerations in nonsyndromic midline craniosynostoses: a study of twins and their families. J Neurosurg. 2005;103:353–6.
6. Fishman RS. Unilateral coronal craniosynostosis in Abraham Lincoln and his family. J Craniofac Surg. 2010;21(5):1542–6.
7. Sun PP, Persing JA. Craniosynostosis. In: Albright AL, Pollack IF, Adelson PD, editors. Principles and practice of pediatric neurosurgery. New York, NY: Thieme Medical; 1999. p. 219–42.
8. Sismets EM, Hatch NE. Cranial neural crest cells and their role in the pathogenesis of craniofacial anomalies and coronal craniosynostosis. J Devel Biol. 2020;8(18):1–27.
9. Timberlake AT, Choi J, Zaidi S, et al. Two locus inheritance of non-syndromic midline craniosynostosis via rare SMAD6 and common BMP2 alleles. ELife5. 2016;5:e20125.
10. Nah HD, Pacifici M, Gerstenfeld LC, Adams SL, Kirsch T. Transient chondrogenic phase in the intramembranous pathway during nor-mal skeletal development. J Bone Miner Res. 2000;15(3):522–33.
11. Gong SG. Cranial neural crest: migratory cell behaviour and regula-tory networks. Exp Cell Res. 2014;325(2):90–5.
12. Slater BJ, Lenton KA, Kwan MD, Gupta DM, Wan DC, Longaker MT. Cranial sutures: a brief review. Plast Reconstr Surg. 2008;121(4):170e–8.

13. Morriss-Kay GM, Wilkie AO. Growth of the normal skull vault and its alteration in craniosynostosis: insights from human genetics and experimental studies. J Anat. 2005;207(5):637–53.
14. Lattanzi W, Barba M, Di Pietro L, Boyadjiev SA. Genetic advances in craniosynostosis. Am J Med Genet A. 2017;173(5):1406–29.
15. Thaller SR, Hoyt J, Tesluk H, Holmes R. The effect of insulin growth factor-1 on calvarial sutures in a Sprague-Dawley rat. J Craniofac Surg. 1993;4(1):35–9.
16. Opperman LA, Moursi AM, Sayne JR, Wintergerst AM. Transforming growth factor-beta 3(Tgf-beta3) in a collagen gel delays fusion of the rat posterior interfrontal suture in vivo. Anat Rec. 2002;267(2):120–30.
17. Anderson PJ, Cox TC, Roscioli T, Elakis G, Smithers L, David DJ, Powell B. Somatic FGFR and TWIST mutations are not a common cause of isolated non-syndromic single suture craniosynostosis. J Craniofac Surg. 2007;18(2):312–4.
18. Paznekas WA, Cunningham ML, Howard TD, Korf BR, Lipson MH, Grix AW, Feingold M, Goldberg R, Borochowitz Z, Aleck K, Mulliken J, Yin M, Jabs EW. Genetic heterogeneity of Saethre-Chotzen syndrome, due to TWIST and FGFR mutations. Am J Hum Genet. 1998;62(6):1370–80.
19. Connerney J, Andreeva V, Leshem Y, Mercado MA, Dowell K, Yang X, Lindner V, Friesel RE, Spicer DB. Twist1 homodimers enhance FGF responsiveness of the cranial sutures and promote suture closure. Dev Biol. 2008;318(2):323–34.
20. Merrill AE, Bochukova EG, Brugger SM, Ishii M, Pilz DT, Wall SA, Lyons KM, Wilkie AO, Maxson RE Jr. Cell mixing at a neural crest-mesoderm boundary and deficient ephrin-Eph signaling in the pathogenesis of craniosynostosis. Hum Mol Genet. 2006;15(8):1319–28.
21. Virchow R. Uber den Cretinismus, namentlich in Franken, und uber pathologische Schadelformen. Verh Phys Med Gesell Wurzburg. 1851;2:230–71.
22. Fearon JA, Singh DJ, Beals SP, et al. The diagnosis and treatment of single-sutural synostoses: are computed tomographic scans necessary? Plast Reconstr Surg. 2007;120:1327–31.
23. Duan M, Skoch J, Pan BS, Shah V. Neuro-ophthalmological manifestations of craniosynostosis: current perspectives. Eye Brain. 2021;13:29–40.
24. Luo W, Chen X, Zhang Y, et al. Ophthalmological outcomes of unilateral coronal synostosis in young children. BMC Ophthalmol. 2020;20(318):1–11.
25. Tay T, Martin F, Rowe N, et al. Prevalence and causes of visual impairment in craniosynostotic syndromes. Clin Experiment Ophthalmol. 2006;34(5):434–40.
26. van de Beeten SDC, Cornelissen MJ, van Seeters RM, van Veelen MC, Versnel SL, Loudon SE, Mathijssen IMJ. Papilledema in unicoronal synostosis: a rare finding. J Neurosurg Pediatr. 2019;24(2):139–44.
27. Vannier MW, Hildebolt CF, Marsh JL, et al. Craniosynostosis: diagnostic value of three-dimensional CT reconstruction. Radiology. 1989;173(3):669–73.
28. Ulma RM, Ranganathan KL, Vercler CJ, Garton HJL, Maher CO, Muraszko KM, Buchman SR. Weighing in on the controversy: preoperative imaging in unicoronal craniosynostosis leads to strategic changes in surgical care. Plast Reconstr Surg. 2021;147(5):1133–9.
29. Guzman R, Looby JF, Schendel SA, et al. Fronto-orbital advancement using an en bloc frontal bone craniotomy. Neurosurgery. 2011;68(Suppl 1):68–74.
30. Moderie C, Govshievich A, Papay F, Fearon J, Gosain A, Doumit G. Current trends in management of nonsyndromic unilateral coronal craniosynostosis: a cross-sectional survey. Plast Reconstr Surg Glob Open. 2019;7(5):e2229.
31. Varidel A, Marucci D. Tranexamic acid in craniosynostosis surgery: a systematic review and meta-analysis. J Craniofac Surg. 2022;33(1):146–50.
32. Martin JP, Wang JS, Hanna KR, Stovall MM, Lin KY. Use of tranexamic acid in craniosynostosis surgery. Plast Surg. 2015;23(4):247–51.
33. Barone CM, Jimenez DF. Endoscopic approach to coronal craniosynostosis. Clin Plast Surg. 2004;31(3):415–22.
34. Han RH, Nguyen DC, Bruck BS, Skolnick GB, Yarbrough CK, Naidoo SD, Patel KB, Kane AA, Woo AS, Smyth MD. Characterization of complications associated with open and endoscopic craniosynostosis surgery at a single institution. J Neurosurg Pediatr. 2016;17(3):361–70.
35. Jimenez DF, Barone CM. Early treatment of coronal synostosis with endoscopy-assisted craniectomy and postoperative cranial orthosis therapy: 16-year experience. J Neurosurg Pediatr. 2013;12(3):207–19.
36. MacKinnon S, Proctor MR, Rogers GF, Meara JG, Whitecross S, Dagi LR. Improving ophthalmic outcomes in children with unilateral coronal synostosis by treatment with endoscopic strip craniectomy and helmet therapy rather than fronto-orbital advancement. J Am Assoc Pediatr Ophthalmol Strabismus. 2013;17(3):259–65.
37. Yan H, Abel TJ, Alotaibi NM, Anderson M, Niazi TN, Weil AG, et al. A systematic review of endoscopic versus open treatment of craniosynostosis. Part 2: the nonsagittal single sutures. J Neurosurg Pediatr. 2018;22(4):361–8.
38. Chan JW, Stewart CL, Stalder MW, Hilaire HS, McBride L, Moses MH. Endoscope-assisted versus open repair of craniosynostosis: a comparison of perioperative cost and risk. J Craniofac Surg. 2013;24(1):170–4.
39. Arts S, Delye H, van Lindert EJ. Intraoperative and postoperative complications in the surgical treatment of craniosynostosis: minimally invasive versus open surgical procedures. J Neurosurg Pediatr. 2018;21(2):112–8.
40. Esparza J, Hinojosa J. Complications in the surgical treatment of craniosynostosis and craniofacial syndromes: apropos of 306 transcranial procedures. Childs Nerv Syst. 2008;24:1421–30.

10 Lambdoid Sutures Synostosis: Key Points for the Neurosurgeons, Management Principles (Diagnosis, Surgical Principles and Their Rationale, Timing)

Matthieu Vinchon

10.1 Introduction

Long held as an exceptional occurrence, lambdoid synostosis (LSy) is increasingly recognized as being not so exceptional, and often a key element of a complex problem. The true prevalence of LSy has long been occulted by a large number of positional head deformations (PHD), a haystack in which just a few needles are to be found. Unlike other craniosynostoses which have a tell-tale morphology or are part of a typical syndromic association, LSy is often inconspicuous, involving the rear of the head and masked by hair, and has a protean presentation.

LSy can be either isolated, uni- or bilateral; associated with other synostoses, most notably of the sagittal suture (the aptly named "Mercedes-Benz" syndrome) [1]; or be part of an ever-increasing nebula of very rare syndromes [2].

Little is known of the pathogenesis and pathophysiology of LSy, and the diagnosis may be challenging, with some cases masquerading as tonsillar herniation, or idiopathic intracranial hypertension [2]. Because it is now acknowledged that LSy has a potential for serious complications, it has become increasingly a surgical concern. Several surgical solutions can be proposed, including craniectomy, cranioplasty, osteogenic distraction, and foramen magnum decompression. However, the indications for surgery, the choice of these different techniques, and their results are unclear. In this chapter, we shall focus on isolated LSy, uni- or bilateral, and study their pathogenesis, pathophysiology, diagnosis, and surgical management.

M. Vinchon (✉)
Service de Neurochirurgie Pédiatrique, Hôpital Femme-Mère-Enfant, Bron, France
e-mail: matthieu.vinchon@chu-lyon.fr

F. Di Rocco, J. Kestle (eds.), *Neurosurgical Aspects of Craniosynostosis*,
https://doi.org/10.1007/978-3-031-69386-1_10

10.2 Anatomy and Physiology

10.2.1 Embryology

The lambdoid suture (LSu), extending from the lambdoid to the asterion fontanelles, is the remnant of the mesodermal soft tissue after the appearance and spread of the parietal and interparietal ossification centers medially (membranous ossification), and the exo-occipital and petrous-temporal bones inferiorly (enchondral ossification) [3]. The LSu is also tightly intricated with the underlying dura mater; it thus sits at the junction between the membranous cranium and the chondrocranium, between derivatives of the mesoderm and the cranial neural crest [4].

10.2.2 Functions of the Lambdoid Suture

The most obvious function of the LSu is calvarial growth, although to which extent it contributes to the overall development, and at which period of life it is at play are unclear. The rarity of incidental findings of LSy suggests that this function is of crucial importance for the harmonious calvarial growth, and the onset of clinical manifestations during childhood and until adolescence suggests that its functions continue to be necessary late during development.

Owing to its peculiar geometry, the LSu provides calvarial growth in the three dimensions; superposition of 3D-CT scanners in LSy with an age-matched normal skull helps understand *a contrario* the function of the LSu, which enlarges the posterior calvaria following a postero-inferior vector, following a pattern similar to the growth of conch shells (Fig. 10.1).

Another, poorly documented function of the LSu is the transmission of strains from muscular contraction; studies in reptiles have shown that the sutures play a role in the repartition of strains during biting [5]. In this perspective, it may be interesting to note that the LSus are placed at the crossroads between the most powerful of craniocervical muscular systems: the sternocleidomastoid (rotation), the nuchal (craniocervical extension and head support in the erect position), and the temporal muscles (biting). These power-

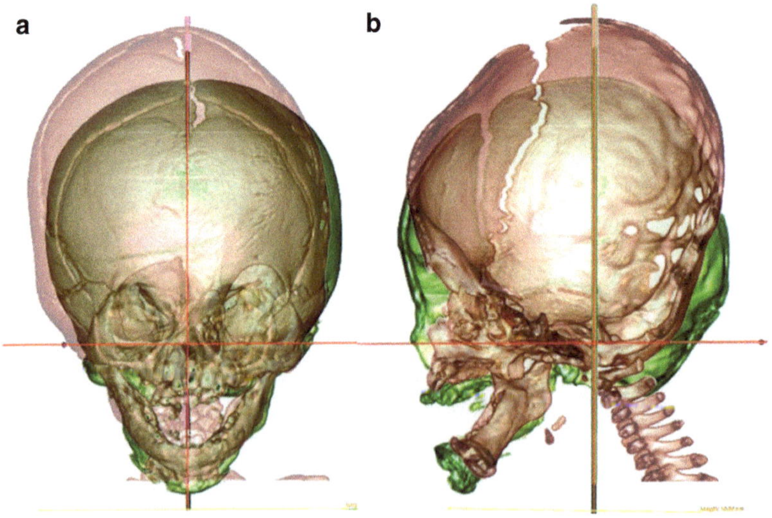

Fig. 10.1 (**a**, **b**) Vestibule-oriented CT scanner 3D CT scanners of a 5-month female, FGRF2 muted, with closure of both lambdoid and the left coronal sutures, superposed with age-matched male control (head injury), showing the pattern of deformity and compensation in bilambdoid synostosis; shaded green: growth deficit; shaded red: compensation growth. The posterior green area shows a contrario of the role of the lambdoid suture in the posterior extension of the calvaria following a postero-inferior vector. Courtesy of pr Philippe Pellerin

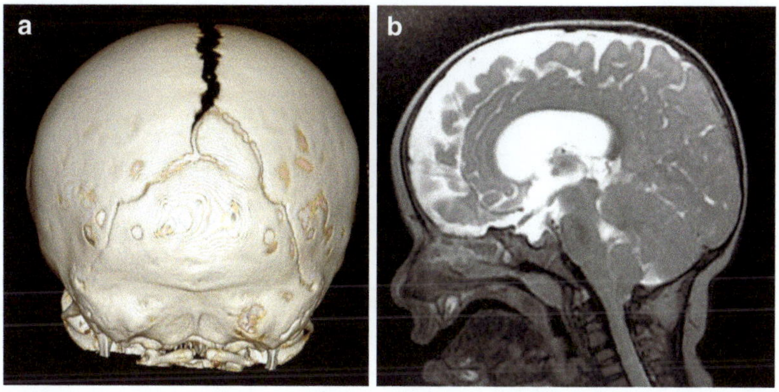

Fig. 10.2 Female infant with Crouzon syndrome caused by FGFR2 mutation. (**a**) CT scanner at 9 months showing bilambdoid synostosis, all other sutures being patent; note the epactal bone, attesting overstimulation of the lambdoid suture, and split sagittal suture, attesting raised intracranial pressure. (**b**) MRI at 9 months shows tonsillar herniation, causing severe central sleep apneas (23/h). She underwent posterior fossa decompression, aged 24 months with good results on sleep apneas

ful strains may account for the many variations in shape and number of the epactal bones developing from the lambdoid suture (Fig. 10.2a).

10.3 Pathology and Pathophysiology

10.3.1 Closure of the Lambdoid Suture

Synostosis of the LSu is a developmental condition, the timing being either pre- or postnatal. LSy can develop as an isolated craniosynostosis, or as part of a multisutural disease, or as a sporadic as well as a syndromic condition [2]. When LSy is unilateral, Shahinian and other authors have reported a right-sided predominance [2, 6], which mirrors the right-sided predominance of unicoronal synostosis. These asymmetries can be put in relation with the asymmetry of the physiological closure of the coronal and lambdoid sutures with age [7].

In multisuture synostosis, the different sutures often do not close synchronously, meaning that with time, an initially isolated LSy can become a complex, multisutural synostosis (Fig. 10.3). It is estimated that, in syndromic synostoses, in due course, LSy will develop almost constantly [8].

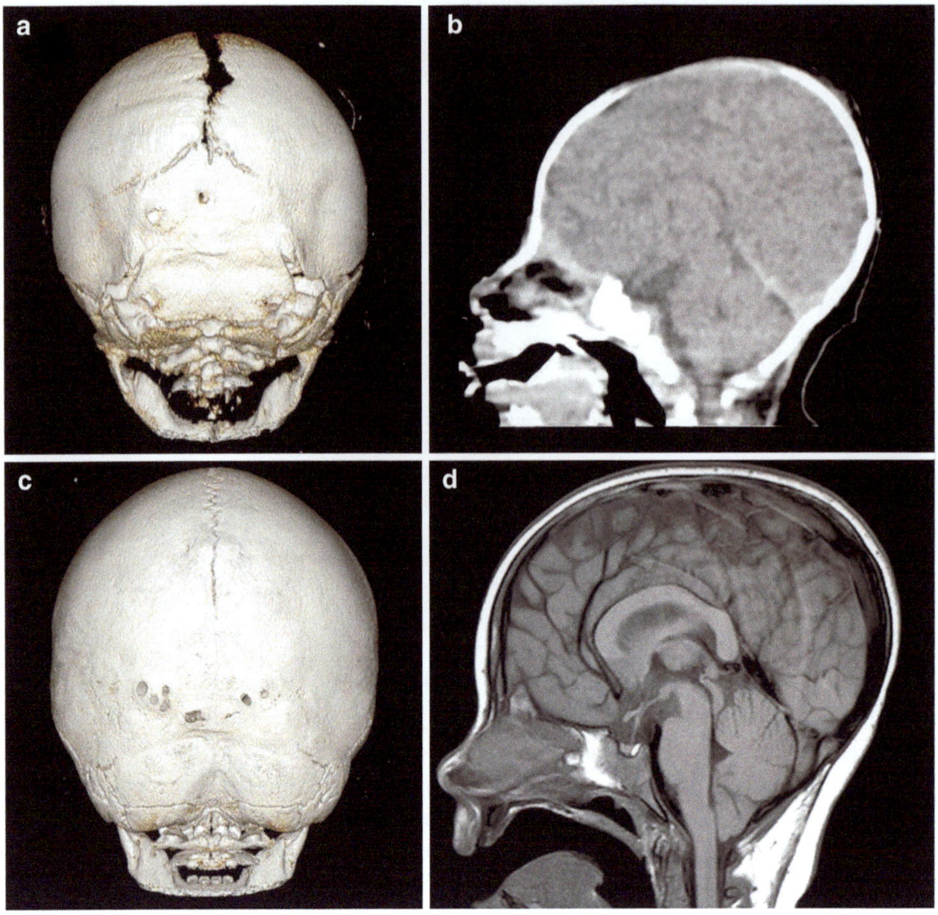

Fig. 10.3 (**a**, **b**) Newborn female, CT performed because of dystocic birth: bilambdoid synostosis with patent coronal and sagittal sutures. (**c**) CT aged 15 months: secondary closure of the sagittal sutures. (**d**) MRI, aged 4 years, showing acquired prolapse of the cerebellar tonsils. Genetic evaluation was negative

10.3.2 Determinants of the Closure

The etiologies of LSy are diverse, some being inborn genetic diseases, others possibly environmental [2]. Some authors considered that antenatal mechanical compression or traumatic birth can cause LSy [6], an attempt to bridge the conceptual gap between synostotic and positional posterior plagiocephaly [9]. However, with increasing prenatal diagnosis, it is now well known that birth difficulties are more likely the result of craniosynostosis than its cause [2]. The prenatal compression hypothesis has also lost momentum since we now know that a genetic disease is found in three-quarters of patients with LSy, although this mostly applies to LSy associated with multisuture synostosis. LSy is also often present in multisuture synostoses developing in shunted patients; however, we consider that overall, cases of acquired, non-genetic LSy are marginal.

Genetic causes of LSy are very diverse, being associated with a variety of mutations or chromosomal imbalances with gene disruption [10]. Some molecular determinants of the closure are now documented, like in a rodent model of Gli3-deficient mice, in which LSy was explained by a downregulation of Twist1, resulting in an expansion of the population of osteogenic precursors of the suture, with osteoblastic differentiation leading to a bony bridge; interestingly, this molecular disturbance could be rescued by FGF2 [11].

10.3.3 Impact on Calvarial Growth

In unilambdoid synostosis (ULSy), the local flattening on the synostotic side is compounded with compensatory bulging taking place in the contralateral LSu, the ipsilateral upper parietal squama, and the mastoid region (Fig. 10.4). The lambdoid bulge is responsible for the downward displacement of the ear lobe, while the posterior tether displaces it backward. When severe, ULSy can even impact facial morphology on account of frontal retrusion [12], with mandibular malalignment [13]. This is unlike the PHD, where the ear lobe is displaced upward and anteriorly, and some frontal advancement is often perceptible (Fig. 10.5). In addition, in ULSy, the nonsynostotic LSu is overstimulated and commonly develops several epactal bones (Fig. 10.4a). ULSy is mostly a morphological concern, and often has little or no impact on health, as attested by the long survival of a premodern human with ULSy [14].

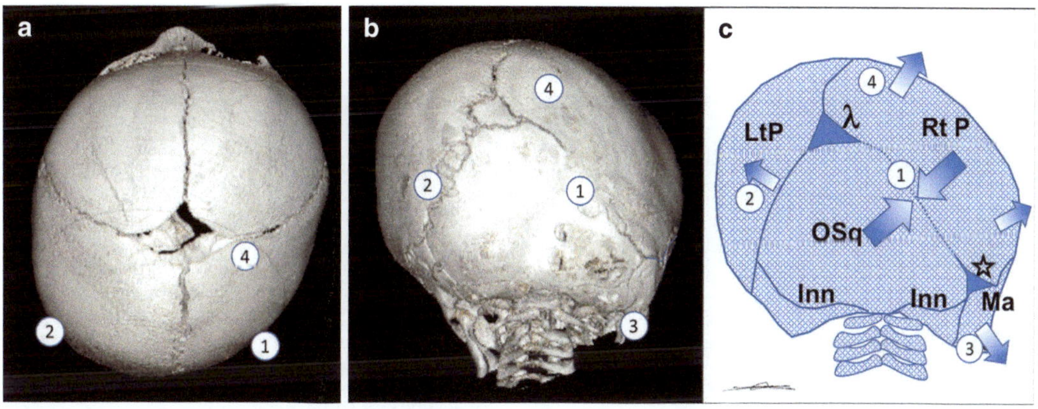

Fig. 10.4 Twelve-months male with right-sided unilambdoid synostosis, without syndromic context. (**a**) bird's eye view, (**b**) posterior inferior view, (**c**) line diagram of **b** unilambdoid synostosis causes (1) parietal flattening on the synostotic side; (2) compensatory contralateral parietal bulging (note extensive epactal bones on **b**); (3) mastoid overgrowth by stimulation of the asterion fontanel (☆); and (4) compensatory bulging near the vertex

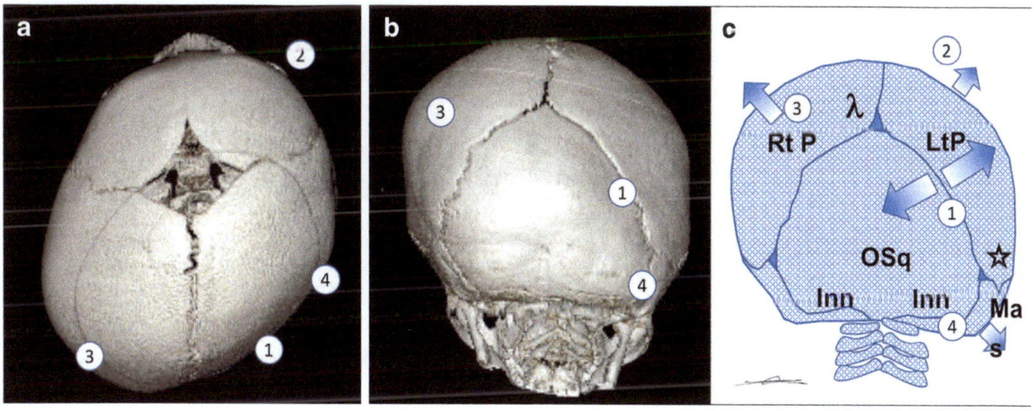

Fig. 10.5 Ten-months female with positional occipital deformation. (**a**) bird's eye view, (**b**) posterior inferior view, (**c**) line diagram of **b**. Excessive asymmetrical occipital compression causes (1) posterior flattening with overstimulation of the lambdoid; (2) ipsilateral frontal bulging; (3) contralateral parietal bulging; (4) ipsilateral mastoid advancement. *Inn* innominate suture, *LtP* left parietal bone, *Mas* mastoid, *OSq* occipital squamma, *RtP* right parietal bone

In bilambdoid synostosis (BLSy), the occiput is symmetrically flattened, the compensation growth being spread over the sagittal and coronal sutures, resulting in an overall harmonious face and forehead, with a brachycephalic tendency. Superposition of a synostotic skull with a normal age-matched control in vestibular orientation (Fig. 10.1) illustrates the pattern of malformation and compensation in BLSy [8].

Impaired calvarial growth results in intracranial hypertension, mostly in BLSy, but also in ULSy, with local bone imprinting, or holocranial intracranial hypertension.

10.3.4 Associated Lesions

Tonsillar herniation is commonly associated with all types of synostosis [15], but appears especially prevalent in LSy, in particular BLSy when it is associated with sagittal synostosis [1]. It is also prevalent in pure LSy, mostly bilateral (Figs. 10.3, 10.6, and 10.7), but also unilateral; we present an observation of ULSy with symptomatic tonsillar herniation and syringomyelia (Fig. 10.8). Tonsillar descent appears to result from intracranial hypertension due to restricted calvarial growth rather than from closure of the

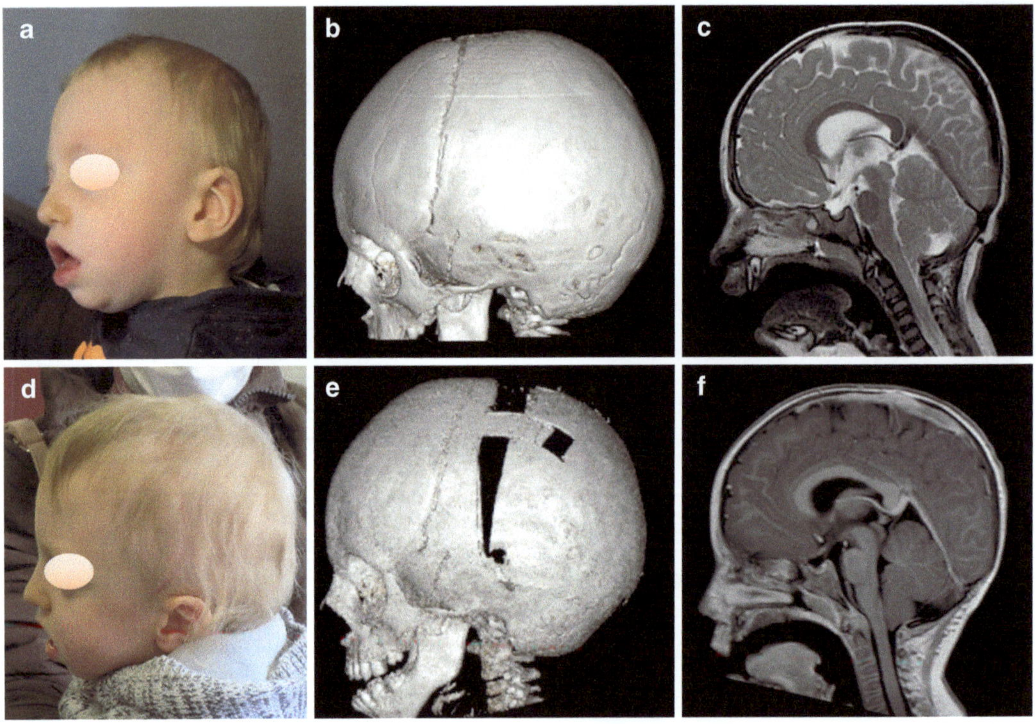

Fig. 10.6 (**a**) Twent-three-month male with Crouzon syndrome, hypotonia, papilledema stagnating head circumference, and mild faciostenosis; (**b**) CT scan shows patent coronal suture, (**c**) MRI shows tonsillar herniation. Parieto-occipital cranioplasty with bone flap rotated backward and fixated with a tongue-and-groove construct. (**d**, **e**) Postoperative morphology and CT scanner; (**f**) MRI shows partial reduction of tonsillar herniation. The patient was markedly improved neurologically. Midfacial distraction-osteogenesis is to be scheduled later on. Reprinted with permission

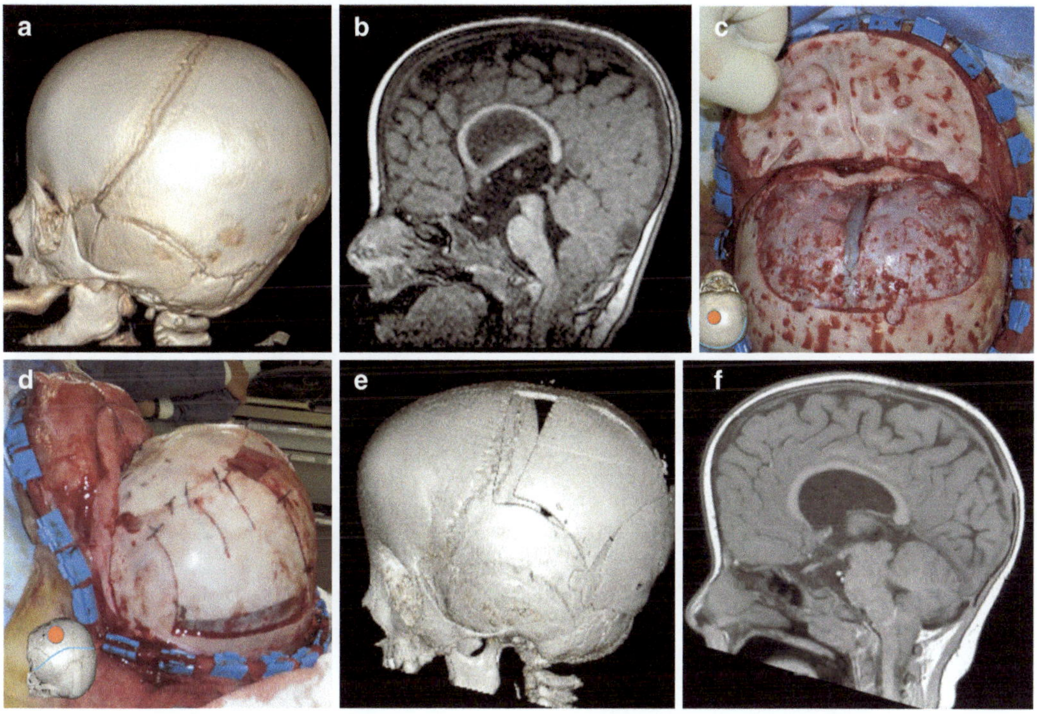

Fig. 10.7 Fourteen-month female with chromosomal rearrangement inactivating GJA5 and ELP4 genes, presenting with developmental delay, occipital flattening, head circumference −1.5 SD, CI96, and papilledema. (**a**) CT scanner shows bilateral lambdoid synostosis. (**b**) MRI shows severe tonsillar herniation with deformed medulla. We decided to perform posterior decompression. (**c**) Occipital bone flap; note the fingerprinting and embedded sagittal sinus. (**d**, **e**) Transposed occipital bone flap buttressed by the parietal fan-shaped flaps transposed following a curvilinear vector. The parietal flaps are trapezoidal, and wider at their anterior aspect, displacing them backward and spreading apart the midline crest and the temporal squamma, contributing to expanding the posterior pole. After surgery, she is feeding better and catching up on development, HC has increased to 0SD, and CI decreased to 91. (**f**) MRI shows a less crowded foramen magnum, although tonsils are still low

skullbase synchondroses [16]. Impaired venous drainage can also play a role; however, hydrocephalus is a rare feature in isolated LSy [2].

In a previous study [2], we also found that a majority of ULSy were associated with hypoplasia or agenesis of the ipsilateral transverse sinus. We also observed a patient with atretic cephalocele, who developed ULSy (Fig. 10.8). The association of anomalies of the bone, meninges end venous sinuses suggests that LSy is a regional disorder of the pericerebral tissues, rather than just a bone disorder. By contrast, the brain is generally intact and development appears normal [17], unless the LSy is part of a systemic, genetic, or chromosomal disorder.

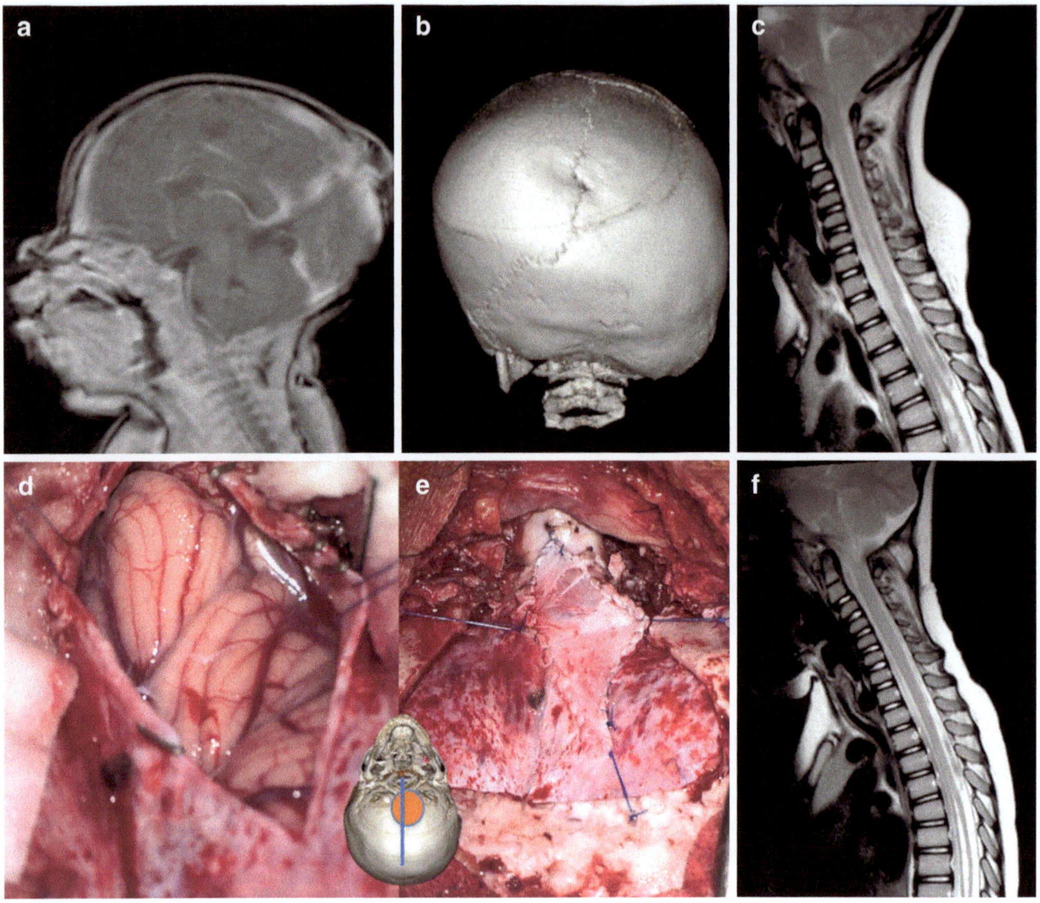

Fig. 10.8 (**a**) A female patient operated at birth for atretic cephalocele, initial MRI (T1, lateral view) shows mild tonsillar herniation without syrinx. Aged 5 years, she presents again because of increasing headache, poor sleep, and falls. (**b**) CT scanner, posterior 3D view, show right-sided unilambdoid stenosis (note that the persistent midline defect of the cephalocele is cephalad to the lambda). (**c**) MRI (T2, lateral view) shows significant occipital foramen crowding with syringomyelia. (**d, e**) we performed posterior fossa decompression (note tonsillar protrusion on dural opening) and duraplasty with periosteum. Postoperatively, she developed a mild subdural collection, which regressed spontaneously, then showed marked improvement regarding pain, walking, and sleep. (**f**) control MRI (T2, lateral view) shows good occipital decompression and regression of syrinx. This observation presents notable features: the association between atretic cephalocele, unilambdoid synostosis, and ipsilateral agenesis of transverse sinus, suggesting a regional developmental disorder; tonsillar herniation with syringomyelia showing intracranial hypertension in unilambdoid synostosis; and efficient decompression by posterior fossa approach alone

10.4 Clinical Diagnosis

10.4.1 Positive and Differential Diagnosis of Unilambdoid Synostosis

The diagnosis of ULSy is generally straightforward, made on gross asymmetrical deformation of the posterior aspect of the calvaria (Fig. 10.9) with, on the synostotic side, the ear lobe attracted backward and downward, the parietal bone elevated and no frontal swelling [18]. Facial asymmetry can be present, on account of fontal retrusion [13, 19]. Head circumference is generally normal in isolated LSy, while the cephalic index tends to be above normal values [2]. The prevalence of torticollis in this population appears to be high and may require specific management [19]. Rarely, ULSy can cause brain compression resulting in symptomatic tonsillar herniation (Fig. 10.8).

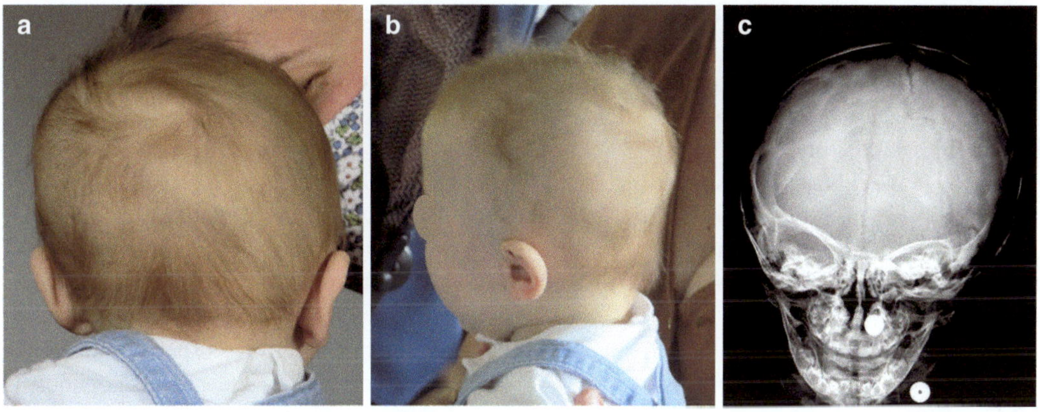

Fig. 10.9 Four months male, with marked occipital deformation; however, clinical examination could not exclude positional flattening with certainty, because of apparent flattening and ear lobe advancement on the non-synostotic side (**a**), although the lateral view shows loss of posterior volume of the calvaria (**b**). Plain X-rays (**c**) brought an unequivocal diagnosis of unilambdoid synostosis with marked imprinting of the calvaria

The main differential diagnosis of ULSy is with PHD, because of the profusion of PHD while LSy are so few, all the more since both entities have at times been considered as extremes of a continuum [9]. The confusion is often made and may have introduced some uncertainty in the medical literature: "The current evidence is difficult to navigate because of deformational plagiocephaly being misdiagnosed as unilateral lambdoid synostosis" [17]. In theory, the diagnosis of PHD is generally easy when watching from above (Fig. 10.5a) and from behind (Fig. 10.5b). However, in some cases of ULSy, compensatory excessive growth of the patent contralateral lambdoid suture can mimic PHD (Fig. 10.4); combined with the lower-set ear on the synostotic side (Fig. 10.9a), this can create confusion with PHD.

10.4.2 Positive and Differential Diagnosis of Bilambdoid Synostosis

BLSy can be more difficult to spot because of the absence of asymmetry, especially when hair is abundant. The inspection of the lateral aspect usually discloses the telltale flat occiput (Fig. 10.6a), but overall, the deformation may go unnoticed, the child does not suffer bullying at school, and his parents are often not in great demand for morphological correction. Synostotic brachycephaly is unmistakable because of its typical turricephalic appearance, with a wide, tall, and flat forehead with a major morphological impact, very much unlike BLSy. Positional nonsynostotic brachycephaly, by contrast, is associated with normal facial features and is remarkable only for the shortness of the head viewed from the lateral aspect, showing a regular parieto-occipital flattening, compensated by parietal widening [20], while in BLSy the depression sits much lower, and the parietal region is not widened (Figs. 10.3b and 10.6a).

Being a bi-sutural craniosynostosis, BLSy can cause focal or holocranial compression, and these patients are diagnosed because of signs and symptoms of tonsillar herniation or intracranial hypertension. In these cases, masquerading as Chiari malformation or pseudotumor [2], it is important to search systematically for bone anomalies, and, whenever in doubt, to complete the MRI with a CT scanner.

10.4.3 Other Clinical Findings

Other anomalies should be looked for, especially indicating a faciostenosis, as well as stigma of FGFR (Fig. 10.6), or Twist, or Twist-related mutations, in the child and his family, since many cases of LSy are syndromic. Finally, some cases of LSy, more often bilateral, are asymptomatic and diagnosed during a screening for syndromic diseases.

10.5 Explorations

In most cases, the diagnosis is made on clinical examination; in some cases, however, plain X-rays or ultrasound may be necessary to confirm the diagnosis, and differentiate ULSy from PHD (Fig. 10.9c). Preoperative evaluation requires a high-quality CT scanner, in order to analyze all the sutures, the cranio-cervical junction, locate bone lacunae, emissary veins, and encased venous sinuses, and also get preliminary information on the presence or not of hydrocephalus and tonsillar herniation. It is important to take into account the persistent sutures and epactal bones, which are points of intense adherence to the dura mater and can make surgery tricky (Cf. infra).

MRI is also necessary, in order to evaluate brain compression, hydrocephalus, tonsillar descent, and associated brain anomalies. Careful analysis of the venogram is very important, on account of venous sinus compression, encasement, and large emissary veins; moreover, hypoplasia or agenesis of a transverse sinus, which is found in a majority of ULSy, warrants special care during surgery for ULSy.

Neuro-ophthalmological examination with fundoscopy, and, whenever possible, evoked potentials and optical coherence tomography, are necessary. ICP monitoring can be discussed, especially in older children, for example, if they complain of symptoms while the fundoscopy remains normal while head circumference appears to progress along normal values. Genetic evaluation should also be proposed systematically in these patients.

10.6 Surgical Management

10.6.1 Rationale

The rationale of surgery for LSy is mostly morphological correction and cerebral decompression; functions are little if ever impacted by LSy, even when asymmetrical. Shape correction is a valid justification for surgery especially in ULS; however, morphology is often mildly impacted by this posterior deformity, especially in BLSy. Regarding morphology, the parents' opinion is thus determinant in the surgical decision.

The most imperative indication for surgery is thus decompression, which can be urgent, but is more generally slowly evolving. BLSy, like most multisutural synostoses, is likely to cause intracranial hypertension in the long run, causing visual and developmental problems, and it is generally accepted that early surgery is indicated [17], especially if imaging shows tonsillar herniation. In ULSy, as reported above, brain compression can already be present in an asymptomatic child, both local (Fig. 10.10c) and holocranial, resulting in tonsillar herniation (Fig. 10.8). However, data on visual and developmental outcomes in isolated ULSy are scant and insufficient to mandate preventive decompressive surgery. On the other hand, the evidence is a little clearer in other monosutural synostoses. As a last resort, it is a matter of clinical judgment, and most pediatric neurosurgeons will deem reasonable to perform decompressive surgery for ULS, especially in a young infant [13].

In the case of clinically eloquent or radiologically severe posterior fossa crowding, a decision has to be made regarding surgery and the choice of the approach. Both calvarial expansion and occipital foramen decompression can be indicated, depending on clinical presentation, severity of posterior fossa crowding, presence of syringomyelia, syndromic context, age of the patient, and expertise of the surgeon.

In the case of abstention, there is no consensus on the modalities of follow-up of nonoperated patients, however, the possibility of long-term decompensation and nonsynchronous closure of other sutures certainly warrants prolonged clinical and ophthalmological follow-up.

10.6.2 Surgical Techniques

10.6.2.1 Linear Craniectomy

Craniectomy is the simplest technique, and the only one practicable in very young infants, when they require emergency decompression [21]. However, this indication applies mostly to multisutural synostoses, and almost never pure LSy [22]. The aim is to free the occipital and parietal squammae by restoring sutural lines. The dissection is subgaleal in order to minimize bleeding and to avoid dural tear through bone lacunae. The fused sutures are removed piece-meal, taking great care to elevate the bone from the dura before biting in order to avoid dural tears, progressing by "tango steps" (two steps forward, one step backward). Several variants of this technique have been proposed, like direct incision along the fused LSu with a "meander-shaped" craniotomy, spread and maintained with plates [23]; or minimally invasive technique, with the use of the endoscope followed by helmet molding [24], or open technique through narrow portals, followed by helmet molding [25]. Whatever the technique, linear craniectomy is mostly indicated in young infants [13, 22], where it can be a salvage surgery; however its long-term effect may be inferior to other techniques [17].

10.6.2.2 Posterior Calvarial Remodeling

This technique, also named posterior pole reshaping, can be indicated both in ULSy and BLSy [26, 27]. In ULSy, like in unicoronal synostosis, there is no normal side, only a synostotic (flat) and a nonsynostotic (bulging) side. The simplest technique consists of a roughly quadrangular bone flap, turned 180° in order to expand the synostotic side and flatten the bulging side (Fig. 10.10). The parietal region can be reshaped with barrel-staves, using Tessier's bone-bender, in order to avoid a parieto-occipital gap, and also to redirect the thrust of the brain posteriorly in order to optimize posterior expansion (Fig. 10.10e). The risk of dural tear should not be underestimated in ULSy, because of the tight dural adhesion of the LSu on

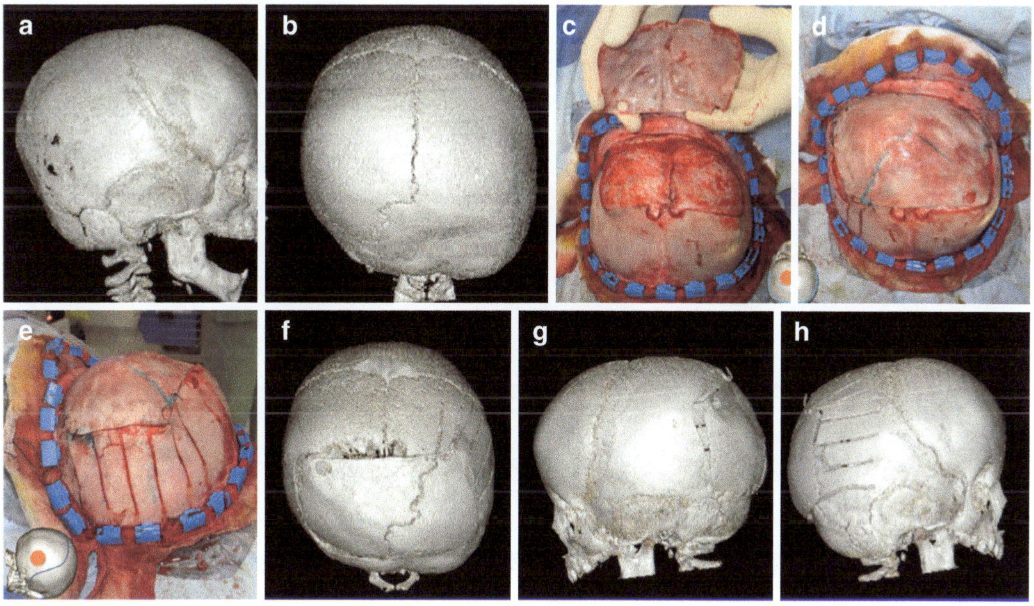

Fig. 10.10 Same patient as Fig. 10.9, operated aged 13 months, in the prone position. (**a, b**) Preoperative CT scanner. (**c**) Bilateral occipital bone flap; the inner aspect shows marked imprinting. (**d**) Bilateral occipital bone flap exposing the transverse sinuses, repositioned turned 180° and fixated with slow-resorption sutures (note the inverted situation of the persistent lambdoid). (**e**) The parietal bulge on the synostotic side is remodeled with barrel staves, shaped using Tessier bone-bender. (**f–h**) Postoperative CT scanner showing good cranial expansion with correction of the deformity

the nonsynostotic side, which is also, incidentally, the side of the hypertrophic persistent transverse sinus (Fig. 10.11).

In BLSy, we trace a tongue-and-groove craniotomy line (Fig. 10.6e) which allows to swivel the flap back along a curvilinear vector (mimicking the growth of the lambdoid, Cf. Fig. 10.1). The inferior limit of the craniotomy usually runs along or below the transverse sinus (Fig. 10.7c). A variant of this technique includes fan-shaped parietal flaps, which are used (mostly in young children) to buttress the occipital bone flap and contribute to expanding the posterior calvaria (Fig. 10.7d, e). Other authors have described a "bucket-handle" bandeau parallel to the coronal suture, inverted in order to correct unilateral flattening, and swiveled 90° in order to cover the occipital region [28]. When tonsillar herniation is present, extending the approach down the nape gives access to the occipital foramen, which can be enlarged during the same session [29]. Reliable bone flap fixation can be achieved using slow-resorption sutures and stabilizing it with sutures (Fig. 10.7d); we think the use of foreign material is unnecessary and should be minimal because it can lead to extrusion [30], which is all the more menacing in this region of the calvaria on which the child's head rests.

The main drawback of this technique is that expansion of the posterior pole is limited to 1.5–2 cm, because excessive scalp tension during closure can cause necrosis and skin breakdown [31]. Scalp expansion using subgaleal inflatable balloons in the weeks before craniotomy is an option, in order to achieve greater cranial expansion.

10.6.2.3 Distraction

Distraction osteogenesis has gained wide acceptance in the management of all types of craniosynostoses, and in particular in LSy [32]. Although the distraction period of several weeks and the need for reoperation in order to remove the hardware are a drawback, cranial expansion with distraction is especially appealing, because osteotomy is performed after subgaleal dissection, limiting blood loss, and progressive distraction can achieve considerable calvarial expansion [31], with anteroposterior diameter increase of up to 3 cm. Extending the craniotomy down to the

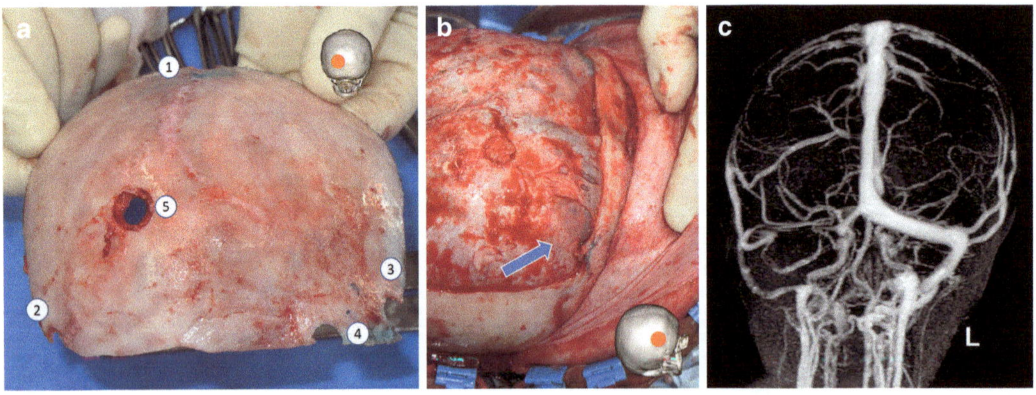

Fig. 10.11 (**a**) Multiple burr holes may be necessary in order to elevate the bone from the tight dural adhesions. Additional burr holes [4, 5] may be necessary; even so, elevation of the dura may be perilous because of additional sutures and epactal bones in the region of the lambdoid and asterion fontanelle. (**b**) Split dura due to tight adherence of the dura to the persistent suture on the left, nonsynostotic side; note the size of the left transverse sinus, in relation to agenesis on the right, synostotic side. A more complete dural tear would have created in a dire situation. (**c**) MR angiogram showing agenesis of the right transverse sinus in the same patient

foramen magnum allows the distraction to act directly on the posterior fossa crowding, rather than indirectly by reducing intracranial hypertension. The direction of the vector of distraction, descendant, or ascendant, is debated [31, 32]. Complications of distraction are a concern, mostly related to "interaction of the device with the dura, device extrusion, and infection" [33].

10.6.2.4 Foramen Magnum Decompression

When tonsillar herniation is present and causes craniocervical compression, in particular syringomyelia, occipital foramen decompression can be discussed (Fig. 10.8). We think it is indicated in older children when the LSy has otherwise a mild impact on morphology and intracranial pressure. These indications have to be balanced with the results obtained with distraction techniques. The advantages and disadvantages of posterior calvarial remodeling, craniectomy, distraction, and posterior fossa decompression are discussed in Table 10.1.

Technique: Tricks, Traps, and Pearls

- Scalp incision should be versatile, in case an anterior approach might be needed later; a bitragal incision allows both a posterior access, which can be extended to the foramen magnum, and an anterior approach down to the floor of the orbits.
- Sub-periosteal dissection incurs the risk of dural effraction on account of cranial lacunae, which require meticulous dissection.
- Subgaleal dissection is less hemorrhagic, a key factor in very young infants, and an argument in favor of distraction in older children.
- Dural adherence to persistent sutures and epactal bones in the region of the lambda and asterion fontanels incurs the risk of dural tear and lesion of an enlarged transverse sinus (Fig. 10.11).
- When elevating the midline bone flap, caution should be taken with the sagittal sinus which can be embedded.
- Emissary veins, especially posterior parietal and of the torcular, can be large and bleed a lot when the bone is stripped of its periosteum; hemostasis is obtained with wax, then, when the bone is elevated, the venous stumps can be easily coagulated.

10.7 Postoperative Follow-Up

After surgery, prolonged follow-up is necessary, because of the risk of recurrence, and also of asynchronous multisuture synostosis. Overall, the reoperation rate is evaluated between 5% and 8% [17, 27]. Functional impairment with persistent refractory torticollis can also be a concern in ULSy, with a prevalence estimated at 37% [19]. By contrast, it is estimated that LSy have no cognitive impact [17], although this has to be confirmed in long-term studies. Genetic reevaluation may become necessary by the time the child becomes adult, on account of rapid advances in this domain.

Table 10.1 Comparison of linear craniectomy, posterior calvarial reshaping, and foramen magnum decompression, regarding indications, advantages, and disadvantages

	Linear craniectomy	Posterior calvarial cranioplasty	Occipital distraction	Foramen magnun decompression
Age	Neonate, infant	>12 months	>12 months	Older child
ULS	+	++	±	±
BLS	++	++	++	+
Chiari	±	±	++	++
Syrinx	±	+	+	++
Advantage	Ultra-early surgery	One-shot	Less invasive	Less invasive
Drawback	Blood loss in young babies, Dural tear	Invasive	Ditraction, removal of distractor	Herniation if hydrocephalus

10.8 Conclusions

LSy is a complex condition which is difficult to apprehend, on account of its rare occurrence, its being easily confused with PHD, and because of its association with synostosis of other sutures, at the time of diagnosis of later in time, as well as with a dazzling variety of very rare conditions. The different techniques developed to treat the different aspects of this rare condition allow satisfactory decompression and morphological correction; however, a long follow-up is required.

References

1. Chivoret N, Arnaud E, Giraudat K, O'Brien F, Pamphile L, Meyer P, Renier D, Collet C, Di Rocco F. Bilambdoid and sagittal synostosis: report of 39 cases. Surg Neurol Int. 2018;11(9):206. https://doi.org/10.4103/sni.sni_454_17. PMID: 30386676; PMCID: PMC6194734
2. Vinchon M, Guerreschi P, Karnoub MA, Wolber A. Synostosis of the lambdoid suture: a spectrum. Childs Nerv Syst. 2021a;37:1991–2000. https://doi.org/10.1007/s00381-020-05003-9. Epub 2021 Jan 6
3. Rice DP. Developmental anatomy of craniofacial sutures. craniofacial sutures. Development, disease and treatment. Front Oral Biol. 2008;12:1–21.
4. Morriss-Kay GM, Wilkie AO. Growth of the normal skull vault and its alteration in craniosynostosis: insights from human genetics and experimental studies. J Anat. 2005;207:637–53. https://doi.org/10.1111/j.1469-7580.2005.00475.x. PMID: 16313397; PMCID: PMC1571561
5. Curtis N, Jones MEH, Evans SE, O'Higgins P, Fagan MJ. Cranial sutures work collectively to distribute strain throughout the reptile skull. J R Soc Interface. 2013;10:20130442. https://doi.org/10.1098/rsif.2013.0442.
6. Shahinian HK, Jaekle R, Suh RH, Jarrahy R, Aguilar VC, Soojian M. Obstetrical factors governing the etiopathogenesis of lambdoid synostosis. Am J Perinatol. 1998;15:281–6. https://doi.org/10.1055/s-2007-993943.
7. Zivanović S. A note on the effect of asymmetry in suture closure in mature human skulls. Am J Phys Anthropol. 1983;60:431–5. https://doi.org/10.1002/ajpa.1330600404.
8. Pellerin P, Vinchon M, Dhellemmes P, Guerreschi P. Crouzon syndrome: posterior fossa volume studies in vestibular orientation. Childs Nerv Syst. 2021;37:3105–11. https://doi.org/10.1007/s00381-021-05186-9. Epub 2021 Apr 27
9. Dias MS, Klein DM. Occipital plagiocephaly: deformation or lambdoid synostosis? II. A unifying theory regarding pathogenesis. Pediatr Neurosurg. 1996;24:69–73. https://doi.org/10.1159/000121019.
10. Hing AV, Click ES, Holder U, Seto ML, Vessey K, Gruss J, Hopper R, Cunningham ML. Bilateral lambdoid and sagittal synostosis (BLSS): a unique craniosynostosis syndrome or predictable craniofacial phenotype? Am J Med Genet A. 2009;149A:1024–32. https://doi.org/10.1002/ajmg.a.32782.
11. Rice DP, Connor EC, Veltmaat JM, Lana-Elola E, Veistinen L, Tanimoto Y, Bellusci S, Rice R. Gli3Xt-J/Xt-J mice exhibit lambdoid suture craniosynostosis which results from altered osteoprogenitor proliferation and differentiation. Hum Mol Genet. 2010;19(17):3457–67. https://doi.org/10.1093/hmg/ddq258. Epub 2010 Jun 22. PMID: 20570969; PMCID: PMC2916710
12. Smartt JM Jr, Reid RR, Singh DJ, Bartlett SP. True lambdoid craniosynostosis: long-term results of surgical and conservative therapy. Plast Reconstr Surg. 2007;120:993–1003. https://doi.org/10.1097/01.prs.0000278043.28952.e8.
13. Goodrich JT, Argamaso R. Lambdoid stenosis (posterior plagiocephaly) and craniofacial asymmetry: long-term outcomes. Childs Nerv Syst. 1996;12:720–6. https://doi.org/10.1007/BF00366157.
14. Gracia A, Martínez-Lage JF, Arsuaga JL, Martínez I, Lorenzo C, Pérez-Espejo MA. The earliest evidence of true lambdoid craniosynostosis: the case of "Benjamina", a Homo heidelbergensis child. Childs Nerv Syst. 2010;26:723–7. https://doi.org/10.1007/s00381-010-1133-y.
15. Cinalli G, Spennato P, Sainte-Rose C, Arnaud E, Aliberti F, Brunelle F, Cianciulli E, Renier D. Chiari malformation in craniosynostosis. Childs Nerv Syst. 2005;21:889–901. https://doi.org/10.1007/s00381-004-1115-z. Epub 2005 May 5
16. Calandrelli R, D'Apolito G, Panfili M, Massimi L, Caldarelli M, Colosimo C. Role of "major" and "minor" lambdoid arch sutures in posterior cranial fossa changes: mechanism of cerebellar tonsillar herniation in infants with multisutural craniosynostosis. Childs Nerv Syst. 2016;32:451–9. https://doi.org/10.1007/s00381-015-2956-3. Epub 2015 Nov 16
17. Al-Jabri T, Eccles S. Surgical correction for unilateral lambdoid synostosis: a systematic review. J Craniofac Surg. 2014;2014:1266–72. https://doi.org/10.1097/SCS.0000000000000961.
18. Haas-Lude K, Wolff M, Will B, Bender B, Krimmel M. Clinical and imaging findings in children with non-syndromic lambdoid synostosis. Eur J Pediatr. 2014;173:435–40. https://doi.org/10.1007/s00431-013-2186-1.
19. Borad V, Cordes EJ, Liljeberg KM, Sylvanus TS, Lim PK, Wood RJ. Isolated lambdoid craniosynostosis. J Craniofac Surg. 2019;30:2390–2. https://doi.org/10.1097/SCS.0000000000006058.
20. Graham JM Jr, Kreutzman J, Earl D, Halberg A, Samayoa C, Guo X. Deformational brachycephaly in supine-sleeping infants. J Pediatr. 2005;146:253–7. https://doi.org/10.1016/j.jpeds.2004.10.017.

21. Vinchon M, Guerreschi P, Karnoub MA, Wolber A. Linear craniectomy for early posterior decompression in craniosynostoses: technique and results. Childs Nerv Syst. 2021b;37:3113–8. https://doi.org/10.1007/s00381-021-05117-8. Epub 2021 Mar 13
22. Tamburrini G, Offi M, Massimi L, Frassanito P, Bianchi F. Posterior vault "free-floating" bone flap: indications, technique, advantages, and drawbacks. Childs Nerv Syst. 2021;37:3143–7. https://doi.org/10.1007/s00381-021-05281-x. Epub 2021 Jul 15. PMID: 34268594; PMCID: PMC8510901
23. Wilbrand JF, Howaldt HP, Reinges M, Christophis P. Surgical correction of lambdoid synostosis—new technique and first results. J Craniomaxillofac Surg. 2016;44:1531–5. https://doi.org/10.1016/j.jcms.2016.07.031. Epub 2016 Aug 6
24. Zubovic E, Woo AS, Skolnick GB, Naidoo SD, Smyth MD, Patel KB. Cranial Base and posterior cranial vault asymmetry after open and endoscopic repair of isolated lambdoid craniosynostosis. J Craniofac Surg. 2015;26:1568–73. https://doi.org/10.1097/SCS.0000000000001891. PMID: 26114505; PMCID: PMC4500679
25. Olshinka A, Har-Shai L, Novitski I, Lev S, Ad-El DD, Kershenovich A. Suturectomies assisted by cranial orthosis remodeling for the treatment of craniosynostosis can be performed without an endoscope. J Craniofac Surg. 2021;32:2774–8. https://doi.org/10.1097/SCS.0000000000007943.
26. Ros B, Iglesias S, Selfa A, Ruiz F, Arráez MÁ. Conventional posterior cranial vault expansion: indications and results-review of the literature. Childs Nerv Syst. 2021;37:3149–75. https://doi.org/10.1007/s00381-021-05318-1. Epub 2021 Oct 4
27. Sgouros S, Goldin JH, Hockley AD, Wake MJ. Posterior skull surgery in craniosynostosis. Childs Nerv Syst. 1996;12:727–33. https://doi.org/10.1007/BF00366158.
28. Fearon JA, Dimas V, Ditthakasem K. Lambdoid craniosynostosis: the relationship with Chiari deformations and an analysis of surgical outcomes. Plast Reconstr Surg. 2016;137:946–51. https://doi.org/10.1097/01.prs.0000480014.18541.d8.
29. Cinalli G, Chumas P, Arnaud E, Sainte-Rose C, Renier D. Occipital remodeling and suboccipital decompression in severe craniosynostosis associated with tonsillar herniation. Neurosurgery. 1998;42:66–71; discussion 71-3. https://doi.org/10.1097/00006123-199801000-00013.
30. Thaller SR, Hoyt J, Boggan J. Surgical correction of unilateral lambdoid synostosis: occipital rotation flap. J Craniofac Surg. 1992;3:12–7; discussion 18–9. https://doi.org/10.1097/00001665-199207000-00006.
31. Derderian CA, Bastidas N, Bartlett SP. Posterior cranial vault expansion using distraction osteogenesis. Childs Nerv Syst. 2012;28:1551–6. https://doi.org/10.1007/s00381-012-1802-0. Epub 2012 Aug 8
32. Komuro Y, Shimizu A, Shimoji K, Miyajima M, Arai H. Posterior cranial vault distraction osteogenesis with barrel stave osteotomy in the treatment of craniosynostosis. Neurol Med Chir (Tokyo). 2015;55:617–23. https://doi.org/10.2176/nmc.ra.2014-0401. Epub 2015 Jul 28. PMID: 26226978; PMCID: PMC4628152
33. Greives MR, Ware BW, Tian AG, Taylor JA, Pollack IF, Losee JE. Complications in posterior cranial vault distraction. Ann Plast Surg. 2016;76:211–5. https://doi.org/10.1097/SAP.0000000000000518.

11 Bilambdoid and Sagittal Craniosynostosis (BLSS)

Tilmann Schweitzer Würzburg
and Wolfgang Wagner Mainz

11.1 Introduction

Bilambdoid and sagittal (cranio-) synostosis (BLSS) is a trisutural craniosynostosis, described iconically as Mercedes-Benz syndrome or Mercedes-Benz synostosis due to the characteristic occipital bony ridges that resemble the Mercedes-Benz logo. Its incidence is reported in the range of 0.3–0.7% of all craniosynostoses [1, 2] (Fig. 11.1).

BLSS occurs as isolated type as well as a rare fusion pattern in the course of a syndromic multisutural disease—in this case with a reported incidence of 3% of the complex multisutural craniosynostoses [1]. These facts underline the need for a genetic testing in every type of craniosynostosis that includes one or both lambdoid sutures. As syndromal pansynostoses are described elsewhere, this chapter focuses on the isolated form and its specific management.

This chapter conveys the general information but also reasonable diagnostic steps as well as management strategies be it surgical or important follow-ups.

11.2 Key Points for the Neurosurgeon

Historically Moore et al. employed the descriptive term "Mercedes-Benz syndrome" in 1998 [3]. However, this specific fusion pattern was already described earlier and named "craniofacial dyssynostosis" by Neuhäuser et al. in 1976.

Isolated BLSS is a rare entity of a trisutural craniosynostosis that mainly affects males (4:1). If the lambdoid suture is part of the craniosynostotic pattern, a syndromic context should always be excluded. Even if intracranial abnormalities are rare in isolated BLSS the shortage of space in the posterior fossa might cause a Chiari malformation. Reports on minor mental delays exist, although most of the patients develop within normal limits.

T. S. Würzburg (✉)
Pediatric Neurosurgery, Center for Craniofacial Malformations, University Clinic of Neurosurgery, Würzburg, Germany
e-mail: Schweitzer_T@ukw.de

W. W. Mainz
Pediatric Neurosurgery, University Clinic of Neurosurgery, Mainz, Germany

F. Di Rocco, J. Kestle (eds.), *Neurosurgical Aspects of Craniosynostosis*,
https://doi.org/10.1007/978-3-031-69386-1_11

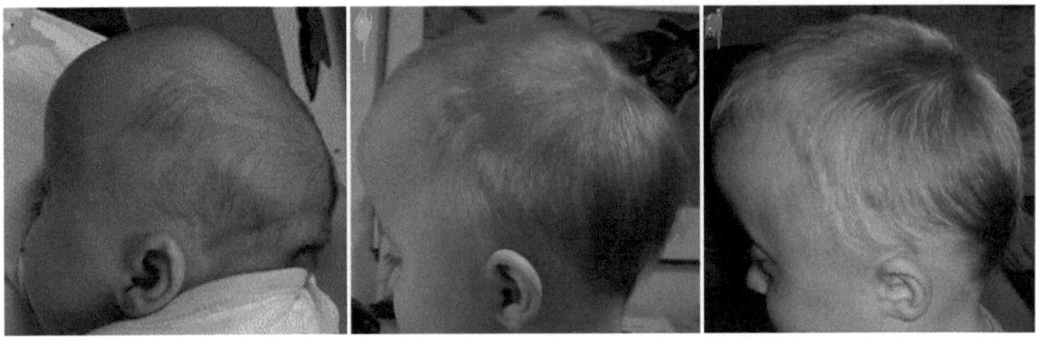

Fig. 11.1 Lateral photographs and mid-sagittal MR of a baby with BLSS. Typical head shape before surgery (left) at the age of 19 months (middle) and 1.5 years (right) postoperatively (W. Wagner)

11.3 Diagnosis

Moore et al. described morphology with a narrow posterior cranial vault, a frontal bossing and posteriorly angulated, patent coronal sutures [3]. The head shape in BLSS is described as anterior turricephaly with mild brachycephaly [4]. In a series of 31 isolated cases of BLSS, Chivoret et al. describe a flat occiput in more than 70%. Nevertheless, the authors distinguish between over 70% with a so-termed "short BLSS," with narrow occiput and almost 30% of a "long BLSS" with dolichocephaly and occipital bossing [5]. A sudden angulation of the occipital skull might resemble a scythe's cut and is therefore described as "coup de serpe" [4]. As both lambdoid sutures are involved the ears appear symmetric but low set.

For diagnosis, the abnormal head shape is suspicious for further investigation. Palpable bony ridges are often a clear hint for synostosis, while involuted sutures usually appear in positional skull deformations. Within the first year of life an ultrasound examination helps to differentiate between patent and fused sutures [6]. If the situation remains unclear, plain skull radiographs with lacking patency or reduced serration of the fused sutures will help to set up a proper diagnosis [7]. These radiographs will also help to depict digital impressions, suggestive of elevated intracranial pressure. However, some experience is needed to differentiate these digital impressions from signs of bone immaturity. A CT scan will clearly demonstrate fused sutures unfortunately; however, it is associated with radiation exposure and possible malignancies, especially in the very young [8–10]. Although some authors strongly recommend a preoperative CT scan in order to detect possible bony defects from previous operations or caused by emissary veins, we are persuaded that any indication for CT diagnostics should be very strict. The argument of a possible intracranial or vascular abnormality justifies an MRI with MRangiography [11]. By combining plain skull radiographs and an MRI with MRangiography, our group gets the same information with far less radiation exposure. Advances in MRI techniques (ultra-fast sequence MR, black bone MRI) with better illustration or depiction of bony structures will help to optimize these strategies.

The premature fusion of both lambdoid sutures restricts the space in the posterior fossa, possibly causing a tonsillar herniation with its sequelae. This fact as well as the association with brain anomalies is not yet diagnosed complex craniosynostoses justify an MRI. As the altered posterior fossa might also cause a pathologic venous drainage pattern, this MRI should include an MRangiography, depicting not only the arterial supply but also the venous drainage above the jugular foramen. A second MRI at the age of 4–6 years serves to rule out a secondary tonsillar herniation (which might develop during the first

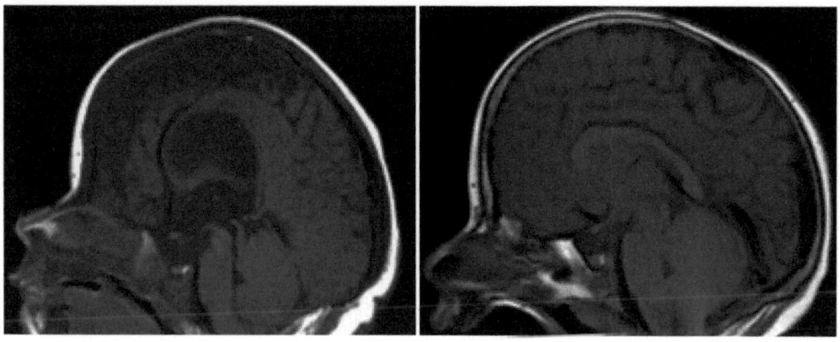

Fig. 11.2 MR before surgery at the age of 3.5 months and 2 years after surgery (W. Wagner)

years of life) or its evolution as well as to judge hydrocephalus, possible syrinx development or any other specific brain abnormalities and should therefore be part of the strategy (Fig. 11.2).

Tonsillar herniation is reported in almost two-thirds of the patients. However, symptomatic cases are rare [4, 5]. The cerebellar tonsillar herniation and its impairment of the CSF outflow might lead to dilated ventricles/hydrocephalus and entail a discussion on subsequent foramen magnum decompression.

Major advances in genetic diagnostics have and will continuously close our knowledge-gap and enable us to characterize more and more mutations and associated phenotypes of craniosynostoses [12].

11.4 Surgical Principles and General Considerations

It is not useful to present a timetable including the different surgical therapies, as the distinctive options should not follow a general algorithm but should be based upon individual decisions considering the individual combination of problems. Especially the premature fusion of the lambdoid sutures, frequently associated with restricted space in the posterior fossa hosting the brain stem, medulla and cerebellum calls for individual and thorough strategies of care. This includes consideration of the possible problems arising from the structures in the posterior fossa or from impaired CSF-circulation but also esthetic topics. Although not automatically required in every case of BLSS, surgery might become an issue. Goals of a surgical intervention therefore consist of increasing intracranial volume and consecutive lowering of elevated ICP, improving a possible tonsillar herniation and its sequelae and/or correcting a striking deformity. Different principles have to be taken into account.

The positioning of the child depends on the strategy and goals. While most procedures addressing the lambdoid suture and the direction toward the foramen magnum are performed in prone position, some strategies allow either prone or supine positioning, which is mentioned in the specific paragraph.

Pre- as well as intraoperatively marking of the sagittal and both transverse sinuses both at skin and at the surface of the skull by using a neuronavigation device will help to prevent life-threatening sinus injuries.

The dural matrix is the decisive matrix for bone formation. Therefore, the surgeon should meticulously take great care of the dural layer, which should always be kept moist. The use of bipolars on the dura should be restricted to short and punctual usage if ever. Noteworthy the reossification will also restore the pre-existing fusion status of the sutures of a BLSS—a fact that should be remembered in every treatment strategy.

The reduced intracranial volume and an existing deformation as well as the explicit surgeon's experience will strongly influence the choice of the technique. Another aspect is the needed extent of intracranial volume gain. Nowinski et al. analyzed different expansion techniques in respect to achievable volume gain with the distraction osteogenesis (see below) being superior to the rest [13].

11.4.1 Different Surgical Strategies Exist

11.4.1.1 Posterior Decompression

Due to the very potent osteoplasticity of the dural layer in the first 7–8 months of life, a pure parieto-occipital decompression is a possible first strategy.

A curved incision posterior to the coronal suture, periosteal dissection and bone removal after meticulous dissection between internal lamina and dural layer through burr holes is performed. The sagittal synostosis might be addressed by an enlarged median craniectomy in the same intervention—surgery in this case might also be performed in supine position.

In case of dilated ventricles or even hydrocephalus, it can be discussed to address this circumstance after the primary decompression: the dilated ventricles might serve as a biological expander in order to enlarge the skull size in between the relatively “short” time span of 8–10 weeks until reossification takes place. If still needed, the correction of disturbed CSF flow can be addressed another 3 months later after renewed diagnostics.

A free-floating parieto-occipital cranial vault release uses a craniotomy in front of both lambdoid sutures leading either to the lambdoid suture or even downwards under the torcula to the foramen magnum. Intrinsic brain growth then is the driving force for gradual occipital displacement of the free-floating bone flap [13].

In case of an associated Chiari malformation, one might even perform an enlargement of the decompression downwards to the direction of the foramen magnum. Due to the large sinus as well as the general hemorrhagic situation in those young infants, a foramen magnum decompression is not a suitable strategy. As the key issue of surgery consists of posterior or even occipital cranial vault release, a patient is usually placed in prone or semi-sitting position.

11.4.1.2 Occipito-Parietal Remodeling

An active repositioning is an option in children older than 12 months. Positioning may be either prone or supine, depending on the surgical planning. Bicoronal curved skin incision, periosteal dissection, burr holes and dissection between dural and internal bony lamina are performed. The surgeon must be aware of tight dural adhesions especially at the site of the fused sutures. Especially in syndromic children deeply embedded bony spiculae on the inner surface need attention and meticulous preparation. Our center usually uses the fixed posterior cranial vault expansion as described by Di Rocco and colleagues [14]. A parietal coronal bone strip with a width of 1.5–5 cm is mobilized, tilted and newly fixated at the occipital bone rim. This bony bandeau, enabling stable overcorrection and harmonization of existing asymmetries, serves as basis in order to fix and rebuild the occipital bone segments. Depending on the operative strategy, defined parietal and occipital osteotomies are drawn and a whole posterior calvarial bone flap is removed. This bone flap might reach up to or even beyond the transverse sinus. The occipital bone flap may be rotated and/or provided with additional barrel-stave incisions for further remodeling [14]. For fixation of bone segments resorbable plates, titanium plates or resorbable sutures may be deployed [15]. Titanium plates have to be removed in a further surgery to prevent transosseus migration. The authors held resorbable sutures for a very good option, as they enable stable fixation at very low costs without another surgery.

Wagner and colleagues describe a very suitable technique for posterior calvarial augmentation by creating intersecting calvarial tongues through a meander-shaped craniotomy followed by subsequent distraction. Fixating resorbable sutures (Vicryl 2.0) substitute plates and screws Fig. 11.3 [16].

Modifications of this technique describe intersecting tongues perpendicular to the sagittal sinus with the basis of these intersecting tongues shifted to the side, where more expansion is needed. This approach enables asymmetric elevation of the calvarium in order to address an asymmetrical occipital skull shape [17].

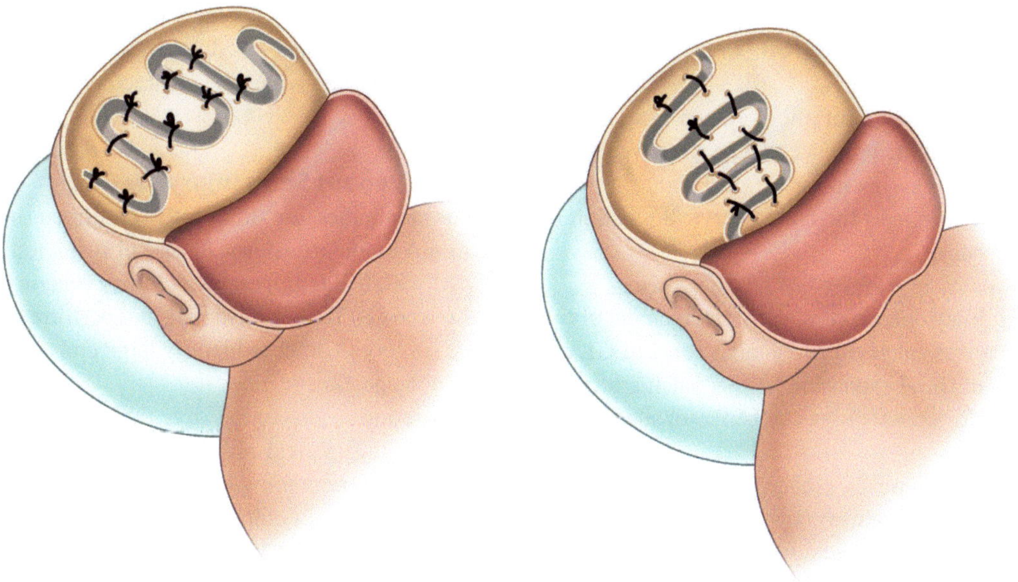

Fig. 11.3 Schematic drawings of the intersecting tongues for calvarial augmentation [16, 17]

11.4.2 Posterior Skull Distraction

A parieto-occipital remodeling enables a significant enlargement mainly in the sagittal plane. For craniotomy a supratorcular, an infratorcular as well as a combined supra- and infratorcular craniotomy may be applied. Special care has to be taken above the sagittal and both transverse sinuses—these regions being separated last—if necessary even using a piezoelectric drill. Distraction osteogenesis is supported by external or internal distractors or is spring assisted. All these distractors need a second surgery for removal of the implanted devices. As the distraction period bears possible risks of infection, regular and close controls of the entry points of the distractors are recommended. Our group usually uses one distractor on each side and another close to the vertex in order to be able to correct asymmetrics by modulating and adjusting distraction "speed" on each side individually. After active distraction of 0.5–1 mm per day for 2–4 (6) weeks, distractors are removed after another 6-week period without any further active distraction. A possible decompressive effect on a Chiari malformation is reported by McMillan et al., who described improvements of a Chiari situation after posterior calvarial distraction in several cases [18].

Preoperative printing of individual 3D-skull-prototypes for planning of the osteotomy lines, the optimal trajectories and suitable distraction devices can be helpful. Distractors itself should have the right size to pass the osteotomy line, set at the right position for the planned trajectory with its activation arms as close as possible to the skull.

11.4.2.1 Endoscopic Suturectomy

An endoscopically assisted suturectomy may be performed, especially if the dolichocephalic aspect is not too prominent. Surgery is performed at 3–4 months of age. Patient is placed in prone position. Burr holes are placed at the former small fontanelle and at each side in the course of both lambdoid sutures. Although this approach is reported to have decreased time of surgery and less blood transfusion rates, the result is more often suboptimal. Due to the early time of surgery reclosure and relapse of the abnormal head shape appears frequently no matter, whether an additional external orthosis was employed or not [19].

11.4.3 Foramen Magnum Decompression

A decompression of the foramen magnum is advisable in the presence of a progressive hydrocephalus or syrinx in the cervical spine. We plan decompression of the cranio-cervical junction in three steps:

First: Bony decompression by enlargement of the foramen magnum and laminectomy of C1.
Second: Dural expansion (with a patch graft).
Third: Resection of the cerebellar tonsils.

The decision to proceed to the next step is made intraoperatively by ultrasound examination. Even if a plastic dural expansion surgery is performed a recurrence of the bony compression can occur, especially if surgery was performed very early. Therefore, an additional MRI should be planned [20].

11.4.3.1 Complications of Surgery

Dural Lacerations

In contrast to syndromic synostosis, where the surgeon might encounter dysplastic areas as signs of bone immaturity with bony spiculae extending deep into the sulci, the isolated types usually only demonstrate areas of digital impressions if associated with reduced intracranial volume. Careful preparation is indeed mandatory, as dural lacerations may occur anyway. In these cases, the surgeon should try to achieve a watertight dural closure, in order to repair the CSF space and preserve the dural layer as supplying matrix for the bone and sutures.

Infection

For surgery, we generally recommend an antibiotic prophylaxis, according to the hospitals' strategy. Commonly used precautions for general wound care are self-understood, especially in those cases where distractors are used.

We experienced one case of relevant superficial infection at an external distractor entry point at the skull after a posterior skull distraction. Meticulous wound care and regular blood samples prevented an abortion and removal of the devices before planned schedule. We recommend regular follow-up, while the distractors are in situ.

11.4.3.2 Venous Sinus Injury

Venous anomalies are frequently described in syndromic craniosynostosis. In case of suspicion, an MRI with MRangiography including imaging of the venous drainage should be performed before surgery in order to identify large emissary veins in the galea.

Preparation or dissection over the sagittal or transverse sinus should always be the last step, after the other craniotomy lines have been set, in order to be able to compress the sinus directly and take care for the bleeding. Knowledge of pathologic venous drainage and emissary veins through the galea are obvious requirements before starting any surgery.

11.5 General Strategy

As BLSS is a multisutural condition that might lead to elevated intracranial pressure, a strategic follow-up is mandatory. Although problems usually arise only after some time, it is crucial to realize a possible development early enough to define a specific (surgical) strategy. The follow-up should assess the changing dynamics of brain growth, therefore an ophthalmologic surveillance every 6 months seems reasonable as well as annual clinical follow-ups in the first 6 years of life, then every 2 years until the age of 12, when brain tissue stops to grow.

In case of clinical suspicion of a BLSS, ultrasound clarifies suture status and excludes striking intracranial abnormalities. Additional plain skull radiographs confirm the suture status as well as depict digital impressions as possible signs of elevated intracranial pressure. An MRI will depict a cerebellar tonsillar herniation and possible CSF-circulation problems due to an outflow restriction inside the posterior fossa. In order to detect an altered venous drainage and pathologic emissary veins, an additional MRangiography (including imaging of the venous drainage above jugular foramen level) in the first 6 months of life is highly recommended. In contrast to existing recommendations, a CT scan is avoidable in many cases [21].

Independent of performed surgical therapies ophthalmoscopic surveillance every 6 months to rule out papillary edema should be routinely planned in the first 12 years. Regular follow-ups every year for the first 4 years and every 2–3 years until 12 years of life seem reasonable.

At these outpatient clinic appointments, plain skull radiographs in lateral projection should be performed to rule out possible signs of elevated intracranial pressure. Routine imaging surveillance must include a second MRI during the first 4 years of life.

A cranio-facial center and expertise should include an experienced pediatric neurosurgeon, a cranio-maxillo-facial surgeon, a (neuro-) pediatrician, an ophthalmologist (at the center as well as at home), a sensible and reliable radiological work-up and experienced specialists (such as pediatric anesthesiology and ICU teams) in case of surgery.

References

1. Sloan GM, et al. Surgical treatment of craniosynostosis: outcome analysis of 250 consecutive patients. Pediatrics. 1997;100(1):E2.
2. Chumas PD, et al. Classification of previously unclassified cases of craniosynostosis. J Neurosurg. 1997;86(2):177–81.
3. Moore MH, et al. Bilambdoid and posterior sagittal synostosis: the Mercedes Benz syndrome. J Craniofac Surg. 1998;9(5):417–22.
4. Balestrino A, et al. Pure bilateral lambdoid and posterior sagittal synostosis (Mercedes-Benz syndrome): case report and literature review. World Neurosurg. 2019;128:77–82.
5. Chivoret N, et al. Bilambdoid and sagittal synostosis: report of 39 cases. Surg Neurol Int. 2018;9:206.
6. Regelsberger J, et al. Ultrasound in the diagnosis of craniosynostosis. J Craniofac Surg. 2006;17(4):623–5; discussion 626–8
7. Schweitzer T, et al. Diagnostic features of prematurely fused cranial sutures on plain skull X-rays. Childs Nerv Syst. 2015;31(11):2071–80.
8. Pearce MS, et al. Radiation exposure from CT scans in childhood and subsequent risk of leukaemia and brain tumours: a retrospective cohort study. Lancet. 2012;380(9840):499–505.
9. Berrington de Gonzalez A, et al. Relationship between paediatric CT scans and subsequent risk of leukaemia and brain tumours: assessment of the impact of underlying conditions. Br J Cancer. 2016;114(4):388–94.
10. Miglioretti DL, et al. The use of computed tomography in pediatrics and the associated radiation exposure and estimated cancer risk. JAMA Pediatr. 2013;167(8):700–7.
11. Salokorpi N, et al. Posterior vault distraction technique: how I do it. Childs Nerv Syst. 2021;37(10):3127–36.
12. Fitzpatrick DR. Filling in the gaps in cranial suture biology. Nat Genet. 2013;45(3):231–2.
13. Nowinski D, et al. Posterior cranial vault expansion in the treatment of craniosynostosis. Comparison of current techniques. Childs Nerv Syst. 2012;28(9):1537–44.
14. Di Rocco F, et al. Fixed posterior cranial vault expansion technique. Childs Nerv Syst. 2021;37(10):3137–41.
15. Linz C, et al. Stable fixation with absorbable sutures in craniofacial surgery. J Craniomaxillofac Surg. 2016;44(5):622–5.
16. Wagner W, et al. Posterior calvarial augmentation in premature craniosynostosis: a technique avoiding foreign implants or free bone flaps. Childs Nerv Syst. 2010;26(11):1549–53.
17. Schulz M, et al. Results of posterior cranial vault remodeling for plagiocephaly and brachycephaly by the meander technique. Childs Nerv Syst. 2014;30(9):1517–26.
18. McMillan K, et al. Experiences in performing posterior calvarial distraction. J Craniofac Surg. 2017;28(3):664–9.
19. Reardon T, et al. Management of Lambdoid Craniosynostosis: a comprehensive and systematic review. Pediatr Neurosurg. 2021;57:1–16.
20. Linz C, et al. Occipital plagiocephaly: unilateral lambdoid synostosis versus positional plagiocephaly. Arch Dis Child. 2015;100(2):152–7.
21. Schweitzer T, et al. Avoiding CT scans in children with single-suture craniosynostosis. Childs Nerv Syst. 2012;28(7):1077–82.

12 Oxycephaly

José Hinojosa Mena-Bernal
and María Victoria Becerra Castro

12.1 Introduction and Definitions

Isolated oxycephaly (from Greek ὀξύς, "sharp, pointed") is a late-appearing form of non syndromic craniosynostosis characterized by premature fusion of both the coronal and sagittal sutures, and, in some cases, of one or both lambdoid sutures [1–4].

Its prevalence and etiology are unknown, and it is not usually congenital as isolated oxycephaly is never diagnosed at birth [2].

Compensating growth in the anterior fontanel region results in the formation of a pointed or cone-shaped skull. In oxycephaly, the sagittal suture is typically fused, and lambdoid sutures may or may not be involved. The continuation of the coronal suture into the cranial base (i.e., the sphenofrontal suture) may be also prematurely fused, while the synchondroses of the cranial base appear to be normal. Sutures of the orbit and the maxillary complex are typically not involved or fused [3].

Isolated oxycephaly is often unrecognized because of its late onset, but it is responsible for insidious intracranial hypertension (ICH), with loss of visual acuity that can lead to blindness, headaches, and cognitive delay if not treated on time.

Described since antiquity and often confused with brachycephaly or other multisuture craniosynostoses, the term oxycephaly was initially coined by Graig [3, 5], although Galen had already used the term *oxycephalus* for a head in the shape of a tower [6, 7]. According to Shimoji, Graig would have considered acrocephaly a misnomer and *tower-skull*, harsh and inelegant [3, 5]. The terms acrocephaly and oxycephaly have been used interchangeably although inconsistently in the past. For some authors, oxycephaly refers to the premature fusions of all the sutures; for others, these terms are used to mean stenosis of the coronal plus one other suture [8–11]. A relative consensus has been reached to accept the term oxycephaly for a premature synostosis of both coronal and sagittal sutures [3, 4, 10, 12, 13] and *isolated* oxycephaly, when this condition occurs without a concurrent craniofacial syndrome, such as Crouzon or Pfeiffer. In literature, related synonyms such as hypsi- or hypsocephaly (gr. ὕψος height, top), pyrgocephaly (gr. Πύργος, tower), or turricephaly may be found.

In this chapter, we will address isolated oxycephaly as a non-syndromic form of late craniosynostosis characterized by the premature fusion of coronal and sagittal sutures.

J. H. Mena-Bernal (✉) · M. V. B. Castro
Department for Neurosurgery, Hospital Sant Joan de Déu, Barcelona, Spain
e-mail: jose.hinojosa@sjd.es; jhinojosa@sjdhospitalbarcelona.org; mariavictoria.becerra@sjd.es

F. Di Rocco, J. Kestle (eds.), *Neurosurgical Aspects of Craniosynostosis*,
https://doi.org/10.1007/978-3-031-69386-1_12

12.2 Oxycephaly in History and Arts

Craniosynostoses have been known since ancient times. In the past, identification of two pre-Columbian skulls with scaphocephaly (dated between 6000 and 250 BC) due to early synostosis of the sagittal suture [14], confirm that craniosynostoses have accompanied human beings since the beginning of time. The Egyptian pharaoh Tutankhamun and his father Amenophis IV were depicted with a dolichocephalic skull, and it is believed that the pharaoh Akhenaten may have suffered from craniosynostosis [15, 16]. The ancient gods of good fortune and long life in traditional Eastern culture, Fukurokuju and Shou Lao were depicted with domed heads with high and wide foreheads [5, 17] as a sign of intelligence and superiority.

Perhaps the first literary reference to a craniosynostosis in the form of an oxycephaly is that of Thersites, in the Iliad, whose behavior—he opposed the right of the Achaean nobles to receive all the spoils of war—was criticized by Homer (Iliad, book II, CCXV) [18]. The poet mocks the "erroneous" (ignoble) attitude of Thersites –which could be explained by a cognitive delay in the context of a craniofacial syndrome—with a bitter description of his physical defects: "the most horrendous man–*aiskistos*—that the walls saw from Troy... he was cross-eyed and lame in one foot; his hunched shoulders sank against his chest, and his head was pointed and covered in sparse hair. Achilles and Odysseus hated him alike...."

Vulgar, obscene, and somewhat dull witted, Thersites disrupts the rallying of the Greek army:

> *He got up in the assembly and attacked Agamemnon in the words of Achilles [calling him greedy and a coward] ... Odysseus then stood up, delivered a sharp rebuke to Thersites, which he coupled with a threat to strip him naked, and then beat him on the back and shoulders with Agamemnon's scepter; Thersites doubled over, a warm tear fell from his eye, and a bloody welt formed on his back; he sat down in fear, and in pain gazed helplessly as he wiped away his tear; but the rest of the assembly was distressed and laughed .... There must be a figuration of wickedness as self-evident as Thersites—the ugliest man who came to Troy—who says what everyone else is thinking* [19].

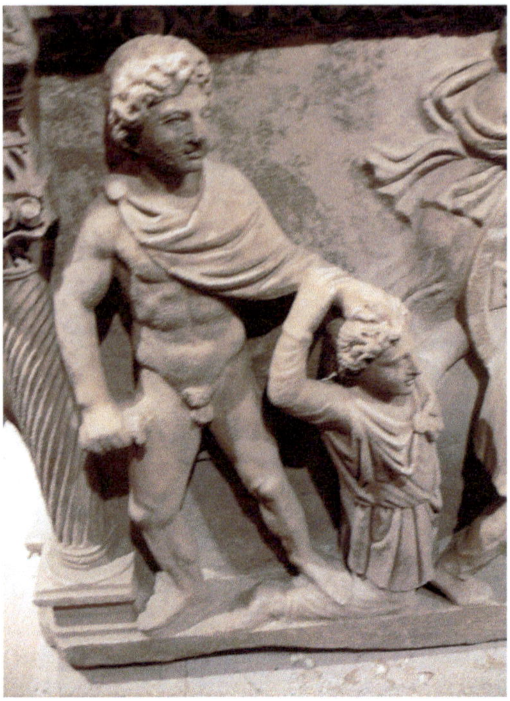

Fig. 12.1 Relief from the sarcophagus of Aurelia Botania Demetria, preserved in the Archaeological Museum of Antalya (Turkey): Achilles beating Thersites (second century AD)

He is not mentioned elsewhere in the *Iliad*, but it seems that in the lost *Aethiopis*, Achilles eventually killed him "for having torn out the eyes of the Amazon Penthesilea that the hero had just killed in combat" [20] (Fig. 12.1). He was represented by Polygnotus at the Porch (λέσχη) of the Cnidians (located at Delphi) playing dice with Palamedes [21, 22].

12.3 Description and Clinical Patterns

The name oxycephaly meaning "pointed head" refers to the "clown's hat" found at the site of the ossified bulging bregmatic fontanel. Compensating growth in the anterior fontanel region results in the formation of a pointed or cone-shaped skull [3, 4] (Fig. 12.2).

Secondary to premature synostosis of the coronal and sagittal sutures, oxycephaly is defined by a receding forehead especially tilted back in continuity with the nasal bridge (Fig. 12.3).

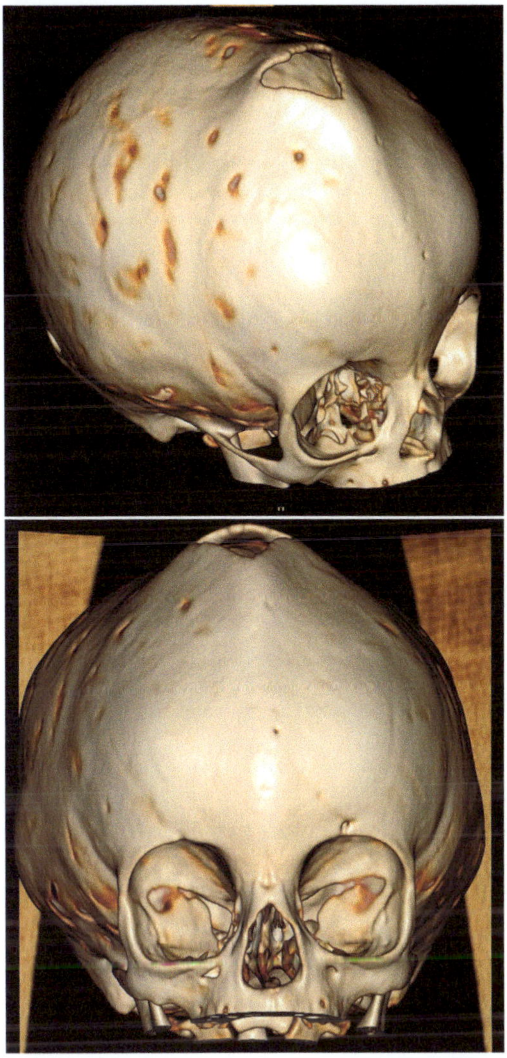

Fig. 12.2 Bicoronal and metopic or sagittal synostosis, together with a compensating growth in the anterior fontanel region, results in the formation of a pointed or skull-shaped cone ("clown's hat") at the site of the ossified bulging bregmatic fontanel

The calvaria is characterized by a high, steep forehead often with a depression of the supraorbital region. The sagittal diameter is short, and the head may appear pointed in the bregmatic region. The cephalic index is usually increased (brachycephaly) and the head circumference decreased, with microcephaly being common. The anterior cranial base is short: the greater wing of the sphenoid is protruded, and the lesser wing exhibits a steep upward and lateral slope with a frontalization of the orbital roof [3, 23].

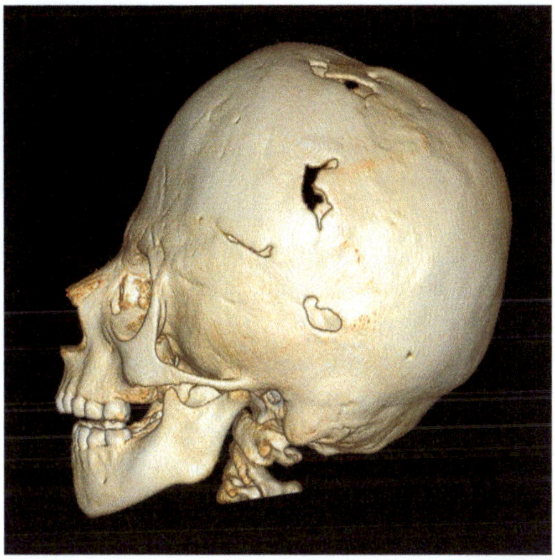

Fig. 12.3 Oxycephaly is defined by a receding forehead, tilted back in continuity with the nasal bridge

The vertical development of the face is characterized by increased anterior and decreased posterior face height, typically narrow and surmounted by a median projection located at the level of the bregmatic fontanel. The facial bone is normal in this type of craniosynostosis. The altered jaw relations, which can be related to the marked flattening of the cranial base, may lead to a malocclusion with frontal open bite, extreme maxillary overjet, and distal molar occlusion. Because of the marked flattening of the cranial base, the head is carried in an extended position in relation to the cervical column [23]. Longitudinal radiographic and roentgen cephalometric studies have shown that the growth of the calvaria is markedly eccentric, with diminished forward growth of the frontal bone and concomitant increased vertical development [24]. Pronounced frontal bossing may be seen in infancy but becomes reduced by virtue of continued increments of the growth in the glabella area combined with decreased growth of the supraglabellar region [23]. In fact, isolated oxycephaly very often goes unnoticed in childhood due to the harmony of the cranial morphology by the end of youth and tends to be diagnosed lately when the child presents with visual loss or signs of intracranial hypertension [3, 25]. A reason for this could be the late fusion of bicoronal and sagittal sutures that may cause symptoms later than in other conditions.

12.3.1 Clinical Forms

Often in the past [1, 2, 5, 13, 26], the term oxycephaly became a synonym of multisutural craniostenosis characterized by a brachycephaly [27, 28] or severe forms of craniostenosis affecting multiple sutures, mostly in the newborn [2, 29]. All these forms should be differentiated from the isolated oxycephaly.

Mantaut and Striker described three types of oxycephaly [30, 31]: type I acrocephaly or turricephaly with a verticalized and receding forehead; type II, *true* oxycephaly, with a receding forehead plus a bregmatic protrusion responsible for a pointed skull; and the type III, an oxycephaly without deformity but with a small skull reduced in all its diameters. This classification has been subjected to criticism. Type I (Fig. 12.4a) corresponds in fact to a brachycephaly in which the age of onset and management are completely different [2]. This distinction is significant, as functional risks and treatment options in oxy-

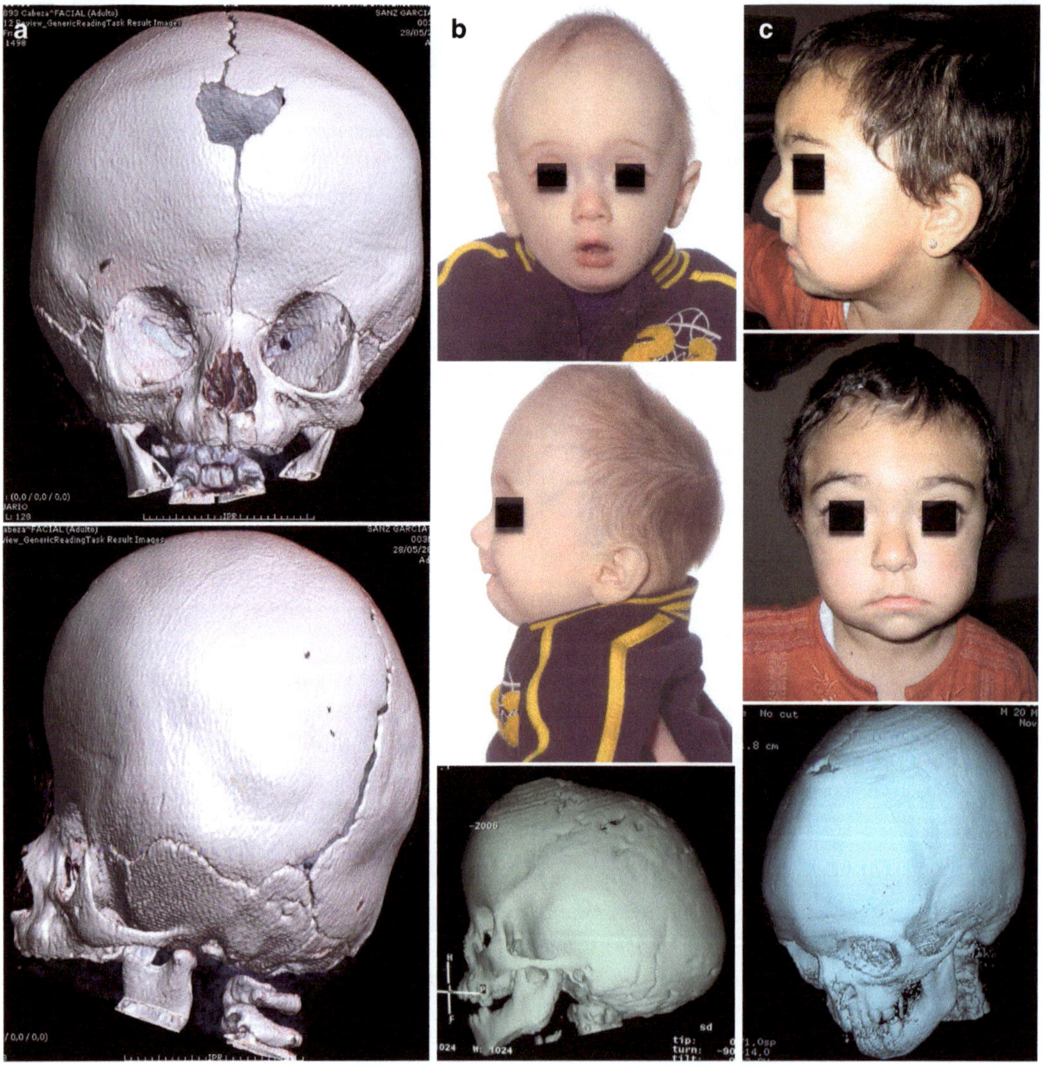

Fig. 12.4 Clinical patterns of oxycephaly. (**a**) Type I acrocephaly or turricephaly corresponds to a bicoronal synostosis (brachycephaly) and should be excluded from this term; (**b**) Type II oxycephaly is the typical case with a pointed skull tilted back in continuity with the nasal bridge and ending in a bregmatic bump; (**c**) Type III is a harmonious form with closure of multiple sutures and without any visible dysmorphism. This girl had an ophthalmological debut at the age of 4 years

cephaly are completely different from those in brachycephaly [32]. Type II is the *true* oxycephaly (*Oxus* = pointed) with a pointed skull tilted back in continuity with the nasal bridge and a bregmatic bump (Fig. 12.4b). The frontonasal angle is wide open giving an impression of exorbitism. Type III has a harmonious shape of the skull, which appears rounded and has no visible dysmorphism, despite multiple sutures being closed (Fig. 12.4c).

Some cases of isolated oxycephaly present at birth or even prenatally with gross dysmorphism and severe brachycephaly; others present later in life with harmonious restriction of intracranial volume and are at risk for neurodevelopment and vision. At the same time, some forms evolve from initially unisutural synostoses [3].

12.4 Epidemiology

Oxycephaly is often diagnosed lately due to harmonious morphology of the skull and, perhaps, postnatal suture closure [2, 3]. Prevalence is unknown, but it has been shown to be under 1/1,000,000 live newborns.

The largest evaluation of the frequency of nonsyndromic craniosynostosis from Paris [2] reported that the incidence of oxycephaly had been decreasing during their 20 years analysis period. From 1975 to 1995, 1483 patients with craniosynostosis were hospitalized in the neurosurgery department of the Hospital des Enfants-Malades in Paris. Among these, 129 patients (8.7%) had nonsyndromic oxycephaly, including 86 boys (66.7%) and 43 girls (33.3%) with ages between 1 and 22 years old (average: 6 years old, average: 4 years 9 months). An anomaly of the calcium phosphate metabolism was found in 22 observations: two cases of hypophosphatasia (in two brothers) and 20 antecedents of rickets (15.5%) [2]. A recent series from the same group reported 1.2% of all the patients with oxycephaly in 2007, compared with 8.8% in 1988. This reduction might be due to better care that is provided to these patients in their countries or to a reduction in the prevalence of this subtype of craniosynostosis [33]. The improvement of the standard of living and the socioeconomic and nutritional conditions can also play a role in this sense.

Although isolated oxycephaly is common in North Africa [2, 25], it is a rare craniosynostosis among Caucasian–European patients. Oxycephaly would be more frequent on the periphery Mediterranean, where it could represent up to 40% of craniostenosis [2, 8, 31], while it would represent only 6–13% in the northern American series [34].

12.5 Physiopathology

Oxycephaly is a common manifestation of different diseases involving premature fusion of coronal and sagittal sutures. Typically, isolated oxycephaly is of late onset, and it is never diagnosed before the age of three [2], which differentiates it from other non-syndromic craniosynostosis evident at birth. There are reports of children that presented with a typical oxycephaly at the age of 4 years and have been studied in the past with a normal x-R at the age of one [2, 35]. Certain elements are specific to this particular type of craniosynostosis. The average age is much later than in other nonsyndromic craniosynostosis, and no cases are usually observed during the first year of life [2, 3].

Oxycephaly, as discussed before, may be also a feature of certain syndromes like Crouzon or Pfeiffer syndrome. The syndromic and nonsyndromic forms can be distinguished by the absence of limb and/or facial anomalies in nonsyndromic forms.

12.5.1 Chiari Malformation in Oxycephaly

The association between Chiari malformation (CM) and premature craniofacial synostosis was first noted by Saldino et al. [36] in 1972 in one patient with Pfeiffer syndrome. Since then, numerous authors have reported the incidence of chronic tonsillar herniation in multiple suture craniosynostosis [37–43], and it is a frequent finding in syndromic and multisuture craniosynostosis, characterized by early fusion of lambdoid sutures and cranial base synchondroses. The incidence of CM has been reported as high as 70% in Crouzon syndrome [2, 42, 43], 75% in nonsyndromic oxycephaly [2], 50% in Pfeiffer syndrome, and 100% in kleeblattschädel deformity [44]. In the series from Renier [2], of the 16 children in whom an MRI was performed, Chiari type I malformation was present in 12 (75%), one of them associated to hydrocephalus. CM has been found in other types of syndromic craniosynostosis, in some cases of nonsyndromic complex craniosynostosis involving the lambdoid suture, and in some rare cases of scaphocephaly [42, 45].

The frequency of Chiari malformation in the oxycephaly is elevated, and it approaches that observed in Crouzon's syndrome [2, 44] (Fig. 12.5). In this syndrome, Cinalli et al. have shown that chronic involvement of the cerebellar tonsils is probably an acquired anomaly and not an associated congenital malformation, and that this anomaly was probably related to a decrease in volume of the posterior cerebral fossa due to a premature synostosis of lambdoid sutures [39] or a decreased intracranial volume motivated by the closure several sutures in the anterior region [46].

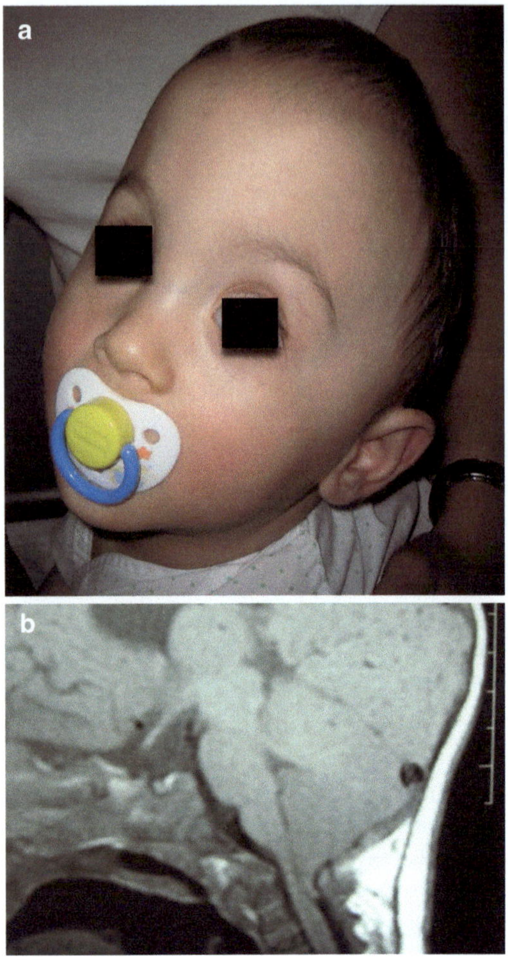

Fig. 12.5 Chiari malformation is a frequent finding in multisutural craniosynostoses. The incidence has been reported as high as 75% in oxycephaly. (**a**) Phenotipic appearance in an 18-month-old boy; (**b**) Chiari malformation is present at first diagnosis

Downward herniation of neural tissue through the foramen magnum is usually an acquired malformation in craniosynostosis and may be secondary to a disproportion between the posterior fossa and the growing hindbrain structures [39, 47]. In most cases of craniosynostosis, hindbrain herniation is not present at birth; rather, it develops in response to the changes in the skull base and posterior fossa secondary to premature closure of the lambdoid and cranial base sutures, supporting the pathogenetic hypothesis of overcrowding of the posterior fossa secondary to premature suture fusion [43, 44, 48]. The rest of the sutures (lambdoid, sagittal, coronal, and metopic) also play a role in the development of CM. In the setting of a postnatal (or in utero) closure of sagittal and coronal sutures, a cephalocranial disproportion in the supratentorial compartment occurs early, forcing the neural growth to be directed posteriorly and inferiorly and pushing down the tentorium. This can induce a lower attachment of the tentorium (near the foramen magnum), reducing the size of the posterior fossa and increasing the risk of CM, especially if premature lambdoid synostosis is also involved. More than one-third of patients with hindbrain herniation become symptomatic for CM or develop syringomyelic cavities. Usually, the onset of symptoms occurs late in life, but they may be dramatic, especially in very young children [39]. Careful radiologic and clinical follow-up is needed in patients with syndromic or complex craniosynostosis to assess the presence and evolution of CM. MRI with venous angiography is the gold standard for the evaluation of these patients [49].

12.6 Etiology

The cause of oxycephaly is unclear, but it has been demonstrated a clear relationship between rickets and the development of craniostenosis [2, 50–52]. In the past, a frequent history of rickets, including involvement in oxycephaly, has been reported by different groups [2, 25, 31, 52]. Reilly et al. [52] have shown that about one-third of children with rickets were susceptible to develop cranlostenosis and that this was related to the severity of rickets. The observation of cases of oxycephaly complicating hypophosphatasia also favors a metabolic cause, and points to a postnatal physiopathological mechanism of this craniostenosis.

The advances of genetics also lead to the discovery of new genetic entities. Unlike synostoses involving the sagittal system (sagittal and metopic sutures), which are most likely idiopathic or secondary to environmental causes, synostoses involving the coronal system are often genetic and warrant systematic genetic evaluation [12, 53].

In some patients, the evolution toward craniofaciostenosis and the diagnosis of other syndromic features or other familial cases are often delayed [4, 54, 55]. The diagnosis is often provisional since closure of the coronal suture is often the first element of a craniofaciostenosis [4, 12]. On the other hand, some patients diagnosed initially with a sagittal or unicoronal synostosis will evolve into an oxycephaly or brachycephaly. The diagnosis of isolated oxycephaly is thus often provisional or retrospective.

12.6.1 Genetic Syndromes Associating Oxycephaly

Isolated oxycephaly is usually sporadic, but familial cases have been reported.

Craniosynostosis-6 (CRS6) is a bicoronal form associated with bony defects in the sagittal, metopic, or lambdoid sutures [56]. Twigg et al. identified a third-generation family in which two affected individuals had bicoronal synostosis and two had a calvarial abnormality (brachycephaly or plagiocephaly). All affected individuals had some degree of impaired intellectual development; one lived in a supervised environment at age 19, two had mildly delayed development, and one had a full-scale IQ of 89 on formal psychological testing. One affected individual had a Dandy-Walker malformation as well as spina bifida occulta, sensorineural hearing loss, and LHRH deficiency; several others had more subtle abnormalities in the conformation of the posterior fossa. The transmission pattern of CRS6 was consistent with autosomal dominant inheritance. The underlying molecular genetics likely correspond to a heterozygous missense mutation in the ZIC1 gene. Human ZIC1 (zinc finger protein of cerebellum 1), one of five homologs of the Drosophila pair-rule gene odd-paired, encodes a transcription factor previously implicated in vertebrate brain development. Recent studies have shown that pathogenic variants in ZIC1 have deleterious effect in developing human central nerves system and skull bone. ZIC1 related clinical conditions are reported and include cerebellum malformation, Dandy-Walker malformation, spinal dysraphism, microcephaly, and craniosynostosis with associated intellectual disability [57, 58]. The diagnosis of a ZIC1 mutation has significant implications for prognosis, and genetic testing for this condition has been recommended, when common causes of coronal synostosis have been excluded.

Oxycephaly is also a common finding in different diseases involving premature fusion of the cranial sutures as a secondary event such as TOLCAS or craniorhiny [12, 59–64].

Mindikoglu et al. (1991) published the first cases of craniosynostosis combined with unusual nasal abnormalities. The skull shape was oxycephalic with recessed forehead and lack of nasofrontal angle. The nasal changes consisted of wide nose, anteverted nostrils, and nasal hirsutism. Bilaterally symmetrical spherical cyst-like formations with fistulas were present just below the nose. This condition was termed craniorhiny [65].

12.6.2 TOLCAS Syndrome

Tolchin-Le Caignec syndrome (TOLCAS) is caused by heterozygous mutation in the SOX6 gene on chromosome 11p15. TOLCAS is a developmental disorder characterized by mildly to moderately impaired intellectual development and behavioral problems, such as autism, attention deficit (ADHD), labile mood, and aggressive episodes. Many patients have bony abnormalities, including osteochondroma, craniosynostosis, dysmorphic facies, arachnodactyly, and large head circumference. Rarely, additional congenital anomalies may also be observed [66]. Clinical depiction of these patients revealed dysmorphic features, including prominent occiput, high forehead, micrognathia, hypertelorism, bitemporal narrowing, broad nasal bridge, large or low-set ears, and full eyebrows.

The heterozygous mutations in the SOX6 gene that were identified in most patients with TOLCAS occurred de novo. However, 2 families showed autosomal dominant transmission of the disorder. Tolchin et al. (2020) noted that SOX6 plays a role in neurogenesis and chondrogenesis, which could explain the phenotypic features [66].

12.7 Management and Surgical Treatment

Isolated oxycephaly is a non-syndromic form of late onset craniostenosis, responsible for insidious intracranial hypertension that can lead, if not treated early, to unnoticed progressive blindness or other related severe complications. Unlike sagittal or metopic synostoses, which do not cause intracranial hypertension and for which the aim of surgery is above all the restoration of normal shape, intracranial hypertension is the rule in oxycephaly [2, 4]. For this reason, decompressive surgery is needed even in newborns when signs of increased intracranial pressure are found. During childhood, it should be performed as soon as the clinical diagnosis has been established. The high prevalence of visual loss caused by optic nerve atrophy and the number of children with oxycephaly and developmental delay confirm that for many of these patients, surgery is not optional [25].

Cranial expansion surgery is essential for relieving intracranial pressure and stabilizing intellectual deficit which, in the absence of treatment, becomes significantly more profound. Following surgery, the intracranial pressure returns to normal, papilledema usually resolves, and the intellectual deficit seems to stabilize. However, secondary surgery is more commonly required in oxycephaly than in patients with a single suture craniosynostosis.

The timing of surgery and the surgical technique used for correction will depend primarily on the patient's age at presentation. The aim of the surgery is mainly to expand intracranial volume trying to achieve a proper ratio between skull and brain, providing adequate aesthetic correction at the same time.

In infants and older children, fronto-orbital advancement with frontoparietal remodeling is the technique of choice, providing good cranial decompression and satisfactory morphological results.

However, decompressive surgery may be needed soon after birth. In the newborn with soft bones, no cranioplasty is possible. For this reason, different techniques including endoscopic assisted suturectomies or open perifrontal craniectomy have been described and will be later discussed.

12.7.1 Early Surgery. Newborns

12.7.1.1 Perifrontal Craniectomy (Peri-Fronto-Orbital Craniectomy)

The French group in Lille introduced Peri-Fronto-Orbital Craniectomy (PFOC) for early treatment of nonsyndromic oxycephaly and brachycephaly [4, 67]. This technique has been used in newborns requiring emergency decompression, and it would be indicated for children below the age of 4 months.

A conventional bicoronal incision is performed and a frontal scalp elevated in a subgaleal fashion. A 2-cm wide strip of the periosteum is removed along the coronal sutures and the orbital rim on both sides. The craniectomy (Fig. 12.6) removes the coronal suture down to the temporal fossa on each side, taking out the pterional bone,

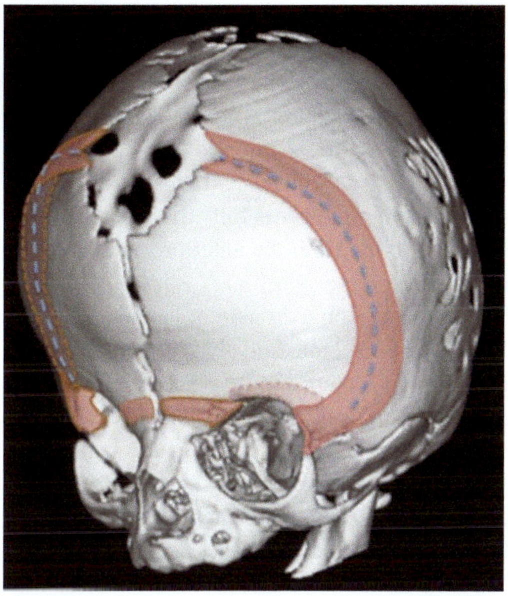

Fig. 12.6 Perifronto-orbital craniectomy, a technique used in newborns requiring emergency decompression. The craniectomy removes the coronal suture down to the fronto-malar suture, the roof of the orbit behind the supraorbital rim, and extends to the fronto-nasal suture. The frontal bone is, in this way, set free and allows the growing brain to remodel the skull. (Taken from Vinchon et al. [4] with permission)

which is usually very thick in this type of pathology [67] and reaches the fronto-malar suture The resection is carried on to the lateral orbital wall and along the orbital roof, removing almost all of it. Osteotomies continue medially to the roof of the orbit behind the orbital rim and extend to the fronto-nasal suture. These craniotomies join on the nasion, which is resected as well. The released frontal bone, only maintained by a thin sagittal bridge, is then able to respond to the brain's growth stimulation [3, 4]. In addition, coagulation is applied to the dura mater along the site of the coronal suture to prevent early ossification and to initiate the formation of a neosuture, as published earlier [68].

Great care must be exerted to avoid tearing the dura mater, especially near the midline (because of the risk of venous bleeding) and in the temporal region because the temporal squama is swiveled into the frontal plane, and the dural folds are intricated with the sphenoid ridge [4]. PFOC technique has the advantage that the bone flap is left undissected from the dura: this preserves its vascular supply and avoids unnecessary bleeding [67].

There are important issues regarding the surgical technique for a satisfactory outcome:

1. The child must be younger than 4 months.
2. The craniectomy should take away not only the periosteum and the frontoparietal fused suture but also the sphenoid wing and a bony strip all around the frontal bone flap along the orbital roofs and the nasion, opening the superior orbital fissure. This is a point to bear in mind when discussing endoscopic approaches.
3. The dissection of the dura must be exclusively limited to the site of the craniectomy to preserve the frontal bone flap vascular supply, and
4. The dura should be gently coagulated along the coronal suture to avoid bony reossification [67].

12.7.1.2 Endoscopic-Assisted Suturectomies

Minimally invasive surgery, involving endoscopic suturectomy combined with cranial molding with helmets, has been advocated for multiple suture craniosynostoses. While craniectomy in a newborn is a large surgery, which requires expertise from both surgeon and anesthetist, other "less invasive" techniques have been reported for the treatment of oxycephaly in infants, below the age of 3–4 months [69, 70].

Given the satisfactory long-term results reported with endoscopy for young infants with single-suture synostosis [69], some groups have started treating infants with nonsyndromic multiple-suture calvarial synostosis using the same principles of minimally invasive endoscopy: assisted craniectomies followed by postoperative cranial orthotic treatment. For most authors, endoscopic technique must be followed by the use of cranial orthesis [69, 71]. The goal of the helmet is to redirect cranial growth and achieve normal head shape and size after releasing osteotomies.

In a series from Jimenez [69], every patient presenting with nonsyndromic multiple-suture synostosis and who were under 6 months of age were selected for endoscopic treatment achieving excellent results. In all patients, the cephalic indices decreased an average of 26% after surgery. Antimongoloid orbital slant was corrected to produce a normal orbital alignment as well as the bitemporal widening seen with brachycephaly. Helmet therapy following release of the stenosed coronal sutures led to internal distraction and forward movement of the nasoorbital complex. None of their cases needed a secondary bifrontal orbital advancement due to proptosis or corneal compromise. Furthermore, longitudinal analysis of their entire cohort demonstrated that all the patients' measurements followed standard population isocurves appropriate for each patient and therefore, there were no cases in which head or brain growth was restricted. The mean preoperative cephalic index was 98 (range 82–111), and the median was 97. Late postoperative cephalic index (≥1 year) was 83 (range 79–92), and the median was 82. Overall, there was a 15% decrease from preoperative baseline [69].

12.7.1.3 Endoscopic Assisted Suturectomies in Oxycephaly Technique

Access to a stenosed coronal suture is reached with a 2- to 3-cm incision located over the coronal suture at the level of the stephanion [69]. Subgaleal dissection is performed between the anterior fontanel and the squamosal suture behind the pterion. If needed, the metopic suture is reached using a new 2- to 3-cm incision located over the metopic suture in front of the anterior fontanel with subgaleal dissection between the nasofrontal suture and the anterior fontanel. Finally, the sagittal suture is reached via two incisions. The first is made over the anterior fontanel, and the second immediately in front of the lambda. The dissection plane proceeds between the galea and pericranium, using monopolar electrocautery. Thus, the loose areolar tissue is separated in a completely bloodless fashion.

Then, a pediatric 7-mm craniotome is used to create a bur hole at each incision. The bur hole is enlarged longitudinally along the suture axis when the coronal, metopic, or lambdoid sutures are involved. In the case of sagittal involvement, the bur hole is placed at the lateral edge of the incision and an osteotomy is carried across the midline to the other side, to a symmetrical distance from the suture. A 4-mm rigid 0° or 30° angled endoscope is inserted into the epidural space for visualization and dissection of the space. The dura mater is fully dissected from the overlying bone from the anterior fontanel to the nasofrontal suture (metopic), squamosal suture behind the pterion (coronal), or lambda (sagittal). In the case of lambdoid involvement, epidural dissection is undertaken between the lambda and asterion. Removal of bone is done with a combination of angled Kerrison rongeurs, bone (pituitary type) rongeurs, and Mayo scissors. The craniectomy size for the metopic, coronal, and lambdoid sutures averages 7 mm (range 5–10 mm) and 50 mm (range 40–60 mm) for sagittal involvement. Osseous hemostasis is obtained using a suction-monopolar unit. The bone is cauterized under direct visualization until all oozing and bleeding stops. The incisions are closed with 4–0 Monocryl (Ethicon, Inc.), and the dermis sealed with Ethibond (Ethicon, Inc.). A custom-made helmet is fitted on the sixth postoperative day and kept for 12–18 months postoperatively.

12.7.1.4 Controversies

The concept of surgery at a very early age may look appealing in severe cases of uni- or bicoronal synostosis diagnosed at birth. Based on the success of strip craniectomies as a simple and efficient method routinely used for treatment of sagittal synostosis, some authors have extended this indication to multisutural (nonsyndromic) craniosynostosis. The very invasive nature of the conventional calvarial remodeling techniques used in most craniofacial centers requires that these patients are treated at later stages (at 6–12 months of age). Invariably, such delay in treatment leads to changes in skull base, nasal, and orbital morphology and alignment that cannot be easily corrected with the use of subsequent surgical procedures. The end result tends to be suboptimal, particularly when more than two sutures are involved.

The goal in approaching these patients with minimally invasive endoscopic techniques at a very early age intends to halt, and even significantly reverse, the progression of associated craniofacial deformities [69]. By releasing the stenosed sutures early, adequate brain growth takes place, which in turn leads to cephalic normalization. Extensive surgeries (mostly fronto-orbital advancement) could then not be needed and could save the children all the risks associated with open procedures.

However, for many authors [4, 17, 45, 67, 71], the deformation of the skull base in multisutural synostosis affecting the anterior fossa requires a more invasive approach in order to obtain a definitive correction.

Oxycephaly has a more complicated pathology compared with bilateral coronal suture synostosis. Linear craniectomies in the region of the coronal suture early in infancy have been shown to have a very limited effect on the growth pattern of the calvaria in most of the patients with oxycephaly [24, 72]. Coronal craniectomy per se does little to alter the pattern of growth in the frontal region over the long term [24, 73]. Simple suturectomy was abandoned in coronal synostosis in the past due to early bony reclosure and failure to achieve satisfactory cranial shape [4, 67]. This could be explained because the coronal suture, in association with the frontosphenoidal and sphenoethmoidal sutures, makes up the largest cranial suture complex [28]. Anderson et al. had described that synostosis of this complex cannot be compensated for by the other sutures [8]. For this reason, Seeger and Gabrielsen had recommended that the coronal strip craniectomies should be extended downward and inward, to include the heavily overgrowth sphenoid ridge [71]. This is one of the main concerns about endoscopic coronal suturectomy: a single incision over the lateral portion of the suture does not allow osteotomies on the orbital roof and resection of the lesser wing of the sphenoid.

Probably more data are needed on the results obtained with minimally invasive surgery, especially on long-term follow-up. In any case, whatever the technique selected for the correction of this malformation is, a close follow-up of these patients is mandatory in a short and long term to recognize early signs of recurrence and increased intracranial pressure.

12.7.2 Late. 6–12 Months. Early Childhood

Since Tessier's innovative work in 1967, the principles of craniofacial surgery established fronto-orbital advancement as an acceptable treatment for craniosynostosis, and it remains the standard for anterior unilateral or multisutural synostoses [72]. This surgery, usually performed within the first year of life to correct the bony deformity and improve cosmetic appearance, involves excision of the fused suture and remodeling/repositioning of the frontal bone and orbits.

Fronto-orbital advancement with frontoparietal remodeling is the technique of choice and provides good cranial decompression and morphological results in oxycephaly. Tessier's tongue-in-groove advancement of the orbital bandeau (supraorbital rim together with roof of the orbits) followed by remodeling and osteosynthesis of the reconstructed forehead bone remains one of the most commonly reported techniques [3].

There are multiple variations of this procedure, but all techniques typically include the resection of the affected sutures and the expansion of the anterior fossa by means of projecting a fronto-orbital bandeau.

Based on the observation by Seeger and Gabrielsen [71] that the sphenofrontal suture (together with the coronal) is also prematurely fused in brachycephaly, the concept of the surgery led to release the sutures of the anterior cranial base, with advance of the supraorbital rim [74–76], and the creation of free-floating flaps in the frontal region [35, 77]. These techniques have been shown to lead to marked improvement in calvarial growth [78].

Hoffman and Mohr used Tessier's method combined with their own technique for advancing the lateral canthal segments of the supraorbital region for the treatment of metopic synostosis [74]. Soon after, Marchac and Renier published the "floating forehead" technique, later combined with a fronto-orbital bandeau remodeling. Marchac advised the use of the floating forehead technique for children under 6 months of age, while for children older than 6 months, he used a horizontal tongue-in-groove advancement [1, 2,

13, 32, 35, 79–81]. In the floating forehead technique, they removed the orbital bar and advanced it by 2 cm after remodeling. This bar was fixed only to the frontal process of the zygoma. The frontal bone was wired to the supraorbital bar leaving a wide craniectomy behind. This allowed the brain to push freely on the forehead [13]. To provide support, a small bone graft was placed between the root of the nose and the advanced supraorbital bar [80]. Although theoretically feasible, their floating forehead technique resulted in temporal hollowing and craniolacuniae and, for this reason, different techniques have been reported since then [4, 68, 81–83].

Since oxycephaly is due to both coronal sutures and an additional sagittal suture synostosis, the forehead is recessed and tilted backward in continuity with the nasal dorsum (frontonasal angle). The supraorbital rim is recessed, producing an impression of exophthalmos. Therefore, Renier et al. modified their surgical technique for the treatment of brachycephaly [13]. They lifted and repositioned the superior orbital bar with an anterior rotation and transposed the upper forehead and lower forehead to obtain better aesthetic results (Fig. 12.7).

The tongue-in-groove procedure is not easily adapted to repositioning the supraorbital bar when rotation in the coronal plane (sagittal axis) is required. Whitaker et al. published their own technique on the correction of craniofacial dysostosis in which three-fourths of the abnormal orbit is osteotomized and advanced to become level with the normal orbit [84]. They used a lateral bone graft between the advanced orbit and the temporal bone to maintain the newly advanced position. Some years later, they published a modified technique in which the orbit advancement was completed with a bony Z-plasty at the lateral orbit or by a tongue-in-groove procedure to reassure the bone firmly positioned (Whitaker 1980) (Fig. 12.8).

Persing et al. stated that the most difficult cranial dimension to correct is excessive skull height [85]. He described a one-staged procedure for turricephaly, made possible largely by using modified prone position. This position allows simultaneous access to both the anterior and posterior cranium. In summary, bifrontal and biparietooccipital "quadrant" craniotomies are

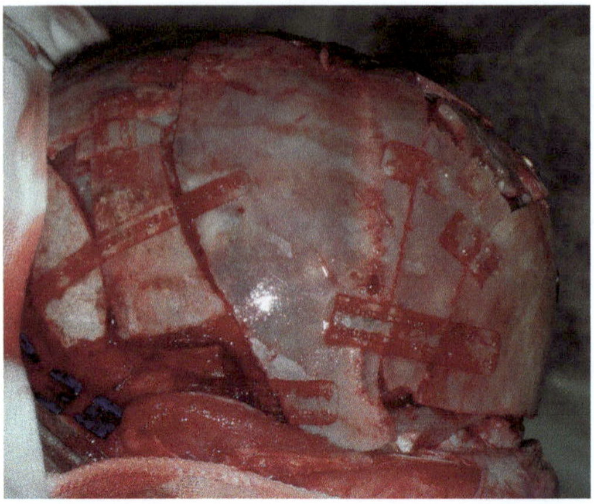

Fig. 12.7 Modification of the Renier fronto-orbital advancement technique for brachycephaly. Their technique advances the superior orbital bar with an anterior rotation and transposes the upper and lower forehead to improve the aesthetic results

performed. A bone plate remains at the vertex of the skull and over the superior sagittal sinus to avoid its injury. The lowering of the vertex and thus, shortening in heights is accomplished by bone resection from the caudal ends of the anterior and the lateral bony struts. Parallel vertical cuts are made into the bone of the basal cranium and occipital osteotomies are carried out down to the foramen magnum. After the reshaping of the bone flaps by the "quadrant" craniotomies, they are replaced and the scalp flap are returned to their normal position. Although this method seems to be very aggressive, the barrel stave osteotomies would act to decrease the resistance of the vertical compression of the skull and increase the capacity of the cranium [3].

Vinchon et al. [4] reported a modification of the bandeau with a two-tongue bone cut: a temporofrontal anterior tongue, a part of the bandeau which is translated and kyphosed; and a posterior tongue, which prolongs the temporoparietal region, on which the anterior tongue is rigidly fixed. This technique is able to withstand the pressure, when the scalp is reapproximated and allows significant frontal advancement providing great stability [4]. However, it may be inapplicable for older children with a thick and rigid bone. In these cases, remodeling of the frontoparietal region will require cutting and remodeling frontal and parietal bone flaps. Repositioning of the parietal flaps laterally and

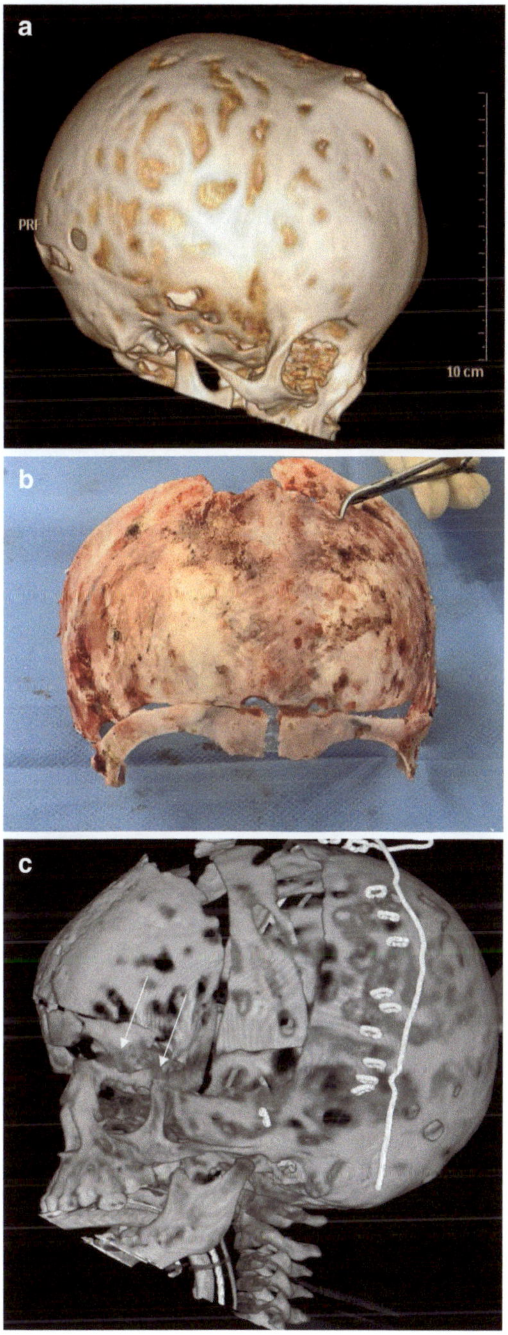

Fig. 12.8 (**a**) Preoperative CT; (**b**) Fronto-orbital remodeling. (**c**) Intraoperative image obtained with the image guided therapy platform Azurion (Philips): observe the distance between the lateral wall of the orbit and the fronto-malar suture corresponding to an advancement of 1.4 mm (white arrows)

anteriorly provides advancement and widening of the calvaria; in addition, "fan-like" anterior rotation provides a reliable buttress to secure the advancement of the fronto-orbital construct.

Another important technical detail is the correction of the bulging temporal squama to narrow excessively wide interparietal diameter. This usually requires resection in the temporal squama, remodeling with barrel staves, or inversion of a temporal bone flap [53].

Shen et al. had described their surgical method in a case report. This consisted in a multiple bone flap rotation-reposition technique to reconstruct the calvaria with the osteotomy bone flaps rotated, repositioned, and fixed in a design to reduce the cranial height [86].

12.7.3 Other Treatments

More radical procedures of subtotal calvariectomy for oxycephalic patients with multiple synostosis have been used in the past [87, 88]. Hanson et al. proposed a wide excision of the bony calvarium from the supraorbital ridge to near the foramen magnum including the entire area of the coronal sutures. They saw a regeneration of the calvarium occurring from 2 to 12 weeks by the presence of the "neosutures" in their usual location. This radical procedure had allowed for normal brain growth without reoperation up to 2 years old. Also, neurologic and intellectual performance was satisfactory, and the cosmetic results appeared to be preferable to those obtained by more limited surgery. These techniques have been mostly abandoned and left for the most severe forms of cloverleaf skulls (kleeblattschädel) or complex craniosynostosis, which need emergent decompression in the first weeks of life [89].

Distracting procedures have been advocated to increase cranial volume and used in the treatment of brachycephaly [90]. The advantages of osteogenic cranial distraction would be the lack of a dead space just after surgery because the distraction is applied gradually and equally to the dura, skin, and soft tissues with simultaneous expansion of bone and soft tissues. It is also very unlikely a bone resorption because blood supply is not hindered during surgery. The amount of blood loss and the duration of surgery also decreases because the release of the membrane from the bone is minimal. The main disadvantage for these techniques would be the limitation of the vectors of the distraction (impossibility for three dimensional vectors) and the necessity for an additional second surgery to remove the device.

Uemura et al. described three-dimensional cranial expansion using distraction osteogenesis to treat oxycephaly [91]. In his technique, a bifrontal craniotomy is extended laterally downward on both sides, including supraorbital rim and orbital roofs. A biparietal bone flap is designed to apply the lateral expanding devices. The frontal expansion device is attached to the bilateral lower area of the frontal bone, including the orbital roof. The bilateral expansion device is attached further backward from the parietal area of the bone flap, supported by the bilateral lower temporal area (Fig. 12.9). Osteogenic distraction is initiated after 5 days after surgery, and the dis-

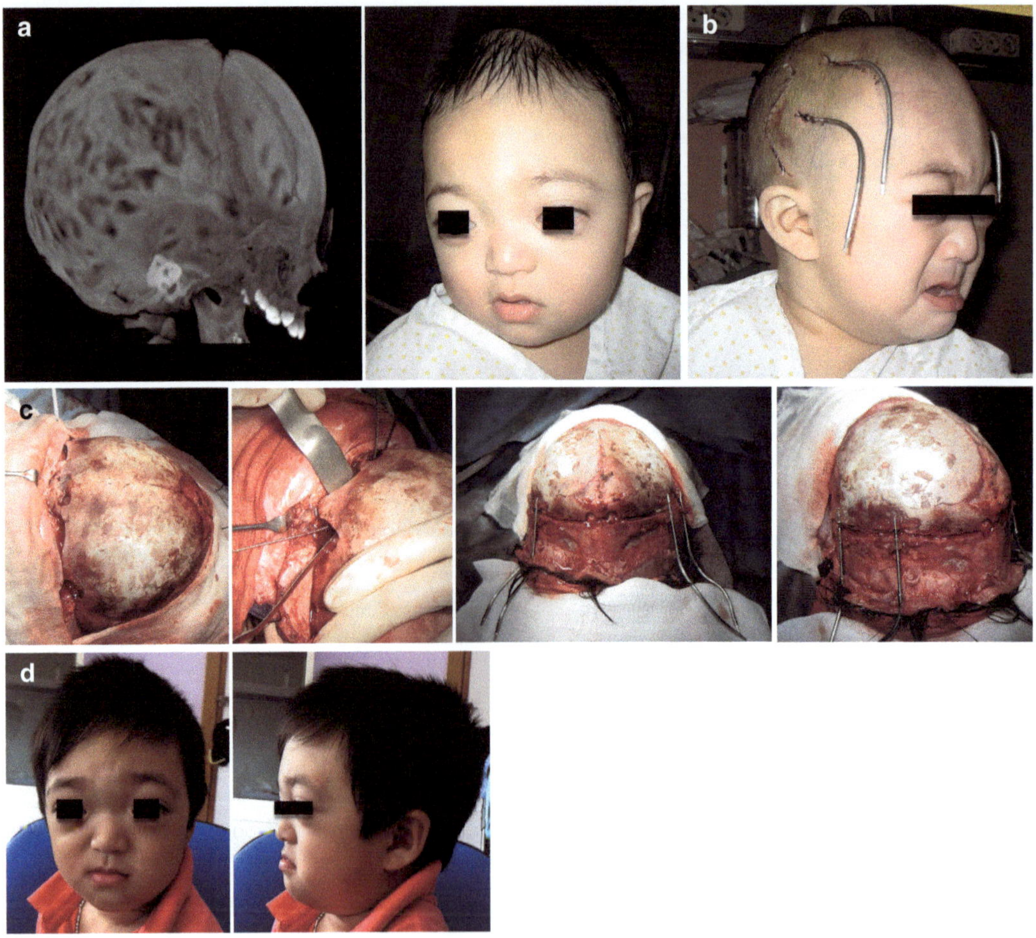

Fig. 12.9 The debut of this patient consisted of a profound alteration of vision at the age of 5. Funduscopy revealed severe papilledema. His father became blind at the age of 16 in his country of origin, without a clear diagnosis. On his arrival at our institution, an oxycephalia was clear and treatment (ICP monitoring and CT/MR studies) was offered, but he refused due to lack of symptoms, other than his long-standing bilateral amaurosis. Treatment in her son's case began with a posterior parieto-occipital distraction, followed by a fronto-orbital advancement, which proved to be very effective in controlling his symptoms and from a cosmetic point of view. His papilledema resolved, and he has been free of symptoms since the first surgery. (**a**) CT and phenotypic appearance at initial diagnosis. (**b**) Posterior (parieto-occipital) advancement. (**c**) "Monobloc" fronto-orbital distraction. Hirabayashi technique [98]. (**d**) Final appearance of the boy, 1 year after the completion of both procedures

traction devices activated simultaneously 1 mm per day. The devices were removed after a consolidation period of 3–5 months.

12.8 Outcome of Oxycephaly

Isolated oxycephaly is a form of multisutural non-syndromic craniosynostosis characterized by premature fusion of both the coronal and sagittal sutures. Elevated intracranial pressure is a common clinical feature (affecting more than 60% of the patients) leading to frequent ophthalmologic complications (papilledema) and moderate to severe intellectual deficit, although individuals may have a completely normal cognitive outcome [92]. When left untreated, it is responsible for insidious intracranial hypertension that can lead to severe related complications.

Intracranial hypertension (ICH) is the rule in oxycephaly, and it will definitely appear at some point in life [4, 93, 94]. For this reason, decompressive surgery is needed even in newborns when signs of increased intracranial pressure are found or as soon as a clinical diagnosis has been established. Cranial expansion is essential for relieving intracranial pressure and stabilizing intellectual deficit. Usually, intracranial pressure returns to normal after proper surgery, and papilledema resolves. However, secondary surgeries are more commonly required in oxycephaly compared with patients with a single suture craniosynostosis.

There are several publications describing outcomes in simple brachycephaly. In the Lille group report [67], patients who underwent peri-fronto-orbital craniectomy before the age of 4 months reached school age and attended normal school programs [4]. None of them presented signs of developmental delay, and no visual deterioration was encountered. From a morphological point of view, peri-fronto-orbital craniectomy allowed a satisfactory improvement in most of their cases (83%). For this reason, their report insisted on the importance of an early surgery.

In a series of 99 children with isolated non-syndromic bicoronal synostosis followed prospectively to study mental outcome, Arnaud et al. reported also a statistically significant difference between the group that underwent surgery before 1 year of age and those who underwent surgery after 1 year of age. Before surgery, mental status was also statistically lower in the group of older than 1 year [3, 95].

However, there are not many reports describing the outcome of oxycephaly. Due to a late diagnosis in this insidious form of harmonic multisutural craniosynostosis [2, 25], there is a higher risk of increased intracranial pressure and mental retardation compared with brachycephaly. Raised intracranial pressure is characteristic of this pathology and leads frequently to ophthalmological complications (even blindness) and moderate or severe intellectual disability [96]. In a series of 646 patients, the proportion of normal mental development in non-syndromic craniosynostosis ranged from 67% to 86%, except for oxycephaly, where it was 42% [1]. The main factor for this ICH is the reduction in cranial volume that can be harmonious, without visible dysmorphism.

The severity of oxycephaly is related to ICH, which is present in 61.6% of cases, with papilledema in only 10% of cases (!) but with a 13% of an optic atrophy at diagnosis [2, 28]. It is necessary to insist on the frequent dissociation that exists between intracranial pressure and the funduscopy, which remain normal in almost two-thirds of children who have ICH, despite its chronic nature [2]. According to Renier et al. [2], in their review of 129 cases, papilledema disappeared and the intracranial pressure returned to normal in all cases with preoperative increased intracranial pressure. The mental level seemed to stabilize; the mean postoperative IQ being strongly correlated with the preoperative level. In non-operated patients, the mental level worsened significantly [2, 3].

In the series of Vinchon et al., although it is a combined series of brachycephaly and oxycephaly, 28 patients out of 61 patients (including 30 patients suffering from brachycephaly and 31 from oxycephaly) had shown signs and symptoms of increased intracranial pressure. Thirteen patients had shown ophthalmological abnormalities. There were four cases of oxycephaly that had developmental delay at the time of diagnosis. Thirteen oxycephalic patients had cognitive and/or behavioral problems. The mean age at surgery was 50.6 months in oxycephalic patient compared with 20.4 months in brachycephalic patients [4]. The higher age in oxycephalic cases can show that this is a late appearing craniosynostosis, which Renier had also posted [2].

From a cosmetic point of view, most of the surgical procedures reported an acceptable aesthetic result, as described previously [1, 2, 13, 35, 68, 75–81, 84, 87, 88, 97].

12.9 Conclusion

Oxycephaly is a late-appearing form of non-syndromic craniosynostosis characterized by the premature fusion of both the coronal and sagittal sutures. It is a rare and serious condition that can pass unnoticed exposing these patients throughout their lives to risks of chronic and insidious ICH. This may result in severe optic atrophy and blindness or cognitive delay if not treated on time. Sudden decompensation can also occur following an intercurrent disease, including a head trauma. A high index of suspicion must be bear in mind since, due to the harmonic microcephaly often associated, its diagnosis that can go unnoticed.

For this reason, decompressive surgery is needed when signs of increased intracranial pressure are found or as soon as a clinical diagnosis has been established. Different techniques for cranial expansion have been described, and all of them have been proved to relieve intracranial pressure and stabilize cognitive decline. Intracranial pressure usually returns to normal after surgery and papilledema resolves. Good results can be obtained also from a cosmetic point of view. However, secondary surgeries are more commonly required in oxycephaly compared with patients with a single suture craniosynostosis to achieve a definitive control of the disease.

The timing of surgery and the most appropriate technique, including the benefits and results of minimally invasive procedures, are still a matter of debate.

References

1. Renier D, Marchac D. Oxycephaly: an often complex diagnosis with a review of surgical management. In: Goodrich J, Hall O, editors. Craniofacial anomalies: growth and development from a surgical perspective. New-York, NY: Thieme Medical Publishers; 1995. p. 56–64.
2. Renier D, Cinalli G, Lajeunie E, Arnaud E, Marchac D. Oxycephaly, a severe craniosynostosis: apropos of a series of 129 cases. Arch Pediatr. 1997;4:722–9.
3. Shimoji K, Miyajima M, Arai H. Nonsyndromic plurisutural synostoses (oxycephaly, Mercedes Benz pattern synostosis). In: Di Rocco C, Pang D, Rutka J, editors. Textbook of pediatric neurosurgery. Cham: Springer; 2018. https://doi.org/10.1007/978-3-319-31512-6_62-1.
4. Vinchon M, Pellerin M, Baroncini M, Wolber A, Dhellemmes P. Non-syndromic oxycephaly and brachycephaly: a review. Childs Nerv Syst. 2012;28:1439–46. https://doi.org/10.1007/s00381-012-1800-2.
5. Greig DM. Oxycephaly. Edinburgh Med J. 1926;33:189–376.
6. Günther H. der Turnchädel als Konstitutionanomalie und als kliniches Symptoms. Ergeb Inn Med Kinderheilkd. 1931;40:40–135.
7. Galen. Comment. Hippocraitis lib 6. Galen commentary on Hippocrates' epidemics book I parts I–III. De Gruyter Akademie forschung. Berlin: Walter de Gruyter; 2014.
8. Anderson FM, Geiger L. Craniosynostosis: a survey of 204 cases. J Neurosurg. 1965;22:339–240.
9. Cohen MM Jr. Genetic perspectives on craniosynostosis and syndromes. J Neurosurg. 1977;47:886–98.
10. Cohen MM Jr. History, terminology, and classification of craniosynostosis. In: Cohen MM, Maclean RE, editors. Craniosynostosis. 2nd ed. New York, NY: Oxford University Press; 2000.
11. Lemire RJ, Loeser SD, Leech RW, et al. Normal and abnormal development of the human nervous system. Hagarstown: Harper and Row; 1975.
12. Di Rocco F, Baujat G, Arnaud E, Renier D, Laplanche JL, Cormier Daire V, Collet C. Clinical spectrum and outcomes in families with coronal synostosis and TCF12 mutations. Eur J Hum Genet. 2014;22:1413–6.
13. Renier D, Lajeunie E, Arnaud E, et al. Management of craniosynostoses. Childs Nerv Syst. 2000;16:645–58.
14. Wilkie AO, Byren JC, Hurst JA, et al. Prevalence and complications of single gene and chromosomal disorders in craniosynostosis. Pediatrics. 2010;126:e391–400.
15. Arensburg B, Hershkovitz I. Cranial deformation and trephination in the middle east. Bull Mem Soc Anthroplogie Paris. 1988;3:139–50.
16. Dingwall EJ. Artificial cranial deformation: a contribution to the study of ethnic mutilations. London: John Bale, Sons & Danielsson Ltd; 1931.

17. Mena-Bernal JH. Tratamiento endoscópicamente asistido de la sinostosis sagital precoz (escafocefalia). [Tesis doctoral]. Universidad Complutense de Madrid; 2016.
18. Laitinen L. Craniosynostosis. Premature fusion of the cranial sutures. Helsinki: Weilin & Ooos; 1956. p. 1–130.
19. Benardete S. The rhetoric of morality and philosophy. Plato's Gorgias and Phaedrus. The Chicago University Press; 1991. p. 100–1.
20. Quinto de Esmirna, I, 768–823; Tzetzes: About Licofrón, 999.
21. Pausanias: Descripción de Grecia, X.31.1.
22. Sófocles: Filoctetes, 442.
23. Kreiborg S. Postnatal growth and development of the craniofacial complex in premature craniosynostosis. In: Cohen MM, Maclean RE, editors. Craniosynostosis. 2nd ed. New York, NY: Oxford University Press; 2000.
24. Kreiborg S, Pruzansky S. Craniofacial growth in patients with premature craniosynostosis. Scand J Plast Reconstr Surg. 1981;15:171–86.
25. Bou-Salah A, Galli I, Ouahes A, Azzal S, Craniosténoses en Algérie. Indications opératoires et résultats d'une technique personnelle. Neurochirurgie. 1984;30:417–21.
26. Fletcher HM. On oxycephaly. Quant J Med. 1910–1911;4:385–98.
27. Faber HK, Towne EG. Early craniectomy as a preventive measure in oxycephaly and allied conditions. Am J Med Sci. 1927;173:701–11.
28. Bertelsen TI. The premature synostosis of the cranial sutures. Acta Ophthalmol. 1958;suppl 51:1–76.
29. Mori K. Craniosynostosis. In: Anomaly of tile central nervous system. Stuttgart-Thieme; 1985. p. 13–9.
30. Montaut J, Stricker M, André JM. Les dysmorphies craniofaciales: les synostoses prématurées (crâniosténoses et faciosténoses). Société de Neurochirurgie de Langue Française, 27e Congrès Annuel, Nice, 24–25 Mai. Neurochirurgie; Supplément; Neurochirurgie. Paris: Masson; 1977.
31. Rifi L, Barkat A, El Ouahabi A. La plaie craniocérébrale chez l'oxycéphale: ¿quelle précaution prendre pour le traiter? Pan Afr Med J. 2015;22:112. https://doi.org/10.11604/pamj.2015.22.112.7366.
32. Renier D. Intracranial pressure in craniosynostosis pre- and postoperative recordings: correlation with functional results. In: Persing JA, Edgerton MT, Jane JA, editors. Scientific foundations and surgical treatment of craniosynostosis. Baltimore, MD: Williams and Wilkins; 1989. p. 263–9.
33. Di Rocco F, Arnaud E, Renier D. Evolution in the frequency of nonsyndromic craniosynostosis. J Neurosurg Pediatr. 2009;4:21–5.
34. Shilito J Jr, Matson DO. Craniosynostosis: a review of 519 surgical patients. Pediatrics. 1968;41:829–53.
35. Marchac D, Renier D. Chirurgie cranio-faciale des craniosténoses. Paris: Médecine et sciences internationales; 1982.
36. Saldino RM, Steinbach HL, Epstein CJ. Familial acrocephalosyndactyly (Pfeiffer syndrome). AJR. 1972;116:609–22.
37. Cinalli G, Renier D, Sebag G, Sainte-Rose C, Arnaud E, Pierre-Kahn A. La "malformation" de Chiari dans le syndrome de Crouzon. Arch Pediatr. 1996;3:433–9.
38. Cinalli G, Chumas P, Arnaud E, et al. Occipital remodeling and suboccipital decompression in severe craniosynostosis associated with tonsillar herniation. Neurosurgery. 1998;42:66–73.
39. Cinalli G, Spennato P, Sainte-Rose C, et al. Chiari malformation in craniosynostosis. Childs Nerv Syst. 2005;21:889–901.
40. Francis PM, Beals S, Rekate HL, et al. Chronic tonsillar herniation and Crouzon's syndrome. Pediatr Neurosurg. 1992;18:202–6.
41. Frim DM, Jones D, Goumnerova L. Development of symptomatic Chiari malformation in a child with craniofacial dysmorphism. Pediatr Neurosurg. 1990;16:228–31.
42. Mulliken JB, Steinberger D, Kunze S, et al. Molecular diagnosis of bilateral bicoronal synostosis. Plast Reconstr Surg. 1999;104:1603–15.
43. Sainte-Rose C, Arnaud E, Pierre-Kahn A. Chronic tonsillar herniation in Crouzon and Apert syndrome: the role of the premature synostosis of the lambdoid suture. J Neurosurg. 1995;83:575–82.
44. Cinalli G, Renier D, Sebag G, et al. Chronic tonsillar herniation in Crouzon's and Apert's syndromes: the role of premature synostosis of the lambdoid suture. J Neurosurg. 1995;83:575–82.
45. Goodrich JT. Skull base growth in craniosynostosis. Child's Nervs Syst. 2005;21:871–9.
46. Di Rocco C, Velardi F. Acquired Chiari type I malformation managed by supratentorial cranial enlargement. Childs Nerv Syst. 2003,19:800–7. https://doi.org/10.1007/s00381-003-0837-7. Epub 2003 Oct 28
47. Nishikawa M, Sakamoto H, Hakuba A, et al. Pathogenesis of Chiari malformation: a morphometric study of the posterior cranial fossa. J Neurosurg. 1997;86:40–7.
48. Cinalli G, Sainte-Rose CH, Kollar EM, et al. Hydrocephalus and craniosynostosis. J Neurosurg. 1998;88:209–14.
49. Rollins N, Booth T, Shapiro K. MR venography in children with complex craniosynostosis. Pediatr Neurosurg. 2000;32:308–15.
50. Gebre-Medhin M. Rickets. In: Jelliffe, Stanfield, ells. Diseases of children in the subtroplcs and tropics. 3rd ed. London: Edward Arnold; 1978. p. 239–42.
51. Gault DT, Renier D, Marchac D, et al. Intracranial volume in children with craniosynostosis. J Craniofac Surg. 1990;1:1–3.
52. Reilly BI, Leeming JM, Fraser D. Craniosynostosis in the rachitic spectrum. J Pedlatr. 1964;64:396–405.
53. Renier D, El Ghouzi V, Bonaventure J, le Merrer M, Lajeunie E. Fibroblast growth factor receptor 3 mutation in nonsyndromic coronal synostosis: clinical spectrum, prevalence, and surgical outcome. J Neurosurg. 2000;92:631–6.

54. Connolly JP, Gruss J, Seto ML, Whelan MF, Ellenbogen R, Weiss A, Buchman SR, Cunningham ML. Progressive postnatal craniosynostosis and increased intracranial pressure. Plast Reconstr Surg. 2004;113:1313–23.
55. Greene CS. Pancraniosynostosis after surgery for single sutural craniosynostosis. Pediatr Neurosurg. 1998;29:127–32.
56. Twigg SRF, Forecki J, Goos JAC, Richardson ICA, Hoogeboom AVM, et al. Gain-of-function mutations in ZIC1 are associated with coronal craniosynostosis and learning disability. Am J Hum Genet. 2015;97:378–88.
57. Sasaki E, Byrne AT, Murray DJ, Reardon W. Caput membranaceum: a novel clinical presentation of ZIC1 related skull malformation and craniosynostosis. Am J Med Genet A. 2020;182:2994–8. https://doi.org/10.1002/ajmg.a.61882.
58. Fitzpatrick DR. Filling in the gaps in cranial suture biology. Nature Genet. 2013;45:231–2.
59. Armanda T, Schaeferb E, Di Rocco F, Edery P, Collet C, Rossia M. Craniosynostosis: State of the Art 2019. Genetic bases of craniosynostoses: an update. Neurochirurgie. 2019;65:196–201.
60. Lattanzi W, Barba M, Di Pietro L, Boyadjiev SA. Genetic advances in craniosynostosis. Am J Med Genet A. 2017;173:1406–29.
61. Ursitti F, Fadda T, Papetti L, et al. Evaluation and management of nonsyndromic craniosynostosis. Acta Paediatr. 2011;100:1185–94. https://doi.org/10.1111/j.1651-2227.2011.02299.x.
62. Passos-Bueno MR, Fanganiello RD, Jehee FS. Craniosynostosis and chromosomal alterations. Craniosynostoses. 2011;19:152–64.
63. Durham EL, Howie RN, Cray JJ. Gene/environment interactions in craniosynostosis: a brief review. Orthod Craniofac Res. 2017;20(Suppl 1):8–11.
64. Wilkie AO. Craniosynostosis: genes and mechanisms. Hum Mol Genet. 1997;6(10):1647–56. Review.
65. Mindikoglu AN, Erginel A, Cenani A. An unknown syndrome of nose deformity, oxycephaly, aplasia of the nasolacrimal ducts, and symmetrical cyst formation on the upper lip in siblings: craniorhiny. Plast Reconst Surg. 1991;88:699–702.
66. Tolchin D, Yeager JP, Prasad P, Dorrani N, Russi AS, et al. De novo SOX6 variants cause a neurodevelopmental syndrome associated with ADHD, craniosynostosis, and osteochondromas. Am J Hum Genet. 2020;106:830–45.
67. Schouman T, Vinchon M, Ruhin-Coupet B, et al. Isolated bilateral coronal synostosis: early treatment by peri-fronto-orbital craniectomy. J Craniofac Surg. 2008;19:40–4.
68. Dhellemmes P, Lejeune JP, Hladky R, et al. Linear coagulation of the dura in the treatment of craniosynostosis. Childs Nerv Syst. 1994;10:410.
69. Jimenez DF, Barone CM. Multiple-suture nonsyndromic craniosynostosis: early and effective management using endoscopic techniques. J Neurosurg Pediatr. 2010;5:223–31.
70. Rivero-Garvía M, Márquez-Rivas J, Giménez-Pando J. Letter to the editor: craniosynostosis. J Neurosurg Pediatr. 2011;7:218–9. https://doi.org/10.3171/2010.8.PEDS10298.
71. Seeger JF, Gabrielsen TO. Premature closure of the frontosphenoidal suture in synostosis of the coronal suture. Radiology. 1971;101:631–5.
72. Rougerie J, Tessier P. Craniosynostosis and craniofacial dysmorphia. A study of 335 cases with reference to neurosurgery and craniofacial surgery. Z Kinderchir. 1981;34:179–83.
73. Moss ML. The pathogenesis of premature cranial synostosis in man. Acta Anat (Basel). 1960;37:351–70.
74. Hoffman HJ, Mohr G. Lateral canthal advancement of the supraorbital margin: a new corrective technique in the treatment of coronal synostosis. J Neurosurg. 1976;45:376–81.
75. McCarthy JG, Coccaro PJ, Epstein F, et al. Early sketal release in the infant with craniofacial dysostosis. The role of the sphenozygomatic suture. Plast Reconstr Surg. 1978;62:335–46.
76. McCarthy JG, Wood-Smith D. Symposium on diagnosis and treatment of craniofacial anomalies. St Louis, MO: CV Mosby Co. 1979; p. 407–11.
77. Marchac D. Radical forehead remodeling for craniostenosis. Plast Reconstr Surg. 1978;61:823–35.
78. Coccaro PJ. Midface advancement in craniofacial dysostosis. In: Converse JM, McCarthy JG, Wood-Smith D, editors. Symposium on diagnosis and treatment of craniofacial anomalies. CV Mosby Co: St Louis, MO; 1979. p. 407–11.
79. Marchac D, Renier D. The "floating forehead" early treatment of craniofacial stenosis. Ann Chir Plast. 1979;24:121–6.
80. Marchac D, Renier D, Jones BM. Experience with the "floating forehead". Br J Plast Surg. 1988;41:1–15.
81. Marchac D, Renier D, Broumand S. Timing of treatment for craniosynostosis and facio-craniosynostosis: a 20-year experience. Br J Plast Surg. 1994;47:211–22.
82. Öcal E, Sun PP, Persing JA. Craniosynostosis. In: Albright AL, Adelson PD, Pollack IF, editors. Principles and practice of pediatric neurosurgery. 2nd ed. New York, NY: Thieme; 2007. p. 265–88.
83. Persing JA, Jane JA, Delashaw JB. Treatment of bilateral coronal synostosis in infancy: a holistic approach. J Neurosurg. 1990;72:171–5.
84. Seal SK, Steinbok P, Courtemanche DJ. The cranial orbital buttress technique for nonsyndromic unicoronal and metopic craniosynostosis. Neurosurg Focus. 2015;38(5):E4. https://doi.org/10.3171/2015.2.FOCUS14844.
85. Persing JA, Edgerton MT, Park TS, et al. Barrel stave osteotomy for correction of turribrachycephaly craniosynostosis deformity. Ann Plast Surg. 1987;18:488–93.
86. Shen W, Cui J, Chen J, Wang G. A method for calculating cranial height reduction for orbital advancement and treatment of oxycephaly using a multiple bone flap rotation-reposition technique. Plast Reconstr Surg. 2012;129:180e–2e.

87. Powiertowski H, Matlosz Z. Effects du traitement de la craniosténosis par résection de la voute du cráne. Ann Chir. 1970;24:1175–80.
88. Hanson JW, Sayers MP, Knopp LM, et al. Subtotal neonatal calvariectomy for severe craniosynostosis. J Pediatr. 1977;91:257–60.
89. Venes JL. Arnold-Chiari malformation in an infant with kleeblattschädel: an acquired deformity? Neurosurgery. 1998;23:360–2.
90. Kim SW, Shim KW, Plesnila N, Kim YO, Choi JU, Kim DS. Distraction vs remodeling surgery for craniosynostosis. Childs Nerv Syst. 2007;23:201–6.
91. Uemura T, Hayashi T, Satoh K, et al. Three-dimensional cranial expansion using distraction osteogenesis for oxycephaly. J Craniofac Surg. 2003;14:29–36.
92. Zanello M, Arnaud E, Di Rocco F. The mysteries of Blaise Pascal's sutures. Childs Nerv Syst. 2015;31:503–6. https://doi.org/10.1007/s00381-015-2622-9.
93. Renier D, Brubet L, Marchac D. IQ and craniostenosis: evolution in treated and untreated cases. In: Marchac D, editor. Craniofacial surgery. Berlin/Heidelberg/New York, NY: Springer; 1987. p. 114–7.
94. Renier D, Marchac D. Le pronostic des craniosténoses opérées. Ann Pediatr. 1995;42:533–40.
95. Arnaud E, Meneses P, Lajeunie E, et al. Postoperative mental and morphological outcome for nonsyndromic brachycephaly. Plast Reconstr Surg. 2002;110:6–12.
96. Paillas JE, Guillot P, Duplay J, Cain J. Etude neuro-ophtalmologique de 15 observations d'oxycephalies. Rev ONO. 1949;21:70–9.
97. Tamburrini G, Caldarelli M, Massimi L, Gasparini G, Pelo S, Di Rocco C. Complex craniosynostoses: a review of the prominent clinical features and the related management strategies. Childs Nerv Syst. 2012;28:1511–23. https://doi.org/10.1007/s00381-012 1819-4.
98. Hirabayashi S, Sugawara Y, Sakurai A, Harii K, Park S. Frontoorbital advancement by gradual distraction. Technical note. J Neurosurg. 1998;89:1058–61. https://doi.org/10.3171/jns.1998.89.6.1058.

13 Multiple Sutures Synostosis: Key Points for the Neurosurgeons and Management Principles

Dale Swift

13.1 Introduction

The involvement of multiple cranial sutures renders care of the patient with craniosynostosis significantly more complicated. In addition to a more complex deformity of the skull, these patients are more likely to develop brain dysfunction related to progressive structural abnormalities. Persons with multiple cranial suture synostosis are more likely to have raised intracranial pressure, hydrocephalus, cerebellar tonsil herniation, and syringomyelia (Fig. 13.1). It is not only incumbent upon the neurosurgeon to be able to perform appropriate surgical interventions but also to anticipate the development of these conditions in order to minimize their ultimate impact.

As part of a dedicated craniofacial team, the neurosurgeon must be able to identify those patients most at risk for the development of specific neurologic complications (e.g., intracranial hypertension). Thus, the neurosurgeon should have a working knowledge of the expected course for each type of multisuture craniosynostosis and can be able to choose the appropriate technique executed at the appropriate time in order to maximize efficacy and minimize surgical complications and long-term sequelae.

Many forms of multisuture craniosynostosis are described by various eponymous craniofacial syndromes. Syndromic forms of craniosynostosis include Apert, Crouzon, Pfeiffer, Muenke, Saethre-Chotzen as well as others. There are reportedly over 180 different syndromes associated with scraniosynostosis [1]. These syndromes are usually associated with some variant of FGFR mutation [1]. Individual craniosynostosis syndromes may also be associated with noncranial somatic malformations such as syndactyly in Apert syndrome and sensorineural hearing loss in Muenke syndrome. Comprehensive care of these patients in a multidisciplinary setting will allow timely attention to these associated conditions. For example, the prevalence of intestinal malrotation is significantly elevated in patients with FGFR-associated craniosynostosis and may be diagnosed and treated before intestinal complications occur [2].

Sporadic, nonsyndromic forms of multisuture craniosynostosis may fall into recognized patterns such as the trisutural "Mercedes Benz" craniosynostosis [3, 4] or may consist of an apparently random association of suture involvement. It must be suspected that these conditions will ultimately be found to have genetic alterations as well. Ultimately, abnormalities of skull growth and subsequent effects upon the brain depend on the pattern of suture involvement, including sutures of the skull

D. Swift (✉)
Department of Neurosurgery, University of Texas Southwestern Medical Center, Dallas, TX, USA
e-mail: dale.swift@utsouthwestern.edu

F. Di Rocco, J. Kestle (eds.), *Neurosurgical Aspects of Craniosynostosis*,
https://doi.org/10.1007/978-3-031-69386-1_13

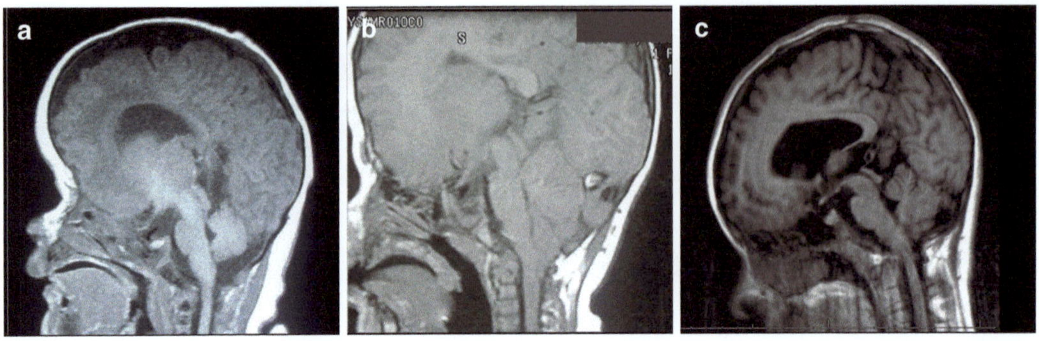

Fig. 13.1 Effect of ventricular shunting on the posterior fossa. (**a**) Sagittal MRI before VPS. (**b**) Sagittal MRI after VPS. (**c**) Sagittal MRI after shunt ligation. This now adult patient had a VPS placed at 8 months of age for progressive ventriculomegaly. Her clinical diagnosis at that time was Crouzon syndrome. Post-operatively she developed CTH. After cranial vault remodeling the shunt was removed. With the availability of genetic testing her diagnosis was changed to Muenke syndrome. This historical case is presented for instructive purposes to illustrate the potential effect of ventricular shunting in complex craniosynostosis

base as well as the calvarium. Although patterns of suture closure tend to follow the syndrome, there is variability within groups [5]. Perhaps, genetic or epigenetic markers may help to distinguish further subgroups of patients in the future.

Due to the relative infrequent prevalence of these conditions, many publications group multiple craniofacial syndromes together. As experience is gained and genetic identification advances, we look forward to more syndrome and morphology-specific investigations. To that end, many groups are now utilizing genetic markers instead of eponyms [6] and recategorizing syndromes based on genetics [7]. For example, Crouzon and Pfeiffer syndromes, both of which usually have FGFR2 mutations, are increasingly considered part of a spectrum [7].

For this chapter, syndromic and multisuture craniosynostosis will be referred to as "complex craniosynostosis" and abbreviated "CCS." The terms "Type 1 Chiari malformation," "hindbrain herniation," "cerebellar tonsil ectopia," "tonsillar prolapse," "chronic tonsillar herniation," and "cerebellar tonsil herniation" will all be considered the same entity and referred to as "cerebellar tonsil herniation" with the abbreviation "CTH."

13.2 Intracranial Hypertension

Although relatively rare in single-suture synostosis, elevated intracranial pressure (ICP) is common in syndromic and multisuture craniosynostosis [8–11]. Despite variations in methodology and patient selection, published incidences of intracranial hypertension (ICH) are consistently higher in syndromic patients and increase with the number of involved sutures [9–11]. The incidence of ICH appears to increase with age in untreated patients [10], although some claim that newly elevated ICP occurs rarely after the age of 8 years [12].

Particularly, informative are the reports of ICP measurements in patients managed expectantly. In these unoperated patients, ICH was reported in 61% of patients with Crouzon syndrome [13] and 83% of patients with Apert syndrome [14]. A recent scoping review of ICH in syndromic synostosis identified 18 studies using invasive ICP monitoring as part of routine prospective screening in patients without signs or symptoms of ICH and reported ICH in 41% [15].

The diagnosis of ICH in patients with CCS may be made definitively with invasive ICP monitoring or inferred by noninvasive methods. The "gold standard" for determining intracranial pressure is invasive intraparenchymal pressure monitoring. Although there are no accepted standards for normal ICP in children of different ages, the values proposed by Renier in 1982 [8] (normal <10 mmHg; abnormal >15 mmHg) are generally accepted today [15]. We aim to obtain 48–36 h of continuous tracing to ensure that there are no effects of anesthesia and that normal sleep and variations in daily activities are recorded. As experience is gained with noninvasive means of ICH detection in this patient population, invasive monitoring is used less frequently [13].

In some patients, the diagnosis of elevated ICP is visually obvious. Patients with a Kleeblattschädel phenotype often demonstrate marked bony construction in some areas with tense dural bulging through cranial defects in other areas. These patients usually exhibit a beaten copper appearance on skull X-rays which is also commonly considered an indicator of elevated ICP [15].

Papilledema is a highly specific indicator of raised intracranial pressure, but is not necessarily sensitive [15]. Sensitivity is significantly higher in patients 8 years or older [16]. Other ophthalmologic measures, such as optical coherence tomography, optic nerve sheath diameter, and visual evoked potentials, have received less widespread use [15].

Simple head growth measurements may be difficult to interpret in CCS patients. Interpretation must consider the patient's surgical history. Fronto-occipital circumference (FOC) has been highly correlated to intracranial volume, and an arrest in FOC growth has been associated with ICH only in patients who have undergone prior cranial expansion [17, 18]

13.2.1 Etiology of Intracranial Hypertension

Four separate physiologic conditions are considered to contribute to elevated ICP in patients with CCS: cranial growth restriction, intracranial venous hypertension, hydrocephalus, and hypoventilation secondary to upper airway obstruction. The contributions of each of these conditions will vary with each syndrome and each patient and must be ascertained individually in each case. A brief description of each of these contributory conditions follows. Hydrocephalus will be described in a later section. Doerga et al. provide a comprehensive review and concise summary of the pertinent literature [15].

13.2.2 Growth Restriction

It seems intuitive that premature closure of multiple cranial sutures would result in restricted growth of the cranium. Normal rapid brain growth in infancy in the setting of restricted cranial growth may therefore be envisioned to be the cause of elevated intracranial pressure. Interestingly, however, measurements of intracranial volume in CCS have demonstrated normal values in most syndromes and increased ICV in Apert syndrome [15, 19–21]. Similarly, brain volume in patients with CCS is reported to be normal [22]. Thus other explanations apart from a simple mechanistic theory of restricted cranial growth are required.

Simple single-suture craniosynostosis has long been known to redistribute the convexity CSF in predictable patterns [23]. Thus, synostosis could reduce skull compliance while maintaining normal volume. This could result in altered pulse pressures leading to elevated pressure. Although this concept has not been explicitly addressed, increased intracranial pulse pressures with normal ICV and elevated ICP have been reported in CCS [21]. Thus, the empiric observation that ICP decreases after cranial vault expansion may be explained by an increase in skull compliance and not necessarily an increase in intracranial volume. Indeed, the description of craniosynostosis as "premature" suture fusion may be a simplistic understanding of a more complex pathology.

13.2.3 Intracranial Venous Hypertension

Intracranial venous hypertension in patients with CCS was first noted only in patients with hydrocephalus and was localized angiographically to the narrowing of the jugular foramen [24]. Subsequently, stenosis or occlusion of the jugular foramina has been found to be a consistent finding in CCS, especially Apert, Crouzon–Pfeiffer, and Saethre-Chotzen syndromes [25–28]. Jugular foramen stenosis has been found to be more severe in CCS patients with ICH even in the absence of hydrocephalus [25, 26, 28]. The etiology of jugular foramen stenosis in CCS is presumed secondary to premature closure of the skull base synchondroses [29].

In addition to bony stenosis of the jugular foramen, varying degrees of collateral vein development surrounding the foramen are consistently observed [25, 30]. Demonstration by MR angiography has replaced conventional catheter angiography in more recent studies [25, 30]. It is theorized that as venous collaterals develop in response to jugular foramen stenosis, intracranial venous hypertension is relieved. The degree of collateral formation does not, however, consistently correlate with the development of ICH [27]. Nonetheless, venous collateral formation may at least partially account for the observation that primary ICH in CCS rarely develops after 6–8 years of age [12, 25].

If intracranial venous hypertension due to jugular foramen stenosis is a major contributor to the ICH observed in CCS, it would seem desirable to address this pathology directly. Attempts at venous bypass initially reported in 1984 have not been subsequently repeated [24]. Indeed, venous bypass graft patency may be difficult to maintain, especially in very young children. In another condition notable for jugular foramen stenosis and achondroplasia, surgical decompression of the jugular foramen has been reported once without follow-up [31]. Certainly, one must be concerned that a surgical approach to this region may disrupt potentially beneficial collateral venous drainage. As yet there are no endovascular options and angioplasty or stenting seems impractical if bony stenosis of the foramen magnum is indeed the primary cause of intracranial venous hypertension.

Thus, cranial expansion remains the procedure of choice for ICH in CCS even when intracranial venous hypertension is a major contributor despite the fact that it does not directly address the problem. Knowledge of abnormal venous anatomy is important during any cranial procedures in these patients as the sinuses may be occluded, deeply embedded in the cranial bone, or even extracranial. Accessory venous drainage must be anticipated as interruption of these collaterals may result in severe cerebral edema [32]. The fact that cranial expansion does not address the venous issue may explain the rapid recurrence of ICH which can be seen in these patients [33].

13.2.4 Upper Airway Obstruction

Obstructive sleep apnea (OSA) is common in patients with syndromic CS [15, 34, 35]. OSA is caused by midface hypoplasia and therefore occurs mostly in the relevant syndromes. Thus, OSA occurs most often in Apert syndrome (80%), Crouzon–Pfeiffer's syndromes (68%), and to a lesser degree in Saethre-Chotzen and Muenke syndromes [35, 36]. The severity of OSA in these syndromes is maximal during the first 3 years of life [34].

OSA has been found to correlate with ICH [37] and indeed to be a predictor of ICH [18]. In addition, marked differences in ICH between quiet sleep and active sleep have been observed with active sleep resulting in increased ICP [37, 38]. These active sleep periods are associated with OSA on polysomnograms and result in significant ICH plateau waves and reductions in cerebral perfusion pressure (CPP) [38]. Although CO_2 levels were not measured in this study, marked hypoxemia was documented [38].

Airway surgery, usually consisting of tonsillectomy and adenoidectomy, improves sleep architecture but has not been documented to obviate the need for cranial vault expansion [34, 36]. Often, the result is incomplete, and nocturnal oxygen with or without continuous positive airway pressure is required to maintain safe arterial oxygen levels during sleep. In the most severely affected children, especially those with Pfeiffer syndrome, tracheostomy may be lifesaving and should be considered early [39]. Ultimately, however, midface advancement may be beneficial for both esthetic, dental, and respiratory concerns. Craniofacial surgeons differ regarding the optimal age and technique for midface distraction, but when successful, patients should be able to be decannulated from any prior tracheostomy [39, 40].

13.2.5 Consequences of Intracranial Hypertension

The consequences of chronic intracranial hypertension in patients with complex craniosynostosis include vision loss and cognitive impairment. Vision loss may occur in the absence of other signs or symptoms [41]. Khan reported that 40% of 141 children with a syndromic form of craniosynostosis had visual impairment sufficient to preclude them from obtaining a driver's license in the UK [42]. Often vision loss is associated with delayed presentation to medical attention. Visual acuity with papilledema may improve with effective ICP treatment but does not when optic atrophy is present [43]. It is essential that CCS therefore receives regular ophthalmologic assessment.

The causative influence of intracranial hypertension on cognition is less as well substantiated. A few studies suggest that elevated ICP is associated with cognitive impairment and that earlier treatment results in improved cognitive outcomes (Renier,1982) [44]. As there are many confounding variables, the causation of this association remains to be proven [45]. Supporting evidence is provided by the observation that decreased cerebral cortical thickness is correlated with papilledema and hydrocephalus independently in patients with CSS [46]. In the end, this author agrees with the concept put forth by Hayward in 2015; *"the neurosurgeon's default position must always be to assume that raised ICP left untreated can indeed impair developmental outcome"* [12].

13.2.6 Treatment

13.2.6.1 Timing

The decisions of if, when, and how to surgically intervene are highly intertwined. It is well established that early (less than 6 months) surgical calvarial expansion and reconstruction will inevitably require further procedures. However, later (over 1 year of age) procedures may expose the patient to prolonged deleterious effects of elevated ICP. In an effort to minimize surgical procedures and maximize functional and esthetic outcomes, each patient must be considered individually, anticipating growth tendencies based on the patient's genotype. At this point in time, "There is no clear consensus on the ideal operative window for syndromic craniosynostosis" [47].

13.2.6.2 Technique

Cranial procedures designed to relieve ICH can be divided into two broad groups, "passive" and "active." [48] Passive procedures consist of bone removal and decompression of the dura and brain. Active procedures include cranial vault expansion and remodeling as well as cranial distraction osteogenesis techniques which aim to reshape the skull to increase intracranial volume. Both types of procedures are carefully planned together by craniofacial and neurosurgeons to consider esthetic as well as neurosurgical concerns.

During "passive" procedures, variable amounts of cranial bone are removed without reconstruction. These procedures are usually performed at less than 3 months of age, in patients with documented or suspected ICH. These decompressive craniectomies have traditionally involved a bicoronal scalp incision and removal of large portions of the calvarium which at this age can reliably be expected to re-ossify. In fact, calvarial regrowth usually reconstitutes the previous pattern of suture pathology. These "passive" procedures are not definitive and nearly always require additional surgery at a later date [48].

Although conceptually simple, these procedures pose considerable surgical risk in this population. Apart from airway and general anesthetic concerns, excessive blood loss is always a concern in neonates. Continuous diligent protection of the dura and underlying brain during the procedure is mandatory. The bone is markedly thin in places and often completely deficit. In other areas, especially at the involved sutures, the bone may be thickened and embedded in the dura. Often spicules of bone deeply embedded in the dura are surrounded by outpouchings of the dura and brain. Even with careful dissection of the bone, often the underlying dura is attenuated and the incidental durotomy is frequent. At times, complete bone removal may not be possible due to severe ingrowth of bone around a dural venous sinus. In that case, the bone may be liberated from all surrounding bones, resulting in a "floating island" of bone, which then assumes a new decompressed position. The author rarely uses a craniotome in this situation for fear of dural injury. At all times, care must be taken to protect the soft infant brain. Often encephalomalacia is apparent on postoperative neuroimaging in areas of most severe compression and may be related to surgical technique. At the completion of the decompression, some of the pieces of bone may be laid on the dura without fixation, or the bone may be omitted. Postoperatively, patients should be carefully positioned to protect the incision, pressure points on the scalp, and the underlying unprotected brain.

The Kleeblattschädel skull deformity represents the most severe manifestation of cranial growth restriction. It consists of synostosis of the coronal, squamosa, and lambdoid sutures and is generally associated with Pfeiffer, Crouzon's, or Apert syndrome. The Kleeblattschädel phenotype is one instance in which early decompressive craniectomy is indicated.

With the development of minimally invasive treatment of single-suture synostosis, endoscopic suturectomy in CCS has also been described [49, 50]. These early reports have few patients, are not syndrome-specific, and report limited follow-up. However, with a 50% durotomy incidence and high recurrence, the practicality of this technique appears limited [50]. Apart from a shorter scalp incision with potentially less blood loss, there is no expectation in multisuture CCS that further surgery would not be required.

Cranial Vault Procedures

In older patients (>1 year) with structurally sufficient cranial bone, open cranial vault expansion and remodeling have been the mainstay of treatment of intracranial hypertension in complex craniosynostosis. Both anterior and posterior cranial vault expansions and remodelings have been used with the dual goals of decreasing ICP and improving cosmetic appearance. The choice has often been surgeon-dependent depending upon the individual cranial and orbital morphology [40]. Due to the pioneering work of Paul Tessier in the 1970s [51], for many years attention was predominantly concentrated on anterior cranial expansion. This approach, which includes forehead advancement, allowed a reduction in ICP with an improvement in apparent proptosis when present [40]. The benefits of anterior cranial vault reconstruction, however, appear to be short-lived in CCS as elevated ICP often recurs [18, 52]. Recurrence may be rapid and evidenced only by persistent or recurrent papilledema [33].

From an esthetic standpoint, multiple operations involving the anterior cranial may lead toward irregular growth and an unacceptable appearance of the orbits and forehead. Accordingly, many craniofacial surgeons began using posterior vault expansion as the first intervention, reserving anterior reconstruction until skeletal maturity and a more durable anterior contour could be anticipated [53, 54]. Posterior expansion was also found to provide a greater increase in head circumference and a diminished tendency toward papilledema and progressive CTH and anterior procedures [54].

Despite this apparent improvement in surgical technique, intracranial hypertension recurs in a substantial proportion of cases [27]. Despite what appears to be rigid reconstruction in an expanded position, maintenance of this expansion may be inhibited by a lack of scalp elasticity exacerbated by patient positioning.

Distraction osteotomy was initially developed as a limb-lengthening technique in the 1950s. Application to the facial skeleton was developed in the 1990s first to the mandible and midface. In 1998, Sugawara reported applying the distraction technique to the anterior cranium [55]. In 2009, White published the first cases of posterior cranial vault distraction osteogenesis (PCVDO) reporting resolution of intracranial hypertension and improved head shape [56]. Since that time, the techniques have been refined and the procedure has become widely accepted with numerous published results [57–63] (Fig. 13.2).

Multiple theoretical advantages of PCVDO have been proposed. Since the cranial bone is not removed from the dura, vascularity to the bone is

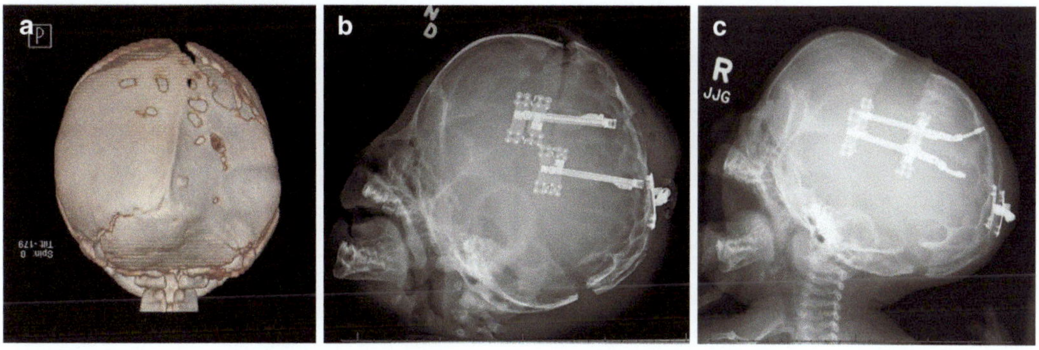

Fig. 13.2 Male patient with sagittal and lambdoid synostosis (Mercedes Benz pattern) who underwent PCVDO with foramen magnum decompression. (**a**) CT at 10 days of age. (**b**) Skull X-ray at beginning of distraction. (**c**) Skull X-ray at completion of distraction

maintained and an epidural dead space is avoided. This should promote growth and minimize infection. In addition, gradual expansion with bone formation in the osteotomy gap should allow a more durable expansion. In practice, PCVDO has been shown to provide a greater increase in intracranial volume than traditional cranial expansion [64–66]. Patients operated at less than 1 year of age experience an even greater proportional increase [67, 68]. Interestingly, PCVDO in patients with turricephaly also appears to improve the anterior bossing deformity [56].

The complication rate of PCVDO is relatively high but appears to be diminishing consistently as multiple craniofacial centers adopt and perfect the technique. Meta-analysis of complications reports aggregate rates of 25–30% with most being device failures and CSF leaks [69, 70]. Device failure is decreasing as the hardware design improves and is standardized. Infection rates were 4.9–6.9% mostly consisting of local infections at the device exit site [69, 70]. Presumably due to the presence of a transcutaneous device, shunt infections are more frequent after PCVDO than traditional posterior vault remodeling [71].

Although the emergence of PCVDO has been primarily driven by the craniofacial community, the role of the neurosurgeon remains integral to safe surgery with minimal complications. Craniotomy cuts must be carefully planned and executed to avoid dural or venous sinus lacerations. Often a high-speed cutting burr should be used instead of a craniotome to cut a trough along the craniotomy path. This should minimize the risk of dural or venous sinus injury and create a furrow wide enough to prevent premature bone fusion during the distraction phase. The neurosurgeons should carefully monitor device placement for potential dural perforations. All dural lacerations should be repaired as CSF leakage is to be expected in these patients with elevated ICP. Even partial thickness dural tears should be addressed as the rent may extend as distraction proceeds [69]. In patients with ventricular shunts, the subgaleal path of the shunt should be assessed and rerouting is considered if the shunt will be subjected to bacterial contamination from the distraction device [72]. PCVDO has also been found to improve the radiographic appearance of CTH as will be discussed later. Thus, the neurosurgeon will continue to be crucial to success as indications for cranial distraction expand.

13.3 Hydrocephalus

13.3.1 Incidence

Whereas the occurrence of hydrocephalus in children with single-suture craniosynostosis is not increased over the general population, hydrocephalus is commonly seen in multisuture and syndromic craniosynostosis [73–75]. The incidence of hydrocephalus in complex craniosynostosis varies with each particular syndrome and

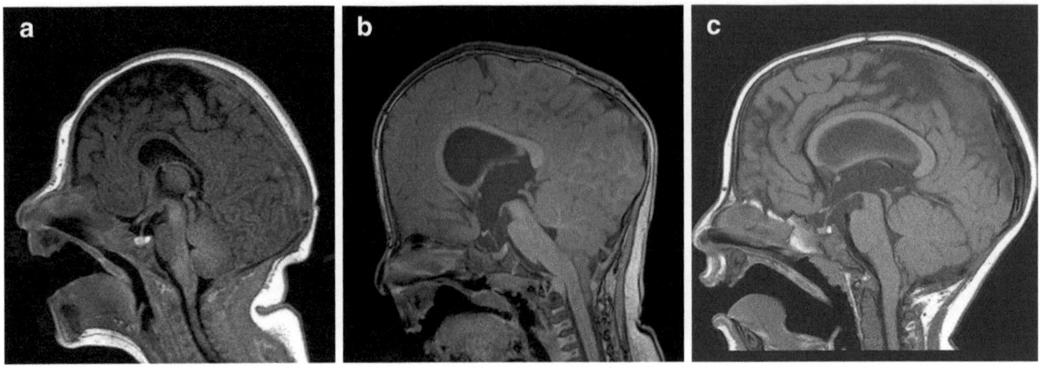

Fig. 13.3 Mid sagittal MRIs of patient in Fig. 13.2. (**a**) MRI at 10 days of demonstrated a small posterior fossa without CTH. (**b**) MRI at 7 months demonstrates the acquisition of significant CTH. (**c**) MRI at 17 months of age, 6 months after removal of distractors demonstrates significant improvement in head shape and CTH

with the patterns of suture involvement. Hydrocephalus appears to occur more often when the lambdoid sutures are involved and when CTH is present [73, 76] (Fig. 13.3).

The published incidences of hydrocephalus in CCS vary widely and must be considered only approximations due to differences in patient referrals and variable definitions of hydrocephalus and ventriculomegaly. The overall rate, however, may be considered to be around 15% [77]. By syndrome, hydrocephalus necessitating intervention has been reported in 47% of patients with Pfeiffer syndrome, 20% of patients with Crouzon syndrome, 8% of patients with Apert syndrome [74], and essentially 100% of patients with a Kleeblattschädel skull deformity [73, 76, 78, 79].

Although hydrocephalus has been reported to be present "at onset," [7] in the author's experience hydrocephalus is not present if neuroimaging is obtained around the time of birth. Thereafter, serial neuroimaging generally reveals progressive ventricular dilatation during the first few months of life which may stabilize (and thus be considered "ventriculomegaly") or progress. Patients with Apert syndrome are more likely to demonstrate stable ventriculomegaly than patients with Crouzon/Pfeiffer syndrome [73]. In patients followed closely during the first years of life, it may be difficult to determine at what point ventricular enlargement becomes sufficiently severe to warrant surgical intervention. Hydrocephalus necessitating treatment, however, is generally apparent within the first 2–3 years of life.

Occasionally, especially in patients with the Kleeblattschädel phenotype, hydrocephalus becomes apparent only after cranial vault decompression and may progress rapidly [80]. Early postoperative neuroimaging is thus recommended in infants after cranial decompressive and expansion procedures. Patients with Apert syndrome may demonstrate increased extra-axial CSF after cranial expansion which usually resolves spontaneously [73].

13.3.2 Etiology

The etiology of hydrocephalus in complex craniosynostosis is likely multifactorial. The two main pathophysiologic mechanisms which have been considered are (1) dural venous hypertension, resulting in a communicating type of hydrocephalus, and (2) fourth ventricle CSF outflow obstruction (from posterior fossa crowding and cerebellar tonsil herniation) resulting in an obstructive hydrocephalus. The relative contribution of each of these pathologies may vary with each syndrome and may change with age. Indeed, the consequences of dural venous hypertension and cerebellar tonsil herniation may influence each other [24, 81].

Understanding of hydrocephalus associated with CCS has evolved with advances in neuroimaging. Early investigations were performed using pneumoencephalography, angiography, or first-generation computed tomography [24, 82, 83]. Angiographic findings revealed jugular foramen stenosis (as discussed in the previous section on *Intracranial Venous Hypertension*), and the resulting increased dural venous pressure was thought to impair CSF absorption [24]. In 1984, Sainte-Rose et al. simultaneously measured pressures in the lateral ventricles, superior sagittal sinuses, and jugular veins of children with various forms of hydrocephalus, including many with craniosynostosis [24]. In patients with craniosynostosis and presumed stenosis of the jugular foramen, elevated pressure in the dural venous sinuses persisted after the removal of CSF from the ventricle. By contrast, in patients without presumed dural sinus obstruction, the venous sinus pressure decreased with CSF removal. It was therefore concluded that hydrocephalus in CSS was the result of impaired CSF absorption due to dural venous hypertension. This communicating type of hydrocephalus would not ostensibly be amenable to endoscopic third ventriculostomy [24] [74]. Some investigators consider this vascular pathophysiology to be similar than that seen in achondroplasia [24]. In achondroplasia, it is currently believed that intracranial-to-extracranial venous collaterals develop in response to jugular foremen stenosis and stabilize intracranial pressure, albeit perhaps slightly above normal.

With the development of MR imaging, it was found that many patients have a "crowded" appearing posterior fossa with herniation of the cerebellar tonsils. In these patients, although there is an open aqueduct of Sylvius, there appears to be resistance to CSF outflow from the fourth ventricle. The fourth ventricle is often small, the aqueduct is flared, and the floor of the third ventricle is bowed outward. This appearance has led to an obstructive theory of hydrocephalus in complex craniosynostosis.

The correlation of hydrocephalus with cerebellar tonsil herniation in complex craniosynostosis is quite high. In Crouzon/Pfeiffer syndrome, it appears that nearly all patients with hydrocephalus also have cerebellar tonsil herniation [7, 84]. In contrast, only 53% of patients with cerebellar tonsil herniation were found to have hydrocephalus [84]. Thus, it appears that in patterns of craniosynostosis that involve premature closure of the lambdoid sutures (most commonly Crouzon/Pfeiffer syndrome), cerebellar tonsil herniation may add an obstructive component to extant communicating hydrocephalus due to venous hypertension.

13.3.3 Treatment

The decision to treat hydrocephalus in the setting of complex craniosynostosis must not be made without careful consideration. Seemingly minor complications such as CSF leaks often result in prolonged hospitalizations, multiple surgeries, cerebrospinal fluid infections, and consequent central nervous system sequelae. There are no universally accepted indications for hydrocephalus intervention in this complicated patient population. Because the ventricles are normal size at birth, ventricular enlargement must be due to some increased CSF resistance—unless due to cerebral atrophy. Although many publications differentiate between ventriculomegaly and "active" hydrocephalus, there are no accepted measurements which distinguish these two entities, and enlarged ventricles which stabilize may still be under abnormally high pressure, especially in patients with impaired cranial growth. Ventricular dilatation probably represents a spectrum of abnormal CSF resistance. Intuitive surgical indications include obviously large ventricles with periventricular edema and tense bulging cranial defects/fontanelles in patients with large ventricles. Other clinical indications such as poor feeding or decreased activity levels are less obvious in this population.

Especially in infancy, the timing of CSF diversion in relation to cranial vault decompression is variable [85]. In the author's experience, cranial vault remodeling generally precedes CSF diversion, however, as previously mentioned, rapid ventricular expansion can appear after cranial decompression. Cranial vault surgery does not generally improve hydrocephalus [59, 76, 80]. This fact should be considered when planning the sequence of surgical procedures. Posterior cranial vault distraction, however, has the potential to improve cerebellar tonsil herniation [59, 60, 62] and with further experience may potentially prove to influence hydrocephalus. In cases in which the optimal sequence of procedures is not clear, we have occasionally performed ETV concomitantly with cranial vault remodeling or distraction. It is not, however, advised to perform shunting procedures simultaneously with cranial expansion procedures as there may be an increased risk of shunt infection and/or migration in the presence of large postoperative subgaleal fluid collections.

Currently, treatment options for hydrocephalus in these patients consist of CSF diversion either via ventricular shunting (usually peritoneal) or endoscopic third ventriculostomy. Lumboperitoneal shunts were in use in the 1960s but were found to have a high incidence of cerebellar tonsil herniation [86–88]. Indeed, in this population, diversion of CSF from the spinal intrathecal space carries a high risk of inducing or worsening hindbrain herniation and may increase mortality from brainstem compression [89] (Fig. 13.4).

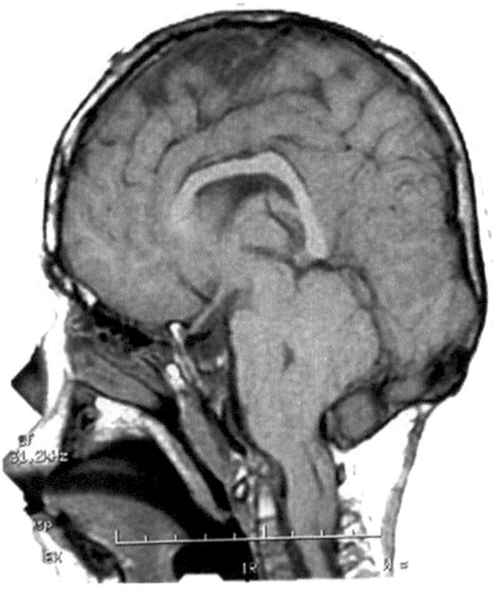

Fig. 13.4 Severe hindbrain herniation with brainstem compression in a 14 year-old male with Crouzon syndrome and a ventricular shunt

13.3.4 Ventricular Shunting

For many years, the only treatment available was VPS. The limitations and frustrations of ventricular shunts are well known to all neurosurgeons. However, shunts in patients with complex craniosynostosis manifest an additional complement of concerns. Ventricular shunting is known to induce premature cranial suture fusion, cranial deformity, and impair cranial growth even in patients without craniosynostosis [90]. Thus, in patients with complex craniosynostosis, the lack of normal outward dural pressure may result in a more irregular cranial shape and impaired cranial growth following cranial reconstruction surgery. Although this is a common observation amongst craniofacial surgeons, this interface of neurosurgery and esthetics has received little academic attention. One study, however, has claimed improved esthetic outcomes in patients with programmable shunt valves compared to fixed pressure valves [85]. Another concern of craniofacial surgeons is the potential for epidural and cranial bone infection from a large epidural dead space in shunted patients. Although not documented in cranial reconstruction for complex craniosynostosis, an increased infection rate in patients with ventricular shunts has been observed in cranioplasty following decompressive craniectomy [91].

One interesting complication that may occur in patients with complex craniosynostosis after extrathecal CSF shunting is the development or worsening of cerebellar tonsil herniation [92]. Although not subject to systematic analysis, the degree of cerebellar tonsil herniation has been observed to be worse in patients with ventricular shunts [92, 93]. This may seem counterintuitive since CSF shunting should decrease ICP and potential downward pressure on the cerebellar tonsils. However, in the presence of increased venous pressure, diversion of CSF may result in relative venous congestion of the brain which encourages hindbrain herniation in an anatomically small posterior fossa [92]. A similar pathophysiologic mechanism has been described in patients with achondroplasia in whom ventricular shunting is notoriously complicated [94].

Thus, we see that ventricular shunting should be carefully considered in patients with complex craniosynostosis. As an alternative, endoscopic third ventriculostomy (vide infra) should be highly considered. Nonetheless, there are situations where a ventricular shunt is the only option and must be provided to control hypertensive hydrocephalus. In these situations, we alter our usual surgical technique in order to minimize expected complications. Although in other types of hydrocephalus, we generally place frontal shunts, in complex craniosynostosis we insert the ventricular catheter from an occipital approach in order to avoid hardware exposure during repeated craniofacial surgeries. The hole-bearing segment of the ventricular catheter is positioned in the frontal horn either endoscopically or with stereotactic guidance. We utilize a burr hole style valve in order to avoid positioning any bulky hardware below the superior nuchal line where muscular action may result in disconnection. We also attempt to plan the subgaleal shunt path under the most robust scalp possible and avoid areas where the overlying scalp might be at risk for breakdown.

The use of programmable or high-resistance valves in this setting is advisable for a few reasons. Although in infancy the valve pressure may need to be relatively low, ultimately shunt valve resistance should be as high as tolerated to avoid many of the complications mentioned previously. We have often observed changes in the level of the cerebellar tonsils with adjustments in shunt valve resistance. In addition, some patients with complex CS and hydrocephalus become shunt-independent with age. Occasionally, ventricular shunting is used to control CSF fistulae [95]. In these situations, programmable valves can provide low pressure initially to close the CSF leak. Later, the valve resistance can be increased with potential shunt removal.

13.3.5 Endoscopic Third Ventriculostomy

The observation that hydrocephalus associated with complex craniosynostosis is triventricular appears to invite the consideration of ETV. Given the well-described vascular theory, ETV has been slow to be accepted as a viable option [74]. Di Rocco reported 11 children in whom ETV was performed with a success rate of 60% [77]. The children were operated on at a mean of 20 months with some as young as 3 months of age [77]. The group was selected based on anatomical features which suggested CSF obstruction in the posterior fossa. Most had Crouzon or Pfeiffer syndrome. Anatomic features such as tonsillar ectopia and outward distention of the floor of the fourth ventricle did not reliably predict success. Importantly, success was achieved in two-thirds of patients with jugular stenosis [77]. Since this initial report, some have suggested ETV as an alternative to VPS [96, 97], while others reject ETV in favor of extrathecal CSF diversion [85].

The author's experience with ETV has a similar success rate of 65% [98]. Our selection criteria include crowding of the posterior fossa and outward bowing of the third ventricle. Initial failures were predominantly due to CSF leakage and as such we now perform watertight dural closure after ETV. It is presumed that ETV can only improve one of the multiple causes of elevated intracranial pressure seen in complex craniosynostosis. Thus, even after successful ETV, some degree of intracranial hypertension may persist. Care must be taken in the postoperative period to anticipate residual elevated ICP and minimize risks of CSF leak and subgaleal fluid collections. In severe cases, a ventricular reservoir may be placed at the time of ETV followed by serial aspirations to minimize the risk of CSF leak as success of the ETV is established.

The treatment of hydrocephalus in patients with complex craniosynostosis must be considered in the totality of care. Simply placing a shunt may not be the best course of action in the long term. The observed success of ETV argues against a purely vascular etiology of hydrocephalus in patients with favorable posterior fossa anatomy. Apart from failure requiring shunt placement, ETV in these patients has not been associated with significant adverse effects. Thus, it is recommended that ETV can be considered primarily when treating hydrocephalus associated with complex craniosynostosis. In the event that ventricular shunting is required, specific modifications to standard techniques should be considered to minimize complications.

13.4 Cerebellar Tonsil Herniation

Cerebellar tonsil herniation in association with craniofacial syndrome was first noted in 1972 [99] and postulated to be an acquired condition in 1988 [100]. With advances in neuroimaging, the prevalence of CTH in the various craniofacial syndromes has been defined. Along with airway obstruction, CTH with brainstem compression represents one of the leading causes of morbidity in complex craniosynostosis. As with CTH in general, syringomyelia and its attendant complications and disabilities may also result. The CTH seen in CSS may be anticipated and its effects minimized with appropriate surgical care. Given the observation that CTH is usually acquired, the condition is best referred to as a postnatal "deformity" than a malformation [93].

13.4.1 Incidence

In the absence of involvement of the lambdoid suture, single-suture synostosis is rarely associated with cerebellar tonsil herniation [101, 102]. CTH is, however, common in multisuture craniosynostosis [101, 103]. The incidence varies with the syndrome and pattern of suture involvement. It is highly correlated with premature lambdoid suture closure [84]. About 75% of patients with Crouzon/Pfeiffer's develop hindbrain herniation, whereas it occurs in less than 5% of patients with Apert syndrome [39, 84]. CTH is rare in bicoronal synostosis, and Muenke and Saethre-Chotzen syndromes in which early lambdoid suture closure is not usually a feature [93, 104]. In apparently random associations of multiple suture fusion, CTH depends upon the involvement of the lambdoid sutures and tonsil herniation may involve only the affected side. The so-called "Mercedes Benz" pattern of bilateral lambdoid and posterior sagittal synostosis appropriately has a high incidence of CTH of at least 60% [10, 53]. With respect to cranial phenotype, essentially all patients with a Kleeblattschädel skull shape develop hindbrain herniation [103] and about 60% with oxycephaly [106].

Similar to hydrocephalus, in patients with complex craniosynostosis, CTH is an acquired condition; thus, estimations of incidence will depend upon the age at which neuroimaging is obtained. Neuroimaging obtained in the neonatal period usually reveals a relatively normal-appearing cerebellum. The time course over which CTH develops has not been fully elucidated but appears to be during the first few months of life and precedes the development of hydrocephalus.

As in patients with other forms of CTH (Chiari I Malformation), syringomyelia is observed frequently in the setting of CCS. The true incidence is not known but in Crouzon patients with CTH has been observed to be about 20% [84]. The pathophysiology of syringomyelia resulting from CTH has been extensively investigated in patients without craniosynostosis [107]. Although presumed to be similar, syringomyelia observed in complex craniosynostosis may also have genetic influences [108].

13.4.2 Etiology

As seen with the development of intracranial hypertension and hydrocephalus, herniation of the cerebellar tonsils in CCS appears to be the result of multiple predisposing forces. These primarily include growth restriction and dural venous hypertension but can be modified by CSF forces.

Hindbrain herniation occurs most commonly in syndromes which exhibit prematurely lambdoid suture closure [103]. Thus, it appears as though growth restriction is a major driver of cerebellar tonsillar herniation. Indeed, in unilateral lambdoid synostosis, there is often asymptomatic herniation of the cerebellar tonsil on the affected side. Volumetric studies of the posterior fossa reveal mixed results with some showing decreased volumes [109] and others showing more normal posterior fossa volumes [110, 111]. Interestingly, one of the studies of unoperated Crouzon patients reported normal posterior fossa volumes despite documenting premature closure of the lambdoid suture and skull base synchondroses [110]. Another study of children with CCS measured posterior fossa and cerebellar volumes and found both to be normal [111]. The ratio of cerebellar volume to posterior fossa volume was, however, found to be increased in patients with CTH [111]. Thus, as discussed in the section on intracranial hypertension, simple growth restriction fails to adequately explain the observed hindbrain herniation.

The role of venous hypertension must again be emphasized as a potential factor in CTH. Venous engorgement of the cerebellum due to elevated dural venous sinus pressure from jugular foramen stenosis may result in engorgement of the cerebellum resulting in cerebellar tonsil herniation. An interesting study of infants with a vein of Galen malformations (without craniosynostosis) revealed CTH which correlated with dural venous hypertension and congestion within the cerebellar veins [81]. CTH reduced after embolization resulted in improved cerebellar venous outflow [81]. The authors also noted that CTH was not the result of raised intraventricular pressure [81]. Others have reported CTH with syringomyelia in adult patients with high-flow AVMs which have reduced after embolization [112, 113]

Thus, there may be some interplay between the effect of premature suture closure and increased venous resistance that predisposes toward CTH. The fact that CTH nearly always develops early in life may be attributable to the exuberant growth demonstrated by the cerebellum in the neonatal period. It is well known that brain growth is rapid during the first year of life. Growth, however, is disproportionate with cerebral hemisphere volume increasing by 90% and cerebellar volume by 240% [114].

Although some consider CTH to be a CSF disorder [6], it is unlikely that hydrocephalus is the main cause of CTH seen in CCS [93]. As mentioned in the section on hydrocephalus, CTH seems to be a prerequisite for hydrocephalus, but hydrocephalus does not necessarily result in CTH. Nonetheless, hydrocephalus may exacerbate brainstem-related symptoms resulting from hindbrain herniation as is commonly observed in patients with Chiari II malformations and myelodysplasia. Thus, control of intracranial and intraventricular hypertension should be achieved in conjunction with craniovertebral decompression. Unintuitively, however, the treatment of hydrocephalus with extrathecal CSF diversion in these patients may worsen or incite cerebellar herniation [92, 93]. As mentioned in the section on hydrocephalus, all efforts should be made to minimize the adverse effects of CSF overdrainage in these patients by either performing ETV or utilizing programmable or high-resistance shunt valves.

13.4.3 Treatment

In patients with CCS, clinical symptoms of CTH may be more difficult to detect than in patients without craniosynostosis. Perhaps, due to the presence of chronic illness, these patients often do not admit to classic tussive occipital or cervical pain. Chronic respiratory obstruction may mask central or obstructive sleep apnea from brainstem compression. We routinely obtain sleep studies in patients with significant CTH on MRI to assess for central sleep apnea even if a tracheostomy is in place.

It is estimated that surgery is indicated for 30% of CSS patients with CTH by virtue of either clinical symptoms or the discovery of syringomyelia [103]. Since syringomyelia is present in 20% of patients and may be asymptomatic, routine MRI of the spine is recommended in patients with known CTH [103]. Despite the high prevalence of CTH in CSS, most patients with radiographic CTH do not require surgical attention. The symptoms are notoriously insidious, and all members of the care team as well as the patients' families should be aware of this potential.

Surgical approaches to CTH in this population may be divided into two groups: traditional direct neurosurgical procedures and more craniofacially oriented combined procedures. Direct approaches are the same as performed in patients without craniosynostosis while combined approaches typically include remodeling of the posterior cranial vault with or without suboccipital decompression. The recent technique of distraction osteogenesis which is rapidly displacing traditional cranial vault remodeling is also providing another option for CTH treatment.

The options for surgical treatment of patients with typical type 1 Chiari malformations *without craniosynostosis* are controversial and continue to be debated [115]. The mainstay of surgery is suboccipital decompression with or without duroplasty and potential intradural reduction of the cerebellar tonsils [115]. This standard approach is associated with a higher failure rate in patients with craniosynostosis [116]. Accordingly, the author often performs subpial resection of herniated cerebellar tonsils in order to more effectively reduce brainstem compression and reestablish the patency of the cisterna magna. Obviously, extreme care must be taken when manipulating the intradural structures so as not to damage the brainstem and to minimize intradural scarring postoperatively. This technique has proven effective and safe in patients without CSS [115].

In patients with CCS, direct decompressive surgery is often much more challenging. Although large studies in CCS are lacking, bony decompression and duraplasty are often insufficient to provide durable improvement. Bone usually regrows over intact dura at the level of the foramen magnum; hence, we nearly always attempt duraplasty. In the presence of dural venous hypertension, opening the dura, especially in infants may be accompanied by significant blood loss. Dilated and aberrant venous collaterals, while an irritant in the subcutaneous tissues, may be life-threatening in the bone and dura [32]. Careful planning with a review of dural venous sinus imaging is advised. Routine surgical approaches may need to be modified when large dural venous collaterals are encountered. For example, a typical dural opening crossing the craniovertebral junction may be complicated by the presence of large marginal and occipital sinuses. In this situation, we have had success by opening the spinal dura in the midline to the level of the foramen magnum and then subpially resecting the cerebellar tonsils from this approach.

Given the observation that hindbrain herniation is worsened by ventricular shunting, we attempt to minimize the effects of CSF diversion when planning surgical intervention in these patients. This usually entails changing an existing shunt valve to a programmable version and then increasing the resistance as high as tolerated. The absolute need for the shunt is seriously investigated toward a goal of shunt removal if possible. ETV may be required. With this aggressive minimization of CSF diversion accompanied by careful microscopic cerebellar tonsil resection, we have had success in alleviating syringomyelia in patients who have previously had multiple unsuccessful surgeries.

Surgery for CTH associated with complex craniosynostosis, although potentially more difficult, has more options than direct decompression with its variants. Multiple craniofacial combined approaches have been assessed. Even anterior cranial vault expansion alone has been observed to improve Chiari symptoms and radiographic appearance [100, 117]. As noted in the section on intracranial hypertension, anterior and posterior cranial expansion/remodeling procedures have been utilized for years with success in ameliorating ICH and often improving CTH [101]. The durability of this result, however, has proven insufficient. Progression of CTH, especially in the first 2–3 years of life, in Crouzon/Pfeiffer patients occurs despite posterior cranial vault expansion procedures [7, 80].

Posterior cranial vault expansion has also been performed with concomitant suboccipital decompressive craniectomy and even upper cervical laminectomy from a bicoronal scalp incision with patients in a prone position [118, 119]. Long-term results are not reported, but the procedure appears safe and could be added to standard posterior cranial vault procedures to potentially minimize the progression of CTH even in asymptomatic patients.

Posterior calvarial vault distraction osteogenesis (PCVDO) in CCS was first reported in 2009 [56]. Although not specifically intending to treat

CTH, they reported an improvement in the degree of tonsillar herniation observed on MRI in one patient [56]. Further series have consistently reported radiographic improvement in CTH following PCVDO [59, 60, 62, 120]. Interestingly, improvement appears to result even when the distracted calvarium is supratentorial. In fact, using routine anterior-posterior vectors, a distraction which incorporates calvarium below the torcula appears less efficient than a distraction above the tentorium—perhaps indicating a constricting effect of the tentorium on potential dural expansion [61]. This may explain the authors' observations that PCVDO generally decompresses the superior aspect of the posterior fossa, but often the cerebellar tonsils remain herniated.

Many technical details remain to be perfected in distraction osteogenesis of the calvarium, and modifications can be made to specifically address the posterior fossa and CTH [121]. Park, in 2021, described "complete" PCVDO in which a foramen magnum decompression is performed and the osteotomy extends to the foramen magnum [62]. Four distractors are used instead of the usual two in order to provide an additional vector of distraction to the infratentorial skull [62]. In this study, all patients demonstrated ascent of the cerebellar tonsils postdistraction with nearly 50% achieving complete reduction [62]. Improvement in syringomyelia after PCVDO has also been reported [60, 122, 123].

Ostensibly, the mechanism by which PCVDO improves CTH is simply by increasing intracranial volume. Cinalli, however, has recently observed that dural sinus volume increased after PCVDO, and measurements of dural venous obstruction improved [123]. Since the jugular foramen was not manipulated, the authors concluded that much of the venous hypertension observed in CSS may be due to compression of the dural sinuses between the skull and the compressed underlying brain—especially in the posterior fossa [123]. This concept may have important consequences and the role of the jugular foramen may have to be revisited with more modern imaging techniques.

Since CTH is known to be acquired in the early postnatal period, it should be anticipated. Appropriate identification and surveillance of these at-risk patients should be the mandate of the craniofacial team. Although more experience is needed, early PCVDO may potentially prove to be of benefit in actually preventing the development of CTH in patients at risk [54, 59].

References

1. Sawh-martinez R, Steinbacher DM. Syndromic craniosynostosis. Clin Plast Surg. 2023;46:141–55.
2. Hibberd CE, et al. FGFR-associated craniosynostosis syndromes and gastrointestinal defects. Am J Med Genet A. 2016;170:3215–21.
3. Rhodes JL, Kolar JC, Fearon JA. Mercedes benz pattern craniosynostosis. Plast Reconstr Surg. 2010;125:299–304.
4. Balestrino A, et al. Pure bilateral lambdoid and posterior sagittal synostosis (Mercedes–Benz syndrome): case report and literature review. World Neurosurg. 2019;128:77–82.
5. Udayakumaran S, Krishnadas A, Subash P. Multisuture and syndromic craniosynostoses: simplifying the complex. J Pediatr Neurosci. 2022;17:29.
6. Coll G, et al. Hydrocephalus and Chiari malformation pathophysiology in FGFR2-related faciocraniosynostosis: a review. Neurochirurgie. 2019;65:264–8.
7. Doerga PN, De Planque CA, Erler NS, Van Veelen MLC, Mathijssen IMJ. The course and interaction of ventriculomegaly and cerebellar tonsillar herniation in Crouzon syndrome over time. Plast Reconstr Surg Glob Open. 2022;10:E3979.
8. Renier D, Sainte-Rose C, Marchac D, Hirsch J-F. Intracranial pressure in craniostenosis. J Neurosurg. 1982;57:370–7.
9. Tamburrini G, Caldarelli M, Massimi L, Santini P, Di Rocco C. Intracranial pressure monitoring in children with single suture and complex craniosynostosis: a review. Childs Nerv Syst. 2005;21:913–21.
10. Kalmar CL, et al. Elevated intracranial pressure with craniosynostosis: a multivariate model of age, syndromic status, and number of involved cranial sutures. J Neurosurg Pediatr. 2021;28:716–23.
11. Thompson DNP, et al. Subdural intracranial pressure monitoring in craniosynostosis: its role in surgical management. Childs Nerv Syst. 1995;11:269–75.
12. Hayward R. Craniofacial syndromes. In: Albright AL, Pollack IF, Adelson PD, editors. Principles and practice of pediatric neurosurgery. Thieme; 2015. p. 249–66.
13. Abu-Sittah GS, Jeelani O, Dunaway D, Hayward R. Raised intracranial pressure in Crouzon syndrome: incidence, causes, and management. J Neurosurg Pediatr. 2016;17:469–75.

14. Marucci DD, Dunaway DJ, Jones BM, Hayward RD. Raised intracranial pressure in apert syndrome. Plast Reconstr Surg. 2008;122:1162–8.
15. Doerga PN, et al. What we know about intracranial hypertension in children with syndromic craniosynostosis. J Craniofac Surg. 2023;34:1903–14.
16. Tuite GF, et al. The effectiveness of papilledema as an indicator of raised intracranial pressure in children with craniosynostosis. Neurosurgery. 1996;38:272–8.
17. Breakey RWF, et al. Intracranial volume and head circumference in children with unoperated syndromic craniosynostosis. Plast Reconstr Surg. 2018;142:708E–17E.
18. Spruijt B, et al. Algorithm for the management of intracranial hypertension in children with syndromic craniosynostosis. Plast Reconstr Surg. 2015;136:331–40.
19. Fok H, Jones BM, Gault DG, Andar U, Hayward R. Relationship between intracranial pressure and intracranial volume in craniosynostosis. Br J Plast Surg. 1992;45:394–7.
20. Sgouros S. Skull vault growth in craniosynostosis. Childs Nerv Syst. 2005;21:861–70.
21. Langvatn EA, Frič R, Due-Tønnessen BJ, Eide PK. Intracranial volume versus static and pulsatile intracranial pressure values in children with craniosynostosis. J Neurosurg Pediatr. 2019;24:66–74.
22. De Jong T, Rijken BFM, Lequin MH, Van Veelen MLC, Mathijssen IMJ. Brain and ventricular volume in patients with syndromic and complex craniosynostosis. Childs Nerv Syst. 2012;28:137–40.
23. Chadduck WM, Chadduck JB, Boop FA. The subarachnoid spaces in craniosynostosis. Neurosurgery. 1992;30:867–71.
24. Sainte-Rose C, LaCombe J, Pierre-Kahn A, Renier D, Hirsch J. Intracranial venous sinus hypertension: cause or consequence of hydrocephalus in infants? J Neurosurg. 1984;60:727–36.
25. Taylor WJ, et al. Enigma of raised intracranial pressure in patients with complex craniosynostosis: the role of abnormal intracranial venous drainage. J Neurosurg. 2001;94:377–85.
26. Rich PM, Cox TCS, Hayward RD. The jugular foramen in complex and syndromic craniosynostosis and its relationship to raised intracranial pressure. Am J Neuroradiol. 2003;24:45–51.
27. Florisson JMG, et al. Venous hypertension in syndromic and complex craniosynostosis: the abnormal anatomy of the jugular foramen and collaterals. J Cranio Maxillofac Surg. 2015;43:312–8.
28. Copeland AE, et al. Clinical significance of venous anomalies in syndromic craniosynostosis. Plast Reconstr Surg Glob Open. 2018;6:e1613.
29. Coll G, et al. Pattern of closure of skull base synchondroses in Crouzon syndrome. World Neurosurg. 2018;109:e460–7.
30. Rollins N, Booth T, Shapiro K. MR venography in children with complex craniosynostosis. Pediatr Neurosurg. 2000;32:308–15.
31. Lundar T, Bakke SJ, Nornes H. Hydrocephalus in an achondroplastic child treated by venous decompression at the jugular foramen: case report. J Neurosurg. 1990;73:138–40.
32. Thompson DNP, Hayward RD, Harkness WJ, Bingham RM, Jones BM. Lessons from a case of kleeblattschadel: case report. J Neurosurg. 1995;82:1071–4.
33. Pollack IF, Losken HW, Biglan AW. Incidence of increased intracranial pressure after early surgical treatment of syndromic craniosynostosis. Pediatr Neurosurg. 1996;24:202–9.
34. Driessen C, et al. How does obstructive sleep apnoea evolve in syndromic craniosynostosis? A prospective cohort study. Arch Dis Child. 2013;98:538–43.
35. Inverso G, Brustowicz KA, Katz E, Padwa BL. The prevalence of obstructive sleep apnea in symptomatic patients with syndromic craniosynostosis. Int J Oral Maxillofac Surg. 2016;45:167–9.
36. de Goederen R, et al. Improvement in sleep architecture is associated with the indication of surgery in syndromic craniosynostosis. Plast Reconstr Surg Glob Open. 2019;7(e2419)
37. Gonsalez S, Hayward R, Jones B, Lane R. Upper airway obstruction and raised intracranial pressure in children with craniosynostosis. Eur Respir J. 1997;10:367–75.
38. Hayward R, Gonsalez S. How low can you go? Intracranial pressure, cerebral perfusion pressure, and respiratory obstruction in children with complex craniosynostosis. J Neurosurg Pediatr. 2005;102:16–22.
39. Fearon JA, Rhodes J. Pfeiffer syndrome: a treatment evaluation. Plast Reconstr Surg. 2009;123:1560–9.
40. Taylor JA, Bartlett SP. What's new in syndromic craniosynostosis surgery? Plast Reconstr Surg. 2017;140:82e–93e.
41. Bartels MC, Vaandrager JM, de Jong THR, Simonsz HJ. Re: visual loss Xin syndromic craniosynostosis with papilledema but without other symptoms of intracranial hypertension. J Craniofac Surg. 2004;15:1019–22.
42. Khan SH, Nischal KK, Dean F, Hayward RD, Walker J. Visual outcomes and amblyogenic risk factors in craniosynostotic syndromes: a review of 141 cases. Br J Ophthalmol. 2003;87:999–1003.
43. Stavrou P, et al. Visual failure caused by raised intracranial pressure in craniosynostosis. Childs Nerv Syst. 1997;13:64–7.
44. Arnaud E, et al. Postoperative mental and morphological outcome for nonsyndromic brachycephaly. Plast Reconstr Surg. 2002;110:6–12.
45. Hayward R, Britto J, Dunaway D, Jeelani O. Connecting raised intracranial pressure and cognitive delay in craniosynostosis: many assumptions, little evidence. J Neurosurg Pediatr. 2016;18:242–50.
46. Wilson AT, et al. Intracranial hypertension and cortical thickness in syndromic craniosynostosis. Dev Med Child Neurol. 2020;62:799–805.

47. Utria AF, et al. The importance of timing in optimizing cranial vault remodeling in syndromic craniosynostosis. Plast Reconstr Surg. 2015;135:1077–84.
48. Grosser JA, et al. The need for additional surgery after passive versus active approaches to syndromic craniosynostosis: a meta-analysis. Plast Reconstr Surg Glob Open. 2023;11:E4891.
49. Rivero-Garvía M, Marquez-Rivas J, Rueda-Torres AB, Ollero-Ortiz Á. Early endoscopy-assisted treatment of multiple-suture craniosynostosis. Childs Nerv Syst. 2012;28:427–31.
50. Hersh DS, Hoover-Fong JE, Beck N, Dorafshar AH, Ahn ES. Endoscopic surgery for patients with syndromic craniosynostosis and the requirement for additional open surgery. J Neurosurg Pediatr. 2017;20:91–8.
51. Tessier P. The definitive plastic surgical treatment of the severe facial deformities of craniofacial dysostosis: Crouzon's and Apert's diseases. Ann Plast Surg. 1987;18:330–51.
52. McCarthy JG, et al. Twenty-year experience with early surgery for craniosynostosis: II. The craniofacial synostosis syndromes and pansynostosis—Results and unsolved problems. Plastic Reconstr Surg. 1995;96:284–98.
53. Ros B, Iglesias S, Selfa A, Ruiz F, Arráez MÁ. Conventional posterior cranial vault expansion: indications and results—review of the literature. Childs Nerv Syst. 2021;37:3149–75.
54. Spruijt B, et al. First vault expansion in Apert and Crouzon-pfeiffer syndromes: front or back? Plast Reconstr Surg. 2016;137:112e–21e.
55. Sugawara Y, Hirabayashi S, Sakurai A, Harii K. Gradual cranial vault expansion for the treatment of craniofacial synostosis: a preliminary report. Ann Plast Surg. 1998;40:554–65.
56. White N, et al. Posterior calvarial vault expansion using distraction osteogenesis. Childs Nerv Syst. 2009;25:231–6.
57. Wiberg A, et al. Posterior calvarial distraction in craniosynostosis—an evolving technique. J Craniomaxillofac Surg. 2012;40:799–806.
58. Pandey S, Reddy GS, Chug A, Dixit A. Posterior cranial vault distraction osteogenesis: a systematic review. J Oral Biol Craniofacial Res. 2022;12:823–32.
59. Lin LO, et al. Onset and resolution of Chiari malformations and hydrocephalus in syndromic craniosynostosis following posterior vault distraction. Plast Reconstr Surg. 2019;144:932–40.
60. Lo WB, et al. Posterior calvarial distraction for complex craniosynostosis and cerebellar tonsillar herniation. J Neurosurg Pediatr. 2020;26:421–30.
61. Sharman J, et al. Supratentorial vs infratentorial posterior calvarial distraction osteogenesis for the increase of ICV in children with syndromic or multisuture craniosynostosis: a retrospective cohort study. Childs Nerv Syst. 2021;37:1677–85.
62. Park H, Oh S, Woo Choi J, Shin Ra Y. Complete posterior cranial vault distraction osteogenesis to correct Chiari malformation type I associated with craniosynostosis. J Neurosurg Pediatr. 2022;29:298–304.
63. Carlson AR, Taylor JA. Posterior vault distraction osteogenesis: indications and expectations. Childs Nerv Syst. 2021;37:3119–25.
64. Nowinski D, et al. Posterior cranial vault expansion in the treatment of craniosynostosis. Comparison of current techniques. Child's Nerv Syst. 2012;28:1537–44.
65. Choi M, Flores RL, Havlik RJ. Volumetric analysis of anterior versus posterior cranial vault expansion in patients with syndromic craniosynostosis. J Craniofac Surg. 2012;23:455–8.
66. Derderian CA, et al. Volumetric changes in cranial vault expansion: comparison of fronto-orbital advancement and posterior cranial vault distraction osteogenesis. Plast Reconstr Surg. 2015;135:1665–72.
67. Goldstein JA, et al. A craniometric analysis of posterior cranial vault distraction osteogenesis. Plast Reconstr Surg. 2013;131:1367–75.
68. Ter Maaten NS, et al. Craniometric analysis of frontal cranial morphology following posterior vault distraction. J Craniofac Surg. 2018;29:1169–73.
69. Greives MR, et al. Complications in posterior cranial vault distraction. Ann Plast Surg. 2016;76:211–5.
70. Hassan AM, et al. Posterior cranial vault distraction (PCVD): common complication rates and strategies of prevention and management. J Craniofac Surg. 2021;32:62–6.
71. Azzolini A, et al. Ventricular shunt complications in patients undergoing posterior vault distraction osteogenesis. Childs Nerv Syst. 2020;36:1009–16.
72. Di Rocco F, et al. Results and limits of posterior cranial vault expansion by osteotomy and internal distractors. Surg Neurol Int. 2018;9:217.
73. Cinalli G, et al. Hydrocephalus and craniosynostosis. J Neurosurg. 1998;88:209–14.
74. Collmann H, Sörensen N, Krauß J. Hydrocephalus in craniosynostosis: a review. Childs Nerv Syst. 2005;21:902–12.
75. Noetzel MJ, Marsh JL, Palkes H, Gado M. Hydrocephalus and mental retardation in craniosynostosis. J Pediatr. 1985;107:885–92.
76. Machado G, et al. Cloverleaf skull deformity and hydrocephalus. Childs Nerv Syst. 2011;27:1683–91.
77. Di Rocco F, Jucá CE, Arnaud E, Renier D, Sainte-Rose C. The role of endoscopic third ventriculostomy in the treatment of hydrocephalus associated with faciocraniosynostosis: clinical article. J Neurosurg Pediatr. 2010;6:17–22.
78. Schulz M, Spors B, Haberl H, Thomale UW. Results of posterior cranial vault remodeling for plagiocephaly and brachycephaly by the meander technique. Childs Nerv Syst. 2014;30:1517–26.
79. Jarrahy R, et al. Three tenets for staged correction of kleeblattschädel or cloverleaf skull deformity. Plast Reconstr Surg. 2009;123:310–8.
80. Thompson DNP, Jones BM, Harkness W, Gonsalez S, Hayward RD. Consequences of cranial vault

expansion surgery for craniosynostosis. Pediatr Neurosurg. 1997;26:296–303.
81. Girard N, Lasjaunias P, Taylor W. Reversible tonsillar prolapse in vein of Galen aneurysmal malformations: report of eight cases and pathophysiological hypothesis. Childs Nerv Syst. 1994;10:141–7.
82. Fishman MA, Hogan GR, Dodge PR. The concurrence of hydrocephalus and craniosynostosis. J Neurosurg. 1971;34:621–9.
83. Hogan GR, Bauman ML. Hydrocephalus in Apert's syndrome. J Pediatr. 1971;79:782–7.
84. Cinalli G, et al. Chronic tonsillar herniation in Crouzon's and Apert's syndromes: the role of premature synostosis of the lambdoid suture. J Neurosurg. 1995;83:575–82.
85. Tcherbbis Testa V, Jaimovich S, Argañaraz R, Mantese B. Management of ventriculomegaly in pediatric patients with syndromic craniosynostosis: a single center experience. Acta Neurochir. 2021;163:3083–91.
86. Hoffman HJ, Tucker WS. Cephalocranial disproportion. A complication of the treatment of hydrocephalus in children. Childs Brain. 1976;2:167–76. https://doi.org/10.1159/000119612.
87. Payner TD, Prenger E, Berger TS, Crone KR. Acquired Chiari malformations: incidence, diagnosis, and management. Neurosurgery. 1994;34:429–34.
88. Chumas PD, et al. Tonsillar herniation: the rule rather than the exception after lumboperitoneal shunting in the pediatric population. J Neurosurg. 1993;78:568–73.
89. Chumas PD, et al. Death from chronic tonsillar herniation in a patient with lumboperitoneal shunt and Crouzon's disease. Br J Neurosurg. 1992;6:595–9.
90. Doorenbosch X, Molloy CJ, David DJ, Santoreneos S, Anderson PJ. Management of cranial deformity following ventricular shunting. Childs Nerv Syst. 2009;25:871–4.
91. Rocque BG, et al. Complications following pediatric cranioplasty after decompressive craniectomy: a multicenter retrospective study. J Neurosurg Pediatr. 2018;22:225–32.
92. Francis PM, et al. Chronic tonsillar herniation and Crouzon's syndrome. Pediatr Neurosurg. 1992;18:202–6.
93. Thompson DNP, Harkness W, Jones BM, Hayward RD. Aetiology of herniation of the hindbrain in craniosynostosis. Pediatr Neurosurg. 1997;26:288–95.
94. Rekate HL. Pathogenesis of hydrocephalus in achondroplastic dwarfs: a review and presentation of a case followed for 22 years. Childs Nerv Syst. 2019;35:1295–301.
95. Munarriz PM, et al. Apert syndrome: cranial procedures and brain malformations in a series of patients. Surg Neurol Int. 2020;11:361.
96. Bonfield CM, et al. Hydrocephalus treatment in patients with craniosynostosis: an analysis from the hydrocephalus clinical research network prospective registry. Neurosurg Focus. 2021;50:1–7.
97. Frassanito P, Palombi D, Tamburrini G. Craniosynostosis and hydrocephalus: relevance and treatment modalities. Childs Nerv Syst. 2021;37:3465–73.
98. Swift DM, Nagy L. Endoscopic third ventriculostomy in hydrocephalus associated with complex multisutural craniosynostosis. In: Proceedings of the 36th Annual Meeting of the International Society for Paediatric Neurosurgery, Cape Town, South Africa, 12–16 October 2008; Child's Nervous System 24, 1235; 2008.
99. Saldino RM, Steinbach HL, Epstein CJ. Familial acrocephalosyndactyly (Pfeiffer syndrome). Am J Roentgenol Radium Therapy Nucl Med. 1972;116:609–22.
100. Venes J. Arnold-Chiari malformation in an infant with Kleeblattschadel: an acquired malformation? Neurosurgery. 1988;23:360–2.
101. Strahle J, et al. Chiari malformation associated with craniosynostosis. Neurosurg Focus. 2011;31:3–10.
102. Engel M, et al. Chiari malformation in nonsyndromal single craniosynostosis-much ado about nothing? Acta Neurochir. 2012;154(1803–1807):1803–7.
103. Cinalli G, et al. Chiari malformation in craniosynostosis. Childs Nerv Syst. 2005;21:889–901.
104. Den Ottelander BK, et al. Saethre–Chotzen syndrome: long-term outcome of a syndrome-specific management protocol. Dev Med Child Neurol. 2021;63:104–10.
105. Chivoret N, et al. Bilambdoid and sagittal synostosis: report of 39 cases. Surg Neurol Int. 2018;9:206.
106. Renier D, Cinalli G, Lajeunie E, Arnaud E, Marchac D. Oxycephaly, a severe craniosynostosis. Apropos of a series of 129 cases. Arch Pediatr. 1997;4:722–9.
107. Heiss JD, et al. Elucidating the pathophysiology of syringomyelia. J Neurosurg. 1999;91:553–62.
108. Fujisawa H, Hasegawa M, Kida S, Yamashita J. A novel fibroblast growth factor receptor 2 mutation in Crouzon syndrome associated with Chiari type I malformation and syringomyelia. J Neurosurg. 2002;97:396–400.
109. Sgouros S, Natarajan K, Hockley AD, Goldin JH, Wake M. Skull base growth in craniosynostosis. Pediatr Neurosurg. 1999;31:281–93.
110. Coll G, et al. The growth of the posterior cranial fossa in FGFR2-induced faciocraniosynostosis: a review. Neurochirurgie. 2019;65:221–7.
111. Rijken BFM, et al. The role of the posterior fossa in developing Chiari I malformation in children with craniosynostosis syndromes. J Cranio Maxillofac Surg. 2015;43:813–9.
112. Rodesch G, Otto B, Mouchamps M, Born J. Reversible tonsillar prolapse and syringomyelia after embolization of a tectal arteriovenous malformation: case report and review of the literature. J Neurosurg. 2007;107:412–5.
113. Iampreechakul P, et al. Acquired Chiari malformation type I and holocord syringomyelia associated with a high-flow supratentorial fistulous arterio-

venous malformations: a case report and literature review. Surg Neurol Int. 2022;13:217.

114. Knickmeyer RC, et al. A structural MRI study of human brain development from birth to 2 years. J Neurosci. 2008;28:12176–82.
115. Braga BP, et al. Cerebellar tonsil reduction for surgical treatment of Chiari malformation type I in children. J Neurosurg Pediatr. 2023:1–10. https://doi.org/10.3171/2023.1.PEDS22222.
116. Sacco D, Scott RM. Reoperation for Chiari malformations. Pediatr Neurosurg. 2003;39:171–8.
117. Fearon JA, Swift DM, Bruce DA. New methods for the evaluation and treatment of craniofacial dysostosis-associated cerebellar tonsillar herniation. Plast Reconstr Surg. 2001;108:1855–61.
118. Cinalli G, Chumas P, Arnaud E, Sainte-Rose C, Renier D. Occipital remodeling and suboccipital decompression in severe craniosynostosis associated with tonsillar herniation. Neurosurgery. 1998;42:66–71; discussion 71–3.
119. Scott WW, Fearon JA, Swift DM, Sacco DJ. Suboccipital decompression during posterior cranial vault remodeling for selected cases of Chiari malformations associated with craniosynostosis. J Neurosurg Pediatr. 2013;12:166–70.
120. Raposo-Amaral CE, Raposo-Amaral CA, Adams JW, Ghizoni E. Posterior vault distraction outcomes in patients with severe Crouzon syndrome resulting from Ser347Cys and Ser354Cys mutations. J Craniofac Surg. 2022;33:1545–8.
121. Marji FP, et al. Posterior cranial vault distraction osteogenesis utilizing a posterior—superior distraction vector in the treatment of Mercedes Benz pattern craniosynostosis. J Craniofac Surg. 2021;32:2059–63.
122. Ahmad F, et al. Amelioration of Chiari type 1 malformation and syringomyelia following posterior calvarial distraction in Crouzon's syndrome-a case report. Childs Nerv Syst. 2014;30:177–9. https://doi.org/10.1007/s00381-013-2202-9.
123. Cinalli G, et al. Changes in venous drainage after posterior cranial vault distraction and foramen magnum decompression in syndromic craniosynostosis. J Neurosurg Pediatr. 2022;30:330–41.

14 Controversies in the Indications for Surgery

Jenny F. Yang, Daniel Sasson, John Smetona, and John A. Persing

14.1 Genetic Basis of Neurologic Dysfunction

In recent years, advancements in genomic sequencing have permitted research on the genes and pathways that contribute to craniosynostosis. Indeed, uncommon Mendelian mutations in syndromic craniosynostosis (mostly in FGFR and TWIST1 genes) have been identified as causal in these forms of craniosynostosis [1, 2]. These mutations commonly cause increased signaling of Wnt, BMP, Ras/ERK, ephrin, hedgehog, STAT, or retinoic acid pathways, which converge on shared nuclear targets that promote bone formation [3, 4].

Nonsyndromic craniosynostoses (NSC), on the other hand, are more genetically heterogenous. Patients show variable neurodevelopmental outcome; however, nearly half of the patients are ultimately diagnosed with some form of neurocognitive dysfunction despite timely and comprehensive surgical intervention [5, 6]. Given that the sutures, meninges, and parenchyma of the forebrain and midbrain have shared neural crest cell origin, this raises a potential role for a genetic injury affecting these early cell lines to affect the sutures and intrinsic brain function concurrently.

FGFR3 has been known to occur with high frequency in nonsyndromic coronal craniosynostosis [7]. The more recent advent of genomic sequencing has allowed identification of several other mutations. Sharma et al. [2] performed exome sequencing on patients with different types of craniosynostosis, and found TCF12 mutations in 32% of bilateral coronal and 10% of unilateral coronal craniosynostosis cases. No TCF12 mutations were seen in sagittal, metopic, or lambdoid craniosynostosis. TCF12 encodes a partner protein of TWIST1 which has been found to be critical for coronal suture development, and combined TCF12 and TWIST1 mutations result in more severe cases of coronal synostosis [2]. Similarly, Justice et al.'s genome wide association study in nonsyndromic metopic synostosis patients found mutations in SPRY3, BMP7, PCDH11X, and upstream from TGIF2LX [8].

J. F. Yang
Mayo Clinic, Plastic and Reconstructive Surgery, Jacksonville, FL, USA
e-mail: yang.jenny2@mayo.edu

D. Sasson
Rochester Regional Health, Interventional Radiology, Rochester, NY, USA
e-mail: daniel.sasson@rochesterregional.org

J. Smetona
Advocate Health, Chicago, IL, USA
e-mail: john.smetona@aah.org

J. A. Persing (✉)
Yale University, Plastic and Reconstructive Surgery, New Haven, CT, USA
e-mail: john.persing@yale.edu

F. Di Rocco, J. Kestle (eds.), *Neurosurgical Aspects of Craniosynostosis*,
https://doi.org/10.1007/978-3-031-69386-1_14

Timberlake et al. performed exome sequencing of genes within the highest quartile of expression in the developing brain in 404 trios with sporadic sagittal, metopic, lambdoid, and combined sagittal and metopic NSC [9]. The authors sequenced the genes that were identified to have a high probability of intolerance to loss of function and found that a striking 34% of their cohort had damaging de novo mutations in these intolerant genes. All NSC patients in this cohort underwent surgical correction, but those who had the high-risk genotypes had a two-fold greater incidence of neurodevelopmental delay, 20-fold greater incidence of intellectual disability, and 3.6-fold higher incidence of persistent delays after 5 years of age compared to NSC patients who did not harbor these mutations. These comparisons were based on patient-reported incidence of diagnosed developmental delays including intellectual disability, and motor, speech, or language delay. Though the findings of this study are likely to be strengthened by in depth standardized neurologic testing, it provides initial compelling evidence of a genetic contribution to neurologic outcome in NSC that may not be completely corrected with surgery. Table 14.1 provides a summary of known genetic mutations in NSC.

Further evidence for the role of genetics in neurocognitive dysfunction in NSC is the identification of loss of function (LOF) mutations in negative regulators of Wnt, BMP, and Ras/ERK signaling in NCS patients [8, 11–13]. Precise regulation of these pathways is crucial for bone formation as well as normal brain development. The most common of these studied mutations is in SMAD6, which accounts for 5% of all midline NSC cases (13% of individuals with metopic NSC and 3% of those with sagittal NSC) [11]. SMAD6 is a negative regulator of SMAD signaling via the BMP pathway, and loss of SMAD6 leads to uninhibited transcription of genes that promote osteoblast differentiation. This cascade plays a role in the development of the bony cranial vault and leads to closure of cranial sutures. Interestingly, genomic analyses on intellectual disability identified SMAD6 as a locus involved in poor intellectual ability; however, the presence or absence of craniosynostosis was not noted in this study [14]. Wu et al. subsequently demonstrated that NSC patients with SMAD6 mutations performed significantly worse on intellectual tasks including numerical operations, performance IQ, full scale IQ, visuomotor integration, and motor coordination compared to their matched controls with NSC without SMAD6 mutation [15].

Taken together, knowledge of high-risk genotypes can be useful for identifying children who are most likely to benefit from surgery. However, NSC can also be influenced by complex polygenic and epigenetic factors. For example, the

Table 14.1 Summary of genetic mutations in nonsyndromic craniosynostosis (NSC)

Study	Sequencing method	Type of NSC	Genes implicated
Moloney et al. (1997) [16]	PCR sequencing	Coronal	FGFR3
Renier et al. (2000) [7]	PCR sequencing	Bilateral coronal, unilateral coronal	FGFR3
Sharma et al. (2013) [2]	Exome sequencing	Bilateral coronal, unilateral coronal	TCF12
Justice et al. (2012) [10]	GWAS	Sagittal	BMP2
Timberlake et al. (2016) [11]	Exome sequencing	Sagittal	SMAD6
Ye et al. (2016) [12]	Sanger sequencing	Sagittal	TWIST1, FGFR1
Timberlake et al. (2017) [13]	Exome sequencing	Sagittal	AXIN1, DVL3, MESP1, NPHP4, RASAL2, SMAD6, SPRY1, SPRY4
		Metopic	ARAP3, PSMC2, PSMC5, SMAD6, SMURF1
Justice et al. (2020) [8]	GWAS	Metopic	SPRY3, BMP7, PCDH11X, upstream from TGIF2LX

SMAD6 mutation demonstrates strikingly variable penetrance, and is dramatically influenced by a common risk allele near BMP2 [10, 11]. An LOF mutation in SMAD6 plus the common BMP2 risk allele conferred 100% risk of NSC, whereas SMAD6 mutation without the BMP2 risk allele only resulted in a 19% risk. BMP2 is an inducer of osteogenesis via SMAD signaling, and it is therefore postulated that this risk allele might increase the penetrance of SMAD6 mutations by increasing BMP2, leading to accelerated and uninhibited SMAD signaling. This two-locus inheritance pattern demonstrates the complexity of epigenetic interplay, and suggests that identification (or lack) of any specific mutation alone should not dictate whether a child with NSC receives surgical intervention.

14.2 Bony Constriction and Neurologic Consequences

Virchow's law states that skull growth is restricted perpendicular to the fused suture and enhanced parallel to it, and it is postulated that constricted growth poses a risk to the developing brain. The detection of elevated intracranial pressure is a frequent indication for surgical intervention; however, the degree to which intracranial hypertension (ICH) affects neurological development outcome remains unclear. Indeed, 61–83% of patients with syndromic craniosynostoses have clinically significant ICH [17–19], yet there is no direct correlation between ICH and IQ.

Cerebral cortical thickness has emerged as a promising indicator of cognitive ability [20–22]. While cortical thickness is an indicator of neuronal density, dendritic arborization, and glial support [23], cortical thinning has been correlated with decreased IQ [20–24]. A recent study used FreeSurfer MRI analysis of cortical thickness evaluated common manifestations of ICH as risk factor for cortical thinning [25]. The authors found that only papilledema and hydrocephalus are associated with thinning of the neural cortex. Other clinical markers of ICH such as tonsillar herniation, obstructive sleep apnea (OSA), and occipitofrontal circumference were not associated with abnormal reduction in cortical depth. The study did not find gender differences; however, it did note a higher rate of neurologic deficit in Apert syndrome compared to other syndromes. Overall, this study suggests that the frequency of neurologic deficit may be more limited, and advocates for timely intervention in the setting of papilledema and prolonged hydrocephalus.

Interestingly, MRI studies of syndromic patients with FGFR mutations after vault expansion procedures in fact demonstrated greater intracranial volume (ICV) in patients compared to normal controls [26]. But despite having seemingly adequate volume, the cerebral cortex in FGFR-mediated craniosynostosis shows abnormal development, as evidenced by reduced cortical surface area, due to decreased cortical folding that is normally driven by grey matter expansion and white matter tension. This reduced surface area was most notable in the parietal and occipital regions, even though the synostosis was along the coronal suture [26]. The parietal cortex plays a role in several measures of intelligence, including working memory, processing speed, and perceptual organization, while the occipital cortex is involved in visual processing ability. When impaired, these could manifest as reading disability and reduced scholastic potential. Furthermore, structural MRI studies demonstrated that syndromic craniosynostosis patients show apparent morphologic deformities at near and distant areas of the brain, including the corpus callosum, septum pellucidum, hippocampus, cortex, cerebellum, and ventricular system [27–31]. Taken together, these findings link brain maldevelopment to the observed neurocognitive dysfunction in syndromic craniosynostosis. However, the pathology remains to be elucidated, and contributions from genetic and compressive forces are expected.

Patients with NSC, on the other hand, rarely present with increased ICP, with reported rates ranging between 6 and 20% [17, 32, 33]. Despite the lack of overt signs of intracranial hypertension, infants with single suture NSC were found to have significantly higher cerebral perfusion and increased cerebral glucose metabolism after surgical release, detected by pre- and post-operative single positron computed tomography (SPECT) [34] and positron emission tomography (PET) scans [35]. Glucose metabolism increases were most consistent in the occipital region, the area of visual development and visuospatial coordination [35].

Structural brain data in NSC patients have also been found to have fundamentally different patterns of morphologic malformation compared to syndromic patients. Untreated NSC patients demonstrate abnormal distances between brain structures that strongly correlate with the phenotype of the particular suture fusion [36–39]. Diffusion tensor imaging (DTI) studies in rabbit models show abnormal changes in white matter tracts that showed signs of subsequent normalization after early suturectomy [40].

Functional MRI (fMRI) has become a very important tool for revealing different aspects of micro- and macrostructures as well as white matter tracts. Cabrejo et al. recently published fMRI study followed patients with isolated sagittal craniosynostosis from infancy to adolescence using fMRI to document aberrancies compared to age and gender matched controls [41]. The test subjects in this cohort underwent whole vault cranioplasty by a single surgeon before 12 months of age. While the pre-operative fMRI demonstrated different connections in most of the defined cerebral networks compared to their matched controls, much of the abnormal network connections corrects by adolescence. Specifically, these positive changes in the brain microstructure were demonstrated as increased connectivity in the insula, putamen, and inferior frontal gyrus, increased anisotropy and connectivity in the putamen and insula. These findings correlate surgery with normalization of brain microstructure and connectivity, which may improve neural function [41, 42]. Table 14.2 provides a summary of structural brain changes in NSC.

Table 14.2 Summary of structural brain changes in nonsyndromic craniosynostosis (NSC)

Study	Imaging modality	Type of NSC	Key findings
David et al. (1996) [34]	SPECT	Infants with sagittal, metopic, coronal, lambdoid NSC	Increased cerebral perfusion after cranial reconstructive surgery
David et al. (1999) [35]	PET	Infants with sagittal, metopic, unicoronal NSC	Increased cerebral glucose metabolism in occipital region after cranial reconstructive surgery
Aldridge et al. (2002) [36]	MRI	Infants with sagittal, metopic NSC	Distinct cortical and subcortical features in sagittal and metopic craniosynostosis, suggesting skeletal and underlying brain structure abnormalities
Aldridge et al. (2005) [38]	MRI	Infants with sagittal NSC	Improved scaphocephaly after surgical intervention, but persistent subcortical abnormalities
Bonfield et al. (2015) [40]	MRI, DTI	Rabbits with coronal NSC	White matter tract abnormalities, worsening with age, improved after strip craniectomy.
Beckett et al. (2014) [39]	fMRI, DTI	Adolescents with sagittal NSC	Altered neocortical structural and functional connectivity in adolescents that persist after surgical treatment during infancy
Brooks et al. (2016) [42]	fMRI, DTI	Infants and adolescents with sagittal NSC	Substantial normalization of brain morphology in adolescents treated with cranial vault surgery during infancy. Some effects of cranial vault may persist especially at frontoparietal and temporal regions
Cabrejo et al. (2021) [41]	fMRI, DTI	Infants and adolescents with sagittal NSC	Normalization of cerebral network connectivity in adolescents treated with cranial vault surgery during infancy

14.3 Timing of Surgery

14.3.1 Sagittal Craniosynostosis

Sagittal NSC is the most common form of NSC and is the most studied. Although there remains conflicting opinion in the literature regarding the optimal treatment period in a young patient's life [43, 44], recent systematic reviews have highlighted the neurocognitive advantages of early surgical intervention (before 7 months of age) for sagittal craniosynostosis [45]. Patients undergoing early surgery have been documented to have 10–20-point IQ increases than their later/no-surgery counterparts.

From an anatomical perspective, the decision to operate early dramatically increases the selection of procedures, as many might require major modification in older patients (greater than 12 months of age) due to mineralization of the calvaria. Decreased pliability of the skull at later stages of development creates the necessity for weakening kerfs or channels, in the bone to allow more extensive remodeling, and stabilization of the skull bone(s). Additionally, defects left in the bone structure, such as burr holes, will often heal without intervention in younger patients but can require a form of bone replacement in older patients with decreased regenerative capabilities.

For these reasons, it is often recommended that surgical intervention take place in the first few months of life, with variation in timing, given the type of surgical procedure to be done (e.g., linear craniectomy <3 months versus whole vault cranioplasty <6 months, with or without spring aided expansion) and appropriate indications and acceptable risk for blood loss and operative time.

14.3.2 Metopic and Unicoronal Craniosynostosis

Unlike in sagittal craniosynostosis, no study to date has compared the neurologic outcomes for early versus late surgery. Most surgeons favor surgery between 3 and 9 months of age [46–48]. In the absence of pressing issues like increased ICP, some surgeons advocate waiting until 4–6 months of age, when the bone is easier to work with and rigid enough to maintain a stable reconstruction. Ophthalmologic data suggest that binocular vision is fully developed by approximately 6 months of age, and it has also been advocated that surgery for nonsyndromic metopic and unicoronal craniosynostosis patients after 6 months of age may increase the risk for abnormal visual function such as astigmatism and strabismus [49].

In the case of metopic craniosynostosis, timely diagnosis and referral to a craniofacial center may be delayed given that the metopic suture can be physiologically fused 30% at 3 months of age, 60% at 6 months of age, and 90% at 9 months of age [46]. While phenotypic presentation remains a common indication of pathologic versus physiologic fusion, objective measurements to quantify the severity, such as that of the endocranial bifrontal angle, have garnered attention [50–52]. Objective measurements, including these, can greatly support a surgeon's decision regarding the need for intervention.

14.3.3 When Is It Too Late?

Treatment of delayed presentation of craniosynostosis is different because the bulk of brain growth has been completed. Nearly 90% of peak adult brain mass develops by the age of 3 [53]; therefore, benefits to the developing brain, including allowing space for normal growth and geometric spatial arrangement, IQ, and behavioral or emotional regulation, is lessened. A child with no concomitant problems related to this pathology could be counseled that the indication to treat is primarily aesthetic, although this is not known for sure. To date, no substantive testing has been done to clarify whether there is benefit to this type of late surgery in asymptomatic patients. However, other sequelae may drive these later presentations: Headaches, increased ICP, or Chiari malformations. These presentations may require treatment just as they would for those presenting at an earlier age.

In the US, unrepaired craniosynostosis after 1 year of age is rare. Several small case series of mixed types of NSC reported that untreated patients over the age of 1 year have high rates of headaches, developmental delay, Chiari malformation, elevated ICP, and abnormal head shape [54, 55]. The authors note that this high rate may reflect the ultimate result of restricted suture growth, or it may be due to selection bias for symptomatic patients, and currently it is not known what the incidence is of asymptomatic individuals with similar skull deformities.

In contrast, an extensive series from the University of Pittsburg consisting of 52 patients with untreated isolated sagittal synostosis over 1 year of age at presentation reported that only a minority of patients (17%) required surgery [56]. Indications for surgery in this group were severe scaphocephaly and abnormal ophthalmologic exam. Non-operative patients were managed by maintaining serial follow-up and ophthalmologic evaluation with fundoscopic exam and visual evoked potentials, which were recommended to continue until growth maturity (at least 18 years old for males, 16 years old for females). Authors reported that these patients were late-presenting due to mild, missed, or late-developing synostosis.

While larger children may allow for a lesser risk anesthetic, and the well-developed diploic space allows for split calvarial bone grafting, the osteogenic potential of the dura is largely lost after the age of 1 year, implying a lesser ability to heal bony defects spontaneously. However, the periosteum is still influential in some bone regeneration in early to mid-infancy. In addition, there is reduced potential for smoothing of contour irregularities or residual shape deformity with further brain and skull growth. Older patients, therefore, often require more extensive cranial remodeling procedures. Despite these concerns, it has been demonstrated that children presenting at an older age can be safely treated with cranioplasty, albeit they may not derive the same functional benefits. There was no significant difference in postoperative transfusion and hospital stay length in older patients undergoing craniosynostosis repair versus those who underwent repair under 12 months [54–56]. Furthermore, they do not appear to have an unacceptably high rate of bony defects or contour problems. Long term outcome data regarding cosmesis, bony defects, and the need for revisions are scant. Neurocognitive testing to assess for changes in mental functioning is yet to be undertaken, but would be essential to determine whether this approach should be adopted.

14.4 Type of Surgery

14.4.1 Sagittal Craniosynostosis

Historically, the decision to operate on patients presenting with sagittal craniosynostosis has been contingent upon the degree to which head shape is affected from a psychosocial perspective. Another factor to consider is the extent of the synostosis itself, affecting the suture along its total length or a specific portion of it. There are several surgical techniques, and the unique benefits and drawbacks of different surgical treatments must be balanced when deciding to operate.

14.4.2 Strip Craniectomy with Helmet Therapy

When treating single suture sagittal craniosynostosis in patients less than 3 months of age, strip craniectomy with subsequent helmet therapy may be the chosen technique due to limited incision size and reduced blood loss [57, 58]. These benefits are further enhanced when endoscopic techniques are utilized. Helmet therapy is necessary, however, often for prolonged periods to enable the skull to heal optimally. More recent analysis indicates that variability of outcome may be more contingent on helmet design than previously thought. Compared with more invasive procedures, patients undergoing strip craniectomy also have shorter hospital length of stay, less ICU stay, and lower hospital costs. A drawback associated with strip craniectomy, however, is its limited scope of effectiveness for patients more than 3 months of age, after which cranial stiffness has begun to limit effectiveness of helmet therapy. A second drawback is that suturectomy only achieves regional release at the time of surgery, and an additional 8–14 months of postoperative helmet therapy may be required on average to gradually achieve adequate correction of skull shape [59]. This additional course of active cranial molding coincides with crucial periods of postnatal brain development. Between birth and 24 months postnatally, the brain undergoes significant cortical maturation processes such as synaptogenesis, synaptic pruning, dendritic arborization, and myelinization of intracortical white matter, which are all essential for achieving normal brain connectivity [60, 61]. Thus, incomplete correction during this time may yield inexact neural connections, ultimately leading to dysfunction of the brain circuitry.

14.4.3 Cranial Vault Reconstruction

Unlike strip craniectomy, cranial vault reconstruction (CVR) can be used at any age regardless of calvarial mineralization, assuming low risk for major blood loss, lung maturation, and the ability to monitor and treat appropriately for volume changes intra and post operatively. For patients 3 months or more, CVR is considered first-line definitive therapy to restore skull morphology to normality. CVR has also been associated with significant IQ and visuomotor integration increases compared to strip craniectomy or spring-assisted cranioplasty [62, 63].

Despite advancements, CVR is a more invasive procedure, with higher risk of blood loss and subsequent need for blood transfusions. Efforts to raise the patients' baseline hematocrit or lessen intraoperative blood loss are commonly employed [64].

14.4.4 Spring-Assisted Cranioplasty

Spring-assisted cranioplasty can also allow for the dynamic and gradual reshaping of the cranium compared to other techniques, such as CVR, which generate more complete and timely changes. However, certain variables, such as spring strength, are difficult to predict without significant experience and are contingent upon age, bone thickness, and synostosis location. Springs are often custom-made and can require close monitoring using imaging to ensure appropriate distraction. However, downsides include univector expansion, migration of the foot plates through younger bone, erosion through bone, and unpredictability of final lengthening [65]. It should be noted that expansion plateaus at around 50 days after spring placement, and begins to restrict growth after approximately 60 days in an animal experimental model. A final downside to this procedure is that a second operation is required to remove the springs and complete closure of the calvarium.

14.4.5 Metopic Craniosynostosis

Trigonocephaly is characterized by a triangular or wedge-shape forehead resulting from suture fusion and supraorbital retrusion, with a wide range of severity. Patients often also demonstrate deficient lateral orbital rims, bitemporal indentations, and hypocanthus. Teardrop shaped orbits and ethmoidal hypoplasia are additional radiological findings, and 55% of cases have prematurely closed anterior fontanels [66].

In addition to phenotypic abnormalities, there is increasing evidence across multiple modalities revealing long-term neurocognitive deficits. Neurodevelopmental dysfunction in patients with metopic craniosynostosis range from 15 to 61%, with reported deficits in speech/language, attention, and behavior, as well as high incidence of attention deficit hyperactivity disorder [66, 67]. The metopic suture overlies the frontal lobe, which is intricately connected with the cingulate gyrus and the limbic system—structures that are responsible for executive function, impulse inhibition, and personality.

Notably, infant event-related potential (ERP) measurements of neurodevelopment and neurocognitive testing in childhood and adolescence have all been demonstrated to correlate with radiographic severity as measured by the preoperative endocranial bifrontal angle [51, 52].

Historically, the first reports of surgical treatment for trigonocephaly described simple strip craniectomies. In present day, limited suturectomy is considered by most to be insufficient to correct the three-dimensional sequelae of metopic craniosynostosis [66, 68, 69]. Marchac published his landmark technique using the "floating forehead technique" combined with remodeling of the supra-orbital bandeau in 1978. Modifications of this technique have evolved to address post operative temporal hollowing, but the general concept still continues to be the standard.

For correction of hypocanthus, a sagittal osteotomy with or without bone grafting are options. Distraction osteogenesis with conventional screws or with springs has also been proposed, and has gained some popularity. However, there is controversy regarding whether hypotelorism really needs to be directly corrected. Fearon noted improvement in intercanthal distance in his cohort without any deliberate attempt at surgical correction [70]. Careful measurements revealed that patients who underwent surgery earlier (before 6 months of age) had greater improvement than those treated after 6 months of age, and those with more severe initial hypotelorism showed significantly more improvement than their milder counterparts within a mean of 21 months of follow up. Opponents of direct surgical correction of hypocanthus argue that doing so would only widen the nasal bones without increasing the interorbital distance.

14.4.6 Unicoronal Craniosynostosis

Unicoronal craniosynostosis (UCS) results in a complex set of craniofacial dysmorphologies affecting the fronto-orbital region, skull base, and facial symmetry. In addition to the cognitive and aesthetic concerns shared with other forms of NSC, as many as 89% of UCS patients have exotropia or vertical deviation of the ipsilateral globe. A series of studies by Ricci et al. found that patients experience high incidences of ocular abnormalities in both eyes—including strabismus, atypical eye movements, astigmatism, and visual field deficits [71]. Formal visual testing is a critical element in evaluating UCS patients, and ocular anomalies are an essential indication for surgical correction.

Open cranial vault remodeling with fronto-orbital advancement is the conventional technique for correcting unicoronal synostosis and remains the most common approach. Alternative techniques such as endoscopic strip craniectomy, distraction osteogenesis, and spring-assisted cranioplasty offer shorter operating time and shorter hospital stays. Another proposed benefit is improved craniofacial growth due to maintenance of blood supply to the cranial bones and limited scarring of the soft tissue [72, 73].

14.4.7 Fronto-Orbital Advancement

Despite being the most commonly used method, long term results of fronto-orbital advancement (FOA) for UCS are mixed. Many studies' outcomes report significant asymmetry at long term follow up even with some initial overcorrection [72]. Poor long term outcome scores are often due to temporal hollowing and supraorbital retrusion with the appearance of "relapse." This has led some to propose hypercorrection as a variation in traditional FOA. The group led by Dr. Buchman at University of Michigan reported on a cohort of 40 patients followed for an average of 4.75 years after hypercorrection [74]. They noted that the hypercorrection appearance persisted for 6–8 months and gradually normalized. However, it is unclear whether in the short term the hypercorrection is more or less displeasing to the child and parents.

14.4.8 Distraction Osteogenesis

The first described use of distraction osteogenesis for forehead distraction in UCS was in 1999 by Kobayashi [75]. Since then, this technique has been known for achieving good improvements in cranial volume and cephalic index, with minimal bleeding and bony defect, short operative time, and no dural tears. Distraction of the cranial base was also successful in improving the angulation of the anterior and posterior cranial fossa.

Compared to FOA, distraction osteogenesis was shown to have advantages of shorter hospital stay and lower incidence of postoperative strabismus [72, 76].

14.4.9 Endoscopic Strip Craniectomy

Though the endoscopic strip technique is characterized by short operative time, low transfusion rates, and low perioperative morbidity [77], the downside of this option is that it does not directly address the concern about cranial base and brain distortion caused by bony constriction as rapidly or completely in the critical time periods for brain growth. Another concern is the limited ability to address the degree of asymmetry of the orbit and temporal region.

14.4.10 Spring-Assisted Cranioplasty

Yet another surgical option that can be used is the spring-assisted coronal strip craniectomy. Shortfalls of this technique for UCS are similar to those for sagittal patients—namely, the unpredictability of final correction, unidirectional vector, and the need for a secondary procedure to remove the springs.

14.4.11 Bicoronal Craniosynostosis

Bilateral coronal craniosynostosis results in turribrachycephaly, which is characterized by a tower-shaped calvarium that is shortened in the anteroposterior dimension and tall in the vertical dimension. Turribrachycephaly is more frequently seen as a feature of syndromic multisuture craniosynostosis such as in Crouzon's and Apert's syndromes, but may be present without a syndrome [78]. The most challenging aspect in the treatment of turribrachycephaly is correction of the excess skull height. Due to its difficulty, the excess height was initially not addressed, and patients underwent staged procedures to address the anterior and posterior cranial vault. In 1987, Persing et al. popularized using barrel stave osteotomies to vertically reduce the skull while increasing the capacity of the cranium [79]. The authors described a modified prone position that allowed access to the anterior and posterior cranial vault in a single procedure.

14.4.12 Posterior Vault Distraction Osteogenesis

First described for treatment of multisuture craniosynostosis in 2009 [80], posterior vault distraction osteogenesis (PVDO) has become widely used as a first step in treatment of turribrachycephaly, especially for syndromic craniosynostosis cases. Though multiple procedures are required, it has been suggested that PVDO provides a larger volumetric increase compared to anterior vault remodeling procedures, and may delay the need for frontal surgery [81].

14.5 Perioperative Safety

14.5.1 Limiting Blood Loss

Cranial surgery is an invasive procedure, with attendant blood loss and subsequent need for blood transfusions, even with minimally invasive techniques. Efforts to raise the patients' baseline hematocrit or lessen intraoperative blood loss have been studied.

Among these approaches, iron supplementation, EPO, intraoperative cell saver devices, acute normovolemic hemodilution (ANH), preoperative autologous blood donation, and tranexamic acid (TXA) have been studied [82, 83]. Preoperative EPO and administration protocols have been found to increase the preoperative Hct and reduce the rate of transfusion from 100% to 64%. Studies on cell saver and ANH as sole means to avoid transfusion have shown mixed efficacy; however, when these methods are combined with EPO, Velardi et al. demonstrated only a 15% rate of transfusion [84]. Use of the antifibrinolytic agent and TXA agent has been studied extensively in craniosynostosis and facial trauma patients. Multiple studies have found that perioperative TXA reduces amount of blood loss and the need for blood transfusions in craniosynostosis patients [83–87]. Furthermore, the effects of TXA and EPO appear to be additive [85]. Dadure et al. performed a randomized control trial and found that patients receiving both agents had a 37% rate of perioperative transfusion, compared to 70% in the EPO only group [85].

There is currently no consensus regarding the optimal dosage for using TXA for CVR for craniosynostosis surgery. A recent study by Goobie et al. showed no difference in blood loss and blood transfusion rates between a "high" loading dose of 50 mg/kg compared to a "low" loading dose of 10 mg/kg, both followed by 5 mg/kg/h [83]. No differences in adverse effects related to TXA were observed. Another study investigated the length of time the TXA was continued, and found no difference in blood loss, hemoglobin levels, need for transfusion, and length of ICU stay between a 4 h continuous drip of TXA versus a 24 h continuous drip [86]. No differences in untoward events related to TXA were noted. The lower dosages of TXA were, however, associated with significantly lower cost.

Risks associated with EPO include thrombosis, thrombocytosis, hypertension, and death, and are usually associated with long term use in adults or chronically ill patients. The risk profile of TXA is also related to thrombosis, and again usually seen in adults. To date, thrombotic events have not been found to be associated with use in the craniosynostosis population. It is felt that this may be due to the lower baseline risk for thrombosis in the pediatric population.

14.5.2 Post Operative Monitoring

At many centers, cranial vault surgery is generally managed postoperatively in the intensive care unit (ICU). However, overutilization of the ICU can result in lower volume of patient care due to lack of space in the ICU. A recent report from McGill University demonstrated a safe 8-year experience with routine postoperative management of healthy NSC patients on the regular surgical floor [88]. Only 2% of patients in their cohort required transfer to the ICU due to adverse intraoperative events. Subsequent studies have identified factors that increase the risk for post operative events that require ICU admission, including <10 kg body weight, ASA status 3 or 4, intraoperative transfusion >60 cc/kg, and significant intraoperative complication [89]. Taken together, these studies may promote use of risk stratification pathways to determine the optimal usage of hospital resources.

References

1. Wilkie AOM, Johnson D, Wall SA. Clinical genetics of craniosynostosis. Curr Opin Pediatr. 2017;29(6):622–8.
2. Sharma VP, Fenwick AL, Brockop MS, McGowan SJ, Goos JAC, Hoogeboom AJM, et al. Mutations in TCF12, encoding a basic helix-loop-helix partner of TWIST1, are a frequent cause of coronal craniosynostosis. Nat Genet. 2013;45(3):304–7.
3. Twigg SRF, Vorgia E, McGowan SJ, Peraki I, Fenwick AL, Sharma VP, et al. Reduced dosage of ERF causes complex craniosynostosis in humans and mice and links ERK1/2 signaling to regulation of osteogenesis. Nat Genet. 2013;45(3):308–13.
4. Twigg SRF, Wilkie AOM. A genetic-pathophysiological framework for craniosynostosis. Am J Hum Genet. 2015;97(3):359–77.
5. Magge SN, Westerveld M, Pruzinsky T, Persing JA. Long-term neuropsychological effects of sagittal craniosynostosis on child development. J Craniofac Surg. 2002;13(1):99–104.
6. Choi JW, Lim SY, Shin HJ. Craniosynostosis in growing children: pathophysiological changes and neurosurgical problems. J Korean Neurosurg Soc. 2016;59(3):197–203.
7. Renier D, El-Ghouzzi V, Bonaventure J, Le Merrer M, Lajeunie E. Fibroblast growth factor receptor 3 mutation in nonsyndromic coronal synostosis: clinical spectrum, prevalence, and surgical outcome. J Neurosurg. 2000;92(4):631–6.
8. Justice CM, Cuellar A, Bala K, Sabourin JA, Cunningham ML, Crawford K, et al. A genome-wide association study implicates the BMP7 locus as a risk factor for nonsyndromic metopic craniosynostosis. Hum Genet. 2020;139(8):1077–90.
9. Timberlake AT, Junn A, Flores R, Staffenberg DA, Lifton RP, Persing JA. Genetic influence on neurodevelopment in non-syndromic craniosynostosis. Plast Reconstr Surg. 2022;149(5):1157–65.
10. Justice CM, Yagnik G, Kim Y, Peter I, Jabs EW, Erazo M, et al. A genome-wide association study identifies

susceptibility loci for nonsyndromic sagittal craniosynostosis near BMP2 and within BBS9. Nat Genet. 2012;44(12):1360–4.
11. Timberlake AT, Choi J, Zaidi S, Lu Q, Nelson-Williams C, Brooks ED, et al. Two locus inheritance of non-syndromic midline craniosynostosis via rare SMAD6 and common BMP2 alleles. elife. 2016;5:e20125.
12. Ye X, Guilmatre A, Reva B, Peter I, Heuze Y, Richtsmeier JT, et al. Mutation screening of candidate genes in patients with nonsyndromic sagittal craniosynostosis. Plast Reconstr Surg. 2016;137(3):952–61.
13. Timberlake AT, Furey CG, Choi J, Nelson-Williams C, Loring E, Galm A, et al. De novo mutations in inhibitors of Wnt, BMP, and Ras/ERK signaling pathways in non-syndromic midline craniosynostosis. Proc Natl Acad Sci USA. 2017;114(35):E7341–7.
14. Lelieveld SH, Reijnders MRF, Pfundt R, Yntema HG, Kamsteeg EJ, de Vries P, et al. Meta-analysis of 2,104 trios provides support for 10 new genes for intellectual disability. Nat Neurosci. 2016;19(9):1194–6.
15. Wu RT, Timberlake AT, Abraham PF, Gabrick KS, Lu X, Peck CJ, et al. SMAD6 genotype predicts neurodevelopment in nonsyndromic craniosynostosis. Plast Reconstr Surg. 2020;145(1):117e–25e.
16. Moloney DM, Wall SA, Ashworth GJ, Oldridge M, Glass IA, Francomano CA, et al. Prevalence of Pro250Arg mutation of fibroblast growth factor receptor 3 in coronal craniosynostosis. Lancet. 1997;349(9058):1059–62. https://doi.org/10.1016/s0140-6736(96)09082-4. PMID: 9107244
17. Gault DT, Renier D, Marchac D, Jones BM. Intracranial pressure and intracranial volume in children with craniosynostosis. Plast Reconstr Surg. 1992;90(3):377–81.
18. Marucci DD, Dunaway DJ, Jones BM, Hayward RD. Raised intracranial pressure in Apert syndrome. Plast Reconstr Surg. 2008;122(4):1162–8.
19. Abu-Sittah GS, Jeelani O, Dunaway D, Hayward R. Raised intracranial pressure in Crouzon syndrome: incidence, causes, and management. J Neurosurg Pediatr. 2016;17(4):469–75.
20. Karama S, Ad-Dab'bagh Y, Haier RJ, Deary IJ, Lyttelton OC, Lepage C, et al. Positive association between cognitive ability and cortical thickness in a representative US sample of healthy 6 to 18-year-olds. Intelligence. 2009;37(2):145–55.
21. Burgaleta M, Johnson W, Waber DP, Colom R, Karama S. Cognitive ability changes and dynamics of cortical thickness development in healthy children and adolescents. NeuroImage. 2014;84:810–9.
22. Romano A, Cornia R, Moraschi M, Bozzao A, Chiacchiararelli L, Coppola V, et al. Age-related cortical thickness reduction in non-demented Down's syndrome subjects. J Neuroimaging. 2016;26(1):95–102.
23. Duncan NW, Gravel P, Wiebking C, Reader AJ, Northoff G. Grey matter density and GABAA binding potential show a positive linear relationship across cortical regions. Neuroscience. 2013;235:226–31.
24. Girault JB, Cornea E, Goldman BD, Jha SC, Murphy VA, Li G, et al. Cortical structure and cognition in infants and toddlers. Cereb Cortex. 2020;30(2):786–800.
25. Wilson AT, Den Ottelander BK, De Goederen R, Van Veelen MLC, Dremmen MHG, Persing JA, et al. Intracranial hypertension and cortical thickness in syndromic craniosynostosis. Dev Med Child Neurol. 2020;62(7):799–805.
26. Wilson AT, Den Ottelander BK, Van Veelen MLC, Dremmen MHG, Persing JA, Vrooman HA, et al. Cerebral cortex maldevelopment in syndromic craniosynostosis. Dev Med Child Neurol. 2021;64:118–24.
27. Quintero-Rivera F, Robson CD, Reiss RE, Levine D, Benson CB, Mulliken JB, et al. Intracranial anomalies detected by imaging studies in 30 patients with Apert syndrome. Am J Med Genet A. 2006;140(12):1337–8.
28. Collmann H, Sörensen N, Krauss J. Hydrocephalus in craniosynostosis: a review. Childs Nerv Syst. 2005;21(10):902–12.
29. Proudman TW, Clark BE, Moore MH, Abbott AH, David DJ. Central nervous system imaging in Crouzon's syndrome. J Craniofac Surg. 1995;6(5):401–5.
30. Yacubian-Fernandes A, Palhares A, Giglio A, Gabarra RC, Zanini S, Portela L, et al. Apert syndrome: analysis of associated brain malformations and conformational changes determined by surgical treatment. J Neuroradiol. 2004;31(2):116–22.
31. Kannu P, Aftimos S. FGFR3 mutations and medial temporal lobe dysgenesis. J Child Neurol. 2007;22(2):211–3.
32. Cohen SR, Persing JA. Intracranial pressure in single-suture craniosynostosis. Cleft Palate Craniofac J. 1998;35(3):194–6.
33. Thompson DN, Malcolm GP, Jones BM, Harkness WJ, Hayward RD. Intracranial pressure in single-suture craniosynostosis. Pediatr Neurosurg. 1995;22(5):235–40.
34. David LR, Wilson JA, Watson NE, Argenta LC. Cerebral perfusion defects secondary to simple craniosynostosis. J Craniofac Surg. 1996;7(3):177–85.
35. David LR, Genecov DG, Camastra AA, Wilson JA, Argenta LC. Positron emission tomography studies confirm the need for early surgical intervention in patients with single-suture craniosynostosis. J Craniofac Surg. 1999;10(1):38–42.
36. Aldridge K, Marsh JL, Govier D, Richtsmeier JT. Central nervous system phenotypes in craniosynostosis. J Anat. 2002;201(1):31–9.
37. Richtsmeier JT, Aldridge K, DeLeon VB, Panchal J, Kane AA, Marsh JL, et al. Phenotypic integration of neurocranium and brain. J Exp Zool B Mol Dev Evol. 2006;306(4):360–78.
38. Aldridge K, Kane AA, Marsh JL, Yan P, Govier D, Richtsmeier JT. Relationship of brain and skull in pre- and postoperative sagittal synostosis. J Anat. 2005;206(4):373–85.
39. Beckett JS, Brooks ED, Lacadie C, Vander Wyk B, Jou RJ, Steinbacher DM, et al. Altered brain con-

nectivity in sagittal craniosynostosis. J Neurosurg Pediatr. 2014;13(6):690–8.
40. Bonfield CM, Foley LM, Kundu S, Fellows-Mayle W, Hitchens T, Rohde G, et al. The influence of surgical correction on white matter microstructural integrity in rabbits with familial coronal suture craniosynostosis. Neurosurg Focus. 2015;38(5):E3.
41. Cabrejo R, Lacadie C, Sun A, Chuang C, Yang J, Brooks E, et al. Functional network development in sagittal craniosynostosis treated with whole vault cranioplasty. J Craniofac Surg. 2021;32(5):1721–6.
42. Brooks ED, Yang J, Beckett JS, Lacadie C, Scheinost D, Persing S, et al. Normalization of brain morphology after surgery in sagittal craniosynostosis. J Neurosurg Pediatr. 2016;17(4):460–8.
43. Bellew M, Mandela RJ, Chumas PD. Impact of age at surgery on neurodevelopmental outcomes in sagittal synostosis. J Neurosurg Pediatr. 2019;23:434–41.
44. Patel A, Yang JF, Hashim PW, Travieso R, Terner J, Mayes LC, et al. The impact of age at surgery on long-term neuropsychological outcomes in sagittal craniosynostosis. Plast Reconstr Surg. 2014;134(4):608e–17e.
45. Mandela R, Bellew M, Chumas P, Nash H. Impact of surgery timing for craniosynostosis on neurodevelopmental outcomes: a systematic review. J Neurosurg Pediatr. 2019;23(4):442–54.
46. Jaskolka MS. Current controversies in metopic suture craniosynostosis. Oral Maxillofac Surg Clin North Am. 2017;29(4):447–63.
47. Moderie C, Govshievich A, Papay F, Fearon J, Gosain A, Doumit G. Current trends in management of nonsyndromic unilateral coronal craniosynostosis: a cross-sectional survey. Plast Reconstr Surg Glob Open. 2019;7(5):e2229.
48. Yee ST, Fearon JA, Gosain AK, Timbang MR, Papay FA, Doumit G. Classification and management of metopic craniosynostosis. J Craniofac Surg. 2015;26(6):1812–7.
49. Denis D, Genitori L, Conrath J, Lena G, Choux M. Ocular findings in children operated on for plagiocephaly and trigonocephaly. Childs Nerv Syst. 1996;12(11):683–9.
50. Beckett JS, Chadha P, Persing JA, Steinbacher DM. Classification of trigonocephaly in metopic synostosis. Plast Reconstr Surg. 2012;130(3):442e–7e.
51. Yang JF, Brooks ED, Hashim PW, Reuman HS, Travieso R, Terner J, et al. The severity of deformity in metopic craniosynostosis is correlated with the degree of neurologic dysfunction. Plast Reconstr Surg. 2017;139(2):442–7.
52. Gabrick KS, Wu RT, Singh A, Persing JA, Alperovich M. Radiographic severity of metopic craniosynostosis correlates with long-term neurocognitive outcomes. Plast Reconstr Surg. 2020;145(5):1241–8.
53. Dekaban AS, Sadowsky D. Changes in brain weights during the span of human life: relation of brain weights to body heights and body weights. Ann Neurol. 1978;4(4):345–56.
54. Iyengar RJ, Klinge PM, Chen WS, Boxerman JL, Sullivan SR, Taylor HO. Management of craniosynostosis at an advanced age: controversies, clinical findings, and surgical treatment. J Craniofac Surg. 2016;27(5):e435–41.
55. Rottgers SA, Kim PD, Kumar AR, Cray JJ, Losee JE, Pollack IF. Cranial vault remodeling for sagittal craniosynostosis in older children. Neurosurg Focus. 2011;31(2):E3.
56. Ruane EJ, Garland CB, Camison L, Fenton RA, Nischal KK, Pollack IF, et al. A treatment algorithm for patients presenting with sagittal craniosynostosis after the age of 1 year. Plast Reconstr Surg. 2017;140(3):582–90.
57. Chong S, Wang KC, Phi JH, Lee JY, Kim SK. Minimally invasive suturectomy and postoperative helmet therapy: advantages and limitations. J Korean Neurosurg Soc. 2016;59(3):227.
58. Gociman B, Marengo J, Ying J, Kestle JRW, Siddiqi F. Minimally invasive strip craniectomy for sagittal synostosis. J Craniofac Surg. 2012;23(3):825–8.
59. Iyer RR, Ye X, Jin Q, Lu Y, Liyanage L, Ahn ES. Optimal duration of postoperative helmet therapy following endoscopic strip craniectomy for sagittal craniosynostosis. J Neurosurg Pediatr. 2018;22(6):610–5.
60. Huttenlocher PR, Dabholkar AS. Regional differences in synaptogenesis in human cerebral cortex. J Comp Neurol. 1997;387(2):167–78.
61. Kostović I, Judas M, Petanjek Z, Simić G. Ontogenesis of goal-directed behavior: anatomo-functional considerations. Int J Psychophysiol. 1995;19(2):85–102.
62. Hashim PW, Patel A, Yang JF, Travieso R, Terner J, Losee JE, et al. The effects of whole-vault cranioplasty versus strip craniectomy on long-term neuropsychological outcomes in sagittal craniosynostosis. Plast Reconstr Surg. 2014;134(3):491–501.
63. Alperovich M, Runyan CM, Gabrick KS, Wu RT, Morgan C, Park SE, et al. Long-term neurocognitive outcomes of spring-assisted surgery versus cranial vault remodeling for sagittal synostosis. Plast Reconstr Surg. 2021;147(3):661–71.
64. Oppenheimer AJ, Ranganathan K, Levi B, Levi B, Strahle JM, Kapurch J, et al. Minimizing transfusions in primary cranial vault remodeling: the role of aminocaproic acid. J Craniofac Surg. 2014;25(1):82–6.
65. Fearon JA. Discussion: spring-assisted cranioplasty for the correction of nonsyndromic scaphocephaly: a quantitative analysis of 100 consecutive cases. Plast Reconstr Surg. 2017;140(1):135–6.
66. van der Meulen J. Metopic synostosis. Childs Nerv Syst. 2012;28(9):1359–67.
67. Bottero L, Lajeunie E, Arnaud E, Marchac D, Renier D. Functional outcome after surgery for trigonocephaly. Plast Reconstr Surg. 1998;102(4):952–8; discussion 959–960
68. Aryan HE, Jandial R, Ozgur BM, Hughes SA, Meltzer HS, Park MS, et al. Surgical correction of metopic synostosis. Childs Nerv Syst. 2005;21(5):392–8.

69. Ozlen F, Kafadar AM, Abuzayed B, Ulu MO, Isler C, Dashti R, et al. Surgical treatment of trigonocephaly: technique and long-term results in 48 cases. J Neurosurg Pediatr. 2011;7(3):300–10.
70. Fearon JA, Kolar JC, Munro IR. Trigonocephaly-associated hypotelorism: is treatment necessary? Plast Reconstr Surg. 1996;97(3):503–9; discussion 510–511
71. Ricci D, Vasco G, Baranello G, Salerni A, Amante R, Tamburrini G, et al. Visual function in infants with non-syndromic craniosynostosis. Dev Med Child Neurol. 2007;49(8):574–6.
72. Alford J, Derderian CA, Smartt JM. Surgical treatment of nonsyndromic unicoronal craniosynostosis. J Craniofac Surg. 2018;29(5):1199–207.
73. Kalantar Hormozi A, Daryani A, Zali A, Mohammadi HR, Shahverediani R, Eskandarloo M. Surgical treatment of unicoronal synostosis: a simplified technique without orbital osteotomy. J Craniofac Surg. 2018;29(1):66–71.
74. Mesa JM, Fang F, Muraszko KM, Buchman SR. Reconstruction of unicoronal plagiocephaly with a hypercorrection surgical technique. Neurosurg Focus. 2011;31(2):E4.
75. Kobayashi S, Honda T, Saitoh A, Kashiwa K. Unilateral coronal synostosis treated by internal forehead distraction. J Craniofac Surg. 1999;10(6):467–71; discussion 472
76. McKee RM, Carbullido MK, Ewing E, Kamel GN, Ryan J, Zaldana-Flynn MV, et al. Orbital volumetric analysis in patients with unicoronal craniosynostosis: a comparison between distraction osteogenesis and fronto-orbital advancement. Ann Plast Surg. 2021;86(5S Suppl 3):S367–73.
77. Jimenez DF, Barone CM. Early treatment of coronal synostosis with endoscopy-assisted craniectomy and postoperative cranial orthosis therapy: 16-year experience. J Neurosurg Pediatr. 2013;12(3):207–19.
78. Sawh-Martinez R, Steinbacher DM. Syndromic craniosynostosis. Clin Plast Surg. 2019;46(2):141–55.
79. Persing JA, Edgerton MT, Park TS, Jane JA. Barrel stave osteotomy for correction of turribrachycephaly craniosynostosis deformity. Ann Plast Surg. 1987;18(6):488–93.
80. White N, Evans M, Dover MS, Noons P, Solanki G, Nishikawa H. Posterior calvarial vault expansion using distraction osteogenesis. Childs Nerv Syst. 2009;25(2):231–6.
81. Zapatero ZD, Kalmar CL, Kosyk MS, Carlson AR, Swanson JW, Bartlett SP, et al. Craniometric and volumetric analysis of posterior vault distraction osteogenesis: 10-year update. J Craniofac Surg. 2021;32(7):2379–83.
82. Escher PJ, Tu A, Kearney S, Wheelwright M, Petronio J, Kebriaei M, et al. Minimizing transfusion in sagittal craniosynostosis surgery: the Children's Hospital of Minnesota Protocol. Childs Nerv Syst. 2019;35(8):1357–62.
83. Goobie SM, Zurakowski D, Isaac KV, Taicher BM, Fernandez PG, Derderian CK, et al. Predictors of perioperative complications in paediatric cranial vault reconstruction surgery: a multicentre observational study from the paediatric craniofacial collaborative group. Br J Anaesth. 2019;122(2):215–23.
84. Velardi F, Di Chirico A, Di Rocco C. Blood salvage in craniosynostosis surgery. Childs Nerv Syst. 1999;15(11–12):695–710.
85. Dadure C, Sauter M, Bringuier S, Bigorre M, Raux O, Rochette A, et al. Intraoperative tranexamic acid reduces blood transfusion in children undergoing craniosynostosis surgery: a randomized double-blind study. Anesthesiology. 2011;114(4):856–61.
86. Kurnik NM, Pflibsen LR, Do A, Bristol R, Singh DJ. Craniosynostosis surgery and the impact of tranexamic acid dosing. J Craniofac Surg. 2018;29(1):96–8.
87. Martin JP, Wang JS, Hanna KR, Stovall MM, Lin KY. Use of tranexamic acid in craniosynostosis surgery. Plast Surg (Oakv). 2015;23(4):247–51.
88. Chocron Y, Azzi A, Galli R, Alnaif N, Atkinson J, Dudley R, et al. Routine postoperative admission to the intensive care unit following repair of nonsyndromic craniosynostosis: is it necessary? J Craniofac Surg. 2019;30(6):1631–4.
89. Goobie SM, Zurakowski D, Proctor MR, Meara JG, Meier PM, Young VJ, et al. Predictors of clinically significant postoperative events after open craniosynostosis surgery. Anesthesiology. 2015;122(5):1021–32.

Part III

CSF, ICP and Hemodynamics Alterations

Ventricular and Pericerebral Cerebrospinal Fluid Accumulation in Craniosynostosis

15

Federico Di Rocco

15.1 Introduction

Alterations of cerebrospinal fluid (CSF) dynamics leading to hydrocephalus and increased intracranial pressure are common features of complex craniosynostoses while they are uncommon in simple craniosynostoses. Indeed, the incidence of hydrocephalus in simple craniosynostoses does not apparently differ from that of the general pediatric population although the studies concerning this specific point are rare [1–3]. In 1998 Cinalli et al. reported a 0.28% rate of hydrocephalus though the series they evaluated included a few children with oxycephaly and brachycephaly that nowadays the modern genetic analysis would probably identify as complex forms [4]. Increased intracranial pressure may be detected in about 15–20% of subjects with simple craniosynostoses often associated with moderate ventriculomegaly and enlargement of the subarachnoid spaces. In many cases the phenomenon may remain clinically silent and escape even to the fundus oculi examination, to be recognized only by means of prolonged intracranial pressure recordings [5]. The presence of papilledema, which is commonly thought to be a reliable indicator of chronically increased intracranial pressure, does not seem to have a good sensitivity in children with craniosynostosis [6]. Two main explanations have been provided, the first of them takes into account the great compliance of unfused normal sutures of the immature cranium that can protect the optic nerve from the raised intracranial pressure, thereby reducing the incidence of papilledema in infant. The second explanation postulates a reduced communication of the subarachnoid spaces with the optic nerve sheath in the very young [6].

However, several studies have demonstrated that the incidence of abnormally high intracranial pressure in craniosynostosis can be underestimated especially in infants when only the clinical and radiographic findings are utilized. In a series of 45 children with craniosynostosis, whose intracranial pressure was recorded preoperatively, abnormally high values (>15 mmHg) were recorded in 24 subjects (53%). However, only 4 (8.9%) of them had papilledema on preoperative funduscopic examination [7].

15.2 Abnormal Dilatation of the Subarachnoid Spaces

An abnormal dilatation of the subarachnoid spaces is often detected in cases of early fusion of the metopic and sagittal sutures as well as in unicoronal synostosis [8] (Figs. 15.1, 15.2, and 15.3).

F. Di Rocco (✉)
Pediatric Neurosurgery, French Referral Center for Craniosynostosis of Lyon, Lyon, France

INSERM 1033, Université de Lyon, Hôpital Femme Mère Enfant, Hospices Civils de Lyon, Lyon, France
e-mail: federico.dirocco@chu-lyon.fr

F. Di Rocco, J. Kestle (eds.), *Neurosurgical Aspects of Craniosynostosis*,
https://doi.org/10.1007/978-3-031-69386-1_15

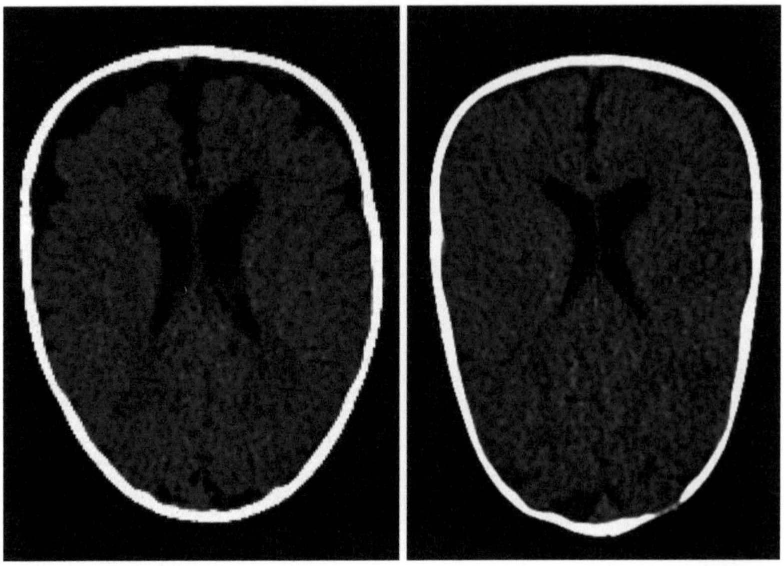

Fig. 15.1 Axial CT scan in two infants with sagittal synostosis. Note the ventriculomegaly associated with an abnormal dilation of the frontal subarachnoid space (left)

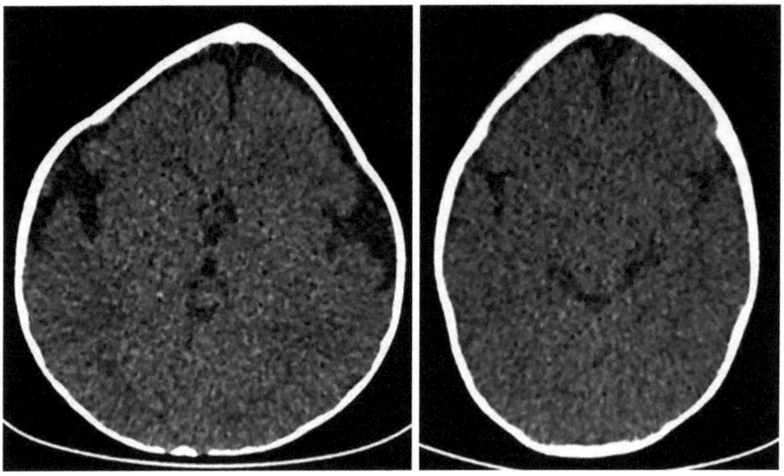

Fig. 15.2 Axial CT scan in two infants with metopic synostosis. Note the abnormally enlarged frontal and sylvian subarachnoid space (left)

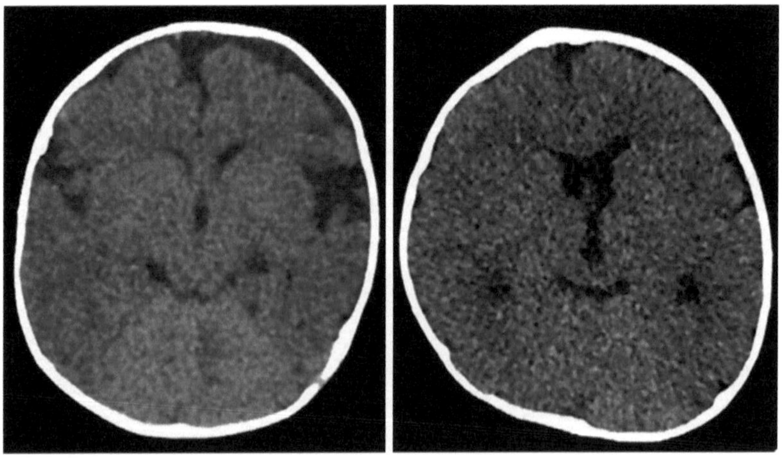

Fig. 15.3 CT scan in two infants with unicoronal synostosis. Note the asymmetrical enlarged subarachnoid space in the non-affected hemicranium (left)

The pathogenesis and the possible role in the evolution and morphological appearance of the skull possibly exerted by the focal enlargements of the subarachnoid spaces are not completely understood yet. An impaired CSF absorption related to the possible compression, focal stenoses, and limited elasticity to expand of the superior sagittal sinus in an abnormally narrow bone groove, created by the premature fusion of the overlying suture, has been proposed to explain the genesis of these fluid accumulations and the enlargement of the subarachnoid spaces [4]. Such an interpretation is supported by the results of the lumbar subarachnoid constant-infusion manometric test which demonstrates an impaired fluid absorption at the low intracranial pressures, that could account for the intracranial abnormal fluid accumulations, and an enhanced ability for fluid absorption at high intracranial pressures, which could have an important role in preventing the occurrence of a frank intracranial hypertension [9, 10]. The absence of warning signs of increased intracranial pressure such as headache and vomiting in the presence of a full or tense anterior fontanel in sagittal synostosis could be explained on these grounds. As a consequence, the occurrence of chronically high intracranial pressure may be underestimated in infants with simple craniosynostosis [11]. A direct damage of the arachnoid granulations induced by the bony changes secondary to the early fusion of the sagittal suture has also been suggested to be the cause of impaired fluid absorption in scaphocephaly and elevated intracranial pressures [12]. However, no definitive correlation has been established between such increases in intracranial pressure and neurocognitive development yet [13]. In general, the degree of abnormally high intracranial pressure in simple craniosynostosis is related to the number of precociously fused suture.

Intracranial hypertension is more frequently observed in syndromic patients than in simple craniosynostoses with a prevalence of 30–40% [5]. Several factors are known to contribute to a pathological increase in intracranial pressure (ICP) in these patients besides the number of fused suture. Though the cephalo-cranial disproportion induced by the early fusion of multiple sutures is regarded as one of the main pathogenic mechanisms, since the early 1990s, several studies have highlighted the lack of a predictable correlation between intracranial volume and ICP [14, 15]. Such lack of correlation between intracranial volume and intracranial pressure in some subjects with complex craniosynostosis has been confirmed by recent studies [16] and explains the failure to reduce intracranial hypertension in these patients by the mere cranial expansive surgical cranial vault reconstruction [17]. Intracranial hypertension in complex craniosynostoses has a multifactorial genesis that may vary in various syndromes, in different subjects, and also in relation to the age. The main factors, besides the reduced skull volume, should be identified in venous anomalies leading to defective CSF absorption, abnormal hypoplasic, and malformed foramen magnum resulting in impaired CSF movements, respiratory abnormalities, related to the possible associated facial malformation, responsible for elevated levels of CO_2, the presence of hydrocephalus and hindbrain malformations, pre-existing to the cranial vault expansive remodeling or developing after the surgical operation. The correct recognition of these pathogenetic factors and the specific role exerted in the single subject is crucial for the successful management of the condition.

15.3 Hydrocephalus in Complex Craniosynostoses

It is well established that hydrocephalus in complex craniosynostoses frequently requires CSF diversion procedures, and in most of the cases already in the first months after birth. In a great proportion of cases, hydrocephalus associated with complex craniosynostosis is multifactorial and progressive. Hydrocephalus is commonly encountered in Pfeiffer and Crouzon syndromes, where it is detected in almost half of the affected subjects usually requiring a prompt surgical treatment. However, nonprogressive ventriculomegaly can also be noted in a minority of children with Crouzon syndrome. On the other hand, nonprogressive hydrocephalus, which rarely needs

CSF shunting procedures, is an almost constant characteristic of Apert's syndrome. It represents a maldevelopmental process rather than an active process in the majority of the affected children.

15.3.1 Apert Syndrome (OMIM#101200)

Among the multiple anomalies harbored by subjects with Apert syndrome, ventriculomegaly is a common feature. The larger expansion of the cerebral ventricles occurs at the side of cranial expansive compensatory growth and can be accompanied by enlarged subarachnoid spaces. However, the brain volume itself is normal and the ventriculomegaly tends to remain stable over time (Fig. 15.4).

At the end of the last century, CSF shunting procedures were considered to be necessary for managing this ventricular enlargement in subjects with Apert syndrome. For example, in 1993 at the Sick Children Hospital in Toronto Hendricks and co-workers operated on 10 out of 44 children with Apert syndrome, whose computed tomography (CT) scans or pneumoencephalograms had revealed a ventriculomegaly. The authors performed a spino-lumbar CSF shunt in seven cases and a ventriculo-peritoneal CSF shunt in the remaining three subjects. In six patients, the CSF shunts were carried out immediately after a decompressive cranial procedure because of post-operative CSF leakage (five cases) or subgaleal fluid collection (one Case). On this ground they propounded an underlying CSF absorption deficit [18]. It is worth to note that the same authors did not find a relation between the volume of the ventricular enlargement and the mental development. Pre- and post-operative (after decompressive cranial procedures) subarachnoid fluid collections were also observed by other authors who proposed an alternative explanation of the phenomenon that they interpreted on the grounds of a defective and slow brain enlargement after the operation rather than an impaired CSF absorption [4].

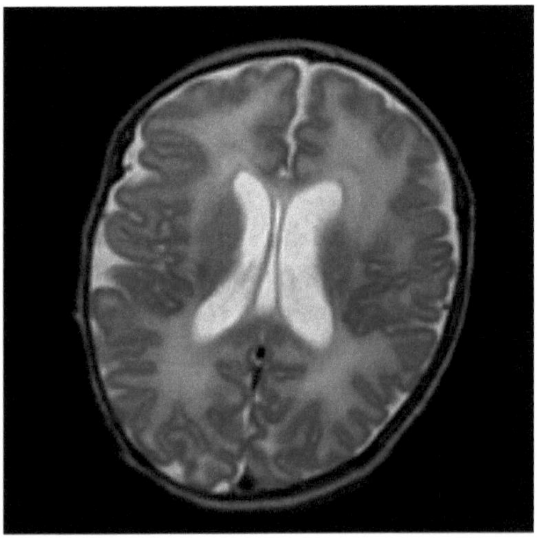

Fig. 15.4 Axial brain MR image of an infant with Apert syndrome. To note the co-existence of a dilated ventricles and enlarged peripheral subarachnoid space

In 1993, Hanieh and David reporting on 33 cases of the syndrome treated in the Australian Craniofacial Unit at the Adelaide Children's Hospital emphasized that mild ventricular dilation was common among their patients but without associated intracranial hypertension. The ventricular dilation was severe only in one child. A further support to the stability of the ventricular dilation was given by the observation that after cranial decompression the obtained new intracranial volume was occupied by the expansion of the cerebral parenchyma without any further dilation of the cerebral ventricular cavities [19].

Cinalli et al. (1995) performed a CSF shunting procedure because of progressive hydrocephalus only in 4 patients out of a series of 65 patients with Apert syndrome. They pointed out that only 1.9% of their cases had chronic herniation of the cerebellar tonsils in contrast with the 72.7% of patients with Crouzon syndrome [20]. Cranial neuroimaging studies performed by Quintero-Rivera et al. (2006) in 30 patients with Apert syndrome showed ventriculomegaly in 76% of patients but showed an active hydrocephalus only in 13% of the cases. The authors also reported on associated cerebral malformations, Namely, complete absence of the septum pellucidum (17%), partially absent septum pellucidum (23%), and defects of the corpus callosum (23%) that could account for mental retardation independent of the ventricular dilation. The same authors focused on other abnormalities that could also impact on CSF dynamics such as jugular foraminal stenosis (28 cases), Chiari I malformation (5 cases), or low-lying cerebellar tonsils (5 cases) [21].

A higher rate of active hydrocephalus requiring CSF diversion procedures was recently reported by Munarriz et al. (2020) who placed an extra-thecal CSF shunt device in a quarter (24.3%) of their subjects with Apert syndrome. A further 8.1% of patients required decompressive surgery for Chiari malformation. In this series, 18 patients (48.7%) presented a normal ventricular size, with an Evans' index from 0.15 to 0.28. Ten patients (27%) harbored nonprogressive ventriculomegaly, with an Evan's index ranging from 0.31 to 0.44 [22].

The prenatal ultrasonographic diagnosis of non-evolutive ventriculomegaly in Apert syndrome supports the malformative nature of the phenomenon in majority of the cases. When its progression after birth occurs, it is related to the impact of factors that may impair CSF dynamics such as the craniostenosis itself, the jugular foramen stenosis, and the possible insufficient cranial blood venous discharge [23–25]. On the other hand, patients who do not develop an active form of hydrocephalus are characterized by normal size of both jugular foramina, normal course of both jugular veins, absence of compensatory emissary veins, and patent cranial lambdoid sutures.

The observation of patients with Apert syndrome harboring ventriculomegaly without a concomitant craniosynostosis further support the possible primary nature of the hydrocephalus in this syndrome [26].

15.3.2 Pfeiffer Syndrome

Pfeiffer syndrome (PS, OMIM #101600) is an inherited craniofacial disorder that is associated with primary craniosynostosis, midface hypoplasia, broad thumbs and great toes, and soft tissue syndactyly of hands (usually second and third digits) and feet of varying severity. It is also defined as Type V acrocephalosyndactity, the other types being Apert syndrome (Type I), Vogt/Crouzon syndrome (Type II), Saethre–Chotzen syndrome (Type III), and Waardenburg syndrome (Type IV).

The premature closure of the coronal and lambdoid sutures accounts for the cloverleaf appearance of the skull which characterizes the type II Pfeiffer syndrome, usually associated with hydrocephalus. Pfeiffer syndrome type III share the cranial and extracranial malformations of type II except for the cloverleaf modification of the skull and is associated with mental retardation as type II. On the contrary, type I is associated with normal intelligence.

Increased intracranial pressure is a common finding of all types of the syndrome mainly due to the reduced intracranial volume resulting from the hypoplastic skull base and the premature fusion of the cranial sutures (Fig. 15.5).

Actually, hydrocephalus in cloverleaf skull deformity is invariably associated with bilateral lambdoid stenosis while it is absent in unilateral or absent lambdoid stenosis [27].

Further contributing factors to CSF dynamics anomalies is the abnormal development of the air pathways which results in respiratory problems and secondary increase in cerebral vascular CO_2 content in several affected children and the tracheal cartilaginous sleeve, that accounts for respiratory complications in some cases of Apert and Crouzon syndromes.

The frequently associated hydrocephalus is often related to a concomitant aqueduct stenosis [28, 29]. However, the pathogenesis of the phenomenon should be considered multi-factorial resulting from the restricted volume of the basal and cerebral convexities subarachnoid spaces, posterior fossa hypoplasia, anatomical and functional anomalies of the cranial venous outflow, as well as the development of a caudal herniation of the cerebellar vermis and tonsils (Fig. 15.6).

15.3.3 Crouzon Syndrome

Crouzon syndrome (OMIM # 123500) is characterized by craniosynostosis resulting in secondary anomalies of the facial bones and facial structure. The syndrome includes ventriculomeg-

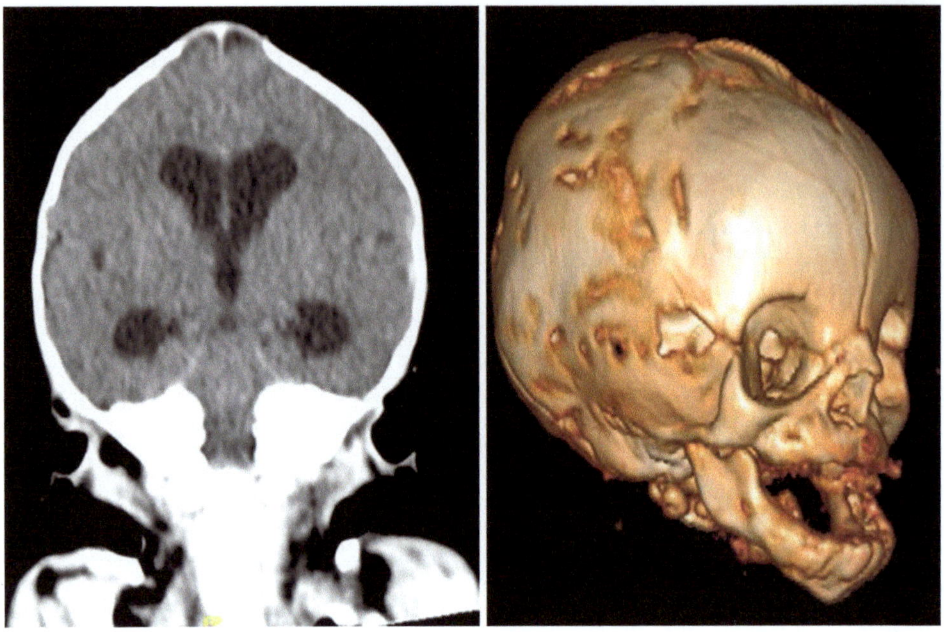

Fig. 15.5 CT scan of a 3-month-old infant with a Pfeiffer syndrome. To note the restricted skull base, the enlarged transverse diameter and the acrocephaply. The ventricular system is dilated while the peripheral subarachnoid space is effaced

aly and hydrocephalus among the other common features, namely, hypertelorism, exophthalmos and external strabismus, parrot-beaked nose, short upper lip, hypoplastic maxilla, and a relative mandibular prognathism. Approximately 30%–40% of individuals with Crouzon syndrome develop hydrocephalus and increased intracranial pressure early in life. Besides hydrocephalus, intracranial hypertension depends on a variety of pathogenic factors, namely, the reduced intracranial volume, secondary to the early fusion of cranial sutures, the constriction of pericerebral subarachnoid spaces, the posterior fossa hypoplasia, the impaired venous circulation, the effect of upper airways obstructions, and the caudal herniation of cerebellar vermis and tonsils that can lead to a syringomyelia (Fig. 15.7). Indeed, in Pfeiffer and Crouzon syndromes with cerebellar tonsils descent, an MRI of the spine should be performed in order to rule out the development of an associated syringomyelia.

More than a quarter of the 68 individuals with Crouzon syndrome described by Cinalli et al. (1995) required a CSF shunting procedures because of progressive hydrocephalus. In most of these subjects, hypertensive hydrocephalus was associated with cerebellar tonsils herniation. Four patients presented syringomyelia confirming the complex pathogenesis of the CSF dynamic alterations that occur in the syndrome [20].

Hydrocephalus is even more frequent in Crouzon subjects with acanthosis nigricans involving approximately 40% of the cases. In early life, these patients show ventriculomegaly, ocular proptosis, midface hypoplasia, and choanal atresia whereas the cutaneous anomalies become clinically evident only during childhood. The association of hydrocephalus and choanal atresia in a subject with Crouzon syndrome should arise the suspicion of Crouzon with acanthosis nigricans even prior to the appearance of the typical cutaneous stigmata [30–33].

The early fusion of the lambdoid suture within the first 2 years of age has been proposed to account for the major incidence of hydrocephalus in Crouzon than in Apert syndrome [20, 34]. The precocious closure of this suture together with other basal synchondroses would be responsible

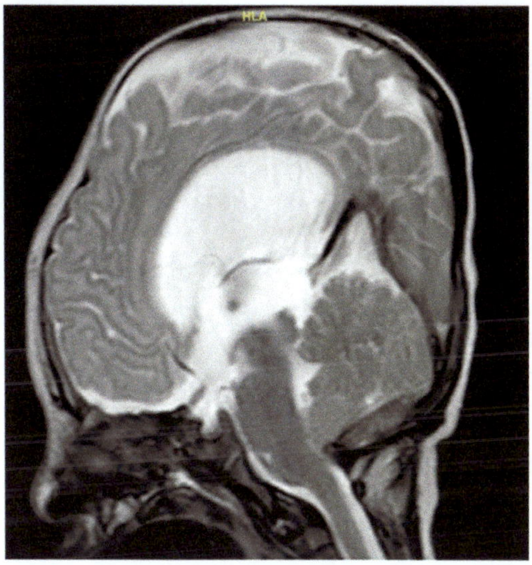

Fig. 15.6 Sagittal brain MR image of a 5-month-old infant with Pfeiffer syndrome showing an obvious triventricular dilation of the ventricular system associated with aqueductal stenosis, hypoplasic posterior cranial fossa with the disappearnce of the cisterna magna, and to an initial caudal displacement of the inferior cerebellar vermis. The volume of the subarachnoid spaces of the cerebral convexities is altered alternating area of focal dilations and compression from the overlying bone structures. The CSF subarachnoid circulation is impaired by the presence of skull bone spicule indentating the membrane coverings

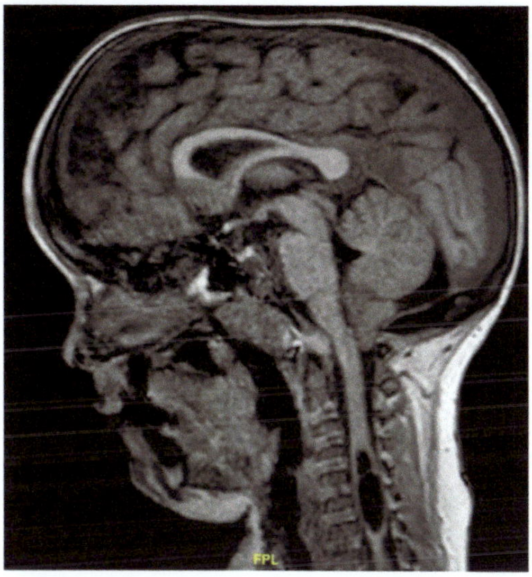

Fig. 15.7 Sagittal MR in an infant with Crouzon syndrome. To note the elongated sagittal diameter, the macrocrania and frontal bossing related to the anomalies in CSF dynamics involving both the ventricular system and the peripheral subarachnoid spaces. The inferior cerebellar vermis is caudally dislocated causing a local obstacle on CSF circulation at the cranio-cervical junction leading to syringomyelia

for the hypoplastic posterior cranial fossa and the possible stenosis of the jugular vein foramina, commonly observed in patients with Crouzon syndrome [34, 35]. Both phenomena concur in subjects with Crouzon syndrome to cause a Chiari type I anomaly, that in turn would add its obstructive effects on CSF dynamics.

Also, the size and the shape of the foramen magnum, that in the Crouzon syndrome differ as compared to controls, may have a role in the occurrence of the Chiari type I anomaly and in determining its clinical severity. Indeed, among all groups, FGFR related syndromes, especially Crouzon syndrome, show reduced anteroposterior diameter as compared to controls ($p = 0.005$) [36, 37].

As previously mentioned, cerebellar tonsils' descent may further alter the CSF dynamics resulting in the development of a syringomyelia.

On the one side, these observations highlight the importance of a routine clinical and radiological examination, in order to search for signs and symptoms related to the tonsil's descent or to the syrinx. On the other side, they also underline the complex physiopathology of CSF disorder in these patients associating with the craniocerebral disproportion, focal alterations in CSF dynamics at the craniovertebral junction level, and increased venous pressure through dural sinuses and jugular veins.

15.4 Surgical Management of Intracranial Hypertension, Focal CSF Collections, Hydrocephalus in Craniosynostosis

A strict collaboration of a large team of specialists that comprise neurosurgeons, cranio-facial surgeons, plastic surgeons, pediatric care intensivists, pediatricians, ENT surgeons, ophthalmologists, orthodontics, and specialized nurses is necessary for the appropriate management of children with complex craniosynostoses. However, the decision on when and how to correct intracranial hypertension and associated CSF dynamics alterations should to be taken by the pediatric neurosurgeon. Consequently, the appropriate treatment requires that the neurosurgeon is familiar with the specific pathophysiological mechanisms that have caused the intracranial hypertension in the single individual.

15.4.1 The Correction of Focal Enlargement of the Subarachnoid Spaces and Intracranial Hypertension in Simple Craniosynostoses

Focal CSF collections are frequently found in sagittal, metopic, and unicoronal synostoses developing in specific anatomical sites related to the precociously fused sutures (Figs. 15.1, 15.2, and 15.3).

In nearly all the cases, these focal enlargements of the subarachnoid spaces appear to be well tolerated and do not require specific surgical corrective measures even though they appear to play a certain role, at least in scaphocephaly, in defining the resulting morphology of the skull. For example, in scaphocephaly, the pericerebral fluid collection in the frontal region contributes to enlarge the bulging forehead and modifies the frontonasal angle (Figs. 15.1 and 15.8) [62].

A correlation with the shape of the fused suture overlying the superior sagittal sinus and the presence of CSF collections has also been found: the abnormal CSF collections are found more commonly in children with an "omega" type configuration of the fused sagittal synostosis [61] (Fig. 15.9).

These findings may suggest that the CSF collection results from a focal venous resorption impairment, but such hypothesis needs to be confirmed. However, the presence of focal frontal

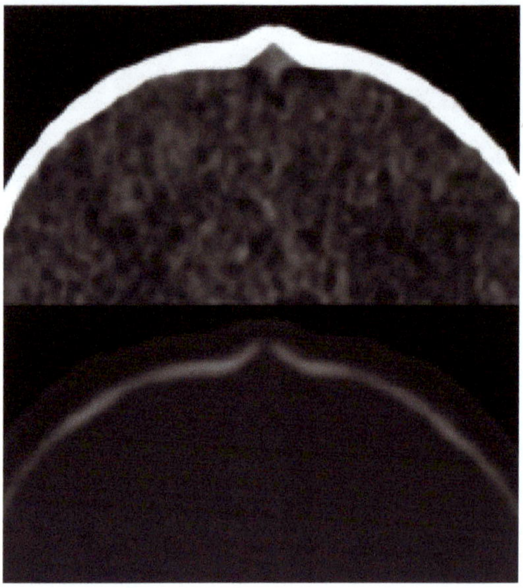

Fig. 15.9 Pattern of bone ridge commonly associated with pericerebral CSF collection. Adapted from Ref. [62]

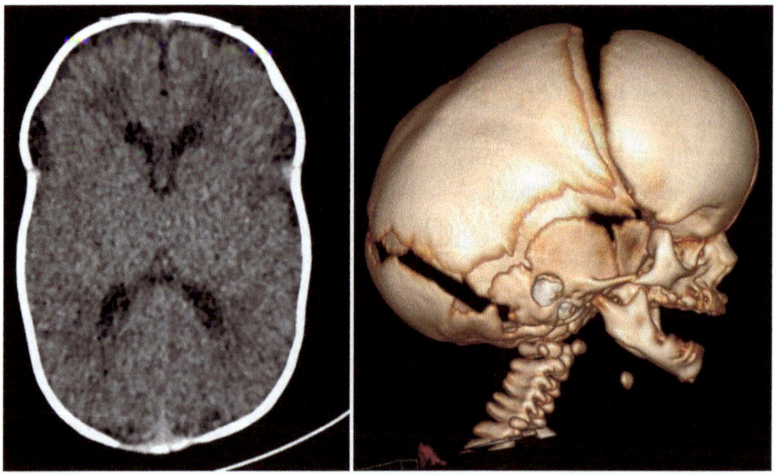

Fig. 15.8 Axial and 3D reconstruction in a 1-month-old infant with scaphocephaly demonstrating the effect of the frontal subarachnoid fluid accumulation on the shape and spatial positioning of the anterior skull

collection in unicoronal synostosis seems to suggest that venous sinus compression is not the sole mechanism for such subarachnoid space enlargement (Fig. 15.3). The expansive remodeling of the skull vault is usually followed by the volumetric reduction of pericerebral fluid collections and finally by their complete or nearly complete disappearance.

The preoperative presence of the enlarged CSF spaces (ventricular or periventricular) seems to play a role in the early post-operative course, at least in cases of endoscopic sagittal suturectomies where the immediate post-operative parietal expansion is greater in case of enlarged CSF spaces. However, the potential impact of such CSF collection on functional results remains unknown.

Bilateral expanding craniotomies induces total relief from the symptoms and signs of raised intracranial pressure even in older children with mild forms of craniosynostosis that were not treated in infancy [38]. Actually, chronically increased intracranial pressure and ocular fundi anomalies are a frequent finding in older children with untreated mild craniosynostosis which are investigated because of neurocognitive delay. Late cranial vault expansive cranioplasty proved to be effective in these patients [39]. The risk of under-evaluating intracranial hypertension in subjects with sagittal synostosis was pointed out by Wall et al., in 2014 [11]. The authors recorded the intraparenchymal pressure in 39 children (mean age: 58 months) whose surgical treatment had been considered to be not indicated on the grounds of the minimal cranial deformity and the absence of clinical manifestations of increased intracranial pressure or refused by the parents. When re-examined at an older age, 16 out of the 39 (41%) individuals presented with marked dolichocephaly, 11 (28%) with mild scaphocephaly and 12 (31%) with a near normal skull shape. Raised intracranial pressure was recorded in 14 (44%) out of the 39 children without any significant difference in incidence among the three groups and in the absence of clinical symptoms and signs and ophthalmological or radiological anomalies that could have suggested intracranial hypertension. The same team of scientists, in 2015 [40], challenged the efficacy of the modified strip craniectomy versus the calvarial remodeling in normalizing the intracranial pressure in sagittal synostosis suggesting the need for a long-term observation, especially for those that had undergone linear craniectomies. They recorded the intracranial pressure in 217 children that had undergone one or two surgical procedures, either a modified strip craniectomy or a calvarial remodeling. Abnormally high-pressure values were found in 6.9% of the cases (mean post-operative period: 51 months), more commonly in subjects treated with modified strip craniectomy (13 out of 89 patients, 14.6%) than with cranial remodeling (2 out of 128 subjects, 1.6%). Most of the children operated on by strip craniectomy were less than 1 year of age at the time of the operation. These data should not be overlooked when considering the recent shift toward strip craniectomy as the result of the introduction of the endoscopic techniques.

A retrospective study on 284 patients with isolated non-syndromic sagittal craniosynostosis operated by cranial vault reconstruction provided a figure of 7.07% of children requiring a second surgical procedure because of the recurrence of abnormally high intracranial pressure, with a double incidence in subjects operated on before 6 months of age compared with those treated later on [41]. Unfortunately, no information on the CSF spaces was provided.

15.4.2 The Management of CSF Disorders Associated with Complex Craniosynostosis

The management of hydrocephalus, and in particular, the timing of a CSF shunting procedure, in children with syndromic craniosynostoses has been and still is a subject of discussion. The early occurrence and rapid progression of ventricular dilation in subjects with Pfeiffer syndrome and, less frequently, Crouzon syndrome may challenge the most common attitude to perform CSF draining procedures only after cranial decompression [42, 43]. Indeed, the insertion of a CSF shunting device to treat immediately the intracranial hypertension may allow to postpone the cranial reconstruction so decreasing the risks of postoperative complications (excessive bleeding, wound infection, meningitis, seizure, pneumonia) that can weigh the very early cranial remodeling of the trilobar skull in case of Pfeiffer and Crouzon syndromes. Actually, after controlling the hypertensive hydrocephalus by means of a ventriculo-peritoneal CSF shunt in the neonatal period, the calvarial remodeling (fronto-orbital advancement or posterior vault enlargement) can be made at 3–6 months and further remodeling at 1 year of age with major safety [35].

In subjects, who appear to tolerate the hydrocephalus relatively well, most of the authors are reluctant to proceed with an immediate insertion of a CSF extrathecal shunt device. Such a cautious attitude is based on three main considerations. First of all, the observation that the expansive calvarial reconstruction may be sufficient to control the hydrocephalus in some cases. Then, the concern that the action of the inserted CSF draining device may reduce the expansive force of the intracranial content necessary to allow the adequate post-operative skull growth. Finally, the high incidence of CSF shunting complications in the pediatric population with craniosynostosis. An incidence of 59% complications rate associated with the extrathecal CSF shunting leading to further surgical procedures has been reported in a recent study [44].

The reluctance to insert a CSF draining device in infants with Crouzon disease and hydrocephalus is further justified by the observation of ventriculomegaly, even quite significant in size, that tends to remain stable in some patients without any CSF shunt diversion procedure [42]. This is the case for the frequent non evolutive ventriculomegaly associated with Apert syndrome for which an intrinsic abnormality in the embryological development of the brain has been postulated [45].

The rate of hydrocephalus regression following the mere expansive remodeling of the cranial vault, that is, the correction of the "constrictive" forces impairing CSF circulation and absorption, cannot be evaluated by the analysis of the literature. Indeed, such an evenience depends on the variable equilibrium of many variables that can play a specific role in the single individual such as an impaired CSF absorption related to the restricted volume of the subarachnoid spaces, venous anomalies, and aqueduct stenosis. Actually, some of the just mentioned pathogenic factors can continue to exert a role even after cranial vault remodeling accounting for the progression of hydrocephalus that can be observed in some infants even after the surgical expansion of the skull.

The still persisting debate on the most appropriate managing of the hydrocephalus associated with complex craniosynostosis continues the discussion about its physiopathogenesis, that can be recognized already in the first proposal of the "constrictive" hypothesis by Rieping, more than a century ago that indicated the mechanical compression exerted by the hypoplasic posterior fossa as the mechanism leading to the impairment in CSF absorption [46]. The hypothesis of an impaired venous discharge resulting in a defective CSF absorption was first propounded by Günther in 1936 [47] and subsequently accepted by a wide number of scientists that pointed on the obstacles in venous circulation exerted by the bony anomalies of the posterior cranial fossa, in particular at the level of the jugular foramina [48, 49]. Sainte-Rose and coworkers individuated in the structural obstruction of the sigmoid sinus as the pathogenic anomaly responsible for the hydrocephalus on the grounds of the pressure variations that they recorded in the sagittal superior sinus, jugular vein, and lateral cerebral ventricles simultaneously following CSF withdrawal and re-injection tests. Based on these tests and the results of sonography, the authors carried on a venous bypass between the lateral sinus and a jugular vein in three patients, a procedure that did not become popular [50].

Cerebellar tonsils caudal herniation is commonly associated with the premature fusion of the lambdoid suture in subjects with Crouzon disease. It can be not obvious in the neonatal period becoming obvious during the first year of life. Such a low position of the cerebellar tonsils is often referred to as "Chiari type I malformation." Indeed, rather than a "malformation," the caudal herniation of the hindbrain structures should be regarded in subjects with Crouzon syndrome as an acquired alteration depending on the cranio-cerebral disproportion brought about by the reduced volume of the posterior cranial fossa secondary to the premature fusion of the lambdoid sutures. Indeed, it is often associated with an upward migration of the upper cerebellar vermis into the pre-vermian cistern that indicates the hypoplasic posterior cranial fossa as the cause of both phenomena, having become the structure unable to accommodate for the growing cerebellum. The possible cerebellar turgor induced by a concomitant local venous hypertension should be considered a further factor accounting for such dynamic events [51].

The caudal herniation of the cerebella tonsils and its clinical manifestations can be precipitated by the pressure "from above" exerted by the further dilatation of the supratentorial ventricular system that can occur because of a functional stenosis of the aqueduct and the block in the CSF circulation at the level of the cranio-vertebral junction. Such a block interferes not only with the CSF upward movements toward the major sites for its absorption into the superior sagittal sinus but also precludes its downward circulation so limiting its absorption by the meninges of the spinal cord and the ependyma of the central spinal canal. In other words, the caudal herniation of the cerebellar structures may result in a functional dissociation between the cranial and spinal compartments so creating a pressure gradient that constitutes a further pathogenic factor for the progression of the hydrocephalus.

The morphology of the foramen magnum also appears to play an important role in both the genesis and the clinical presentation of the acquired caudal descent of the cerebellar tonsils [36]. The foramen magnum area is reduced in size in subjects with Crouzon syndrome and hydrocephalus, with diminished sagittal diameter ($p = 0.023$), sagittal posterior diameter ($p = 0.0173$), and transversal diameter ($p = 0.03985$) as compared to the normal population [52, 53]. The reduced area of the foramen magnum does not only differentiate individuals with Crouzon and Pfeiffer syndrome from the normal population but also from subjects with Apert, Saethre-Chotzen, or isolated bicoronal synostosis ($p = 0.37$, $p = 0.71$, $p = 0.40$, respectively) [37, 54].

In recent years, endoscopic third-cisternostomy (ETV) has been in subjects with craniofacial synostosis, caudal herniation of the cerebellar structures, and hypertensive hydrocephalus proposed in the attempt to avoid the insertion of an extrathecal CSF drainage. Out of 11 patients (Crouzon syndrome 5, Pfeiffer syndrome 3, and unclassifiable syndrome 3) the hydrocephalus was controlled in 7 cases, whereas the remaining 4 patients required a ventriculo-peritoneal CSF shunt at a variable temporal distance ranging from 1 week to 6 months, consequently, demonstrating the necessity of a strict prolonged monitoring of the operated-on patients [55]. The posterior cranial fossa bone decompression seems effective in decreasing the incidence of late failure of the ETV [44]. The effectiveness of ETV in treating the hydrocephalus associated with the caudal herniation of the cerebellar tonsils in a good percentage of cases has been demonstrated by several studies and proposed as a measure to post-pone the skull reconstruction for a few months in order to decrease the surgical risk and select the most appropriate age for the operation [56–59]. The same approach has been suggested for the rare cases of isolated cranial synostosis, namely, sagittal synostosis, presenting with hydrocephalus and hindbrain structures descent [60].

In conclusion, the accurate evaluation of the morphology of the CSF spaces and the CSF dynamics aimed at identifying the pathogenic mechanisms of the hydrocephalus associated with craniosynostosis is mandatory to decide for a timely surgical correction and to select the appropriate surgical procedure, as well as, to recognize those subjects whose ventricular dilation is likely to not progress or being controlled by the mere cranial remodeling.

References

1. Collmann H, Sörensen N, Krauss J, Mühling J. Hydrocephalus in craniosynostosis. Childs Nerv Syst. 1988;4(5):279–85. https://doi.org/10.1007/BF00271924. PMID: 3242797
2. Collmann H, Sörensen N, Krauss J. Hydrocephalus in craniosynostosis: a review. Childs Nerv Syst. 2005;21:902–12.
3. Frassanito P, Palombi D, Tamburrini G. Craniosynostosis and hydrocephalus: relevance and treatment modalities. Childs Nerv Syst. 2021;37(11):3465–73. https://doi.org/10.1007/s00381-021-05158-z. Epub 2021 Apr 7
4. Cinalli G, Sainte-Rose C, Kollar EM, Zerah M, Brunelle F, Chumas P, Arnaud E, Marchac D, Pierre-Kahn A, Renier D. Hydrocephalus and craniosynostosis. J Neurosurg. 1998;88(2):209–14. https://doi.org/10.3171/jns.1998.88.2.0209. PMID: 9452225
5. Tamburrini, Caldarelli M, Massimi L, Santini P, Di Rocco C. Intracranial pressure monitoring in children with single suture and complex craniosynostosis: a review. Childs Nerv Syst. 2005;21:913.
6. Tuite GF, Chong WK, Evanson J, Narita A, Taylor D, Harkness WF, Jones BM, Hayward RD. The effectiveness of papilledema as an indicator of raised intracranial pressure in children with craniosynostosis. Neurosurgery. 1996;38(2):272–8. https://doi.org/10.1097/00006123-199602000-00009.
7. Judy BF, Swanson JW, Yang W, Storm PB, Bartlett SP, Taylor JA, Heuer GG, Lang S-S. Intraoperative intracranial pressure monitoring in the pediatric craniosynostosis population. J Neurosurg Pediatr. 2018;22(5):475–80. https://doi.org/10.3171/2018.5.PEDS1876.
8. Di Rocco F, Garcia-Gonzalez O, Szathmari A, Chauvel-Picard J, Beuriat PA, Paulus C, Gleizal A, Mottolese C. Emissary veins and pericerebral cerebrospinal fluid in trigonocephaly: do they define a specific subtype? Childs Nerv Syst. 2021;37(4):1159–65. https://doi.org/10.1007/s00381-020-04982-z. Epub 2021 Jan 6. PMID: 33409617
9. Caldarelli M, Di Rocco C, Rossi GF. Lumbar subarachnoid infusion test in paediatric neurosurgery. Dev Med Child Neurol. 1979;21(1):71–82. https://doi.org/10.1111/j.1469-8749.1979.tb01582.x. PMID: 43738
10. Di Rocco C, Iannelli A, Velardi F. Early diagnosis and surgical indication in craniosynostosis. Childs Brain. 1980;6(4):175–88. https://doi.org/10.1159/000119902. PMID: 7371441
11. Wall SA, Thomas GP, Johnson D, Byren JC, Jayamohan J, Magdum SA, McAuley DJ, Richards PG. The preoperative incidence of raised intracranial pressure in nonsyndromic sagittal craniosynostosis is underestimated in the literature. J Neurosurg Pediat. 2014;14(6):674–81. https://doi.org/10.3171/2014.8.PEDS1425. Epub 2014 Sep 2
12. Hassler W, Zentner J. Radical osteoclastic craniectomy in sagittal synostosis. Neurosurgery. 1990;27(4):539–43. https://doi.org/10.1097/00006123-199010000-00006.
13. Thiele-Nygaard AE, Foss-Skiftesvik J, Juhler M. Intracranial pressure, brain morphology and cognitive outcome in children with sagittal craniosynostosis. Childs Nerv Syst. 2020;36(4):689–95. https://doi.org/10.1007/s00381-020-04502-z. Epub 2020 Feb 3
14. Fok H, Jones BM, Gault DG, Andar U, Hayward R. Relationship between intracranial pressure and intracranial volume in craniosynostosis. Br J Plast Surg. 1992;45(5):394–7. https://doi.org/10.1016/0007-1226(92)90013-n.
15. Gault DT, Renier D, Marchac D, Jones BM. Intracranial pressure and intracranial volume in children with craniosynostosis. Plast Reconstr Surg. 1992;90(3):377–81. https://doi.org/10.1097/00006534-199209000-00003.
16. Langvatn EA, Frič R, Due-Tønnessen BJ, Eide PK. Intracranial volume versus static and pulsatile intracranial pressure values in children with craniosynostosis. J Neurosurg Pediatr. 2019;24(1):66–74. https://doi.org/10.3171/2019.2.PEDS18767. PMID: 31003225
17. Thompson DN, Jones BM, Harkness W, Gonsalez S, Hayward RD. Consequences of cranial vault expansion surgery for craniosynostosis. Pediatr Neurosurg. 1997;26(6):296–303. https://doi.org/10.1159/000121209.
18. Murovic JA, Posnick JC, Drake JM, Humphreys RP, Hoffman HJ, Hendricks EB. Hydrocephalus in Apert syndrome: a retrospective review. Pediatr Neurosurg, 1993. 19(3):151–5. https://doi.org/10.1159/000120720).
19. Hanieh A, David DJ. Apert's syndrome. Childs Nerv Syst. 1993;9(5):289–91. https://doi.org/10.1007/BF0030627.
20. Cinalli G, Renier D, Sebag G, Sainte-Rose, Arnaud E, Pierre-Kahn A. Chronic tonsillar herniation in Crouzon's and Apert's syndromes: the role of premature synostosis of the lambdoid suture. J Neurosurg. 1995;83:575–82.
21. Quintero-Rivera F, Robson CD, Reiss RE, Levine D, Benson CB, Mulliken JB, Kimonis VE. Intracranial anomalies detected by imaging studies in 30 patients with Apert syndrome. (Letter). Am J Med Genet. 2006;140A:1337–8.
22. Munarriz PM, Pascual B, Castaño-Leon AM, García-Recuero I, Redondo M, de Aragón AM, Romance A. Apert syndrome: cranial procedures and brain malformations in a series of patients. Surg Neurol Int. 2020;11:361.
23. Respondek-Liberska M, Smigiel R, Zielinski A, Sasiadek MM. Progressive development of sonographic features in prenatal diagnosis of Apert syndrome--case report and literature review. Ginekol Pol. 2010;81(12):935–9.

24. Driessen C, van Veelen MLC, Joosten KF, Versnel SL, van Nieuwenhove CA, Wolvius EB, et al. Apert syndrome: the Paris and Rotterdam philosophy. Expert Opin Orphan Drugs. 2017;5(7):599–605.
25. Tamburrini G, Caldarelli M, Massimi L, Di Rocco C. Complex craniosynostoses: a review of the prominent clinical features and the related management strategies. Child's Nervous Syst. 2012;28(9):1511–2.
26. de Ângelis Ramos D, Matushita H, Cardeal DD, Nascimento CN, Teixeira MJ. Apert syndrome without craniosynostosis. Child Nerv Syst. 2019;35(3):565–7.
27. Machado G, Di Rocco F, Sainte-Rose C, Meyer P, Marchac D, Macquet-Nouvion G, Arnaud E, Renier D. Cloverleaf skull deformity and hydrocephalus. Childs Nerv Syst. 2011;27(10):1683–91. https://doi.org/10.1007/s00381-011-1508-8. Epub 2011 Sep 17
28. Fearon J, Rhodes J. Pfeiffer syndrome: a treatment evaluation. Plast Reconstr Surg. 2009;123(5):1560–9.
29. Moore MH, Hanieh A. Hydrocephalus in Pfeiffer syndrome. J Clin Neurosci. 1994;1(3):202–4.
30. Orlow SJ. Cutaneous findings in craniofacial malformation syndromes. Arch Dermatol. 1992;128:1379–86.
31. Schweitzer DN, Graham GM Jr, Lachman RS, Jabs WS, Okajima K, Przylepa KA, Shanske A, Chen K, Neidich JA, Wilcox WR. Subtle radiographic findings of achondroplasia in patients with Crouzon syndrome with acanthosis nigricans due to an Ala391Glu substitution in FGFR3. Am J Med Genet. 2001;98(1):75–91.
32. Arnaud-Lopez L, Fragoso R, Mantilla-Capacho J, Barros-Nunez P. Crouzon with acanthosis nigricans: further delineation of the syndrome. Clin Genet. 2007;72:405–10.
33. Di Rocco F, Collet C, Legeai-Mallet L, Arnaud E, Le Merrer M, Hadj-Rabia S, Renier D. Crouzon syndrome with acanthosis nigricans: a case-based update. Childs Nerv Syst. 2011;27(3):349–54. https://doi.org/10.1007/s00381-010-1347-z. Epub 2010 Dec 7. PMID: 2113606
34. Protzenko T, Bellas A, Ribeiro CMC, Gonzalez SMC, Horovitz DDG. Venous anomalies in hypoplastic posterior fossa: unsolved questions. Childs Nerv Syst. 2021;37(10):3177–87. https://doi.org/10.1007/s00381-021-05315-4. Epub 2021 Aug 18
35. Coll G, El Ouadih Y, Abed Rabbo F, Jecko V, Sakka L, Di Rocco F. Hydrocephalus and Chiari malformation pathophysiology in FGFR2-related faciocraniosynostosis: a review. Neurochirurgie. 2019;65(5):264–8. https://doi.org/10.1016/j.neuchi.2019.09.001. Epub 2019 Sep 13
36. Coll G, Lemaire JJ, Di Rocco F, Barthélémy I, Garcier JM, De Schlichting E, Sakka L. Human foramen magnum area and posterior cranial fossa volume growth in relation to cranial base synchondrosis closure in the course of child development. Neurosurgery. 2016;79(5):722–35. https://doi.org/10.1227/NEU.0000000000001309. PMID: 273
37. Assadsangabi R, Hajmomenian M, Bilaniuk LT, Vossough A. Morphology of the foramen magnum in syndromic and non-syndromic brachycephaly. Childs Nerv Syst. 2015;31(5):735–41. https://doi.org/10.1007/s00381-015-2639-0. Epub 2015 Feb 17
38. Martínez-Lage JF, Alamo L, Poza M. Raised intracranial pressure in minimal forms of craniosynostosis. Childs Nerv Syst. 1999;15(1):11–5; discussion 16. https://doi.org/10.1007/s003810050319. PMID: 10066015.
39. Inagaki T, Kyutoku S, Seno T, Kawaguchi T, Yamahara T, Oshige H, Yamanouchi Y, Kawamoto K. The intracranial pressure of the patients with mild form of craniosynostosis. Childs Nerv Syst. 2007;23(12):1455–9. https://doi.org/10.1007/s00381-007-0436-0. Epub 2007 Aug 7. PMID: 17680250 DOI: 10.1007/s00381-007-0436-0
40. Thomas GP, Johnson D, Byren JC, Judge AD, Jayamohan J, Magdum SA, Richards PG, Wall SA. The incidence of raised intracranial pressure in nonsyndromic sagittal craniosynostosis following primary surgery. J Neurosurg Pediatr. 2015;15(4):350–60. https://doi.org/10.3171/2014.11.PEDS1426. Epub 2015 Jan 10. PMID: 25559921
41. Moore MH, Chaisrisawadisuk S, Prasad V, Santoreneos S, Molloy CJ. Secondary raised Intracranial pressure after cranial vault remodeling for isolated sagittal craniosynostosis. J Craniofac Surg. 2021,32(8):2651–5. https://doi.org/10.1097/SCS.0000000000007886. PMID: 34238873
42. Hanieh A, Sheen R, David DJ. hydrocephalus in Crouzon's syndrome. Childs Nerv Syst. 1989;5(3):188–9.
43. Golabi M, Edwards MS, Ousterhout DK. Craniosynostosis and hydrocephalus. Neurosurgery. 1987;21:63–7.
44. Grant J, Jagadeesan J, Gallo P, Rodrigues D. Evaluation and management of patients with hydrocephalus in craniosynostosis. Neurol India. 2021;69(Suppl S2):357–61.
45. Noetzel MJ, Marsh JL, Palkes H, Gado M. Hydrocephalus and mental retardation in craniosynostosis. J Pediatr. 1985;107:885–92.
46. Rieping A. Zur Pathogenese des Turmschädels. Deutsche Zeitschrift für Chirurgie. 1919;148:1–51.
47. Günther H. The turricephaly as constitutional anomaly and as a clinical symptom. Ergebnisse of Internal Medicine and Pediatrics. 1931:40–135.
48. Gross H. Relationship between the brain and meninges in turricephalic craniostenotic dysostoses. Virchows Arch Pathol Anat Physiol Clin Med. 1957;330:365–83.
49. Hoffman HJ, Hendrick EB. Early neurosurgical repair in craniofacial dysmorphism. Neurovascular surgery. Berlin, Heidelberg: Springer; 1979. p. 117–24.
50. Sainte-Rose C, LaCombe J, Pierre-Kahn A, Renier D, Hirsch JF. Intracranial venous sinus hypertension: cause or consequence of hydrocephalus in infants? J Neurosurg. 1984;60:727–36.
51. Di Rocco C, Frassanito P, Massimi L, Peraio S. Hydrocephalus and Chiari type I malformation. Childs Nerv Syst. 2011;27(10):1653–64. https://doi.org/10.1007/s00381-011-1545-3. Epub 2011 Sep 17

52. Coll G, Arnaud E, Selek L, Brunelle F, Sainte-Rose C, Collet C, Di Rocco F. The growth of the foramen magnum in Crouzon syndrome. Childs Nerv Syst. 2012;28(9):1525–35. https://doi.org/10.1007/s00381-012-1805-x. Epub 2012 Aug 8
53. Coll G, Arnaud E, Colle C, Brunelle F, Sainte-Rose C, Di Rocco F. Skull base morphology in fibroblast growth factor receptor type 2-related faciocraniosynostosis: a descriptive analysis. Neurosurgery. 2015;76(5):571–83.; discussion 583. https://doi.org/10.1227/NEU.0000000000000676.
54. Di Rocco F, Dubravova D, Ziyadeh J, Sainte-Rose C, Collet C, Arnaud E. The foramen magnum in isolated and syndromic brachycephaly. Childs Nerv Syst. 2014;30(1):165–72. https://doi.org/10.1007/s00381-013-2245-y. Epub 2013 Oct 18. PMID: 24136083
55. Di Rocco F, Jucá CE, Arnaud E, Renier D, Sainte-Rose C. The role of endoscopic third ventriculostomy in the treatment of hydrocephalus associated with faciocraniosynostosis. J Neurosurg Pediatr. 2010;6:17–22.
56. Mohanty A, Suman R, Shankar SR, Satish S, Praharaj SS. Endoscopic third ventriculostomy in the management of Chiari I malformation and syringomyelia associated with hydrocephalus. Clin Neurol Neurosurg. 2005;108(1):87–92. https://doi.org/10.1016/j.clineuro.2004.11.017. Epub 2005 Jan 12
57. Massimi L, Pravatà E, Tamburrini G, Gaudino S, Pettorini B, Novegno F, Colosimo C Jr, Di Rocco C. Endoscopic third ventriculostomy for the management of Chiari I and related hydrocephalus: outcome and pathogenetic implications. Neurosurgery. 2011;68(4):950–6. https://doi.org/10.1227/NEU.0b013e318208f1f3. PMID: 21221038
58. Massimi L, Pennisi G, Frassanito P, Tamburrini G, Di Rocco C, Caldarelli M. Chiari type I and hydrocephalus. Childs Nerv Syst. 2019;35(10):1701–9. https://doi.org/10.1007/s00381-019-04245-6. Epub 2019 Jun 21. PMID: 31227858 Review
59. Konar S, Shukla D. Bilateral lambdoid and sagittal craniosynostosis with hydrocephalus: ETV, bifrontal craniotomy, anterior cranial vault remodeling, and posterior cranial vault expansion. Neurol India. 2021;69(3):592–4. https://doi.org/10.4103/0028-3886.319204.
60. Sgulò FG, Spennato P, Aliberti F, Di Martino G, Cascone D, Cinalli G. Contemporary occurrence of hydrocephalus and Chiari I malformation in sagittal craniosynostosis. Case report and review of the literature. Childs Nerv Syst. 2017;33(1):187–92. https://doi.org/10.1007/s00381-016-3189-9. Epub 2016 Jul 22. PMID: 27447182.
61. Usami K, Nicolini F, Arnaud E, Di Rocco F. Cerebrospinal fluid collections in sagittal suture synostosis. Childs Nerv Syst. 2016;32(3):519–25. https://doi.org/10.1007/s00381-015-3011-0. Epub 2016 Jan 15
62. Nicolini F, Arnaud E, Usami K, Vecchione A, Brunelle F, Di Rocco F. Impact of extra-axial cerebrospinal fluid collection in frontal morphology after surgical treatment of scaphocephaly. Surg Neurol Int. 2018;9:215. https://doi.org/10.4103/sni.sni_13_18.

16 Craniocerebral Disproportion, Cerebral Perfusion, and Raised Intracranial Pressure in Craniosynostosis

Jeffrey Nadel and John R. W. Kestle

The timing of intervention in a child with premature fusion of the cranial sutures has long been debated. In part, this debate centers around how craniosynostosis affects brain development and, specifically, whether increased intracranial pressure (ICP) from premature bony fusion is causally related to worse cognitive outcomes. This chapter will discuss the data surrounding craniocerebral disproportion, its effect on cerebral perfusion and ICP, and clinical and cognitive outcomes in children with single-suture, multisuture, and syndromic craniosynostosis.

Not surprisingly, the relationship between premature fusion of the cranial sutures and ICP has long been of concern to neurosurgeons. Indeed, historically, one of the primary drivers of intervention in craniosynostosis has been to avoid secondary brain injury from chronic elevations in ICP. Before reviewing the data on raised ICP in craniosynostosis, it is worth discussing the definition of raised ICP in childhood.

J. Nadel · J. R. W. Kestle (✉)
Department of Neurosurgery, University of Utah, Salt Lake City, UT, USA
e-mail: neuropub@hsc.utah.edu

16.1 Establishing Normative Values

There is a paucity of normative data on ICP in childhood. Because of significant physiologic variation, age-related changes, changes in pressure due to sedation at the time of measurement, and the effects of body mass index and position on ICP, the definition of a normal ICP in childhood has been elusive [1]. Directly measuring ICP in pediatric patients without an intracranial pathology necessitating its measurement (e.g., traumatic brain injury) is challenging. Therefore, medical professionals have largely relied on using lumbar puncture opening pressure in the lateral decubitus position as a surrogate for ICP. In 2010, Avery et al. [2] reported the results of a large, single-center prospective study of children receiving a lumbar puncture as part of their routine clinical care. The purpose of the study was to develop a reference range for normalcy of lumbar puncture opening pressure in children. Abnormally elevated or reduced values were defined a priori as those in the 90th percentile or higher or 10th percentile or lower, respectively. Abnormally elevated opening pressures were determined to be those >28 cm H_2O and abnormally reduced opening pressures were those <11.5 cm H_2O. Statistically significant factors impacting the value of the opening pressure were sedation administered for the procedure and body

F. Di Rocco, J. Kestle (eds.), *Neurosurgical Aspects of Craniosynostosis*, https://doi.org/10.1007/978-3-031-69386-1_16

mass index. Opening pressure was not found to significantly vary across age.

In recent years, several studies have called into question the validity of lumbar puncture opening pressure as a true representation of ICP because of the aforementioned factors [1, 3]. In fact, one study that measured ICP via a bolted intracranial ICP monitor and compared it with lumbar puncture opening pressure performed during the same hospital admission found that lumbar puncture opening pressure significantly overestimated the true ICP value [3]. One historical report argued that normal ICP was approximately 2 mmHg in neonates, 5 mmHg in infants, 6–13 mmHg in children up to 7 years, and less than 20 mmHg in older children and adults [4]. Indeed, understanding how ICP changes across childhood remains a topic of ongoing debate, and true normative data have not been clearly established. Below, we discuss the literature on ICP measurement in patients with craniosynostosis and how the commonly accepted ICP thresholds in children with craniosynostosis were determined.

16.2 Historical Investigations of Raised ICP in Craniosynostosis

The first comprehensive evaluation of ICP in patients with craniosynostosis was performed by Renier et al. [5] in 1982. In a seminal study, they examined 92 cases of craniosynostosis—both single-suture and multisuture—with preoperative and postoperative epidural ICP monitoring. They defined ICP >15 mmHg as elevated, 10–15 mmHg as borderline, and ICP <10 mmHg as normal. On the basis of these criteria, they concluded that preoperative ICP was elevated in approximately one-third of patients, borderline in one-third, and normal in the final third. ICP spikes were frequently observed during REM sleep, and there was a direct, positive relationship between the number of sutures involved and elevation in preoperative ICP. In those patients with preoperative elevated and borderline ICP, ICP progressively returned to normal within weeks after surgery. Notably, in a post hoc analysis, an examination of ICP as a function of age demonstrated that ICP peaked at age 6 years in this population and decreased with increasing age. This work served as the foundation for evaluating ICP in children with craniosynostosis. It is worth noting, however, that not all craniofacial groups adopted this threshold of abnormal ICP values. Instead, it became common to consider elevated ICP as >20 mmHg, borderline ICP as 15–20 mmHg, and normal ICP as <15 mmHg based on values adopted from the traumatic brain injury literature.

Over the next decade, the focus of further research efforts was understanding how craniosynostosis of different etiologies and among distinct patient groups affected ICP. Using subdural ICP monitoring, it was determined that raised ICP was more common in those with syndromic and multisuture craniosynostosis than in those with nonsyndromic and single-suture craniosynostosis [6, 7]. This finding makes intuitive sense. Those with multiple fused sutures have less ability to accommodate brain tissue expansion throughout childhood development. Furthermore, patients with syndromic craniosynostosis generally have multiple fused sutures, worse clinical deformity, and additional pathologies that may predispose them to have increased ICP.

Interestingly, regarding the effect of age on ICP in craniosynostosis, additional studies confirmed the positive relationship between age and ICP that Renier et al. [5] originally described. When fused sutures were discovered later in childhood—even in the setting of single-suture synostosis—it was common for patients to have preoperative elevated ICPs when measured using a ventriculostomy catheter [8]. One reason that patients may come to surgical attention later in childhood is mild or minimal clinical deformity from their synostosis. Nearly 44% of patients older than 12 months with sagittal synostosis but mild or no clinical scaphocephaly had elevated ICPs in the preoperative setting [9]. As such, one cannot assume that a patient with only mild clinical deformity will not have elevated ICP.

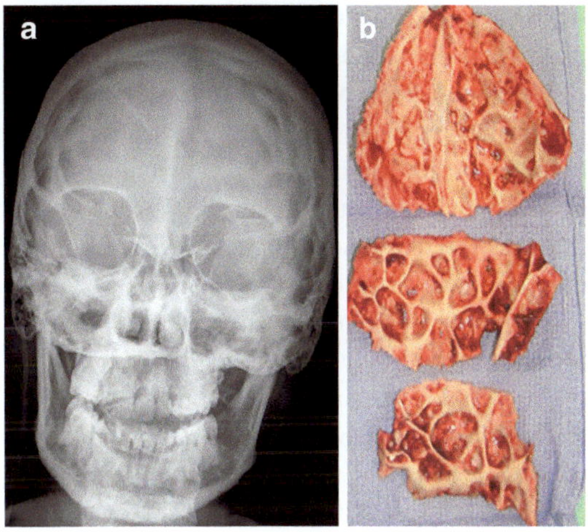

Fig. 16.1 (**a**) Plain radiograph demonstrating the "copper beaten skull" appearance of chronically elevated intracranial pressure. (**b**) Intraoperative photograph demonstrating the anatomic correlation to a radiographic "copper beaten skull," with chronic bony remodeling of the calvaria in response to elevated intracranial pressure

From a radiographic perspective, chronically elevated ICP can lead to the appearance of a "copper beaten skull" [10–13]. This is often seen in the setting of long-standing congenital hydrocephalus but is clearly pertinent in patients with untreated craniosynostosis as well. Specifically, a copper beaten skull is one in which the calvaria has a scalloped appearance on skull X-ray or computed tomography scan, with multiple convolutions and involutions (Fig. 16.1a). It is hypothesized that chronically increased intracranial tension can induce bony remodeling of the calvaria (Fig. 16.1b). The discovery of a copper beaten skull on imaging warrants further investigation into possible causative factors for elevated ICP.

In summary, most pediatric craniofacial surgeons and neurosurgeons today consider an abnormally elevated ICP to be greater than 15–20 mmHg. It is widely accepted that untreated craniosynostosis is associated with elevated ICP, and this relationship strengthens with increasing age. Syndromic and multisuture craniosynostosis are risk factors for elevated preoperative ICP, although even patients with single-suture synostosis and mild or no clinical deformity may have elevated preoperative ICP.

16.3 Etiology of Raised ICP in Craniosynostosis

The cause of elevated ICP in craniosynostosis is complex and multifactorial. As discussed above, restricted skull volume with resulting craniocerebral disproportion is one element that leads to raised ICP, although it is clearly not the only responsible cause [5, 7, 14–16]. Additional factors discussed below include hindbrain herniation through the foramen magnum [17–19], intracranial venous congestion causing venous hypertension or other venous anomalies [14, 17, 20–27], hydrocephalus [28–34], and airway obstruction [26, 35–46]. Each of these factors likely influences the others and, in combination, leads to issues with raised ICP. Further, the majority of these factors are present in syndromic and multisuture craniosynostosis and are therefore part of the reason that these conditions have a higher incidence of raised ICP when compared with nonsyndromic and single-suture synostosis.

Posterior fossa hypoplasia is a common finding in patients with complex craniosynostosis because of skull base developmental abnormalities. The small posterior fossa volume in these patients can lead to higher rates of tonsillar herniation through the foramen magnum and other hindbrain compression syndromes. The literature on Chiari malformation has shown that crowding at the craniocervical junction alters cerebrospinal fluid (CSF) flow dynamics, decreases CSF drainage, and reduces venous outflow from the cranial vault [47–52]. The consequence of this type of mechanical obstruction is elevated ICP. Additionally, because of direct compression onto the adjacent brainstem, tonsillar herniation may lead to central respiratory insufficiency with hypoventilation and CO_2 retention, thereby also leading to an elevation in ICP [17–19].

Intracranial venous congestion leading to venous hypertension is another leading cause of elevated ICP in the setting of complex craniosynostosis. Physiologically, in accordance with the Monro-Kellie doctrine, impaired venous drainage from the cranial vault results in a backup of blood that cannot escape the calvaria. Unless a concomitant decrease in CSF volume or brain tissue is achieved, ICP will rise. In patients with craniosynostosis, the most common reasons that patients might have reduced cerebral venous outflow are congenitally anomalous venous drainage pathways and inborn stenosis of anatomically normal venous outflow channels that worsen with premature fusion of the cranial sutures. Interestingly, several studies have suggested that anomalous venous vasculature in complex craniosynostosis is common. Especially in syndromic craniosynostosis, there are disproportionately elevated rates of patients with angiographically demonstrated venous sinus malformations, stenotic transverse-sigmoid or sigmoid-jugular junctions, large intraosseous draining veins, and intracranial–extracranial venous drainage anomalies such as sinus pericranii (Fig. 16.2) [14, 17, 20–27]. Without normal channels for venous drainage, venous hypertension is common and develops quickly in these patients. This has consequences both for preoperative ICP management as well as for intraoperative planning so as not to inadvertently occlude a primary venous outflow tract causing rapid-onset venous hypertension and ICP crisis [27].

The development of hydrocephalus in craniosynostosis, as in hydrocephalus from other causes, may be due to problems in CSF outflow or CSF malabsorption. As discussed previously, patients with craniosynostosis have craniocerebral disproportion. With brain tissue in excess of what the hypoplastic posterior fossa can accommodate, mechanical obstruction of CSF outflow can result in obstructive hydrocephalus. This is primarily due to osseous constriction. In contrast to CSF outflow obstruction, patients may also develop hydrocephalus from CSF malabsorption. We have previously discussed that venous hypertension is common in patients with craniosynostosis. Venous hypertension creates increased intravascular resistance to the absorption of CSF at arachnoid granulations and can thus impair CSF reabsorption into the systemic venous circulation [28–34]. This may also lead to the development of hydrocephalus. Importantly, some patients with complex craniosynostosis may not have progressive hydrocephalus but instead demonstrate nonprogressive ventriculomegaly from abnormal brain development or the involution of normal brain parenchyma during disordered development [32]. Progressive hydrocephalus requires treatment with either ventricular shunting or endoscopic third ventriculostomy [30], whereas nonprogressive ventriculomegaly may not require CSF diversion. Hydrocephalus in either form, however, can drive elevated ICP in these patients.

Finally, upper airway obstruction is a common finding in patients with complex craniosynostosis. Especially in syndromic children, midface hypoplasia and other congenital anomalies in the formation of caudal face and neck structures can lead to issues with mechanical airway obstruction. Whether while the patient is awake or asleep—such as in the setting of obstructive sleep apnea, airway obstruction leads to an elevation in ICP from mechanical hypoventilation [26, 35–46]. On a physiologic level, with poor respiratory ventilation, the body retains carbon dioxide. Carbon dioxide is a vasodilatory substance, thus increasing the volume of blood in the intracranial compartment. With increased intracranial blood volume, the body must reflexively decrease

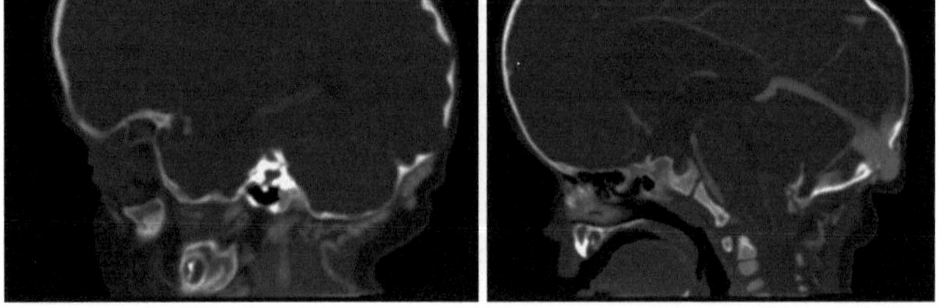

Fig. 16.2 CT venogram in a child with Crouzon syndrome and multisuture synostosis demonstrating (**a**) prominent extracranial venous drainage and (**b**) protruding torcula

intracranial CSF or brain parenchyma to maintain a normal ICP. As reviewed, most patients with craniosynostosis already have a decreased ability to dynamically control CSF flow. Therefore, because of this decreased reserve, obstructive hypoventilation often leads to increased ICP in patients with craniosynostosis. It is worth noting that in sleep studies of patients with craniosynostosis, ICP often peaked during periods of active sleep [53]. Active sleep, compared with passive sleep, is associated with periods of respiratory compromise due to paralysis of the tongue and pharyngeal musculature. Thus, in patients predisposed to have obstructive apnea, active sleep can lead to worsening of their apnea with concomitant increases in measured ICP.

16.4 Clinical Impact of Craniocerebral Disproportion

From the perspective of a practicing clinician, craniocerebral disproportion may significantly impact child development and impede normal central nervous system (CNS) maturation. In normal childhood development, a delayed fusion of the cranial sutures allows for progressive CNS maturation and brain growth without osseous constraint. Premature fusion may disrupt brain perfusion and neuronal plasticity via mechanical compressive forces, thereby impeding normal brain growth, hindering the formation of appropriate neural networks, and negatively affecting a child's special senses (Fig. 16.3).

It is widely accepted that craniosynostosis can negatively affect ophthalmic outcomes and, in some cases, result in devastating loss of vision [54]. The visual system is arguably the part of the CNS most affected in craniosynostosis, whether as a direct result of the premature fusion itself or as a secondary effect of it. As discussed, elevated ICP is common in single-suture and multisuture synostosis. Both acute and chronic elevations in ICP are known to lead to optic disc edema (Fig. 16.4). If persistent, this can eventually result in atrophy of the optic apparatus and worsening

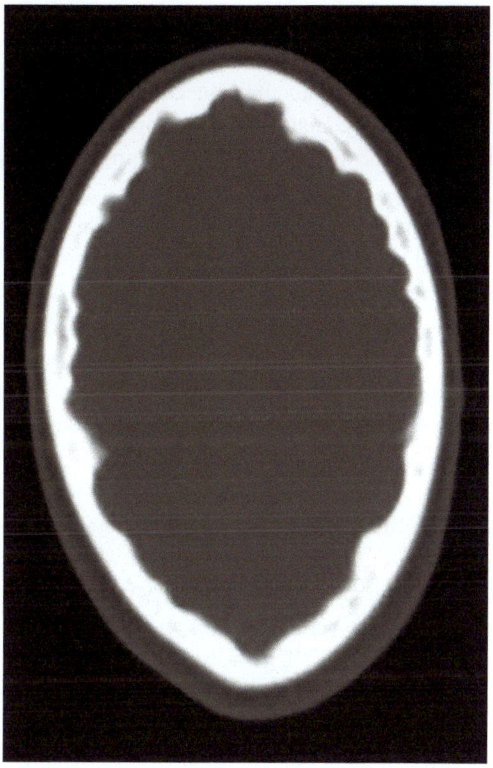

Fig. 16.3 Constrained brain growth due to calvarial restriction from premature fusion of sutures

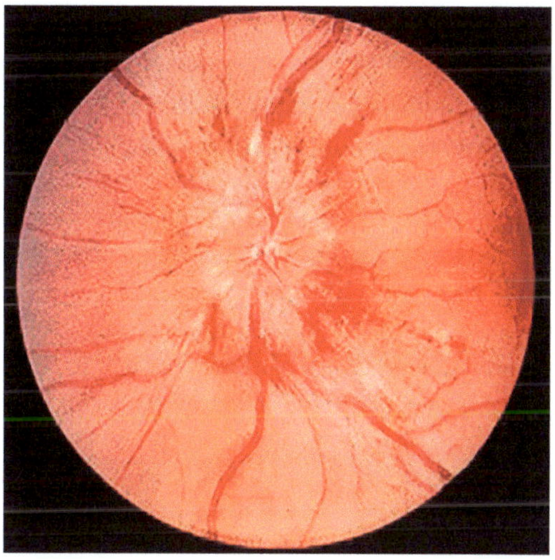

Fig. 16.4 Retinal photograph demonstrating papilledema and optic nerve edema in response to chronically elevated intracranial pressure

visual dysfunction over time. Further, extraocular ophthalmic issues may arise in craniosynostosis. These include extraocular muscle entrapment by abnormal bony maturation, strabismus, ptosis, proptosis, and resultant corneal exposure issues [54–56]. Initial consultation with ophthalmology and, in many cases, long-term surveillance are essential to prevent permanent loss of vision and enable early intervention for treatable visual sequelae.

As previously mentioned, airway obstruction is a common finding in craniosynostosis. This may lead to significant sleep disturbance and disrupted sleep architecture due to obstructive sleep apneas or central hypoventilation [38, 46]. The chronic effects of poor sleep and sleep deprivation are out of the scope of this review; however, it has been demonstrated that respiratory compromise during active sleep in children with craniosynostosis can result in transiently decreased cerebral perfusion [53]. Over time, the cumulative effects of such decreased perfusion may contribute to the ophthalmic and psychomotor disability seen in this disease.

A discussion of clinically relevant aspects of craniosynostosis would be incomplete without considering how craniosynostosis impacts cerebral perfusion. Premature skull vault maturation can not only lead to elevated ICP but also affects brain perfusion. Indeed, this hypothesis led investigators in the mid-1990s to study local and global cerebral perfusion in patients with craniosynostosis as a means to fully understand the physiologic impact of the disease. At the time, these studies were performed using positron emission tomography and single-photon emission computed tomography and aimed to examine cerebral perfusion and cerebral metabolism. Unsurprisingly, it was determined that brain perfusion under a fused suture is hypoperfused relative to adjacent brain tissue because of mechanical compressive forces [9, 23, 53, 57–61]. Importantly, this perfusion deficit is seen along the spectrum of disease severity. Specifically, local hypoperfusion is seen in both nonsyndromic, single-suture craniosynostosis and syndromic, multisuture synostosis. Thus, mild cases of single-suture synostosis cannot be presumed to be completely benign. Surgical intervention for craniosynostosis was also successful in relieving this perfusion deficit in many cases.

The long-term effects of a chronic cerebral perfusion deficit in children are unclear. Adequate cerebral perfusion is essential for proper brain development, early neural plasticity, and formation of neural networks [62–66]. Research on adult traumatic brain injury has shown that a persistent perfusion deficit, even in the absence of frank ischemia, can lead to poor cerebral reserve, compromised neurologic recovery, and worse neurologic and neuropsychologic outcomes [67, 68]. It would not be surprising that failure to relieve a perfusion deficit may have negative effects on overall neurologic development and outcome. Thus, in addition to relief of elevated ICP, improvement in local cerebral perfusion is another compelling argument for early surgical intervention.

16.5 Impact of Craniocerebral Disproportion on Cognitive Development

The relationship between craniocerebral disproportion and cognitive development is complex and contentious. In 1982, Renier et al. [5] first suggested that elevated preoperative ICP from craniocerebral disproportion might be related to low intellectual quotient (IQ), because they found a significant statistical relationship between the two in their seminal work. They qualified this assertion by stating that increased ICP and low IQ might be two consequences of a third variable. Since that time, there has been significant debate regarding how craniocerebral disproportion itself—i.e., the constrained skull alone—impacts neuropsychological and cognitive outcomes in patients with craniosynostosis and raised ICP.

By way of background, across the spectrum of disease, patients with craniosynostosis are at increased risk for developmental delays, lower intellectual attainment, poorer cognitive performance, and psychological and linguistic problems. The type and severity of craniosynostosis likely have a significant impact on cognitive and developmental outcomes. In many series, more than 50% of patients with syndromic, multisuture craniosynostosis score lower on metrics of infant developmental outcome preoperatively and have persistent developmental delays in childhood and poorer eventual neurocognitive outcomes when compared with their age-matched counterparts [26, 41, 69–73]. The landscape of cognitive outcomes in patients with nonsyndromic, single-suture craniosynostosis is somewhat less clear [9, 74–90]. Numerous studies have demonstrated that patients with idiopathic single-suture synostosis, even with intervention early in infancy, remain at risk for developmental delays and cognitive and learning disability during childhood and have higher rates of these issues than age-matched counterparts; however, many of the early studies were plagued by small sample sizes and nonstandardized methodologies, making it difficult to generalize the results. Recent systematic reviews and meta-analyses do suggest that children with idiopathic, single-suture synostosis warrant increased surveillance and screening for developmental delay and neuropsychological impairments because of their disproportionate likelihood of having these problems [79, 80, 86]. There is also inconclusive evidence to suggest that earlier surgery may be beneficial in preventing negative developmental outcomes in the setting of single-suture synostosis [88, 89].

The cause of cognitive and neuropsychological impairments in craniosynostosis is widely debated. It should be stated that there is no controversy about whether patients with craniosynostosis have craniocerebral disproportion with frequently elevated ICP, locally compromised cerebral perfusion, and concomitant poor cognitive and neuropsychological outcomes. Rather, the debate centers on whether there is a causal relationship between restricted skull volume and neurocognitive impairment. In a controversial 2014 editorial, Hayward and colleagues argued that the data directly linking restricted skull volume/high ICP with neurocognitive impairments are sparse [91]. Historically, the rationale for surgically expanding the cranial vault centered on relieving elevated ICP and thereby preventing the secondary brain injury that causes neurocognitive impairments. Although this is a rational assumption, Hayward et al. asserted that the data only partly support this claim and that what data exist are poor in quality. As they noted, this mattered because if there is no clear evidence linking elevated ICP and neurocognitive development, then infants may be subjected to operations that are unnecessary and carry significant risk.

Although restricted skull volume and craniocerebral disproportion are factors, other variables may also affect neurocognitive development in patients with craniosynostosis. Whether these variables mediate or simply contribute to the relationship among craniocerebral disproportion, elevated ICP, and cognitive impairment remains unclear. In syndromic craniosynostosis, one such factor is the genetic cause of the disease. In addition to the dysmorphic craniofacial anatomy, genetic alterations in the disease process may directly affect neuronal development, capacity for neuronal plasticity, development of neural networks, and the function of neurons on a cellular level [26, 69–71, 84, 91]. As such, it is feasible that neurocognitive impairments in syndromic patients may be inborn and at least in part a result of abnormal cellular brain development. Additional variables, some of which have been discussed previously at length, include coexistent hydrocephalus; chronic respiratory obstruction and insufficient oxygenation during sleep and wakefulness; feeding difficulties from midface hypoplasia leading to failure to thrive; a lack of stimulation from impaired vision or hearing that results in delayed cognitive development; the ill-effects of surgical intervention in infancy including exposure to prolonged anesthesia; and low familial and societal expectations due to the craniofacial deformity that lead to fewer enriching opportunities in early childhood [29–34, 37, 38, 43, 45, 46, 53, 91–102].

In reality, it is likely that the cause of cognitive impairment in children with craniosynostosis is multifactorial and quite individualized. For the practicing craniofacial surgeon, it is important to understand that this topic is nuanced and that appropriate preoperative counseling with parents should include a discussion about the downstream development of potential neurocognitive abnormalities, even in the setting of early surgical intervention.

16.6 Conclusion

In summary, many children with craniosynostosis will present with elevated preoperative ICP by any definition of ICP thresholds. Craniocerebral disproportion with restricted skull volume is a driving force for elevated ICP, although other factors that may lead to high ICP in this group of patients include posterior fossa hypoplasia and hindbrain herniation through the foramen magnum; anomalous intracranial venous drainage, venous congestion, and venous hypertension; hydrocephalus; and chronic airway obstruction. Clinically, craniocerebral disproportion can manifest in ophthalmic compromise, local hypoperfusion of the brain beneath the affected suture(s), and neurocognitive impairment. There is no clear, causative link between neurocognitive impairment in these patients and restricted skull volume. Rather, neurocognitive impairment in craniosynostosis is multifactorial and may be related to craniocerebral disproportion/elevated ICP, abnormal cellular brain development due to genetic or chromosomal anomalies, hydrocephalus, chronic respiratory insufficiency, failure to thrive, poor cognitive stimulation in development due to impairment of the CNS special senses, exposure to surgical intervention in early infancy, and low societal expectations leading to a paucity of enriching opportunities during development. Further research is warranted to better understand these relationships, as they may influence the timing and extent of surgery.

References

1. Avery RA. Interpretation of lumbar puncture opening pressure measurements in children. J Neuroophthalmol. 2014;34(3):284–7.
2. Avery RA, Shah SS, Licht DJ, Seiden JA, Huh JW, Boswinkel J, et al. Reference range for cerebrospinal fluid opening pressure in children. N Engl J Med. 2010;363:891–3.
3. Cartwright C, Igbaseimokumo U. Lumbar puncture opening pressure is not a reliable measure of intracranial pressure in children. J Child Neurol. 2015;30(2):170–3.
4. Minns RA. Intracranial pressure monitoring. Arch Dis Child. 1984;59(5):486–8.
5. Renier D, Sainte-Rose C, Marchac D, Hirsch JF. Intracranial pressure in craniostenosis. J Neurosurg. 1982;57(3):370–7.
6. Thompson DNP, Malcolm GP, Jones BM, Harkness WJ, Hayward RD. Intracranial pressure in single-suture craniosynostosis. Pediatr Neurosurg. 1995;22(5):235–40.
7. Thompson DNP, Harkness W, Jones B, Gonsalez S, Andar U, Hayward R. Subdural intracranial pressure monitoring in craniosynostosis: its role in surgical management. Childs Nerv Syst. 1995;11(5):269–75.
8. Seruya M, Oh AK, Boyajian MJ, Posnick JC, Keating RF. Treatment for delayed presentation of sagittal synostosis: challenges pertaining to occult intracranial hypertension: clinical article. J Neurosurg Pediatr. 2011;8(1):40–8.
9. Wall SA, Thomas GPL, Johnson D, Byren JC, Jayamohan J, Magdum SA, et al. The preoperative incidence of raised intracranial pressure in nonsyndromic sagittal craniosynostosis is underestimated in the literature: clinical article. J Neurosurg Pediatr. 2014;14(6):674–81.
10. Bogdanović M, Radnić B, Savić S, Popović V, Durmić T. Copper-beaten skull appearance as a response of chronically increased intracranial pressure. Am J Forensic Med Pathol. 2019;40(1):58–60.
11. Ittyachen AM, Anand R. Copper beaten skull. BMJ Case Rep. 2019;12(8):e230916.
12. van der Meulen J, van der Vlugt J, Okkerse J, Hofman B. Early beaten-copper pattern: its long-term effect on intelligence quotients in 95 children with craniosynostosis. J Neurosurg Pediatr. 2008;1(1):25–30.
13. Poonia A, Giridhara P, Sheoran D. Copper beaten skull. J Pediatr. 2019;206:297–297.e1.
14. Bristol RE, Lekovic GP, Rekate HL. The effects of craniosynostosis on the brain with respect to intracranial pressure. Semin Pediatr Neurol. 2004;11(4):262–7.
15. Gault DT, Renier D, Marchac D, Jones BM. Intracranial pressure and intracranial volume in children with craniosynostosis. Plast Reconstr Surg. 1992;90(3):377–81.
16. Langvatn EA, Frič R, Due-Tønnessen BJ, Eide PK. Intracranial volume versus static and pulsatile intracranial pressure values in children with craniosynostosis. J Neurosurg Pediatr. 2019;24(1):66–74.
17. Francis PM, Beals S, Rekate HL, Pittman HW, Manwaring K, Reiff J. Chronic tonsillar herniation and Crouzon's syndrome. Pediatr Neurosurg. 1992;18(4):202–6.
18. Hayward R, Harkness W, Kendall B, Jones B. Magnetic resonance imaging in the assessment of craniosynostosis. Scand J Plast Reconstr Surg Hand Surg. 1992;26(3):293–9.
19. den Ottelander BK, Dremmen MHG, de Planque CA, van der Oest MJW, Mathijssen IMJ, van Veelen MLC. Does the association between abnormal anatomy of the skull base and cerebellar tonsillar position also exist in syndromic craniosynostosis? J Plast Reconstr Aesthetic Surg. 2021;75:797.

20. Bento RA, Rodrigues D, Levy J, Eça T, Oliveira V, Luís L. Bilateral severely stenotic jugular foramen: diagnosis and management from the otologist/neurotologist point of view. Case Rep Otolaryngol. 2020;2020:1530310.
21. Sainte-Rose C, LaCombe J, Pierre-Kahn A, Renier D, Hirsch JF. Intracranial venous sinus hypertension: cause or consequence of hydrocephalus in infants? J Neurosurg. 1984;60(4):727–36.
22. Protzenko T, Bellas A, Ribeiro CMC, Gonzalez SMC, Horovitz DDG. Venous anomalies in hypoplastic posterior fossa: unsolved questions. Childs Nerv Syst. 2021;37(10):3177–87.
23. Doerga PN, Lequin MH, Dremmen MHG, den Ottelander BK, Mauff KAL, Wagner MW, et al. Cerebral blood flow in children with syndromic craniosynostosis: cohort arterial spin labeling studies. J Neurosurg Pediatr. 2019;25(4):340–50.
24. Cornelissen MJ, de Goederen R, Doerga P, Cuperus I, van Veelen ML, Lequin M, et al. Pilot study of intracranial venous physiology in craniosynostosis. J Neurosurg Pediatr. 2018;21(6):626–31.
25. Copeland AE, Hoffman CE, Tsitouras V, Jeevan DS, Ho ES, Drake JM, et al. Clinical significance of venous anomalies in syndromic craniosynostosis. Plast Reconstr Surg Glob Open. 2018;6(1):e1613.
26. Sakamoto H, Matsusaka Y, Kunihiro N, Imai K. Physiological changes and clinical implications of syndromic craniosynostosis. J Korean Neurosurg Soc. 2016;59(3):204–13.
27. Taylor WJ, Hayward RD, Lasjaunias P, Britto JA, Thompson DNP, Jones BM, et al. Enigma of raised intracranial pressure in patients with complex craniosynostosis: the role of abnormal intracranial venous drainage. J Neurosurg. 2001;94(3):377–85.
28. Tcherbbis Testa V, Jaimovich S, Argañaraz R, Mantese B. Management of ventriculomegaly in pediatric patients with syndromic craniosynostosis: a single center experience. Acta Neurochir. 2021;163(11):3083–91.
29. Frassanito P, Palombi D, Tamburrini G. Craniosynostosis and hydrocephalus: relevance and treatment modalities. Childs Nerv Syst. 2021;37(11):3465–73.
30. Bonfield CM, Shannon CN, Reeder RW, Browd S, Drake J, Hauptman JS, et al. Hydrocephalus treatment in patients with craniosynostosis: an analysis from the Hydrocephalus Clinical Research Network prospective registry. Neurosurg Focus. 2021;50(4):E11.
31. Cinalli G, Sainte-Rose C, Kollar EM, Zerah M, Brunelle F, Chumas P, et al. Hydrocephalus and craniosynostosis. J Neurosurg. 1998;88(2):209–14.
32. Collmann H, Sörensen N, Krauss J. Hydrocephalus in craniosynostosis: a review. Childs Nerv Syst. 2005;21(10):902–12.
33. Golabi M, Edwards MS, Ousterhout DK. Craniosynostosis and hydrocephalus. Neurosurgery. 1987;21(1):63–7.
34. Fishman MA, Hogan GR, Dodge PR. The concurrence of hydrocephalus and craniosynostosis. J Neurosurg. 1971;34(5):621–9.
35. Couloigner V, Ayari Khalfallah S. Craniosynostosis and ENT. Neurochirurgie. 2019;65(5):318–21.
36. Mathews F, Shaffer AD, Georg MW, Ford MD, Goldstein JA, Jabbour N, et al. Airway anomalies in patients with craniosynostosis. Laryngoscope. 2019;129(11):2594–602.
37. Calandrelli R, Pilato F, Massimi L, Panfili M, D'Apolito G, Gaudino S, et al. Quantitative evaluation of facial hypoplasia and airway obstruction in infants with syndromic craniosynostosis: relationship with skull base and splanchnocranium sutural pattern. Neuroradiology. 2018;60(5):517–28.
38. Spruijt B, Mathijssen IMJ, Bredero-Boelhouwer HH, Cherian PJ, Corel LJA, van Veelen ML, et al. Sleep architecture linked to airway obstruction and intracranial hypertension in children with syndromic craniosynostosis. Plast Reconstr Surg. 2016;138(6):1019e–29e.
39. Cielo CM, Montalva FM, Taylor JA. Craniofacial disorders associated with airway obstruction in the neonate. Semin Fetal Neonatal Med. 2016;21(4):254–62.
40. Tan HL, Kheirandish-Gozal L, Abel F, Gozal D. Craniofacial syndromes and sleep-related breathing disorders. Sleep Med Rev. 2016;27:74–88.
41. Helman SN, Badhey A, Kadakia S, Myers E. Revisiting Crouzon syndrome: reviewing the background and management of a multifaceted disease. Oral Maxillofac Surg. 2014;18(4):373–9.
42. Driessen C, Joosten KFM, Florisson JMG, Lequin M, van Veelen MLC, Dammers R, et al. Sleep apnoea in syndromic craniosynostosis occurs independent of hindbrain herniation. Childs Nerv Syst. 2013;29(2):289–96.
43. Hardin KA. Syndromic craniosynostosis: complicated airway obstruction calls for progressive strategies in surgical management. Expert Rev Respir Med. 2010;4(3):315–9.
44. Tamburrini G, Caldarelli M, Massimi L, Santini P, Di Rocco C. Intracranial pressure monitoring in children with single suture and complex craniosynostosis: a review. Childs Nerv Syst. 2005;21(10):913–21.
45. Lo LJ, Chen YR. Airway obstruction in severe syndromic craniosynostosis. Ann Plast Surg. 1999;43(3):258–64.
46. Gonsalez S, Hayward R, Jones B, Lane R. Upper airway obstruction and raised intracranial pressure in children with craniosynostosis. Eur Respir J. 1997;10(2):367–75.
47. Langridge B, Phillips E, Choi D. Chiari malformation type 1: a systematic review of natural history and conservative management. World Neurosurg. 2017;104:213–9.
48. Saletti V, Farinotti M, Peretta P, Massimi L, Ciaramitaro P, Motta S, et al. The management of Chiari malformation type 1 and syringomyelia in

children: a review of the literature. Neurol Sci. 2021;42(12):4965–95.
49. Strahle J, Muraszko KM, Garton HJL, Smith BW, Starr J, Kapurch JR, et al. Syrinx location and size according to etiology: identification of Chiari-associated syrinx. J Neurosurg Pediatr. 2015;16(1):21–9.
50. Strahle J, Smith BW, Martinez M, Bapuraj JR, Muraszko KM, Garton HJL, et al. The association between Chiari malformation type I, spinal syrinx, and scoliosis. J Neurosurg Pediatr. 2015;15(6):607–11.
51. Hale AT, Adelson PD, Albert GW, Aldana PR, Alden TD, Anderson RCE, et al. Factors associated with syrinx size in pediatric patients treated for Chiari malformation type I and syringomyelia: a study from the Park-Reeves Syringomyelia Research Consortium. J Neurosurg Pediatr. 2020;25(6):629–39.
52. Yilmaz TF, Toprak H, Sari L, Oz II, Kitis S, Kaya A, et al. Chiari type 1 malformation: CSF flow dynamics and morphology in the posterior fossa and craniocervical junction and correlation of these findings with syrinx formation. Neurochirurgie. 2022;68:595.
53. Hayward R, Gonsalez S. How low can you go? Intracranial pressure, cerebral perfusion pressure, and respiratory obstruction in children with complex craniosynostosis. J Neurosurg Pediatr. 2005;102(1):16–22.
54. Newman SA. Ophthalmic features of craniosynostosis. Neurosurg Clin N Am. 1991;2(3):587–610.
55. Kajdic N, Spazzapan P, Velnar T. Craniosynostosis—recognition, clinical characteristics, and treatment. Bosn J Basic Med Sci. 2018;18(2):110–6.
56. Ganesh A, Edmond J, Forbes B, Katowitz WR, Nischal KK, Miller M, et al. An update of ophthalmic management in craniosynostosis. J AAPOS. 2019;23(2):66–76.
57. Martini M, Röhrig A, Wenghoefer M, Schindler E, Messing-Jünger AM. Cerebral oxygenation and hemodynamic measurements during craniosynostosis surgery with near-infrared spectroscopy. Childs Nerv Syst. 2014;30(8):1367–74.
58. David LR, Wilson JA, Watson NE, Argenta LC. Cerebral perfusion defects secondary to simple craniosynostosis. J Craniofac Surg. 1996;7(3):177–85.
59. Satoh M, Ishikawa N, Enomoto T, Takeda T, Yoshizawa T, Nose T. Study by I-123-IMP-SPECT before and after surgery for craniosynostosis. Kaku Igaku. 1990;27(12):1411–8.
60. Barik M, Bajpai M, Das RR, Malhotra A, Panda SS, Sahoo MK, et al. Role of 99mTc-ECD SPECT in the management of children with craniosynostosis. Biomed Res Int. 2014;2014:172646.
61. Sen A, Dougal P, Padhy AK, Bhattacharya A, Kumar R, Bal C, et al. Technetium-99m-HMPAO SPECT cerebral blood flow study in children with craniosynostosis. J Nucl Med. 1995;36(3):394–8.
62. Milona E, Rallis D, Mitsiakos G, Goutsiou E, Hatziioannidis E, Tsakalidis C, et al. Evaluation of cerebral oxygenation and perfusion in small for gestational age neonates and neurodevelopmental outcome at 24–36 months of age. J Perinat Med. 2020;48(3):280–8.
63. Yadav BK, Hernandez-Andrade E, Krishnamurthy U, Buch S, Jella P, Trifan A, et al. Dual-imaging modality approach to evaluate cerebral hemodynamics in growth-restricted fetuses: oxygenation and perfusion. Fetal Diagn Ther. 2020;47(2):145–55.
64. Kehrer M, Krägeloh-Mann I, Goelz R, Schöning M. The development of cerebral perfusion in healthy preterm and term neonates. Neuropediatrics. 2003;34(6):281–6.
65. Paniukov D, Lebel RM, Giesbrecht G, Lebel C. Cerebral blood flow increases across early childhood. NeuroImage. 2020;204:116224.
66. Hales PW, Kawadler JM, Aylett SE, Kirkham FJ, Clark CA. Arterial spin labeling characterization of cerebral perfusion during normal maturation from late childhood into adulthood: normal "reference range" values and their use in clinical studies. J Cereb Blood Flow Metab. 2014;34(5):776–84.
67. Metting Z, Spikman JM, Rödiger LA, van der Naalt J. Cerebral perfusion and neuropsychological follow-up in mild traumatic brain injury: acute versus chronic disturbances? Brain Cogn. 2014;86:24–31.
68. Bendinelli C, Cooper S, Evans T, Bivard A, Pacey D, Parson M, et al. Perfusion abnormalities are frequently detected by early CT perfusion and predict unfavourable outcome following severe traumatic brain injury. World J Surg. 2017;41(10):2512–20.
69. Wang JC, Nagy L, Demke JC. Syndromic craniosynostosis. Facial Plast Surg Clin N Am. 2016;24(4):531–43.
70. Fernandes MBL, Maximino LP, Perosa GB, Abramides DVM, Passos-Bueno MR, Yacubian-Fernandes A. Apert and Crouzon syndromes—cognitive development, brain abnormalities, and molecular aspects. Am J Med Genet A. 2016;170(6):1532–7.
71. Kennedy-Williams P, Care H, Dalton L, Horton J, Kearney A, Rooney N, et al. Neurodevelopmental, cognitive, and psychosocial outcomes for individu als with pathogenic variants in the TCF12 gene and associated craniosynostosis. J Craniofac Surg. 2021;32(Suppl 3):1263–8.
72. Maximino LP, Ducati LG, Abramides DVM, Corrêa CC, Garcia PF, Fernandes AY. Syndromic craniosynostosis: neuropsycholinguistic abilities and imaging analysis of the central nervous system. Arq Neuropsiquiatr. 2017;75(12):862–8.
73. Renier D, Arnaud E, Cinalli G, Sebag G, Zerah M, Marchac D. Prognosis for mental function in Apert's syndrome. J Neurosurg. 1996;85(1):66–72.
74. Millichap JG. Cognitive development of children with craniosynostosis. Pediatr Neurol Briefs. 2015;29(6):47.
75. Thiele-Nygaard AE, Foss-Skiftesvik J, Juhler M. Intracranial pressure, brain morphology and cognitive outcome in children with sagittal craniosynostosis. Childs Nerv Syst. 2020;36(4):689–95.

76. Proctor MR, Meara JG. A review of the management of single-suture craniosynostosis, past, present, and future. J Neurosurg Pediatr. 2019;24(6):622–31.
77. Kljajić M, Maltese G, Tarnow P, Sand P, Kölby L. The cognitive profile of children with nonsyndromic craniosynostosis. Plast Reconstr Surg. 2019;143(5):1037e–52e.
78. Becker DB, Petersen JD, Kane AA, Cradock MM, Pilgram TK, Marsh JL. Speech, cognitive, and behavioral outcomes in nonsyndromic craniosynostosis. Plast Reconstr Surg. 2005;116(2):400–7.
79. Osborn AJ, Roberts RM, Mathias JL, Anderson PJ, Flapper WJ. Cognitive, behavioral and psychological functioning in children with metopic synostosis: a meta-analysis examining the impact of surgical status. Child Neuropsychol. 2019;25(2):263–77.
80. Knight SJ, Anderson VA, Spencer-Smith MM, Da Costa AC. Neurodevelopmental outcomes in infants and children with single-suture craniosynostosis: a systematic review. Dev Neuropsychol. 2014;39(3):159–86.
81. Kapp-Simon KA, Wallace E, Collett BR, Cradock MM, Crerand CE, Speltz ML. Language, learning, and memory in children with and without single-suture craniosynostosis. J Neurosurg Pediatr. 2016;17(5):578–88.
82. Lekovic GP, Bristol RE, Rekate HL. Cognitive impact of craniosynostosis. Semin Pediatr Neurol. 2004;11(4):305–10.
83. Mathijssen I, Arnaud E, Lajeunie E, Marchac D, Renier D. Postoperative cognitive outcome for synostotic frontal plagiocephaly. J Neurosurg Pediatr. 2006;105(1):16–20.
84. Mathijssen I, de Goederen R, Versnel SL, Joosten KFM, van Veelen MLC, Tasker RC. Letter to the Editor. Raised intracranial pressure and cognitive delay in craniosynostosis. J Neurosurg Pediatr. 2017;20(5):498–502.
85. Speltz ML, Collett BR, Wallace ER, Kapp-Simon K. Behavioral adjustment of school-age children with and without single-suture craniosynostosis. Plast Reconstr Surg. 2016;138(2):435–45.
86. Bellew M, Chumas P. Long-term developmental follow-up in children with nonsyndromic craniosynostosis. J Neurosurg Pediatr. 2015;16(4):445–51.
87. Arnaud E, Renier D, Marchac D. Prognosis for mental function in scaphocephaly. J Neurosurg. 1995;83(3):476–9.
88. Bellew M, Mandela RJ, Chumas PD. Impact of age at surgery on neurodevelopmental outcomes in sagittal synostosis. J Neurosurg Pediatr. 2019;23(4):434–41.
89. Bellew M, Liddington M, Chumas P, Russell J. Preoperative and postoperative developmental attainment in patients with sagittal synostosis: 5-year follow-up: clinical article. J Neurosurg Pediatr. 2011;7(2):121–6.
90. Kulkarni AV, Donnelly R. Editorial. Neurodevelopmental outcome and sagittal synostosis. J Neurosurg Pediatr. 2019;23(4):432–3.
91. Hayward R, Britto J, Dunaway D, Jeelani O. Connecting raised intracranial pressure and cognitive delay in craniosynostosis: many assumptions, little evidence. J Neurosurg Pediatr. 2016;18(2):242–50.
92. Pereira V, Sacher P, Ryan M, Hayward R. Dysphagia and nutrition problems in infants with apert syndrome. Cleft Palate Craniofac J. 2009;46(3):285–91.
93. Green MA, Resnick CM. Feeding considerations for infants with craniofacial malformations. Semin Fetal Neonatal Med. 2021;26(6):101280.
94. Shipster C, Hearst D, Dockrell JE, Kilby E, Hayward R. Speech and language skills and cognitive functioning in children with Apert syndrome: a pilot study. Int J Lang Commun Disord. 2002;37(3):325–43.
95. Shipster C, Hearst D, Somerville A, Stackhouse J, Hayward R, Wade A. Speech, language, and cognitive development in children with isolated sagittal synostosis. Dev Med Child Neurol. 2003;45(1):34–43.
96. Wong-Gibbons DL, Kancherla V, Romitti PA, Tyler MC, Damiano PC, Druschel CM, et al. Maternal reports of satisfaction with care and outcomes for children with craniosynostosis. J Craniofac Surg. 2009;20(1):138–42.
97. van der Vlugt JJB, van der Meulen JJNM, Creemers HE, Willemse SP, Lequin ML, Okkerse JME. The risk of psychopathology in children with craniosynostosis. Plast Reconstr Surg. 2009;124(6):2054–60.
98. Cloonan YK, Collett B, Speltz ML, Anderka M, Werler MM. Psychosocial outcomes in children with and without non-syndromic craniosynostosis: findings from two studies. Cleft Palate Craniofac J. 2013;50(4):406–13.
99. Naumann HL, Haberkern CM, Pietila KE, Birgfeld CB, Starr JR, Kapp-Simon KA, et al. Duration of exposure to cranial vault surgery: associations with neurodevelopment among children with single-suture craniosynostosis. Paediatr Anaesth. 2012;22(11):1053–61.
100. Starr JR, Kapp-Simon KA, Cloonan YK, Collett BR, Cradock MM, Buono L, et al. Presurgical and postsurgical assessment of the neurodevelopment of infants with single-suture craniosynostosis: comparison with controls. J Neurosurg. 2007;107(2 Suppl):103–10.
101. Starr JR, Collett BR, Gaither R, Kapp-Simon KA, Cradock MM, Cunningham ML, et al. Multicenter study of neurodevelopment in 3-year-old children with and without single-suture craniosynostosis. Arch Pediatr Adolesc Med. 2012;166(6):536–42.
102. Cohen SR, Cho DC, Nichols SL, Simms C, Cross KP, Burstein FD. American society of maxillofacial surgeons outcome study: preoperative and postoperative neurodevelopmental findings in single-suture craniosynostosis. Plast Reconstr Surg. 2004;114(4):841–7; discussion 848–9.

17 Non-invasive Assessment of ICP and Perfusion in Craniosynostosis

Llewellyn Padayachy

17.1 Introduction

Raised ICP is a common finding in children with craniosynostosis. The frequency in single suture synostosis is between 15% and 20% [1–3] and is higher in complex craniosynostosis with a described prevalence of 30–40% [4, 5]. The clinical signs and symptoms associated with raised ICP in craniosynostosis can be quite subtle with a slow, progressive clinical course and therefore may be of limited diagnostic value. Radiological features consistent with raised ICP are also observer-dependent and have a variable diagnostic accuracy [6]. The rates of post-operative raised ICP, especially in syndromic craniosynostosis, even in aesthetically successful corrective procedures, also appear to be unclear due to the lack of reliable indicators of raised ICP [7].

The value of a reliable non-invasive diagnostic technique to detect raised ICP in children with craniosynostosis is also underscored by the current limitations related to invasive ICP monitoring [8]. Continuous advancements in technology have also made.

L. Padayachy (✉)
Department of Neurosurgery, University of Pretoria, Pretoria, South Africa

Steve Biko Academic Hospital, Pretoria, South Africa
e-mail: LC.Padayachy@up.ac.za

17.2 Methods for Detecting Raised ICP

17.2.1 Clinical Assessment

Neurological evaluation and accurate history-taking remain the mainstay of diagnosis and monitoring. Careful history-taking is of paramount importance when making a diagnosis of raised ICP. Symptoms suggestive of raised ICP include headache, nausea and vomiting, visual impairment, altered level of consciousness and developmental delay.

The clinical presentation due to raised ICP differs in neonates and older children. In neonates, where the anterior fontanelle is still patent, an increasing head circumference, bulging of the anterior fontanelle, an upward gaze palsy, distended scalp veins, a thin, shiny scalp and, depending on the type of craniosynostosis, splaying of the sutures, remain the most prominent clinical findings. In older children and adults, the findings related to raised ICP can be more difficult to elicit. On fundoscopic examination, papilledema, loss of spontaneous venous pulsation or optic atrophy (depending on the duration of the raised ICP) are helpful findings. Palsies of the third and sixth cranial nerves and abnormalities of gaze (specifically Parinaud's syndrome) are consistent with severely raised ICP. Cushing's response of hypertension, bradycardia and abnormal respiration usually signal impending hernia-

F. Di Rocco, J. Kestle (eds.), *Neurosurgical Aspects of Craniosynostosis*,
https://doi.org/10.1007/978-3-031-69386-1_17

tion, requiring urgent treatment. In diagnosing raised ICP, good history and proper examination cannot be highlighted enough.

17.2.2 Neuro-Ophthalmologic Findings in Craniosynostosis

Visual complications related to craniosynostosis are common and include optic neuropathy, especially papilledema or optic atrophy due to raised ICP, strabismus, refractive errors, exposure keratopathy due to exorbitism and amblyopia. These ophthalmological conditions have been described more frequently in syndromic craniosynostosis [9]. Visual field deficits are also common, highlighting the value of ophthalmological assessment and monitoring of visual function in the diagnosis of raised ICP in craniosynostosis patients [10].

17.2.3 Radiological Markers

Imaging in children with raised ICP forms a cornerstone of decision-making. The spectrum of imaging modalities available ranges from X-rays to magnetic resonance imaging (MRI).

X-rays: Skull X-rays have limited value in the modern imaging armamentarium. The appreciation of the 'copper-beating' of the skull and erosion of the clinoid process are still valuable in detecting chronically raised ICP [11].

Ultrasound: The usefulness of bedside imaging and the benefit of being radiation-free, portable and easy-to-use, have made ultrasound an attractive tool for confirming the diagnosis of craniosynostosis and positional plagiocephaly, especially in the outpatient department [12]. In addition, ultrasound can be used as a prenatal diagnostic technique to detect cranial malformation during the third trimester [13]. For experienced operators, ultrasound has even been suggested as the first-line imaging tool where craniosynostosis is suspected, especially for infants aged 8–12 months [14]. Transorbital imaging of the ONSD and transcranial Doppler (TCD) have also made use of ultrasound as a screening modality for raised ICP in craniosynostosis, but these will be discussed in more detail later in the chapter.

CT scan: This imaging modality remains the most widely used for diagnosing craniosynostosis and suspected cases of raised ICP. The features on the CT scan which are suggestive of raised ICP include—midline shift, enlarged ventricles, transependymal fluid shift, presence of a space-occupying lesion/haematoma, effacement of the basal cisterns, loss of grey/white differentiation, CSF volume in the subarachnoid space (can be either enlarged or decreased, depending on the condition) [15–17]. 3D-CT imaging and reconstruction have emerged as valuable diagnostic and surgical planning tools [18, 19]. Despite the widespread use of CT scans in children with craniosynostosis and raised ICP, the exposure of the developing brain to repeated, high doses of radiation has been criticised and the indications should be carefully considered [20]. CT angiography and perfusion studies are valuable.

MRI: The role of MRI in brain imaging has become almost indispensable. The exquisite structural and functional detail that it provides, has become fundamental to our decision-making. The features on standard T1- and T2-weighted images related to raised ICP are somewhat similar to those assessed on CT scan. Vascular imaging using MR angiography and venography (MRA and MRV) are widely used for, but their value in the context of ICP assessment is unclear.

The change in apparent diffusion coefficient (ADC) in the frontal white matter measured on diffusion MRI before and after surgery for craniosynostosis indicates that it may reflect change in ICP and could therefore provide a useful non-invasive technique for assessing ICP [21].

Arterial spin labelling sequences provide an attractive non-invasive imaging method for assessing cerebral blood flow (CBF). This non-invasive MR perfusion technique utilises arterial blood water as a diffusible endogenous tracer to quantitatively assess absolute CBF. While still considered a research tool, several advances and descriptions of its utility in clinical conditions such as hypoxic-ischaemic encephalopathy, paediatric cerebrovascular disease, e.g. moyamoya disease, paediatric brain tumours, infection, traumatic brain injury and hydrocephalus [22]. The applicability of this technique in certain craniosynostosis procedures to establish and perhaps quantify perfusion pre- and post-surgery, certainly provides an interesting value proposition.

A strong relationship between ICP and brain elastance has been described using the MRI-derived elastance index. This is a technique using cine phase-contrast pulse sequences to estimate blood and CSF flow in the brain by calculating changes in intracranial volume based on arterial inflow, venous outflow and CSF flow between the brain and spine [23]. This technique demonstrated a good correlation with shunt valve opening pressures in children with hydrocephalus [24].

17.3 Non-invasive Techniques for Assessing ICP

Estimating ICP and especially detecting and diagnosing raised ICP remains a challenge for the paediatric neurosurgeon. Invasive techniques for measuring ICP and other haemodynamic and perfusion parameters have role to play in traumatic brain injury patients, especially in the neurocritical care unit. While an overall benefit of invasive ICP monitoring has been described in a population of children with craniosynostosis [25], several publications describe higher complication rates in adults and children [26, 27], especially in TBI.

The appeal of reliable non-invasive methods of assessing ICP, which are portable, easy-to-use, reproducible, cost-effective and radiation-free, is therefore quite clear.

The most relevant of these non-invasive methods in craniosynostosis patients will be discussed here.

17.3.1 Optic Nerve Sheath Diameter (ONSD) Measurement

The relationship between CSF pressure in the intracranial space and CSF pressure in the optic nerve sheath, as well as the association with oedema of the optic disc, was described by Hayreh in the 1960s [28]. Since then several publications have supported the association of an increase in the optic nerve sheath diameter (ONSD) and raised ICP, and the measurement of the (ONSD) has been widely described as a useful non-invasive technique for assessing ICP in a wide variety of conditions [29]. The applicability of this technique in adults and children as well as its relative reproducibility have made it an attractive option for non-invasive assessment [30]. Transorbital ultrasound measurement of the ONSD is the most widely reported imaging technique in children, as it provides a radiation-free, portable, cost-effective, easy-to-use and reproducible alternative [31]. The issue of an optimal cut-off value for detecting raised ICP remains contentious, though. Studies comparing ONSD measurement to directly measure ICP in children suggest that where the anterior fontanelle is closed, a measurement of above 5.5 cm is consistent with an ICP above 15 mmHg, and an ONSD above 5.8 cm suggests ICP above 20 mmHg [32, 33]. Other studies reporting on this technique describe normative age-related values, 4.5 mm in patients over 1 year of age and 4.0 mm in children less than 1 year old [34]. Limitations of this technique include inter-rater variability, hyperechoic artefacts and variation in described ONSD cut-off values for detecting raised ICP [35]. Despite these limitations, this technique demonstrates promise as a non-invasive marker of raised ICP.

17.3.2 Optical Coherence Tomography (OCT)

OCT is a non-invasive imaging technique using infrared light, that provides high-resolution images of the retina and optic nerve in seconds. It can be used to measure and segment the retinal nerve fibre layers as well as the optic nerve head [36]. The use of OCT to measure total retinal thickness has demonstrated favourable diagnostic accuracy for the detection of papilledema in raised ICP when compared to conventional fundoscopy, especially in lower-grade abnormalities [37]. A described limitation of this technique, especially in young children, has been the table-mounted nature of the equipment, which required that patients be taken to the ophthalmology department where the equipment was located. A recent publication describing the use of OCT in children with craniosynostosis undergoing surgery found the technique to be a potentially sensitive marker of raised ICP [38]. As a screening tool for children with craniosynostosis, the use of OCT may not yet have enough evidence to support its role [39].

The feasibility of a portable OCT system for assessing raised ICP in children with craniosynostosis was recently described and appears promising [40, 41].

17.3.3 Pupillometry

Quantitative measurement of changes in pupil size in response to light stimulus using infrared pupillometry. The pupil size decreases by around 34% in response to a standard light stimulus. In patients with ICP > 20 mmHg, this response is reduced to 10% [42, 43]. The appeal of this portable technique is its ease of use in children; however, the clinical applicability and repeatability of this technique still requires further investigation.

17.3.4 Intraocular Pressure (IOP)

The use of handheld tonometers require very little in the way formal training and can easily be performed by junior members of the team. This makes the technique appealing as a rapid screening tool for detecting raised ICP. The described relationship between IOP and increased ICP was demonstrated at quite high values of around 46.8 mmHg [44]. While the relationship between an increase in IOP and raised ICP appears useful, the pooled diagnostic accuracy is not enough to predict individual patient ICP [45].

17.3.5 Visual Evoked Potentials (VEP)

Disturbances of the visual pathways can be recorded from electrodes placed over the occipital scalp [46]. Use of the N2 latency during flash-evoked VEPs has demonstrated a good correlation with ICP in children with hydrocephalus [47]. The inter-subject variability however, is a limitation of this technique [48]. Pattern reversal VEPs are useful in monitoring visual pathway function, as a proxy for raised ICP in children with craniosynostosis [49]. Combining pattern reversal VEP and fundoscopy to assess for papilledema appears to improve the diagnostic accuracy for detecting raised ICP in children with craniosynostosis [50].

17.3.6 Transcranial Doppler (TCD) Sonography

The use of TCD to assess blood flow through major intracranial vessels is based on the 'Doppler effect', which determines the difference between incident and reflected waves to estimate the speed of blood flow [51]. The technique has been described extensively to measure intracranial CBF velocity. The most commonly described parameters include the pulsatility index (PI), the resistance index (RI) and the peak systolic and diastolic velocity. The PI, in particular, has demonstrated a good correlation with ICP in adults [52]. In children however, this relationship appears less consistent when compared to absolute ICP values [53], but may serve as a good screening tool to identify patients requiring invasive ICP monitoring [54]. For craniosynostosis, TCD may be used to assess patients with decreased intracranial compliance due to raised ICP and to monitor the effects of surgery [55].

17.3.7 Near Infrared Spectroscopy (NIRS)

This technique is useful for assessing regional cerebral blood volume (CBV) and cerebral blood oxygen saturation (rSO_2). Variation in the absorption of infrared light allows the detection of changes in oxyhaemoglobin and deoxyhaemoglobin concentration as a marker of rSO_2, which demonstrated a significant difference in TBI patients with raised and normal ICP [56]. Limitations of this technique are that is presently does not provide an estimation of absolute ICP, or changes in ICP [57]. Detecting regional compromise of cortical metabolism and CBF in craniosynostosis patients provides very useful information pre- and post-operatively [58].

There are several other techniques which have been described in the quest for developing a reliable non-invasive method for assessing ICP. These include tympanic membrane displacement, otoacoustic emissions, venous ophthalmodynamometry and spectral analysis electroencephalography (EEG). Combinations of techniques have also been used to improve diagnostic accuracy [59].

Several of the techniques described in this chapter show promise in terms of demonstrating a relationship with increasing ICP. Currently however, there is no standalone non invasive technique the provides sufficient diagnostic accuracy to guide the diagnosis and treatment regimen for raised ICP, especially in children with craniosynostosis. The most attractive solutions appear to be methods aimed at combining certain static and dynamic parameters to refine the overall user-friendliness and diagnostic accuracy [60].

References

1. Tamburrini G, Caldarelli M, Massimi L, Santini P, Di Rocco C. Intracranial pressure monitoring in children with single suture and complex craniosynostosis: a review. Childs Nerv Syst. 2005;21:913–21.
2. Cohen SR, Persing JA. Intracranial pressure in single-suture craniosynostosis. Cleft Palate Craniofac J. 1998;35(3):194–6.
3. Renier D. Intracranial pressure in craniosynostosis: pre-and postoperative recordings—correlation with functional results. In: Persing JA, Edgerton MT, Jane J, editors. Scientific foundations and surgical treatment of craniosynostosis. Baltimore: Williams and Wilkins; 1989. p. 263–9.
4. Eide PK, Helseth E, Due-Tønnessen B, Lundar T. Assessment of continuous intracranial pressure recordings in childhood craniosynostosis. Pediatr Neurosurg. 2002;37(6):310–20.
5. Thompson DN, Malcolm GP, Jones BM, Harkness WJ, Hayward RD. Intracranial pressure in single-suture craniosynostosis. Pediatr Neurosurg. 1995;22(5):235–40.
6. Kayhanian S, Young AM, Piper RJ, Donnelly J, Scoffings D, Garnett MR, Fernandes HM, Smielewski P, Czosnyka M, Hutchinson PJ, Agrawal S. Radiological correlates of raised intracranial pressure in children: a review. Front Pediatr. 2018;6:32.
7. Thomas GP, Johnson D, Byren JC, Judge AD, Jayamohan J, Magdum SA, Richards PG, Wall SA. The incidence of raised intracranial pressure in nonsyndromic sagittal craniosynostosis following primary surgery. J Neurosurg Pediatr. 2015;15(4):350–60.
8. Padayachy LC, Figaji AA, Bullock MR. Intracranial pressure monitoring for traumatic brain injury in the modern era. Childs Nerv Syst. 2010;26:441–52.
9. Duan M, Skoch J, Pan BS, Shah V. Neuro-ophthalmological manifestations of craniosynostosis: current perspectives. Eye Brain. 2021;13:29–40.
10. Liasis A, Nischal KK, Walters B, Thompson D, Hardy S, Towell A, Dunaway D, Jones B, Evans R, Hayward R. Monitoring visual function in children with syndromic craniosynostosis: a comparison of 3 methods. Arch Ophthalmol. 2006;124(8):1119–26.
11. Tuite GF, Evanson J, Chong WK, Thompson DN, Harkness WF, Jones BM, Hayward RD. The beaten copper cranium: a correlation between intracranial pressure, cranial radiographs, and computed tomographic scans in children with craniosynostosis. Neurosurgery. 1996;39(4):691–9.
12. Regelsberger J, Delling G, Tsokos M, Helmke K, Kammler G, Kränzlein H, Westphal M. High-frequency ultrasound confirmation of positional plagiocephaly. J Neurosurg Pediatr. 2006;105(5):413–7.
13. Miller C, Losken HW, Towbin R, Bowen AD, Mooney MP, Towbin A, Faix RS. Ultrasound diagnosis of craniosynostosis. Cleft Palate Craniofac J. 2002;39(1):73–80.
14. Proisy M, Bruneau B, Riffaud L. How ultrasonography can contribute to diagnosis of craniosynostosis. Neurochirurgie. 2019;65(5):228 31.
15. Eisenberg HM, Gary HE, Aldrich EF, Saydjari C, Turner B, Foulkes MA, Jane JA, Marmarou A, Marshall LF, Young HF. Initial CT findings in 753 patients with severe head injury: a report from the NIH Traumatic Coma Data Bank. J Neurosurg. 1990;73(5):688–98.
16. Miller MT, Pasquale M, Kurek S, White J, Martin P, Bannon K, Wasser T, Li M. Initial head computed tomographic scan characteristics have a linear relationship with initial intracranial pressure after trauma. J Trauma Acute Care Surg. 2004;56(5):967–73.
17. Eide PK. The relationship between intracranial pressure and size of cerebral ventricles assessed by computed tomography. Acta Neurochir. 2003;145:171–9.
18. Parisi M, Mehdizadeh HM, Hunter JC, Finch IJ. Evaluation of craniosynostosis with three-dimensional CT imaging. J Comput Assist Tomogr. 1989;13(6):1006–12.
19. Kotrikova B, Krempien R, Freier K, Mühling J. Diagnostic imaging in the management of craniosynostoses. Eur Radiol. 2007;17:1968–78.
20. Schweitzer T, Böhm H, Meyer-Marcotty P, Collmann H, Ernestus RI, Krauß J. Avoiding CT scans in chil-

dren with single-suture craniosynostosis. Childs Nerv Syst. 2012;28:1077–82.
21. Takahashi Y, Hori M, Shimoji K, Miyajima M, Akiyama O, Arai H, Aoki S. Changes in delta ADC reflect intracranial pressure changes in craniosynostosis. Acta Radiol Open. 2017;6(9):2058460117728535.
22. Narayanan S, Schmithorst V, Panigrahy A. Arterial spin labeling in pediatric neuroimaging. In: Seminars in pediatric neurology, vol. 33. WB Saunders; 2020. p. 100799.
23. Alperin NJ, Lee SH, Loth F, Raksin PB, Lichtor T. MR-intracranial pressure (ICP): a method to measure intracranial elastance and pressure noninvasively by means of MR imaging: baboon and human study. Radiology. 2000;217(3):877–85.
24. Glick RP, Niebruegge J, Lee SH, Egibor O, Lichtor T, Alperin N. Early experience from the application of a noninvasive magnetic resonance imaging-based measurement of intracranial pressure in hydrocephalus. Neurosurgery. 2006;59(5):1052–61.
25. Ma R, Rowland D, Judge A, Calisto A, Jayamohan J, Johnson D, Richards P, Magdum S, Wall S. Complications following intracranial pressure monitoring in children: a 6-year single-center experience. J Neurosurg Pediatr. 2018;21(3):278–83.
26. Rosner MJ, Becker DP. ICP monitoring: complications and associated factors. Neurosurgery. 1976;23:494–519.
27. Anderson RC, Kan P, Klimo P, Brockmeyer DL, Walker ML, Kestle JR. Complications of intracranial pressure monitoring in children with head trauma. J Neurosurg Pediatr. 2004;101(2):53–8.
28. Hayreh SS. Pathogenesis of oedema of the optic disc (papilloedema): a preliminary report. Br J Ophthalmol. 1964;48(10):522.
29. Robba C, Santori G, Czosnyka M, Corradi F, Bragazzi N, Padayachy L, Taccone FS, Citerio G. Optic nerve sheath diameter measured sonographically as non-invasive estimator of intracranial pressure: a systematic review and meta-analysis. Intensive Care Med. 2018;44:1284–94.
30. Khan MN, Shallwani H, Khan MU, Shamim MS. Noninvasive monitoring intracranial pressure—a review of available modalities. Surg Neurol Int. 2017;8:51.
31. Driessen C, Bannink N, Lequin M, van Veelen MLC, Naus NC, Joosten KF, Mathijssen IM. Are ultrasonography measurements of optic nerve sheath diameter an alternative to funduscopy in children with syndromic craniosynostosis? J Neurosurg Pediatr. 2011;8(3):329–34.
32. Padayachy LC, Padayachy V, Galal U, Gray R, Fieggen AG. The relationship between transorbital ultrasound measurement of the optic nerve sheath diameter (ONSD) and invasively measured ICP in children: Part I: Repeatability, observer variability and general analysis. Childs Nerv Syst. 2016;32:1769–78.
33. Kerscher SR, Schöni D, Hurth H, Neunhoeffer F, Haas-Lude K, Wolff M, Schuhmann MU. The relation of optic nerve sheath diameter (ONSD) and intracranial pressure (ICP) in pediatric neurosurgery practice—Part I: Correlations, age-dependency and cut-off values. Childs Nerv Syst. 2020;36:99–106.
34. Newman WD, Hollman AS, Dutton GN, Carachi R. Measurement of optic nerve sheath diameter by ultrasound: a means of detecting acute raised intracranial pressure in hydrocephalus. Br J Ophthalmol. 2002;86(10):1109–13.
35. Ballantyne J, Hollman AS, Hamilton R, Bradnam MS, Carachi R, Young DG, Dutton GN. Transorbital optic nerve sheath ultrasonography in normal children. Clin Radiol. 1999;54(11):740–2.
36. Driessen C, Eveleens J, Bleyen I, van Veelen ML, Joosten K, Mathijssen I. Optical coherence tomography: a quantitative tool to screen for papilledema in craniosynostosis. Childs Nerv Syst. 2014;30:1067–73.
37. Scott CJ, Kardon RH, Lee AG, Frisén L, Wall M. Diagnosis and grading of papilledema in patients with raised intracranial pressure using optical coherence tomography vs clinical expert assessment using a clinical staging scale. Arch Ophthalmol. 2010;128(6):705–11.
38. Swanson JW, Xu W, Ying GS, Pan W, Lang SS, Heuer GG, Bartlett SP, Taylor JA. Intracranial pressure patterns in children with craniosynostosis utilizing optical coherence tomography. Childs Nerv Syst. 2020;36:535–44.
39. Rufai SR, Bowman R, Bunce C, Panteli V, McLean RJ, Teli S, Gottlob I, Thomas MG, Proudlock FA. Feasibility and repeatability of handheld optical coherence tomography in children with craniosynostosis. Transl Vis Sci Technol. 2021;10(8):24.
40. Purohit R, Rufai SR, Patel CK, Thomas GP, Jeelani NUO, Johnson D, Lawrence TP. Feasibility of a portable optical coherence tomography system in children with craniosynostosis. Eye. 2023;37(3):576–7.
41. Rufai SR, McLean RJ. Early recognition of raised intracranial pressure in craniosynostosis using optical coherence tomography. J Craniofac Surg. 2021;32(1):201.
42. Taylor WR, Chen JW, Meltzer H, Gennarelli TA, Kelbch C, Knowlton S, Richardson J, Lutch MJ, Farin A, Hults KN, Marshall LF. Quantitative pupillometry, a new technology: normative data and preliminary observations in patients with acute head injury. J Neurosurg. 2003;98(1):205–13.
43. Boev AN, Fountas KN, Karampelas I, Boev C, Machinis TG, Feltes C, Okosun I, Dimopoulos V, Troup C. Quantitative pupillometry: normative data in healthy pediatric volunteers. J Neurosurg Pediatr. 2005;103(6):496–500.
44. Lehman RA, Krupin T, Podos SM. Experimental effect of intracranial hypertension upon intraocular pressure. J Neurosurg. 1972;36(1):60–6.
45. Li Z, Yang Y, Lu Y, Liu D, Xu E, Jia J, Yang D, Zhang X, Yang H, Ma D, Wang N. Intraocular pressure vs intracranial pressure in disease conditions: a prospective cohort study (Beijing iCOP study). BMC Neurol. 2012;12(1):1–4.

46. Liasis A, Thompson DA, Hayward R, Nischal KK. Sustained raised intracranial pressure implicated only by pattern reversal visual evoked potentials after cranial vault expansion surgery. Pediatr Neurosurg. 2003;39(2):75–80.
47. York DH, Pulliam MW, Rosenfeld JG, Watts C. Relationship between visual evoked potentials and intracranial pressure. J Neurosurg. 1981;55(6):909–16.
48. Andersson L, Sjölund J, Nilsson J. Flash visual evoked potentials are unreliable as markers of ICP due to high variability in normal subjects. Acta Neurochir. 2012;154:121–7.
49. Thompson DA, Liasis A, Hardy S, Hagan R, Hayward RD, Evans RD, Nischal KK. Prevalence of abnormal pattern reversal visual evoked potentials in craniosynostosis. Plast Reconstr Surg. 2006;118(1):184–92.
50. Rufai SR, Marmoy OR, Thompson DA, van de Lande LS, Breakey RW, Bunce C, Panteli V, Schwiebert K, Mohamed S, Proudlock FA, Gottlob I. Electrophysiological and fundoscopic detection of intracranial hypertension in craniosynostosis. Eye. 2023;37(1):139–45.
51. Aaslid R, Markwalder TM, Nornes H. Noninvasive transcranial Doppler ultrasound recording of flow velocity in basal cerebral arteries. J Neurosurg. 1982;57(6):769–74.
52. Bellner J, Romner B, Reinstrup P, Kristiansson KA, Ryding E, Brandt L. Transcranial Doppler sonography pulsatility index (PI) reflects intracranial pressure (ICP). Surg Neurol. 2004;62(1):45–51.
53. Figaji AA, Zwane E, Fieggen AG, Siesjo P, Peter JC. Transcranial Doppler pulsatility index is not a reliable indicator of intracranial pressure in children with severe traumatic brain injury. Surg Neurol. 2009;72(4):389–94.
54. Melo JRT, Di Rocco F, Blanot S, Cuttaree H, Sainte-Rose C, Oliveira-Filho J, Zerah M, Meyer PG. Transcranial Doppler can predict intracranial hypertension in children with severe traumatic brain injuries. Childs Nerv Syst. 2011;27:979–84.
55. Westra SJ, Stotland MA, Lazareff J, Anderson CT, Sayre JW, Kawamoto H. Perioperative transcranial Doppler US to evaluate intracranial compliance in young children undergoing craniosynostosis repair surgery. Radiology. 2001;218(3):816–23.
56. Kampfl A, Pfausler B, Denchev D, Jaring HP, Schmutzhard E. Near infrared spectroscopy (NIRS) in patients with severe brain injury and elevated intracranial pressure: a pilot study. In: Brain Edema X: Proceedings of the Tenth International Symposium San Diego, California, October 20–23, 1996. Vienna: Springer; 1997. p. 112–4.
57. Kristiansson H, Nissborg E, Bartek J Jr, Andresen M, Reinstrup P, Romner B. Measuring elevated intracranial pressure through noninvasive methods: a review of the literature. J Neurosurg Anesthesiol. 2013;25(4):372–85.
58. Martini M, Röhrig A, Wenghoefer M, Schindler E, Messing-Jünger AM. Cerebral oxygenation and hemodynamic measurements during craniosynostosis surgery with near-infrared spectroscopy. Childs Nerv Syst. 2014;30:1367–74.
59. Müller SJ, Henkes E, Gounis MJ, Felber S, Ganslandt O, Henkes H. Non-invasive intracranial pressure monitoring. J Clin Med. 2023;12(6):2209.
60. Padayachy LC. Non-invasive intracranial pressure assessment. Childs Nerv Syst. 2016;32:1587–97.

Venous Anomalies in Craniosynostosis

18

Tatiana Protzenko, Antônio Bellas, and José Francisco M. Salomão

18.1 Introduction

In the world of craniofacial surgery, patients with syndromic craniosynostosis represent some of the most complex and challenging conditions to manage. They are usually submitted to multiple surgical procedures, including skull vault posterior expansion, fronto-orbital advancement, monobloc advancement, decompression of the posterior fossa, and/or treatment of hydrocephalus. Anomalous intracranial venous anatomy is a well-described phenomenon in these patients and interruption of important collateral drainage routes during surgery can lead to massive hemorrhage and intractable intracranial hypertension, and the study of the venous outflow is nowadays recognized as essential in the preoperative planning [1–3]. However, there is still controversy about the origin of collateral venous circulation and its relation to the skull base morphology. The authors discuss here the pathophysiology and the study findings in different syndromes.

T. Protzenko (✉) · A. Bellas · J. F. M. Salomão
Division of Pediatric Neurosurgery, Department of Pediatric Surgery, National Institute of Health for Women, Children and Adolescents Fernandes Figueira, Oswaldo Cruz Foundation (IFF-Fiocruz), Rio de Janeiro, Brazil

18.2 Pathophysiology

Abnormal intracranial venous anatomy is described in patients with syndromic craniosynostosis and is of significant importance in terms of surgical morbidity [1, 4, 5]. Literature reports suggest that dural venous sinus stenosis occurs due to changes in the skull base (jugular foramen stenosis), which would lead to the development of compensatory collateral circulation or persistence of fetal venous sinuses [6].

The jugular foramen is a gap between the occipital and the temporal bone that contains the sigmoid sinus and the jugular bulb, the inferior petrosal sinus, meningeal branches of a pharyngeal and an occipital artery, the glossopharyngeal nerve, the vagus nerve and the accessory nerve, the tympanic branch of the glossopharyngeal nerve (Jacobson's nerve), the auricular branch of the vagus nerve (Arnold's nerve), and finally the cochlear aqueduct [7]. Thus, it would not be difficult to imagine that the stenosis of this foramen could lead to stenosis of the drainage pathways. Asymmetries between the two jugular foramina were observed in postmortem studies, with the right jugular foramen being larger than the left in 68% of cases, the same size in 12% of cases, and smaller in 20% of cases [8].

However, in patients with syndromic craniosynostosis, jugular foramen stenosis is a reality and is related to the hypoplastic skull base. In the 1970s, Hoffmann was the first to describe the

F. Di Rocco, J. Kestle (eds.), *Neurosurgical Aspects of Craniosynostosis*,
https://doi.org/10.1007/978-3-031-69386-1_18

posterior fossa as small in patients with syndromic craniosynostosis, and Saldino in 1972 associated Chiari I malformation with Pfeiffer syndrome [9, 10]. Cinalli et al. also demonstrated that the posterior fossa is small in FGFR2-related craniosynostosis, and these authors associated this hypoplastic posterior fossa with the early closure of lambdoid sutures and synchondrosis of the skull base [11]. Martinez-Perez et al. proposed through a case report of a patient with Crouzon syndrome and acanthosis nigricans that bilateral atresia of the jugular foramen was the cause of intracranial hypertension, venous hypertension, and dilatation of the scalp veins [12]. Other authors [1, 13] have associated venous alterations with the state of intracranial hypertension, thus being considered a compensatory mechanism.

On the other hand, other authors described that evidence of venous outflow obstruction may not be indicative of significant intracranial venous hypertension, even in intriguing cases presenting venous obstruction, hydrocephalus, and tonsillar herniation [14, 15]. This lack of relationship between venous obstruction and intracranial hypertension was also proposed by Cinalli et al. [16]. In an angiographic study of patients with syndromic craniosynostosis, only 1/3 of them had unilateral or bilateral stenosis of the jugular foramen and intracranial hypertension.

The results presented by Florisson et al. [2] agree with those found by Cinalli. Although they found small jugular foramina in all patients with syndromic craniosynostosis, the number of collaterals were not different between groups with and without papilledema and are therefore not considered related to intracranial hypertension.

Although most literature publications agree that the jugular foramen is restricted in syndromic craniosynostosis, Coll et al. reported that, in their population, the only patients with a truly narrow jugular foramen were the Apert syndrome group [17]. Then, if collateral circulation is associated with jugular foramen stenosis, it would be obvious to admit that these patients would have the greatest number of collaterals. However, a prospective series showed that, in Apert syndrome, the venous anomalies are generally less exuberant than in Pfeiffer and Crouzon patients [1]. This makes us wonder if the stenosis of the jugular foramen is directly related to the venous anomalies or if an intrinsic trouble could be associated.

A possible intrinsic theory is based on a primary vascular abnormality resulting from a similar dysplastic process that occurs in the bones of the skull. FGFR gene expression products have been detected in cranial vascular endothelium—as well as present in synostotic sutures—in patients with syndromic craniosynostosis by immunohistochemical examination [18, 19]. Premature endothelial proliferation may cause stenosis of these vessels. Tischfield et al. also support this theory and describe that cerebral venous malformations can result from loss of expression of the Twist 1 gene [20]. The presence of collaterals in inborn patients found in a retrospective series also imply that collateral development could be an intrinsic disorder [2]. Therefore, the true origin of collateral venous circulation, whether it is related to stenosis of the jugular foramen or whether intrinsic mechanisms exist and when it plays a role in intracranial hypertension, remains a mystery in the literature. Probably intracranial hypertension has a multifactorial origin, and prospective studies based on molecular analysis may clarify the true role of genetic mutations in these patients.

Regardless of the mechanism of abnormal venous outflow, studies are increasingly focused on its study in preoperative planning, since the rupture of this circulation can have fatal consequences.

18.3 How to Study: How Do I Do It

The study of venous outflow in patients with complex craniosynostosis has been previously documented using cerebral arteriography, venography, computed tomography (CT)-venography, and magnetic resonance (MR)-venography [1–3,

13, 14, 21, 22]. Although cerebral arteriography is considered "gold standard," it is a very invasive exam, being reserved for special cases. MR venography has the advantage of being a noninvasive method but with problems with saturation effects, especially in newborns and young children [14]. CT venography, despite the inconvenience of exposure to irradiation, is able to show cerebral veins or smaller venous sinuses with low flow and its relationship to the skull bones and skull base foramina and, for this reason, it has been used by many authors [1–3].

From our ongoing prospective study, we agree with the use of CT venography to study the venous outflow in patients with syndromic craniosynostosis. CT venography allows us to visualize the true relationship between collateral veins and bone foramina, allowing safer surgical planning. Figure 18.1 shows the outstanding difference between MR venography and CT venography in the same patient.

The available studies consider the following collateral veins, as proposed by Jeevan et al. [3]: parietal emissary vein from the superior sagittal sinus, occipital emissary vein from the transverse sinus or torcula, mastoid emissary veins from the transverse or sigmoid sinus, condylar emissary vein from sigmoid sinus or jugular sinus to the deep cervical vein, occipital sinus from the margin of the falx cerebelli, the marginal sinus at the rim of the foramen magnum, and venous collaterals from the ophthalmic vein. The intracranial sinuses are also studied: sagittal, transverse, sigmoid, jugular bulb complex, and straight sinus. In addition, the inferior sagittal sinus, pericallosal vein, and pterygoid sinus plexus were studied by Florisson et al. [2]. Figure 18.2 shows the different collateral circulation that can be found.

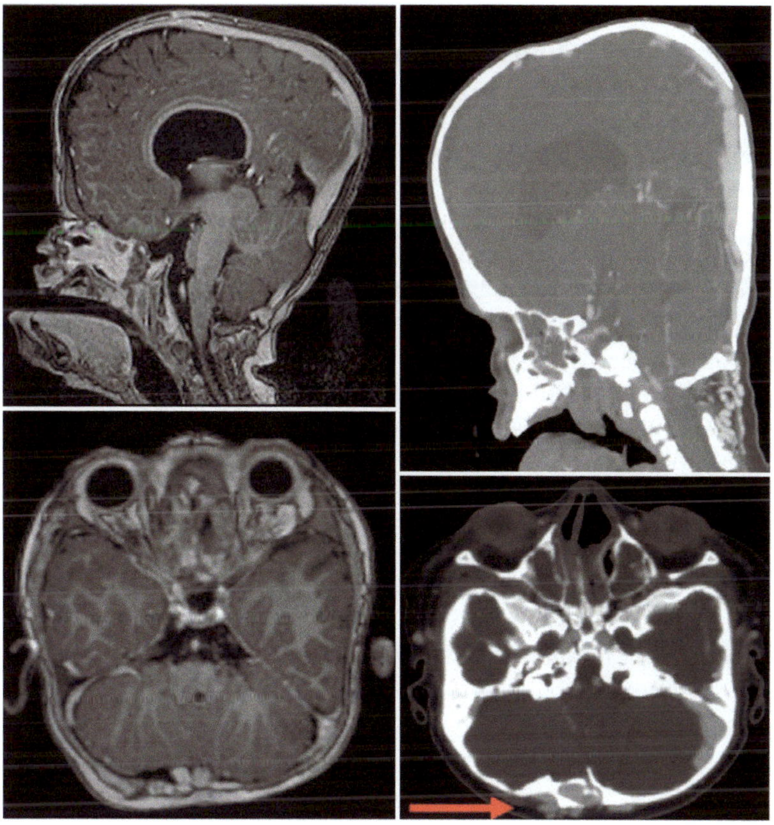

Fig. 18.1 Difference between MR venography (left) and CT venography (right) in the same patient. The occipital transosseous veinous drainage (red arrow) is not explicit in MR venography

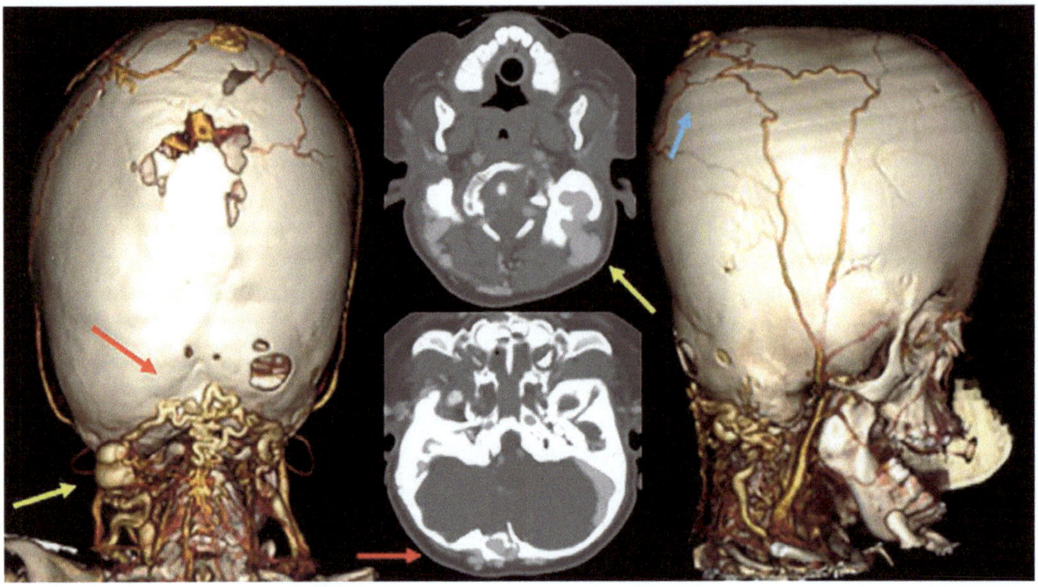

Fig. 18.2 Example case of abnormal venous outflow. CT venography reconstruction with enlarged condylar emissary vein (yellow arrow), occipital transosseous emissary vein (red arrow), and parietal transosseous emissary vein (blue arrow)

18.4 Presentation in Different Syndromes

Few papers compare collateral circulation among the different syndromes presented. Rollins et al. describe that functional stenosis of the jugular foramen occurs in 100% of patients with Pfeiffer syndrome, 62% in Crouzon syndrome, 50% in Apert syndrome, and 83% in complex craniosynostosis [14]. Today, these data make us wonder if these patients with complex craniosynostosis really did not have any associated syndrome, since molecular studies modified the identification of mutations not previously found. This interpretation may also extend to other case reports on complex nonsyndromic craniosynostosis [15, 22]. Florisson et al. reported that collateral venous outflow is more frequent in Apert syndrome, followed by Crouzon-Pfeiffer syndrome and Saerthre-Chotzen syndrome, and the most important route of drainage was the condylar emissary vein [2]. On the other hand, Copeland et al. described that emissaries were found in 100% of patients with Pfeiffer syndrome, 74% in Crouzon, 36% in Apert, 33% in Saerthre-Chotzen, and 0% in Muenke. Occipital and mastoid emissaries were most common [1].

In our experience, patients with Crouzon and Pfeiffer syndromes have the highest number of collaterals, followed by Apert syndrome (Fig. 18.3). Patients with Muenke and Saerthre-Chotzen syndromes have a more benign course. Interestingly, many patients have a large jugular foramen and still important collateral circulation, making us agree with the relationship between venous anomalies and intrinsic problems of the syndrome.

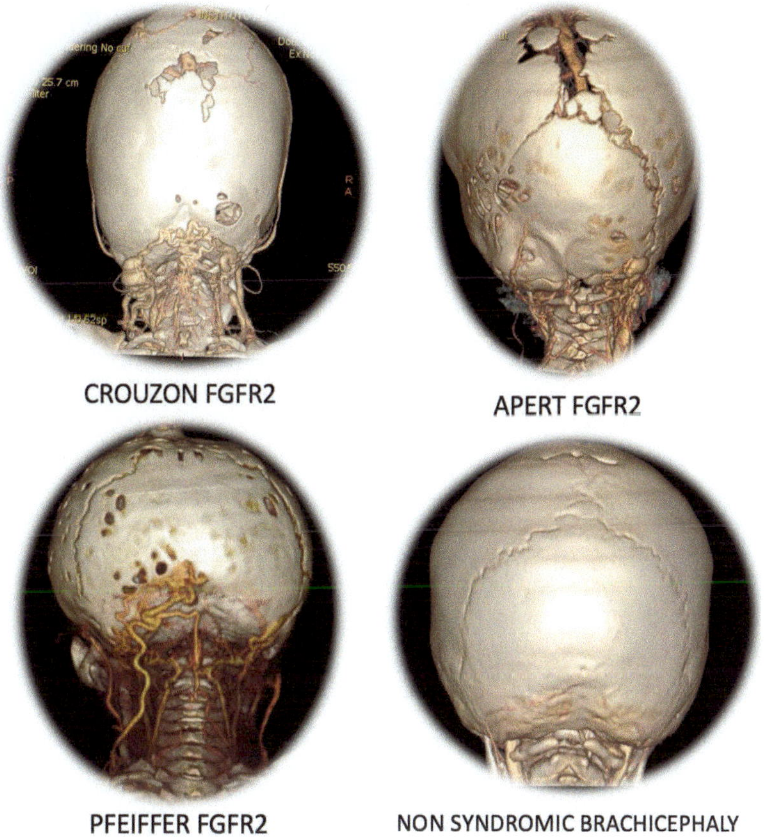

Fig. 18.3 Differences in CT-venogram reconstruction between Crouzon, Pfeiffer, Apert syndromes and nonsyndromic brachycephaly

18.5 Venous Outflow in Clinical Practice

The importance of the venous study in children with syndromic craniosynostosis was described in a remarkable case in the literature, in which a transosseous circulation was, in fact, the main route of cranial venous outflow [5]. Other authors described that the venous analysis allowed the modification of the surgical approach or even the decision of conservative treatment to avoid disastrous consequences [1, 3, 21, 23]. In reality, it is not only the presence of anomalous circulation that seems to prevent surgery but whether this circulation is the main route of venous outflow to determine a surgical decision.

The literature is clear about the use of posterior vault expansion to control intracranial hypertension and correction of Chiari 1 malformation, as a first approach to the syndromic patient. In Fig. 18.4, the authors present a case of a patient with Pfeiffer syndrome and Chiari 1 malformation, whose approach performed consisted of posterior vault expansion using springs. The presence of collateral circulation was previously studied in order to avoid large drainage veins, which could lead to massive hemorrhage, and a craniotomy was defined in the supratorcular region, avoiding collateral circulation in the mastoid and suboccipital region. Note the important increase in the volume of the posterior fossa, resolution of the Chiari 1, without the need to approach the infratentorial skull, being a simpler surgery, with little blood loss and, undoubtedly, safer.

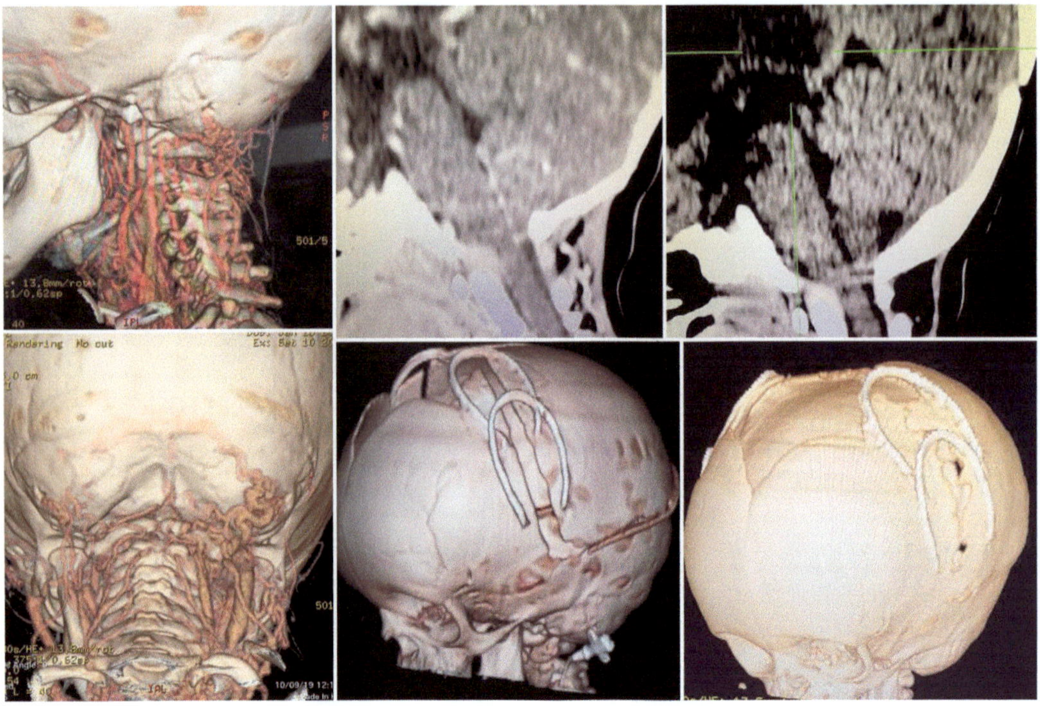

Fig. 18.4 Venous analysis of Pfeiffer syndrome patient and surgical approach. Important collateral circulation is shown on a 3D CT venogram (mastoid emissary vein, condylar vein, and occipital circulation). A posterior vault expansion was performed with 8N springs. Pre- and post-op CT scans show tonsillar herniation improvement with the increase in posterior fossa volume

18.6 Should We Study All Complex Types of Craniosynostosis?

Whether genetic mutation plays a role or not in the formation of collateral circulation has already been discussed in the scope of this chapter. According to the literature, important studies show that the jugular foramen is reduced in complex and syndromic craniosynostosis, and thus, both can develop collateral circulation [1, 2, 6, 14, 15]. Some cases reported in the literature of unclassified complex craniosynostosis demonstrate an exuberant collateral circulation [22, 23]. In such cases, it is possible that a mutation not previously identified is associated. Regardless, all multisutural craniosynostosis has the risk of presenting changes in the skull base and, consequently, changes in venous outflow. Copeland et al. claim that, in small sample groups of syndromes, it is not possible to determine the risk of venous anomalies, like in Saerthre-Chotzen and Muenke syndrome [1]. Thus, the study of all syndromic patients is still recommended. We can extend this statement to all patients with suspected syndromes. Further molecular investigation will probably help us to solve this question and to improve our current protocols.

References

1. Copeland AE, Hoffman CE, Tsitouras V, Jeevan DS, Ho ES, Drake JM, et al. Clinical significance of venous anomalies in syndromic craniosynostosis. Plast Reconstr Surg Glob Open. 2018;6(1):e1613.
2. Florisson JMG, Barmpalios G, Lequin M, van Veelen MLC, Bannink N, Hayward RD, et al. Venous hypertension in syndromic and complex craniosynostosis: the abnormal anatomy of the jugular foramen and collaterals. J Craniofac Surg. 2015;43(3):312–8.
3. Jeevan DS, Anlsow P, Jayamohan J. Abnormal venous drainage in syndromic craniosynostosis

and the role of CT venography. Childs Nerv Syst. 2008;24(12):1413–20.
4. Hayward R, Gonsalez S. How low can you go? Intracranial pressure, cerebral perfusion pressure, and respiratory obstruction in children with complex craniosynostosis. J Neurosurg Pediatr. 2005;102(1):16–22.
5. Thompson DNP, Hayward RD, Harkness WJ, Bingham RM, Jones BM. Lessons from a case of kleeblattschädel. J Neurosurg. 1995;82(6):1071–4.
6. Robson CD, Mulliken JB, Robertson RL, Proctor MR, Steinberger D, Barnes PD, et al. Prominent basal emissary foramina in syndromic craniosynostosis: correlation with phenotypic and molecular diagnoses. AJNR Am J Neuroradiol. 2000;21(9):1707–17.
7. Rhoton AL. Jugular foramen. Neurosurgery. 2000;47(Suppl_3):S267–85.
8. Rhoton AL, Buza R. Microsurgical anatomy of the jugular foramen. J Neurosurg. 1975;42(5):541–50.
9. Hoffman HJ, Tucker WS. Cephalocranial disproportion. A complication of the treatment of hydrocephalus in children. Childs Brain. 1976;2(3):167–76.
10. Saldino RM, Steinbach HL, Epstein CJ. Familial acrocephalosyndactyly (Pfeiffer syndrome). Am J Roentgenol. 1972;116(3):609–22.
11. Cinalli G, Renier D, Sebag G, Sainte-Rose C, Arnaud E, Pierre-Kahn A. Chronic tonsillar herniation in Crouzon's and Apert's syndromes: the role of premature synostosis of the lambdoid suture. J Neurosurg. 1995;83(4):575–82.
12. Martinez-Perez D, Vander Woude DL, Barnes PD, Scott M, Mulliken JB. Jugular foraminal stenosis in Crouzon syndrome. Pediatr Neurosurg. 1996;25(5):252–5.
13. Taylor WJ, Hayward RD, Lasjaunias P, Britto JA, Thompson DNP, Jones BM, et al. Enigma of raised intracranial pressure in patients with complex craniosynostosis: the role of abnormal intracranial venous drainage. J Neurosurg. 2001;94(3):377–85.
14. Rollins N, Booth T, Shapiro K. MR venography in children with complex craniosynostosis. Pediatr Neurosurg. 2000;32(6):308–15.
15. Sanchez R, Ward K, St. Hilaire H, Mussell J. Basicranial venous anomalies associated with complex nonsyndromic craniosynostosis in a child. J Craniofac Surg. 2013;24(6):1970–3.
16. Cinalli G, Sainte-Rose C, Kollar EM, Zerah M, Brunelle F, Chumas P, et al. Hydrocephalus and craniosynostosis. J Neurosurg. 1998;88(2):209–14.
17. Coll G, Arnaud E, Collet C, Brunelle F, Sainte-Rose C, Di Rocco F. Skull base morphology in fibroblast growth factor receptor type 2-related faciocraniosynostosis. Neurosurgery. 2015;76(5):571–83.
18. Gray JL, Kang SS, Zenni GC, Kim DU, Kim PI, Burgess WH, et al. FGF-1 affixation stimulates ePTFE endothelialization without intimal hyperplasia. J Surg Res. 1994;57(5):596–612.
19. Ignelzi MA, Wang W, Young AT. Fibroblast growth factors lead to increased Msx2 expression and fusion in calvarial sutures. J Bone Miner Res. 2003;18(4):751–9.
20. Tischfield MA, Robson CD, Gilette NM, Chim SM, Sofela FA, DeLisle MM, et al. Cerebral vein malformations result from loss of Twist1 expression and BMP signaling from skull progenitor cells and dura. Dev Cell. 2017;42(5):445–461.e5.
21. Al-Otibi M, Jea A, Kulkarni AV. Detection of important venous collaterals by computed tomography venogram in multisutural synostosis: case report and review of the literature. J Neurosurg Pediatr. 2007;107(6):508–10.
22. Anderson PJ, Harkness WJ, Taylor W, Jones BM, Hayward RD. Anomalous venous drainage in a case of non-syndromic craniosynostosis. Childs Nerv Syst. 1997;13(2):97–100.
23. Sandberg DI, Navarro R, Blanch J, Ragheb J. Anomalous venous drainage preventing safe posterior fossa decompression in patients with Chiari malformation Type I and multisutural craniosynostosis: report of two cases and review of the literature. J Neurosurg Pediatr. 2007;106(6):490–4.

19 Cerebellar Tonsils Herniation and Syringomyelia in Craniosynostoses

Luca Massimi

19.1 Introduction

The hypoplasia of the posterior cranial fossa (PCF) is an issue often addressed by embryologists and physicians when dealing with children with craniosynostosis. Actually, the physiopathological changes occurring in this subset of patients, especially in case of syndromic synostoses, are investigated with the goal to explain and prevent not only the signs/symptoms related to the craniosynostosis but also the possible consequences of these changes, as the secondary chronic tonsillar descent and the syringomyelia. Moreover, the continuously increasing number of tonsillar caudal ectopia and/or syringomyelia diagnoses among the pediatric population gives reason for the great attention payed by the Scientific Community to these entities and to their proper management. Therefore, to rule out the presence of a craniosynostosis has become a mandatory step for the correct management of a child with hindbrain herniation and syringomyelia as well as the occurrence of the latter conditions is constantly taken into account for the appropriate treatment of craniosynostosis.

L. Massimi (✉)
Pediatric Neurosurgery, Fondazione Policlinico Universitario A. Gemelli IRCCS, Rome, Italy

Università Cattolica del Sacro Cuore, Rome, Italy
e-mail: luca.massimi@policlinicogemelli.it

This chapter is focused on the pathophysiological and clinical relationship between craniosynostoses and chronic tonsils herniation/syringomyelia and on their management.

19.2 Pathophyslology

19.2.1 Cerebellar Tonsils Herniation (CTH)

Phylogenetically, human PCF would have been originated from an increase of the supratentorial brain volume combined with the acquisition of the bipedal stance that has led to a progressive weight redistribution. The prominence of the human tentorium would have played a crucial role in this redistribution, bearing the cerebral weight and distributing the resulting load to the skull. Therefore, the downward rotation of the fetal tentorium would be the intracranial response to a disproportion between the human cerebrum and cerebellum [1]. On the other hand, the bony response would be represented by the two phases of PCF growth. The first step occurs during the early childhood, when PCF grows in length mainly alongside the intra-occipital, petro-occipital, and spheno-occipital synchondrosis, while the second step takes place during the puberty, when PCF enlarges mainly following the spheno-occipital growth [2]. These two different patterns of growth are favored by the initial

F. Di Rocco, J. Kestle (eds.), *Neurosurgical Aspects of Craniosynostosis*,
https://doi.org/10.1007/978-3-031-69386-1_19

absence of ossification of the petro-occipital, the occipitomastoid, and the spheno-occipital synchondroses. The time for PCF to grow is shorter and faster in girls compared with boys [3]. In spite of that, boys show a bigger PCF at the end of the development because of the smaller PCF at birth in girls [4].

Some hypotheses have been formulated so far to explain the genesis of CTH in craniosynostosis, starting from the evidence of the increased rate of CTH in children with an early fusion of the posterior sutures. The most accepted theory is based on the cephalo-cranial disproportion (between a normal or enlarged neural tissue and a narrowed PCF) induced by the progressing, premature fusion of the lambdoid arch sutures [5]. It is an acquired disorder, which is not present at birth and which develops in the first months of life (namely, between the third and the sixth month), as soon as the lambdoid sutures start closing. The venous engorgement, resulting from the occlusion of the jugular foramina, and the associated hydrocephalus, which are common in syndromic craniosynostoses, can further increase such a cranio-cerebral disproportion because of the subsequent brain turgor. Moreover, in this subset of patients, the brain turgor is exacerbated by the chronic CO_2 retention due to the upper airway's obstruction [6]. The cranio-cerebral disproportion has been proposed by Cinalli and coworkers as the main causal factor for the tonsillar descent [2]. This hypothesis is supported by the progressive appearance of CTH/syringomyelia in craniosynostosis depending on the time of suture closure: the earlier the premature suture fusion, the higher the risk of CTH. As known, children affected by early closure of the lambdoid arch (e.g., Crouzon patients) are more prone to develop (early) CTH than those where these sutures close later (e.g. Apert patients) (Figs. 19.1 and 19.2). The disappearance of hindbrain herniation following cra-

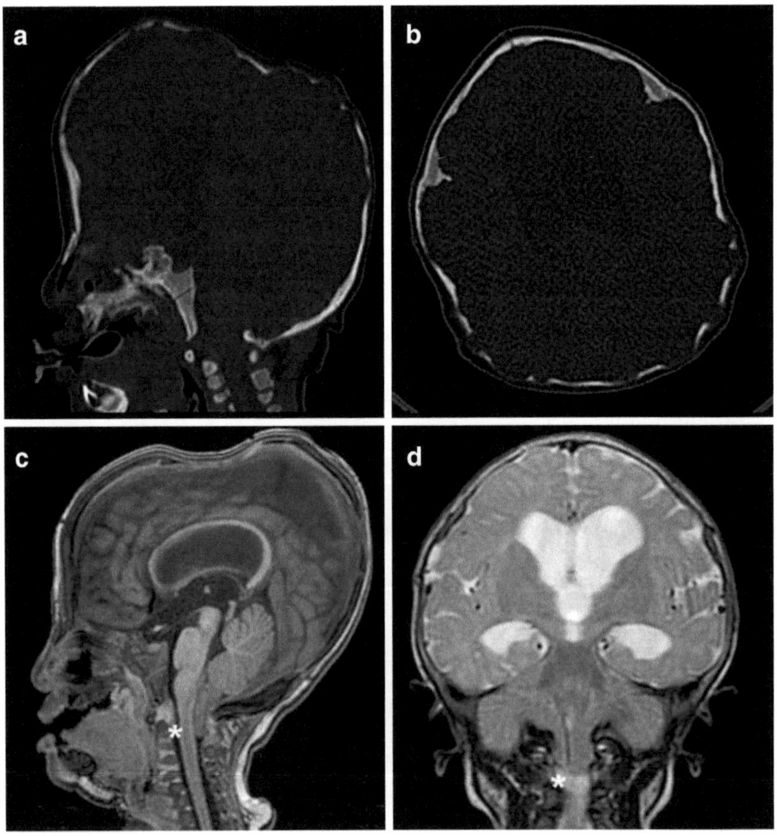

Fig. 19.1 Seven-month-old girl with Crouzon syndrome: (**a**, **b**) CT scan showing the early and severe pansynostosis with fingerprintings and sellar deformation of the cranial vault; (**c**, **d**) The MRI shows the severe hypoplasia of PCF with early CTH (**c**) and ventriculomegaly (**d**). The anteroposterior diameter of the foramen magnum is minimally reduced (**c**, asterisk), while the latero-lateral is reduced (**d**, asterisk)

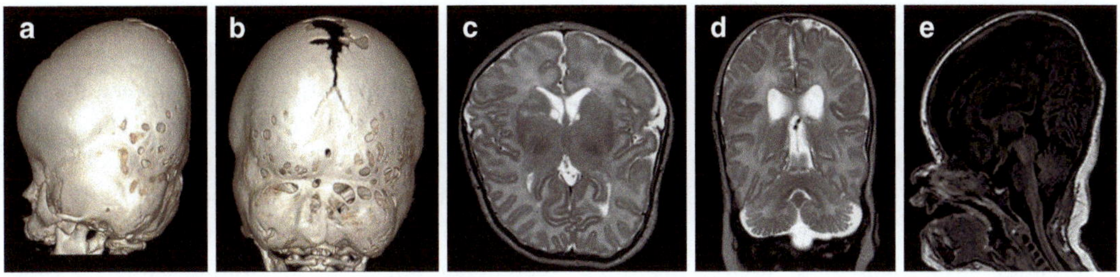

Fig. 19.2 Eight-month-old boy with Apert syndrome: (**a**, **b**) 3D CT scan showing acrocephaly and brachicephaly with partial fusion of the coronal and lambdoid sutures, fingerprintings and compensatory bilaterale mastoid bossing. (**c**–**e**) The MRI shows severe PCF hypoplasia, brachicephaly, mild ventriculomegaly but absence of CTH. The missing hindbrain herniation, compared with the Crouzon syndrome in Fig. 19.1, could depend on the incomplete closure of lambdoid sutures, the compensatory mastoid bossing and the large cisterna magna

nial vault expansion is another robust argument in favor of this theory [7].

Coll and colleagues enlarged the spectrum of etiologic factors by considering also the CSF in the occurrence of disproportion. The authors postulated that the presence of a small PCF would result in a mechanical increase in resistance to the CSF flow, which is complicated by the venous hypertension determined by the jugular foramina stenosis and by the foramen magnum stenosis with subsequent subarachnoid CSF blockage [3, 8]. This theory would explain also the occurrence of hydrocephalus in children with craniosynostosis and CTH. Accordingly, the following timeline should be considered. (a) progressive fusion of the lambdoid suture with secondary skull base alteration (the age below 2 years is critical because of the physiologically enlarged cerebellum compared with the forebrain); (b) stenosis of the jugular foramina; (c) growth of hypoplasic PCF; (d) cerebellar herniation; (e) venous hypertension; (f) crowding of the posterior fossa; and (g) CSF hydrodynamics alteration. Some basic and clinical genetic observations allow us to better understand the differences that can be found among syndromic children. For example, FGFR2 mutations involving exons 3a and 3c are more frequently encountered in craniosynostotic patients developing CIM [2, 4, 9]. Moreover, in spite of the shared FGFR2 involvement, Apert patients tend to have an enlarged basiocciput, while the Crouzon ones tend to show a narrowed one (and expanded supero-inferiorly rather than antero-posteriorly) with subsequent normal volume PCF in Apert syndrome and hypoplasic PCF in Crouzon syndrome [2, 10].

19.2.2 Radiological Findings

To further understand the PCF changes leading to CTH and their clinical implications, several bidimensional parameters have been investigated and their relationships have been studied. The main measures are represented by (1) PCF cephalic index: ratio between skull width (measured between the orifices of the right and left internal auditory canals) and skull length (measured from the posterior edge of the clivus to the inner table of the occiput); (2) tentorial angle: angle between the tentorium and a line running from the internal occipital protuberance to the tuberculum sellae; (3) occipital angle: angle between the tentorium and a line running from internal occipital protuberance to opisthion. According to some studies, CTH is more like to occur in syndromic and bicoronal synostoses than in single suture synostoses because of the brachycephalic skull and the vertical tentorium (high PCF cephalic index and large tentorial and occipital angle) [2, 11, 12]. In spite of the small PCF, in sagittal synostosis, the risk of CTH is inferior compared with the previous conditions because of the flat tentorium. Overall, craniosynostostic children with CTH have been found to show a significantly shorter anteroposterior PCF length than those without CTH (33.4 mm versus 36.7 mm) [13]. The PCF cross-sectional area too is significantly reduced in CTH children (654.1 versus 764.9 mm^2). As a result, the foramen magnum cross-sectional area in CTH children is about 88% of no-CTH children.

Additional information comes from the volumetric analysis of PCF. The study of Calandrelli et al. on children (both syndromic and non-syndromic) with lambdoid arch synostosis, showed an involvement of the lambdoid sutures alone (major sutures) in 40% of cases, of the minor sutures alone (occipito-mastoid and occipito-petrosal sutures) in another 40% of cases, and of both major and minor sutures in the remaining 20% of cases [14]. The comparison with healthy age-matched controls revealed normal measurements (included PCF volume, PCF brain volume, PCF volume/PCF brain volume ratio, cerebellum and CSF volume) except for the exocciput lengths and the anteroposterior diameter of the foramen magnum (significantly reduced) and the tentorial angle (significantly increased) in case of major sutures involvement. On the other hand, in case of minor sutures involvement, a significant increase of the tentorial angle and a significant decrease of meatus-opisthion lengths, diameters of the foramen magnum (both anteroposterior and latero-lateral) and jugular foramina area were found (once again, the volumetry as normal). These findings suggest that as follows: (1) In case of major sutures synostosis of the lambdoid arch, the PCF hypoplasia depends on a reduced exocciput length; therefore, the cerebellum is forced to growth both rostrally and caudally and, due to a normal anteroposterior diameter of the foramen magnum, early CTH occurs (80% of children with this condition harbored CTH) (Fig. 19.1). These data would explain also the higher incidence of CTH in isolated major suture involvement (e.g. asymmetrical, ipsilateral tonsillar herniation in lambdoid synostosis) than in minor one, even though both conditions are characterized by PCF hypoplasia; (2) In case of closure of minor lambdoid arch sutures, PCF is hypoplasic because of the reduced length of the two hemifossae; therefore, the cerebellum is allowed to growth mainly rostrally. Such a rostral growth of the cerebellum together with a complete reduction of the area of the foramen magnum gives reason for the absence of CTH in this subset of patients (CTH may occur later on, when the tentorium reaches its maximum slope). The combination between skull base anomalies and size of the foramen magnum has been recently confirmed to be crucial for the final position of the cerebellar tonsils in syndromic subjects, especially in Crouzon syndrome (largest foramen magnum) [15].

A mismatch between the reduced compliance of the skull base and the compensatory increase of the supratentorial cranial volume has been identified as the possible cause of CTH in children with severe sagittal synostosis [16]. Accordingly, anterior, middle and posterior cranial fossae are symmetric as well as the anterior and middle length of the skull base are increased in all scaphocephalic children. Similarly, the lengths of the posterior fossae are comparable in all children, independently form the severity of their sagittal synostosis (assessed by cephalic index). Nevertheless, the compensatory enlargement of the anterior fossae is relevant only in case of mild or moderate sagittal synostosis. On these grounds, it has been postulated that a spontaneous calvarial remodeling drives the anterior and middle skull base enlargement probably because the central section of the sagittal suture is the first to fuse. Subsequently, in case of the severe scaphocephaly, the minor elongation of the skull base would result from an earlier fusion of the sagittal suture. Under a volumetric point of view, this corresponds to a major compensatory intracranial volume in mild scaphocephalic forms compared with the severe ones. Actually, in spite of the normal overall PCF volume found in all scaphocephalic children, patients with moderate and severe groups showed a significant reduction of PCF volume/PCF brain volume ration and infratentorial CSF volume, thus revealing a "brain constriction" that leads to the hindbrain herniation in the more severe cases of sagittal synostosis.

The volumetric analysis also explains some apparently paradoxical findings, as the more frequently occurrence of CTH in some bicoronal synostosis than some bi-lambdoid ones. In the study provided by Rijken and coworkers, for example, children with Muenke syndrome showed both a bigger cerebellar (CV) and PCF volume (PFV) than those with Apert syndrome (in whom only PCF volume was larger than normal) [17]. For these reasons (together with the higher frequency of mega cisterna magna in Apert syndrome), Apert children show a significantly lower CV/PFV ratio and, therefore, a lower risk of CTH. The author proposed the CV/PFV ratio as a reliable indicator of PCF crowding because, even in case of significant PCF hypoplasia, CTH does not occur if also the cerebellum is hypoplasic.

It is worth noting that the volumetric analyses usually point out a normal volume of PCF in children with craniosynostosis and CTH. Therefore, CTH would result from the PCF overcrowding rather than PCF hypoplasia. A support to this theory comes from a study on the whole exome sequencing of 232 CIM families (668 patients), where CHD3 and CHD8 genes (chromodomain genes) were hypothesized to contribute to CTH genesis [18]. These genes are demonstrated to cause macrocephaly in zebrafishes and macrocephaly was predominant in the families enrolled for this study. Thus, one could conclude that CTH is the result of an excessive brain growth rather than a too small PCF. Moreover, also the presence of venous obstruction can help in justifying the occurrence of CTH and the differences among the various craniosynostoses and syndromes. Actually, the stenosis of the jugular foramina is an additional factor causing the increased risk of CTH in syndromic subjects (compared with non-syndromic ones) as well as the increased risk of CTH in Crouzon and Pfeiffer patients (higher incidence of jugular stenosis and more extensive venous collaterals) compared with Apert and Saethre-Chotzen ones [19, 20].

19.2.3 Altered CSF Dynamics

The aforementioned observations provide the basis to better understand the changes in the CSF dynamics possibly leading to hydrocephalus and syringomyelia, two diseases often associated with craniosynostosis-related CTH. The physiopathology of these two conditions is complex and not completely understood yet. The current theories, in particular, cannot explain why, starting from a similar anatomical picture, only some subjects develop hydrocephalus and/or syringomyelia.

Hydrocephalus is found in about 12–15% of syndromic craniosynostosis and up to 90% of hydrocephalic children with syndromic synostosis are affected by CTH too (Fig. 19.3) [21]. The impaired CSF circulation causing hydrocephalus in syndromic synostoses results from a vitious circle including all factors involved in the genesis of CTH: PCF hypoplasia, basilar invagination, foramen magnum overcrowding, compression of the IV ventricle, jugular foramina stenosis [2, 22]. Such a multifactorial etiology origins from the impairment of CSF circulation at level of the fourth ventricle (direct compression due to PCF

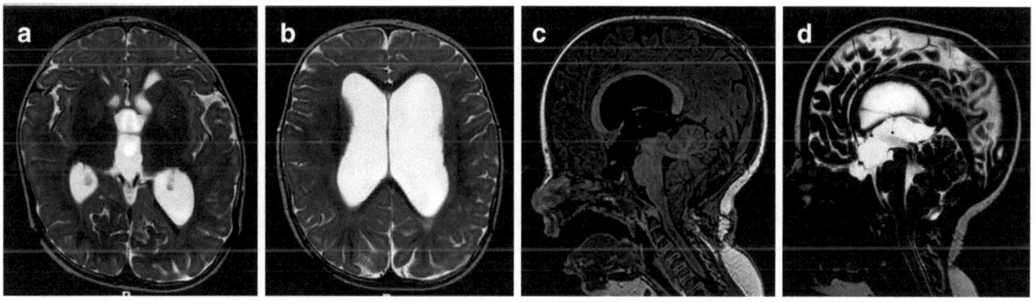

Fig. 19.3 MRI showing the typical features of supratentorial hydrocephalus in Crouzon syndrome (1 year-old boy). Note the enlargement of the third (**a**) and lateral ventricles (**b**) and the PCF hypoplasia with CTH (**c**). The posterior recess of the third ventricle is enlarged, the aqueduct is patent, and the CSF spaces of PCF are completely effaced (**d**): these findings suggest a CSF obstruction at level of IV ventricle/foramen magnum

overcrowding because of the cephalo-cranial disproportion and subsequent obstruction of the fourth ventricle outlets) and at level of the foramen magnum (limited CSF flow due to the overcrowding of the foramen magnum because of CTH). The raised ICP resulting from the impaired CSF circulation starts the vitious circle by worsening the foramen magnum overcrowding. At the same time, the stenosis of the jugular foramina enhances the vitious circle through the venous engorgement, which produces cerebellar edema (thus worsening the PCF overcrowding), raised intracranial pressure (by increasing the upward venous hypertension) and decreased CSF readsorption. When these mechanisms are activated, hydrocephalus occurs. The stenosis of the jugular foramina alone can induce hydrocephalus, even in case of normal PCF.

The prevented CSF outflow from the cranial compartment at level of an overcrowded foramen magnum would be responsible for the occurrence of syringomyelia. More in details, the foramen magnum overcrowding would generate an intra-extracranial CSF pressure gradient pulsating with the cardiac cycle. The resulting abnormal pressure waves would force the CSF to penetrate into the perivascular spaces of the spinal cord generating the syringomyelia [23], independently from the severity of the overcrowding and the tonsillar ectopia [24, 25]. In this context, the platybasia could play a role in favoring the syringomyelia and in differentiating CTH subjects with and without syringomyelia. Yan and coworkers hypothesized that the CSF turbulences and flow alterations occurring in the anterior aspect of the foramen magnum would be responsible for the syringomyelia formation [26]. Indeed, patients with more pronounced platybasia show a reduced pre-pontine and pre-bulbar cisternal space with consequent local turbulences in the anterior PCF compartment. The authors did not find differences in their 67 CTH patients as far as the PCF parameters were concerned (clival length, posterior fossa length and height, supraocciput length) apart from the clival gradient defining the platybasia (anterior angle between the clivus and McRae's line). Interestingly, the clival gradient of CTH patients without syringomyelia was similar to normal controls. The indirect CSF flow measurement by MRI cine sequences confirmed that the most relevant alterations of CSF flow occur in the anterior portion of the foramen magnum of CTH patients, in particular, some unilateral or bilateral small regions of the anterior quadrants [23]. The faster the CSF velocity flow in these regions, the higher the risk of syringomyelia. The decrease of CSF velocity flow in these regions after surgery accounts for the syringomyelia reduction or disappearance.

19.3 Peculiar Clinical Aspects

19.3.1 Non-syndromic Craniosynostosis

The aforementioned pathophysiological studies are useful to explain the occurrence of CTH in some types of not syndromic synostosis. As expected, the highest incidence is found in multisutural synostosis like Mercedes syndrome (60%) (Fig. 19.4) and oxycephaly (80–100%) [27, 28]. Among single suture synostosis, lambdoid craniosynostosis is the most involved one (60% of the affected children present CTH) followed by sagittal craniosynostosis (3–5%) [29–31]. Unicoronal craniosynostosis shows a higher incidence of CTH than sagittal synostosis in some series (6%) [31]. This is because of the secondary anterior attraction and shortening of one posterior hemi-fossa in this apparently less predisposing synostosis. However, a reason for the relatively low incidence of CTH in sagittal synostosis could be represented by the missed diagnosis of this craniosynostosis among CTH patients (Fig. 19.5). For example, Valentini et al. reported on 48 scaphocephalic children who received the diagnosis of CTH (mean age: 9 years) before the diagnosis of their previously unrecognized synostosis (mean age: 10.5 years) [32]. Interestingly, 21 children were completely asymptomatic (43%; mean tonsillar descent: 5–6 mm) and did not receive any treatment, while only 3 out of the remaining 27 subjects showed symptoms related to the craniosynostosis and were managed by cranial vault remodeling (24

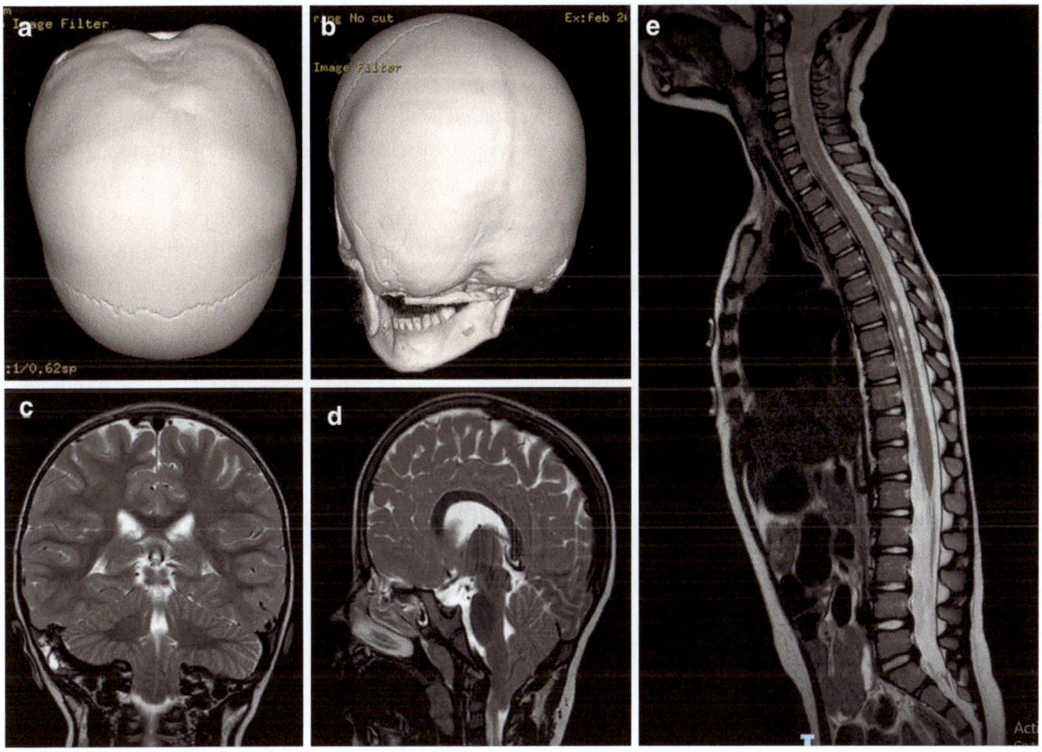

Fig. 19.4 Eight-month-old girl with Mercedes syndrome: (**a**, **b**) 3D CT scan showing the early sagittal and bi-lambdoid fusion with PCF indentation. The MRI demonstrates the bilateral CTH (**c**) with PCF hypoplasia (**d**) and dorsal syringomyelia (**e**)

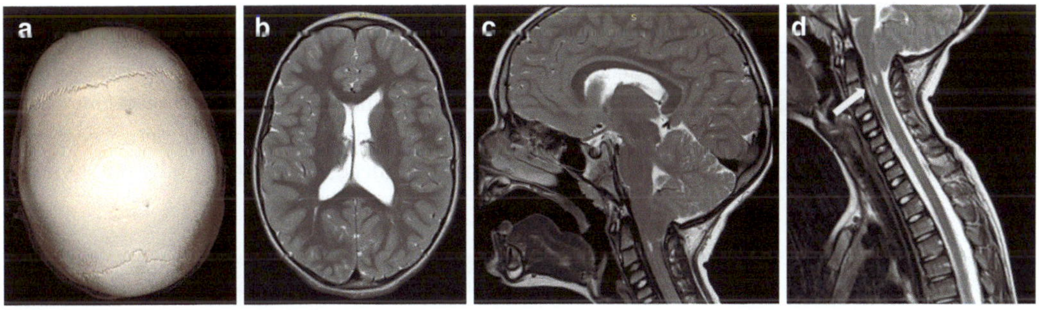

Fig. 19.5 Radiological picture of a 7-year-old boy with delayed diagnosis of sagittal synostosis. 3D CT scan shows the closure of the sagittal synostosis and a spontaneous bi-parietal expansion (**a**). MRI demonstrates a mild ventriculomegaly (**b**), moderate PCF hypoplasia with CTH (**c**) and a focal hydromyelic spot in the upper cervical spinal cord (**d**). The child, who presents symptoms of Chiari I without signs of raised ICP, is candidate to PCF decompression alone

children received surgery for CTH/syringomyelia; mean tonsillar descent: 12 mm). A further, possible cause of low incidence of CTH in non-syndromic craniosynostosis at diagnosis is the still incomplete expression of the clinical picture. Indeed, according to the largest series available in the literature about this topic (377 scaphocephalic children), the incidence of CTH was 1% among children with early diagnosis (2/161) versus 9.2% among those with delayed diagnosis

(20/216) [33]. As expected, the incidence was statistically significantly higher also in operated on patients (7%) compared with not operated on children (4.5%). Another typical example of delayed expression is the late appearance of CTH due to the delayed occurrence of a pansynostosis in children initially treated for a single suture synostosis and without genetic alterations [34]. The occurrence of CTH and syringomyelia in patients with delayed diagnosis of craniosynostosis has been reported even in adults [35].

CTH in non-syndromic subjects meanly varies from 5 to 12 mm [30] (Valentini et al. 2019). As far as the laterality of the tonsillar herniation is concerned, an asymmetry between the two sides is usually observed in the clinical practice, with a predominance to the synostotic suture side in asymmetric synostoses [28].

With regards to the primary clinical picture, it is hard to demonstrate symptoms of CTH/syringomyelia in children with single suture synostosis. Actually, if treated for the craniosynostosis within the standard rage of time (3–8 months), most of the patients tend to be asymptomatic both at the diagnosis (short clinical history) and at follow-up (CTH/syringomyelia are likely to have disappeared or improved). Moreover, if treated at the time of a delayed diagnosis of craniosynostosis, some symptoms can be confused with those caused by the synostosis (namely, headaches). Finally, most case of single suture synostosis are likely to present just a tonsils descent rather than a symptomatic Chiari I malformation. In the aforementioned series provided by Davies and coworkers, 27% of children with CTH in sagittal synostosis (6 out of 22) required treatment for their Chiari malformation [33]. In the series provided by Chivoret et al. on bi-lambdoid-sagittal synostosis, only 2 out of 19 subjects presented a symptomatic CTH [27]. Anyway, based on the clinical experiences reported in the literature, the most common signs or symptoms attributable to CTH/syringomyelia are headache, scoliosis, neck pain, gait disorders, dizziness, hydrocephalus, sleep apneas, and dysesthesias in the hands and feet [36–38] (Valentini et al. 2019).

19.3.2 Syndromic Craniosynostosis

The rate of CTH in syndromic subjects is as high as 2–10% in Apert syndrome, 50% in Pfeiffer syndrome, 70–75% in Crouzon syndrome and 100% in cloverleaf skull, Saethre-Chotzen syndrome being the less affected one (<2%) thanks to the enlarged cisterna magna [39, 40] (Fig. 19.6). Overall, the incidence of CTH in syndromic synostosis is around 14% (versus 1% in the general population) [41]. The reasons for such an incidence and such differences have been discussed in Sect. 19.2. Here, it is important to remind that CTH and the possibly associated syringomyelia are intrinsic part of the complex clinical picture of these patients and have to be considered for their appropriate management. Indeed, CTH is one of the predominant

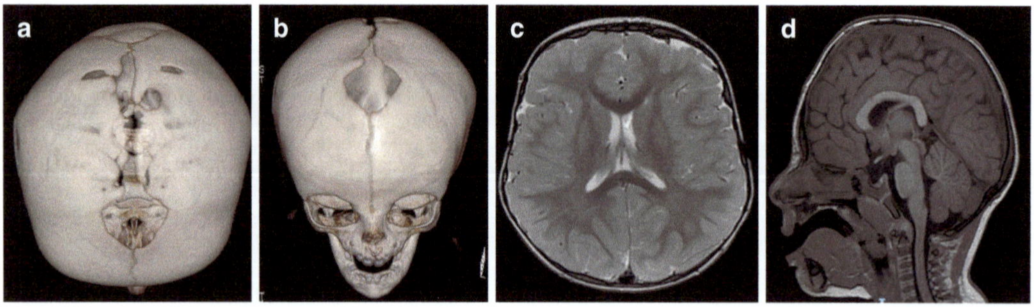

Fig. 19.6 Six-month-old boy with Saethre-Chotzen syndrome. 3D CT scan shows the premature bicoronal fusion with compensatory enlargement of anterior fontanel and sagittal suture (**a**, **b**). In spite of the subsequent brachicephaly, visible on MRI (**c**), CTH does not occur thanks to the large cisterna magna (**d**), which is a distinctive characteristic of this syndrome

clinical signs, together with facial dysmorphism, speech and language delay, learning difficulties, and behavioral problems even in recently detected syndromes, like the ERF-related craniosynostosis [42]. This entity arises from mutations in the ERF gene, which codes for ETS2 repressor factor. It is characterized by a sagittal and bi-lambdoid sutural pattern with late expression (mean age: 42 months), a Crouzon-like facial dysmorphology and frequent speech delay. CTH is the rule when the complete multisutural pattern is expressed. Another typical association between craniosynostosis and CTH can be found in patients with X-linked hypophosphatemic rickets. Accordingly, about 60% of these patients show a complete or partial sagittal synostosis and one-fourth of them present CTH [43].

As far as the clinical symptoms are concerned, the occurrence of neurological deficits seems to correlate with the presence of the synostosis rather with CTH/syringomyelia. This is mainly because of two reasons: (1) the diagnosis of the synostosis is generally obtained before the occurrence or the diagnosis of CTH, thus preventing the appearance of CTH symptoms thanks to the management of the synostosis in many cases (of course, CTH can persist even after the surgical treatment of the synostosis and can become symptomatic later on). The diagnosis of CTH before the syndromic synostosis has been exceptionally reported [44]; (2) The facio-cranial dysmorphism is basically more symptomatic at diagnosis than CTH (ocular proptosis, obstructive apnea syndrome, psychomotor delay, and so on). In the historical series by the Necker Hospital in Paris, indeed, only 6 out of 44 Crouzon patients and none out of 51 Apert patients showed CTH-related neurological symptoms [45]. In a recent study on 63 children with syndromic synostosis specifically addressing this topic, Doerga et al. did not find any difference between patients with and those without CTH/syringomyelia as far as the neurological symptoms were concerned [46]. Twenty out of 63 patients showed CTH and/or syringomyelia (32%), with a typical distribution: 16/34 with Crouzon syndrome, 2/11 with Muenke syndrome, 2/12 with Apert syndrome, and no cases out of 7 with Saethre-Chotzen syndrome. The neurological deficits (cerebellum: motor delay and coordination deficits; cranial nerve: nystagmus, pharyngeal asymmetry, and dysphagia; sensory-motor pathways: pyramidal syndrome, sensory dysfunction, and motor dysfunction) were present in 73% of cases, but there was no relationship between neurological picture and CTH/syringomyelia in any combinations matching the types of symptoms and CTH and/or syringomyelia. Only 3 out of 23 children undergoing surgery (all with Crouzon syndrome and presenting severe pyramidal syndrome and gait problems) harbored CTH and/or syringomyelia.

Also in syndromic subjects, CTH/syringomyelia typically cause headache, neck pain, ataxia, muscle weakness, altered sensation (paresthesia and dysesthesia), dysphagia, hydrocephalus, scoliosis, and obstructive apneas. The problem of central sleep apneas could be underestimated because of the predominant occurrence of obstructive sleep apneas. In their recent study on 89 syndromic children undergoing polysomnography and MRI, den Ottelander et al. did not find a significant rate of cervical cord compression by the odontoid process (compared with controls), but they detected an increased rate of compression at level of the foramen magnum in Crouzon children [47]. Such compressions as well as the age of the patients did not correlate with the obstructive apneas, while the age correlated with the central apneas. The authors concluded that the prevalence of central sleep apneas is low in this subset of patients (compared with obstructive apneas), and it is not associated with cervical spinal cord compression, but polysomnography is indicated in any case as important part of the clinical work-up. Central apneas usually improve significantly after foramen magnum decompression [48].

19.4 Preoperative Radiological Screening

The rationale for a radiological assessment in syndromic synostosis is quite obvious. Neuroimaging is actually required to define timing and modality of surgery and to define the optimal follow-up. Moreover, it is necessary to detect possible anomalies characterizing the clinical phenotype, such as extracranial (midface retrusion, high-arched palate or cleft lip and palate, widely spaced eyes, ptosis, proptosis…) or body anomalies (vertebral fusion, ankylosis, syndactyly, polydactyly, and heart malformation). However, a crucial reason to perform 3D CT scan of the skull, angio-MRI of the brain and MRI of the spinal cord in these subjects is to rule out associated diseases such as hydrocephalus (40–70% of cases), venous anomalies, callosum hypoplasia, syringomyelia, and CTH, the latter being the most common one (70–75%) [49].

The matter is more complicated in non-syndromic children with single suture craniosynostosis. Actually, some authors question the need for a neuroimaging screening in this subset of patients. Engel et al. emphasized that only one asymptomatic child with lambdoid synostosis out of 89 of their patients with isolated synostosis harbored CTH (1.1%), thus suggesting the avoidance of routine brain MRI in these patients unless symptomatic [50]. In spite of the limitation of this study (only 89 out of 215 children composing the entire series were investigated by MRI), this position could be acceptable when dealing with low-risk patients, as those with metopic or sagittal synostosis. However, in spite of the same low rate of CTH (1.2%) in their 80 patients with non-syndromic craniosynostosis, Magge and coworkers found other incidental findings (prominent extra-axial cerebrospinal fluid, ventriculomegaly, choroid fissure cyst, cavum septum pellucidum) in more than 50% of cases, 6.25% of them requiring an additional management just because of these findings [51]. The authors recommended the use of preoperative radiological screening. In their series of 121 non-syndromic children (most of them were scaphocephalic), all investigated by MRI, Hukki et al. found brain anomalies in 18% of cases [52]. The rate of CTH was 9%. These figures suggest, once again, that a preoperative imaging is useful also in single suture synostoses. On these grounds, the main problem would not concern the utility of preoperative neuroimaging but rather the use of preoperative MRI, which is burdened by the risk of anesthesia in young children. In the author's center, all non-syndromic children are screened by low-dose CT scan (according to pediatric protocols) and, if possible, by cerebral ultrasounds and doppler: only those with brain anomalies undergo preoperative (angio) MRI.

Instead, in case of lambdoid synostosis, the use of MRI has been demonstrated to be mandatory because of the high incidence of CTH (45–60% in single suture synostosis, 71% in complex synostosis) and PCF venous anomalies (36%), the possible occurrence of syringomyelia (4.5%), and the need to plan an appropriate management (e.g., simultaneous cranial vault remodeling and posterior fossa decompression) [29, 53]. Moreover, some synostoses require a radiological assessment by definition. This is the case, for example, of the craniosynostosis of the coronal arch, where CT scan is used to rule out the involvement of minor sutures (spheno-squamous and spheno-petrosal sutures) or to confirm the differential diagnosis (e.g., coronal suture synostosis versus fronto-sphenoidal synostosis), to correctly plan the surgical operation and to formulate a reliable prognosis based on the deformation of the skull base [54–56]. In these instances, CT scan can be utilized also to detect CIM (which, as mentioned, is not infrequent in coronal synostosis), thus driving the following use of MRI.

Furthermore, it is worth mentioning that, in several centers, a radiological assessment may be required not only for planning surgery but also for legal purposes. Of course, in these cases, the diagnosis can be first obtained by skull X-rays or ultrasounds, the use of CT scan or MRI being limited to doubtful cases [57]. However, "black bone" MRI, a peculiar sequence of fast MRI developed to investigate sutures, has been proposed to avoid CT scan-related radiation in these patients [58, 59]. Its modification could represent another useful tool to rule out CTH in this subset of patients without radiation (and sedation). In any case, once CTH is diagnosed, the presence of syringomyelia must be evaluated by MRI of the whole spinal cord.

19.5 Surgical Management

The management of CTH/syringomyelia still misses guidelines, also when associated with craniosynostosis. However, according to the recently published results of the International Consensus Conference on Chiari malformation and Syringomyelia held in 2019, most of the issues on the management of these conditions in children reached a significant agreement among the 34 international experts who were called to address this topic [60]. Those of interest for this chapter can be summarized as follows: (1) In CTH children with non-syndromic craniosynostosis, the craniosynostosis should be treated before CTH (agreement: 100%); (2) In infants with syndromic craniosynostosis and CTH, surgery should first aim at increasing the cranial volume, with a proper cranial vault remodeling for each syndrome (agreement: 90.9%); (3) In case of persistent CTH in children already treated for their syndromic craniosynostosis, the surgical management depends on syndrome, cranial volume obtained by previous operations, posterior fossa volume, and CTH symptoms/associated syringomyelia (agreement: 100%); (4) In symptomatic children with CTH and hydrocephalus, hydrocephalus should be treated first to relieve raised intracranial pressure and to avoid postoperatory complications. CTH can be treated afterwards if symptoms do not disappear (agreement: 90.9%).

19.5.1 The Craniosynostosis Should Be Treated First by Increasing the Cranial Volume

The indication to surgery in children with craniosynostosis and CTH/syringomyelia is provided according to the clinical picture (presence of symptomatic synostosis and/or CTH/syringomyelia and/or progressing syringomyelia) and the need to prevent of the PCF narrowing [2, 17]. To treat CTH/syringomyelia, independently from the synostosis, could be a valid option in subjects with symptomatic CTH/syringomyelia and stabilized synostosis [61, 62]. As for the rest, there is a wide agreement on to address the treatment of the craniosynostosis as first step because of the secondary character of CTH, which results from the synostosis and its consequences (PCF hypoplasia, venous engorgement and so on). The rationale of the initial treatment, therefore, is to perform a cranial decompression aiming at protecting the brain structures (especially the vital ones of the PCF), decompressing the venous outflows, and preventing at the same time the occurrence or the worsening of hydrocephalus and/or CTH/syringomyelia.

In case of exclusive involvement of lambdoid arch sutures, the gold standard management is represented by the posterior cranial vault expansion. This can be realized through a fixed bi-occipital expansion or by a posterior distraction advancement [63]. The description of the techniques goes beyond the goals of this paragraph, since they are reported in other chapters. Here, it is important to remind that the technique should be tailored on each patient's characteristics. The posterior distraction, for example, has the advantage of shorter operative times and lower rate of blood transfusion (because of the reduced manipulation of bones and dural sinuses) compared with fixed occipital expansion but, at the same time, it is burdened by the risk of skull fractures due to the implants, breaking or dislocations of the distractors, and by the need of a second operation to remove the implants themselves [5]. Although some of these limits can be overcome by resorbable distractors, the posterior distraction should be used in children not too small and with an enough thick bone. On the other hand, the fixed posterior expansion is not limited by the use of mechanical tools but by the need to detach the bone from the dura that, often, takes long operation times and a risk of significant blood losses. Therefore, this option is considered mainly in small infants, where the distractor devices cannot be utilized. To reduce the morbidity resulting from the blood losses, a posterior expansion obtained by free bone flaps is successfully used in many centers in infants with honeycomb bones to achieve a good decompression and to gain time for the anterior vault advancement [64].

In case of involvement of other sutures or pansinostosis already at the diagnosis, as not infrequently happens in Crouzon subjects, a total calvarial remodeling is advised to manage CTH/syringomyelia [27, 31, 40]. The discussion, in this instance, concerns the use of the total cranial vault expansion versus the use of the posterior distraction alone, the concurrent performance of a suboccipital decompression and, in case of suboccipital decompression, the need to open the dura and to perform a cervical decompression. The total vault reconstruction is of course the most "radical" approach, which ensures good results not only on the synostosis but also on CTH [65]. It is usually indicated in children with the most severe picture of synostosis, where an (early) fronto-orbital advancement is needed. The total vault remodeling can be realized by a single procedure, using the prone position with hyperextension of the head to manage both the occipital expansion and the front-orbital advancement [66]. However, in children with CTH, it seems more reasonable to avoid such a prolonged hyperextension of the neck and to realize the operation in two steps, by alternating the prone (occipital expansion) and the supine position (fronto-orbital advancement). The two steps approach offers also the advantage to include the treatment of hydrocephalus, if required [37].

Currently, however, the posterior calvarial distraction alone is more and more proposed, even in children with syndromic pansynostosis, to manage CTH and syringomyelia. This approach is actually indicated mainly in patients, where CTH/syringomyelia (and the hypoplasic PCF) represent the main clinical problem. Nevertheless, the posterior distraction has been proved to increase not only the PCF volume but also the supratentorial volume, thus providing an advantage also on the overall management of the synostosis. Actually, Lo et al. observed that only 2 out of their 16 cases managed by posterior distraction needed a fronto-orbital advancement later (one of them only for cosmetic purposes), as result of the increased supratentorial volume [67]. The series was composed of 14 children with pansynostosis (8 of them were syndromic subjects) and 2 cases of bi-lambdoid synostosis. CTH meanly improved from 9.3 to 6.0 mm, while syringomyelia was reduced from 7.9 to 3.1 mm in thickness and from 203 to 136 mm in length (all these results were statistically significant). Hydrocephalus needed a separate treatment in two cases. In their series of 72 children with craniosynostosis (64.3% with syndromes), Lin and coworkers found a major protection against the new appearance of CTH in children undergoing posterior cranial distraction (1 out of 49 cases) compared with those receiving total vault reconstruction (4 out of 23 cases) [68]. No significant differences were detected between the two techniques about the occurrence of hydrocephalus.

A further point of discussion concerns the "direct" increase of PCF volume by the use of PCF suboccipital decompression in addition to total cranial vault remodeling or posterior cranial distraction. The rationale of a focused PCF decompression in the context of a wide decompression of the skull is to give the PCF an immediate relief from their constriction, namely in children with clear CTH/syringomyelia symptoms or, if asymptomatic, with significant hindbrain herniation/constriction and/or large and progressing syringomyelia. However, in several centers, such an indication is extended to every craniosynostotic patient with CTH/syringomyelia because of the possibility to reduce the occurrence or progression of CTH with a one-step operation carried out for the synostosis [29, 69]. Scott et al., for example, combined the posterior vault remodeling with the suboccipital decompression in 34 children (80% were syndromic) just because of the coexistence of synostosis and CTH [70]. The procedure was effective (only two patients require a further treatment of CTH, 19 and 36 months after the first surgery) and the authors did not detect intraoperative problems or relevant complications. Other authors, instead, question the usefulness of this approach due to the effectiveness of the posterior remodeling/distraction alone in improving CTH [71]. To avoid the suboccipital decompression allows also to reduce the operation times and morbidity. In the author of this chapter's experience, the suboccipital decompression is combined to the posterior expansion whenever possible, but it is not carried out at any cost. More in details, in case of posterior expansion, the skin flap is designed to expose and decompress also the foramen magnum so that the procedure is realized with a single surgical field. When the anatomical conditions or the kind of operation are not favorable to realize a single wound incision, a second, suboccipital skin incision is performed but only if the PCF decompression is clinically necessary and the need to perform a C1 laminectomy is expected. In case of profuse dural bleeding during the posterior expansion, the suboccipital decompression is not performed or, if necessary, it is postponed, waiting for the improvement of the intracranial hypertension and the venous engorgement.

Generally, the dural opening and the duraplasty are not routinely required (unless the clinical and/or radiological picture is severe: e.g., significant brainstem compression); they are even contraindicated in several patients because of the copious bleeding from the dural sinuses [31, 40].

19.5.2 Persistent CTH

As mentioned above, old children with stabilized synostosis and previously asymptomatic CTH are managed following as for Chiari malformation and syringomyelia, if they have become symptomatic (Fig. 19.5). Accordingly, a suboccipital PCF decompression alone versus a dural opening with or without shrinkage of the cerebellar tonsils are considered according to the clinical and radiological picture. On the other hand, if an adequate cranial volume has not been achieved after the previous cranial vault expansion and/or signs and symptoms of raised intracranial pressure are still present, CTH/syringomyelia are better managed by performing a new skull expansion [31, 36]. Once again, the surgical technique (posterior expansion or distraction versus total cranial vault remodeling) should be tailored on the patient's characteristics.

19.5.3 Hydrocephalus Should Be Treated First

Significant venous anomalies and ventriculomegaly/hydrocephalus are found in 35% and 52% of children with craniosynostosis and CTH, respectively [31]. Although the venous anomalies are crucial in the pathogenesis (namely, the stenosis of the jugular foramina), their management is limited to the diagnostic work-up, an operative approach being usually unnecessary or even contraindicated [72]. Actually, if the attempt at decreasing the venous engorgement by cranial vault expansion is the rule, the direct bony decompression of venous outflows is risky and often insufficient.

On the other hand, hydrocephalus represents a common operative issue. The indication to treat the hydrocephalus first originates from the association between this condition and Chiari I malformation. In CTH subjects, indeed, hydrocephalus is likely to result from the impaired CSF circulation due to the compression of the fourth ventricle. Such hydrocephalus is "obstructive" and, therefore, it can be successfully treated by endoscopic third ventriculostomy (ETV) in the great majority of cases [73] (Fig. 19.3). It is treated first because usually more symptomatic than CTH and also to prevent a cerebellar ptosis in case of suboccipital decompression (and persistent hydrocephalus). In children with synostosis and CTH-related hydrocephalus, however, the matter is a little different. First of all, it has to be considered that hydrocephalus complicated very rarely the clinical course of single suture synostoses; therefore, the management of these subjects is tailored according to etiology and the clinical picture of each patient. Once again, it is advisable to treat the hydrocephalus before the surgical correction of the synostosis to normalize the intracranial pressure before opening the cranial sutures and to reduce CSF-related complications [74]. ETV or ventriculoperitoneal shunt (VPS) are proposed according to the type of hydrocephalus. Second, in multisutural synostoses of syndromic children, where hydrocephalus is common, the symptomatic hydrocephalus should be differentiated by the non-tense ventriculomegaly. The latter condition, usually found in Apert subjects, can be managed by clinical and radiological monitoring. The active hydrocephalus, present in 12–15% of cases (up to more than 80% in some syndromes, like Pfeiffer II), on the other side, may require an operative approach [75]. In these instances, if the hydrocephalus is not clinically predominant, it is advisable to start the surgical treatment by cranial vault expansion with the twin goal to relieve from intracranial pressure and to avoid a worsening of the cranio-cerebral disproportion (that could lead to an increase of CTH/syringomyelia). Moreover, the cranial vault expansion (namely, the increased volume of PCF) has been proved to stabilize the hydrocephalus itself, thanks to the re-opening of the fourth ventricle outlets, at least in the early follow-up [5]. On the contrary, if hydrocephalus is clinically prominent, it has to treated first because of the aforementioned reasons. A successful treatment of hydrocephalus is expected to improve also the associated alterations of CSF dynamics, like syringomyelia. Once again, ETV, if feasible, is the first option for the treatment of this kind of hydrocephalus because it offers a good rate of success (about 65%) and allows to avoid the worsening of the cranio-cerebral disproportion [76]. If ETV is not feasible or has failed, extrathecal CSF shunting remains the last resource. VPS does not represent the first option, indeed, because it favors the cranial shrinkage (working in contrast to the cranial vault expansion) and because of its well-known complications. The use of self-regulating valves and antisyphon devices can help in reducing the risk of slit ventricles syndrome/increased cranio-cerebral disproportion. Third, it is worth noting that hydrocephalus may progress from ventriculomegaly, often after cranial vault expansion/PCF decompression [40, 75]. In these instances, it is mandatory to carry on a clinical and radiological monitoring and, in doubtful cases, to perform a measurement of the intracranial pressure to identify the candidate to ETV or VP shunt.

References

1. Jeffery N. Differential regional brain growth and rotation of the prenatal human tentorium cerebelli. J Anat. 2002;200(Pt 2):135–44.
2. Cinalli G, Spennato P, Sainte-Rose C, Arnaud E, Aliberti F, Brunelle F, Cianciulli E, Renier D. Chiari malformation in craniosynostosis. Childs Nerv Syst. 2005;21:889–901.
3. Coll G, Lemaire J-J, Di Rocco F, Barthélémy I, Garcier J-M, De Schlichting E, Sakka L. Human foramen magnum area and posterior cranial fossa volume growth in relation to cranial base synchondrosis closure in the course of child development. Neurosurgery. 2016;79:722–35.
4. Coll G, Abed Rabbo F, Jecko V, Sakka L, Di Rocco F, Delion M. The growth of the posterior cranial fossa in FGFR2-induced faciocraniosynostosis: a review. Neurochirurgie. 2019;65:221–7.
5. Tamburrini G, Caldarelli M, Gasparini G, Pelo S, Di Rocco C. Complex craniosynostoses: a review of the prominent clinical features and the related management strategies. Childs Nerv Syst. 2012;28:1511–23.
6. Thompson DNP. Chiari I malformation and associated syringomyelia. In: Di Rocco C, Pang D, Rutka JT, editors. Textbook of pediatric neurosurgery. Cham: Springer; 2020. p. 2709–32.
7. Winston KR, Stence NV, Boylan AJ, Beauchamp KM. Upward translation of cerebellar tonsils following surgical expansion of supratentorial cranial vault: a unified biomechanical explanation of Chiari type I. Pediatr Neurosurg. 2015;50:243–9.
8. Coll G, El Ouadih Y, Abed Rabbo F, Jecko V, Sakka L, Di Rocco F. Hydrocephalus and Chiari malformation pathophysiology in FGFR2-related faciocraniosynostosis: a review. Neurochirurgie. 2019;65:264–8.
9. Fujisawa H, Hasegawa M, Kida S, Yamashita J. A novel fibroblast growth factor receptor 2 mutation in Crouzon syndrome associated with Chiari type I malformation and syringomyelia. J Neurosurg. 2002;97:396–400.
10. Richtsmeier JT. Comparative study of normal, Crouzon, and Apert craniofacial morphology using finite element scaling analysis. Am J Phys Anthropol. 1987;74:473–93.
11. Beez T, Koppel D, Sangra M. Morphometric analysis of the posterior cranial fossa in syndromic and nonsyndromic craniosynostosis. J Craniofac Surg. 2017;28:e484–8.
12. Coll G, Arnaud E, Collet C, Brunelle F, Sainte-Rose C, Di Rocco F. Skull base morphology in fibroblast growth factor receptor type 2-related faciocraniosynostosis: a descriptive analysis. Neurosurgery. 2015;76:571–83.

13. Leikola J, Haapamäki V, Karppinen A, Koljonen V, Hukki J, Valanne L, Koivikko M. Morphometric comparison of foramen magnum in non-syndromic craniosynostosis patients with or without Chiari I malformation. Acta Neurochir. 2012;154:1809–13.
14. Calandrelli R, D'Apolito G, Panfili M, Massimi L, Caldarelli M, Colosimo C. Role of "major" and "minor" lambdoid arch sutures in posterior cranial fossa changes: mechanism of cerebellar tonsillar herniation in infants with multisutural craniosynostosis. Childs Nerv Syst. 2016;32:451–9.
15. den Ottelander BK, Dremmen MHG, de Planque CA, van der Oest MJW, Mathijssen IMJ, van Veelen MC. Does the association between abnormal anatomy of the skull base and cerebellar tonsillar position also exist in syndromic craniosynostosis? J Plast Reconstr Aesthet Surg. 2021;22:S1748–6815.
16. Calandrelli R, Pilato F, Massimi L, Panfili M, Colosimo C. A systematic quantitative morpho-volumetric analysis in infants with sagittal craniosynostosis and relationship with the severity of scaphocephalic deformity. Radiol Med. 2020;125:585–94.
17. Rijken BFM, Lequin MH, van der Lijn F, van Veelen-Vincent M-LC, de Rooi J, Hoogendam YY, Niessen WJ, Mathijssen IMJ. The role of the posterior fossa in developing Chiari I malformation in children with craniosynostosis syndromes. J Craniomaxillofac Surg. 2015;43:813–9.
18. Sadler B, Wilborn J, Antunes L, Kuensting T, Hale AT, Gannon SR, McCall K, Cruchaga C, Harms M, Voisin N, Reymond A, Cappuccio G, Brunetti-Pierri N, Tartaglia M, Niceta M, Leoni C, Zampino G, Ashley-Koch A, Urbizu A, Garrett ME, Soldano K, Macaya A, Conrad D, Strahle J, Dobbs MB, Turner TN, Shannon CN, Brockmeyer D, Limbrick DD, Gurnett CA, Haller G. Rare and de novo coding vari ants in chromodomain genes in Chiari I malformation. Am J Hum Genet. 2021;108(2):368.
19. Ghali GZ, Zaki Ghali MG, Ghali EZ, Srinivasan VM, Wagner KM, Rothermel A, Taylor J, Johnson J, Kan P, Lam S, Britz G. Intracranial venous hypertension in craniosynostosis: mechanistic underpinnings and therapeutic implications. World Neurosurg. 2019;127:549–58.
20. Protzenko T, Bellas A, Cunha Ribeiro CM, de Carvalho Gonzalez SM, Gandelman Horovitz DD. Venous anomalies in hypoplastic posterior fossa: unsolved questions. Childs Nerv Syst. 2021;7:3177–87.
21. Massimi L, Pennisi G, Frassanito P, Tamburrini G, Di Rocco C, Caldarelli M. Chiari type I and hydrocephalus. Childs Nerv Syst. 2019;35:1701–9.
22. Di Rocco C, Frassanito P, Massimi L, Peraio S. Hydrocephalus and Chiari type I malformation. Childs Nerv Syst. 2011;27:1653–64.
23. Iskandar BJ, Quigley M, Haughton VM. Foramen magnum cerebrospinal fluid flow characteristics in children with Chiari I malformation before and after craniocervical decompression. J Neurosurg. 2004;101(2 Suppl):169–78.
24. McGirt MJ, Atiba A, Attenello FJ, Wasserman BA, Datoo G, Gathinji M, Carson B, Weingart JD, Jallo GI. Correlation of hindbrain CSF flow and outcome after surgical decompression for Chiari I malformation. Childs Nerv Syst. 2008;24:833–40.
25. Shaffer N, Martin BA, Rocque B, Madura C, Wieben O, Iskandar BJ, Dombrowski S, Luciano M, Oshinski JN, Loth F. Cerebrospinal fluid flow impedance is elevated in type I Chiari malformation. J Biomech Eng. 2014;136:021012.
26. Yan H, Han X, Jin M, Liu Z, Xie D, Sha S, Qiu Y, Zhu Z. Morphometric features of posterior cranial fossa are different between Chiari I malformation with and without syringomyelia. Eur Spine J. 2016;25:2202–9.
27. Chivoret N, Arnaud E, Giraudat K, O'Brien F, Pamphile L, Meyer P, Renier D, Collet C, Di Rocco F. Bilambdoid and sagittal synostosis: report of 39 cases. Surg Neurol Int. 2018;9:206.
28. Karppinen A, Koljonen V, Valanne L, Leikola J. Asymmetric laterality of Chiari type I malformation in patients with non-syndromic single-suture craniosynostosis. Acta Neurochir. 2012;154:2103–7.
29. Fearon JA, Dimas V, Ditthakasem K. Lambdoid craniosynostosis: the relationship with Chiari deformations and an analysis of surgical outcomes. Plast Reconstr Surg. 2016;137:946–51.
30. Leikola J, Koljonen V, Valanne L, Hukki J. The incidence of Chiari malformation in nonsyndromic, single suture craniosynostosis. Childs Nerv Syst. 2010;26:771–4.
31. Strahle J, Muraszko KM, Buchman SR, Kapurch J, Garton HJL, Maher CO. Chiari malformation associated with craniosynostosis. Neurosurg Focus. 2011;31:E2.
32. Valentini LG, Saletti V, Erbetta A, Chiapparini L, Furlanetto M. Chiari 1 malformation and untreated sagittal synostosis: a new subset of complex Chiari? Childs Nerv Syst. 2019;35(10):1741–53. https://doi.org/10.1007/s00381-019-04283-0. Epub 2019 Jul 21
33. Davis AA, Zuccoli G, Haredy MM, Runkel L, Losee J, Pollack IF, Tamber MS, Tyler-Kabara E, Goldstein JA, Nischal KK. The incidence of Chiari malformations in patients with isolated sagittal synostosis. Plast Reconstr Surg Glob Open. 2019;7:e2090.
34. Poggi J, Chen WS, Taylor HO, Sullivan S, Woo AS, Klinge PM. Revisiting the resolution of Chiari malformation in nonsyndromic craniosynostosis: a case of posterior cranial vault reconstruction in secondary pan-suture synostosis. World Neurosurg. 2020;143:158–62.
35. Sano M, Yoshimura J, Fujii Y. Adult Chiari type 1 malformation with holocord syringomyelia associated with sagittal synostosis. NMC Case Rep J. 2018;5:27 30.
36. Feller C, Jensen JN, Lew SM. Chiari malformation Type 1 and syringomyelia in a patient with prior surgically-treated sagittal synostosis effectively

treated with posterior cranial vault distraction osteogenesis. J Craniofac Surg. 2021;32:2110–3.
37. Konar S, Shukla D. Bilateral lambdoid and sagittal craniosynostosis with hydrocephalus: ETV, bifrontal craniotomy, anterior cranial vault remodeling, and posterior cranial vault expansion. Neurol India. 2021;69:592–4.
38. Pouratian N, Sansur CA, Newman SA, Jane JA Jr, Jane JA Sr. Chiari malformations in patients with uncorrected sagittal synostosis. Surg Neurol. 2007;67:422–7.
39. de Jong T, Rijken BF, Lequin MH, van Veelen ML, Mathijssen IM. Brain and ventricular volume in patients with syndromic and complex craniosynostosis. Childs Nerv Syst. 2012;28:137–40.
40. Hinojosa J. Syndromic craniosynlstosis. In: Di Rocco C, Pang D, Rutka JT, editors. Textbook of pediatric neurosurgery. Springer; 2020. p. 1–31.
41. Jansen PR, Dremmen M, van den Berg A, Dekkers IA, Blanken LME, Muetzel RL, Bolhuis K, Mulder RM, Kocevska D, Jansen TA, de Wit M-CY, Neuteboom RF, Polderman TJC, Posthuma D, Jaddoe VWV, Verhulst FC, Tiemeier H, van der Lugt A, White TJH. Incidental findings on brain imaging in the general pediatric population. N Engl J Med. 2017;377:1593–5.
42. Glass GE, O'Hara J, Canham N, Cilliers D, Dunaway D, Fenwick AL, Jeelani NO, Johnson D, Lester T, Lord H, Morton JEV, Nishikawa H, Noons P, Schwiebert K, Shipster C, Taylor-Beadling A, Twigg SRF, Vasudevan P, Wall SA, Wilkie AOM, Wilson LC. ERF-related craniosynostosis: the phenotypic and developmental profile of a new craniosynostosis syndrome. Am J Med Genet A. 2019;179:615–27.
43. Rothenbuhler A, Fadel N, Debza Y, Bacchetta J, Diallo MT, Adamsbaum C, Linglart A, Di Rocco F. High incidence of cranial synostosis and Chiari I malformation in children with X-linked hypophosphatemic rickets (XLHR). J Bone Miner Res. 2019;34:490–6.
44. Canpolat A, Akçakaya MO, Altunrende E, Ozlü AM, Duman H, Ton T, Akdemir O. Chiari type I malformation yielded to the diagnosis of Crouzon syndrome. J Neurosci Rural Pract. 2014;5:81–3.
45. Cinalli G, Renier D, Sebag G, Sainte-Rose C, Arnaud E, Pierre-Kahn A. Chronic tonsillar herniation in Crouzon's and Apert's syndromes: the role of premature synostosis of the lambdoid suture. J Neurosurg. 1995;83:575–82.
46. Doerga PN, Rijken BFM, Bredero-Boelhouwer H, Joosten KFM, Neuteboom RF, Tasker RC, Dremmen MHG, Lequin MH, van Veelen MLC, Mathijssen IMJ. Neurological deficits are present in syndromic craniosynostosis patients with and without tonsillar herniation. Eur J Paediatr Neurol. 2020;28:120–5.
47. den Ottelander BK, de Goederen R, de Planque CA, Baart SJ, van Veelen MLC, Corel LJA, Joosten KFM, Mathijssen IMJ, Dremmen MHG. Cervical spinal cord compression and sleep-disordered breathing in syndromic craniosynostosis. Am J Neuroradiol. 2021;42:201–5.
48. Addo NK, Javadpour S, Kandasamy J, Sillifant P, May P, Sinha A. Central sleep apnea and associated Chiari malformation in children with syndromic craniosynostosis: treatment and outcome data from a supraregional national craniofacial center. J Neurosurg Pediatr. 2013;11:296–301.
49. Massimi L, Bianchi F, Frassanito P, Calandrelli R, Tamburrini G, Caldarelli M. Imaging in craniosynostosis: when and what? Childs Nerv Syst. 2019;35:2055–69.
50. Engel M, Castrillón-Oberndorfer G, Hoffmann J, Orakcioglu B, Rohde S, Seeberger R, Freudlsperger C. Chiari malformation in nonsyndromal single craniosynostosis—much ado about nothing? Acta Neurochir. 2012;154:1803–7.
51. Magge KT, Magge SN, Keating RF, Myseros JS, Boyajian MJ, Sauerhammer TM, Rogers GF, Oh AK. Incidental findings on preoperative computed tomography for nonsyndromic single suture craniosynostosis. J Craniofac Surg. 2014;25:1327–30.
52. Hukki A, Koljonen V, Karppinen A, Valanne L, Leikola J. Brain anomalies in 121 children with nonsyndromic single suture craniosynostosis by MR imaging. Eur J Paediatr Neurol. 2012;6:671–5.
53. Ranganathan K, Rampazzo A, Hashmi A, Muraszko K, Strahle J, Vercler CJ, Buchman SR. The role of preoperative imaging in the management of nonsyndromic lambdoid craniosynostosis. J Craniofac Surg. 2018;29:36–9.
54. Calandrelli R, D'Apolito G, Massimi L, Gaudino S, Visconti E, Pelo S, Di Rocco C, Colosimo C. Quantitative analysis of craniofacial dysmorphology in infants with anterior synostotic plagiocephaly. Childs Nerv Syst. 2016;32:2339–49.
55. Calandrelli R, Pilato F, Massimi L, Panfili M, Di Rocco C, Colosimo C. Quantitative analysis of cranial-orbital changes in infants with anterior synostotic plagiocephaly. Childs Nerv Syst. 2018;34:1725–33.
56. Di Rocco C, Paternoster G, Caldarelli M, Massimi L, Tamburrini G. Anterior plagiocephaly: epidemiology, clinical findings, diagnosis, and classification. Childs Nerv Syst. 2012;28:1413–22.
57. Mathijssen IMJ. Guideline for care of patients with the diagnoses of craniosynostosis: working group on craniosynostosis. J Craniofac Surg. 2015;26:1735–807.
58. Eley KA, Watt-Smith SR, Sheerin F, Golding SJ. "Black bone" MRI: a potential alternative to CT with three-dimensional reconstruction of the craniofacial skeleton in the diagnosis of craniosynostosis. Eur Radiol. 2014;24:2417–26.
59. Low XZ, Lim MC, Nga V, Sundar G, Tan AP. Clinical application of "black bone" imaging in paediatric craniofacial disorders. Br J Radiol. 2021;94:20200061.
60. Massimi L, Peretta P, Erbetta A, Solari A, Farinotti M, Ciaramitaro P, Saletti V, Caldarelli M, Canheu AC, Celada C, Chiapparini L, Chieffo D, Cinalli G, Di Rocco F, Furlanetto M, Giordano F, Jallo G, James S, Lanteri P, Lemarchand C, Messing-Jünger M, Parazzini C, Paternoster G, Piatelli G, Poca MA, Prabahkar P, Ricci F, Righini A, Sala F, Sahuquillo

J, Stoodley M, Talamonti G, Thompson D, Triulzi F, Zucchelli M, Valentini L, International Experts—Jury of the Chiari & Syringomyelia Consensus Conference, "Milan, November 11–13, 2019". Diagnosis and treatment of Chiari malformation type 1 in children: the International Consensus Document. Neurol Sci. 2021; https://doi.org/10.1007/s10072-021-05317-9.
61. Aransay-Garcia A, Villarejo-Ortega F. Treatment of syringomyelia in patients with Chiari malformation and craniosynostosis. A case report and review of the literature. Rev Neurol. 2016;63:455–9. [Spanish].
62. Sakamoto H, Matsusaka Y, Kunihiro N, Imai K. Physiological changes and clinical implications of syndromic craniosynostosis. J Korean Neurosurg Soc. 2016;59:204–13.
63. Nowinski D, Di Rocco F, Renier D, SainteRose C, Leikola J, Arnaud E. Posterior cranial vault expansion in the treatment of craniosynostosis. Comparison of current techniques. Childs Nerv Syst. 2012;28:1537–154.
64. Tamburrini G, Offi M, Massimi L, Frassanito P, Bianchi F. Posterior vault "free-floating" bone flap: indications, technique, advantages, and drawbacks. Childs Nerv Syst. 2021;37:3143–7.
65. Esparza J, Hinojosa J. Complications in the surgical treatment of craniosynostosis and craniofacial syndromes: a propos of 306 transcranial procedures. Childs Nerv Syst. 2008;24:1421–30.
66. Pollack IF, Losken HW, Hurwitz DJ. A combined frontoorbital and occipital advancement technique for use in total calvarial reconstruction. J Neurosurg. 1996;84:424–9.
67. Lo WB, Thant KZ, Kaderbhai J, White N, Nishikawa H, Dover MS, Evans M, Rodrigues D. Posterior calvarial distraction for complex craniosynostosis and cerebellar tonsillar herniation. J Neurosurg Pediatr. 2020;10:1–10.
68. Lin LO, Zhang RS, Hoppe IC, Paliga JT, Swanson JW, Bartlett SP, Taylor JA. Onset and resolution of Chiari malformations and hydrocephalus in syndromic craniosynostosis following posterior vault distraction. Plast Reconstr. 2019;144:932–40.
69. Sofos SS, Robertson B, Duncan C, Sinha A. Delayed presentation of isolated sagittal synostosis with raised intracranial pressure and secondary Chiari malformation with cervical syringomyelia. J Craniofac Surg. 2017;28:1334–6.
70. Scott WW, Fearon JA, Swift DM, Sacco DJ. Suboccipital decompression during posterior cranial vault remodeling for selected cases of Chiari malformations associated with craniosynostosis. J Neurosurg Pediatr. 2013;12:166–70.
71. Levitt MR, Niazi TN, Hopper RA, Ellenbogen RG, Ojemann JG. Resolution of syndromic craniosynostosis-associated Chiari malformation type I without suboccipital decompression after posterior cranial vault release. J Neurosurg Pediatr. 2012;9:111–5.
72. Frassanito P, Massimi L, Tamburrini G, Caldarelli M, Pedicelli A, Di Rocco C. Occipital sinus pericranii superseding both jugular veins: description of two rare pediatric cases. Neurosurgery. 2013;72:E1054–8.
73. Massimi L, Pravatà E, Tamburrini G, Gaudino S, Pettorini B, Novegno F, Colosimo C Jr, Di Rocco C. Endoscopic third ventriculostomy for the management of Chiari I and related hydrocephalus: outcome and pathogenetic implications. Neurosurgery. 2011;68:950–6.
74. Sgulò FG, Spennato P, Aliberti F, Di Martino G, Cascone D, Cinalli G. Contemporary occurrence of hydrocephalus and Chiari I malformation in sagittal craniosynostosis. Case report and review of the literature. Childs Nerv Syst. 2017;33:187–92.
75. Frassanito P, Palombi D, Tamburrini G. Craniosynostosis and hydrocephalus: relevance and treatment modalities. Childs Nerv Syst. 2021;37:3465–73.
76. Di Rocco F, Jucà CE, Arnaud E, Renier D, Sainte Rose C. The role of endoscopic third ventriculostomy in the treatment of hydrocephalus associated with faciocraniosynostosis. J Neurosurg Pediatr. 2010;6:17–22.

Part IV

The Multidisciplinary Team and the Neurosurgeon

20 Antenatal Diagnosis of Craniosynostosis

Mona Massoud, Jean-Philippe Bault, and Sara Cabet

Abbreviations

CT Computed tomography
MRI Magnetic resonance imaging
US Ultrasound

20.1 Introduction

During normal human embryogenesis, skull development starts with the formation of bone centers within the membranous anlage and enlarges by ongoing ossification at the edges [1, 2]. Skull sutures start to develop at the sites where the bones come in close proximity and consist of the main site of skull growth [1, 2]. The premature closure of one or multiple sutures defining craniosynostosis is known to start during the early second trimester of pregnancy, starting 15 weeks of gestation (WG) for trigonocephaly and 18 WG for scaphocephaly [2, 3]. Skull sutures may be visualized as echo-free linear structures as early as 15 weeks of gestation [2] (Fig. 20.1). The classification of skull deformation in craniosynostosis is based on the suture involved (Fig. 20.2). Premature closure of the sagittal, coronal, and metopic sutures is associated with scaphocephaly (Fig. 20.3) or dolichocephaly, brachycephaly, and trigonocephaly (Fig. 20.4), respectively. Plagiocephaly develops when only one coronal or lambdoid suture is closed. Craniosynostosis constitutes a group of heterogeneous conditions with often distinct clinical, genetic, and molecular characteristics. They are classified into syndromic craniosynostosis when associated with other abnormalities (15%) and nonsyndromic when they are isolated (85%). Prenatal diagnosis of craniosynostosis remains rare and challenging, its detection in the prenatal period is difficult, in nonsyndromic forms or in the absence of family history. Its diagnosis is made late during the third trimester of pregnancy [3–8] and in a large majority of these cases, the positive diagnosis of craniosynostosis is made

M. Massoud (✉)
Obstetrics and Fetal Medicine Unit, Centre Hospitalier Lyon Sud, Hospices Civils de Lyon, Lyon, France

Equipe FLUID, Lyon Neurosciences Research Center, INSERM U1028, CNRS UMR5292, Lyon-1 University, Lyon, France
e-mail: mona.massoud@chu-lyon.fr

J.-P. Bault
Fetal Medicine Department, Centre Hospitalier Intercommunal de Poissy, Saint Germain en Laye, Lumière Foundation, Necker Hospital, Assistance Publique Hôpitaux de Paris, Paris, France

S. Cabet
Department of Antenatal and Pediatric Imaging, HFME, Hospices Civils de Lyon, Lyon, France

Institut NeuroMyoGène, CNRS UMR5292, INSERM U1028, Université Claude Bernard Lyon 1, Lyon, France
e-mail: sara.cabet@chu-lyon.fr

F. Di Rocco, J. Kestle (eds.), *Neurosurgical Aspects of Craniosynostosis*,
https://doi.org/10.1007/978-3-031-69386-1_20

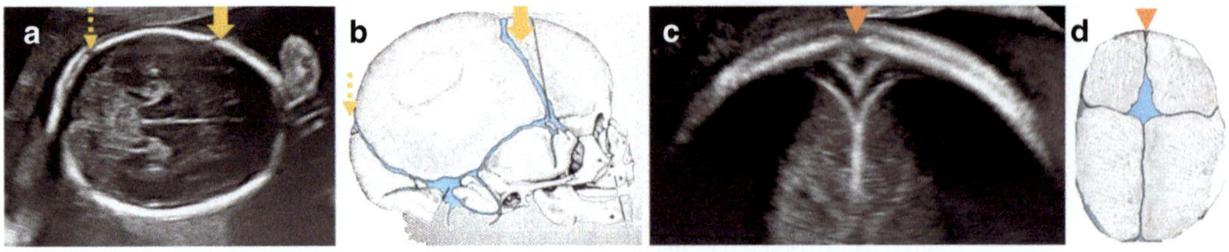

Fig. 20.1 Transabdominal 2D-US of normal fetal head showing the cranial sutures on transverse axial view (**a**) and figure (**b**), (coronal suture (yellow arrow) and lambdoid suture (yellow dotted arrow)); and the metopic suture visualized on a coronal view (**c**) with the head arrow and the figure (**d**)

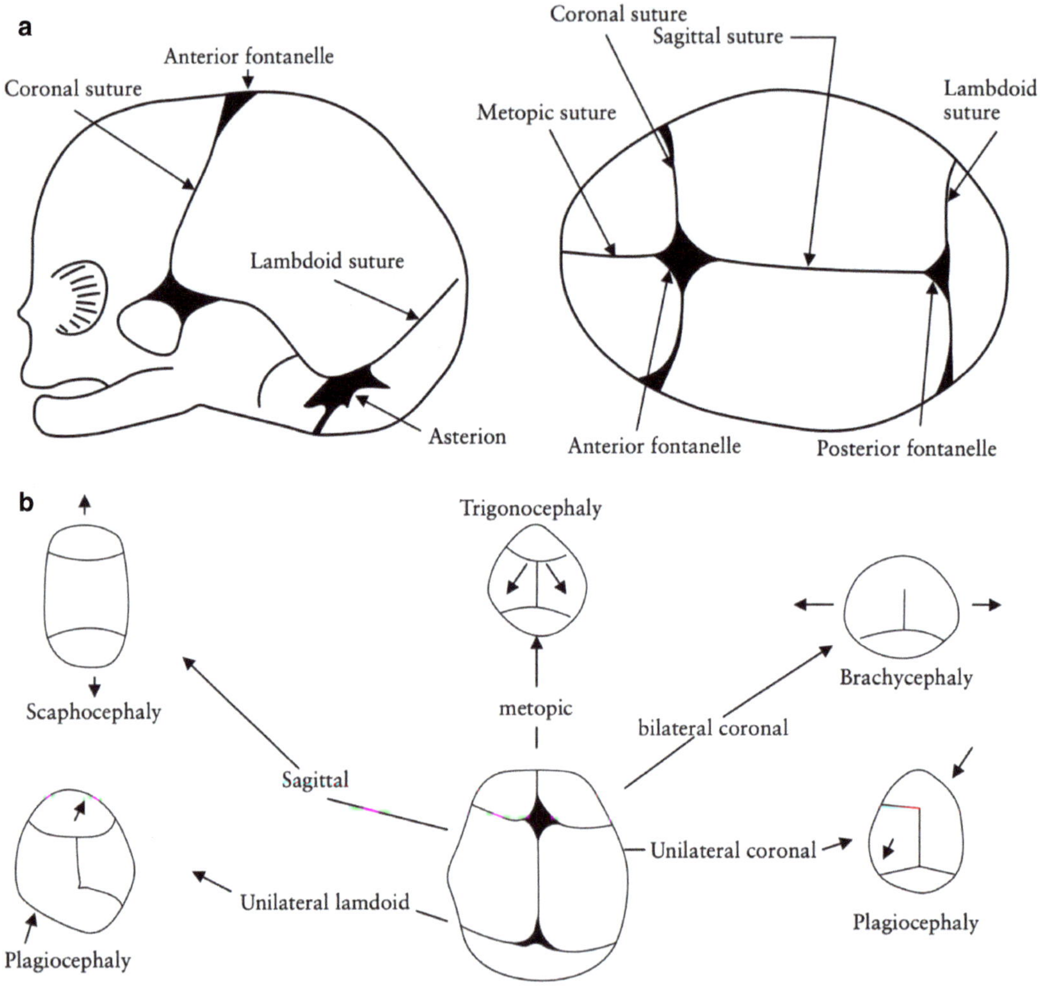

Fig. 20.2 (**a**) Major sutures involved in craniosynostosis and (**b**) skull deformities based on the suture involved. (Figure adapted from Keating et al. [9])

postnatally, during the first year of life [1, 2]. The commonest isolated forms are scaphocephaly and trigonocephaly. In this chapter, we will discuss how we assess prenatal diagnosis of craniosynostosis. We will describe prenatal imaging findings and the different imaging modalities, additional anomalies that should be sought in case of syndromic craniosynostosis and finally,

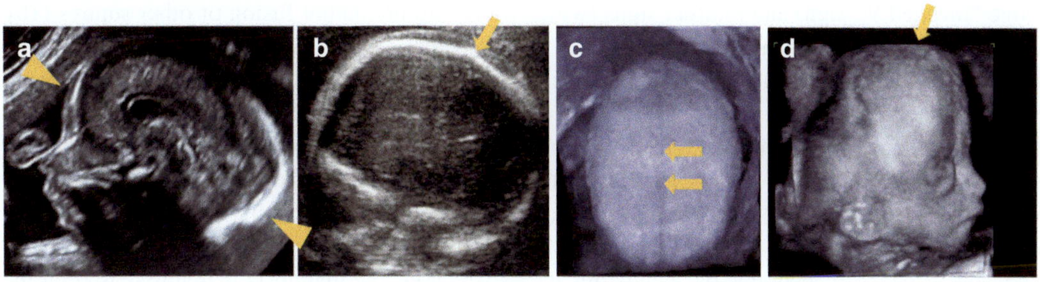

Fig. 20.3 A case of isolated scaphocephaly. Elongated skull and an occipital bulging, (**a**—heads of arrow) on 2D-US. Fusion of the sagittal suture on a coronal view in 2D-US (**b**—single arrow) and on 3D-US (**c**—double arrow). Closure of the sagittal suture with irregular thickened margin (**d**—arrow)

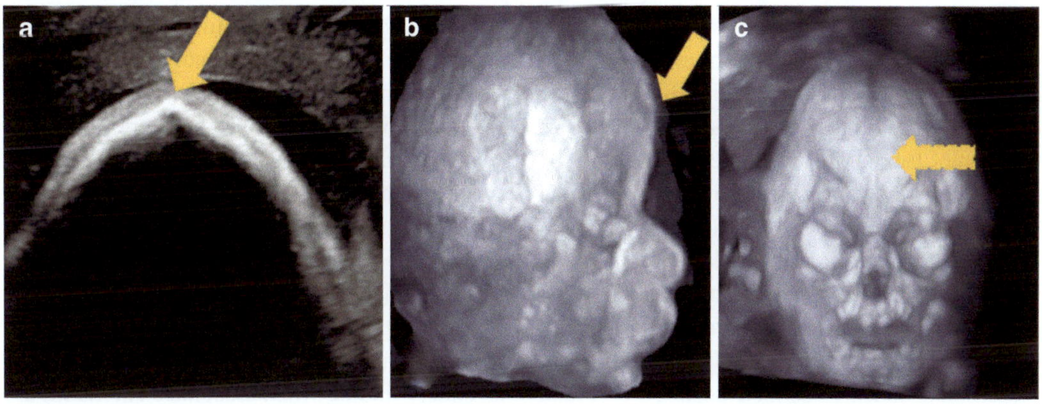

Fig. 20.4 An isolated case of trigonocephaly showing an abnormal skull shape with a narrow and pointed forehead, a fusion and loss of the hypoechogenicity of the metopic suture on a 2D-US axial view (**a**—arrow), an abnormal facial profile with a direct visualization of the metopic synostosis on a 3D-US profile view (**b**) and a coronal view (**c**)

we will focus on prenatal counseling in case of prenatal diagnosis of craniosynostosis.

20.2 Prenatal 2D-Ultrasound Findings in Craniosynostosis

Ultrasound (US) imaging using the 2D mode is the reference tool in many countries for fetal exploration since it is an easy, nonradiating, and commonly available imaging modality. While prenatal detection is straightforward when distinguishing cranial shape abnormalities, such as cloverleaf skull, there are conditions that cause minimum cranial shape deformity making prenatal diagnosis of craniosynostosis challenging, especially in single-suture fusion which are detected only sporadically during pregnancy and, if so, almost invariably during the third trimester [5–7]. Therefore, prenatal diagnosis of isolated cases of craniosynostosis is relatively rare and the majority of the described cases are syndromic as shown by Harada et al. in their cohort of 41 newborns with a prenatal diagnosis of craniosynostosis, in which the detection rate was of 61%; however, 73% (30 cases) were syndromic craniosynostosis, 7% (3 cases) were secondary craniosynostosis of chromosomal deletion syndromes, and only 20% (8 cases) were isolated [4]. Several authors have reported characteristic US findings for the prenatal diagnosis of craniosynostosis in 2D-US to increase the detection rate of this condition. These signs are divided into direct (loss of hypoechogenicity of the skull suture, a bony ridge "inverted V" sign) and indirect signs (wide concurrent open sutures, abnormal skull shape, brain shadowing sign, abnormal fetal face, and ventriculomegaly).

During routine mid-trimester fetal US scan, sonographers examine the fetal head in order to realize the cephalic measurements (biparietal diameter (BPD) and head circumference (HC)) and check the head anatomy by evaluating its size, shape, integrity, and density. The coronal and lambdoid sutures can be visualized clearly in this cephalic view as well as the normally oval shape of the skull (Fig. 20.1). In routine US examination, prenatal diagnosis of craniosynostosis relies mainly on the abnormal shape of the fetal skull [9] not always straightforward to detect [5, 7]. Skull deformity results from a combination of lack of growth perpendicularly to the fused suture and compensatory overgrowth at the open sutures [3, 4, 10]. Skull shape is partly and objectively appreciated by the cephalic index which is the ratio between the biparietal and the occipitofrontal diameters, which is automatically calculated by most US devices. Normal range of the cephalic index is defined between 0.75 and 0.85 [4]. An increased cephalic index was thought to be a reliable marker of brachycephaly secondary to bilateral coronal synostosis with a sensitivity of 95%, which is helpful during the third trimester [3, 4, 6, 11, 12]. A reduction in the biparietal diameter curve with a subsequent decrease of the cephalic index is found in fetuses with scaphocephaly, starting at 20 WG and being an ongoing process for which a repeated measurement could be informative [6, 13]. Bilateral bulging of the temporal, occipital, and frontal lobes, and a high cranial vault (acrocephaly) are seen in a cloverleaf skull (*Kleeblattschädel*) secondary to coronal and lambdoid synostosis, and often result in an increased cephalic index [11, 12]. In sagittal synostosis, growth of the lambdoid sutures leads to an elongated skull with decreased biparietal diameter and cephalic index, and an occipital bulging [12, 14]. Sagittal synostosis is of variable onset and can occur from the late first trimester to the early postnatal period [15]. It can affect only a segment or the whole length of the suture and may be either isolated or in association with premature fusion of other sutures [16]. However, these objective measurements have several limits. The standard prenatal biometric parameters are not reliable to diagnose prenatal craniosynostosis in all cases, as for example, in cases of trigonocephaly, cephalic measurements do not differ significantly from control cases as well as in cases of partial sagittal synostosis. In such cases, the diagnosis is mainly based on the subjective assessment of the abnormal skull shape during the US examination [3, 6]. The metopic synostosis leads to a narrowed and pointed forehead with bitemporal narrowing (trigonocephaly) [8]. Premature fusion of a single coronal (frontoparietal or frontosphenoid) suture results in an ipsilateral cranial flattening or plagiocephaly with elevation and posterior displacement of the ipsilateral orbit and anterior displacement of the ipsilateral ear canal [11]. Premature fusion of a single lambdoid suture is less common and leads to parieto-occipital plagiocephaly [16] (Fig. 20.2).

Despite these tools, the rate of prenatal diagnosis of craniosynostosis is low, it is mainly a secondary finding when associated anomalies are identified. Thus, when facing abnormal cephalic biometry, the patient should be referred for a more detailed US examination. Notably, direct observation of a fused cranial suture with loss of hypoechogenicity of the synostotic suture is possible after 4–16 weeks of the skull deformity [4, 5, 17]. Other US findings of great value in the assessment of the cranial sutures are the presence of an "inverted V" ridge, corresponding to a bony ridge and wide orthogonal open sutures [3]. Sutures have to be examined along their entire length because only a short segment of the suture needs to be fused for the entire suture to be functionally closed [5, 18]. In 2D-US, the acoustic beam is directed tangentially to the skull surface, then moved along the long axis of the suture back and forward from the metopic to the sagittal suture, and finally turned into 90° to explore the coronal and lambdoid sutures [5]. Direct 2D-US examination of the sutures shows an excellent negative predictive value contrary to isolated skull shape abnormalities [5]. However, such direct exploration of the sutures is not a routine practice and requires expert skills in ultrasound fetal exploration. The "brain shadowing sign" was described in craniosynostosis due to the sutures obliteration [3] that leads to the absence of penetration of US beam through the fetal cranial vault, creating an acoustic shadow on the underlying brain tissue that may be either complete or partial according to the degree of synostosis [3]. The brain shadowing sign corresponds to the difficulty in obtaining a proper transthalamic axial view in 2D-US due to acoustic shadow which persists despite repeated tilting movements of the probe [7]. One should note that an incorrect position of the transducer over the fetal head to scan the brain may cause misinterpretation of this finding because insonation through calcified skull bones always provides acoustic shadows that should not be mistaken for the brain shadowing sign [3]. So, the identification of this sign depends on the sonographer's expertise in fetal neurosonography and in fetal position [3]. Dall Hasta et al., have reported this sign starting at 24 WG in the absence of obvious abnormality of the skull shape. Its detection should lead to a direct examination of the fetal suture to exclude overlapping sutures and head molding (false-positive diagnosis of craniosynostosis) [3]. Although sensitive, this sign does not allow the detection of all cases of craniosynostosis, especially if sutures other than the coronal and the lambdoid are concerned [7]. Ventriculomegaly was also described as an indirect sign of craniosynostosis, it is the third most common 2D-US sign found in syndromic craniosynostosis as noted by Harada et al. in 41% of their series in association with skull deformation [4, 19]. Ventriculomegaly may be helpful in detecting craniosynostosis when skull deformation is minimal [4]. However, if isolated, this is not a reliable specific sign [4]. Dysmorphism was also described as an indirect sign of craniosynostosis [5, 7], thus in the case of turricephaly, the midsagittal view of the fetal profile is abnormal [7]. Proptosis and frontal bossing have been reported in fetuses with bilateral coronal suture synostosis [3, 4]. Interestingly, Harada et al. have reported three cases of craniosynostosis who presented with proptosis and ventriculomegaly without abnormal skull shape or abnormal cephalic index or biometry [4]. Hypertelorism (defined as an interorbital diameter exceeding the diameter of one globe) or hypotelorism was also observed in cases of brachycephaly and trigonocephaly, respectively [15, 16].

20.3 What Is the Additional Value of the Other Imaging Modalities?

In a selected high-risk population of craniosynostosis, there is a high-positive predictive value of the direct examination of the sutures using a 2D-US, however, the specificity of such an exploration is low in low-risk populations [12, 20]. In such cases, 3D-US, magnetic resonance imaging (MRI), or computed tomography (CT) may be of a good help to investigate prenatal diagnosis of craniosynostosis (Table 20.1) [5, 21–23].

Although 3D-US requires some skills and devices for high-definition rendering, this imaging modality can be useful to visualize the skull sutures as early as 13–15 WG, showing closure, irregularly thickened inner sutural margin with a high-negative predictive value for the diagnosis of craniosynostosis (Fig. 20.5) [3, 5, 16, 21, 24, 25]. It represents also a potential complementary tool for the measurement of the bony gaps of the uninvolved sutures with the multiplanar mode, contributing to the differential diagnosis between craniosynostosis and overriding sutures in severe fetal head molding [3, 7, 21, 26, 27]. Krakow et al. have demonstrated the superiority of 3D-US over 2D-US in a case of fetal molding which was initially thought to be an isolated craniosynostosis, by showing the open suture [28]. Some authors have also reported better visualization of fetal facial dysmorphism using this technique [21, 24, 29]. However, in their series of 60 craniofacial malformations, while admitting that 3D-US helped parental understanding and medical communication, Ghi et al. have noted no objective diagnostic benefit compared to 2D-US [30]. In conclusion, 3D-US can be a useful additional tool associated with 2D-US during paren-

Table 20.1 Summary of the advantages and limits of different imaging modalities in the exploration of direct and indirect signs of craniosynostosis

Imaging modalities	Advantages	Limits
2D-US	Accessibility Dynamic exploration Direct visualization of sutures	Brain shadowing Fetal position
3D-US	Three-plane exploration Direct visualization of sutures Evaluation of the bony gaps of uninvolved sutures Visualization of fetal face dysmorphism Help of parental understanding	Skills required Adapted devices
MRI	Three-plane exploration Brain exploration Extremities exploration Independent of fetal position High negative predictive value	Absence of direct visualization of sutures Lack of accessibility
CT scan	Three-plane exploration Direct visualization of sutures Visualization of the entire length of the sutures Assessment of skull shape Exploration of other skeletal abnormalities	Irradiation

Abbreviations: *2D-US* two-dimensional ultrasonography, *3D-US* three-dimensional ultrasonography, *MRI* magnetic resonance imaging, *CT scan* computed tomography scan

tal counseling that may help parental–fetal bonding [24, 31, 32].

Reports on prenatal MR examination of craniosynostosis are rare in the literature. The fetal skull sutures are not directly visualized by MRI but this modality facilitates the evaluation of brain abnormalities or small changes in hands and feet [4]. Fjørtoft et al. presented the first evaluation of fetal MRI in a series of patients with suspicion of craniosynostosis [33]. They noted that the MRI showed abnormal skull shape, bone thickening, and slight skull indentations at the level of the closed sutures with a high-negative predictive value in their series [16, 33, 34]. For example, temporal indentations, which were also visible in the US, were correlated with coronal synostosis [33], the "lampshade" sign reflecting the bulging of the temporal regions, the undeveloped frontal lobes, and the turricephaly were more easily assessed on coronal MRI sequences than on 2D-US [35]. Boog et al. showed that MRI contributes to additional findings during the imaging assessment of craniosynostosis, such as verticalization of the clivus and the flattened angle of the skull base during the second trimester [23]. However, the great advantage of MRI concerns the better assessment of brain abnormalities that might be associated with craniosynostosis such as ventriculomegaly and agenesis of the corpus callosum, especially because US exploration is limited by suture synostosis [33, 35, 36]. MRI could be of good help in the assessment of facial fetal abnormalities such as proptosis which is defined as a protrusion of more than 50% of the ocular globe beyond the orbital rim [35]. Thus, the contribution of fetal MRI to the diagnosis of isolated craniosynostosis seems minimal. Therefore, US and MRI should be considered complementary imaging modalities [16].

Prenatal 3D-CT seems to be very useful, as it allows direct visualization of the cranial vault sutures, the skull shape, and all the skeletal abnormalities in syndromic craniosynostosis, which is not possible with MRI [3, 4, 22, 33]. Moreover, it allows the exploration of the entire length of the suture in the three dimensions, which is useful during the assessment of craniosynostosis since even though a tiny segment of the suture is fused, the entire suture could be functionally closed [5].

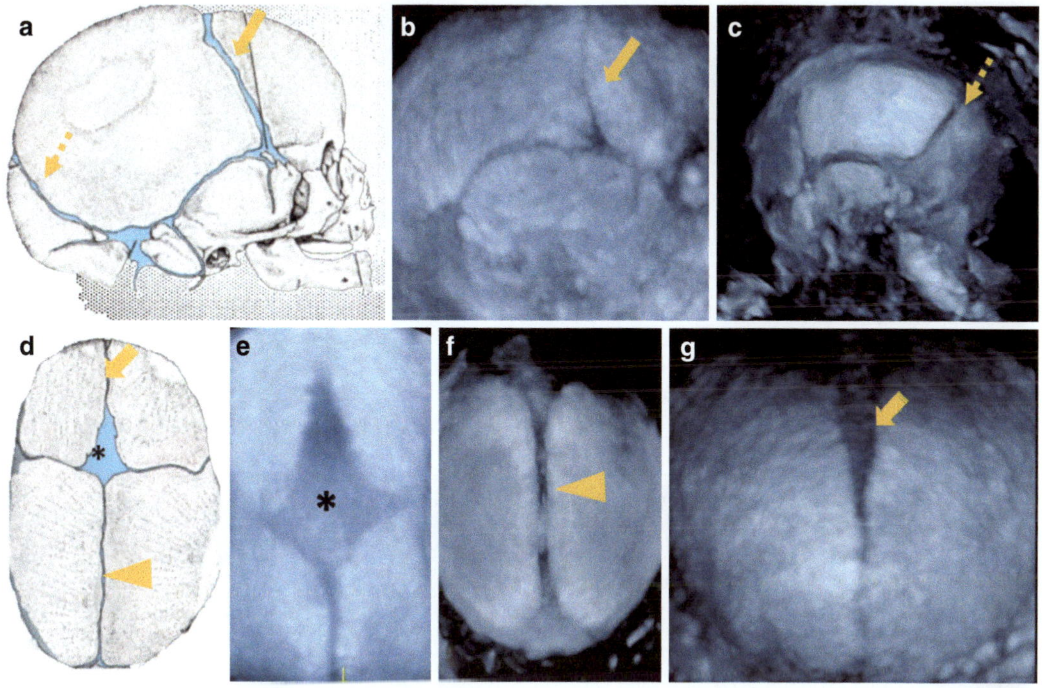

Fig. 20.5 3D-US of the cranial sutures. Major sutures involved in craniosynostosis. Coronal suture(arrow in **a**, **b**), lambdoid suture (dotted arrow in **a**, **c**), the anterior fontanelle (asterisk in **d**, **e**), the sagittal suture (head of the arrow of **d**, **f**), and the metopic suture (arrow on **d**, **g**)

20.4 Syndromic Craniosynostosis: What Should the Sonographer Look for?

Despite the imaging tools at our disposal, prenatal diagnosis of craniosynostosis relies mainly on the skull deformity and the associated anomalies [4, 5, 37]. Distinguishing between isolated and syndromic craniosynostosis during the prenatal period is crucial for appropriate counseling since syndromic cases present generally a higher rate of developmental delay (56% vs. 25% in a series of 41 cases by Harada et al.) [4, 35]. The median gestational age at diagnosis in the context of syndromic craniosynostosis [6, 8, 38] is 25 WG versus 31 WG in cases of isolated ones [3]. An extensive list of syndromes with craniosynostosis includes Antley–Bixler, Apert, Baller-Gerold, Beare–Stevenson, Carpenter, Crouzon, Jackson–Weiss, Meckel–Gruber, Muenke, Pfeiffer, Ruvalcaba, Saethre–Chotzen, Williams, 9p deletions, chondrodysplasia punctata, hypophosphatasia, thanatophoric dysplasia, and cranioectodermal dysplasia or Sensenbrenner syndrome. Distinguishing between these different syndromes of craniosynostosis is difficult during the prenatal period considering the great heterogeneity of the diseases and the overlap of phenotypic features among fetuses with different genetic variants and syndromes [8]. Molecular analysis of fetal DNA can be used in Apert (Fig. 20.6), Crouzon (Fig. 20.7), Pfeiffer and Jackson-Weiss syndromes when the family history is informative. The imaging findings of 15 syndromes with craniosynostosis are described in Table 20.2 [4, 5, 8, 12, 16, 35, 39–51]. Brachycephaly due to bilateral coronal synostosis is typical of, though not specific for, Pfeiffer and Apert syndromes. Coronal synostosis associated with lambdoid synostosis leads to a cloverleaf shape of the skull with bitemporal and bifrontal bulging that is more frequently observed in thanatophoric dwarfism, Pfeiffer, Apert, and Crouzon syndromes [5, 11, 15, 16, 52–55].

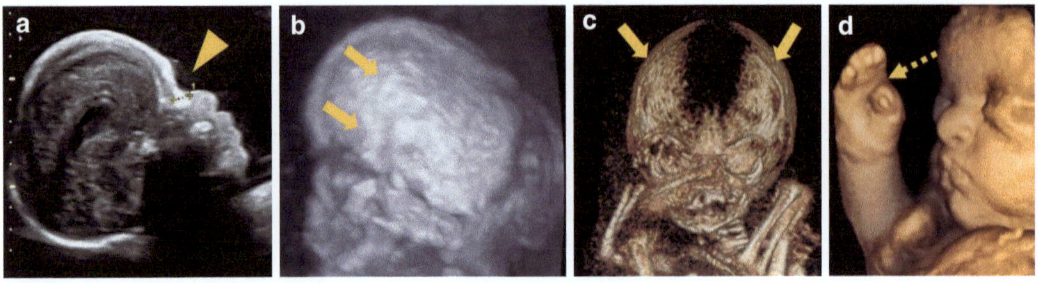

Fig. 20.6 Apert syndrome. Abnormal profile face with a marked nasal bridge (**a**—head of arrow) on a 2D-US. Direct visualization of the fusion of the coronal synostosis on a 3D-US (**b**—double arrow) and on a CT scan that shows the fusion of the bicoronal sutures (**c**—arrows). Abnormal aspect of the hand on a 3D-US with syndactyly and a "mitten-like" hand (**d**—dotted arrow)

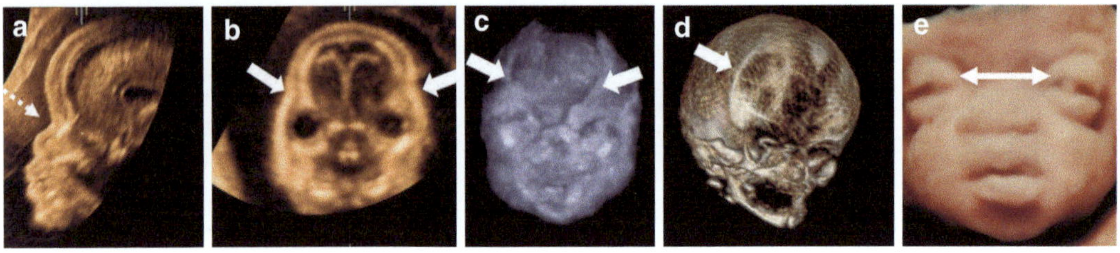

Fig. 20.7 Crouzon syndrome. Abnormal profile face with a midface hypoplasia (**a**—dotted arrow) on a sagittal 2D-US view, a bilateral fusion of the coronal suture (**b**, **c** arrow) on a 3D-US coronal view and on a CT-scan view (**d**). Dysmorphic face with hypertelorism (arrow) on a 3D view, with exophthalmia (**e**)

Crouzon syndrome is the most frequent syndrome with craniosynostosis but is more challenging to diagnose during the prenatal period than Pfeiffer syndrome because of mild skull deformities without any specifically associated anomalies during gestation [4]. Indeed, the fetuses with Pfeiffer syndrome present with more evident and severe skull shape abnormalities that developed earlier during the gestational period than other syndromes [4]. The location of the synostosis varies even within the same syndrome [4, 56], thus, Pfeiffer syndrome is divided into three different subtypes with overlapping features and different skull shapes: mild cases (type 1 with midface hypoplasia and limbs malformations), severe cases (type 2 with cloverleaf skull, limbs malformations, and elbow ankylosis), and intermediate cases (type 3 similar to type 2 but without cloverleaf skull) [8, 35]. Moreover, depending on the degree of suture synostosis, the skull shape abnormalities may be absent or subtle until the third trimester [2], which leads in some cases to the suspicion of the underlying syndrome in the absence of skull shape abnormality [6]. Exploration of the central nervous system during the assessment of suspected craniosynostosis is mandatory using US and MRI if required. In Apert syndrome, temporal lobe dysgyria has been reported in association with agenesis of the corpus callosum and may precede the detection of craniosynostosis [57]. Ventriculomegaly is common in craniosynostosis and can be associated with subtle scalloping of the inner skull table due to the high intracranial pressure [8, 35]. Additional imaging findings of dysmorphism were associated with syndromic craniosynostosis including hyper- or hypotelorism, proptosis, cleft palate, and midface hypoplasia [8, 16]. Proptosis is generally more pronounced in Crouzon syndrome, in association with mild hypertelorism, starting the second trimester [39, 58]. The association of microphthalmia and craniosynostosis is a very rare condition and was reported in Curry-Jones, Gorlin-

Table 20.2 Antenatal imaging findings of 15 syndromes with craniosynostosis

Syndrome	Cephalic abnormalities				Extracephalic abnormalities	
	Suture synostosis	Skull shape	Fetal face	Central nervous system	Skeletal	Other
Antley-Bixler	Coronal, lambdoid	Brachycephaly	Midface hypoplasia, proptosis, frontal bossing, dysplastic ears, choanal stenosis or atresia, depressed nasal bridge		Radiohumeral synostosis, radioulnar synostosis, multiple joint contractures, femoral bowing, ulna bowing, fractures, camptodactyly, narrow iliac wings	Heart malformation, urogenital malformation
Apert	Variable multisutural: often bicoronal synostosis with wide metopic and sagittal sutures	Brachycephaly, turribrachycephaly, oxycephaly, foreshortened anterior cranial fossa, ridging of the coronal sutures, prominent convolutional impressions on the calvarium	Midface hypoplasia, hypertelorism, proptosis, marked nasal bridge, prominent forehead, cleft palate, inner ear malformation	Corpus callosum agenesis, temporal dysgyria	Symmetrical syndactyly of hands and feet, "mitten-like" hands and feet (complete soft tissue syndactyly), broad thumb, broad great toe	Cardiac ventricular septal defect, tracheal cartilaginous sleeve risk
Baller-Gerold	Metopic, coronal	Brachycephaly, trigonocephaly, oxycephaly, thickening of the inferior part of the frontal bone	Micrognathia, proptosis, bulging forehead		Radial hypo/aplasia, short curved ulna, oligodactyly, thumb aplasia or hypoplasia, carpal/metacarpal aplasia	Heart dextroposition, anterior or imperforate anus, growth retardation, urogenital malformation
Beare-Stevenson	Multisutural	Brachycephaly, cloverleaf skull	Midface hypoplasia, low nasal bridge, anteverted nares, smallmouth, cutis gyrata, hypertelorism, proptosis, downslanting palpebral fissures	Ventriculomegaly, distortion of the frontal horn of the lateral ventricle		Anterior anus, urogenital malformation, cutis gyrata

(continued)

Table 20.2 (continued)

Syndrome	Cephalic abnormalities				Extracephalic abnormalities	
	Suture synostosis	Skull shape	Fetal face	Central nervous system	Skeletal	Other
Carpenter	Variable: sagittal, lambdoid, coronal	Brachycephaly, turricephaly, cloverleaf skull		Ventriculomegaly	Postaxial polysyndactyly, brachydactyly of the hands with agenesis of the middle phalanges, broad thumbs, preaxial polysyndactyly of the feet, bowed femora, bowed tibiae, short limbs	Umbilical hernia, situs anomaly, congenital heart malformation, growth retardation, cystic hygroma, polyhydramnios
Crouzon	Variable multisutural: bicoronal, sagittal	Brachycephaly, oxycephaly	Midface hypoplasia, mandibular prognathism, hypertelorism, proptosis, downslanting palpebral fissures, short upper lip, low-set dorsally rotated ears, beaked nose		None	Tracheal cartilaginous sleeve risk, anal atresia
Crouzon with acanthosis nigricans	Variable multisutural: bicoronal, sagittal	Brachycephaly, oxycephaly	Same as Crouzon syndrome + choanal atresia or stenosis, hypoplastic malar bone	Ventriculomegaly, Chiari I malformation	Skeletal findings similar to those of achondroplasia, short vertebra (anteroposterior), short broad metacarpals	
Jackson-Weiss	Coronal, sagittal	Brachycephaly, oxycephaly	Midface hypoplasia		Normal hands, broad great toes, syndactyly of the toes 2 and 3, tarsal/metatarsal coalition	
Muenke	Uni- or bicoronal	Brachycephaly	Midface hypoplasia, hypertelorism, proptosis, marked bulging of the temporal fossae, frontal bossing, short up-turned nose, low-set ears	Ventriculomegaly, corpus callosum agenesis	Thimble-shaped middle phalanges, brachydactyly, carpal fusion, tarsal fusion	Cardiac septal defects, esophageal atresia

Pfeiffer	Variable multisutural: bicoronal, sagittal	Brachycephaly, cloverleaf skull (type 2), foreshortened anterior cranial base	High forehead, frontal bossing, midface hypoplasia, hypoplastic nasal bone, low-set ear, hypertelorism, proptosis (type 2)	Ventriculomegaly	Polysyndactyly, broad radially deviated thumb, broad medially deviated great toe, brachydactyly	Tracheal cartilaginous sleeve risk, increased nuchal-fold thickness, polyhydramnios, heart malformation, anal atresia, hypospadias, bifid scrotum
Saethre-Chotzen	Uni- or bicoronal	Brachycephaly	Flat asymmetric face, high forehead, small low-set posteriorly rotated ears with prominent horizontal crura, hypertelorism, cleft palate		Cutaneous syndactyly of digits 2 and 3, bifid terminal phalanges of digits 2 and 3, coarse hands (hypoplastic distal phalanx), brachydactyly, absence of the first metatarsal, broad toes, radioulnar synostosis, contractures	Heart malformation
Cranioectodermal dysplasia	Sagittal, lambdoid	Scaphocephaly	Hypertelorism, low-set ears, flat nasal bridge, up-turned nares, long smooth philtrum, everted lower lip, high forehead, cleft palate		Short limbs, fractures, polydactyly, brachydactyly, webbed fingers, narrow chest	Cystic hygroma, nephronophthisis, heart malformation, hepatomegaly
Oculofaciocardiodental syndrome	Coronal, lambdoid	Brachycephaly	Microphthalmia, long narrow face, broad bifid nasal tip, cleft palate, midface hypoplasia		Radioulnar synostosis, syndactyly, hammertoes	Cardiac atrial or ventricular septal defect
Craniofrontonasal syndrome	Variable, often coronal	Brachycephaly	Hypertelorism, bifid nasal tip, downslanting palpebral fissures, frontal bossing, facial asymmetry, cleft lip and palate, low-set ears	Ventriculomegaly, corpus callosum agenesis	Broad partially bifid thumbs, syndactyly	Webbed neck, diaphragmatic hernia
Thanatophoric dysplasia	Variable multisutural	Cloverleaf skull	Frontal bossing, flat facies, low nasal bridge, proptosis	Ventriculomegaly, encephalocele	Short limbs, bowed femur (type 1), platyspondyly (type 1), narrow chest with short ribs, brachydactyly	Growth retardation, polyhydramnios

Chaudhry-Moss, and oculo-facio-cardio-dental syndromes [46]. Inner ear anomalies are classic in Apert syndrome [59]. Other sonographic features such as limb abnormalities and hand anomalies are encountered in syndromic craniosynostosis. US observation of fetal "mitten hands" (complete symmetrical syndactyly of the hands and feet seen as smooth oval shapes) is highly characteristic of Apert syndrome that in association with molecular diagnosis allows the prenatal detection of sporadic Apert syndromes during the second trimester [22, 35, 60, 61]. In Baller-Gerold syndrome, radial aplasia or hypoplasia is considered a very evocative finding [62]. Radio-humeral synostosis and joint contractures as well as fractures or bowing of the long bones [63] are suggestive of Antley-Bixler syndrome. Additional malformations can be associated with syndromic craniosynostosis such as diaphragmatic hernias, abdominal wall defects, heart malformations, echogenic kidneys, and abnormal airways with echogenic and hyperexpanded lungs with effusions [3, 35, 64]. MRI is useful for the detailed evaluation of fetal airways and lung changes [35]. In addition to midface hypoplasia that leads to a decrease in nasopharynx and oropharynx diameters, a tracheal cartilaginous sleeve is common in Crouzon, Apert, and Pfeiffer syndromes, and is thought to contribute to premature death in the affected newborns [65, 66].

20.5 Implications of Prenatal Diagnosis of Craniosynostosis in Prenatal Counseling

Once prenatal diagnosis of fetal craniosynostosis is confirmed and considered as isolated or associated with other malformations, fetal genetic assessment including fetal chromosomal microarray on amniotic fluid cells as well as molecular confirmation, when possible, should be recommended and is crucial for prenatal counseling regarding the prognosis [3, 11, 15, 62, 63]. Thus, the risk for cognitive disabilities in the affected infant depends on the underlying syndrome [11]. In cases of isolated brachycephaly and dolichocephaly, Delahaye et al. have found a normal outcome in 80% of these cases and therefore they confirmed that these isolated features are rarely associated with fetal abnormalities. However, some of the nonsyndromic craniosynostosis may have an underlying genetic etiology but less commonly identified antenatally [8]. Regarding high-risk fetuses with a family history of craniosynostosis, future parents are often requested to know if the newborn will be affected or not, irrespective of their willingness to terminate or not the pregnancy [5]. Interestingly, in cases of nonsyndromic craniosynostosis, siblings of an affected child have approximately double the estimated risk of craniosynostosis than the general population [9].

Since most cases of craniosynostosis are compatible with survival, prenatal diagnosis of craniosynostosis allows the careful planning of delivery modality and perinatal care since delivery complications seem to be associated with craniosynostosis [58]. Indeed, an important function of the sutures is to enable molding of the skull when passing through the birth canal and craniosynostosis may avoid this adaptation [59]. Thus, a higher rate of vaginal breech deliveries and secondary cesarean sections have been reported in newborns with craniosynostosis compared to the general population as well as a lower Apgar score and a lower pH value [58]. In addition, a high mortality rate is observed during the neonatal period in some conditions, since infants with craniosynostosis are at increased risk of concomitant abnormalities of the upper airways due to midfacial hypoplasia and may require ventilatory support and delivery in an adequate structure [7, 8, 15, 60]. Moreover, craniosynostosis may be complicated by various types of neurological anomalies including elevated intracranial pressure, and hydrocephaly that may require prompt surgical treatment after birth for which time for referral is critical [6, 15]. Prenatal diagnosis of such conditions requires a multidisciplinary approach to provide optimal care and allow timely decision-making for the newborn [34].

Prenatal diagnosis of fetal craniosynostosis enables psychological support for future parents.

They will be aware of the main treatments that their child may require during the postnatal period and this may decrease the stress caused by the diagnosis of craniosynostosis [61].

20.6 Conclusion

Prenatal diagnosis of craniosynostosis remains challenging in particular in isolated single-suture forms. Abnormal skull shape, abnormal cephalic index, the brain shadowing sign, and ventriculomegaly are the main key features for detecting fetal craniosynostosis in 2D-US. Once craniosynostosis is suspected, patients should be referred to a fetal medicine unit in order to perform a second-level scan by an expert in fetal neurosonography to confirm the diagnosis and to assess the associated malformations. A 3D-US may be an optional additional tool to improve the exploration of the skull sutures and to help future parents visualize the malformation. MRI, as a complementary imaging modality, allows detection and better assessment of central nervous system malformations which may be associated with craniosynostosis. Distinguishing between isolated and syndromic craniosynostosis is crucial during the prenatal period for appropriate counseling, and scrutinizing for fetal limbs and facial anomalies is useful. Once the diagnosis of craniosynostosis is made, fetal chromosomal microarray and molecular analysis should be recommended.

References

1. Mathijssen IM, Vaandrager JM, van der Meulen JC, Pieterman H, Zonneveld FW, Kreiborg S, et al. The role of bone centers in the pathogenesis of craniosynostosis: an embryologic approach using CT measurements in isolated craniosynostosis and Apert and Crouzon syndromes. Plast Reconstr Surg 1996;98(1):17–26.
2. Mathijssen IM, van Splunder J, Vermeij-Keers C, Pieterman H, de Jong TH, Mooney MP, et al. Tracing craniosynostosis to its developmental stage through bone center displacement. J Craniofac Genet Dev Biol. 1999;19(2):57–63.
3. Krajden Haratz K, Leibovitz Z, Svirsky R, Drummond CL, Lev D, Gindes L, et al. The 'brain shadowing sign': a novel marker of fetal craniosynostosis. Fetal Diagn Ther. 2016;40(4):277–84.
4. Harada A, Miyashita S, Nagai R, Makino S, Murotsuki J. Prenatal sonographic findings and prognosis of craniosynostosis diagnosed during the fetal and neonatal periods. Congenit Anom. 2019;59(4):132–41.
5. Delahaye S, Bernard JP, Rénier D, Ville Y. Prenatal ultrasound diagnosis of fetal craniosynostosis. Ultrasound Obstet Gynecol. 2003;21(4):347–53.
6. Cornelissen MJ, Apon I, van der Meulen JJNM, Groenenberg IAL, Kraan-van der Est MN, Mathijssen IMJ, et al. Prenatal ultrasound parameters in single-suture craniosynostosis. J Matern Fetal Neonatal Med. 2018;31(15):2050–7.
7. Dall'Asta A, Paramasivam G, Lees C, Ghi T, Frusca T. The brain shadowing sign: a clue finding for early suspicion of craniosynostosis? Fetal Diagn Ther. 2019;45(5):357–60.
8. Ketwaroo PD, Robson CD, Estroff JA. Prenatal imaging of craniosynostosis syndromes. Semin Ultrasound CT MR. 2015;36(6):453–64.
9. Keating RF. Craniosynostosis: diagnosis and management in the new millennium. Pediatr Ann. 1997;26(10):600–12.
10. Johnson D, Wilkie AOM. Craniosynostosis. Eur J Hum Genet. 2011;19(4):369–76.
11. Miller C, Losken HW, Towbin R, Bowen A, Mooney MP, Towbin A, et al. Ultrasound diagnosis of craniosynostosis. Cleft Palate Craniofac J. 2002;39(1):73–80.
12. Tonni G, Panteghini M, Rossi A, Baldi M, Magnani C, Ferrari B, et al. Craniosynostosis: prenatal diagnosis by means of ultrasound and SSSE-MRI. Family series with report of neurodevelopmental outcome and review of the literature. Arch Gynecol Obstet. 2011;283(4):909–16
13. Agrawal D, Steinbok P, Cochrane DD. Long-term anthropometric outcomes following surgery for isolated sagittal craniosynostosis. J Neurosurg. 2006;105(5 Suppl):357–60.
14. Blaser SI, Padfield N, Chitayat D, Forrest CR. Skull base development and craniosynostosis. Pediatr Radiol. 2015;45(Suppl 3):S485–96.
15. Wong GB, Mulliken JB, Benacerraf BR. Prenatal sonographic diagnosis of major craniofacial anomalies. Plast Reconstr Surg. 2001;108(5):1316–33.
16. Robson CD, Barnewolt CE. MR imaging of fetal head and neck anomalies. Neuroimaging Clin N Am. 2004;14(2):273–91, viii.
17. Lyu KJ, Ko TM. Prenatal diagnosis of Apert syndrome with widely separated cranial sutures. Prenat Diagn. 2000;20(3):254–6.
18. Fernbach SK. Craniosynostosis 1998: concepts and controversies. Pediatr Radiol. 1998;28(9):722–8.
19. Tokumaru AM, Barkovich AJ, Ciricillo SF, Edwards MS. Skull base and calvarial deformities: association with intracranial changes in craniofacial syndromes. AJNR Am J Neuroradiol. 1996;17(4):619–30.

20. Bernard JP, Levaillant JM. Prenatal diagnosis of craniosynostosis. Neurochirurgie. 2006;52(2–3 Pt 2):246–58.
21. Benacerraf BR, Spiro R, Mitchell AG. Using three-dimensional ultrasound to detect craniosynostosis in a fetus with Pfeiffer syndrome. Ultrasound Obstet Gynecol. 2000;16(4):391–4.
22. Mahieu-Caputo D, Sonigo P, Amiel J, Simon I, Aubry MC, Lemerrer M, et al. Prenatal diagnosis of sporadic Apert syndrome: a sequential diagnostic approach combining three-dimensional computed tomography and molecular biology. Fetal Diagn Ther. 2001;16(1):10–2.
23. Boog G, Le Vaillant C, Winer N, David A, Quere MP, Nomballais MF. Contribution of tridimensional sonography and magnetic resonance imaging to prenatal diagnosis of Apert syndrome at mid-trimester. Fetal Diagn Ther. 1999;14(1):20–3.
24. David AL, Turnbull C, Scott R, Freeman J, Bilardo CM, van Maarle M, et al. Diagnosis of Apert syndrome in the second-trimester using 2D and 3D ultrasound. Prenat Diagn. 2007;27(7):629–32.
25. Esser T, Rogalla P, Bamberg C, Kalache KD. Application of the three-dimensional maximum mode in prenatal diagnosis of Apert syndrome. Am J Obstet Gynecol. 2005;193(5):1743–5.
26. Flores-Sarnat L. New insights into craniosynostosis. Semin Pediatr Neurol. 2002;9(4):274–91.
27. Faro C, Chaoui R, Wegrzyn P, Levaillant JM, Benoit B, Nicolaides KH. Metopic suture in fetuses with Apert syndrome at 22–27 weeks of gestation. Ultrasound Obstet Gynecol. 2006;27(1):28–33.
28. Krakow D, Santulli T, Platt LD. Use of three-dimensional ultrasonography in differentiating craniosynostosis from severe fetal molding. J Ultrasound Med. 2001;20(4):427–31.
29. Blaumeiser B, Loquet P, Wuyts W, Nöthen MM. Prenatal diagnosis of Pfeiffer syndrome type II. Prenat Diagn. 2004;24(8):644–6.
30. Ghi T, Perolo A, Banzi C, Contratti G, Valeri B, Savelli L, et al. Two-dimensional ultrasound is accurate in the diagnosis of fetal craniofacial malformation. Ultrasound Obstet Gynecol. 2002;19(6):543–51.
31. Pretorius DH, Gattu S, Ji EK, Hollenbach K, Newton R, Hull A, et al. Preexamination and postexamination assessment of parental-fetal bonding in patients undergoing 3-/4-dimensional obstetric ultrasonography. J Ultrasound Med. 2006;25(11):1411–21.
32. Ji EK, Pretorius DH, Newton R, Uyan K, Hull AD, Hollenbach K, et al. Effects of ultrasound on maternal-fetal bonding: a comparison of two- and three-dimensional imaging. Ultrasound Obstet Gynecol. 2005;25(5):473–7.
33. Fjørtoft MI, Sevely A, Boetto S, Kessler S, Sarramon MF, Rolland M. Prenatal diagnosis of craniosynostosis: value of MR imaging. Neuroradiology. 2007;49(6):515–21.
34. Helfer TM, Peixoto AB, Tonni G, Araujo Júnior E. Craniosynostosis: prenatal diagnosis by 2D/3D ultrasound, magnetic resonance imaging and computed tomography. Med Ultrason. 2016;18(3):378–85.
35. Rubio EI, Blask A, Bulas DI. Ultrasound and MR imaging findings in prenatal diagnosis of craniosynostosis syndromes. Pediatr Radiol. 2016;46(5):709–18.
36. Itoh S, Nojima M, Yoshida K. Usefulness of magnetic resonance imaging for accurate diagnosis of Pfeiffer syndrome type II in utero. Fetal Diagn Ther. 2006;21(2):168–71.
37. Renier D, Lajeunie E, Arnaud E, Marchac D. Management of craniosynostoses. Childs Nerv Syst. 2000;16(10–11):645–58.
38. Derderian C, Seaward J. Syndromic craniosynostosis. Semin Plast Surg. 2012;26(2):64–75.
39. Menashe Y, Ben Baruch G, Rabinovitch O, Shalev Y, Katzenlson MB, Shalev E. Exophthalmus—prenatal ultrasonic features for diagnosis of Crouzon syndrome. Prenat Diagn. 1989;9(11):805–8.
40. Narayan H, Scott IV. Prenatal ultrasound diagnosis of Apert's syndrome. Prenat Diagn. 1991;11(3):187–92.
41. Pooh RK, Nakagawa Y, Pooh KH, Nakagawa Y, Nagamachi N. Fetal craniofacial structure and intracranial morphology in a case of Apert syndrome. Ultrasound Obstet Gynecol. 1999;13(4):274–80.
42. Kaufmann K, Baldinger S, Pratt L. Ultrasound detection of Apert syndrome: a case report and literature review. Am J Perinatol. 1997;14(7):427–30.
43. Filkins K, Russo JF, Boehmer S, Camous M, Przylepa KA, Jiang W, et al. Prenatal ultrasonographic and molecular diagnosis of Apert syndrome. Prenat Diagn. 1997;17(11):1081–4.
44. Chang CC, Tsai FJ, Tsai HD, Tsai CH, Hseih YY, Lee CC, et al. Prenatal diagnosis of Apert syndrome. Prenat Diagn. 1998;18(6):621–5.
45. Chenoweth-Mitchell C, Cohen GR. Prenatal sonographic findings of Apert syndrome. J Clin Ultrasound. 1994;22(8):510–4.
46. Cinnirella G, Taylor RL, Coco C, Piludu F, Vidiri A, Sinibaldi L, et al. Craniosynostosis-microphthalmia syndrome belongs to the spectrum of BCOR-related disorders. Clin Genet. 2020;98(4):413–5.
47. Gripp KW, Stolle CA, Celle L, McDonald-McGinn DM, Whitaker LA, Zackai EH. TWIST gene mutation in a patient with radial aplasia and craniosynostosis: further evidence for heterogeneity of Baller-Gerold syndrome. Am J Med Genet. 1999;82(2):170–6.
48. Seto ML, Lee SJ, Sze RW, Cunningham ML. Another TWIST on Baller-Gerold syndrome. Am J Med Genet. 2001;104(4):323–30.
49. Ashby T, Rouse GA, De Lange M. Prenatal sonographic diagnosis of Carpenter syndrome. J Ultrasound Med. 1994;13(11):905–9.
50. O'Byrne JJ, Laffan E, Murray DJ, Reardon W. Oculo-facio-cardio-dental syndrome with craniosynostosis, temporal hypertrichosis, and deafness. Am J Med Genet A. 2017;173(5):1374–7.
51. Khonsari RH, Delezoide AL, Kang W, Hébert JM, Bessières B, Bodiguel V, et al. Central nervous system malformations and deformations in FGFR2-

related craniosynostosis. Am J Med Genet A. 2012;158A(11):2797–806.
52. Stamm ER, Pretorius DH, Rumack CM, Manco-Johnson ML. Kleeblattschadel anomaly. In utero sonographic appearance. J Ultrasound Med. 1987;6(6):319–24.
53. Weber B, Schwabegger AH, Vodopiutz J, Janecke AR, Forstner R, Steiner H. Prenatal diagnosis of Apert syndrome with cloverleaf skull deformity using ultrasound, fetal magnetic resonance imaging and genetic analysis. Fetal Diagn Ther. 2010;27(1):51–6.
54. Meilstrup JW, Botti JJ, MacKay DR, Johnson DL. Prenatal sonographic appearance of asymmetric craniosynostosis: a case report. J Ultrasound Med. 1995;14(4):307–10.
55. Hill LM, Grzybek PC. Sonographic findings with Pfeiffer syndrome. Prenat Diagn. 1994;14(1):47–9.
56. Cohen MM, Kreiborg S. Suture formation, premature sutural fusion, and suture default zones in Apert syndrome. Am J Med Genet. 1996;62(4):339–44.
57. Stark Z, McGillivray G, Sampson A, Palma-Dias R, Edwards A, Said JM, et al. Apert syndrome: temporal lobe abnormalities on fetal brain imaging. Prenat Diagn. 2015;35(2):179–82.
58. Leo MV, Suslak L, Ganesh VL, Adhate A, Apuzzio JJ. Crouzon syndrome: prenatal ultrasound diagnosis by binocular diameters. Obstet Gynecol. 1991;78(5 Pt 2):906–8.
59. Zhou G, Schwartz LT, Gopen Q. Inner ear anomalies and conductive hearing loss in children with Apert syndrome: an overlooked otologic aspect. Otol Neurotol. 2009;30(2):184–9.
60. Gorincour G, Rypens F, Grignon A, Garel L, Bortoluzzi P, Oligny L, et al. Prenatal diagnosis of cloverleaf skull: watch the hands! Fetal Diagn Ther. 2005;20(4):296–300.
61. Ferreira JC, Carter SM, Bernstein PS, Jabs EW, Glickstein JS, Marion RW, et al. Second-trimester molecular prenatal diagnosis of sporadic Apert syndrome following suspicious ultrasound findings. Ultrasound Obstet Gynecol. 1999;14(6):426–30.
62. Van Maldergem L, Siitonen HA, Jalkh N, Chouery E, De Roy M, Delague V, et al. Revisiting the craniosynostosis-radial ray hypoplasia association: Baller-Gerold syndrome caused by mutations in the RECQL4 gene. J Med Genet. 2006;43(2):148–52.
63. Lee HJ, Cho DY, Tsai FJ, Shen WC. Antley-Bixler syndrome, description of two new cases and review of the literature. Pediatr Neurosurg. 2001;34(1):33–9.
64. Haye D, Collet C, Sembely-Taveau C, Haddad G, Denis C, Soulé N, et al. Prenatal findings in Carpenter syndrome and a novel mutation in RAB23. Am J Med Genet A. 2014;164A(11):2926–30.
65. Lertsburapa K, Schroeder JW, Sullivan C. Tracheal cartilaginous sleeve in patients with craniosynostosis syndromes: a meta-analysis. J Pediatr Surg. 2010;45(7):1438–44.
66. Noorily MR, Farmer DL, Belenky WM, Philippart AI. Congenital tracheal anomalies in the craniosynostosis syndromes. J Pediatr Surg. 1999;34(6):1036–9.

21 Neuroimaging in the Craniosynostoses

Susan Blaser and Charles Raybaud

21.1 Introduction

The craniosynostoses (CS) are usually suspected, diagnosed, and often assessed, by clinical examination only. Confirmation with imaging may be needed to confirm the stenoses and to evaluate the associated skull base, calvarial, brain, and vascular structures, particularly in cases with complex and syndromic craniosynostosis.

Skull shape in the craniosynostoses reflects compensatory growth at patent sutures and lack of growth perpendicular to the fused suture. Brain abnormalities commonly associated with both the simple and complex craniosynostoses (CS) may result from brain deformation reflecting that focal or diffuse constriction of the bony vault. They may also be mediated by the CSF when the venous drainage is impeded by the bony abnormality, as occurs when the craniosynostosis involves the skull base foramina, or they may be developmental, part of the syndromic constellation. While brain deformations related to bone deformities are the most apparent, modern imaging has also revealed cerebral developmental changes that are part of the disease. These associated changes seem logical in syndromic craniosynostoses, but modern imaging demonstrates that it may also occur in seemingly "isolated" single-suture craniosynostoses, suggesting that the developmental disorder that affects the bone may also interfere with brain development. Additional abnormalities such as dentofacial problems (Apert, Crouzon mostly), inner ear (Apert), exoptosis (FGFR mutations), limb anomalies (Apert, Pfeiffer, Saethre-Chotzen, Antley-Bixtler, Muenke, and Baller-Gerold RECQL4 syndromes), and upper airway obstruction (highest in Apert, Crouzon, and Pfeiffer) are imaging clues to aid in phenotype-genotype assessment.

21.2 The Imaging Tools

The choice of imaging modalities required is based on the need to evaluate the calvarium, brain, and CSF for a given clinical presentation. In clinically complex cases, that may also include the assessment of the minor sutures, the skull base and synchondroses, the craniocervical junction, and the upper cervical spine. Assessment of arterial and venous structures is also required in cases where surgical access may be compromised. Imaging tools include Photogrammatic analysis, fetal and postnatal ultrasonography, plain film radiography, CT with 3D surface reconstructions, MRI, and vascular studies on either CT or MRI [1–4].

Photogrammatic analysis, with an overlay of pre-and postoperative scans, has been used to

S. Blaser (✉) · C. Raybaud
Radiology, The Hospital for Sick Children and University of Toronto, Toronto, ON, Canada
e-mail: susan.blaser@sickkids.ca; charles.raybaud@sickkids.ca

F. Di Rocco, J. Kestle (eds.), *Neurosurgical Aspects of Craniosynostosis*,
https://doi.org/10.1007/978-3-031-69386-1_21

objectify calvarial changes in the single-suture synostoses by assessment of cranial length and width, diagonal measurements, quadrant volumes, anterior and posterior asymmetry ratios, and cranial index, but is not able to provide information regarding intracranial contents [5, 6].

Ultrasonography (U/S) is considered an efficient tool to evaluate single-suture stenosis in infants under 8 months of age. It can be used to provide a first postnatal sutural evaluation, as it is relatively cheap, easily available, without radiation, easy to repeat, and can be performed without sedation at the infant's bedside. It also allows a first assessment of the brain and peri-cerebral spaces. Hyperechogenic osseous thickening with external periosteum is seen with bony bridging, while a hypoechogenic gap reflects the unfused suture. Sagittal sutures are shown to have an end-to-end appearance, while the coronal and lambdoid sutures typically have a beveled junction. The metopic suture shows a beaked appearance, whether fused early or at the age-appropriate time [7–13]. Normative values of suture width are available for both US and CT. The measurements should be obtained well away from the fontanels. The average width of the proximal sagittal suture at birth on ultrasound is 0.9–1.4 mm, but 5.0 ± 0.2 mm on CT, decreasing by approximately half at 1 month of age. The difference between modalities may reflect the inclusion of a fibrous portion of the suture. It should be noted that while postnatal U/S readily evaluates the entirety of the sagittal, metopic, and lambdoid sutures, it cannot evaluate the skull base synchondroses in the coronal synostosis, which involve the coronal hemi-ring and skull base, or in complex craniosynostoses. It is strongly operator-dependent, needs to be performed by an experienced professional, and acoustic transmission may be hindered by thick hair [14] (Fig. 21.1).

Calvarial bones appear hyperechoic on *prenatal ultrasound* at or after 9 weeks GA, while cranial sutures are identifiable by focal through-transmission at 15–16 weeks gestation and when the imaging plane is perpendicular to the synostosed suture. Loss of the suture visualization precedes thickening of bone and subsequent indentations or "divets" at the site of the fused suture or minor fontanel. The coronal and lambdoid sutures are more readily accessible on fetal ultrasound than metopic or sagittal sutures, although metopic synostosis is identifiable if trigonocephaly is pronounced. A triangular appearance of the skull is present on axial images in metopic synostosis, while a triangular calvarial appearance may be seen on coronal images of sagittal synostosis. Syndromic cases are usually easier to identify due to the severity as in cases of the cloverleaf skull, abnormal brain imaging, and associated features like limb anomalies. Evidence of calvarial deformity due to constraint by uterine malformations, fibroids, or multiple gestations is easily assessed. Identification of calvarial deformity is furthered by the use of 3D surface reconstructions on both CT and MRI [15–18]. Milder cases of single-suture synostosis may be missed. Additional useful features include an abnormal cephalic index, normally between 75% and 85%, for example in sagittal synostosis, the head circumference remains stable, while the BPD drops centiles. In scaphocephaly, the CI is below 75%, and in brachycephaly above 86%. Syndromic synostosis may be noted at the first anatomy ultrasound scan around 20 weeks of gestation [16, 18, 19]. Additionally, the presence of the "Brain Shadow Sign" with acoustic shadowing due to the failure of sound waves to penetrate a closed suture increases the diagnostic rate [20] (Fig. 21.2).

Plain film radiography was formerly the method of choice to confirm a clinical diagnosis of CS, but not anymore with the advent of more sophisticated techniques. In our institution, infants seen for skull asymmetry are referred instead for an ultrasound if single-suture synostosis is suspected or for ultra-low-radiation dose CT if synostosis appears complicated, syndromic, or the infant is preoperative. While no longer having an important role in the preop evaluation of the craniosynostoses, plain films remain useful in the serial postoperative assessment of surgical apparatus, for example, posterior cranial vault distraction hardware, or to assess the extracranial component of ventricular catheters in the presence of shunt. Plain film radiography may, how-

Fig. 21.1 Coronal US (**a**) in a GA 37 week old newborn demonstrates a patent sagittal suture. The arrows demarcate the bony border of the suture. Coronal US (**b**) in a 17 day old neonate with Apert syndrome shows markedly widened sagittal suture width (arrows) at location well behind the anterior fontanel. Coronal US (**c**) in a 13 day old neonate with Muenke syndrome and unicoronal synostosis reveals the elevated orbital roof (arrow) ipsilateral to the unilateral coronal synostosis. Coronal US (**d**) reveals sagittal synostosis (arrow) in a 5 month old infant with microcephaly

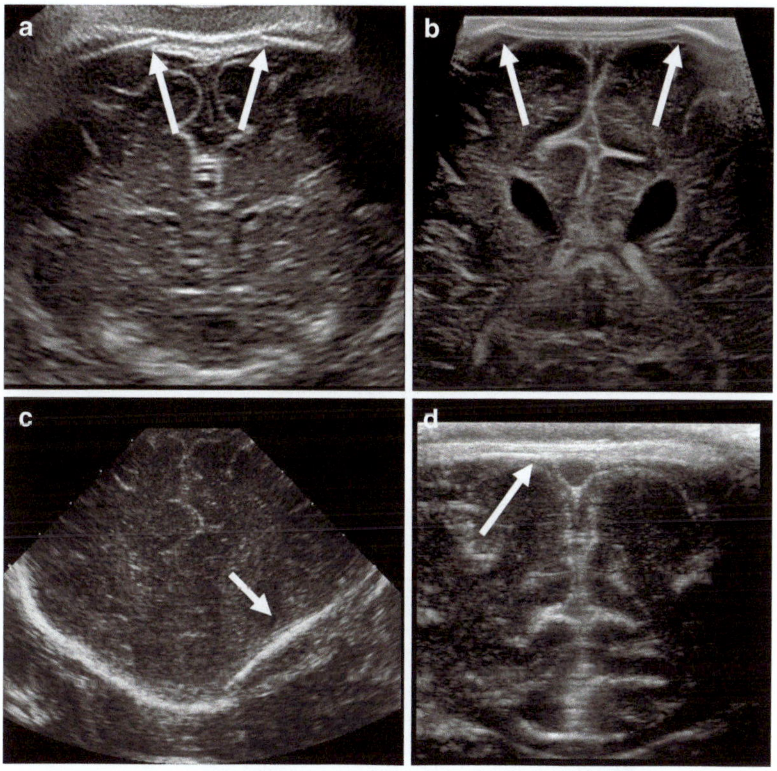

Fig. 21.2 Fetal US. Axial fetal US (**a**) performed at GA 27 + 6 weeks in a pregnancy with maternal FGFR1 Kallmann mutation reveals trigonocephaly (arrow). Follow-up postnatal oblique 3D CT at 7 weeks of age (**b**) confirms beaking and fusion (arrow) of the metopic suture. Axial fetal US (**c**) performed at GA 26 + 0 weeks in confirmed Apert syndrome demonstrates the brain shadow sign, with the shadow (arrow) from the fused coronal sutures obscuring the frontal lobes. Postnatal oblique 3D CT at 6 weeks of age (**d**) confirms bicoronal synostosis (arrow). Note early midface and glabellar retrusion

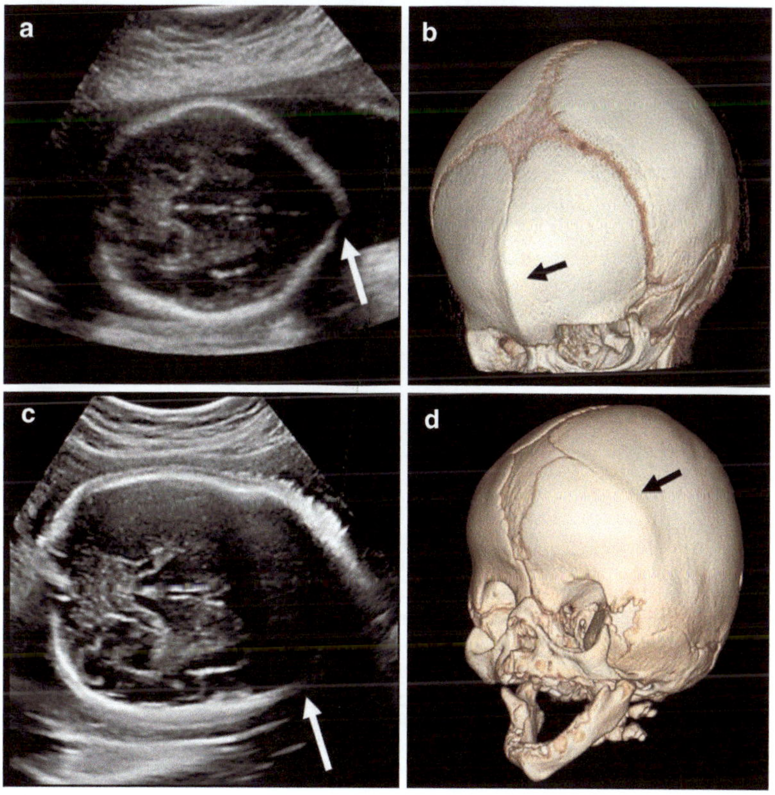

ever, be obtained as part of a skeletal survey for genetic assessment. Low calvarial density in the neonate, blurring of the sutures, inability to assess the minor sutures and basal synchondroses, and the presence of partial fusion render suture assessment on radiography difficult. Absence or straightening of the sutures, bridging or breaking, and sclerotic bands reflecting the fused sutures and pressure-related inner table scalloping or lacunae are classically described. Serrations of the closed coronal, squamosal, sagittal, and lambdoid sutures may remain visible into the fourth decade or later. The metopic suture fuses between 3 and 9 months of age and is the only suture that fuses completely without visible serrations of hydrocephalus (Fig. 21.3).

Computed tomography (*CT*) allows for a fast, ultra-low-radiation dose examination of the skull with 3D-volumic reformatting. Images in this manuscript were performed with 20–30 mAs (DLP of 29.7 with an effective dose of 0.09 mSv). While radiographs can demonstrate many of the salient features of craniosynostoses, such as skull and orbit shape and involvement of the major vault sutures of the cranial vault arches, specific advantages of CT and 3D calvarial and skin surface reconstructions include an exquisite demonstration of the skull base, minor sutures, and synchondroses [21] (Fig. 21.4). The width of the major and minor sutures and synchondroses are easily measured and correlated with published controls of both measurements and the expected timing of

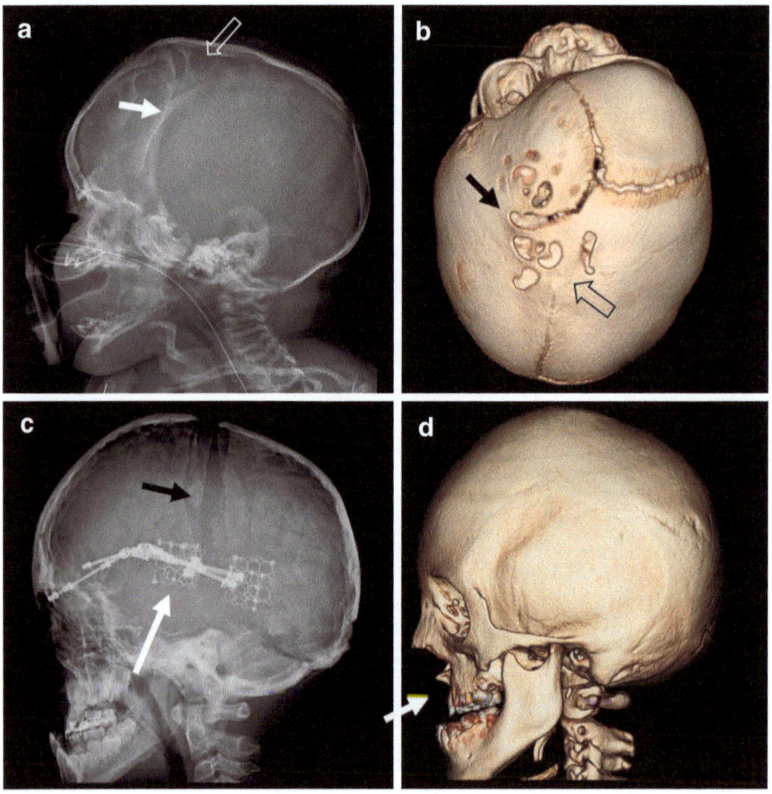

Fig. 21.3 Radiographs. Lateral skull radiograph (**a**) obtained as part of genetic skeletal survey at 5 days of age demonstrates microcephaly and coronal synostosis (arrow). Lacunae are present (open arrow). Ultralow-dose axial 3D CT reconstruction (**b**) performed in the same infant at 30 days shows both sagittal (open arrow) and coronal (white arrow) synostosis and confirms multiple bony lacunae around the fused sutures. 22q11DS mutation was confirmed. Lateral radiograph (**c**) demonstrates posterior distraction apparatus (white arrow) and separation of the operative margins in a nearly 9-year-old child with Alagille syndrome (JAG1 mutation). Preoperative lateral CT 3D reconstruction (**d**) in the same child revealed brachycephaly, pansynostosis, and maxillary retrusion (arrow)

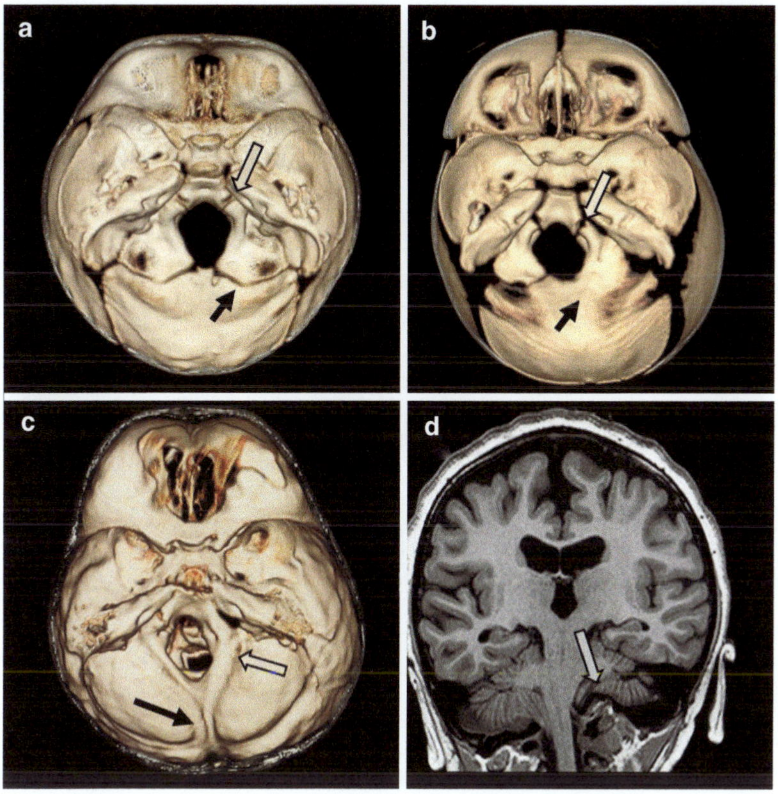

Fig. 21.4 Skull base synchondroses. Axial 3D reconstruction (**a**) in a 4-month-old infant control reveals normal patent anterior intraoccipital synchondroses (open arrow) and patent posterior intraoccipital synchondroses (arrow). A normal Kerkring ossicle has been incorporated into the posterior arc of foramen magnum. Axial 3D reconstruction (**b**) in a different 4-week-old infant with multiple congenital anomalies shows patent anterior intraoccipital synchondroses (open arrow), but unilateral fused posterior intraoccipital synchondrosis (black arrow). Axial 3D reconstruction (**c**) of the child seen in (**b**), now nearly 5 years of age, shows hypertrophied margin of foramen magnum (open arrow) and fused ipsilateral anterior intraoccipital synchondrosis. There is hypertrophy of the inferior occipital crest (black arrow). Coronal T1 (**d**) of the same child shows acquired displacement of the cerebellar hemisphere by the hypertrophied bony protuberance (arrow)

suture closure, confirming the presence or absence of synostosis as the cause of skull and orbit deformity [14]. A common cause of nonsynostotic causes of skull deformity is positional plagiocephaly (Fig. 21.5). An additional cause of plagiocephaly is growth at accessory sutures (Fig. 21.6). Finally, focal calvarial thickening due to bone dysplasia, intraosseous vascular malformations, or neoplasms may simulate synostotic causes of skull deformity (Fig. 21.7). Data obtained from postnatal ultra-low-radiation dose CT can be used for virtual surgical planning (VSP) 3D printed templates, computer-aided design/computer-aided manufacturing (CAD/CAM), and in simulators for surgical training [22–24].

Low and ultra-low dose in vivo *fetal CT and 3D CT*, performed after 20 weeks gestation and using doses as low as 0.5–2 mSv and model-based iterative reconstruction (MBIR), are used in some centers in the evaluation of fetal skeletal dysplasias and anomalies [17, 25–27]. Autopsy-based CT with 3D reconstructions can be very helpful in the evaluation of calvarial sutures and skull base synchondroses. Microfocus-CT (micro-CT) takes considerably less time than UHF-MRI and can be used to evaluate bone and soft tissue structures in fetuses <20 weeks' GA. Evaluation of soft tissues with micro-CT, however, does require iodine-based staining prior to imaging [28–31].

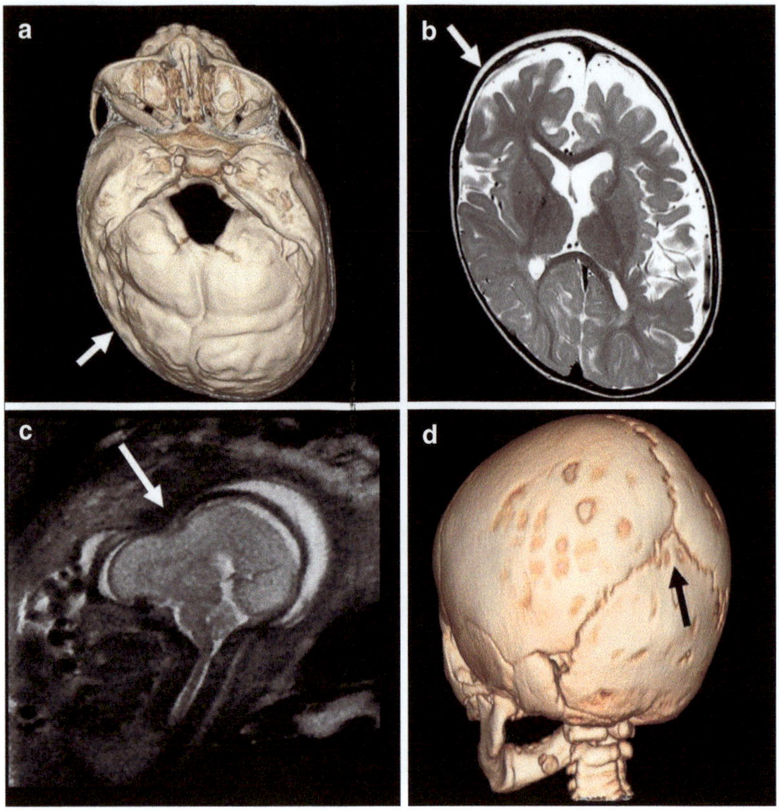

Fig. 21.5 Positional plagiocephaly. Axial 3D CT (**a**) in a 19-month-old hypotonic infant with PIGN mutation shows right posterior positional plagiocephaly (arrow). T2 axial MRI (**b**) demonstrates ipsilateral frontal bossing. Pericerebral CSF is redistributed to the left hemisphere due to right posterior mechanical compression. Sagittal T2-SSFSE (**c**) in a 27-week-old fetus reveals calvarial deformity due to constraint from fibroids and oligohydramnios. Oblique 3D CT (**d**) in a different 3-month-old back sleeper imaged for brachycephaly shows indentation of the lambda point (arrow)

Pre- and postoperative *Vascular Imaging* provides an illustration of the intracranial venous and arterial systems in selected cases utilizing CT venography (CTV) or CT angiography (CTA), both of which require contrast injection and specific postinjection timing and/or MR venography (MRV) and MR angiography (MRA), which require neither. Arterial abnormalities are less common but do occur. *Venous abnormalities* are common in the syndromic or complex craniosynostoses, and include persistent fetal sinuses, dural sinus stenosis or obstruction, aberrant venous drainage, sinus pericranii, collaterals, and dilated emissaries [32–35] (Fig. 21.8). In one study of 41 patients with FGFR mutation-related craniosynostosis, venous abnormalities occurred in 76%. They were universal in Pfeiffer patients and present in 84% of Crouzon patients and 64% of Apert patients [35]. During development, the skull base foramina surround nerve and vascular structures, mesenchyme clearing, condensing, and then ossifying around them. While the shape and size of the skull base foramina during development is dictated by traversing nerves and blood vessels, abnormal skull base ossification, and sutural/synchondrosis fusion in FGFR mutations, for example, can in turn lead to progressive foraminal stenosis with resultant compression and deformity of those traversing structures over time [36–39]. Jugular foraminal stenosis in FGFR mutations leads to dural sinus stenosis at the junction of the sigmoid sinus and internal jugular vein resulting in venous outflow resistance [38, 40–43]. Similarly, MRV studies are suggested in TWIST1-related craniosynostoses due to the progressive nature of foraminal stenosis [44]. Even compression on the flattened side in patients with posterior positional plagiocephaly is associated with a higher incidence of venous abnormalities on that side [45]. Sinovenous sinus volume has been shown to increase following posterior cranial vault distraction plus foramen magnum decompression due to the "dural traction effect" in a small cohort of

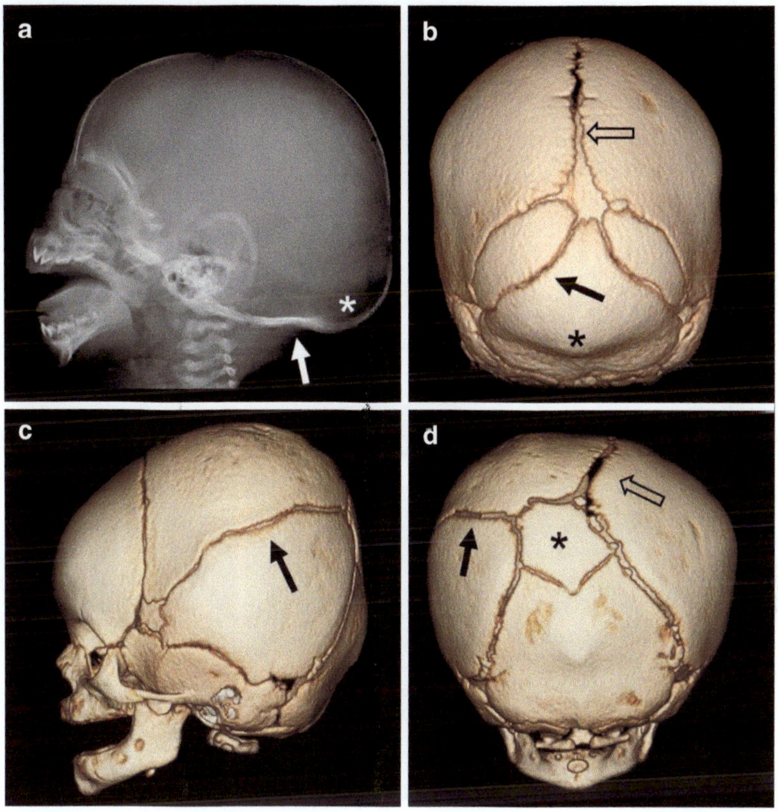

Fig. 21.6 Abnormal skull shape due to accessory sutures. Lateral radiograph (**a**) obtained at 10 weeks of age for dolichocephaly shows an elongated AP skull and a horizontal shelf-like supraoccipital bone (arrow). Posterior CT 3D reconstruction (**b**), however, demonstrates a patent sagittal suture (open arrow). Growth at the patent suture of the accessory supraoccipital os (black arrow) contributes to elongation of the occiput (asterisk) or bathrocephaly (**a**, **b**). Lateral 3D CT (**c**) in a 9-week-old infant with plagiocephaly shows an accessory parietal suture (arrow). Posterior CT 3D reconstruction in the same infant (**d**) shows lateral displacement of the sagittal suture (open arrow) due to growth at the accessory suture (black arrow). An accessory interparietal os (asterisk) is present

children with syndromic synostosis and chronic tonsillar herniation [43]. Imaging features can be used to differentiate between physiologic IJV slenderness and pathologic IJV stenosis or narrowing. Important features of clinically significant IJV stenosis include local stenosis, abnormal venous collaterals, local white matter hyperintense signal, and mismatch between the transverse diameter of IJV and the caliber of the jugular foramina or bony transverse sinus groove on the inner table of the calvarium [46]. While intracranial hypertension in complex or systemic craniosynostosis may reflect venous outflow obstruction, craniocerebral disproportion, Chiari 1 malformation, and obstructive sleep apnea are also implicated [47–49].

Sinus pericranii associated with occipital and cervical venous plexi can be seen with obstruction of the usual outflow foramina and redirected flow. These have been reported in the FGFR2, FGFR3, and TWIST-related syndromes, including Apert, Crouzon, Pfeiffer, Jackson-Weiss, Achondroplasia, and Saethre-Chotzen syndromes, and can also be seen in cases of mutation-unconfirmed complex craniosynostoses. Communication between internal and external compartments can be suggested by a bony defect on CT and must be evaluated with vascular imaging for preoperative planning, as they may significantly compromise access during cranial vault reconstruction. Additionally, as most are the dominant venous drainage, surgical planning

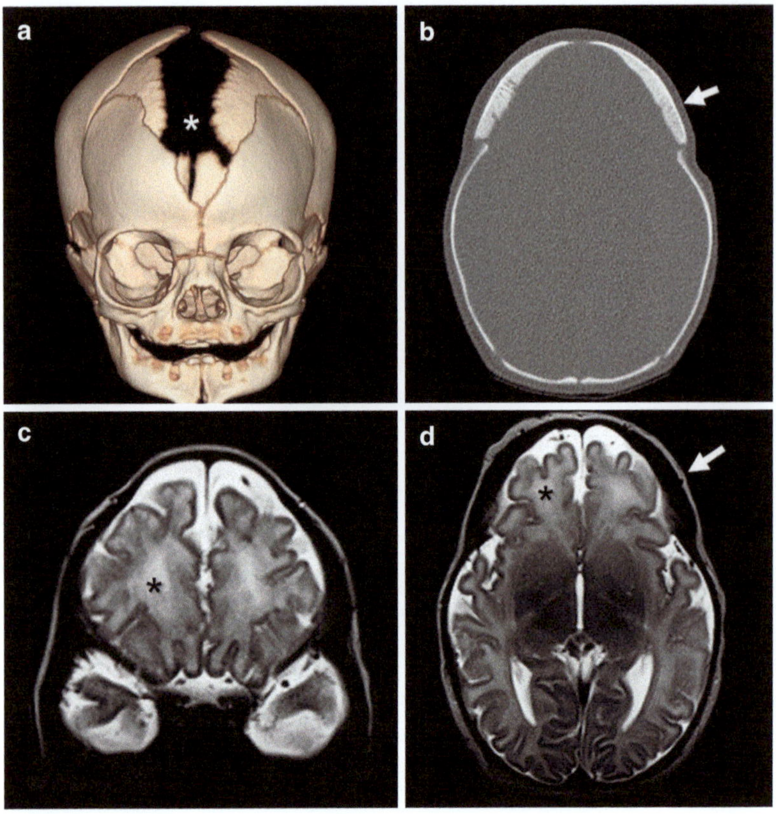

Fig. 21.7 Nonsynostotic trigonocephaly. Frontal 3D CT (**a**) at 12 days of age in newborn with Marshall syndrome (Col11A1), and trigonocephaly reveals bitemporal narrowing, widely patent fontanel, and sagittal suture (asterisk). Axial CT (**b**) shows thickening of the frontal bone (arrow). The metopic suture remains open. Coronal (**c**) and axial (**d**) T2 MRI at 9 days of age demonstrate frontal lobe hypoplasia (asterisk) and calvarial thickening (arrow)

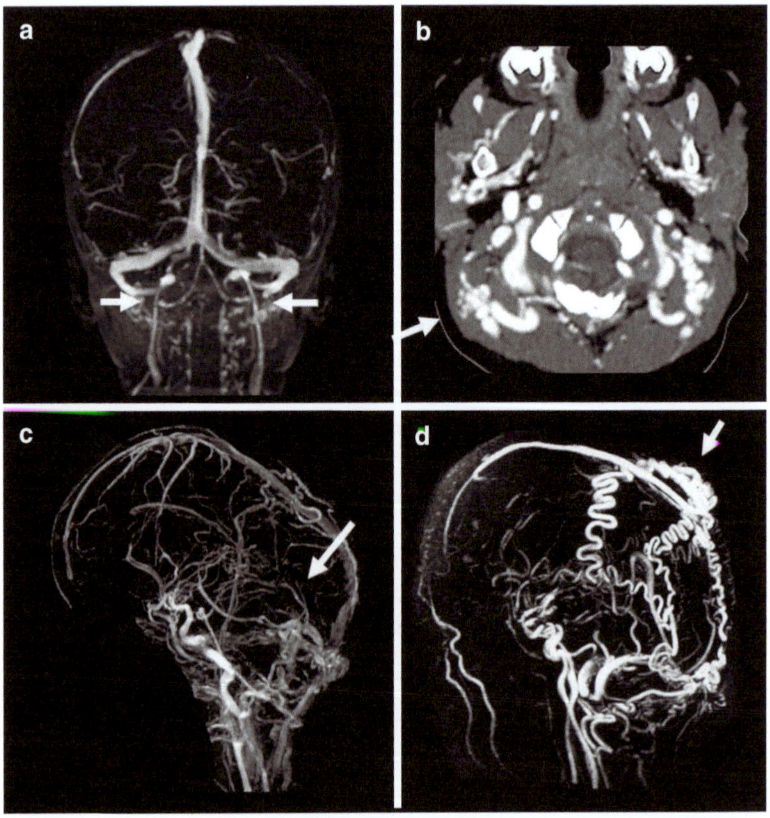

Fig. 21.8 Venous obstruction and collaterals. MRV (**a**) in a 17-month-old toddler with Crouzon syndrome shows bilateral jugular vein stenosis (arrows). CT venogram (**b**) in an 8-month-old infant, also Crouzon syndrome, with jugular vein obstruction reveals extensive suboccipital collateral veins (arrow). MRV (**c**) in a 7-month-old with Crouzon syndrome reveals loss of venous flow in a thrombosed straight sinus (arrow) after shunt placement, but prior to cranial vault reshaping. MRV (**d**) in a 12-year-old child with Crouzon and a history of remote cranial vault reshaping and sinovenous obstruction shows extensive superficial venous collaterals (arrow)

needs to include preservation rather than occlusion of the abnormal venous connection to avoid stroke or fatal outcome [50–56] (Fig. 21.9).

Specific arterial features in the craniosynostoses include those related to the skull base, such as progressive stenosis of the carotid canal following fusion of the contiguous petro-occipital fissure or due to pseudomigration of the juxtasellar carotid arteries following arrested skull base growth due to early fusion of the central skull base synchondroses in the syndromic craniosynostoses with FGFR mutations. Other craniosynostosis syndromes may also exhibit vascular abnormalities. Vasculopathies, both venous and arterial, are present in 30–40% of patients with Alagille syndrome (JAG1 or NOTCH2). Specific arterial abnormalities in Alagille syndrome, such as stenoses, aneurysms, dolichoectasia, and moyamoya are felt to reflect defects in angiogenic vascular remodeling [57–59]. Displaced vessels may interfere with a surgical approach. Intrasphenoid- or intrasellar kissing or contiguous carotid arteries have been reported in association with empty sella syndrome, with dolichoectasia and with acromegaly, but as previously discussed, may be present in the FGFR mutations due to early fusion of the intersphenoidal and spheno-occipital synchondroses [37, 60–64] (Fig. 21.10). Additionally, medially displaced and kissing retropharyngeal carotid arteries and abnormal high or low position of the cervical carotid bifurcations may be seen, for example with 22q11.2 deletions, both in velocardiofacial and DiGeorge patients [65]. Arterial spin labeling (ASL) fused with MRI images may be used to study regional cerebral blood flow in craniosynostosis patients. Frontal lobe CBF in trigonocephaly patients under 18 months of age is normal, while patients under 1 year of age with syndromic craniosynostosis have demonstrated lower panlobar, cortical, and white matter CBF than controls. CBF has been shown to be greater in treated than untreated syndromic craniosynostosis patients, falling into the range of the control

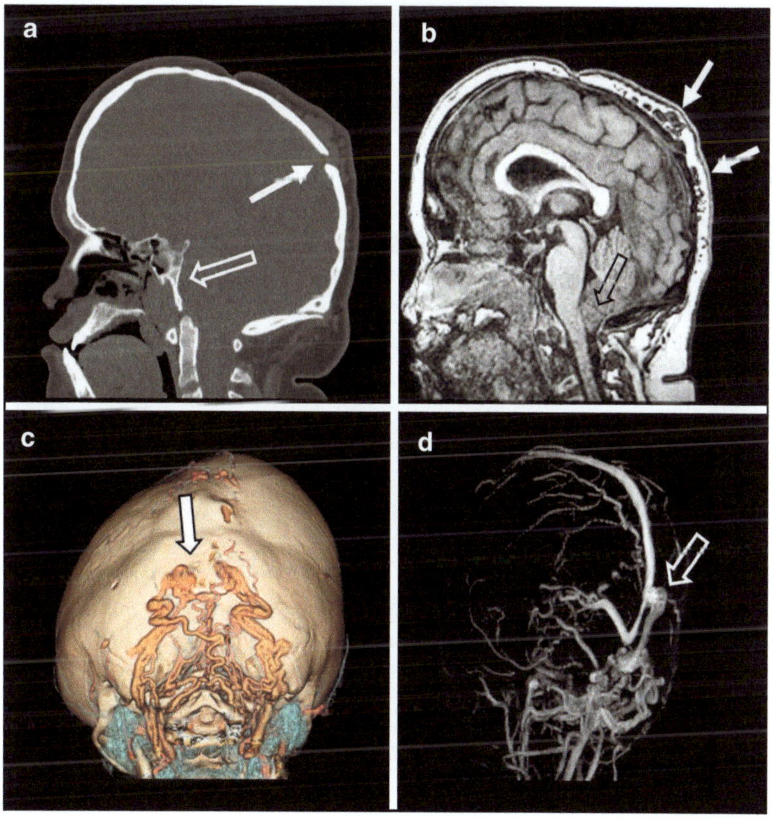

Fig. 21.9 Sinus pericranii. Sagittal CT image (**a**) in a 12-year-old with Crouzon syndrome demonstrates focal skull defect (arrow) and typical scalloped clivus (open arrow). T1 sagittal image (**b**) in same preteen shows multiple flow voids (arrows) from associated sinus pericranii and extracranial collaterals. Note also the Chiari 1 malformation (open arrow). 3D CT venogram (**c**) in a 4-year-old child with pansynostosis reveals a prominent suboccipital venous plexus (arrow). Axial MRV (**d**) in the same child demonstrates the sinus pericranii (open arrow) supplying the extracranial suboccipital venous plexus

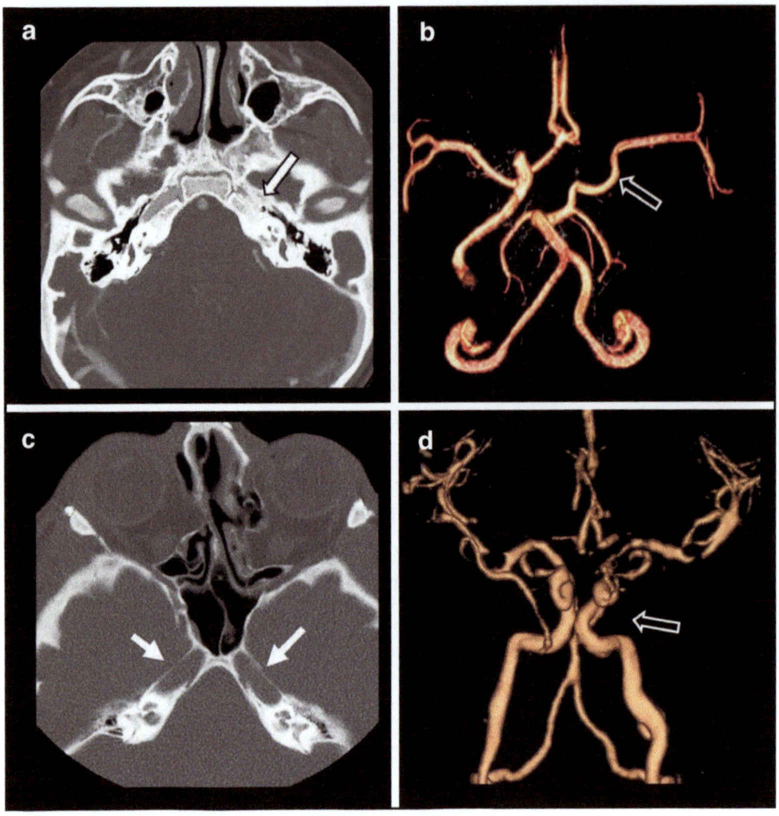

Fig. 21.10 Arterial abnormalities. Axial CTA (**a**) in an 8-year-old with Alagille syndrome and multisuture synostosis reveals absent left carotid canal (arrow). MRA (**b**) confirms absent ICA and origin of the left MCA from the PCA (open arrow). Axial CT (**c**) in a 14-year-old with Crouzon syndrome shows medialized carotid arteries (arrows). MRA (**d**) in a different 12-year-old with Crouzon syndrome shows severe carotid medialization (open arrow) or "kissing carotids"

subjects although the expected CBF childhood peak occurred somewhat later than in controls [66, 67].

Concomitant brain imaging utilizing *routine brain CT doses or magnetic resonance imaging (MRI)* is required when evaluating for syndromic involvement or for perioperative complications, as ultra-low-dose CT does not provide a detailed evaluation of brain anatomy. The presence of microcephaly or marked asymmetry also alerts us to the need for further brain imaging. MRI avoids ionizing radiation but may require sedation or general anesthesia. MR imaging aids in the evaluation of clinical features associated with craniosynostosis such as increased intracranial pressure, hydrocephalus, and vascular anatomy, and may clarify the etiology of headache, epilepsy, and abnormal cognitive development (Fig. 21.11). Routine 3D T1 MRI and particularly 3D T1 spoiled gradient echo-based (T1SGRE) sequences have shown some facility visualizing vault suture and 3D reconstructions are reported with the latter, but visibility is currently inferior to that of CT [68, 69]. With the currently available technology, "black bone" 2D MR prenatally and postnatally, and "CT-like MR-derived" source images postnatally demonstrate the skull and the sutures well, both and fast imaging allows a good appreciation of the fluid-filled spaces [70–73]. The use of "black bone" technology to plan 3D printing CAD/CAM and assisted cranial vault reconstruction has been reported [74, 75]. However, while postprocessed 3D reconstructions of the skin surface and skull shape are possible with MR imaging, 3D demonstration of the minor sutures and actual visualization of the skull base synchondroses is not yet robust (Fig. 21.12).

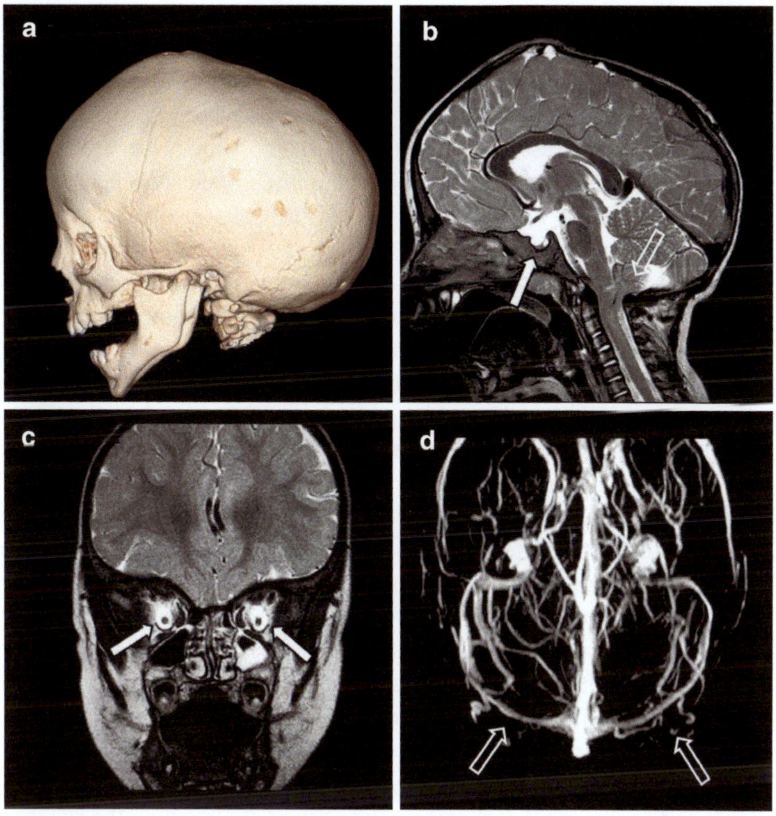

Fig. 21.11 Increased intracranial pressure. Lateral 3D CT (**a**) in a FGFR/TWIST-negative 16-month-old toddler reveals pansynostosis. MRI shows multiple features suggesting increased intracranial pressure. Sagittal T2 (**b**) demonstrates both partially empty sella (white arrow) and Chiari 1 malformation (open arrow). T2-weighted coronal image (**c**) in the same child reveals enlarged optic nerve sheaths (open arrows). MRV (**d**) shows narrowing of the transverse sinuses. Both features reflect increased intracranial pressure

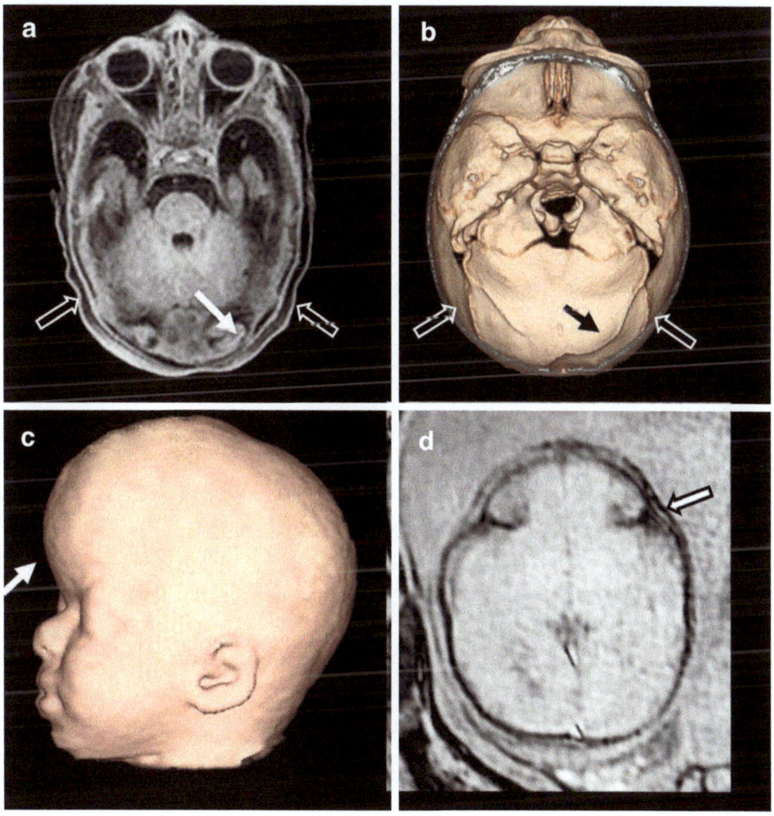

Fig. 21.12 Black bone technique. MRI black bone technique (**a**) in an 8-week-old infant with microcephaly demonstrates normal lambdoid synostoses (open arrows) and additional focal calvarial defect (arrow). Axial 3D CT (**b**) reveals an accessory unfused ossification center (arrow) contiguous with the mendosal suture. Lateral 3D skin surface reconstruction image (**c**) from fetal MRI at 34 weeks' gestation shows frontal bossing (arrow) and brachycephaly. Black bone sequence (**d**) shows the fused pterion (open arrow) in the same fetus with Crouzon syndrome and bicoronal synostosis

21.2.1 Specific Features of the Craniosynostoses

Restricted growth perpendicular to early fused suture or sutures in association with persistent growth and enlargement of the adjacent uninvolved sutures leads to characteristic head and orbital shapes. Patterns of fusion reflect the involvement of the vault arches. The sagittal arch includes the metopic and sagittal sutures, but also the ethmoidofrontal suture. The lambdoid arch includes the lambdoid sutures, but also the occipitopetrosal, occipitomastoid sutures, and sphenooccipital synchondrosis. The parietosquamosal arch consists of the parietosquamous and parietomastoid sutures. The coronal arch consists of the coronal sutures, the anterior branch of which includes the frontosphenoidal and ethmoidosphenoidal synchondroses, while the posterior branch is composed of the sphenosquamous, sphenoparietal, and sphenopetrosal synchondroses [76, 77]. Partial or asymmetric involvement or variation in the timing of fusion of arch components may lead to atypical plagiocephaly and orbital shapes and to skull base scoliosis or endocranial base deflection due to asymmetric shortening of the cranial base [60, 61, 78–81].

Metopic synostosis can present as an isolated single-suture synostosis, or may be involved in syndromic, complex, or pansynostosis. Partial fusion originates at the nasion around 3 months of age, with fusion extending toward the anterior fontanelle. The window of complete closure ranges from 8 to 14 months. Early fusion leads to trigonocephaly with forehead breaking, a narrowed anterior cranial fossa, and hypotelorism are present in *metopic synostosis*. Age-appropriate physiologic metopic fusion occurs without forming the serrated fusion lines seen after fusion of the sagittal, coronal, and lambdoid fusion and may exhibit some midline ridging. Assessment of the fusion site may help confirm early synostosis. A midline endocranial ridge or spur, the "M" sign, is present at the site of physiologic fusion, and an endocranial notch, the "omega sign," is present in synostotic patients, although there is crossover. In addition to the superomedial displacement of the orbits, also known as "quizzical" orbits, there is the medial displacement of the supraorbital foramina. While no single feature was pathognomonic of metopic synostosis, these signs were especially helpful if multiple were present [82–85] (Fig. 21.13).

Scaphocephaly due to *sagittal synostosis* is the result of elongation of the skull in the anterior-posterior direction. Patterns of calvarial deformity are dependent upon the site of sagittal fusion (anterior, central, or posterior), as well as the presence or absence of additional suture and synchondrosis involvement [86]. Early onset of fusion of the *sagittal suture* occurring in the first year of life tends to occur in the posterior third of the suture with small remnants of open suture more pronounced anteriorly than posteriorly. When the metopic suture remains patent, the shape is called sphenocephalic with the typical relative enlargement of the anterior fontanel and frontal bossing [1, 87, 88]. Additional specific features of calvarial shape and facial features in sagittal synostosis are biparietal narrowing or narrowing of the vertex on AP view, occipital bulleting, and a longitudinal "beak and groove" containing the superior sagittal sinus. Less commonly, fusion of the metopic suture concomitant with sagittal synostosis results in a leptocephalic (narrow forehead) shape [89]. Localized fusion originating in the anterior or middle third of the sagittal suture may lead to a retrocoronal vault depression and a saddle-shape deformity known as *clinocephaly*. Children presenting with clinocephaly tend to be slightly older. Early or atypical sagittal fusion or the presence of additional suture involvement requires CT assessment of the minor sutures and skull base synchondroses [90, 91]. The skull base synchondroses are typically spared in isolated sagittal synostosis, however, the foramen magnum often has a smaller volume than normocephalic controls and the transverse and anterior sagittal diameters reflect this [92]. *Bathrocephaly*, a steplike deformity of the occiput due to overgrowth at lambdoid or accessory occipital ossification centers or at mendosal sutures remaining patent past 6 months of age is more common in sagittal synostosis than in controls. Mendosal suture fusion extends centrally to laterally to the asterion, begins in utero,

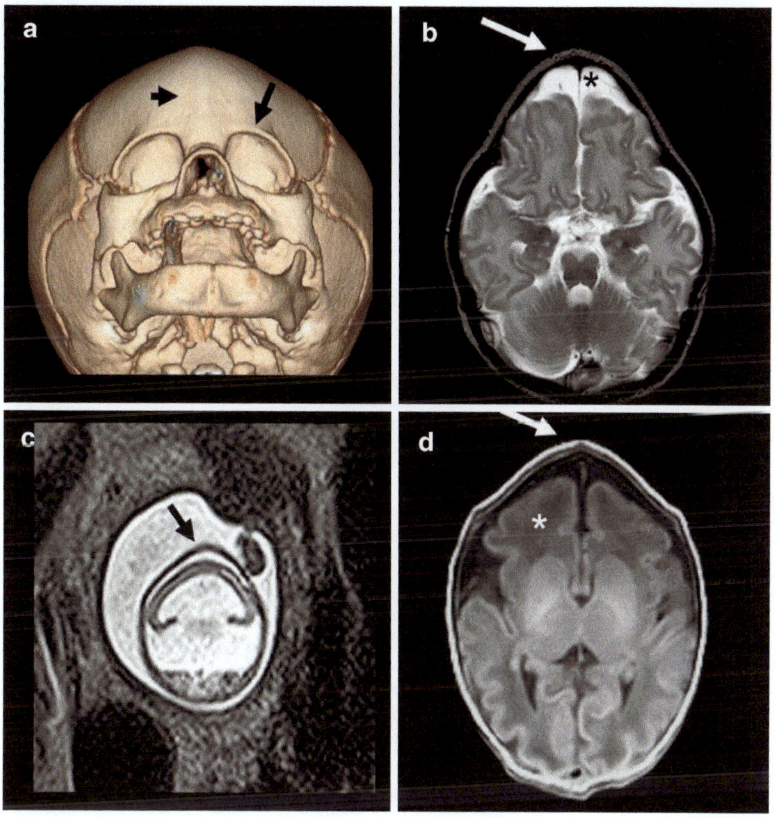

Fig. 21.13 Metopic synostosis. 3D CT (**a**) in a non-syndromic 4-week-old infant shows beaking of the fused metopic suture (short arrow) and medial uptilted ("quizzical") orbits (arrow). Axial T2 (**b**) reveals trigonocephaly (arrow), mild lateral flattening of the frontal lobes, and prominent frontal peri-cerebral fluid (asterisk) in the same infant. SSFSE-T2 fetal MRI (**c**) at GA 19 weeks demonstrates a lobar holoprosencephaly and trigonocephaly. T1 axial image (**d**) in an 8-day-old with microcephaly and trisomy 13 reveals trigonocephaly (arrow) and under-sulcated frontal lobes (asterisk)

and usually completes by 8 months of age, although a delay to 18 months may occur and the presence of lateral mendosal remnants in normal adult skulls has been reported [93–97]. Unless syndromic, intracranial abnormalities other than Chiari 1 are uncommon in isolated sagittal synostosis, however, Chiari 1 malformation is more common with familial cases of sagittal synostosis and with involvement of multiple sutures or skull base synchondroses (Fig. 21.14).

Lambdoid synostosis is relatively uncommon, although imaging may be obtained to differentiate it from posterior positional plagiocephaly. In unilateral lambdoid synostosis cases, ipsilateral mastoid prominence occurs due to growth related to the patent posterolateral fontanel and occipitomastoid synchondrosis and is best shown on frontal or occipitomental (Waters' view). Downward shift of the ipsilateral ear and petrous bone occurs. There may be posterior fontanel deviation and skull base tilting. While ipsilateral forehead flattening occurs in unilateral lambdoid synostosis, contralateral forehead flattening occurs in posterior positional plagiocephaly, leading to a trapezoid configuration in unilateral lambdoid synostosis and a parallelogram configuration on axial CT in posterior positional plagiocephaly (Fig. 21.5). Bilateral lambdoid synostosis is often syndromic, seen in cases of FGFR-related bicoronal synostosis, where Chiari 1 malformations and increased intracranial pressure are common. Syndromic lambdoid synostosis may progress to involve contiguous sutures and synchondroses. Associated mendosal suture synostosis is often present in both unilateral and bilateral lambdoid synostosis. Lambdoid synostosis, brachycephaly, and posterior skull flattening have also been reported in rhombencephalosynapsis [98–100] (Fig. 21.15).

Trisutural fusion of the posterior sagittal suture and both lambdoid sutures with fusion across the posterior fontanel has been called Mercedes-Benz synostosis or bilamdoid and sagittal synostosis (BLSS). This complex craniosyn-

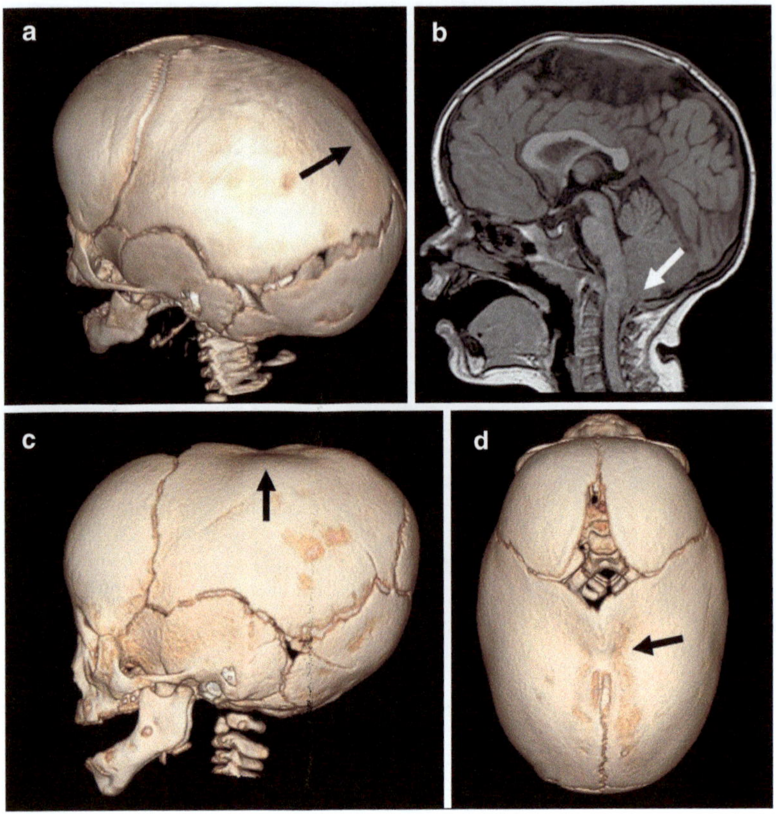

Fig. 21.14 Sagittal synostosis. Sagittal-oblique 3D CT reconstruction (**a**) in a 3-month-old ex-premature multiple birth infant with scaphocephaly demonstrates typical sagittal synostosis with bridging (arrow) of the mid to posterior sagittal suture, bullet-shaped occiput, and frontal bossing. Sagittal T1 (**b**) in the same child at 19 months old reveals normal AP dimension following strip craniectomy, but Chiari 1 protrusion (arrow) of the cerebellar tonsils through foramen magnum. Clinocephaly, saddle-shape depression (arrows) of the retrocoronal vault due to fusion of the anterior or middle third of the sagittal suture is shown on sagittal (**c**) and axial (**d**) 3D CT reconstructions in a 5-month-old with elongated AP calvarium

ostosis blunts the occipital bullet shape and may present with brachycephaly and indentation of the suboccipital bone adjacent to the posterior arc of foramen magnum. Extension to involve the mendosal sutures and posterior intraoccipital synchondroses leads to fusion of the inferior internal occipital crest and to decreased posterior fossa volume. It is associated with Chiari 1 deformation in greater than 50% of involved patients. It also may be an early presentation of pansynostosis [98, 101–103] (Fig. 21.16).

Unlike metopic, sagittal, and lambdoid synostosis, the coronal suture rarely fuses in isolation. The coronal synostoses are more complex due to the involvement of the coronal ring/hemi-ring. In *unilateral coronal synostosis*, an angle forms between the unfused sagittal and metopic sutures, with a fulcrum at the bregma. There is a shallow anterior cranial fossa with flattening of the ipsilateral forehead. Due to the involvement of the facial sutures, the frontomaxillary, nasofrontal, and nasomaxillary sutures, there is facial twisting, and the nasal root points toward the side of the synostosis [104]. Severity of craniofacial change is related to the differential timing of closure [76]. There may be associated skull base scoliosis or endocranial base deflection ipsilateral to the side of the involved coronal suture due to shortening of the ipsilateral zygomatic, sphenoid, and temporal bones along the sphenozygo-

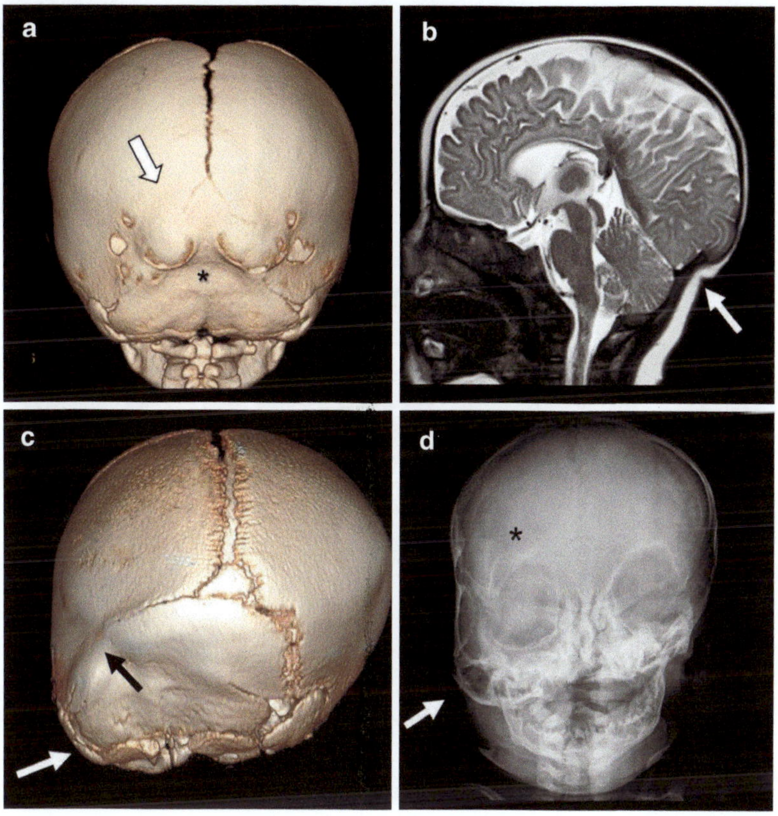

Fig. 21.15 Lambdoid synostosis. Posterior 3D CT (**a**) obtained in a 3-month-old infant without a defined genetic mutation shows an indented skull base (asterisk), bilateral lambdoid synostosis (arrow), closed mendosal sutures, and lacunae. Sagittal T2 MRI (**b**) in same infant confirms parieto-occipital shelf (arrow), but no Chiari 1 malformation at this time. Posterior 3D CT (**c**) in a 30-day-old infant shows unilateral fused lambdoid suture (black arrow) and typical prominent mastoid protrusion (white arrow). Frontal radiograph (**d**) in a different 11-week-old infant demonstrates right forehead depression (asterisk) associated with right lambdoid synostosis and ipsilateral mastoid protrusion (white arrow)

matic, sphenoparietal, and sphenotemporal suture fronts [77, 78, 105] (Fig. 21.17).

Bilateral coronal synostoses result in brachycephaly or brachyturricephaly and narrow bitemporal measurement [1, 87, 88]. Additionally, closure of the posterior branch (sphenoparietal, sphenosquamous sutures, and the sphenopetrosal synchondrosis) of the coronal ring in bilateral craniosynostosis leads to nasal stenosis, and insufficient facial growth. Posterior branch fusion and spheno-occipital synchondroses contribute to maxillary retrusion [106]. Orbital exophthalmos is present in bilateral syndromic synostosis. Involvement of the anterior branch of the coronal ring leads to differences in orbital shape in the coronal synostoses. Coronal suture synostosis begins in the middle of the suture and progresses outward. "Isolated" coronal synostosis is diagnosed at a younger age and there is usual progressive involvement to the lateral frontosphenoidal suture. In a small percentage, variations of this occur, dependent upon the order of involvement of the sutures and synchondroses. Vertex (coronal) to cranial base (frontosphenoidal) vector of fusion involvement is typical, base to vertex less common. With earlier involvement of the frontosphenoidal suture, there is a limitation of the vertical deviation of the greater wing of the sphenoid that gives rise to the taller or "Harlequin" orbit, while the involvement of the frontosphenoidal

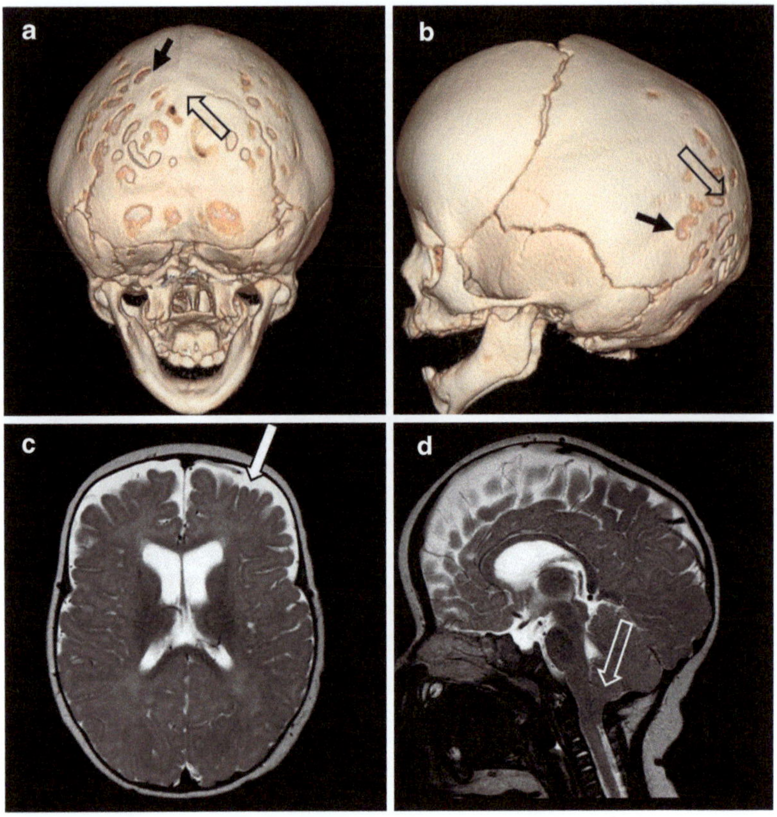

Fig. 21.16 BLSS (Mercedes-Benz) synostosis. Posterior (**a**) and lateral 3D CT reconstructions (**b**) in a 6-month-old infant with frontal bossing and large anterior fontanel show BLSS-type fusion of the lambdoid sutures, lambda point (open arrows), and posterior sagittal suture. Lacunae related to the asymmetric lambdoid fusion are present (black arrows). T2-weighted axial image (**c**) in the same infant reveals prominent frontal pericerebral fluid (arrow) associated with frontal bossing. Sagittal T2 image (**d**) demonstrates Chiari 1 malformation (open arrow)

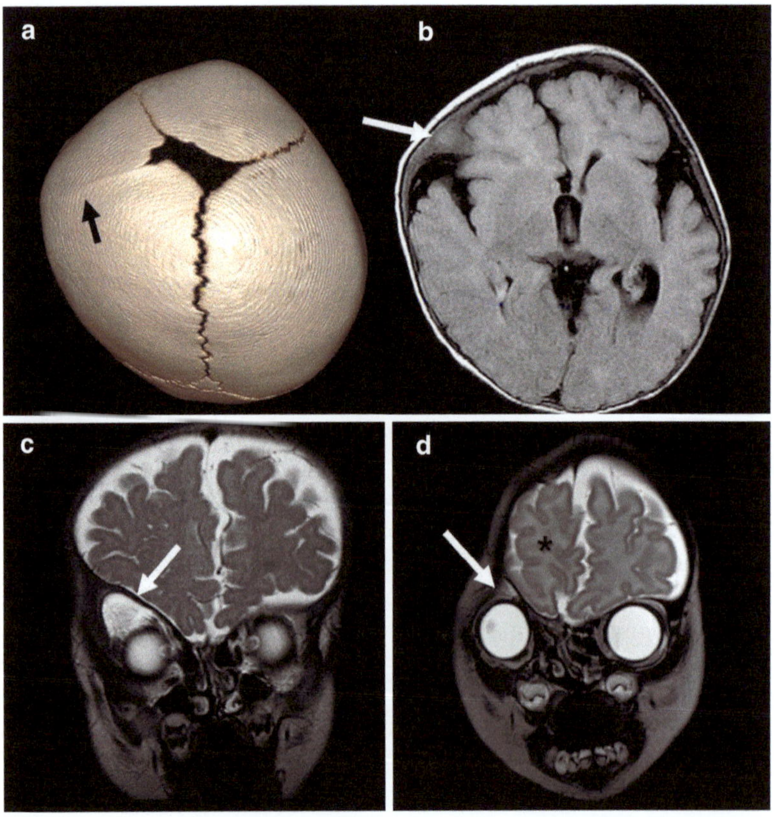

Fig. 21.17 Unicoronal synostosis, brain and CSF deformation. Axial 3D CT (**a**) in a 6-month-old infant with trisomy 9 demonstrates right unilateral coronal synostosis (arrow) resulting in tilted sagittal-metopic angle. Axial FLAIR (**b**) at 9 months of age shows bone buttressing at the site of fusion (arrow) and deformation of the frontal lobes. Coronal T2 (**c**) in the same infant shows prominent fat within "Harlequin" orbit (arrow). Coronal T2-weighted MRI (**d**) in a different 1-month-old infant with 22Q11DS and unilateral coronal synostosis shows frontal lobe dysplasia (asterisk). Lack of anterior falx results in frontal lobe interdigitation. Similar "Harlequin" orbit is present (arrow)

suture leads to a shorter, more oval orbit [77, 78, 107, 108] (Fig. 21.18).

Pansynsostosis or universal synostosis can be acquired or genetic. Pansynostosis may be seen following severe perinatal insult, such as hypoxia with brain atrophy. It may also reflect genetic causes, such as FGFR mutation-related kleeblatschädel, microcephaly, aneuploidy, or hereditary osteodystrophies (Fig. 21.19). For example, premature suture fusion has been seen in up to 20% of children with sickle cell anemia [109]. Progressive postnatal pansynostosis, with normal head shape, a slowly falling head circumference, and increased intracranial pressure, may be idiopathic or may be present as a mild syndromic phenotype [110]. Genetically associated pansynostoses may lead to typical or atypical skull configurations with or without lacunae. While symmetrical progression to cloverleaf or kleeblatschädel with orbital shapes occurs typically with Apert or Crouzon syndromes, asymmetric multisuture involvement has been reported in Muenke syndrome, all of which harbor FGFR mutations (Fig. 21.20).

As previously noted, ultra-low-dose CT excels in the evaluation of the major and minor sutures and synchondroses of the vault arches and skull base. Early fusion of the skull base synchondroses is a clue to potential complex or progressive craniosynostosis and for complications related to the foramen magnum and craniocervical junction. Ventrally, the basioccipital bone joins the

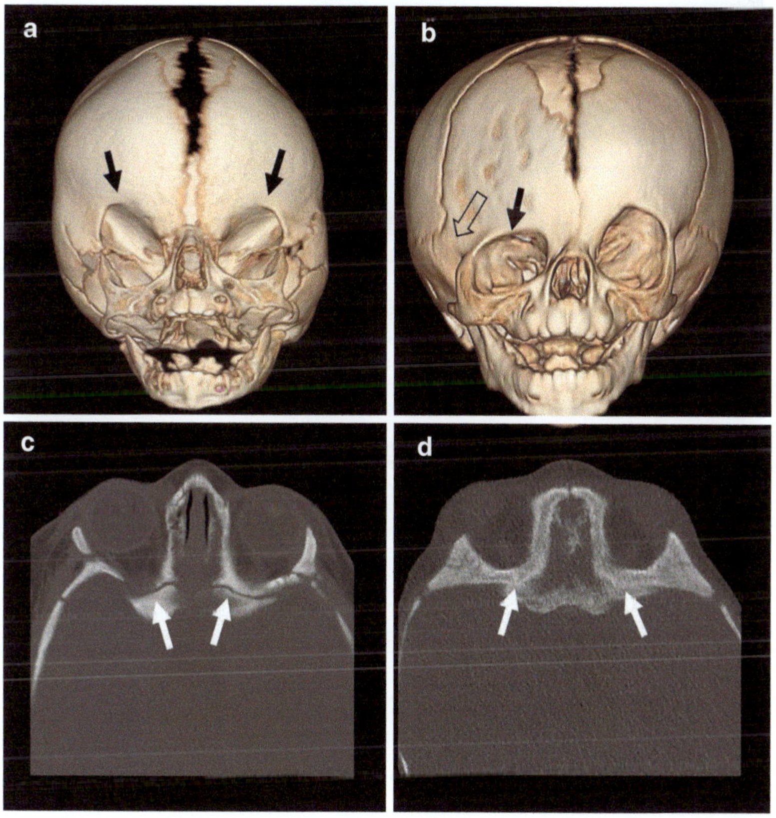

Fig. 21.18 Orbits in coronal synostosis. Coronal 3D CT (**a**) in an 11-week-old infant with FGFR3 mutation and bicoronal synostosis demonstrates bilateral elevation of the lateral bony orbits, "Harlequin" configuration (arrows). Coronal 3D CT (**b**) in an 8-month-old with Noonan syndrome and early involvement of the frontosphenoidal suture (open arrow), part of the coronal hemiring, reveals an oval (arrow) rather than "Harlequin" orbit. Axial ultralow-dose CT (**c**) in a 30-day-old normal control reveals the normal patent frontosphenoidal suture (arrows). Bilateral fusion of the frontosphenoidal sutures (arrows) is shown on axial CT (**d**) in a 3-month-old with Apert syndrome

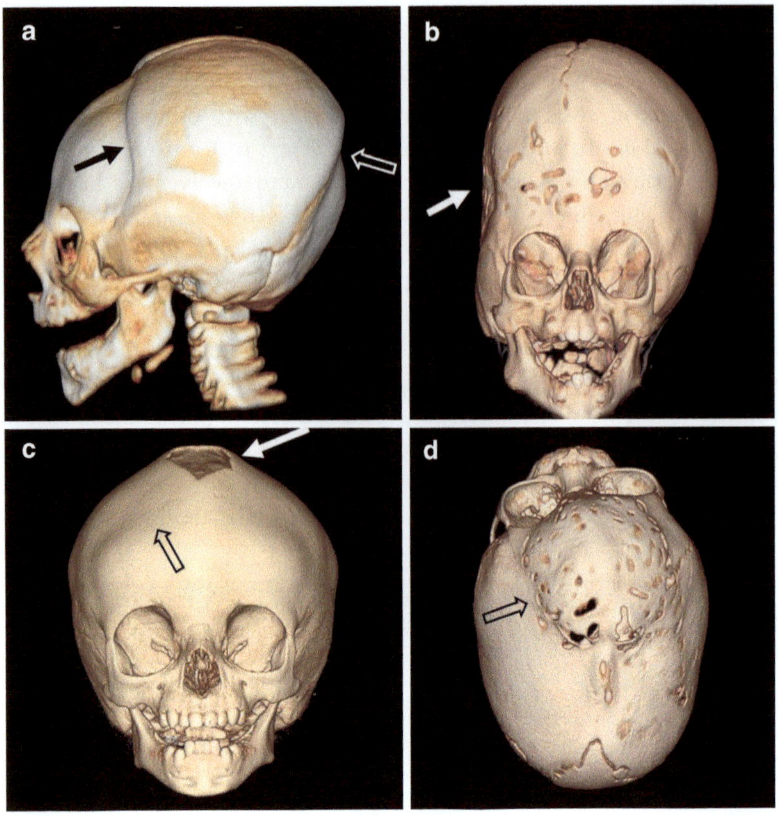

Fig. 21.19 Atypical pansynostosis. Sagittal 3D CT (**a**) in a 3-month-old infant with acquired microcephaly and pansynostosis following severe perinatal hypoxic ischemic encephalopathy shows ridging at the fused coronal (black arrow) and lambdoid (open arrow) sutures. Coronal 3D CT (**b**) in a 5-month-old infant with Chr 7p deletion reveals pansynostosis, lacunae, and indentation of the right parietosquamosal region (arrow). Coronal 3D CT (**c**) in a 14-month-old with an ILR11RA mutation and pansynostosis (open arrow on fused coronal suture). Patent anterior fontanel with everted margins (arrow) leads to a "volcano defect." Axial 3D CT (**d**) in a 4-month-old with a TCF12 mutation demonstrates metopic, sagittal, and coronal synostosis and bulging and lacunae of the calvarium overlying the region of the closed anterior fontanel (open arrow)

basisphenoid at the spheno-occipital synchondrosis, a component of the lambdoid arch. The spheno-occipital synchondrosis is considered a pivot point for craniofacial growth. A dense focal nodule of midline ossification bridging the spheno-occipital synchondrosis is usually visible on axial and sagittal reformats at around 8 years of age. Symmetric ossification centers lateral to this center may be seen within the synchondrosis before fusion and a dense continuous line, or fusion scar, can be seen upon fusion. While fusion is essentially complete in most by 17 years of age, the age range of complete fusion is variable, ranging between 6 and 27 years. Remnants may persist until later. Once fused, the sphenoid sinus reaches the clivus in nearly half [60–62, 79]. The spheno-occipital and intersphenoid synchondroses fuse considerably earlier in patients with FGFR mutations, including Apert, Crouzon, Pfeiffer syndromes, and achondroplasia, correlating with severity of midface hypoplasia and retrusion, and giving rise to a narrow skull base with potential intrasphenoid or intrasellar "kissing" carotid arteries [37, 63, 64, 79, 111] (Fig. 21.10c, d). Surrounding the foramen magnum are the basioccipital, exoccipital, and supraoccipital bones. The basioccipital and exoccipital bones are joined by the anterior intraoccipital synchondroses on each side. The posterior intraoccipital (innominate) synchondroses join the

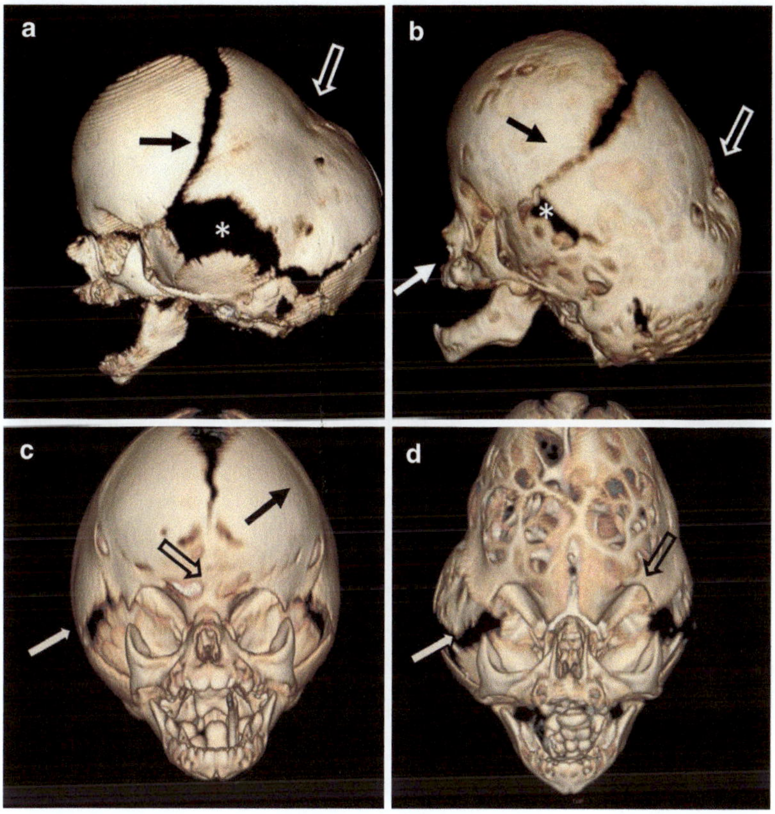

Fig. 21.20 Kleeblattschädel. Sagittal 3D CT reconstructions in infant with FGFR2 (Crouzon with acanthosis nigricans) mutation demonstrate rapid progression of pansynostosis between 7 days (**a**) and 2 months (**b**) of age. There is fusion of the sagittal suture (open arrows) on both images. The coronal (black arrow) and lambdoid sutures are patent at 7 days (**a**) and closing at 2 months (**b**). The squamosal suture is widely patent (asterisk) at 7 days (**a**), contributing to the cloverleaf configuration of the bulging squamosal region, but essentially fused by 2 months (**b**). There is new maxillary retrusion (white arrow). Coronal 3D CT (**c**) in a 2-day-old newborn with Crouzon syndrome reveals bicoronal synostosis (black arrow), metopic synostosis (open black arrow), and bulging squamosa with patent squamosal suture (white arrow). Coronal 3D CT (**d**) in a 15-day-old with Pfeiffer type 2 shows Harlequin orbits (open black arrow), bulging squamosa, and widely patent squamosal sutures (white arrow)

exoccipital and supraoccipital bones bilaterally and fuse. Neither the posterior nor anterior intraoccipital synchondroses belong to the sutural arches. The anterior intraoccipital synchondroses show partial fusion at 3.5 years and complete fusion around 7 to 10 years of age. The posterior intraoccipital synchondroses show partial fusion between 12 and 17 months of age and complete fusion by 4 years of age. Anterior and posterior intraoccipital synchondroses should be compared with age-matched controls, as early fusion may predate progressive cranial synostosis. Foramen magnum restriction can be marked and progressive in the FGFR mutation-related syndromes, including achondroplasia, Crouzon, Pfeiffer, Apert, and Muenke syndromes. Decrease in size of the synchondroses and early closure or ossification in the youngest infants and newborns is associated with foramen magnum coarctation and progression to pansynostosis and kleeblatschädel (Fig. 21.21). Foramen magnum restriction may already be restricted at birth, prior to the development of demonstrable calvarial suture fusion. There are some differences amongst the various syndromic synchondroses. Evaluation of the cranial base in achondroplasia and thanatophoric dysplasia demonstrates earlier bridging of the anterior intraoccipital synchondrosis [112].

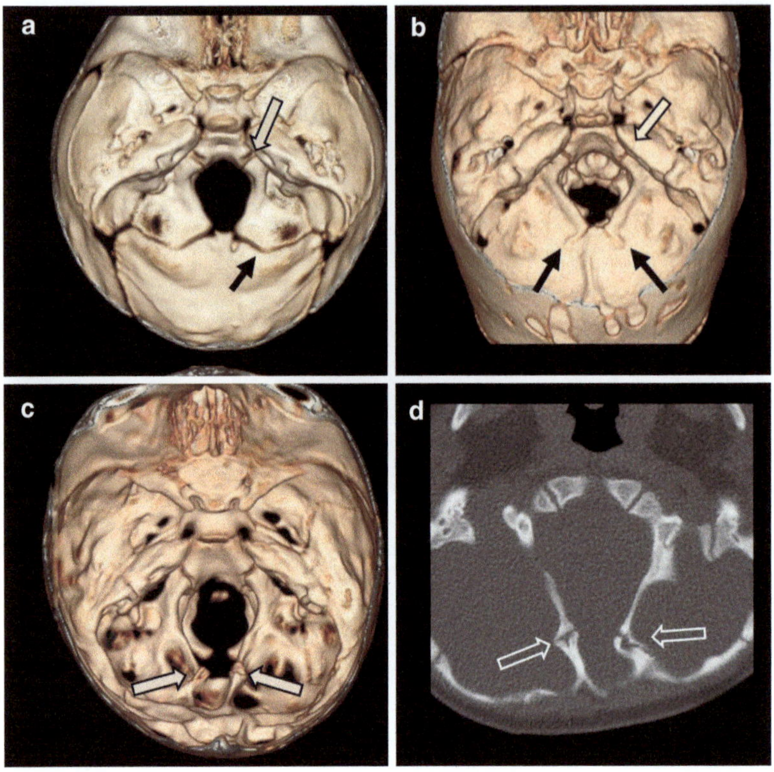

Fig. 21.21 Posterior intraoccipital fusion. 3D reconstruction (**a**) in a 4-month-old infant control reveals normal patent anterior intraoccipital synchondroses (open arrow) and patent posterior intraoccipital synchondroses (arrow). 3D reconstructions (**b**) in a 3-month-old infant with Crouzon syndrome show patent anterior intraoccipital synchondroses (open arrow) and fused posterior intraoccipital synchondroses (arrows). 3D reconstruction (**c**) and axial CT (**d**) in a 6-month-old infant with Loeys-Dietz syndrome demonstrate patent anterior intraoccipital synchondroses, but fused posterior intraoccipital synchondroses (open arrows) and an abnormally shaped foramen magnum. Lacunar defects are identified on both studies

The foramen magnum in achondroplasia narrows rapidly in the first year of life, particularly in the transverse dimension. In Crouzon, the spheno-occipital, petrooccipital, and intraoccipital synchondroses fuse earlier than controls and may completely fuse in the first year of life [113, 114]. Foramen magnum surface area is smaller in Crouzon and Pfeiffer syndromes than Apert, while the transverse diameter of the foramen magnum is smaller in achondroplasia, Crouzon, Pfeiffer, and Apert syndromes. Of the FGFR-related syndromes, Crouzon shows a reduced AP dimension, while Pfeiffer and Apert show elongation. Saethre-Chotzen, related to TWIST-1 mutation, only shows a mild decrease in the foramen magnum area, reflecting a decrease in the AP measurement of the anterior foramen magnum from basion to the posterior margin of the anterior intraoccipital synchondrosis. Not all Muenke cases show early intraoccipital synchondrosis fusion. A similar decrease in the anterior foramen magnum AP dimension is reported in scaphocephalic patients, resulting in a decrease in area, but to a lesser degree than in the brachycephalic patients. The foramen magnum is typically spared in isolated bicoronal synostosis [42, 92, 115–119]. There is also a small Kerckring supraoccipital synchondrosis between the inferior margin of the supraoccipital bone and Kerckring's ossicle, the latter forming the opisthion, or midpoint of the posterior arc of the foramen magnum. Kerckring's ossicle or center may appear ossified in the late third trimester. This ossicle is variably visible in term births, with fusion in the first 3–4 months of postnatal life. Early or delayed incorporation of Kerckring's ossicle leads to stenosis in the former and a keyhole-shaped foramen magnum in the latter [21, 79, 113, 120].

21.3 CNS Abnormalities in the Craniosynchondroses

The first mechanism suggested to explain the clinical manifestations of CS sounded obvious: *brain growth restriction*, based on the then-dominant idea that the skull expanded as an effect of the cerebral growth during the first months of life. Premature fusion of the sutures would thus prevent adaptation to cerebral growth. Modern CT and MR morphometry studies, however, show that the volume of the brain and of the intracranial spaces is normal or even increased in patients with a craniosynostosis of any type, except in the rare cases of pansynostosis. Increased ventricular volume is largest in the syndromic bicoronal synostoses, Apert Syndrome in particular [121–125]. Also, modern data has made it clear that it is not the brain parenchymal volume, but CSF pressure, that drives the expansion of the vault. Neuroimaging demonstrates that the peri-cerebral space can be prominent in the fetus and maintained after birth, and for life, over the supra-Sylvian convexity in normal individuals. Therefore, while the cranial expansion may be prevented locally by an early sutural fusion, the force exerted by the CSF may induce a compensatory enlargement of the skull away from it [126–129], resulting in typical cranial deformities, which in turn allow the commonly observed "deformation" of the brain, as it adapts to the shape of the cranial cavity (Fig. 21.22).

21.3.1 The CSF in Craniosynostoses

Increased *intracranial pressure* (*ICP*) has been suggested as a possible cause for delays in neurodevelopment, by affecting the cerebral (mostly cortical) blood flow, or even by preventing a normal development of the cortex. It may also affect vision and is made worse by the occurrence of obstructive sleep apnea in patients with facial deformities. A high ICP can be identified by clinical evidence, such as increased cranial volume/head circumference, or even papilledema, and can be confirmed and monitored instrumentally. It is quite common in *complex* forms of craniosynostosis: Apert (up to 83%), Crouzon (up to 64%), Saethre-Chotzen (up to 43%), multisuture (up to 67%), and bicoronal (up to 31%) synostosis. It is also observed in a significant number of *single*-suture craniostenosis cases: sagittal (up to 14%) coronal (up to 16%), or metopic (up to 8%) [4, 124, 129, 130]. It may be present without enlarging the head. It may also present as an accumulation of CSF, either due to a deficit of absorption, or with an obstruction the CSF pathways; both absorptive and obstructive (loss of compliance) processes are usually associated. Useful imaging features include inner table scalloping, crowding of the posterior fossa, and distortion or disruption of the venous system.

In infants, a defect of CSF absorption typically results in the pattern of an *external hydrocephalus* (or *benign arachnoid CSF collection*), intracranial accumulation of CSF with macrocephaly. This can appear and develop whenever the arteriovenous compliance is reduced by an increased venous outflow resistance while the CSF absorption is decreased, occurring when the venous outlets are restricted. A study evaluating the utility of MR venograms has shown that the pattern of the dural sinuses is commonly incomplete in young children with external hydrocephalus [45], in a way that is actually often referred to as a "normal anatomic variant," possibly erroneously. Such a process of restriction of the venous outlets is evident in cases of sagittal synostosis when the abnormal growth of the sutural tissue surrounds the superior sagittal sinus. The ridges of the resultant furrow may form an Ω-like overgrowth on either side of the superior sagittal sinus [130, 131], which may impact the CSF absorption by reducing the caliber of the sinus itself, or by partially obstructing the outlets of the cortical veins when they connect with the sinus,

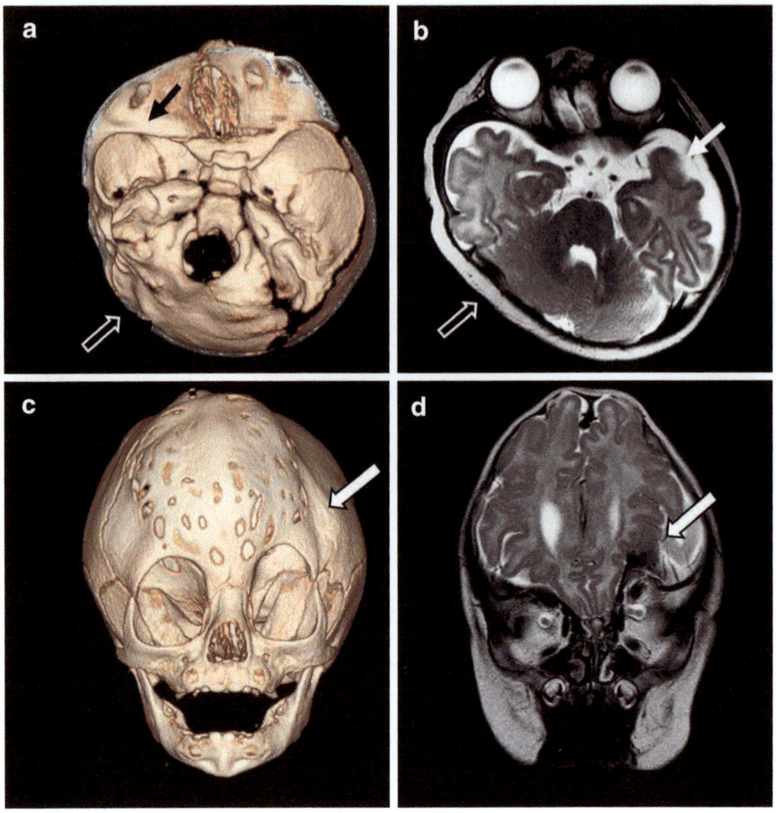

Fig. 21.22 Brain deformation. Axial 3D CT (**a**) reconstruction in a 28-day-old infant with congenital plagiocephaly and skull base deflection demonstrates buttressed right sphenoid greater wing (black arrow) associated with unicoronal synostosis. There is right mendosal and lambdoid synostosis (open arrow). The ipsilateral posterior intraoccipital suture is closed. Axial T2 (**b**) shows right cerebellar compression (open arrow) and enlargement of the left middle cranial fossa CSF (white arrow) contralateral to the synostosed coronal suture. Coronal 3D CT (**c**) in a 4-month-old infant with TCF12 mutation demonstrates metopic fusion, lacunes, and left coronal synostosis (arrow) with Harlequin orbit. Coronal T2 (**d**) in the same infant reveals associated distortion (arrow) of the left frontal lobe

either directly or through the parasagittal dura. The alleged involvement of the arachnoid granulations seems unlikely in infants, as the practice of cranial venography at this age has revealed that they have not really developed yet. In any case, the high venous pressure associated with CSF retention may produce a CSF collection as long as the calvarium is capable of expansion. A similar process of bony overgrowth with venous compromise has been convincingly demonstrated in a series of cases of metopic craniosynostosis, with, in addition, the early development of emissary veins along the anterior sagittal midline correlating with both an Ω-shaped bony ridge and subarachnoid prominence of the CSF spaces [132]. Consequentially, whenever the development of an external hydrocephalus is suspected, neuroimaging must include coronal images in addition to the traditional axial images, to better appreciate the bony changes and the peri-cerebral spaces of the vertex. It should also include imaging of the dural venous sinuses, as low down as the upper cervical region to evaluate the patency of the cranial venous drainage.

By contrast, an *obstructive hydrocephalus* is characterized morphologically by a dilatation of the ventricles with an *effacement* of the pericerebral spaces, clinically by the evidence of intracranial hypertension, clinically by a slowly enlarging head, and on serial (if needed) imaging, by a progressive enlargement of the ventricle. It is important to stress that the ventricular dilatation is not, in itself, a proof of obstructive hydrocephalus. It is present, although usually mild, in nonobstructive hydrocephalus. More importantly, a nonprogressive *ventriculomegaly* is common in complex craniosynostoses, reported in 30–70% of Crouzon/Pfeiffer patients, and in 40–90% of Apert patients [133], and can be explained by a developmental defect of the white matter. Hydrocephalus is considered as probably incidental, when observed in a simple craniosynostosis. In syndromic craniosynostoses, on the contrary, real progressive obstructive hydrocephalus does occur, affecting up to 15% in the whole group of patients, but up to 88% in the group of Pfeiffer type 2 [134]. It is generally closely associated with the presence of a Chiari 1 deformity, which is particularly common in Crouzon, Pfeiffer/Cloverleaf skull, and multisuture synostoses involving the lambdoid suture. Yet, its pathogenesis in complex craniosynostosis is unclear, and it probably results from the occurrence of several separate but convergent actors. Of course, the effacement of the posterior fossa cisterns and the small size of the foramen magnum may play a role, but cannot be the whole story, as in other contexts, a Chiari 1 deformity is typically not associated with hydrocephalus, and a surgical correction of the Chiari 1 in complex craniosynostosis does not necessarily cure the hydrocephalus. The association of the venous factors to the posterior fossa abnormalities is therefore felt to be determinant. This restriction of the venous outflow can convincingly be explained by the severe bony narrowing of the jugular and possibly also, by an abnormal dural proliferation [47, 48]. The effects of this narrowing may be made more severe in the context of the anatomical and physiological changes of the cranial drainage that take place when the standing position is being acquired. Subsequently, with progressive bony restriction of the jugular foramen and jugular vein attenuation, collateral drainage develops via the emissary veins of the posterior fossa [36, 47, 48]. In the meantime, however, three factors are significant: (1) the anatomical restriction of the venous outflow decreases the compliance of the system to the force exerted by the systolic wave, as most of the systolic blood volume goes directly into the veins (continuous systolo-diastolic arterio-venous flow); (2) the high venous pressure opposes the parenchymal and trans-dural absorption of the CSF; (3) the turgor of the venous channels adds its own mass effect the intracranial content. The CSF compliance being at the same time reduced by the effacement of the cisternal spaces and fourth ventricle in the posterior fossa, the addition of those factors may well explain the development of a progressive hydrocephalus. Of note, however, it has been mentioned that hyperactivation of FGFR2 could also be involved in a hydrocephalic process [135].

21.3.2 Brain Abnormalities in Craniosynostosis

The most striking deformity of the neural axis that results from the bony abnormalities is *Chronic Tonsillar Herniation*, also known as a *Chiari 1 deformity*. In syndromic craniosynostosis, hydrocephalus is associated with a Chiari 1 deformity in most of the cases, but only 47% of cases of Chiari 1 deformity are associated with hydrocephalus [99]. It is now admitted that in general, Chiari 1 is not a cerebellar malformation per se (except in very rare instances), but a cerebellar deformation that appears when the cerebellum expands normally into too small a posterior fossa; it is a primarily bony, not neural problem [136]. It is a common finding in the context of some, but not all, syndromic craniosynostosis: 72.7% of Crouzon; 50% of Pfeiffer; 100% of Cloverleaf; but only 1.9% of Apert syndrome. The difference reflects the variation in fusion of the intraoccipital synchondroses [99]. In Crouzon and Pfeiffer syndromes, all spheno-occipital, posterior intraoccipital, and anterior intraoccipital sutures close early as compared with normal individuals; in Apert syndrome, only the spheno-occipital and posterior intraoccipital sutures do so, while the anterior intraoccipital sutures close at a more normal time [118]. This results in the posterior fossa being reduced in all diameters in the two former ones, while remaining transversally preserved in the later. In addition, it was demonstrated [99] that it is the early fusion of the lambdoid suture that precipitates the process of chronic tonsillar herniation through the foramen magnum: this happens much earlier in Crouzon or Pfeiffer syndromes than in Apert syndrome. The anterior fontanel remains enlarged in Apert syndrome well beyond the time of closure in the other bicoronal craniosynostoses [122].

Although the presence of a Chiari 1 is occasionally seen in the presence of an otherwise isolated sagittal suture stenosis, the presence of it should alert to the possibility of either an undiagnosed syndrome or a familial case. In particular, the bony components of the fourth occipital sclerotome should be evaluated. Also, while a Chiari 1 deformity is not usually seen in association with a single-suture metopic, or coronal craniosynostosis, it is found in 25–50% of cases of nonsyndromic bilateral lambdoid synostosis, and in 70% of the cases of nonsyndromic multiple-suture craniosynostosis when the lambdoid suture is involved, against 7% if it is not [4]. On MR imaging, the diagnosis of a Chiari 1 deformity in this context is not different from what it is in other contexts: complete effacement of the cisterna magna, descent of the cerebellar tonsils across the foramen magnum, and depending on the severity, effacement the prepontine cistern and fourth ventricle, within, often, an abnormally shaped bony posterior fossa with a concave clivus and an abnormally oriented tentorium.

Other cerebral deformities are observed in craniosynostoses, but with no, or less significant clinical consequences. As a general rule, cerebral deformation follows the deformity of the skull. A posterior displacement of the parietal lobules was described in dolichocephaly, and a shortening of the anterior frontal lobes in trigonocephaly; the anterior temporal lobes in the cloverleaf phenotype bulge laterally, and the temporal horns may be enlarged as well, following the bulge of the temporal squama. It has been suggested by some authors that these deformations might explain some of the neurodevelopmental defects that are observed in growing children. However, such changes develop progressively, which allows the axons to grow and collaterals to adjust and probably to maintain normal connections with the cortex.

Many children with single-suture craniosynostosis develop intellectually in the low range of normality, and more severe intellectual defects or epilepsy are common in syndromic craniosynostosis, even in the absence of complications like hydrocephalus. If an early corrective surgery improves the situation, there is now ample evidence, pathologically and radiologically, that in most subtypes of craniosynostosis, the bony changes are associated with abnormal brain development. In syndromic craniosynostosis, this is consistent with the fact that Fibroblast Growth Factors FGFs (and their receptors FGFRs) are ubiquitous in the body and are, beyond the development of bone, involved, among others, in the development of the central nervous system (cell proliferation, neuronal differentiation, migration and apoptosis, presynaptic differentiation). Besides FGFR1, 2, and 3, TWIST1 (Saethre-Chotzen) modulates the response of FGFRs to FGF ligands; MSX2 (Boston-type craniosynostosis) modulates the downstream FGF activity; RAB-23 (Carpenter) regulates negatively the Hedgehog signaling in the ventral neural tube [137]. The frontal bone, the coronal suture in part, and the sagittal suture derive from the anterior Neural Crest Cells [138], which also participate in the development of the interhemispheric fissure and of the early commissural plate via *Fgf8*; FGFR1 and 2 mediate the action of *Fgf8*, which acts as an early organizer of the dorsal telencephalon (and of the brainstem); FGRF1 is essential for the early development of the corpus callosum, and acts as a receptor for L1CAM in the process of axonal fasciculation in the brain [139]. The gross malformations that can be observed in syndromic craniosynostoses concern the midline and the mesial temporal structures mostly; radiologically, they are more apparent at the level of the white matter (nonprogressive ventriculomegaly, callosal hypoplasia).

Apert syndrome (*FGFR2; s252w; p253r*) is the most common of the syndromic craniosynos-

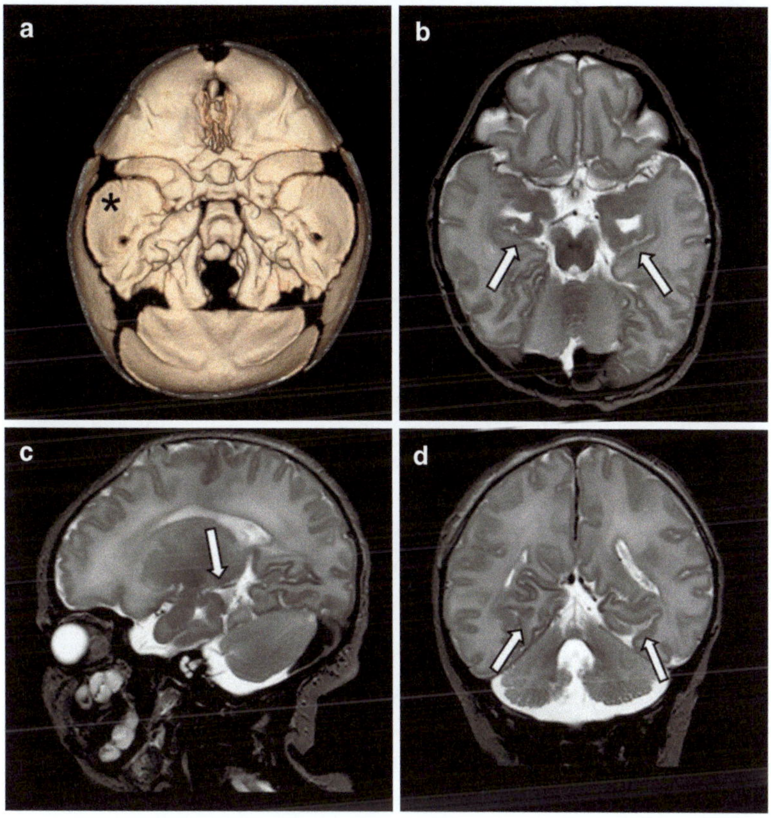

Fig. 21.23 FGFR temporal lobes. Axial 3D CT (**a**) in a 1-day-old with Apert syndrome demonstrates enlargement of the middle cranial fossa. Axial T2 (**b**) reveals overexpansion of the temporal lobes and abnormally shaped temporal horns. There are inferomedial deep transverse fissures (arrows). Abnormal sagittal clefting (arrow) is shown on sagittal T2 (**c**) in the same infant, while oversulcation (arrows) of the medial occipital lobes is revealed on coronal T2 (**d**)

toses, characterized by an early bilateral coronal, spheno-occipital, and posterior intraoccipital synostosis. Most children present with a significant developmental delay. They may present with seizures. The main brain abnormalities are a nonprogressive ventriculomegaly, rather than hydrocephalus, a significant callosal hypoplasia, an absence or attenuation of the septum pellucidum, and an "ammonic hypoplasia," abnormalities of the "rhinencephalon" or "olfactory complex": absence or midline fusion of the olfactory bulbs, tracts and tubercles; hypoplastic cornu ammonis, with triangular section of the temporal horn; prominent temporal lobes with anterior temporal over-convolution (Fig. 21.23) (but the cortex is histologically normal), yet poorly developed white matter; characteristically, there is a prominent abnormal inferior-medial transverse sulcus; All this is already present before the sutural closure in the fetus [140]; Additionally, the pyramidal tracts are incomplete in the brainstem [139–145]. Interestingly similar temporal abnormalities are found in the Pfeiffer syndrome (FGFR2) [140], and in different syndromes related to FGFR3 mutations (thanatophoric dwarfism, achondroplasia, and hypochondroplasia) [146–148]. This combined involvement of the mesial temporal and midline structures suggests the possibility of hyperactivity of the *telencephalic hem*, which corresponds to the lips of the dorsal fusion line of the telencephalon, that is, the embryonic anterior neural ridge [140]. The hem, which persists in adulthood as a medial hemispheric medullary velum that contains the fornix and the septocingulate perforating pathway (septum pellucidum), is in the 4–5-week-old embryo the inducer laterally, of the early telencephalic cortical plate (primordial hippocampus) and medially, of the telencephalic tela choroidea [149].

Crouzon syndrome (*FGFR2, multiple mutations*) is characterized by the early closure of the coronal, then lambdoid, spheno-occipital, and intraoccipital sutures, resulting in a brachycephaly with a small posterior fossa, in addition to the facial anomalies. Patients usually present with a Chiari 1 deformity and hydrocephalus is common, with a venous turgor. Even before hydrocephalus develops, a ventriculomegaly is observed; defects of the corpus callosum and septum pellucidum may be present [139, 145]. Abnormalities of the cortex have been described, as thicker in the frontal, parietal, and occipital lobes and thinner in the temporal, insular, and cingulate regions [150].

Pfeiffer syndrome type I (*FGFR1,2*) is characterized by brachycephaly (coronal synostosis), flat face, and hypertelorism, with a small posterior fossa with a concave clivus. Neurodevelopmentally the patients may be normal, or present a mental deficiency; a passive ventriculomegaly or a Chiari 1 deformity may be observed [139, 151].

Pfeiffer syndrome type 2 (*FGFR2*) is the most spectacular of all syndromic craniosynostoses as it presents with a cloverleaf skull: major brachycephaly and acrocephaly, exophthalmos, a very small posterior fossa with concave clivus, a diffusely dysplastic calvarium, and a massive bulging of the temporal squamae. Clinically, mental deficiency, seizures, and features of severe intracranial hypertension are observed. Morphologically there is a huge hydrocephalus associated with a severe form of Chiari 1 deformity. The septum pellucidum is absent, likely due to hydrocephalus, although a developmental defect cannot be ruled out. Venography would show a venous turgor with stenosis of the jugular foramina. There is a major deformation of the brain structures that results from the abnormal morphology of the calvarium: bulging temporal lobes with ballooning temporal horns, kinking of the brain that may be made apparent by the kinking of the corpus callosum, the occipital lobe being displaced below the third ventricle [139, 151, 152]. Such deformities of course preclude the identification of gross malformations of the mesial temporal lobes in vivo. The typical temporal lobe overfolding may become more apparent following shunting. A pathological study of four fetuses has demonstrated an outgrowth of the temporal lobes with malformation of the hippocampus and amygdala, suggesting that the hyperactivity of FGFR2 could, like in the Apert syndrome, result in hyperactivity of the hemispheric hem with a mesiotemporal dysplasia [135].

Pfeiffer syndrome type 3 (*FGFR2*) doesn't present with a cloverleaf skull, but there is a short anterior cranial fossa and a very small posterior fossa with a concave clivus. The patients present with epilepsy, severe neurodevelopmental deficiencies, high intracranial pressure, and hydrocephalus that can be explained by a Chiari 1 deformity and a stenosis of the venous jugular outlets [136, 151].

Saethre-Chotzen syndrome (*TWIST1*) is uncommon, and there is only scarce literature that describes the brain abnormalities [139, 153]. It is characterized by an acrocephaly/brachycephaly with proptosis and upper lid ptosis and is due to an early closure of the coronal, lambdoid, and metopic sutures, which may be associated with late-closing fontanels however, and parietal foramina. Clinically, affected children are said to be mentally normal, but some degree of mental retardation is often observed. Hypotonia is common, and they may present a pyramidal syndrome (lower limbs). Also, the occurrence of seizures is not exceptional, and slow waves and spikes are reported [153]. Brain imaging may be normal, or show enlarged subarachnoid spaces only, but ventriculomegaly is not mentioned. An abnormal gyration with pachygyria is described in some cases. No mention is made of the corpus callosum either, but in one case at least, it appears short and thickened [139], and "upright" in another report quoted by [153]. A most striking finding, although subtle, is the abnormal signal of the white matter, which may indicate a gliosis or a myelination defect. TWIST1 is an upstream regulator of the FGFR pathways.

Muenke syndrome (*FGFR3, p250r mutation*) is characterized by a premature uni-or bilateral coronal synostosis with a variable phenotype, sensory-neural hearing loss, some intellectual disability, epilepsy, and a special risk of obstructive sleep apnea [154]. Neuroradiological studies in different patients mention a persistent cavum septi pellucidi (finding of uncertain significance), agenesis of the corpus callosum, periventricular hyperintensities (of unclear origin), and hemimegalencephaly [154]. In one report, illustrations of an MR study show ventriculomegaly and a striking bilateral dysplasia of the mesial temporal lobes with a thick, abnormally convoluted cortex, a poorly defined hippocampus and white matter, and a dilated ventricular horns, strikingly similar to what is shown in a fellow case in the same article of a patient with hypochondroplasia, also due to an FGFR3 mutation [155]; the images presented however do not allow a complete comparison with the abnormalities described in other imaging studies of the Apert syndrome [139], thanatophoric dysplasia [146], and hypochondroplasia [147].

Finally, descriptions of the brain abnormalities in the *Carpenter syndrome* (*RAB-23 mutation*) are few as it is a rare syndrome. The affected sutures are the uni- or bilateral coronal, sagittal, and lambdoid sutures. The patients present typically with acrocephaly, but other bony morphotypes, such as a cloverleaf skull, may be encountered. Patients present with an (often) profound developmental delay. A poor, bilateral but asymmetric hemispheric development, an agenesis of the anterior part of the corpus callosum, and an abnormal gyral pattern have been described [156].

There are many additional syndromes associated with craniosynostosis that are worth noting. These include Loeys-Dietz Syndrome, Shprintzen-Goldberg syndrome, velocardiofacial syndrome (22q11DS), and various aneuploidies including Trisomy 13, amongst others.

In *nonsyndromic craniosynostoses*, neural development may be altered, even if only mildly, typically within the lower range of normal [124–129, 157, 158]. The cranial deformity, factors like a high ICP, or even a prolonged hospital environment, may play a role. But even if no specific genetic disorder is usually identified, it is generally considered that the same developmental alteration that resulted in the bony pathology may also have resulted in a cerebral organization disorder. This is confirmed by multiple studies using MRI tractography, and functional MRI. The changes in brain organization seem to depend on the suture involved. In sagittal synostosis, there appears to be a decreased connectivity in the parietal lobes, involved in visuospatial cognition, visuomotor integration, and attention; right coronal synostosis seems to be associated with a decreased connectivity of the prefrontal cortex, involved in executive functions, language fluency, and visual attention [159]. Another study suggested that the changes were not unlike, in their mechanism, those of ADHD, but affected different cortical areas, with decreased connectivity of the primary visual cortex, visual association cortex, and visuospatial integration cortex, with loss of the ability to generate mental images [160]. These troubles may be, at least in part, corrected by an early release of the sutural synostosis [157].

References

1. Massimi L, Bianchi F, Frassanito P, Calandrelli R, Tamburrini G, Caldarelli M. Imaging in craniosynostosis: when and what? Childs Nerv Syst. 2019;35(11):2055–69. https://doi.org/10.1007/s00381-019-04278-x.
2. Brah TK, Thind R, Abel DE. Craniosynostosis: clinical presentation, genetics, and prenatal diagnosis. Obstet Gynecol Surv. 2020;75(10):636–44. https://doi.org/10.1097/OGX.0000000000000830.
3. Cacciaguerra G, Palermo M, Marino L, et al. The evolution of the role of imaging in the diagnosis of craniosynostosis: a narrative review. Children (Basel). 2021;8(9):727. https://doi.org/10.3390/children8090727.
4. Mathijssen IMJ, Working Group Guideline Craniosynostosis. Updated guideline on treatment and management of craniosynostosis. J Craniofac Surg. 2021;32(1):371–450. https://doi.org/10.1097/SCS.0000000000007035.
5. Wilbrand JF, Szczukowski A, Blecher JC, et al. Objectification of cranial vault correction for craniosynostosis by three-dimensional photography. J Craniomaxillofac Surg. 2012;40(8):726–30. https://doi.org/10.1016/j.jcms.2012.01.007.
6. Schaufelberger M, Kühle R, Wachter A, et al. A radiation-free classification pipeline for craniosynostosis using statistical shape modeling. Diagnostics (Basel). 2022;12(7):1516. https://doi.org/10.3390/diagnostics12071516.
7. Soboleski D, McCloskey D, Mussari B, Sauerbrei E, Clarke M, Fletcher A. Sonography of normal cranial sutures. AJR Am J Roentgenol. 1997;168(3):819–21. https://doi.org/10.2214/ajr.168.3.9057541.

8. Sze RW, Parisi MT, Sidhu M, et al. Ultrasound screening of the lambdoid suture in the child with posterior plagiocephaly. Pediatr Radiol. 2003;33(9):630–6. https://doi.org/10.1007/s00247-003-1009-3.
9. Regelsberger J, Delling G, Helmke K, et al. Ultrasound in the diagnosis of craniosynostosis. J Craniofac Surg. 2006;17(4):623–5; discussion 626–8. https://doi.org/10.1097/00001665-200607000-00002.
10. Simanovsky N, Hiller N, Koplewitz B, Rozovsky K. Effectiveness of ultrasonographic evaluation of the cranial sutures in children with suspected craniosynostosis. Eur Radiol. 2009;19(3):687–92. https://doi.org/10.1007/s00330-008-1193-5.
11. Proisy M, Riffaud L, Chouklati K, Tréguier C, Bruneau B. Ultrasonography for the diagnosis of craniosynostosis. Eur J Radiol. 2017;90:250–5. https://doi.org/10.1016/j.ejrad.2017.03.006.
12. Whittall I, Lambert WA, Moote DJ, et al. Postnatal diagnosis of single-suture craniosynostosis with cranial ultrasound: a systematic review. Childs Nerv Syst. 2021;37(12):3705–14. https://doi.org/10.1007/s00381-021-05301-w.
13. Constantine S, Kiermeier A, Anderson P. Sonographic indicators of isolated fetal sagittal craniosynostosis during pregnancy. J Med Imaging Radiat Oncol. 2020;64(5):626–33. https://doi.org/10.1111/1754-9485.13068.
14. Mitchell LA, Kitley CA, Armitage TL, Krasnokutsky MV, Rooks VJ. Normal sagittal and coronal suture widths by using CT imaging. AJNR Am J Neuroradiol. 2011;32(10):1801–5. https://doi.org/10.3174/ajnr.A2673.
15. Ginath S, Debby A, Malinger G. Demonstration of cranial sutures and fontanelles at 15 to 16 weeks of gestation: a comparison between two-dimensional and three-dimensional ultrasonography. Prenat Diagn. 2004;24(10):812–5. https://doi.org/10.1002/pd.988.
16. Rubio EI, Blask A, Bulas DI. Ultrasound and MR imaging findings in prenatal diagnosis of craniosynostosis syndromes. Pediatr Radiol. 2016;46(5):709–18. https://doi.org/10.1007/s00247-016-3550-x.
17. Helfer TM, Peixoto AB, Tonni G, Araujo Júnior E. Craniosynostosis: prenatal diagnosis by 2D/3D ultrasound, magnetic resonance imaging and computed tomography. Med Ultrason. 2016;18(3):378–85. https://doi.org/10.11152/mu.2013.2066.183.3du.
18. Constantine S, Niznik P. Antenatal ultrasound imaging for analysis of human craniosynostosis. Methods Mol Biol (Clifton, NJ). 2022;2403:295–310. https://doi.org/10.1007/978-1-0716-1847-9_20.
19. Harada A, Miyashita S, Nagai R, Makino S, Murotsuki J. Prenatal sonographic findings and prognosis of craniosynostosis diagnosed during the fetal and neonatal periods. Congenit Anom. 2019;59(4):132–41. https://doi.org/10.1111/cga.12308.
20. Krajden Haratz K, Leibovitz Z, Svirsky R, et al. The "Brain Shadowing Sign": a novel marker of fetal craniosynostosis. Fetal Diagn Ther. 2016;40(4):277–84. https://doi.org/10.1159/000444298.
21. Madeline LA, Elster AD. Suture closure in the human chondrocranium: CT assessment. Radiology. 1995;196(3):747–56. https://doi.org/10.1148/radiology.196.3.7644639.
22. Soldozy S, Yağmurlu K, Akyeampong DK, et al. Three-dimensional printing and craniosynostosis surgery. Childs Nerv Syst. 2021;37(8):2487–95. https://doi.org/10.1007/s00381-021-05133-8.
23. Vyas K, Gibreel W, Mardini S. Virtual surgical planning (VSP) in craniomaxillofacial reconstruction. Facial Plast Surg Clin N Am. 2022;30(2):239–53. https://doi.org/10.1016/j.fsc.2022.01.016.
24. Cheng D, Yuan M, Perera I, et al. Developing a 3D composite training model for cranial remodeling. J Neurosurg Pediatr. 2019;24:632. https://doi.org/10.3171/2019.6.PEDS18773.
25. Adler-Levy Y, Yagel S, Nadjari M, Bar-ziv Y, Simanovsky N, Hiller N. Use of low dose computed tomography with 3D reconstructions for the prenatal evaluation of suspected skeletal dysplasia. Isr Med Assoc J. 2015;17(1):42–6.
26. Ketwaroo PD, Robson CD, Estroff JA. Prenatal imaging of craniosynostosis syndromes. Semin Ultrasound CT MR. 2015;36(6):453–64. https://doi.org/10.1053/j.sult.2015.06.002.
27. Victoria T, Zhu X, Lachman R, et al. What is new in prenatal skeletal dysplasias? AJR Am J Roentgenol. 2018;210(5):1022–33. https://doi.org/10.2214/AJR.17.19337.
28. Dawood Y, Strijkers GJ, Limpens J, Oostra RJ, de Bakker BS. Novel imaging techniques to study postmortem human fetal anatomy: a systematic review on microfocus-CT and ultra-high-field MRI. Eur Radiol. 2020;30(4):2280–92. https://doi.org/10.1007/s00330-019-06543-8.
29. Dawood Y, Honhoff C, van der Post AS, et al. Comparison of postmortem whole-body contrast-enhanced microfocus computed tomography and high-field magnetic resonance imaging of human fetuses. Ultrasound Obstet Gynecol. 2022;60(1):109–17. https://doi.org/10.1002/uog.24827.
30. Dawood Y, Buijtendijk MFJ, Shah H, et al. Imaging fetal anatomy. Semin Cell Dev Biol. 2022;131:78–92. https://doi.org/10.1016/j.semcdb.2022.02.023.
31. Simcock IC, Shelmerdine SC, Hutchinson JC, Sebire NJ, Arthurs OJ. Human fetal whole-body postmortem microfocus computed tomographic imaging. Nat Protoc. 2021;16(5):2594–614. https://doi.org/10.1038/s41596-021-00512-6.
32. Al-Otibi M, Jea A, Kulkarni AV. Detection of important venous collaterals by computed tomography venogram in multisutural synostosis. Case report and review of the literature. J Neurosurg. 2007;107(6 Suppl):508–10. https://doi.org/10.3171/PED-07/12/508.

33. Jeevan DS, Anlsow P, Jayamohan J. Abnormal venous drainage in syndromic craniosynostosis and the role of CT venography. Childs Nerv Syst. 2008;24(12):1413–20. https://doi.org/10.1007/s00381-008-0667-8.
34. Costa MA, Ackerman LL, Tholpady SS, Greathouse ST, Tahiri Y, Flores RL. Spring-assisted cranial vault expansion in the setting of multisutural craniosynostosis and anomalous venous drainage: case report. J Neurosurg Pediatr. 2015;16(1):80–5. https://doi.org/10.3171/2014.12.PEDS14604.
35. Copeland AE, Hoffman CE, Tsitouras V, et al. Clinical significance of venous anomalies in syndromic craniosynostosis. Plast Reconstr Surg Glob Open. 2018;6(1):e1613. https://doi.org/10.1097/GOX.0000000000001613.
36. Robson CD, Mulliken JB, Robertson RL, et al. Prominent basal emissary foramina in syndromic craniosynostosis: correlation with phenotypic and molecular diagnoses. AJNR Am J Neuroradiol. 2000;21(9):1707–17.
37. Balboni AL, Estenson TL, Reidenberg JS, Bergemann AD, Laitman JT. Assessing age-related ossification of the petro-occipital fissure: laying the foundation for understanding the clinicopathologies of the cranial base. Anat Rec A Discov Mol Cell Evol Biol. 2005;282(1):38–48. https://doi.org/10.1002/ar.a.20149.
38. Akbareian SE, Pitsillides AA, Macharia RG, McGonnell IM. Occipital foramina development involves localised regulation of mesenchyme proliferation and is independent of apoptosis. J Anat. 2015;226(6):560–74. https://doi.org/10.1111/joa.12304.
39. McGonnell IM, Akbareian SE. Like a hole in the head: development, evolutionary implications and diseases of the cranial foramina. Semin Cell Dev Biol. 2019;91:23–30. https://doi.org/10.1016/j.semcdb.2018.08.011.
40. Rich PM, Cox TCS, Hayward RD. The jugular foramen in complex and syndromic craniosynostosis and its relationship to raised intracranial pressure. AJNR Am J Neuroradiol. 2003;24(1):45–51.
41. Booth CD, Figueroa RE, Lehn A, Yu JC. Analysis of the jugular foramen in pediatric patients with craniosynostosis. J Craniofac Surg. 2011;22(1):285–8. https://doi.org/10.1097/SCS.0b013e3181f7b738.
42. Bosemani T, Orman G, Hergan B, Carson KA, Huisman TAGM, Poretti A. Achondroplasia in children: correlation of ventriculomegaly, size of foramen magnum and jugular foramina, and emissary vein enlargement. Childs Nerv Syst. 2015;31(1):129–33. https://doi.org/10.1007/s00381-014-2559-4.
43. Cinalli G, Russo C, Vitulli F, et al. Changes in venous drainage after posterior cranial vault distraction and foramen magnum decompression in syndromic craniosynostosis. J Neurosurg Pediatr. 2022;30:330. https://doi.org/10.3171/2022.6.PEDS22171.
44. Tischfield MA, Robson CD, Gilette NM, et al. Cerebral vein malformations result from loss of Twist1 expression and BMP signaling from skull progenitor cells and dura. Dev Cell. 2017;42(5):445–61.e5. https://doi.org/10.1016/j.devcel.2017.07.027.
45. Cinalli G, di Martino G, Russo C, et al. Dural venous sinus anatomy in children with external hydrocephalus: analysis of a series of 97 patients. Childs Nerv Syst. 2021;37(10):3021–32. https://doi.org/10.1007/s00381-021-05322-5.
46. Wang M, Wu X, Lan D, et al. Differentiation between anatomical slenderness and acquired stenosis of the internal jugular veins. CNS Neurosci Ther. 2022;28(11):1849–60. https://doi.org/10.1111/cns.13924.
47. Taylor WJ, Hayward RD, Lasjaunias P, et al. Enigma of raised intracranial pressure in patients with complex craniosynostosis: the role of abnormal intracranial venous drainage. J Neurosurg. 2001;94(3):377–85. https://doi.org/10.3171/jns.2001.94.3.0377.
48. Hayward R. Venous hypertension and craniosynostosis. Childs Nerv Syst. 2005;21(10):880–8. https://doi.org/10.1007/s00381-004-1114-0.
49. Cornelissen MJ, de Goederen R, Doerga P, et al. Pilot study of intracranial venous physiology in craniosynostosis. J Neurosurg Pediatr. 2018;21(6):626–31. https://doi.org/10.3171/2018.1.PEDS17480.
50. Mitsukawa N, Satoh K, Hayashi T, et al. Sinus pericranii associated with craniosynostosis. J Craniofac Surg. 2007;18(1):78–84. https://doi.org/10.1097/01.scs.0000249363.48794.2a.
51. Scott AA, Hodge KD, Torres-Martinez W, Dlouhy SR, Smith JL, Weaver DD. Sinus pericranii in achondroplasia: a case report and review of the literature. Clin Dysmorphol. 2017;26(4):252–5. https://doi.org/10.1097/MCD.0000000000000196.
52. Shaw AV, Jayamohan J, Sheerin F, Johnson D. Staged raising of a coronal flap for fronto-orbital advancement and remodeling in Saethre-Chotzen syndrome complicated by sinus pericranii. J Craniofac Surg. 2018;29(7):1956–9. https://doi.org/10.1097/SCS.0000000000004786.
53. Celie KB, Yuan M, Hoffman C, O'Connor A, Bogue J, Imahiyerobo T. Surgical management of complex syndromic craniosynostosis: experience with a rare genetic variant. J Craniofac Surg. 2020;31(1):294–9. https://doi.org/10.1097/SCS.0000000000005949.
54. Tyrell R, Limoges N, Kestle J, Gociman B, Siddiqi F. Sinus pericranii in posterior cranial vault distraction. J Craniofac Surg. 2020;31(7):e715–7. https://doi.org/10.1097/SCS.0000000000006642.
55. Han T, Ji Y, Cui J, Shen W. Surgical management of sinus pericranii with Crouzon syndrome. J Craniofac Surg. 2021;32(3):1068–70. https://doi.org/10.1097/SCS.0000000000007297.
56. Kumari S, Verma SK, Singh PK. Crouzon's syndrome with a dominant sinus pericranii draining transverse sinus: report of a rare association and review of lit-

erature. Pediatr Neurosurg. 2022;57(3):196–201. https://doi.org/10.1159/000524134.
57. Kamath BM, Spinner NB, Emerick KM, et al. Vascular anomalies in Alagille syndrome: a significant cause of morbidity and mortality. Circulation. 2004;109(11):1354–8. https://doi.org/10.1161/01.CIR.0000121361.01862.A4.
58. Carpenter CD, Linscott LL, Leach JL, Vadivelu S, Abruzzo T. Spectrum of cerebral arterial and venous abnormalities in Alagille syndrome. Pediatr Radiol. 2018;48(4):602–8. https://doi.org/10.1007/s00247-017-4043-2.
59. D'Amico A, Perillo T, Cuocolo R, et al. Neuroradiological findings in Alagille syndrome. Br J Radiol. 2022;95(1129):20201241. https://doi.org/10.1259/bjr.20201241.
60. Okamoto K, Ito J, Tokiguchi S, Furusawa T. High-resolution CT findings in the development of the sphenooccipital synchondrosis. AJNR Am J Neuroradiol. 1996;17(1):117–20.
61. McDonald SW, Miller J. When does the spheno-occipital synchondrosis close? Clin Anat. 2022;35(4):512–25. https://doi.org/10.1002/ca.23847.
62. Bassed RB, Briggs C, Drummer OH. Analysis of time of closure of the spheno-occipital synchondrosis using computed tomography. Forensic Sci Int. 2010;200(1–3):161–4. https://doi.org/10.1016/j.forsciint.2010.04.009.
63. Goldstein JA, Paliga JT, Wink JD, Bartlett SP, Nah HD, Taylor JA. Earlier evidence of spheno-occipital synchondrosis fusion correlates with severity of midface hypoplasia in patients with syndromic craniosynostosis. Plast Reconstr Surg. 2014;134(3):504–10. https://doi.org/10.1097/PRS.0000000000000419.
64. McGrath J, Gerety PA, Derderian CA, et al. Differential closure of the spheno-occipital synchondrosis in syndromic craniosynostosis. Plast Reconstr Surg. 2012;130(5):681e–9e. https://doi.org/10.1097/PRS.0b013e318267d4c0.
65. de Almeida JR, James AL, Papsin BC, Weksburg R, Clark H, Blaser S. Thyroid gland and carotid artery anomalies in 22q11.2 deletion syndromes. Laryngoscope. 2009;119(8):1495–500. https://doi.org/10.1002/lary.20281.
66. de Planque CA, Petr J, Gaillard L, et al. Cerebral blood flow of the frontal lobe in untreated children with trigonocephaly versus healthy controls: an arterial spin labeling study. Plast Reconstr Surg. 2022;149(4):931–7. https://doi.org/10.1097/PRS.0000000000008931.
67. Doerga PN, Lequin MH, Dremmen MHG, et al. Cerebral blood flow in children with syndromic craniosynostosis: cohort arterial spin labeling studies. J Neurosurg Pediatr. 2019;25:340. https://doi.org/10.3171/2019.10.PEDS19150.
68. Sreedher G, Gillespie C, Brown M, Ganapathy SS. Cranial suture evaluation on routine pediatric MRI. Curr Probl Diagn Radiol. 2021;50(5):650–5. https://doi.org/10.1067/j.cpradiol.2020.07.003.
69. Saarikko A, Mellanen E, Kuusela L, et al. Comparison of Black Bone MRI and 3D-CT in the preoperative evaluation of patients with craniosynostosis. J Plast Reconstr Aesthetic Surg. 2020;73(4):723–31. https://doi.org/10.1016/j.bjps.2019.11.006.
70. Eley KA, Watt-Smith SR, Sheerin F, Golding SJ. "Black Bone" MRI: a potential alternative to CT with three-dimensional reconstruction of the craniofacial skeleton in the diagnosis of craniosynostosis. Eur Radiol. 2014;24(10):2417–26. https://doi.org/10.1007/s00330-014-3286-7.
71. Eley KA, Delso G. Automated 3D MRI rendering of the craniofacial skeleton: using ZTE to drive the segmentation of black bone and FIESTA-C images. Neuroradiology. 2021;63(1):91–8. https://doi.org/10.1007/s00234-020-02508-7.
72. Kuusela L, Hukki A, Brandstack N, Autti T, Leikola J, Saarikko A. Use of black-bone MRI in the diagnosis of the patients with posterior plagiocephaly. Childs Nerv Syst. 2018;34(7):1383–9. https://doi.org/10.1007/s00381-018-3783-0.
73. Leonhardt Y, Kronthaler S, Feuerriegel G, et al. CT-like MR-derived images for the assessment of craniosynostosis and other pathologies of the pediatric skull. Clin Neuroradiol. 2022;33:57. https://doi.org/10.1007/s00062-022-01182-x.
74. Eley KA, Watt-Smith SR, Golding SJ. "Black Bone" MRI: a novel imaging technique for 3D printing. Dento Maxillo Facial Radiol. 2017;46(3):20160407. https://doi.org/10.1259/dmfr.20160407.
75. Lethaus B, Gruichev D, Gräfe D, et al. "Black bone": the new backbone in CAD/CAM-assisted craniosynostosis surgery? Acta Neurochir. 2021;163(6):1735–41. https://doi.org/10.1007/s00701-020-04445-z.
76. Calandrelli R, D'Apolito G, Gaudino S, et al. Radiological assessment of skull base changes in children with syndromic craniosynostosis: role of "minor" sutures. Neuroradiology. 2014;56(10):863–73. https://doi.org/10.1007/s00234-014-1392-5.
77. Rogers GF, Mulliken JB. Involvement of the basilar coronal ring in unilateral coronal synostosis. Plast Reconstr Surg. 2005;115(7):1887–93. https://doi.org/10.1097/01.prs.0000165073.64309.bd.
78. Dundulis JA, Becker DB, Govier DP, Marsh JL, Kane AA. Coronal ring involvement in patients treated for unilateral coronal craniosynostosis. Plast Reconstr Surg. 2004;114(7):1695–703. https://doi.org/10.1097/01.prs.0000142474.25114.cb.
79. Vu GH, Xu W, Go BC, et al. Physiologic timeline of cranial-base suture and synchondrosis closure. Plast Reconstr Surg. 2021;148(6):973e–82e. https://doi.org/10.1097/PRS.0000000000008570.
80. Eley KA, Thomas GPL, Sheerin F, Cilliers D, Wall S, Johnson D. The significance of squamosal suture

synostosis. J Craniofac Surg. 2016;27(6):1543–9. https://doi.org/10.1097/SCS.0000000000002888.
81. Beiriger JW, Zhu X, Bruce MK, et al. Squamosal suture synostosis: an under-recognized phenomenon. Cleft Palate Craniofacial J. 2022;2022:10556656221100676. https://doi.org/10.1177/10556656221100675.
82. Vu HL, Panchal J, Parker EE, Levine NS, Francel P. The timing of physiologic closure of the metopic suture: a review of 159 patients using reconstructed 3D CT scans of the craniofacial region. J Craniofac Surg. 2001;12(6):527–32. https://doi.org/10.1097/00001665-200111000-00005.
83. Weinzweig J, Kirschner RE, Farley A, et al. Metopic synostosis: defining the temporal sequence of normal suture fusion and differentiating it from synostosis on the basis of computed tomography images. Plast Reconstr Surg. 2003;112(5):1211–8. https://doi.org/10.1097/01.PRS.0000080729.28749.A3.
84. Birgfeld CB, Heike CL, Al-Mufarrej F, et al. Practical computed tomography scan findings for distinguishing metopic craniosynostosis from metopic ridging. Plast Reconstr Surg Glob Open. 2019;7(3):e1944. https://doi.org/10.1097/GOX.0000000000001944.
85. Teager SJ, Constantine S, Lottering N, Anderson PJ. Physiologic closure time of the metopic suture in South Australian infants from 3D CT scans. Childs Nerv Syst. 2019;35(2):329–35. https://doi.org/10.1007/s00381-018-3957-9.
86. Diab J, Flapper W, Grave B, Abou-Hamden A, Anderson P, Moore M. The many faces of sagittal synostosis: a novel classification and approach to diagnosis. J Craniofac Surg. 2022;33(1):192–7. https://doi.org/10.1097/SCS.0000000000008086.
87. Schweitzer T, Kunz F, Meyer-Marcotty P, et al. Diagnostic features of prematurely fused cranial sutures on plain skull X-rays. Childs Nerv Syst. 2015;31(11):2071–80. https://doi.org/10.1007/s00381-015-2890-4.
88. Dias MS, Samson T, Rizk EB, Governale LS, Richtsmeier JT, Section on Neurologic Surgery, Section on Plastic and Reconstructive Surgery. Identifying the misshapen head: craniosynostosis and related disorders. Pediatrics. 2020;146(3):e2020015511. https://doi.org/10.1542/peds.2020-015511.
89. Vinchon M, Pellerin P, Guerreschi P, Baroncini M, Dhellemmes P. Atypical scaphocephaly: a review. Childs Nerv Syst. 2012;28(9):1319–25. https://doi.org/10.1007/s00381-012-1807-8.
90. Wilkinson CC, Stence NV, Serrano CA, et al. Fusion patterns of major calvarial sutures on volume-rendered CT reconstructions. J Neurosurg Pediatr. 2020;25:519. https://doi.org/10.3171/2019.11.PEDS1953.
91. Pfaff MJ, Fenton R, Mittal A, et al. The clinical significance of clinocephaly in late-presentation sagittal craniosynostosis. Cleft Palate Craniofac J. 2022;2022:10556656211064484. https://doi.org/10.1177/10556656211064484.
92. Skadorwa T, Wierzbieniec O. The foramen magnum in scaphocephaly. Childs Nerv Syst. 2022;38(11):2163–70. https://doi.org/10.1007/s00381-022-05624-2.
93. Nakahara K, Utsuki S, Shimizu S, et al. Age dependence of fusion of primary occipital sutures: a radiographic study. Childs Nerv Syst. 2006;22(11):1457–9. https://doi.org/10.1007/s00381-006-0210-8.
94. Nayak SR, Krishnamurthy A, Madhan Kumar SJ, et al. The mendosal suture of the occipital bone: occurrence in Indian population, embryology and clinical significance. Surg Radiol Anat. 2007;29(4):329–32. https://doi.org/10.1007/s00276-007-0216-2.
95. Davanzo J, Samson T, Tubbs SR, Rizk E. Bathrocephaly: a case report of a head shape associated with a persistent mendosal suture. Ital J Anat Embryol. 2014;119(3):263–7.
96. Chaisrisawadisuk S, Moore MH. Posterior cranial vault manifestations in nonsyndromic sagittal craniosynostosis. J Craniofac Surg. 2021;32(7):2273–6. https://doi.org/10.1097/SCS.0000000000007756.
97. Escandón JM, Duarte-Bateman D, Mantilla-Rivas E, et al. Prevalence of mendosal suture patency in infants up to the age of 18 months. Plast Reconstr Surg Glob Open. 2022;10(6):e4383. https://doi.org/10.1097/GOX.0000000000004383.
98. Rhodes JL, Tye GW, Fearon JA. Craniosynostosis of the lambdoid suture. Semin Plast Surg. 2014;28(3):138–43. https://doi.org/10.1055/s-0034-1384809.
99. Cinalli G, Renier D, Sebag G, Sainte-Rose C, Arnaud E, Pierre-Kahn A. Chronic tonsillar herniation in Crouzon's and Apert's syndromes: the role of premature synostosis of the lambdoid suture. J Neurosurg. 1995;83(4):575–82. https://doi.org/10.3171/jns.1995.83.4.0575.
100. Sze RW, Hopper RA, Ghioni V, et al. MDCT diagnosis of the child with posterior plagiocephaly. AJR Am J Roentgenol. 2005;185(5):1342–6. https://doi.org/10.2214/AJR.04.1388.
101. Rhodes JL, Kolar JC, Fearon JA. Mercedes Benz pattern craniosynostosis. Plast Reconstr Surg. 2010;125(1):299–304. https://doi.org/10.1097/PRS.0b013e3181c2a6aa.
102. Chivoret N, Arnaud E, Giraudat K, et al. Bilambdoid and sagittal synostosis: report of 39 cases. Surg Neurol Int. 2018;9(1):206. https://doi.org/10.4103/sni.sni_454_17.
103. Balestrino A, Secci F, Piatelli G, et al. Pure bilateral lambdoid and posterior sagittal synostosis (Mercedes–Benz syndrome): case report and literature review. World Neurosurg. 2019;128:77–82. https://doi.org/10.1016/j.wneu.2019.04.117.
104. Miri S, Mittermiller P, Buchanan EP, Khosla RK. Facial twist (asymmetry) in isolated unilateral coronal synostosis: does premature facial suture fusion play a role? J Craniofac Surg.

2015;26(3):655–7. https://doi.org/10.1097/SCS.0000000000001436.
105. Sakamoto Y, Nakajima H, Tamada I, Miyamoto J, Kishi K. Involvement of the sphenosquamosal suture for unilateral coronal synostosis. J Craniofac Surg. 2012;23(5):1267–9. https://doi.org/10.1097/SCS.0b013e3182519a97.
106. Calandrelli R, Pilato F, Massimi L, et al. Quantitative evaluation of facial hypoplasia and airway obstruction in infants with syndromic craniosynostosis: relationship with skull base and splanchnocranium sutural pattern. Neuroradiology. 2018;60(5):517–28. https://doi.org/10.1007/s00234-018-2005-5.
107. Showalter BM, David LR, Argenta LC, Thompson JT. Influence of frontosphenoidal suture synostosis on skull dysmorphology in unicoronal suture synostosis. J Craniofac Surg. 2012;23(6):1709–12. https://doi.org/10.1097/SCS.0b013e31826beecc.
108. Watts GD, Antonarakis GS, Blaser SI, Phillips JH, Forrest CR. Cranioorbital morphology caused by coronal ring suture synostosis. Plast Reconstr Surg. 2019;144(6):1403–11. https://doi.org/10.1097/PRS.0000000000006256.
109. Manrique M, Toro-Tobon S, Bade Y, et al. Sickle cell disease association with premature suture fusion in young children. Plast Reconstr Surg Glob Open. 2022;10(10):e4620. https://doi.org/10.1097/GOX.0000000000004620.
110. Wood BC, Oh AK, Keating RF, et al. Progressive postnatal pansynostosis: an insidious and pernicious form of craniosynostosis. J Neurosurg Pediatr. 2015;16(3):309–16. https://doi.org/10.3171/2015.1.PEDS14464.
111. Funato N. New insights into cranial synchondrosis development: a mini review. Front Cell Dev Biol. 2020;8:706. https://doi.org/10.3389/fcell.2020.00706.
112. Matsushita T, Wilcox WR, Chan YY, et al. FGFR3 promotes synchondrosis closure and fusion of ossification centers through the MAPK pathway. Hum Mol Genet. 2009;18(2):227–40. https://doi.org/10.1093/hmg/ddn339.
113. Coll G, Lemaire JJ, Di Rocco F, et al. Human foramen magnum area and posterior cranial fossa volume growth in relation to cranial base synchondrosis closure in the course of child development. Neurosurgery. 2016;79(5):722–35. https://doi.org/10.1227/NEU.0000000000001309.
114. Coll G, Abed Rabbo F, Jecko V, Sakka L, Di Rocco F, Delion M. The growth of the posterior cranial fossa in FGFR2-induced faciocraniosynostosis: a review. Neurochirurgie. 2019;65(5):221–7. https://doi.org/10.1016/j.neuchi.2019.09.005.
115. Hecht JT, Horton WA, Reid CS, Pyeritz RE, Chakraborty R. Growth of the foramen magnum in achondroplasia. Am J Med Genet. 1989;32(4):528–35. https://doi.org/10.1002/ajmg.1320320421.
116. Keiper GL, Koch B, Crone KR. Achondroplasia and cervicomedullary compression: prospective evaluation and surgical treatment. Pediatr Neurosurg. 1999;31(2):78–83. https://doi.org/10.1159/000028838.
117. Di Rocco F, Dubravova D, Ziyadeh J, Sainte-Rose C, Collet C, Arnaud E. The foramen magnum in isolated and syndromic brachycephaly. Childs Nerv Syst. 2014;30(1):165–72. https://doi.org/10.1007/s00381-013-2245-y.
118. Rijken BFM, Lequin MH, Van Veelen MLC, de Rooi J, Mathijssen IMJ. The formation of the foramen magnum and its role in developing ventriculomegaly and Chiari I malformation in children with craniosynostosis syndromes. J Craniomaxillofac Surg. 2015;43(7):1042–8. https://doi.org/10.1016/j.jcms.2015.04.025.
119. Assadsangabi R, Hajmomenian M, Bilaniuk LT, Vossough A. Morphology of the foramen magnum in syndromic and non-syndromic brachycephaly. Childs Nerv Syst. 2015;31(5):735–41. https://doi.org/10.1007/s00381-015-2639-0.
120. Lingawi SS. Determination of the chronological age of skull base suture closure using computed tomography. J Basic Appl Sci. 2012;8(1):247–52. https://doi.org/10.6000/1927-5129.2012.08.01.38.
121. Hill CA, Vaddi S, Moffitt A, et al. Intracranial volume and whole brain volume in infants with unicoronal craniosynostosis. Cleft Palate Craniofac J. 2011;48(4):394–8. https://doi.org/10.1597/10-051.
122. de Jong T, Rijken BFM, Lequin MH, van Veelen MLC, Mathijssen IMJ. Brain and ventricular volume in patients with syndromic and complex craniosynostosis. Childs Nerv Syst. 2012;28(1):137–40. https://doi.org/10.1007/s00381-011-1614-7.
123. Choi JW, Lim SY, Shin HJ. Craniosynostosis in growing children: pathophysiological changes and neurosurgical problems. J Korean Neurosurg Soc. 2016;59(3):197–203. https://doi.org/10.3340/jkns.2016.59.3.197.
124. Shim KW, Park EK, Kim JS, Kim YO, Kim DS. Neurodevelopmental problems in non-syndromic craniosynostosis. J Korean Neurosurg Soc. 2016;59(3):242–6. https://doi.org/10.3340/jkns.2016.59.3.242.
125. Aldridge K, Collett B. Structural brain differences in school-age children with and without single-suture craniosynostosis. J Neurosurg Pediatr. 2017;19(4):479–89. https://doi.org/10.3171/2016.9.PEDS16107.
126. Aldridge K, Marsh JL, Govier D, Richtsmeier JT. Central nervous system phenotypes in craniosynostosis. J Anat. 2002;201(1):31–9. https://doi.org/10.1046/j.1469-7580.2002.00074.x.
127. Aldridge K, Kane AA, Marsh JL, et al. Brain morphology in nonsyndromic unicoronal craniosynostosis. Anat Rec A Discov Mol Cell Evol Biol. 2005;285(2):690–8. https://doi.org/10.1002/ar.a.20201.
128. Aldridge K, Kane AA, Marsh JL, Yan P, Govier D, Richtsmeier JT. Relationship of brain and skull in pre- and postoperative sagittal synos-

tosis. J Anat. 2005;206(4):373–85. https://doi.org/10.1111/j.1469-7580.2005.00397.x.
129. Kapp-Simon KA, Speltz ML, Cunningham ML, Patel PK, Tomita T. Neurodevelopment of children with single suture craniosynostosis: a review. Childs Nerv Syst. 2007;23(3):269–81. https://doi.org/10.1007/s00381-006-0251-z.
130. Tamburrini G, Caldarelli M, Massimi L, Santini P, Di Rocco C. Intracranial pressure monitoring in children with single suture and complex craniosynostosis: a review. Childs Nerv Syst. 2005;21(10):913–21. https://doi.org/10.1007/s00381-004-1117-x.
131. Usami K, Nicolini F, Arnaud E, Di Rocco F. Cerebrospinal fluid collections in sagittal suture synostosis. Childs Nerv Syst. 2016;32(3):519–25. https://doi.org/10.1007/s00381-015-3011-0.
132. Di Rocco F, Garcia-Gonzalez O, Szathmari A, et al. Emissary veins and pericerebral cerebrospinal fluid in trigonocephaly: do they define a specific subtype? Childs Nerv Syst. 2021;37(4):1159–65. https://doi.org/10.1007/s00381-020-04982-z.
133. Collmann H, Sörensen N, Krauss J. Hydrocephalus in craniosynostosis: a review. Childs Nerv Syst. 2005;21(10):902–12. https://doi.org/10.1007/s00381-004-1116-y.
134. Frassanito P, Palombi D, Tamburrini G. Craniosynostosis and hydrocephalus: relevance and treatment modalities. Childs Nerv Syst. 2021;37(11):3465–73. https://doi.org/10.1007/s00381-021-05158-z.
135. Khonsari RH, Delezoide AL, Kang W, et al. Central nervous system malformations and deformations in FGFR2-related craniosynostosis. Am J Med Genet A. 2012;158A(11):2797–806. https://doi.org/10.1002/ajmg.a.35598.
136. Raybaud C, Jallo GI. Chiari 1 deformity in children: etiopathogenesis and radiologic diagnosis. Handb Clin Neurol. 2018;155:25–48. https://doi.org/10.1016/B978-0-444-64189-2.00002-0.
137. Senarath-Yapa K, Chung MT, McArdle A, et al. Craniosynostosis: molecular pathways and future pharmacologic therapy. Organogenesis. 2012;8(4):103–13. https://doi.org/10.4161/org.23307.
138. Siismets EM, Hatch NE. Cranial neural crest cells and their role in the pathogenesis of craniofacial anomalies and coronal craniosynostosis. J Dev Biol. 2020;8(3):E18. https://doi.org/10.3390/jdb8030018.
139. Raybaud C, Di Rocco C. Brain malformation in syndromic craniosynostoses, a primary disorder of white matter: a review. Childs Nerv Syst. 2007;23(12):1379–88. https://doi.org/10.1007/s00381-007-0474-7.
140. Stark Z, McGillivray G, Sampson A, et al. Apert syndrome: temporal lobe abnormalities on fetal brain imaging. Prenat Diagn. 2015;35(2):179–82. https://doi.org/10.1002/pd.4515.
141. Maksem JA, Roessmann U. Apert's syndrome with central nervous system anomalies. Acta Neuropathol (Berl). 1979;48(1):59–61. https://doi.org/10.1007/BF00691792.
142. Tokumaru AM, Barkovich AJ, Ciricillo SF, Edwards MS. Skull base and calvarial deformities: association with intracranial changes in craniofacial syndromes. AJNR Am J Neuroradiol. 1996;17(4):619–30.
143. Yacubian-Fernandes A, Palhares A, Giglio A, et al. Apert syndrome: analysis of associated brain malformations and conformational changes determined by surgical treatment. J Neuroradiol. 2004;31(2):116–22. https://doi.org/10.1016/s0150-9861(04)96978-7.
144. Quintero-Rivera F, Robson CD, Reiss RE, et al. Intracranial anomalies detected by imaging studies in 30 patients with Apert syndrome. Am J Med Genet A. 2006;140(12):1337–8. https://doi.org/10.1002/ajmg.a.31277.
145. Fernandes MBL, Maximino LP, Perosa GB, Abramides DVM, Passos-Bueno MR, Yacubian-Fernandes A. Apert and Crouzon syndromes—cognitive development, brain abnormalities, and molecular aspects. Am J Med Genet A. 2016;170(6):1532–7. https://doi.org/10.1002/ajmg.a.37640.
146. Miller E, Blaser S, Shannon P, Widjaja E. Brain and bone abnormalities of thanatophoric dwarfism. AJR Am J Roentgenol. 2009;192(1):48–51. https://doi.org/10.2214/AJR.08.1524.
147. Philpott CM, Widjaja E, Raybaud C, Branson HM, Kannu P, Blaser S. Temporal and occipital lobe features in children with hypochondroplasia/FGFR3 gene mutation. Pediatr Radiol. 2013;43(9):1190–5. https://doi.org/10.1007/s00247-013-2684-3.
148. Manikkam SA, Chetcuti K, Howell KB, Savarirayan R, Fink AM, Mandelstam SA. Temporal lobe malformations in achondroplasia: expanding the brain imaging phenotype associated with FGFR3-related skeletal dysplasias. AJNR Am J Neuroradiol. 2018;39(2):380–4. https://doi.org/10.3174/ajnr.A5468.
149. Raybaud C. Corpus callosum: molecular pathways in mice and human dysgeneses. Neuroimaging Clin N Am. 2019;29(3):445–59. https://doi.org/10.1016/j.nic.2019.03.006.
150. Wilson AT, de Planque CA, Yang SS, et al. Cortical thickness in Crouzon-Pfeiffer syndrome: findings in relation to primary cranial vault expansion. Plast Reconstr Surg Glob Open. 2020;8(10):e3204. https://doi.org/10.1097/GOX.0000000000003204.
151. Mavridis IN, Rodrigues D. Nervous system involvement in Pfeiffer syndrome. Childs Nerv Syst. 2021;37(2):367–74. https://doi.org/10.1007/s00381-020-04934-7.
152. Itoh S, Nojima M, Yoshida K. Usefulness of magnetic resonance imaging for accurate diagnosis of Pfeiffer syndrome type II in utero. Fetal Diagn Ther. 2006;21(2):168–71. https://doi.org/10.1159/000089297.
153. Elia M, Musumeci SA, Ferri R, et al. Saethre-Chotzen syndrome: a clinical, EEG and neuroradiologi-

cal study. Childs Nerv Syst. 1996;12(11):699–704. https://doi.org/10.1007/BF00366154.
154. Agochukwu NB, Solomon BD, Gropman AL, Muenke M. Epilepsy in Muenke syndrome: FGFR3-related craniosynostosis. Pediatr Neurol. 2012;47(5):355–61. https://doi.org/10.1016/j.pediatrneurol.2012.07.004.
155. Grosso S, Farnetani MA, Berardi R, et al. Medial temporal lobe dysgenesis in Muenke syndrome and hypochondroplasia. Am J Med Genet A. 2003;120A(1):88–91. https://doi.org/10.1002/ajmg.a.10171.
156. Taravath S, Tonsgard JH. Cerebral malformations in Carpenter syndrome. Pediatr Neurol. 1993;9(3):230–4. https://doi.org/10.1016/0887-8994(93)90092-q.
157. Brooks ED, Yang J, Beckett JS, et al. Normalization of brain morphology after surgery in sagittal craniosynostosis. J Neurosurg Pediatr. 2016;17(4):460–8. https://doi.org/10.3171/2015.7.PEDS15221.
158. Kapp-Simon KA, Wallace E, Collett BR, Cradock MM, Crerand CE, Speltz ML. Language, learning, and memory in children with and without single-suture craniosynostosis. J Neurosurg Pediatr. 2016;17(5):578–88. https://doi.org/10.3171/2015.9.PEDS15238.
159. Sun AH, Eilbott J, Chuang C, et al. An investigation of brain functional connectivity by form of craniosynostosis. J Craniofac Surg. 2019;30(6):1719–23. https://doi.org/10.1097/SCS.0000000000005537.
160. Cabrejo R, Lacadie C, Brooks E, et al. Understanding the learning disabilities linked to sagittal craniosynostosis. J Craniofac Surg. 2019;30(2):497–502. https://doi.org/10.1097/SCS.0000000000005194.

ENT and Craniosynostosis

22

Romain Luscan and Vincent Couloigner

ENT specialists are primarily involved in two areas of the follow-up and treatment of patients with craniosynostosis (CS): obstructive sleep apnea (OSA) and hearing impairment.

OSA is related to reduced airway patency during sleep. In the case of CS, it is mainly due to hypoplasia of the middle third of the face, with subsequent stenosis of the nasal cavities and narrow rhinopharynx (Fig. 22.1). However, it can also be present in CS forms which do not encompass midface hypoplasia, such as Muenke or Saethre-Chotzen syndromes [1].

Considering the management of nasal obstruction, both medical (nasal washing with saline, topical steroids, antihistamines in case of mucosal inflammation) and surgical treatments can be used. The surgical treatment consists of a bilateral turbinoplasty or turbinectomy (Fig. 22.2). Enlargement of piriform aperture stenosis is sometimes necessary. Nasopharyngeal narrowing can be addressed by an adenoidectomy and a resection of the posterior part of the vomer in order to artificially increase the depth of the nasopharynx.

R. Luscan · V. Couloigner (✉)
Pediatric ENT Department, Hôpital Necker—Enfants Malades, Assistance Publique—Hôpitaux de Paris, Université Paris Cité, Centre de Référence Malformations Rares en ORL (MALO), Paris, France
e-mail: romain.luscan@aphp.fr; vincent.couloigner@aphp.fr

Tonsillar hypertrophy is also frequently involved in CS-related OSA. Tonsillectomy and adenoidectomy decrease the apnea—hypopnea index (AHI) and desaturation index by 5/h and 8.5/h, respectively [2]. It improved OSAS in 60% of cases, but AHI normalization is rare [2].

Drug-induced sleep endoscopy is a very useful procedure to accurately guide the optimal treatment strategy in children with CS and severe OSA [3]. It can be proposed before any treatment or after of adenoidectomy and tonsillectomy.

For patients with very severe OSA and impossibility or failure of surgical treatment, noninvasive ventilation (NIV) can be proposed. When NIV is not insufficiently effective or is not tolerated, a tracheostomy is required.

Tracheal cartilaginous sleeve is another airway disorder that can be observed in patients with CS [4, 5]. This malformation seems to be associated with an increased risk of tracheostomy and an increased risk of morbidity and mortality related to tracheostomy.

Hearing impairment is frequent in CS [6]. The main cause is otitis media with effusion (OME), which is related to the constitutional narrowing of the Eustachian tube linked in these patients. Insertion of ventilation tubes is sometimes necessary to restore normal hearing. Much more rarely, external ear or ossicular malformations can be present [6]. Sensorineural hearing loss is mostly observed in Muenke syndrome [7].

F. Di Rocco, J. Kestle (eds.), *Neurosurgical Aspects of Craniosynostosis*,
https://doi.org/10.1007/978-3-031-69386-1_22

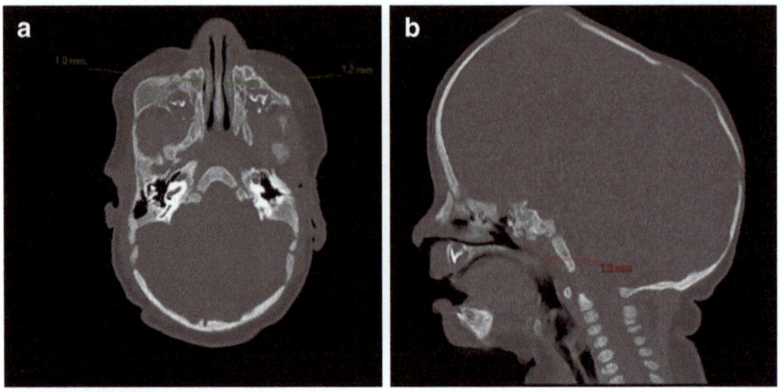

Fig. 22.1 Cranial CT scan in a 2-month-old child with Crouzon syndrome. (**a**) Axial section. Stenosis of the nasal cavities. (**b**) Sagittal section. Narrowing of the nasopharyngeal airway

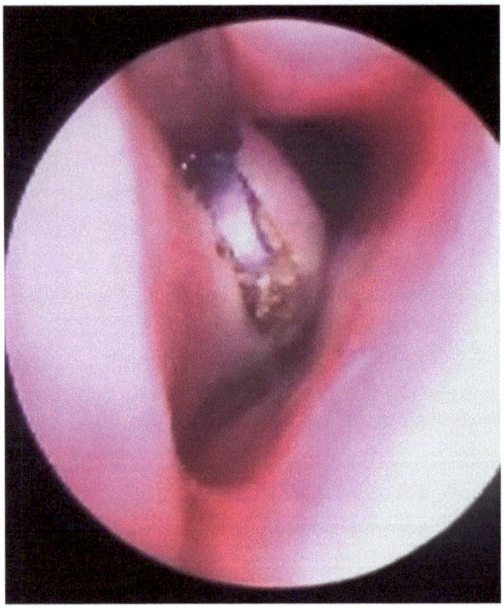

Fig. 22.2 Perioperative endoscopic view of a laser turbinectomy (removal of the inferior turbinates) in a 3-month-old child with Apert syndrome

22.1 Conclusions

Given the frequency and the potential severity of respiratory and auditory disorders in children with CS, yearly ENT visits with wake upper airway endoscopy and hearing tests are recommended. Early ENT assessment may be required in case of neonatal respiratory distress. Additional consultations are sometimes necessary if additional ENT symptoms appear.

References

1. Derderian C, Seaward J. Syndromic craniosynostosis. Semin Plast Surg. 2012;26:64–75.
2. Saengthong P, Chaitusaney B, Hirunwiwatkul P, Charakorn N. Adenotonsillectomy in children with syndromic craniosynostosis: a systematic review and meta-analysis. Eur Arch Otorrinolaringol. 2019;276:1555–60.
3. Leclere JC, Marianowski R, Monteyrol PJ, Akkari M, Chalumeau F, Fayoux P, Leboulanger N, Franco P, Couloigner V, Mondain M. Guidelines of the French Society of Otorhinolaryngology. Role of the ENT specialist in the diagnosis of obstructive sleep apnea hypopnea syndrome (OSAHS) in children. Part 2: Diagnostic investigations apart from sleep studies. Eur Ann Otorhinolaryngol Head Neck Dis. 2019;136:295–9.
4. Noble AR, Cunningham ML, Lam A, Wenger TL, Sie KC, Perkins JA, Dahl JP. Complex airway management in patients with tracheal cartilaginous sleeves. Laryngoscope. 2022;132:215–21.
5. Pickrell BB, Meaike JD, Cañadas KT, Chandy BM, Buchanan EP. Tracheal cartilaginous sleeve in syndromic craniosynostosis: an underrecognized source of significant morbidity and mortality. J Craniofac Surg. 2017;28:696–9.
6. Agochukwu NB, Solomon BD, Muenke M. Hearing loss in syndromic craniosynostoses: otologic manifestations and clinical findings. Int J Pediatr Otorhinolaryngol. 2014;78:2037.
7. de Jong T, Toll MS, de Gier HH, Mathijssen IM. Audiological profile of children and young adults with syndromic and complex craniosynostosis. Arch Otolaryngol Head Neck Surg. 2011;137:775–8.

23 Complications and Long-Term Surgical Outcome in Craniosynostoses

Matthieu Vinchon, Pierre-Aurélien Beuriat, Alexandru Szathmari, and Federico Di Rocco

23.1 Introduction

The life of a child affected by craniosynostosis is impacted in many and highly variable ways, on account of both of his condition and of the surgery it leads to. Craniosynostoses are serious malformations, with often dire consequences, even more so when associated with faciostenosis. On the other hand, despite constant effort to optimize results and decrease morbidity, surgery is always an important undertaking and is associated with a number of unwanted consequences, during operation, in the immediate postoperative course, or later in life. For these reasons, it is important to know the complications of synostoses and of their treatment, in order to inform the decision to the operated, taken conjointly by the surgeon and the child's parents, as well as anticipate surgical difficulties. In the present chapter, we shall review chronologically the different complications of craniosynostoses before, during, and after surgery, and their management and prevention. We shall conclude on the issues of surgical decision and informed consent and the need for consensual quantitative scales to evaluate the morphological results as well as surgical complications.

23.2 Preoperative Complications

23.2.1 Birth Difficulties

The calvarial sutures play an important role in the biomechanics of birth, and their fusion can have dire consequences [1]. In an earlier, unpublished study conducted in Lille during the years 2016–2021, among 233 new cases of craniosynostoses, we found that the overall prevalence of dystocia (difficult or instrumented birth) was 45.5%; among these, 30.5% were delivered by C-section (compared with 20% in the general population in France during that period), 24.4% of them because of fetal distress. The prevalence of C-section was highest among boys, and patients with metopic or multisutural synostosis (Fig. 23.1). Dystocia was the cause of birth trauma in four identified cases: one with sagittal synostosis who developed a large subperiosteal hematoma (Fig. 23.2a, b); one with metopic synostosis who had petrous bone fracture and subdural bleeding associated with forceps delivery (Fig. 23.2c, d); one with unilambdoid synostosis who developed a subdural hemorrhage; and one with complex multi-suture synostosis who

M. Vinchon (✉)
Department of Pediatric Neurosurgery, Hospices Civils de Lyon, Lyon, France

Service de Neurochirurgie Pédiatrique, Hôpital Femme Mère Enfant, Bron, France
e-mail: matthieu.vinchon@chu-lyon.fr

P.-A. Beuriat · A. Szathmari · F. Di Rocco
Department of Pediatric Neurosurgery, Hospices Civils de Lyon, Lyon, France

F. Di Rocco, J. Kestle (eds.), *Neurosurgical Aspects of Craniosynostosis*,
https://doi.org/10.1007/978-3-031-69386-1_23

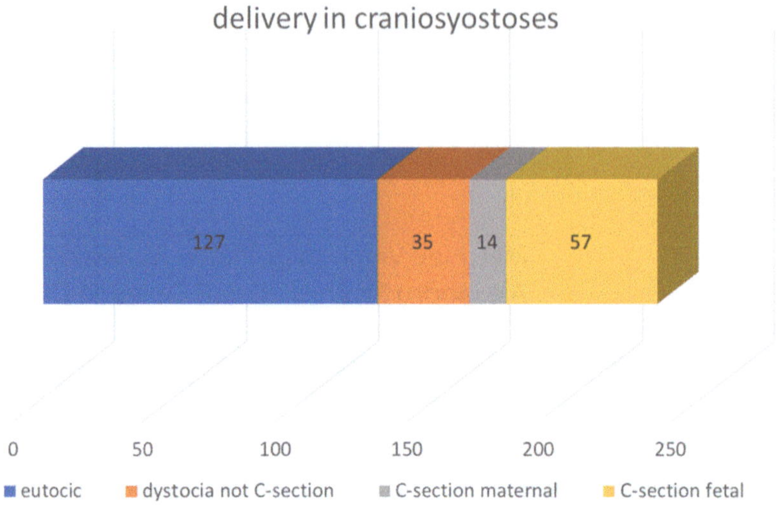

Fig. 23.1 Conditions of birth in 233 cases of craniosynostoses followed during the period 2016–2019 in Lille. Close to half of these children had delivery difficulties, 30.3% born by C-section, 24.4% by C-section for fetal distress. These birth difficulties can be anticipated in case of prenatal diagnosis, and may be a confusion factor regarding the developmental outcome

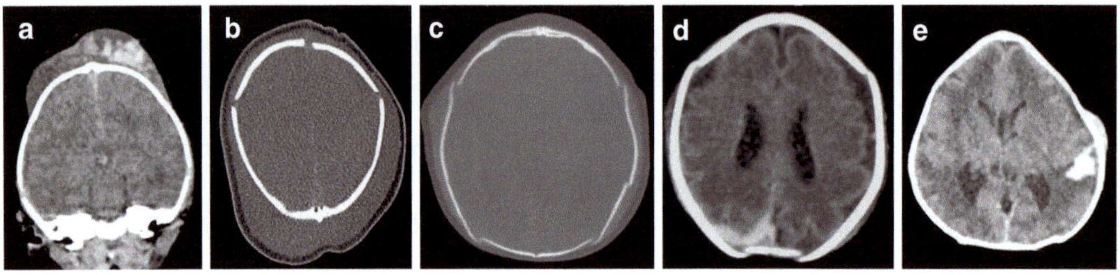

Fig. 23.2 Birth trauma in children with craniosynostosis; (**a** and **b**) Sagittal synostosis, with the characteristic bilateral cephalhematoma, because no periosteal midline adherence limits its spread; (**c** and **d**) Metopic synostosis, with difficult forceps delivery, scalp laceration, fracture of the petrous bone and subdural bleeding; and (**e**) A newborn with complex multi-suture synostosis who developed intracerebral hemorrhage

developed intracerebral hemorrhage (Fig. 23.2e). Although the mechanical trauma was predominantly mild and had no or few consequences, dystocia could also cause fetal distress during and after birth, with potential impact on the patient's later development. Birth difficulties could thus be a confounding factor when studying the developmental impact of brain compression by the synostosis. Although the majority of children with craniosynostosis are delivered by natural vaginal delivery, a prenatal diagnosis should reinforce the vigilance regarding possible dystocia and lower the threshold for cesarean section.

23.2.2 Brain Compression

Brain decompression by calvarial expansion is the cornerstone of surgery for craniosynostoses. However, the relation between reduced intracranial volume and intracerebral pressure is complex, certainly underpinned by poorly understood hydrodynamic mechanisms [2].

Multiple suture synostoses, mostly syndromic, are associated with raised intracranial pressure (ICP), which increases with the number of fused sutures [3]. Calvarial growth restriction is often the main presenting symptom of multisuture craniosynostoses, sometimes present at birth in case of cloverleaf malformation, or later during progression toward oxycephaly, with progressive closure of the different sutures [4].

By contrast, in unisutural synostoses, the initial presentation in early childhood is mostly related to morphological concerns, and the brain is generally not compressed initially. Typically, the closure of the sagittal suture is compensated by the coronal and metopic sutures, giving the child his typical dolichocephalic appearance with a bulging forehead and an above-normal head circumference. However, in older children, sagittal synostosis can mimic pseudotumor cerebri [5], and is a not an uncommon finding in clinically eloquent tonsillar herniation [6]. Similarly, ICP can rise late after correction of unisutural synostosis, because of non-synchronous multisuture synostosis [7].

Regarding metopic synostosis, the occurrence of brain compression and the benefit of decompressive surgery are controversial. While some authors have documented intracranial hypertension [8], others, using sophisticated imaging techniques, found no evidence of brain compression [9]. Better developmental outcomes have been reported in all types of craniosynostoses when surgery was performed before the age of 1 year [10]; however, in this retrospective study, the reason why some children were operated early, and others later, was not analyzed. A more recent study has found that the late surgery was associated with confounding factors susceptible to influence developmental outcome, such as social context, prematurity, and co-morbidities [11].

23.2.3 Psychosocial Impact of Morphological Disgrace

Difficulties can arise during childhood because of the morphological disgrace, leading to problems of self-image, taunting and even harassment by schoolmates (and even occasionally by teachers!). The psychological impact at school age should not be taken lightly. Compounded with the parental stress, which children and infants feel and absorb like sponges, this psychological burden may play a significant role in the future life of these patients. Very rarely, the demand for morphological correction is not expressed until adult age [12]. Moreover, in familial cases, the demand for early morphological correction for their child, coming from affected parents, is revealing.

23.3 Intraoperative Complications

23.3.1 Anesthesia and Installation

Complications of anesthesia and installation are the shared responsibility of the surgeon and the anesthetist. Among these, the risk of complications of venous and arterial catheters, and pressure sores on the scalp or eyeballs (Fig. 23.3) must be decreased by scrupulous attention from both teams.

23.3.2 Bleeding

Intraoperative bleeding occurring, whatever the technique chosen, is the most threatening complication during surgery, with a potential for fatal consequences, and requires blood transfusion in a number of patients. The importance of bleeding relates to the body proportions in infants, with a larger head and a limited blood volume (estimated around 500 ml at 3 months and 750 ml at 9 months) compared to adults. Diffuse bleeding comes from the scalp, the dura-mater (in particular arachnoid villi, which appear around 9 months) and above all from the bone, especially at the skull base. In craniosynostosis surgery, bleeding is increased by enlarged trans-osseous veins and intracranial hypertension. Clotting problems can result from profuse bleeding and hypothermia, so a high degree of vigilance and close interactions between surgeon and anesthetist are warranted, in order to avoid entering a fatal spiral.

Rigorous anesthesia protocols are followed in order to monitor hemodynamics; near-infra red spectroscopy can help to determine if and when transfusion must be decided (Fig. 23.4). In case of profuse bleeding, supplementation with platelets and clotting factors may also be needed. Transfusion following all the security protocols incurs extremely low additional risk, whereas reluctance or delay to transfuse can have fatal consequences. Although all precautions to dimin-

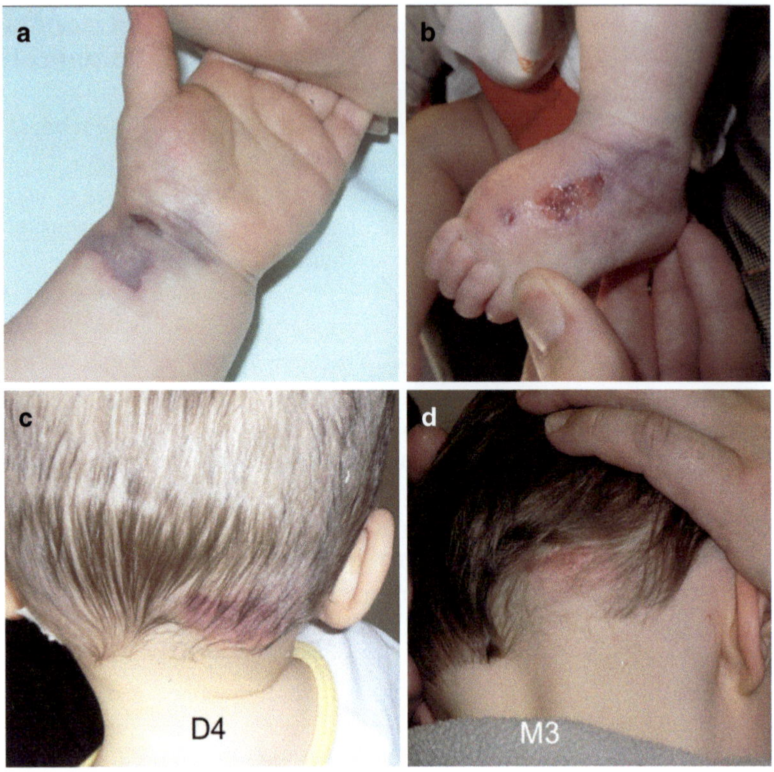

Fig. 23.3 Complications of the arterial catheter (**a**), of peripheral venous catheters (**b**), of positioning (**c** and **d**) are a shared responsibility of the surgeon and anesthetist

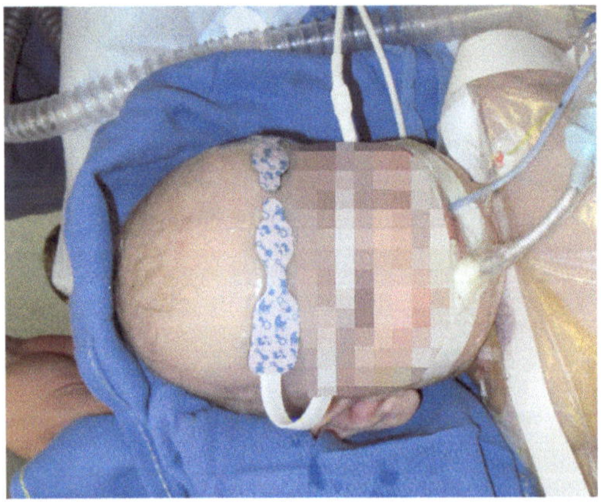

Fig. 23.4 Near infra red spectroscopy can be used when the forehead is not in the operative field (sagittal synostosis and posterior pole surgeries), and helps to determine if and when transfusion is needed

ish the risk of bleeding should be taken, we consider that transfusion should not be regarded as a complication. In consequence, the acceptance from parent that transfusion may be needed is a prerequisite for surgery.

Intraoperative blood loss is anticipated preoperatively by iron supplementation and/or erythropoietin, and mitigated during surgery by hemodilution and volume expansion. Meticulous hemostasis at each stage of the operation requires precise knowledge of where the bleeding comes from, notably the location of trans-osseous veins (Figs. 23.5 and 23.6). Permanent communication between surgeon and anesthetist before, during, and after surgery is vital for the successful management of this potentially lethal complication.

23.3.3 Dural Tear

Even though most dural tears occur at a distance from the venous sinuses, dural lesions, even when involving only the outer layer, increase blood loss, and, if left unattended, can initiate a meningocele. Bleeding can become catastrophic if a dural tear involves a venous sinus (Fig. 23.7). The risk of dural tear is diversely evaluated, because not all authors take note of the minimal splits of the dural outer layer. Endoscopic techniques may not lead to more dural tears [13], but make these more difficult to cope with. The risk of dural tear is higher in newborns, in children with longstanding intracranial hypertension, in craniofacial advancement [14] and in redo surgery [15], especially after previous dural repair. Dural adherences are intense along the sutures, in particular underneath the fontanels and epactal bones, and on the midline of the skull base. Opening of the sagittal sinus is thus at higher risk when the metopic suture is still patent [1]. The adherence of patent sutures to the dura is especially tricky in unilambdoid synostosis, because the lateral sinus is often lacking on the synostotic side [16], and the sinus on the non-synostotic, adherent side is compensatorily enlarged.

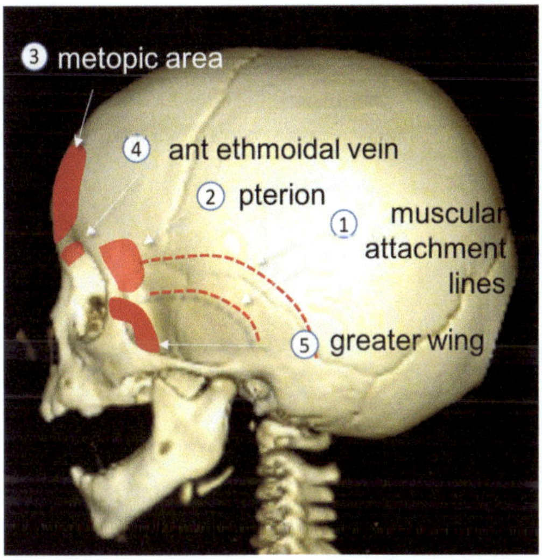

Fig. 23.5 Location of trans-osseous veins in metopic synostosis, numbered according to the timing of their occurrence during fronto-orbital remodeling

Dural tear at the skull base is a not uncommon complication of the different techniques of fronto-orbital advancement in craniofaciosynostoses [14, 17], with a high risk of cerebrospinal fluid leakage and meningeal infection. Although these leaks can often dry spontaneously, intracranial dural repair is sometimes necessary (Fig. 23.8).

Partial dural tears, limited to the outer dural layer, should be reapproximated by a few stitches whenever possible, sometimes completed with fibrin glue. Complete dural tears must be repaired with a running suture as watertight as possible, which may require harvesting an epidural graft.

The prevention of dural tears involves careful dissection of bone from permeable fontanels, and of sutures from the underlying sinuses before using the craniotome. Use of the burr over the pterional and asterial fontanels should be especially cautious. Dissection of the dura from the bone can be tedious, on account of adherences and uneven inner surface of the calvaria, as well as frequent bleeding from the middle meningeal artery or dural veins. In very small infants with cloverleaf malformation, patient dissection of the lacunae and epactal bones, followed by piece-

Fig. 23.6 Parietal emissary veins in sagittal synostosis; (**a**) 3D-CT scanner and (**b**) Operative view of the exposed sagittal sinus, patient in the prone position

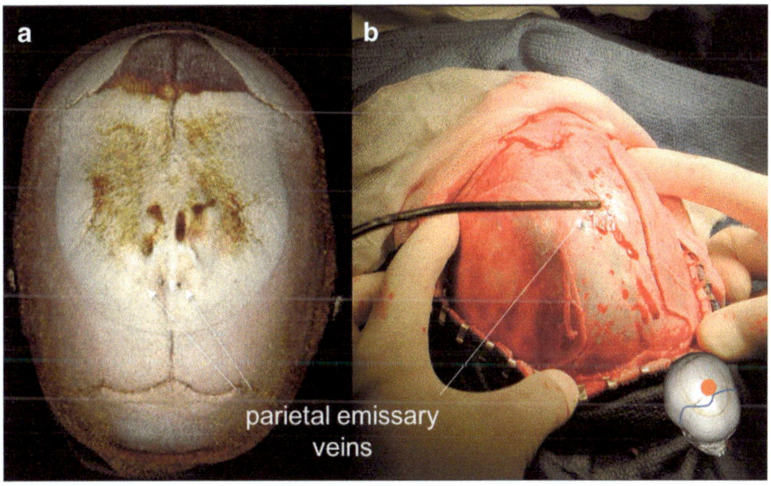

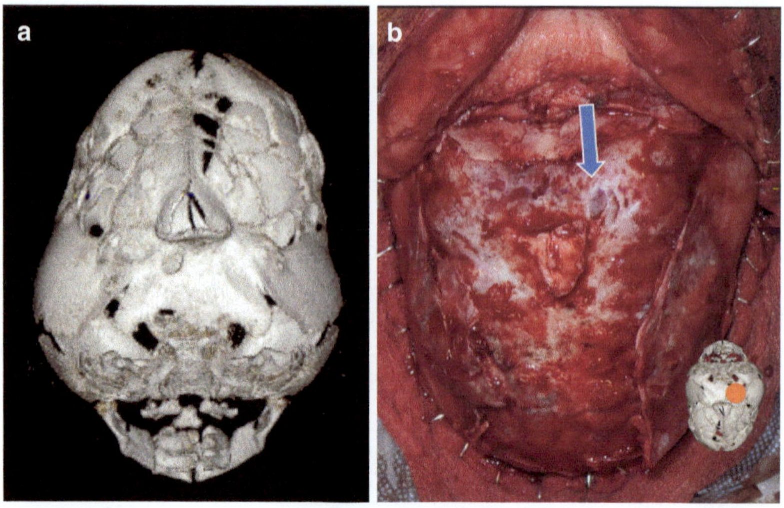

Fig. 23.7 Cloverleaf skull, operated on D5 of life because of life-threatening intracranial hypertension with tonsillar herniation. (**a**) CT-scanner showing the lacunae and complex sutural pattern around the lesser fontanelle. (**b**) Operative view showing limited dural tear close to the posterior fontanel

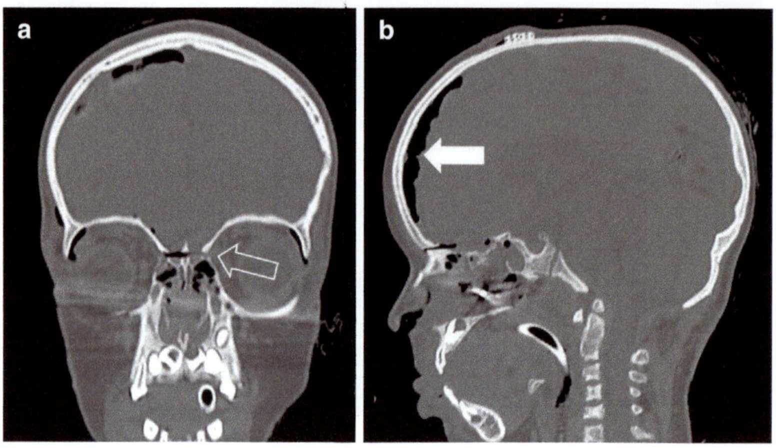

Fig. 23.8 Two-year-old femaleoperated for Crouzon disease with Le Fort 3 osteotomy because of severe sleep apneas (**a**) coronal and (**b**) sagittal view. She developed rhinorrhea because of ethmoidal dural tear (empty arrow); note intradural pneumocephalus (full arrow), which required craniotomy for duraplasty

meal removal of the bone septa, often extending deep between the sulci, is the most delicate time of suturectomy [18].

23.4 Early Postoperative Period

23.4.1 The Emotional Shock

In the immediate postoperative days, parental distress is almost constant [19]. In addition to the child being in pain, or drowsy and feeding poorly on account of opioid medications, he often presents with facial edema, of variable severity but which can be major and complicated by chemosis, and even subluxation of the tarsal cartilage. The child's ordeal appeals to his parent's feelings of guilt over their decision to have him operated, and echoes with the guilt which is very widespread in parents of a child with inborn diseases, especially if genetically determined. When the edema subsides, the change in facial features, which was the purpose of the operation, can be difficult to cope with. The rare complaint "it's not my child anymore" is only the most radical expression of a widespread parental unease. To make things worse, parental stress is absorbed by the child, so that parental and infantile stress amplify each other in a play of mirrors. This often translates into sleepless nights back home, regressive reactions, with often prolonged co-sleeping. This postoperative stress should not be overlooked and must be anticipated. Physical contact, cradling, and cuddling should be encouraged immediately after surgery. Before surgery, parents should be informed of the oncoming physical changes and convinced that the child's appearance will be "more normal," and that he will have "the head he should have had." Contacts with patients' associations can be a precious resource for these parents, who can thus interact with others who "have been through that" before them.

23.4.2 Infection

Infection is a rare complication but can prolong hospital stay and have dire consequences. A sepsis can result of operative site infection (OSI) or venous or urinary catheter. However, aseptic fever is common, on account of the large subcutaneous exposure, and should not lead to untimely antibiotic treatments. By contrast, the reappearance of fever and scalp edema after initial subsidence should raise alarm of OSI.

Operative site infection occurs in up to 7% [20], and can be epidermal, dermal, or deep. OSI is sometimes elicited by the child scratching his wound, or initiated by inflammation caused by absorbable sutures, or skin necrosis due to tension closure associated with ambitious calvarial expansion. It can also be a consequence of incidental respiratory or ocular infection present at the time of surgery; in these cases, it is wise to postpone the scheduled operation, provided that the infection is circumstantial and not chronic, in relation with faciostenosis, and also that the child has no menacing intracranial hypertension. Other potential factors associated with postoperative infection are the long duration of surgery [21], the extended incision, opening of the facial sinuses, the creation of an epidural dead space, skin breakdown, the presence of implanted material, especially external distractors [22] or springs, and prolonged use of venous or urinary catheter.

Whereas superficial scalp infection usually requires only local measures (removal of scabs and remaining sutures plus local antiseptics), superficial suppuration may be aggressive, the scab protecting an ecosystem in which staphylococcus aureus thrives; in addition to scab removal, oral antibiotics may be necessary. Deep suppuration is rare but can be associated with septic signs, and require debridement, drainage, and irrigation in addition to antibiotics [23]. The management of these postoperative empyema should be as conservative as possible, because wide opening and dismantling of the construct would devascularize the bone flaps, and bone necrosis would have catastrophic morphological consequences (Fig. 23.9).

Prevention of local and deep infection implies rigorous asepsis, before, during, and after surgery, and high-quality layered closure without excessive tension. The child must be prevented from scratching his wound, sometimes with the help of antihistamine medications. Prophylactic antibiotics are administered routinely during surgery, justified by the extent of surgery, its duration, and the potential gravity of OSI; however, protocols vary and are mostly tradition-based [24].

23.4.3 Complications of Implants and Fixation Devices

Aseptic subcutaneous granulomas can develop on absorbable sutures and plates, and take months to disappear, but require nothing more than reassuring words. During surgery, simple precautions can decrease these benign but vexing complications, like avoiding to place knots over salient facial features, cutting threads short, and burying the knots in bone perforations. Bone fixation with wires is generally well tolerated but can lead to skin compromise or perforation [23], as well as migrate inward into the dura as the calvaria grows by apposition-resorption, and should be used sparingly (Fig. 23.10). The same happens with much more serious consequences with non-absorbable plates [25], springs, and prosthetic materials [26]. Absorbable plates are generally well tolerated but can also cause aseptic granulomas, and migrate, both inward and outward [27, 28].

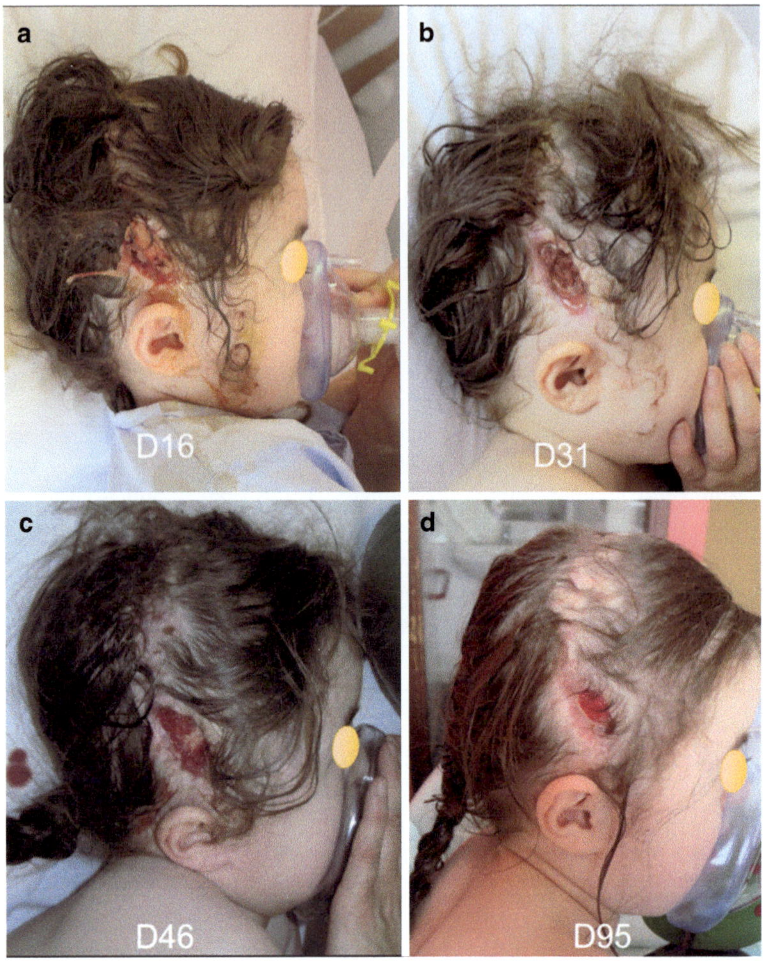

Fig. 23.9 Crouzon syndrome, first operated for posterior pole expansion at 6 months, reoperated at 5 years for fronto-orbital advancement. The child presented with fistulization of an epidural empyema, which was treated with antibiotics, prolonged drainage-irrigation, and directed scarring (at day 16 (**a**), day 31 (**b**), day 46 (**c**) and day 95 (**d**))

23.4.4 Scalp and Calvarial Breakdown

Skin or bone disruption generally results of excessive tension of the scalp, after generous volume expansion; it almost never happens after external trauma.

Skin breakdown occurs mostly in children with multisuture synostosis, especially in older children and after redo surgery. Even when the underlying bone is exposed, it rarely causes serious infection, but may require prolonged directed scarring, or sometimes reoperation. Breakdown is prevented by progressive scalp traction, which is one of the important advances brought about by distraction techniques. Alternately, scalp expansion using a balloon expander can be proposed, provided that the child's calvaria is already rigid enough not to cave in, and surgery can be programmed some time in advance.

Bone dislocation is a rare but worrisome complication. Cranioplasties are at best semi-rigid constructs, especially in young infants, and the mechanical compression by scalp traction can be enough to cause breakdown of construct. The lordosis of the fronto-orbital bandeau is caused by breakage of plates [29] or bone dislocation at the pterion, especially if the coronal suture is incompletely fused (Fig. 23.11). The fronto-malar synfibrosis is also a weak point, where fixation of the lateral orbital pillar can give way. Bone breakdown also occurs in redo

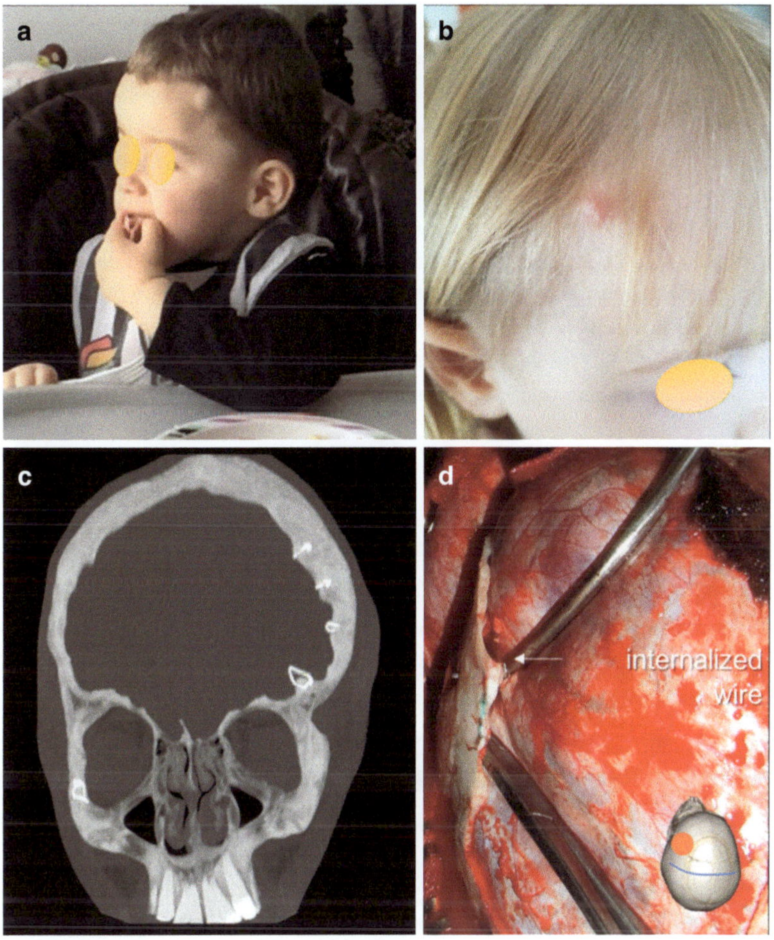

Fig. 23.10 Complications of wires: outward migration of wires (**a** and **b**) can threaten or perforate the scalp (**b**), while their inward migration (**c** and **d**), caused by resorptional calvarial growth, brings these into contact or conflict with the dura (**d**)

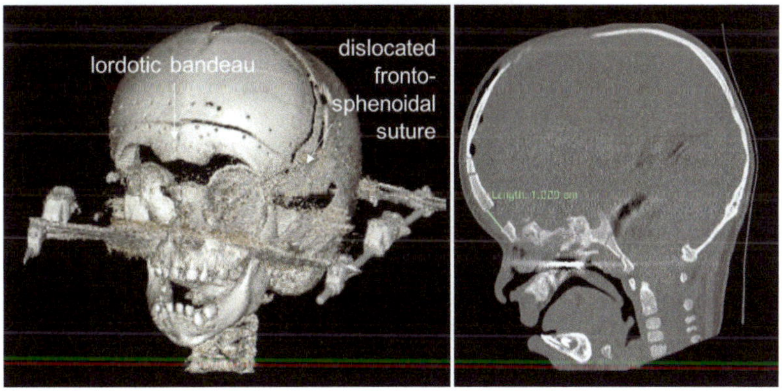

Fig. 23.11 Breakdown of construct caused by dislocation of the fronto-sphenoidal suture under the tension of scalp, resulting in lordosis of the bandeau, lifted 12 mm, with eye exposure and pulsating exophthalmos, and requiring reoperation for refixation of bandeau

surgery, because regenerative bone becomes brittle. The occurrence of "gull-winging" (the uplifting of the parietal bone by disjunction of sutures) happens after posterior distraction [30], as the consequence of distracting a patent or incompletely fused suture. Anterior distraction procedures can also cause skull base dislocation, causing optic neuropathy after monobloc osteotomy [31], or oculomotor paralysis on account of spheno-petrous ("Le Fort 6") dislocation (Fig. 23.12). All these complications impose reoperations and/or reappraisal of the surgical strategy.

23.4.5 Growing Fracture

Postoperative leptomeningeal cysts or growing fractures develop as a result of untended intraoperative dural tear or postoperative dural necrosis, with the brain herniating through the rent and preventing it from healing. It can develop after endoscopic surgery, because dural tear can be unnoticed or because dural repair is most uneasy [32]. The pressure gradient causes focal hydrodynamic disturbance, with enlarged Virchow-Robin spaces [33].

Anatomical repair of the dura and calvaria is necessary (Fig. 23.13). Whenever possible, autologous materials are highly preferable [33, 34]. The management of postoperative leptomeningeal cysts can be challenging because of the tension of the brain (which may require temporary lumbar drainage); of the proximity of the dural defect to the sinuses; of the extent of bone defect requiring a large donor site; of the young age of the child whose thin calvaria is difficult to split. However, modern high-speed motors and piezoelectric saws allow the splitting of calvaria in very young children [35].

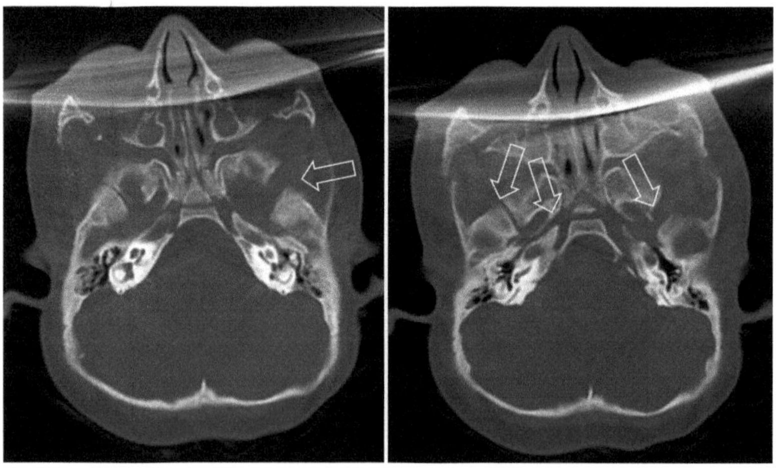

Fig. 23.12 Fifteen-months-old child with Crouzon disease, operated for fronto-orbital advancement with transfacial pin; axial CT scanner performed on D14 of craniofacial distraction because of abducens palsy, showed spheno-temporal ("Le Fort 6") dislocation (arrows)

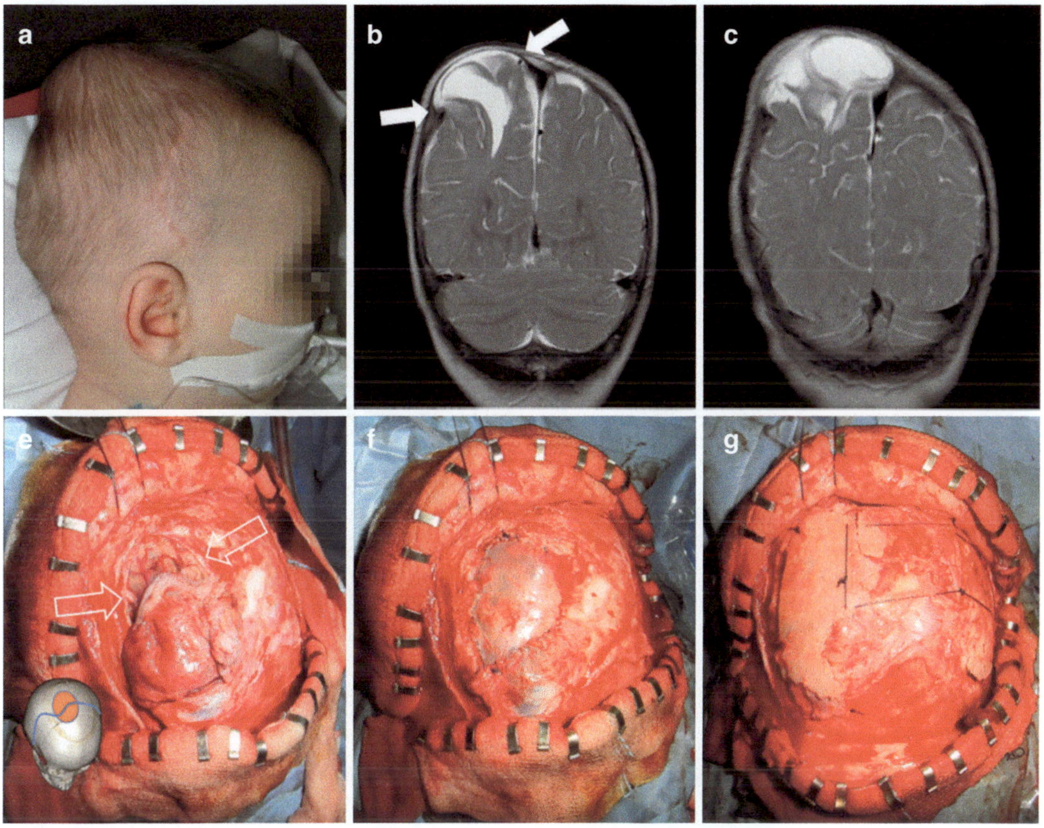

Fig. 23.13 Growing fracture (**a**) Seven-months male operated 2 months earlier for sagittal synostosis (H-craniectomy with linear coagulation of the dura mater and no drainage, causing dural necrosis). (**b**) Note the thickened bone margins (full arrows) due to uplifting of the periosteal tissues; (**b**, **c**) the herniated brain tissue is highly edematous, due to expansion of Virchow-Robin spaces; (**e**) The margins of the dural defect are much retracted (empty arrows), requiring a large pericranial autograft (**f**). The bone defect is bridged with split calvarial autograft (**g**)

23.5 Late Surgical Outcome

23.5.1 The Scar

Whatever the surgery, it leaves a scar. However much, as A. Raimondi quipped, the infant's scalp may be "forgiving," the scar can be a problem for the child's self-image and a source of embarrassment. Its perception is highly variable: while some children shun going to the swimming pool for fear that their scar might show through wet hair, others glorify it with creative hairstyle (Fig. 23.14). Like any bodily imperfection, the scar can be a fixation point for teasing, taunting, and harassment at school age, as well as self-depreciation at adolescence. In order to make the scar as stealthy as possible, its curve should as much as possible keep a 90° orientation relative to the direction of hair. When a father has a receding hairline, his son's incision may need to be more posterior than usual. In complex synostoses, it should be kept in mind that repeated surgeries may be needed in the future, and that the bicoronal incision should be versatile enough to give access to both the posterior and anterior poles. This may be problematic when the initial surgery was endoscopic, with two scars, one very anterior, and the other very posterior.

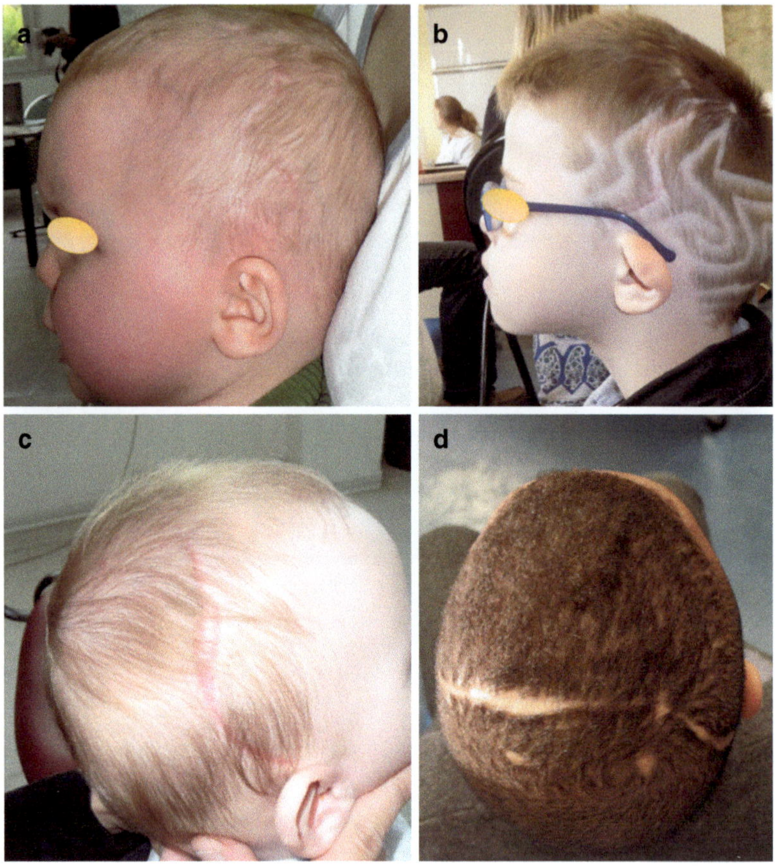

Fig. 23.14 (**a**) Discrete "lazy S" incision, curved in order to stay perpendicular to the natural direction of hair, leaves the most discreet scar; (**b**) "Zig-zag" scar, intended to be easily hidden, but glorified by creative haircut; (**c**) Early, wide, and red scar, destined to whiten with time; (**d**) Persistent Keloid scar of the scalp incision and of the drain

23.5.2 Redo Operations

Reoperations can be needed, sometimes many years after the initial surgery. The larger or lesser importance of these reoperations led Whitaker et al. to propose a grading of surgical results as: (1) not requiring reoperation; (2) minor reoperation proposed; (3) reoperation less than initial surgery necessary; and (4) reoperation as large or more than initial surgery [36]. In addition to the operative complications mentioned above, many of which can require additional surgery, other operations may become necessary during follow-up.

Incomplete reossification of the calvaria leaves pulsating lacunae. These occur in about 5% of the operated cases, and appear to be more frequent in the fronto-orbital advancement [37], and occipital pole remodeling [38]. Lacunae most often sit close to the midline, especially at the vertex, and occur most often after extensive midline bone resection [39], all the more in older children. On account of their location, calvarial lacunae present no risk of traumatic brain injury, and no limitations should be imposed on the child's activities. Lacunae thus present mostly an aesthetic problem, although some children also experience the "syndrome of the trephined," with headaches or learning difficulties, and changes in the cerebral blood flow have been documented in some cases [38]. The surgical management of persistent lacunae can be proposed after the fifth or sixth birthday, and the most desirable technique is autologous graft by split calvaria [35] (Fig. 23.15).

Temporal hollowing is specific problem with metopic synostosis, and can result from atrophy of the temporal muscle compounded with excessive restoration of frontal bosses. The progressive nature of this imperfection, which becomes more apparent with time (Fig. 23.16), suggests that bone growth is focally disturbed by surgery, pos-

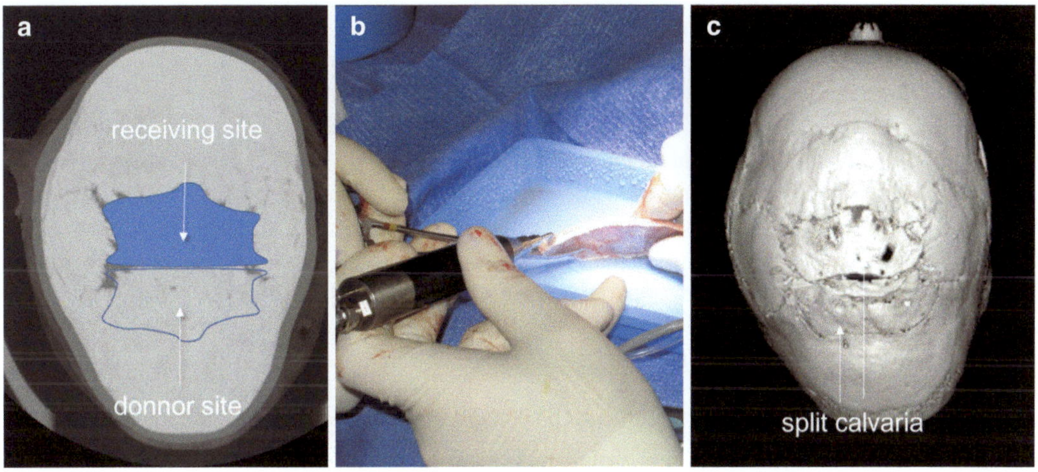

Fig. 23.15 Persisting lacuna at the vertex after craniectomy at 4 months for sagittal synostosis; repair age 4 years, using split calvaria. (**a**) The craniotomy for the donor site is tailored on a template outlined around the limits of the lacuna; (**b**) The flap is then split using the piezoelectric saw; (**c**) Both bone tables are fixed rigidly in place in order to fill the lacuna and the donor site

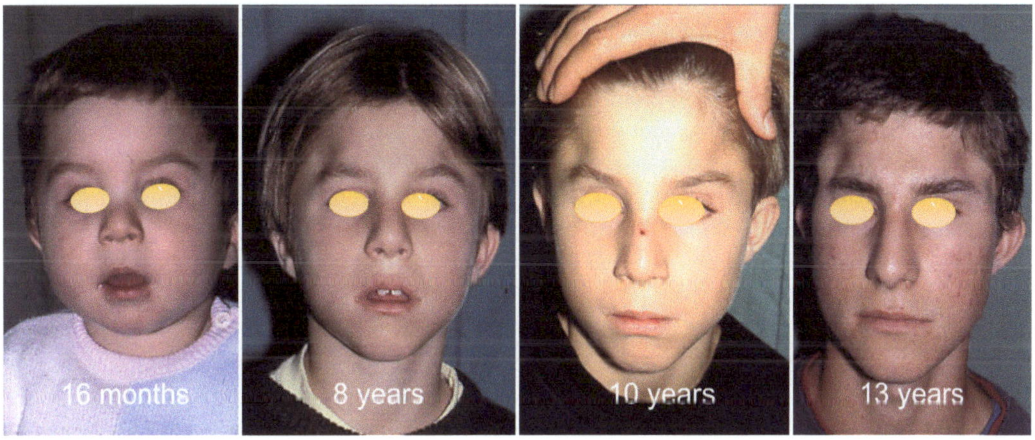

Fig. 23.16 Progressive temporal hollowing after surgery for metopic synostosis

sibly because the greater wing of the sphenoid needs the strain of muscles to sustain its growth. Temporal hollowing can be well accepted, or lead to a demand for esthetic correction; this is easily performed by lipofilling, which can be repeated as needed, but should preferably be delayed until adolescence. Different technical refinements have been proposed in order to reduce the prevalence of temporal hollowing, like large temporal "elephant ears" [40], or tongue-and groove bandeau advancement, with mixed results leaving room for improvement.

23.5.3 Other Craniofacial Operations

Other major craniofacial operations are often needed in craniofaciostenoses, in order to correct midface retrusion or hypertelorism. Secondary multisuture synostosis should be expected in syndromic craniofaciostenoses [4] as well as in lambdoid synostosis [16], but are rare in sagittal synostosis, occurring in about 2% of cases [39], and are almost never found in non-syndromic metopic synostosis. Secondary closure of new sutures attests of the progressive nature of the disease, and these reoperations should not be regarded as complications of surgery. However, this information regarding this evolution should be given to parents as early as the first consultation, in particular in case of prenatal diagnosis.

In addition, other relatively minor operations may be needed, such as onlay grafts, rhinoplasty, removal of facial scars, correction of slant eyes, or of strabismus. Ideally, all these operations, which are mostly destined to improve cosmesis, should be performed at the end of growth and on demand from the patient himself.

The large array of different operations, implicating different surgical specialists, at different ages, underlines the importance of prolonged multidisciplinary follow-up.

23.5.4 Morphological Result

Although the Whitaker classification mentioned above [36] is convenient and widely accepted [41], this classification is focused on reinterventions, not on morphology, and does not quantify the preoperative dysmorphism; for these reasons, it does not evaluate accurately morphological results. Obviously, the objective quantification of something as subjective as morphological disgrace has proved difficult.

The evaluation of results by satisfaction questionnaires filled by the parents may be fraught with complacency, or by the fear of another operation. In one study, parents were generally as satisfied as surgeons on all items, except for syndromic cases [42], where doctors appeared ready to accept suboptimal results, possibly because no good surgical solution exists. Similarly, another study found a better acceptance by doctors, compared with parents, of what is inevitable (the scar, alopecia) or for which they have no good surgical remedy (calvarial asymmetry, bony bumps) [41]. This discrepancy shows a mismatch between surgeons' and parents' expectations; whereas parents might have inordinately high hopes of normalization, surgeons might be more centered on what they can expect from their usual technique. Blinded morphological evaluation by independent surgeons avoids the complacency bias, but not the professional one [43]: the criteria by which surgeons judge may be at odds from what the patients expect. In a self-declarative evaluation by adult patients operated in infancy for non-syndromic craniosynostosis, values regarding self-esteem and depression scores were in the normal range; these patients satisfied themselves with all the imperfections of surgical techniques from a past era, except asymmetry of facial features [44]. A blinded evaluation of "attractiveness" by laypersons confirmed the negative impact of craniofacial asymmetry [45]; the method in this study, enrolling as evaluators independent female professionals of a daycare center, is probably a step in the right direction. All these subjective evaluations would also be more in line with the patients' expectations, with the input of patients' associations.

Multiple efforts have been devoted recently to the creation of pre and postoperative quantitative evaluation scales of the deformity, much-needed tools if we want to scale postoperative results, and compare one technique with another. The Rotterdam team has proposed a score for scaphocephaly, summing semi-quantitative subscores in the same spirit as the long-established Glasgow Coma Scale [39, 46]. The evaluation by an independent panel is necessarily based on documents, and 2D pictures are obviously misleading; for this reason, 3D photogrammetry is a promising tool [47]. We hope that in a near future, a consensus will emerge on quantitative morphological scales adapted to each of the different craniosynostoses.

23.6 Clinical Outcome

23.6.1 Mortality

Overall mortality is very low in craniosynostoses, and it affects almost exclusively syndromic cases [48]. Already from birth, some of these patients are beyond surgical resources, and they die because of breathing and feeding difficulties, and also possibly because of associated tonsillar herniation. Intraoperative mortality is poorly documented in literature, and mostly caused by uncontrolled bleeding; this outcome, although hopefully exceptional, cannot be dismissed.

23.6.2 Development

What is the real influence of cerebral compression on development? As mentioned above, the relation between intracranial volume and brain compression is not linear. Furthermore, intracranial hypertension occurs most regularly in multisuture synostoses, which have almost always a genetic background, so that the two factors cannot be separated. The correlation between developmental outcome and the age at surgery might be an indication of the developmental impact of brain compression [10, 49], but other factors, like a syndromic context, or a lack of parental motivation for surgery are confusing factors [11].

The impact of focal cerebral compression on development is also elusive. The Leeds group found a discrepancy between verbal and performance IQ (VIQ > PIQ) in unisutural craniosynostoses [50], which they ascribed to parietal compression, and which could be reversed by early surgery [49]. On the other hand, other researchers found no correlation between the severity of deformity and cerebral compression in metopic synostosis [8]. Shimoji found even paradoxical results, development being more impaired in milder forms of metopic synostosis [51]; this might suggest different referral patterns, and confirms that the importance of trigonocephalic deformation plays a secondary role, if any role at all in the patient's development. Overall, these studies suggest that the developmental impact of each type of synostosis is a specific problem.

23.6.3 Influence of the Syndromic Context

In syndromic craniosynostoses, gene or chromosomal disorders as well as environmental factors causing the synostosis can have a marked impact on development. In a previous, unpublished series of 188 cases of metopic synostosis operated over 20 years, the only significant and independent variable impacting negatively the development was syndromic context, which was identified in 31%. In FGFR3 mutation, experimental models in mice have shown that a developmental impact existed irrespective of the presence or absence of synostosis, and could be salvaged by targeted therapy by BGj398 [52]. This suggests that the mutation affects brain function directly, and opens exciting new treatment perspectives.

In addition, comorbidities and complications of many syndromic craniosynostoses are susceptible to impact on psychomotor and cognitive development [11]. Tonsillar herniation can cause sleep apneas, predominantly central [53], which can combine with obstructive apneas caused by midface retrusion, compromising wake periods and hindering learning. Hand and foot malformations in Apert syndrome require early management in order to allow psychomotor development [54]. Optic nerve atrophy caused by raised ICP, found in 12.3% of syndromic craniosynostoses, affects predominantly FGFR-related diseases [55], and deafness associated with Muenke syndrome, or resulting from tubal dysfunction in faciostenoses [56], can also both impair learning. In addition, careful brain imaging can disclose alterations of the cerebellar vermis and corpus callosum, which can be the consequence of deformation as well as associated malformations, and can impact on the child's development [57].

23.7 The Operative Decision and the Informed Consent

The decision to operate is taken jointly by the surgeon and the child's parents, based on the expected positive and adverse effects of surgery. The aims of surgery must therefore be clearly defined, and the potential complications well known by the surgeon and exposed to the parents. As mentioned above, much uncertainty surrounds the natural history of unoperated craniosynostoses, while many unknowns lay in the future after surgery, especially in syndromic cases. Unlike in multisuture synostoses, for which consent for surgery is comparatively straightforward, the aim of surgery for unisutural craniosynostosis is in a large part morphological. In that regard, the treatment can be seen as morphological surgery with a risk of severe morbidity and even mortality; few other fields of cranial surgery have such potential benefit-risk imbalance. The expected improvement of morphological appearance and better conformity with the social norm, as well as the potentially traumatic change of their child's facial features contribute to make the decision to operate an agonizing process for the parents.

Although emotions are the substance of which we are made, and society is the medium in which we live, surgeons are often poorly trained in psychology and sociology, often wrongly dismissed as "soft sciences." In addition, their position as professionals, which requires objectivity, sometimes hinders a more heartfelt approach. In this regard also, patients' associations can be a precious resource for these parents, helping them to cope with the mixed feeling and stress associated with decision-making.

23.8 The Future

The invasiveness of classical craniofacial surgery and the potentially high morbidity prompted the development of less invasive techniques and the boom of endoscopic surgery for craniosynostoses. However, the abundant literature published on these techniques appears to focus almost exclusively on easily measured outcome variables, such as transfusion rate and duration of hospital stay, with no indication on the long-term morphological results.

This points to the need for a consensual quantitative morphological rating based on objective criteria, which would allow to compare the patients pre and postoperatively, and one technique with another. A morphological scoring proposed for scaphocephaly allows the comparison of techniques [39, 43], and other scales are in development.

In order to weight the other pan of the scale, we also need a quantitative grading of complications. A classification of complications, sorted by their timing relative to operation, and their consequences for the patient, was proposed by the team in Leeds [58], and should certainly be a source of inspiration.

In order to be meaningful, the two quantitative scales, results, and complications, should not be simple lists of items, but require a ponderation of variables. In that regard, direct interview or collaboration of the patients themselves is invaluable to identify what really matters to them [44]; and here again, the input of patients' associations would be a precious help.

References

1. Vinchon M. The metopic suture: natural history. Neurochirurgie. 2019;65(5):239–45. https://doi.org/10.1016/j.neuchi.2019.09.006. Epub 2019 Sep 25.
2. Langvatn EA, Frič R, Due-Tønnessen BJ, Eide PK. Intracranial volume versus static and pulsatile intracranial pressure values in children with craniosynostosis. J Neurosurg Pediatr. 2019;24(1):66–74. https://doi.org/10.3171/2019.2.PEDS18767.
3. Tamburrini G, Caldarelli M, Massimi L, Santini P, Di Rocco C. Intracranial pressure monitoring in children with single suture and complex craniosynostosis: a review. Childs Nerv Syst. 2005;21(10):913–21. https://doi.org/10.1007/s00381-004-1117-x. Epub 2005 May 3.
4. Pellerin P, Vinchon M, Dhellemmes P, Guerreschi P. Crouzon syndrome: posterior fossa volume studies in vestibular orientation. Childs Nerv Syst. 2021;37(10):3105–11. https://doi.org/10.1007/s00381-021-05186-9. Epub 2021 Apr 27.
5. Martinez-Lage JF, Alamo L, Poza M. Raised intracranial pressure in minimal forms of craniosynostosis. Childs Nerv Syst. 1999;15(1):11–5; discussion 16. https://doi.org/10.1007/s003810050319.
6. Sgulò FG, Spennato P, Aliberti F, Di Martino G, Cascone D, Cinalli G. Contemporary occurrence of hydrocephalus and Chiari I malformation in sagittal craniosynostosis. Case report and review of the literature. Childs Nerv Syst. 2017;33(1):187–92. https://doi.org/10.1007/s00381-016-3189-9. Epub 2016 Jul 22.
7. Vinchon M, Pellerin P, Guerreschi P, Baroncini M, Dhellemmes P. Atypical scaphocephaly: a review. Childs Nerv Syst. 2012;28(9):1319–25. https://doi.org/10.1007/s00381-012-1807-8. Epub 2012 Aug 8.
8. Blum JD, Beiriger J, Kalmar C, Avery RA, Lang SS, Villavisanis DF, Cheung L, Cho DY, Tao W, Whitaker R, Bartlett SP, Taylor JA, Goldstein JA,

Swanson JW. Relating metopic craniosynostosis severity to intracranial pressure. J Craniofac Surg. 2022;33(8):2372–8. https://doi.org/10.1097/SCS.0000000000008748. Epub 2022 Jul 22.
9. de Planque CA, Florisson JMG, Tasker RC, Rijken BFM, van Veelen MLC, Mathijssen IMJ, Lequin MH, Dremmen MHG. A diffusion tensor imaging analysis of white matter microstructures in non-operated craniosynostosis patients. Neuroradiology. 2022;64(12):2391–8. https://doi.org/10.1007/s00234-022-02997-8. Epub 2022 Jun 27.
10. Renier D, Arnaud E, Marchac D. Craniosténoses: résultats fonctionnels et morphologiques post-opératoires [Craniosynostosis: functional and morphologic postoperative results]. Neurochirurgie. 2006;52(2–3 Pt 2):302–10. French. https://doi.org/10.1016/s0028-3770(06)71223-1.
11. Lynn JV, Buchman LK, Breuler CJ, Buchman SR. Surgical timing and neurocognitive development among patients with craniosynostosis: analysis of confounders. Plast Reconstr Surg. 2023;151(4):821–9. https://doi.org/10.1097/PRS.0000000000010004. Epub 2023 Mar 29.
12. Marchac D, Renier D, Arnaud E. Unoperated craniosynostosis patients: correction in adulthood. Plast Reconstr Surg. 2008;122(6):1827–38. https://doi.org/10.1097/PRS.0b013e31818cc388.
13. Arts S, Delye H, van Lindert EJ. Intraoperative and postoperative complications in the surgical treatment of craniosynostosis: minimally invasive versus open surgical procedures. J Neurosurg Pediatr. 2018;21(2):112–8. https://doi.org/10.3171/2017.7.PEDS17155. Epub 2017 Nov 24.
14. Dunaway DJ, Britto JA, Abela C, Evans RD, Jeelani NU. Complications of frontofacial advancement. Childs Nerv Syst. 2012;28(9):1571–6. https://doi.org/10.1007/s00381-012-1804-y. Epub 2012 Aug 8.
15. Wagner CS, Pontell ME, Hitchner MK, Barrero CE, Salinero LK, Swanson JW, Bartlett SP, Taylor JA. Prior fronto-orbital advancement associated with complications from transcranial midface surgery in patients with syndromic craniosynostosis. Childs Nerv Syst. 2023;39:1619. https://doi.org/10.1007/s00381-023-05879-3.
16. Vinchon M, Guerreschi P, Karnoub MA, Wolber A. Synostosis of the lambdoid suture: a spectrum. Childs Nerv Syst. 2021;37(6):1991–2000. https://doi.org/10.1007/s00381-020-05003-9. Epub 2021 Jan 6.
17. Hassan AM, Chappell AG, Murthy N, Stoehr JR, Alden T, Gosain AK. Posterior cranial vault distraction (PCVD): common complication rates and strategies of prevention and management. J Craniofac Surg. 2021;32(1):62–6. https://doi.org/10.1097/SCS.0000000000006980.
18. Vinchon M, Guerreschi P, Karnoub MA, Wolber A. Linear craniectomy for early posterior decompression in craniosynostoses: technique and results. Childs Nerv Syst. 2021;37(10):3113–8. https://doi.org/10.1007/s00381-021-05117-8. Epub 2021 Mar 13.
19. Lim J, Davis A, Tang AR, Shannon CN, Bonfield CM. Caregiver stress in children with craniosynostosis: a systematic literature review. Childs Nerv Syst. 2019;35(2):217–25. https://doi.org/10.1007/s00381-018-3959-7. Epub 2018 Aug 29.
20. Hennedige A, Richardson D, Duncan C, Parks C, Sinha A, Ellenbogen J, Robertson B. Part 1: Surgical correction in 231 trigonocephaly patients—the Alder Hey experience. J Craniofac Surg. 2021;32(6):2123–8. https://doi.org/10.1097/SCS.0000000000007475.
21. Puthumana JS, Lopez CD, Lake IV, Yang R. Evaluation of complications and outcomes in craniosynostosis by age of operation: analysis of the National Surgical Quality Improvement Program-Pediatric. J Craniofac Surg. 2023;34(1):29–33. https://doi.org/10.1097/SCS.0000000000008872. Epub 2022 Aug 11.
22. Goldstein JA, Paliga JT, Taylor JA, Bartlett SP. Complications in 54 frontofacial distraction procedures in patients with syndromic craniosynostosis. J Craniofac Surg. 2015;26(1):124–8. https://doi.org/10.1097/SCS.0000000000001320.
23. Natghian H, Song M, Jayamohan J, Johnson D, Magdum S, Richards P, Wall S. Long-term results in isolated metopic synostosis: the Oxford experience over 22 years. Plast Reconstr Surg. 2018;142(4):509e–15e. https://doi.org/10.1097/PRS.0000000000004768.
24. Holle J, Finger T, Lugonja J, Schmidt F, Schaumann A, Gratopp A, Thomale UW, von Bernuth H, Schulz M. The influence of perioperative antibiotic prophylaxis on wound infection and on the colonization of wound drains in patients after correction of craniosynostosis. Front Pediatr. 2021;9:720074. https://doi.org/10.3389/fped.2021.720074.
25. Mullens Cody L, Grome Luke J, Serrano Cesar A, Rabia Q, Mason AC. Titanium hardware extrusion following pediatric cranioplasty. Int Surg. 2018;13:1–5. https://doi.org/10.1016/j.inat.2018.01.002.
26. Ma IT, Symon MR, Bristol RE, Beals SP, Joganic EF, Adelson PD, Shafron DH, Singh DJ. Outcomes of titanium mesh cranioplasty in pediatric patients. J Craniofac Surg. 2018;29(1):99–104. https://doi.org/10.1097/SCS.0000000000004045.
27. Aldana PR, Wieder K, Postlethwait RA, James HE, Steinberg B. Ultrasound-aided fixation of biodegradable implants in pediatric craniofacial surgery. Pediatr Neurosurg. 2011;47(5):349–53. https://doi.org/10.1159/000337874. Epub 2012 May 9.
28. Yang L, Xu M, Jin X, Xu J, Lu J, Zhang C, Tian T, Teng L. Complications of absorbable fixation in maxillofacial surgery: a meta-analysis. PLoS One. 2013;8(6):e67449. https://doi.org/10.1371/journal.pone.0067449.
29. Hayden Gephart MG, Woodard JI, Arrigo RT, Lorenz HP, Schendel SA, Edwards MS, Guzman R. Using bioabsorbable fixation systems in the treatment of pediatric skull deformities leads to good outcomes and low morbidity. Childs Nerv Syst. 2013;29(2):297–301. https://doi.org/10.1007/s00381-012-1938-y. Epub 2012 Oct 26.

30. Iida C, Sakamoto Y, Miwa T, Yoshida K, Kishi K. Posterior distraction first or fronto-orbital advancement first for severe syndromic craniosynostosis. J Craniofac Surg. 2019;30(1):47–9. https://doi.org/10.1097/SCS.0000000000004897.
31. Alonso N, Goldenberg D, Fonseca AS, Kanashiro E, Matsushita H, Freitas Rda S, Shin JH. Blindness as a complication of monobloc frontofacial advancement with distraction. J Craniofac Surg. 2008;19(4):1170–3. https://doi.org/10.1097/SCS.0b013e318176ac83.
32. Aryan HE, Meltzer HS, Gerras GG, Jandial R, Levy ML. Leptomeningeal cyst development after endoscopic craniosynostosis repair: case report. Neurosurgery. 2004;55(1):235–7; discussion 237–8. https://doi.org/10.1227/01.neu.0000126951.74653.a6.
33. Zemann W, Metzler P, Jacobsen C, Kruse AL, Lübbers HT, Könü D, Obwegeser JA. Growing skull fractures after craniosynostosis repair: risk factors and treatment algorithm. J Craniofac Surg. 2012;23(5):1292–5. https://doi.org/10.1097/SCS.0b013e31825435d5.
34. Rinehart GC, Pittman T. Growing skull fractures: strategies for repair and reconstruction. J Craniofac Surg. 1998;9(1):65–72.
35. Vercler CJ, Sugg KB, Buchman SR. Split cranial bone grafting in children younger than 3 years old: debunking a surgical myth. Plast Reconstr Surg. 2014;133(6):822e–7e. https://doi.org/10.1097/PRS.0000000000000222.
36. Whitaker LA, Bartlett SP, Schut L, Bruce D. Craniosynostosis: an analysis of the timing, treatment, and complications in 164 consecutive patients. Plast Reconstr Surg. 1987;80(2):195–212.
37. Prevot M, Renier D, Marchac D. Lack of ossification after cranioplasty for craniosynostosis: a review of relevant factors in 592 consecutive patients. J Craniofac Surg. 1993;4(4):247–54; discussion 255–6.
38. Szathmari A, Morgado A, Beuriat PA, Petrescu P, Di Rocco F, Mottolese C. Cranioplasty for bone defects after craniosynostosis surgery. Case series with literature review. Neurochirurgie. 2020;66(2):97–101. https://doi.org/10.1016/j.neuchi.2019.10.015. Epub 2020 Feb 24.
39. Vinchon M, Guerreschi P, Karnoub MA, Wolber A. Morphological and surgical results in sagittal synostosis: early craniectomy versus later cranioplasty. Childs Nerv Syst. 2021;37(7):2335–41. https://doi.org/10.1007/s00381-021-05178-9. Epub 2021 Apr 22.
40. Pellerin P, Vinchon M, Dhellemmes P, Wolber A, Guerreschi P. Trigonocephaly: Lille's surgical technique. Childs Nerv Syst. 2013;29(12):2183–8. https://doi.org/10.1007/s00381-013-2229-y. Epub 2013 Jul 31.
41. Messerer M, Cottier R, Vandenbulcke A, Belouaer A, Daniel RT, Broome M, Cossu G. Aesthetic results in children with single suture craniosynostosis: proposal for a modified Whitaker classification. Childs Nerv Syst. 2023;39(1):221–8. https://doi.org/10.1007/s00381-022-05678-2. Epub 2022 Sep 22.
42. Kluba S, Rohleder S, Wolff M, Haas-Lude K, Schuhmann MU, Will BE, Reinert S, Krimmel M. Parental perception of treatment and medical care in children with craniosynostosis. Int J Oral Maxillofac Surg. 2016;45(11):1341–6. https://doi.org/10.1016/j.ijom.2016.03.017. Epub 2016 Apr 23.
43. van Veelen ML, Mihajlović D, Dammers R, Lingsma H, van Adrichem LN, Mathijssen IM. Frontobiparietal remodeling with or without a widening bridge for sagittal synostosis: comparison of 2 cohorts for aesthetic and functional outcome. J Neurosurg Pediatr. 2015;16(1):86–93. https://doi.org/10.3171/2014.12.PEDS14260. Epub 2015 Apr 24.
44. Svalina A, Heikura E, Savolainen T, Serlo W, Sinikumpu JJ, Silvola AS, Salokorpi N. Appearance or attitude: what matters to craniosynostosis patients? Association of self-esteem, depressive symptoms, and facial aesthetics in patients with sagittal and metopic synostosis. Childs Nerv Syst. 2022;38(10):1929–36. https://doi.org/10.1007/s00381-022-05587-4. Epub 2022 Jun 23.
45. Collett BR, Gray KE, Kapp-Simon KA, Birgfeld C, Cunningham M, Rudo-Stern J, Ung D, Buono L, Speltz ML. Laypersons' ratings of appearance in children with and without single-suture craniosynostosis. J Craniofac Surg. 2013;24(4):1331–5. https://doi.org/10.1097/SCS.0b013e3182997885.
46. Van Veelen MC, Kamst N, Touw C, Mauff K, Versnel S, Dammers R, de Jong THR, Prasad V, Mathijssen IM. Minimally invasive, spring-assisted correction of sagittal suture synostosis: technique, outcome, and complications in 83 cases. Plast Reconstr Surg. 2018;141(2):423–33. https://doi.org/10.1097/PRS.0000000000004037.
47. Abdel-Alim T, Kurniawan M, Mathijssen I, Dremmen M, Dirven C, Niessen W, Roshchupkin G, van Veelen ML. Sagittal craniosynostosis: comparing surgical techniques using 3D photogrammetry. Plast Reconstr Surg. 2023;152:675e. https://doi.org/10.1097/PRS.0000000000010441. Epub ahead of print.
48. Vinchon M. What remains of non-syndromic bicoronal synostosis? Neurochirurgie. 2019;65(5):252–7. https://doi.org/10.1016/j.neuchi.2019.09.002. Epub 2019 Sep 13.
49. Bellew M, Mandela RJ, Chumas PD. Impact of age at surgery on neurodevelopmental outcomes in sagittal synostosis. J Neurosurg Pediatr. 2019;23:434. https://doi.org/10.3171/2018.8.PEDS18186. Epub ahead of print.
50. Bellew M, Chumas P. Long-term developmental follow-up in children with nonsyndromic craniosynostosis. J Neurosurg Pediatr. 2015;16(4):445–51. https://doi.org/10.3171/2015.3.PEDS14567. Epub 2015 Jul 24.
51. Shimoji T, Shimabukuro S, Sugama S, Ochiai Y. Mild trigonocephaly with clinical symptoms: analysis of surgical results in 65 patients. Childs Nerv Syst. 2002;18(5):215–24. https://doi.org/10.1007/s00381-002-0568-1. Epub 2002 May 7.

52. Cornille M, Moriceau S, Khonsari RH, Heuzé Y, Loisay L, Boitez V, Morice A, Arnaud E, Collet C, Bensidhoum M, Kaci N, Boddaert N, Paternoster G, Rauschendorfer T, Werner S, Mansour SL, Di Rocco F, Oury F, Legeai-Mallet L. FGFR3 overactivation in the brain is responsible for memory impairments in Crouzon syndrome mouse model. J Exp Med. 2022;219(4):e20201879. https://doi.org/10.1084/jem.20201879. Epub 2022 Mar 7.
53. Rijken BF, Lequin MH, van der Lijn F, van Veelen-Vincent ML, de Rooi J, Hoogendam YY, Niessen WJ, Mathijssen IM. The role of the posterior fossa in developing Chiari I malformation in children with craniosynostosis syndromes. J Craniomaxillofac Surg. 2015;43(6):813–9. https://doi.org/10.1016/j.jcms.2015.04.001. Epub 2015 Apr 14.
54. Kim JS, Block LM, Zhu X, Davit AJ. Management of paronychia in patients with Apert syndrome. Tech Hand Up Extrem Surg. 2020;25(1):30–4. https://doi.org/10.1097/BTH.0000000000000295.
55. Fearon JA, Barrientos S, Ditthakasem K, Herbert M. Optic nerve atrophy in syndromic craniosynostosis. Plast Reconstr Surg. 2022;150(2):381e–6e. https://doi.org/10.1097/PRS.0000000000009367. Epub 2022 Jun 8.
56. Couloigner V, Ayari Khalfallah S. Craniosynostosis and ENT. Neurochirurgie. 2019;65(5):318–21. https://doi.org/10.1016/j.neuchi.2019.09.015. Epub 2019 Sep 27.
57. Aldridge K, Collett BR, Wallace ER, Birgfeld C, Austin JR, Yeh R, Feil M, Kapp-Simon KA, Aylward EH, Cunningham ML, Speltz ML. Structural brain differences in school-age children with and without single-suture craniosynostosis. J Neurosurg Pediatr. 2017;19(4):479–89. https://doi.org/10.3171/2016.9.PEDS16107. Epub 2017 Feb 3.
58. Shastin D, Peacock S, Guruswamy V, Kapetanstrataki M, Bonthron DT, Bellew M, Long V, Carter L, Smith I, Goodden J, Russell J, Liddington M, Chumas P. A proposal for a new classification of complications in craniosynostosis surgery. J Neurosurg Pediatr. 2017;19(6):675–83. https://doi.org/10.3171/2017.1.PEDS16343. Epub 2017 Mar 31.

24 Syndromic Craniosynostosis

Rehan Zahid, Lucia Collar Yagas, and Faizi Siddiqi

24.1 Introduction

During childhood, the skull expands to accommodate the growing brain. This growth occurs at the cranial sutures between different bones. The paired frontal and parietal bones are separated in the midline by the metopic and sagittal sutures, respectively; the frontal and parietal bones are separated by coronal sutures; and the parietal bones are separated from the single occipital bone by lambdoid sutures. Craniosynostosis is defined as the premature fusion of one or more cranial sutures, leading to abnormal skull shape because of a lack of growth perpendicular to the fused sutures and compensatory growth at the nonfused sutures. Incidence of craniosynostosis has been estimated between 1 in 2100 and 1 in 2500 births [1].

The most common presentation is with an unusual head shape in the first year of life. The head may be long and narrow (scaphocephaly), triangular at the front (trigonocephaly), broad and flattened (brachycephaly), or skewed (plagiocephaly).

Craniosynostosis occurring in conjunction with other genetic anomalies is classified as syndromic craniosynostosis. Syndromes commonly associated with craniosynostosis include Apert, Crouzon, Saethre-Chotzen, Pfeiffer, and Muenke syndromes. They are usually associated with the gain of function mutation genes related to the Fibroblast Growth Factor Receptor (FGFR) family. However, they can occur in association with other gene variants and chromosomal abnormalities.

The FGFRs bind to the Fibroblast Growth Factor (FGF), promoting growth and differentiation of mesenchymal and neuroectodermal cells. Animal studies have demonstrated that mutated FGFRs lead to a defective FGF signal transduction which causes growth arrest of the cranium and the midface [2, 3].

These syndromes share common features along with craniosynostosis which lead to certain functional ramifications that must be dealt with in a systematic manner. These patients are usually more complicated than the nonsyndromic craniosynostosis patients and require a multidisciplinary team to take care of their needs [4]. The team often includes a neurosurgeon, plastic surgeon, geneticist, ENT surgeon, sleep specialist, pediatrician, orthodontist, ophthalmologist, speech therapist, audiologist, and psychologist.

R. Zahid (✉)
Division of Plastic Surgery, University of Utah School of Medicine, Salt Lake City, UT, USA

Division of Plastic Surgery, University of Iowa Carver College of Medicine, Iowa City, IA, USA
e-mail: rehan-zahid@uiowa.edu

L. C. Yagas · F. Siddiqi
Division of Plastic Surgery, University of Utah School of Medicine, Salt Lake City, UT, USA
e-mail: faizi.siddiqi@hsc.utah.edu

F. Di Rocco, J. Kestle (eds.), *Neurosurgical Aspects of Craniosynostosis*,
https://doi.org/10.1007/978-3-031-69386-1_24

24.2 General Considerations in Management of Such Patients

Care of neonates and infants with severe craniosynostosis is directed toward maintenance of the airway, support of feeding, eye protection, treatment of raised intracranial pressure (ICP), speech and hearing development, correcting skull deformity, and orthognathic occlusion.

Diagnostic approach for syndromic patients includes a thorough history and physical examination. Emphasis should be given to additional features suggesting an associated syndrome. It's important to evaluate whether the patient requires urgent or elective management. Computed tomographic (CT) scan of the head with three-dimensional reconstruction and CT scan of the brain are useful adjuncts to evaluate the patency or closure of sutures and other cranial abnormalities, as well as any associated intracerebral abnormalities (such as ventriculomegaly or craniocerebral disproportion).

Respiratory difficulty may require urgent sleep study assessment by specialist pediatric respiratory physicians and ear, nose, and throat (ENT) surgeons. Patients may require either continuous positive airway pressure (CPAP) support, nasal stenting, tonsillectomy/adenoidectomy, choanal dilatation, early midface advancement, or tracheostomy, depending on the anatomical cause [1].

Raised ICP associated with craniosynostosis has several different causes, which require different treatments. Noninvasive modalities for monitoring ICP have included radiographs, fundoscopic examination for papilledema, transorbital ultrasound, and visual evoked potentials. Regular follow-ups are necessary to monitor for symptoms of raised ICP.

Elective management includes skull deformity correction, prevention of its progression, and reduction in risk of raised ICP in the future [1]. Early midface advancement may be necessary to address breathing difficulties. Distraction osteogenesis is an effective technique in addition to the more conventional methods of midface advancement. Further description of the management options is discussed later.

24.3 Apert

Apert syndrome is an autosomal dominant disorder that is caused by specific missense mutations of FGFR2 [1]. Incidence is about 1 in 65,000 to 200,000 cases with a predominant Asian prevalence [5]. Apert syndrome is characterized by bicoronal craniosynostosis, midface hypoplasia, and symmetric syndactyly of both hands and feet. Frequently, cleft palate and learning disability are also present requiring special needs.

Typically, the presentation includes an abnormally tall and broad head shape with a prominent forehead (turribrachycephaly), proptosis, hypertelorism, down slanting palpebral fissures, and a flattened nasal bridge with sunken midface. Patients often have shallow orbits and risk of corneal exposure due to restricted frontal and maxillary growth [6]. Oral findings include dental crowding, high-arched narrow palate, and cleft anomalies in about 75% of Apert's patients [7]. Maxillary hypoplasia with class III malocclusion and anterior open bite contribute to breathing difficulty and a high incidence of obstructive sleep apnea. Such patients often have an inability to create sufficient intraoral negative pressure that affects their feeding and swallowing as well.

Apert patients also have characteristic complex syndactyly of bilateral hands and feet. Syndactyly can be categorized into three subtypes which are spade (side-to-side fusion with flat palm), mitten (fusion of fingers resulting in concave palm), and rosebud (fusion of all digits) [5]. Central nervous system abnormalities may exist as well including ventriculomegaly and other structural abnormalities [6]. Furthermore hearing loss occurs in 90% of Apert patients [8]. These patients also have a higher incidence of developmental delay. Extracranial features also include cervical spine abnormalities and acne vulgaris.

Airway compromise, feeding abnormalities, raised ICP, and corneal exposure often need early intervention.

24.4 Crouzon

Crouzon syndrome was first described by Louis Octave Crouzon in 1912. It is caused by mutations in the FGFR2 and FGFR3 genes with an autosomal dominant pattern. Incidence is estimated at 1 in 60,000 newborn patients. Patients with Crouzon syndrome express a wide phenotypic variability. Bicoronal craniosynostosis resulting in brachycephaly, midface hypoplasia, exorbitism, hypertelorism, high-arched constricted palate, beaked nose, anterior open bite, and malocclusion are characteristic features. These patients are typically of normal intelligence.

Crouzon syndrome has been associated with a higher risk of increased intracranial pressure when compared to other craniosynostosis syndromes, with up to 65% incidence. There is a higher incidence of Chiari malformation as well requiring monitoring throughout childhood. Other findings include conductive hearing loss, strabismus, and hydrocephalus. Crouzon syndrome is the milder form of the Crouzon-Pfeiffer spectrum. Initial clinical concerns are similar requiring identification and management of airway compromise, corneal exposure, and raised ICP [4–6, 8, 9].

24.5 Saethre-Chotzen

Saethre-Chotzen syndrome (SCS) is characterized by craniosynostosis, limb deformities, and facial dysmorphism. It was first described in 1931 by Norwegian psychiatrist Haakon Saethre and in 1932 by German psychiatrist Fritz Chotzen.

Inheritance is autosomal dominant and caused by deletions in chromosome 7p21.1 leading to loss of function mutations of the TWIST 1 gene. Saethre-Chotzen syndrome is one of the more common syndromic craniosynostosis with a prevalence of 1:25,000 to 1:50,000 live births, similar to Crouzon syndrome. There is wide phenotypic variability and incomplete penetrance among these patients and this may lead to underdiagnosis.

The most common clinical feature is craniosynostosis and the coronal suture is the most frequently affected, either unilaterally or bilaterally. In some cases, the mildness of the synostosis has resulted in delayed or missed diagnosis.

Among limb anomalies, partial cutaneous syndactyly of the second and third digits of the hands is the most common. Others include radioulnar synostosis, brachydactyly, hallux valgus, bifid distal phalanx of the hallux, and triangular epiphyses of the hallux.

Facial findings include facial asymmetry, especially in unicoronal synostosis, low frontal hairline, small ears with prominent crus, prominent nasal bridge, eyelid ptosis, strabismus, ocular hypertelorism, maxillary hypoplasia, mandibular prognathism and high-arched palate, tear duct stenosis, dystopia canthorum. Other findings include parietal foramina, vertebral anomalies, short stature, obstructive sleep apnea, and increased intracranial pressure. Less common anomalies are hearing loss, renal abnormalities, and congenital heart defects.

Moreover, cognitive development is usually normal, but some patients have a mental disability, which may be related to large genomic deletions in the Twist gene [10–16].

24.6 Pfeiffer

In 1964, Pfeiffer described a three-generation family in which eight individuals had a syndrome consisting of craniosynostosis, broad thumbs and great toes, and partial syndactyly of the hands and feet.

It is caused by mutations in the fibroblast growth factor receptor genes FGFR-1 or FGFR-2. Inheritance is autosomal dominant but is most commonly a result of de novo mutations. Pfeiffer syndrome is rare with a prevalence of 1:100,000 births and affects males and females equally.

Clinical findings include multiple suture craniosynostosis, broad and deviated thumbs and great toes, and partial syndactyly on hands and feet. Occasionally patients present with hydrocephalus, severe ocular proptosis, ankylosed elbows, abnormal viscera, slow development, Chiari type I malformation, and spinal anomalies such as fusion of vertebrae, "butterfly" vertebra, and sacrococcygeal extension. Pfeiffer syndrome is divided into three clinical subtypes based on the severity of the phenotype [17, 18].

24.7 Muenke

Muenke syndrome is caused by a unique point mutation on the FGFR3 gene, that results in Pro 250 to Arg mutation. It has an incidence of 1 in 10,000 and demonstrates an autosomal dominant pattern of inheritance.

Muenke syndrome is characterized by considerable phenotypic variability: features may include coronal synostosis (more often bilateral than unilateral); synostosis of other sutures, all sutures (pansynostosis), or no sutures; or macrocephaly. Bilateral coronal synostosis typically results in brachycephaly (reduced anteroposterior dimension of the skull), although turribrachycephaly (a "tower-shaped" skull) or a cloverleaf skull can be observed. Unilateral coronal synostosis results in anterior plagiocephaly (asymmetry of the skull and face). Other craniofacial findings typically include temporal bossing; widely spaced eyes, ptosis or proptosis (usually mild); midface retrusion (usually mild); and highly arched palate or cleft lip and palate. Strabismus is common. Other findings can include hearing loss (in 33–100% of affected individuals); developmental delay (~33%); epilepsy; intracranial anomalies; intellectual disability; carpal bone and/or tarsal bone fusions; brachydactyly, broad toes, broad thumbs, and/or clinodactyly; and radiographic findings of thimble-like (short and broad) middle phalanges and/or cone-shaped epiphyses [19, 20].

24.8 Surgical Management

Management of syndromic craniosynostosis consists of multiple staged procedures spanning from infancy to skeletal maturity [21]. The goal of surgical treatment for a newly diagnosed syndromic craniosynostosis patient is to increase the intracranial volume to reduce the risk of increased intracranial pressure, as well as improve head shape. In this chapter, we focus on facial dysmorphism and the specific surgical management for syndromic craniosynostosis patients. Cranial vault expansion techniques are described separately.

Airway compromise may need to be addressed if nonsurgical treatment (CPAP and nasopharyngeal airway) is insufficient. Early adenotonsillectomy, tracheostomy, and frontofacial advancement are surgical options that are considered depending on the severity and cause of airway compromise. There should be a high index of suspicion for syndromic patients with close monitoring for snoring and daytime somnolence. Formal sleep study is indicated in most of these patients.

Feeding difficulty usually accompanies airway compromise since these patients are predominantly mouth breathers which makes it difficult to maintain a negative intraoral pressure while feeding. Presence of a cleft palate, enlarged tonsils, or adenoids may worsen the feeding difficulty even further [8]. Gastrostomy tube or nasogastric tube feeding may be needed to prevent failure to thrive. Furthermore, tarsorrhaphy may be required to protect from corneal exposure if needed.

Midface surgery is generally considered later in life, usually after 8–10 years of life; however, it may be indicated earlier in patients to address functional outcomes for airway compromise, obstructive sleep apnea, feeding difficulty, and corneal exposure. Class III malocclusion may be addressed with midface surgery at an earlier age of 4–7 years of life to improve the quality of life; however, a later secondary surgery may be warranted since maxillary growth is innately stunted in such patients leading to recurrent malocclusion.

Midface and orbital surgery may consist of monobloc frontofacial advancement, facial bipartition, Le Fort II and III osteotomies with distraction osteogenesis, or rigid internal fixation. Choice of surgery depends on the midface morphology, age of the patient, previous surgeries carried out, and the main objective of reconstruction, keeping in mind the functional correction, psychosocial benefit, and long-term esthetic outcome.

Evaluation of the midface morphology in syndromic craniosynostosis patients focuses on the position of the orbits and supraorbital ridge when viewed from a sagittal plane, evaluation of the maxillary, nasal, and zygomatic complex and the overall midface concavity (often present in dual—axial and sagittal planes), width and position of the root of the nose, presence of hypertelorism, and dental occlusion [8, 22]. Apert and Crouzon share similar morphological features with Apert being generally more severe with less variation in expression [23].

Le Fort II surgery is generally indicated in patients with midface hypoplasia involving the maxilla and nasal complex with an acceptable position of the zygomatic complex and orbits, whereas Le Fort III is required when the zygomatic complex is involved. Monobloc procedure is preferred when there is a retrusive forehead as well [22]. Various different approaches have been adopted, refined, and described by different surgeons to address the complex abnormalities in the syndromic patient population. The final goal is to customize the management plan according to each patient's clinical presentation and needs.

McCarthy and later Cohen introduced craniofacial distraction osteogenesis in the 1990s [24, 25]. It has become increasingly popular and an adjunct to the conventional advancement procedure with grafting and rigid fixation. Main advantages include producing larger movements, decreased infectious risk, decreased relapse rate, gradual soft tissue expansion, shorter surgery time, and less dissection. General rule is that midface distraction osteogenesis is required for the advancement of more than 10 mm. In this patient population, midface growth is intrinsically inhibited which warrants overcorrection and over distraction to compensate for the overall facial growth. Furthermore, distraction osteogenesis has also become widely popular for cranial vault expansion in patients with craniosynostosis.

Hopper et al. described a technique to address the unique morphological features of Apert, Pfeiffer, and Crouzon syndromes using Le Fort II distraction with simultaneous zygomatic repositioning [25, 26]. This technique involves a single surgery that first repositions and fixates the Le Fort III osteotomy laterally with titanium plates to the lateral orbital wall and frontal bone, followed by osteotomy at the Le Fort II level to allow unrestricted movement of the central nasomaxillary region through distraction osteogenesis. The vertical lengthening and advancement of the central Le Fort II segment not only corrects this biconcave deformity of Apert and Pfeiffer syndromes, but it also creates a desirable lengthening of the nose and downward movement of the medial canthus to improve the periorbital esthetics. The Le Fort II segment is distracted significantly more than the zygoma lengthening the midface and helping to close the anterior open bite. This technique not only helps to correct the dual plane concavity but also preserves the orbito-malar relationship and prevents iatrogenic periorbital deformity.

24.9 Conclusion

Surgical management of syndromic craniosynostosis patients is complex and must be tailored to each patient's skeletal deformity and functional requirement. Regardless of the surgical technique and timing of operative management, the goals are directed toward restoring the patient's airway, increasing the intracranial volume to reduce the risk of increased intracranial pressure, restoring orbital volume, addressing the feeding difficulty, malocclusion, and overall esthetic outcome.

Syndromic craniosynostosis presents a spectrum of clinical challenges. A multidisciplinary team approach is warranted for such patients. An in-depth understanding of each syndrome and the associated clinical problems is essential to formulate a comprehensive long-term treatment plan.

References

1. Johnson D, Wilkie AOM. Craniosynostosis. Eur J Hum Genet. 2011;19:369–76.
2. Passos-Bueno MR, Serti Eacute AE, Jehee FS, Fanganiello R, Yeh E. Craniofacial sutures.

Development, disease and treatment. Front Oral Biol. 2008;12:107–43.
3. Holmes G, Basilico C. Mesodermal expression of Fgfr2S252W is necessary and sufficient to induce craniosynostosis in a mouse model of Apert syndrome. Dev Biol. 2012;368:283–93.
4. Derderian C, Seaward J. Syndromic craniosynostosis. Semin Plast Surg. 2012;26(2):64–75.
5. Christopher D. Conrady. In: Patel BC, Sharma S, editors. Apert syndrome. StatPearls; 2021.
6. O'Hara J, Ruggiero F, Wilson L, James G, Glass G, Jeelani O, Ong J, Bowman R, Wyatt M, Evans R, Samuels M, Hayward R, Dunaway DJ. Syndromic craniosynostosis: complexities of clinical care. Mol Syndromol. 2019;10(1–2):83–97.
7. Peterson SJ, Pruzansky S. Palatal anomalies in the syndromes of Apert and Crouzon. Cleft Palate J. 1974;11:394–403.
8. Posnick JC. Syndromes with craniosynostosis: evaluation and treatment. In: Principles and practice of orthognathic surgery. Elsevier; 2014.
9. Conrady CD, Patel BC. Crouzon syndrome. Treasure Island, FL: StatPearls; 2022.
10. Gallagher ER, Ratisoontorn C, Cunningham ML. Saethre-Chotzen syndrome. GeneReviews® [Internet]. 2003.
11. Reardon W, Winter RM. Saethre-Chotzen syndrome. J Med Genet. 1994;31(5):393–6.
12. Kress W, Schropp C, Lieb G, et al. Saethre-Chotzen syndrome caused by TWIST 1 gene mutations: functional differentiation from Muenke coronal synostosis syndrome. Eur J Hum Genet. 2006;14(1):39–48.
13. Abulezz TA, Allam KA, Wan DC, Lee JC, Kawamoto HK. Saethre-Chotzen syndrome: a report of 7 patients and review of the literature. Ann Plast Surg. 2020;85(3):251–5.
14. Pelc A, Mikulewicz M. Saethre-Chotzen syndrome: case report and literature review. Dent Med Probl. 2018;55(2):217–25.
15. de Los D, Ríos Quintanero B, Gracia Rojas E, Ortiz Movilla R, Cabrejas Núñez MJ, Marín Gabriel MÁ. Síndrome de Saethre-Chotzen: a propósito de un caso [Saethre-Chotzen syndrome: a case report]. Arch Argent Pediatr. 2021;119(2):e129–32.
16. Junn A, Dinis J, Lu X, et al. Facial dysmorphology in Saethre-Chotzen syndrome. J Craniofac Surg. 2021;32(8):2660–5.
17. Vogels A, Fryns JP. Pfeiffer syndrome. Orphanet J Rare Dis. 2006;1(19):1750–172.
18. Harb E, Kran B. Pfeiffer syndrome: systemic and ocular implications. Optometry. 2005;76(7):352–62.
19. Kruszka P, Addissie YA, Agochukwu NB, Doherty ES, Muenke M. Muenke syndrome. GeneReviews® [Internet]. 2006. https://www.ncbi.nlm.nih.gov/books/NBK1415/.
20. Sabatino G, Di Rocco F, Zampino G, Tamburrini G, Caldarelli M, Di Rocco C. Muenke syndrome. Childs Nerv Syst. 2004;20(5):297–301.
21. Forrest CR, Hopper RA. Craniofacial syndromes and surgery. Plast Reconstr Surg. 2013;131(1):86e–109e.
22. Tahiri YTJ. An update on midface advancement using Le Fort II and III distraction osteogenesis. Semin Plast Surg. 2014;28(4):184–92.
23. Posnick JC. The craniofacial dysostosis syndromes. Current reconstructive strategies. Clin Plast Surg. 1994;21(4):585–98.
24. Cohen SR, Rutrick RE, Burstein FD. Distraction osteogenesis of the human craniofacial skeleton: initial experience with new distraction system. J Craniofac Surg. 1995;6(5):368–74.
25. Hopper RA, Kapadia H, Morton T. Normalizing facial ratios in apert syndrome patients with Le Fort II midface distraction and simultaneous zygomatic repositioning. Plast Reconstr Surg. 2013;132(1):129–40.
26. Hopper RA, Wang HD, Mercan E. Le Fort II distraction with simultaneous zygomatic repositioning. Clin Plast Surg. 2021;48(3):487–96.

25 What to Ask to the Geneticist in Craniosynostosis?

Pauline Marzin, Alessandro De Falco, Corine Collet, and Massimiliano Rossi

25.1 Introduction

Craniosynostosis (CS) is defined as a developmental abnormality of the skull caused by premature fusion of one or more cranial sutures; the resulting abnormal head shape depends on the sutures involved in this process [1]. The major sutures in the skull are: the sagittal suture which separates parietal bones; the metopic suture (also known as frontal suture) separating the two halves of the frontal bone; the coronal suture which divides the frontal bone from the parietal bones; the lambdoid suture, located at the posterior part of the skull, which separates the occipital bone from the two parietal bones. The fontanels are mainly two: the anterior fontanel, located at the top of the skull, which is the largest one and the posterior fontanel, at the back of the skull [2].

From the sixth week of life, the fontanels begin to close: the posterior fontanel closes usually within a few months after birth while the anterior fontanel typically closes at the age of 18–24 months. During infancy, sutures allow slight movement between the cranial bones, which is essential for brain growth [3]. A premature fusion of the sutures causes a perpendicular growth defect and a compensatory parallel growth, leading to a specific skull abnormality (principle of Virchow) [1]. CS should be differentiated from positional plagiocephaly, due to a mechanical deformation of the skull.

Among rare diseases (defined as affecting less than 1 in 2000 live births), CS are relatively com-

Pauline Marzin and Alessandro De Falco; Corine Collet and Massimiliano Rossi have contributed equally to this work.

P. Marzin · C. Collet
Centre de Référence pour les Maladies Osseuses Constitutionnelles, Fédération de Génétique, AP-HP, Hôpital Necker-Enfants Malades, Paris, France

Université Paris Cité, INSERM UMR1163, Institut Imagine, Paris, France

A. De Falco
Service de Génétique, Centre de Référence Maladies Osseuses Constitutionnelles, Centre de Référence Anomalies du Développement, Hospices Civils de Lyon, ERN Ithaca, Bron, France

Dipartimento di Scienze Mediche Traslazionali, Università di Napoli Federico II, ERN Ithaca, Naples, Italy

M. Rossi (✉)
Service de Génétique, Centre de Référence Maladies Osseuses Constitutionnelles, Centre de Référence Anomalies du Développement, Hospices Civils de Lyon, ERN Ithaca, Bron, France

INSERM U1028, CNRS UMR5292, Centre de Recherche en Neurosciences de Lyon, GENDEV Team, Université Claude Bernard Lyon 1, Bron, France
e-mail: massimiliano.rossi01@chu-lyon.fr

F. Di Rocco, J. Kestle (eds.), *Neurosurgical Aspects of Craniosynostosis*,
https://doi.org/10.1007/978-3-031-69386-1_25

mon as a group, their incidence being estimated as 1:2000 or 1:2500 [2]..

25.2 Classifications

Various classifications of CS have been proposed, based on different criteria: head morphology and affected sutures; etiology; the association with other developmental abnormalities; and CS as skeletal disorders. These classifications can help in the diagnostic workout.

25.2.1 Head Morphology and Affected Sutures

CS can be classified based on the abnormal head shape caused by the premature fusion of specific sutures: scaphocephaly is due to the premature fusion of the sagittal suture and results in a long and narrow head shape; premature fusion of coronal sutures results in brachycephaly, characterized by a short and wide head shape; trigonocephaly, described as a triangular or pointed forehead often associated with hypotelorism, occurs when there is a premature fusion of the metopic suture; plagiocephaly, characterized by an asymmetrical and flattened head shape, is caused by the premature fusion of lambdoid sutures; premature fusion of multiple sutures may cause a high, tower-like appearance of the skull named turricephaly, which can be cone-shaped (oxycephaly), or a cloverleaf skull [4]. Sagittal sutures are involved in approximately 50% of cases, metopic sutures in about 25% of cases, coronal sutures in about 20%, and lambdoid sutures in less than 5% of cases. Single suture fusion is seen in 78% of cases, and multiple suture fusions in 22% [5].

25.2.2 Etiology

CS can also be classified based on etiology: primary CS are caused by intrinsic genetic factors affecting specifically skull development while secondary CS are due to systemic diseases affecting the developing sutures, such as skeletal disorders (i.e., acrodysostosis; hypophosphatasia; hypophosphatemic rickets) and metabolic diseases with skeletal involvement (i.e., mucopolysaccharidoses).

Various etiologies have been reported for CS. A genetic cause (chromosomal or gene pathogenic variants) is found overall in 25% of cases [6]. Chromosomal abnormalities are found in about 20% of the observed genetic causes, especially in patients showing syndromic trigonocephaly or scaphocephaly and developmental delay [5]. It is important to mention that CS can be caused also by non-genetic etiologies such as prenatal exposure to teratogens (e.g., valproic acid, retinoic acid, hydantoin, and fluconazole) [7].

25.2.3 Association with Other Developmental Abnormalities

CS can be classified as syndromic (SCS), characterized by the presence of multiple congenital abnormalities, or non-syndromic (NSCS) [8, 9]. SCS are rarer and represent around 25–30% of cases, while NSCS account for 70–75% of cases. Neurodevelopmental problems may be observed in both SCS and NSCS, thus blurring the distinction between the two groups [10].

25.2.4 Nosology of Skeletal Disorders

CS are included in the last nosology of skeletal disorders (group 34: Syndromes featuring craniosynostosis), which is based on a dyadic naming system, associating each phenotypic condition with the causing gene, thus taking into account either etiology or clinical manifestations [11].

25.3 Genetic Assessment, Testing, and Diagnosis

Patients with CS should be systematically referred to multidisciplinary teams (MDT) including neurosurgeons, clinical geneticists, molecular geneticists, genetic counsellors and psychologists, in order to provide a patient-tailored appropriate genetic assessment.

The genetic consultation includes an accurate family history and, if necessary, a clinical examination of parents or other relatives. A few SCS and NSCS are characterized by variable expressivity (affected individuals show a wide range of clinical severity) and/or reduced penetrance (some individuals carrying the genetic anomaly are asymptomatic). Proband's history should be accurately assessed including possible prenatal teratogenic exposure, growth, and psychomotor development. An exhaustive clinical examination should be performed, in order to detect possible associated dysmorphic features, notably concerning limbs and extremities. Skull imaging (i.e., 3D CT scan) can be performed to confirm the presence of CS. If a SCS is suspected, cardiac ultrasounds scan (USS), abdominal USS, eye examination, and hearing test can be performed. Skeletal X-rays can be considered if a secondary CS is suspected. Brain MRI can be considered in the presence of micro- or macrocephaly and/or specific neurological signs (i.e., epilepsy; developmental delay) [5]. More than 200 syndromes presenting with craniosynostosis have been reported [5], with various patterns of inheritance. A genetic study should be carried out to confirm the clinical diagnosis and provide appropriate genetic counseling; the molecular assessment depends on the clinical phenotype. Diagnostic tools include Chromosomal microarray (CMA), evaluating the possible presence of chromosomal imbalance (Copy Number Variants/CNV), and next-generation sequencing (NGS), allowing the detection of Single Nucleotide Variants (SNV) and including the analysis of panels of genes causing CS, or whole exome sequencing (WES) or whole genome sequencing (WGS). The genetic assessment of SCS with no specific diagnostic hypothesis including, notably, syndromic trigonocephaly and scaphocephaly, and multiple CS should include CMA and, if negative, NGS. NGS can be the first choice in all other types of CS except isolated non familial scaphocephaly and isolated posterior plagiocephaly in which a molecular assessment is not mandatory because of the low diagnostic rate [12].

If a molecular diagnosis is confirmed in the proband, parents should be tested in order to evaluate possible inheritance, assess the recurrence risk and give appropriate genetic counseling. In this respect, it is important to emphasize that variable intra-familial expressivity has been reported for SCS (i.e., Saethre-Chotzen, Muenke, Crouzon, and Pfeiffer syndromes) and NSCS [13], making genetic counseling difficult.

The diagnosis should be announced in a dedicated consultation by the MDT including ideally the clinical geneticist and the neurosurgeon. The aim is to inform the patient and/or their legal representatives, about the main clinical features of the disease, provide relevant information concerning co-morbidities and prognosis, discuss management and follow-up options, and provide genetic counseling. Psychological support for patients and their families should be systematically proposed. Contact details of Patients' associations should be provided to families. Given the complexity of the information provided, it may be necessary to organize a second consultation a few weeks after the diagnosis announcement, in order to further discuss any outstanding issues with the family, with or without psychological follow-up depending on the family's needs.

The results of CMA and NGS can be difficult to interpret when variants of unknown significance are found. Moreover, a systematic genetic evaluation of NSCS patients can lead to the detection of susceptibility factors with low penetrance, whose interpretation in genetic counseling is difficult. These aspects emphasize the need for a clear rationale for performing genetic tests [14]. We propose a diagnostic flowchart in Fig. 25.1.

Some examples of the main SCS and NSCS are summarized in the following paragraphs.

25.3.1 SCS

SCS represent 25–30% of CS. Multiple congenital abnormalities including dysmorphic features, limb malformations, congenital heart defects,

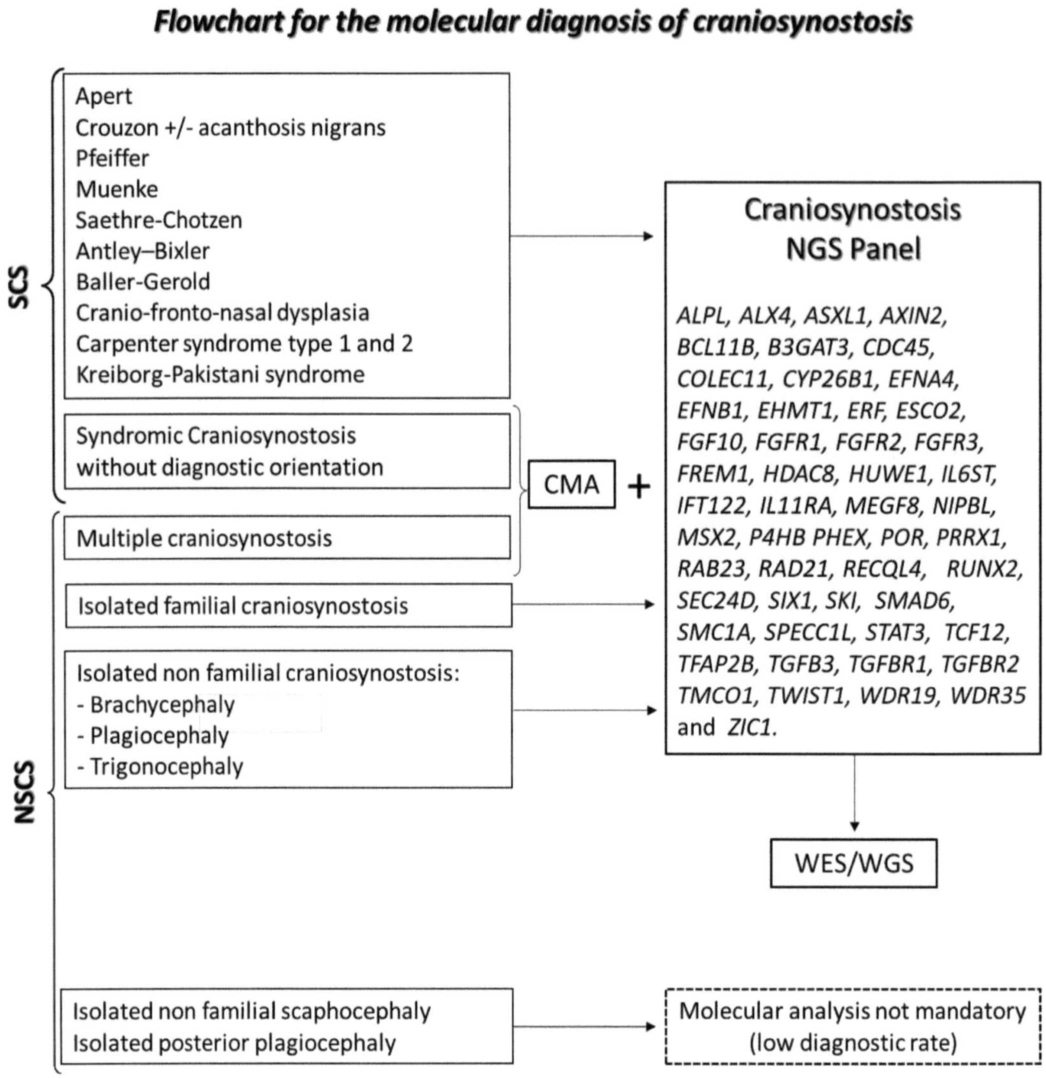

Fig. 25.1 Flowchart for genetic evaluation of patients affected by craniosynostosis. *NGS* next generation sequencing, *WES* whole exome sequencing, *WGS* whole genome sequencing, *SCS* syndromic craniosynostosis, *NSCS* non-syndromic craniosynostosis, *CMA* chromosomal microarray analysis

developmental delay, and intellectual disability can be associated with SCS. SCS can be due to teratogenic exposure (i.e., valproate exposure) or genetic abnormalities: these include monogenic disorders (around 80% of cases), with a predominantly autosomal dominant inheritance, and predominant involvement of the coronal suture, and chromosomal imbalance (around 20%), with a predominant involvement of the metopic or sagittal sutures. The main chromosomal abnormalities causing CS have already been extensively reviewed [15]. The main features of the most frequent monogenic SCS are summarized here.

25.3.1.1 Crouzon Syndrome (# 123500)

Crouzon syndrome is characterized by progressive coronal CS or multiple synostosis with midface hypoplasia, without anomalies of the extremities. Phenotypic features also include hypertelorism, eye proptosis, and inversion of the dental articulation. Synostosis is progressive, so signs may become more evident during infancy. Auditory, olfactory, visual, and neurological complications (hydrocephalus, cerebellar tonsil involvement, intracranial hypertension) are frequent. If craniosynostosis is correctly managed, intellectual disability is rarely observed. Crouzon syndrome is an autosomal dominant disorder, linked to heterozygous pathogenic variations in the *FGFR2* gene. There is a particular form of Crouzon syndrome associated with acanthosis nigricans (# 612247) due to a recurrent mutation in the *FGFR3* gene (p.Ala391Glu). The autosomal recessive Kreiborg-Pakistani syndrome and Craniosynostosis 4 should be considered in the differential diagnosis (see specific paragraphs).

25.3.1.2 Apert Syndrome (# 101200)

Apert syndrome is generally characterized by severe bicoronal CS associated with moderate to severe facial involvement with maxillary hypoplasia, inversion of the dental articulation, hypertelorism, and eye proptosis. Soft tissue and bony syndactyly of fingers and toes are also present, which may be total or partial and can be associated with elbow ankylosis. Moderate to severe intellectual disability is common and cerebral malformations can be observed. Early neurosurgical intervention can improve intellectual prognosis. Apert syndrome is an autosomal dominant disorder, caused by specific heterozygous pathogenic variations in the *FGFR2* gene [16].

25.3.1.3 Pfeiffer Syndrome (# 101600)

Pfeiffer syndrome is characterized by brachycephaly (bicoronal craniosynostosis) or cloverleaf skull (pansynostosis), moderate to severe hypoplasia of the midface, and limb abnormalities including broad and deviated thumbs and hallux, partial syndactyly of fingers and toes, and possible elbow ankylosis. Neurological complications are possible (developmental delay, hydrocephalus, epilepsy). Deafness, choanal atresia, cleft palate, and laryngotracheal anomalies can be observed. Pfeiffer syndrome is an autosomal dominant disorder due to heterozygous pathogenic variations in the *FGFR2* gene in the majority of cases. A less severe form is caused by *FGFR1* mutation p.Pro252Arg [17].

25.3.1.4 Saethre-Chotzen Syndrome (# 101400)

Saethre-Chotzen syndrome is an autosomal dominant disorder, caused by heterozygous pathogenic variations in the *TWIST1* gene or 7p21.1 chromosomal deletions including this gene. In this condition, bicoronal or unicoronal craniosynostosis is generally observed leading to facial asymmetry, a flat and high forehead, eyelid ptosis, possible strabismus, and small ears with prominent crus. Limb abnormalities include brachydactyly and partial cutaneous syndactyly of the second and third fingers. Some patients show hearing loss, and congenital heart diseases can be associated. Intelligence is usually normal but developmental delay can be observed in patients carrying large 7p21.1 chromosomal deletions encompassing *TWIST1*. There is considerable inter- and intra-familial phenotypic variability [18] and mutations in *TWIST1* have also been reported in individuals showing NSCS (isolated Craniosynostosis 1).

25.3.1.5 Muenke Syndrome (# 602849)

Muenke syndrome is characterized by uni- or bilateral coronal craniosynostosis responsible for brachycephaly, possibly associated with macrocephaly, plagiocephaly or premature fusion of multiple sutures. Craniosynostosis may be associated with minor limb abnormalities (brachydactyly, clinodactyly, broad thumbs and great toes, carpal or tarsal fusions). Strabismus and hearing loss can be observed; intelligence is usually normal but speech delay, developmental delay, intellectual disability, and behavioral issues have been reported. Muenke syndrome is an autosomal dominant disorder, linked to a recurrent p.(Pro250Arg) variation in the *FGFR3* gene. There is considerable inter- and intra-familial phenotypic variability [19].

25.3.1.6 Antley–Bixler Syndrome (# 207410–# 201750)

This condition presents with several distinct clinical features including craniosynostosis, trapezoidocephaly, midface hypoplasia, choanal stenosis or atresia, multiple joint contractures, radiohumeral synostosis, and in some cases, internal organ malformations and developmental delay. CS and radiohumeral synostosis are generally considered to be the hallmarks of this condition [20, 21].

Two different forms of Antley–Bixler syndrome have been described. The autosomal recessive form (# 201750) is caused by biallelic mutations in the *POR* gene, encoding P450 oxidoreductase, leading to a disorder in steroidogenesis and cholesterol biosynthesis [20]. Individuals affected by autosomal-recessive Antley–Bixler syndrome typically exhibit less severe craniosynostosis and skeletal manifestations; they may be at risk for adrenal insufficiency and can present genital abnormalities; maternal virilization can be observed during pregnancies with an affected fetus.

Autosomal-dominant Antley–Bixler syndrome (# 207410) is caused by heterozygous mutations of the *FGFR2* gene, showing a phenotypic overlap with Pfeiffer syndrome [21]: this condition is characterized by more severe CS and normal steroidogenesis.

25.3.1.7 Baller-Gerold Syndrome (# 218600)

The main phenotypic features of Baller-Gerold syndrome include coronal craniosynostosis and limb anomalies, mainly radial and thumb hypoaplasia, metacarpal bones malformations, oligodactyly. Patients also show short stature; lower limbs anomalies (absent patellae, genu valgum, club feet), imperforate or anteriorly placed anus, heart and renal malformations, skin involvement including poikiloderma, and facial dysmorphic features. Affected individuals have predisposition to malignancies, in particular osteosarcoma. This condition is inherited with an autosomal recessive pattern, and it is caused by biallelic mutations in the *RECQL4* gene [22].

25.3.1.8 Cranio-Fronto-Nasal Dysplasia (# 304110)

Cranio-fronto-nasal dysplasia is an X-linked dominant syndromic craniosynostosis, in which girls are more severely affected than boys. Affected individuals show coronal craniosynostosis with brachycephaly, fronto-nasal dysplasia (marked hypertelorism, broad nasal root with bifid nasal tip) and longitudinally grooved fingernails. Skeletal malformations may also be present, with Sprengel deformity, scoliosis, short and wide first toes, and brachydactyly. Other malformations have also been described (microcephaly, cleft lip and palate, inner ear anomalies, diaphragmatic hernia, etc.). Boys generally present with mild clinical features and can show only isolated hypertelorism. Cranio-fronto-nasal dysplasia is due to pathogenic variations in the *EFNB1* gene, located on the X chromosome [23].

25.3.1.9 Carpenter Syndrome Type 1 (# 201000) and 2 (# 614976)

Type 1 Carpenter syndrome is characterized by multisuture CS, facial dysmorphic features, limb anomalies (syndactyly of hands and foot, preaxial polydactyly of toes and postaxial polydactlyly in upper limbs, brachydactyly, broad thumbs, coxa valga, coxa vara, genu valgum), obesity, dental abnormalities, possible mixed hearing loss, congenital heart defects, hydronephrosis, genital abnormalities in males (hypogonadism and cryptorchidism), and the possible presence of developmental delay of variable severity. This condition is due to biallelic pathogenic variants in the *RAB23* gene [24].

Pathogenic variants in the *MEGF8* gene cause autosomal recessive type 2 Carpenter syndrome, whose characteristics include metopic craniosynostosis, less frequent involvement of coronal and sagittal sutures, dysmorphic facial features, limb abnormalities, lateralization defects, congenital heart disease, and variable neurodevelopmental delay [25].

25.3.1.10 Kreiborg-Pakistani Syndrome (# 614188)

This autosomal recessive condition is caused by biallelic pathogenic variants in the *IL11RA* gene. Phenotypic spectrum includes premature fusion of metopic and/or coronal sutures; sagittal and lambdoid sutures can also be involved and multisuture CS has been observed. Some affected individuals can have a Crouzon-like appearance (eye proptosis, midface hypoplasia, malocclusion, and prognathism). Dental anomalies including delayed eruption, ectopic, or supernumerary teeth have been reported, as well as minor limb anomalies (cutaneous syndactyly, clinodactyly) [26].

25.3.2 NSCS

NSCS are the most frequent form of CS (69–75%) and involve most often a single suture [5, 27]. Currently, the diagnostic rate of genetic assessment in NSCS is about 13% in unicoronal, 60% in bicoronal, and 13% in metopic synostosis [28]. A few papers suggest a progressively increasing incidence of NSCS, which currently remains unexplained [14, 29]. The availability of NGS diagnostic techniques has led to the molecular characterization of an increasing number of NSCS and to a "reverse" characterization of the phenotypic spectrum of these conditions, which can include associated features such as neurodevelopmental problems and minor limb abnormalities, thus blurring the limit between NSCS and SCS.

Sagittal craniosynostosis is the most frequent among NSCS cases (40–55%), occurring in about 1 in 5000 births [30, 31]. This type of CS predominantly affects males in a ratio of 3.5:1, with most cases being sporadic, although about 6% are speculated to be familial [27]. Various environmental factors have been linked to sagittal NSCS, such as parity, prematurity, intrauterine constraint, maternal tobacco, and nitrosatable drug use [31–34].

Coronal synostosis, the second most common type, constitutes 20–25% of NSCS cases, occurring in roughly 1 in 10,000 births. It occurs more often in females (60–75% of cases) and is more likely to be associated with known genetic syndromes and gene mutations. There is a strong genetic influence noted in non-syndromic coronal synostosis, with 8–15% of patients having a positive family history [27].

Metopic synostosis, accounting for approximately 14% of NSCS cases, presents an incidence rate of about 1 in 15,000 births [27], with a male-to-female ratio of 3.3:1 [27, 30]. Most cases (70%) are isolated without other clinical malformations, although 5–10% have a positive familial history [27, 35].

Lambdoid synostosis represents 3–5% of NSCS cases [27, 35], occurring in about 1 per 33,000 births [27]. Its genetics are largely unknown, and instances of a positive family history are rare [36]. Lambdoid synostosis is hypothesized to have a weaker genetic component.

Complex craniosynostosis, involving two or more distinct sutures, comprises 5% of non-syndromic cases [30]. Patients with complex craniosynostosis often experience increased intracranial pressure, leading to chronic headaches, developmental delays [4], and a higher likelihood of re-synostosis necessitating further surgeries [37].

Overall, recurrence rates of NSCS differ based on suture type and complexity. The genetic contribution to NSCS appears to be suture-specific, and the incidence rate among first-degree relatives varies based on the suture type [27].

The main features of the most frequent monogenic NSCS are summarized here.

25.3.2.1 Craniosynostosis 2: Boston Type (# 604757)

Mutations in *MSX2* cause craniosynostosis 2—Boston type, an autosomal dominant condition characterized by variable expressivity within families and affecting mainly metopic and coronal sutures; a multisuture involvement may occur. Main features of this syndrome include frontal bossing, turricephaly, trigonocephaly, brachycephaly, and cloverleaf skull in severe cases. Craniosynostosis can be associated with brachydactyly; intelligence is usually normal [38].

25.3.2.2 Craniosynostosis 3 (# 615314)

Autosomal dominant mutations in *TCF12* lead to Craniosynostosis 3, characterized by coronal and/or sagittal synostosis possibly associated with mild dysmorphic features including eyelids ptosis, prominent ear crus, malocclusion, and limb abnormalities (brachydactyly, clinodactyly, camptodactyly, and toe syndactyly). Developmental delay and learning difficulties can be observed. Incomplete penetrance (up to 50%) has been reported [39]. This condition should be considered in the differential diagnosis of Muenke and Saethre-Chotzen syndromes.

25.3.2.3 Craniosynostosis 4 (# 600775)

Affected individuals can present with NSCS or Crouzon-like appearance including midface-hypoplasia and eye proptosis. Coronal, sagittal, and lambdoid sutures can be involved and possible multisuture involvement has been observed. Brain imaging can detect non-specific brain abnormalities including Chiari type 1 and dilated ventricles. Intelligence is usually normal but learning difficulties and behavioral problems can be observed as well as minor limb abnormalities (large thumbs, clinodactyly and brachydactyly). This condition is caused by heterozygous pathogenic variants in *ERF* with an autosomal dominant pattern of inheritance [40].

25.3.2.4 Craniosynostosis 5 (# 615529)

ALX4 mutations are considered to be susceptibility factors for the NSCS craniosynostosis 5. Midline involvement is observed, including premature fusion of metopic and/or sagittal sutures. Inheritance is autosomal dominant with incomplete penetrance [41].

25.3.2.5 Craniosynostosis 6 (# 616602)

This condition is due to pathogenic variants in the *ZIC1* gene. Inheritance pattern is autosomal dominant. Clinical phenotype includes premature fusion of coronal sutures (mostly bilateral) leading to brachycephaly; lambdoid suture involvement has also been reported. Associated features include dysmorphic features (eyelid ptosis, strabismus), hearing loss, scoliosis, delayed closure of anterior fontanelle, and skull defects. A neurological involvement has been reported including speech delay, learning difficulties and autistic spectrum disorders. Brain imaging can detect non-specific anomalies including cerebellar anomalies (such as atrophy and Dandy-Walker malformation), pons hypoplasia, dilated ventricles, and corpus callosum abnormalities [42].

25.3.2.6 Craniosynostosis 7 (# 617439)

Heterozygous pathogenic variants in the *SMAD6* gene are associated with susceptibility to craniosynostosis 7. Phenotypic spectrum includes midline craniosynostosis, involving metopic and sagittal sutures, and possible developmental delay. Inheritance pattern is autosomal dominant with reduced penetrance [43].

25.3.2.7 *EFNA4* Defects

EFNA4 variants have been rarely reported in individuals showing coronal NSCS with incomplete penetrance [44].

25.3.3 Genetic Counseling

Depending on molecular results, it is necessary to provide clear information about the mode of transmission to the proband and relatives, and to offer family genetic counseling. The majority of craniosynostosis of genetic origin is transmitted in an autosomal dominant manner, but there are also rare autosomal recessive and X-linked forms.

Concerning autosomal dominant CS, in the case of a *de novo* mutation in the proband, parents have a low risk of recurrence for future pregnancies (estimated at about 1% due to the risk of germline mosaicism).

The proband has a risk of 50%, at each pregnancy, to transmit the pathogenic variant to the offspring but the risk of craniosynostosis in the offspring carrying the pathogenic variant depends on the expressivity and the penetrance.

In autosomal recessive CS, the parents of an affected child are generally heterozygote carriers of one pathogenic variant. Thus, at conception, each sib of the propositus has a 25% chance of being affected, a 50% chance of being an asymptomatic carrier, and a 25% chance of being unaffected and not a carrier. An affected individual will transmit a heterozygous pathogenic variant to all offspring, who will be asymptomatic carriers. The risk that the offspring inherits a second pathogenic variant depends on the genetic status of the reproductive partner and, for rare and ultra-rare CS, can be significant in cases of shared ancestry or close genetic relationships.

Craniofrontonasal dysplasia is inherited in an X-linked dominant manner. Affected females have a 50% risk of transmitting an *EFNB1* gene mutation to offspring. Affected males have a 100% risk of transmitting *EFNB1* mutation to females and no risk of transmitting to males. As previously discussed, females are more severely affected than males.

It is important to emphasize that while in the majority of SCS penetrance is complete, although expressivity can be a variable, several genes causing NSCS are characterized by an incomplete penetrance, thus making genetic counseling challenging for these conditions.

25.3.4 Prenatal Diagnosis

In the prenatal setting, even in reference centers, detection of CS is difficult and thus, the diagnostic rate is lower. In the absence of specific family history, CS are often detected in the third trimester by USS. Further imaging techniques, such as fetal CT or MRI can be performed to better characterize skull morphology and to rule out brain, skeletal, or internal organ abnormalities.

A molecular assessment including CMA and NSG molecular techniques can be considered, depending on the severity of the morphological picture, gestational age and parental request.

In the presence of specific family history with significant recurrence risk, and a well-established molecular diagnosis, pre-implantation or prenatal diagnosis can be considered, based on the severity of CS and parental request. In the absence of a molecular diagnosis, close ultrasound monitoring may be proposed (even if normal ultrasound monitoring does not formally eliminate the risk of CS), followed by a clinical examination of the child at birth. As previously discussed, prenatal diagnosis should be organized within an MDT including gynecologists, midwives, clinical and molecular geneticists, genetic counselors, psychologists, and neurosurgeons.

25.4 Conclusion

The availability of powerful molecular tools like gene panel molecular analysis, whole exome or whole genome sequencing has led to the characterization of an increasing number of CS. The timely identification of secondary CS or SCS is pivotal for managing associated complications and improving prognosis. The genetic characterization of primary CS has shed light on the considerable genetic heterogeneity of these conditions, in some cases blurring the limits between SCS and NSCS. Overall, the current detection rate of the molecular analysis of exhaustive panels of CS causing genes and WES is about 30–40%; this detection rate is extremely variable depending on the type of suture involved and the possible association with other developmental abnormalities.

The molecular characterization of CS not only leads to appropriate genetic counseling and offers pertinent information on associated health issues and prognosis but can also provide a reversed portrayal of the phenotypic spectrum of these conditions. Nevertheless, a systematic genetic assessment of NSCS patients may detect susceptibility factors with low penetrance, making genetic counseling challenging and prompting concerns regarding cost-effectiveness for healthcare systems. These aspects underline the need of a clear rationale when considering molecular testing.

Patients with CS, either syndromic or non-syndromic, should be addressed to experienced MDT, including neurosurgeons, clinical geneticists, molecular geneticists, genetic counsellor, and psychologists, in order to select medically appropriate and patient-tailored indications for performing genetic tests. Additionally, the results of genetic tests should be discussed in multidisciplinary meetings involving clinical and molecular geneticists, genetic counsellors, and the referring neurosurgeon, to assess the pathogenicity and clinical significance of gene variants.

In conclusion, genetic assessment of patients affected by SCS and NSCS should be performed with a multidisciplinary approach and according to a clearly established diagnostic flowchart.

Acknowledgements We would like to acknowledge the French network for rare diseases OSCAR and ERN ITHACA.

References

1. Alden TD, Lin KY, Jane JA. Mechanisms of premature closure of cranial sutures. Childs Nerv Syst. 1999;15(11–12):670–5.
2. Johnson D, Wilkie AOM. Craniosynostosis. Eur J Hum Genet. 2011;19(4):369–76.
3. Sgouros S. Skull vault growth in craniosynostosis. Childs Nerv Syst. 2005;21:861–70.
4. Renier D, Cinalli G, Lajeunie E, Arnaud E, Marchac D. L'oxycephalie, une craniostenose severe. A propos d'une serie de 129 cas. Arch Pediatrie. 1997;4(8):722–9.
5. Ching RC, Palmer SC, Jones KL, Johnson D. Recognising a child with isolated craniosynostosis. BMJ. 2023;381:e073906.
6. Wilkie AOM, Byren JC, Hurst JA, Jayamohan J, Johnson D, Knight SJL, et al. Prevalence and complications of single-gene and chromosomal disorders in craniosynostosis. Pediatrics. 2010;126(2):e391.
7. Rogers GF. Deformational plagiocephaly, brachycephaly, and scaphocephaly. Part II: Prevention and treatment. J Craniofac Surg. 2011;22(1):17–23.
8. Sawh-Martinez R, Steinbacher DM. Syndromic craniosynostosis. Clin Plast Surg. 2019;46:141–55.
9. Durham EL, Howie RN, Cray JJ. Gene/environment interactions in craniosynostosis: a brief review. Orthodont Craniofac Res. 2017;20:8–11.
10. Lattanzi W, Barba M, Di Pietro L, Boyadjiev SA. Genetic advances in craniosynostosis. Am J Med Genet A. 2017;173(5):1406–29.
11. Unger S, Ferreira CR, Mortier GR, Ali H, Bertola DR, Calder A, et al. Nosology of genetic skeletal disorders: 2023 revision. Am J Med Genet A. 2023;191(5):1164–209.
12. Calpena E, Cuellar A, Bala K, Swagemakers SMA, Koelling N, McGowan SJ, et al. SMAD6 variants in craniosynostosis: genotype and phenotype evaluation. Genet Med. 2020;22(9):1498–506.
13. Yapijakis C, Pachis N, Sotiriadou T, Vaila C, Michopoulou V, Vassiliou S. Molecular mechanisms involved in craniosynostosis. In Vivo. 2023;37:36–46.
14. Armand T, Schaefer E, Di Rocco F, Edery P, Collet C, Rossi M. Genetic bases of craniosynostoses: an update. Neurochirurgie. 2019;65:196–201.
15. Passos-Bueno MR, Fanganiello RD, Jehee F. Craniosynostosis and chromosomal alterations. Craniosynostoses. 2011;19:152–64.
16. Wenger TL, Hing AV, Evans KN, Adam MP, Feldman J, Mirzaa GM. Apert Syndrome. GeneReviews® [Internet]. 2019;1993–2023. https://www.ncbi.nlm.nih.gov/books/NBK541728/.
17. Wenger T, Miller D, Evans K, Adam MP, Feldman J, Mirzaa GM. FGFR craniosynostosis syndromes overview. GeneReviews® [Internet]. 1998;1993–2023. https://www.ncbi.nlm.nih.gov/books/NBK1455/.
18. Abulezz TA, Allam KA, Wan DC, Lee JC, Kawamoto HK. Saethre-Chotzen syndrome: a report of 7 patients and review of the literature. Ann Plast Surg. 2020;85:251–5.
19. Kruszka P, Rolle M, Kahle KT, Adam MP, Feldman J, Mirzaa GM. Muenke syndrome. GeneReviews® [Internet]. 2006;1993–2023. https://www.ncbi.nlm.nih.gov/books/NBK1415/.
20. Kelley RI, Kratz LE, Glaser RL, Netzloff ML, Wolf LM, Jabs EW. Abnormal sterol metabolism in a patient with Antley-Bixler syndrome and ambiguous genitalia. Am J Med Genet. 2002;110(2):95–102.
21. McGlaughlin KL, Witherow H, Dunaway DJ, David DJ, Anderson PJ. Spectrum of Antley-Bixler syndrome. J Craniofac Surg. 2010;21(5):1560–4.
22. Van Maldergem L, Piard J, Larizza L. Baller-Gerold syndrome. GeneReviews® [Internet]. 2007;1993–2023. https://www.ncbi.nlm.nih.gov/books/NBK1204/.
23. Bukowska-Olech E, Gawliński P, Jakubiuk-Tomaszuk A, Jędrzejowska M, Obersztyn E, Piechota M, et al. Clinical and molecular characterization of craniofrontonasal syndrome: new symptoms and novel pathogenic variants in the EFNB1 gene. Orphanet J Rare Dis. 2021;16(1):286.
24. Gershoni-Baruch R. Carpenter syndrome: marked variability of expression to include the Summitt and Goodman syndromes. Am J Med Genet. 1990;35(2):236–40.
25. Twigg SRF, Lloyd D, Jenkins D, Elçioglu NE, Cooper CDO, Al-Sannaa N, et al. Mutations in multidomain protein MEGF8 identify a Carpenter syndrome subtype associated with defective lateralization. Am J Hum Genet. 2012;91(5):897–905.
26. Nieminen P, Morgan NV, Fenwick AL, Parmanen S, Veistinen L, Mikkola ML, et al. Inactivation of IL11 signaling causes craniosynostosis, delayed tooth eruption, and supernumerary teeth. Am J Hum Genet. 2011;89(1):67–81.
27. Greenwood J, Flodman P, Osann K, Boyadjiev SA, Kimonis V. Familial incidence and associated symptoms in a population of individuals with nonsyndromic craniosynostosis. Genet Med. 2014;16(4):302–10.
28. Wilkie AOM, Johnson D, Wall SA. Clinical genetics of craniosynostosis. Curr Opin Pediatr. 2017;29:622–8.
29. Santiago GS, Santiago CN, Chwa ES, Purnell CA. Positional plagiocephaly and craniosynostosis. Pediatr Ann. 2023;52(1):e10–7.
30. Slater BJ, Lenton KA, Kwan MD, Gupta DM, Wan DC, Longaker MT. Cranial sutures: a brief review. Plast Reconstr Surg. 2008;121:170e.
31. Zeiger JS, Beaty TH, Hetmanski JB, Wang H, Scott AF, Kasch L, et al. Original articles genetic and environmental risk factors for sagittal craniosynostosis. J Craniofac Surg. 2002;13(5):602–6.

32. Sanchez-Lara PA, Carmichael SL, Graham JM, Lammer EJ, Shaw GM, Ma C, et al. Fetal constraint as a potential risk factor for craniosynostosis. Am J Med Genet A. 2010;152(2):394–400.
33. Gardner JS, Guyard-Boileau B, Alderman BW, Fernbach SK, Greene C, Mangione EJ. Maternal exposure to prescription and non-prescription pharmaceuticals or drugs of abuse and risk of craniosynostosis. Int J Epidemiol. 1998;27:64.
34. Brah TK, Thind R, Abel DE. Craniosynostosis: clinical presentation, genetics, and prenatal diagnosis. Genet Prenat Diagn. 2020;75(10):636–44.
35. Al-Shaqsi S, Ching JA, Novak CB, Forrest CR. Morphometric analysis and outcomes following posterior cranial vault distraction in syndromic and multisuture craniosynostosis. J Plast Reconstr Aesthet Surg. 2023;87:379–86.
36. Fryburg JS, Hwang V, Lin KY. Recurrent lambdoid synostosis within two families. Am J Med Genet. 1995;58:262.
37. Chumas PD, Cinalli G, Arnaud E, Marchac D, Renier D. Classification of previously unclassified cases of craniosynostosis. J Neurosurg. 1997;86:177–81.
38. Florisson JMG, Verkerk AJMH, Huigh D, Hoogeboom AJM, Swagemakers S, Kremer A, et al. Boston type craniosynostosis: report of a second mutation in MSX2. Am J Med Genet A. 2013;161A(10):2626–33.
39. Sharma VP, Fenwick AL, Brockop MS, Mcgowan SJ, Goos JAC, Hoogeboom AJM, et al. Mutations in TCF12, encoding a basic helix-loop-helix partner of TWIST1, are a frequent cause of coronal craniosynostosis. Nat Genet. 2013;45(3):304–7.
40. Twigg SRF, Vorgia E, Mcgowan SJ, Peraki I, Fenwick AL, Sharma VP, et al. Reduced dosage of ERF causes complex craniosynostosis in humans and mice and links ERK1/2 signaling to regulation of osteogenesis. Nat Genet. 2013;45(3):308–13.
41. Yagnik G, Ghuman A, Kim S, Stevens CG, Kimonis V, Stoler J, et al. ALX4 gain-of-function mutations in nonsyndromic craniosynostosis. Hum Mutat. 2012;33(12):1626–9.
42. Twigg SRF, Forecki J, Goos JAC, Richardson ICA, Hoogeboom AJM, Van Den Ouweland AMW, et al. Gain-of-function mutations in ZIC1 are associated with coronal craniosynostosis and learning disability. Am J Hum Genet. 2015;97(3):378–88.
43. Timberlake AT, Choi J, Zaidi S, Lu Q, Nelson-Williams C, Brooks ED, et al. Two locus inheritance of non-syndromic midline craniosynostosis via rare SMAD6 and common BMP2 alleles. Elife. 2016;5:e20125.
44. Merrill AE, Bochukova EG, Brugger SM, Ishii M, Pilz DT, Wall SA, et al. Cell mixing at a neural crest-mesoderm boundary and deficient ephrin-Eph signaling in the pathogenesis of craniosynostosis. Hum Mol Genet. 2006;15(8):1319–28.

26 The Role of a Psychologist on a Craniosynostosis Team

Kathleen Kapp-Simon

26.1 Introduction

Craniosynostosis, occurring in 1 to 2000–2500 live births, encompasses a range of conditions that vary widely in complexity and the types of medical and psychological interventions required. Broadly speaking, 86% of craniosynostosis cases are categorized as non-syndromic, meaning that they do not have a known genetic cause while the remaining cases are complex multi-sutural or syndromic [1]. In its most basic presentation, craniosynostosis involves a single fused suture requiring a single cranial surgery. While many children with nonsyndromic craniosynostosis go on to have typical childhoods requiring few additional medical, psychological, or educational interventions after a single surgery to correct the synostosis, a sizable number of these children (30–50% depending on suture and other factors) require ongoing medical, psychological, or educational interventions [2–7]. Therefore, it is necessary that even children with nonsyndromic craniosynostosis should be followed by their craniosynostosis team until it is clear that no further intervention is needed. Children born with a complex or syndromic craniosynostosis almost always require frequent medical, psychological, and educational interventions throughout childhood [7]. While the specific needs of children with craniosynostosis may vary by diagnosis, the role of the pediatric psychologist working with these children and their families is similar across diagnoses and falls into four broad areas: Family support and education; fostering child social, emotional, and behavioral adjustment; regular screening of development including need for early intervention, school readiness, and academic progress; and formal neuropsychological assessment as needed. In addition to clinical support, pediatric psychologists working in the field of craniofacial conditions may be involved in research that examines precursors or correlates of psychological adjustment; identifies or develops effective interventions for social, emotional, and behavioral problems; and clarifies the neurodevelopmental implications of the various craniosynostosis diagnoses.

26.2 Family Support and Education

A diagnosis of craniosynostosis, regardless of whether it is a single suture craniosynostosis or a complex syndrome, is disruptive to the family. How a family responds to this diagnosis is influenced by their culture; attitudes toward medicine;

K. Kapp-Simon (✉)
Shriners Hospitals for Children, Chicago, IL, USA

Department of Surgery, University of Illinois at Chicago, Chicago, IL, USA
e-mail: kkapps@uic.edu

F. Di Rocco, J. Kestle (eds.), *Neurosurgical Aspects of Craniosynostosis*,
https://doi.org/10.1007/978-3-031-69386-1_26

and family adaptability, cohesion, and emotional health. When a diagnosis is new, families receive a tremendous amount of information. In all but those relatively rare instances of family reoccurrence, family members have never heard the word craniosynostosis before and the idea that there is something wrong with their child's head/brain can be terrorizing. An important role of the psychologist is to help families process the information they have been given, support the emotional reactions they are having, and guide them toward positive actions they can take to support each other and their child. Helping parents to identify their strengths can be critical. For example, is one parent better able to ask questions or process the medical information provided while the other is better at hands on care? Affirmation of differing roles can help parents to feel positive about their individual contributions to their child's treatment.

It is also vital for the psychologist to help families talk about how they handle strong emotions. The first few months, sometimes even years, of the child's life can be extremely hard on a family. Parents may have to make decisions about surgery or other treatments. The child may have frequent or prolonged hospitalizations. Parents may have to implement home treatments such as feeding tubes or apnea monitors. There may be differences in the child's appearance that draw negative attention to the child and family when they are in public. Extended family may or may not be supportive. One or the other of the parents may feel guilty about, or responsibility for, the child's condition. How families process these emotions, the coping strategies they use, and the ways they seek support are all important areas for discussion. A psychologist's role is to help families develop the psychological skills they need to cope with the varying emotions that they are experiencing.

Treatment for craniosynostosis frequently occurs in stages from birth through young adulthood [7]. The initial cranial vault decompression and suture release will generally be completed by the time a child is a year of age. Subsequent procedures are more fluid and are recommended based on "functional, aesthetic, and psychological needs of the patient" ([7], p9S). When there is a functional problem (e.g., increased cranial pressure, obstructive sleep apnea), there is less ambiguity about the need for intervention; however, when a procedure is being considered for esthetic or psychological reasons, families need to decide if the recommended procedure and timing are right for their child. When the child is very young, that decision primarily falls to the parents in consultation with the child's medical providers; however, as the child grows, he or she becomes an important part of the decision-making process [8]. A psychologist who is part of the craniosynostosis team can help facilitate the decision-making process, particularly when there is uncertainty, or differing opinions, as to whether or when a procedure should be undertaken.

Clear communication between parents and medical staff and ultimately between parents, medical staff, and the growing child impacts the decision-making process, as well as long-term satisfaction with outcomes [8]. Craniosynostosis teams that acknowledge the importance of family-centered care recognize that the family is the child's primary source of strength and support. A child's primary caregivers bring expertise to treatment discussions about their child's needs/desires, emotional status, and coping style. Therefore, whenever possible, caregivers' suggestions should be incorporated into treatment plans. The child's perspective should also be recognized. Allowing the child to play an active role in the decision-making process allows them to feel empowered.

Younger children who have already had multiple stages of treatment often want recommended procedure, but are frightened because they know what surgery involves. Children who have had surgery in the past may have specific fears related to needle pricks, anesthesia masks, postsurgery nausea, or waking up alone in the recovery room. The role of the psychologist in this situation is to work with parents to help the child identify the source of their fears and develop coping strategies that enable the child to successfully undergo the desired treatment. Many hospitals provide specialized child support services, called "called child life services," to support young children who are having surgery or in the hospital. If available, the team psychologist can work with the child life therapist to facilitate implementation of the identified coping strategies on the day of surgery.

Older children may have other reasons for resisting recommended treatments. Resistance to a specific procedure may simply be that they just need a break from surgery. If a specific procedure is not time-dependent, a delay may not affect the long-term medical outcome but may allow the child to feel that they have some control over their bodies, which promotes psychological health and may ensure better cooperation from the child when the procedure is scheduled. Likewise, children who have frequent surgeries may find that many of their school breaks are spent preparing for surgery, having surgery, or recovering from surgery and they don't want another ruined vacation. The psychologist role in this situation is to facilitate communication between the child and parent and work toward compromise. It may be better for a child's psychological health to have surgery during the school year rather than always having surgery during the summer or other school breaks.

A more challenging scenario occurs when parent, surgeon, and adolescent have differing perspectives on what constitutes the end of treatment. Many of the last stages of treatment for craniosynostosis, as with many craniofacial conditions, focus on esthetics with possible medical benefits (e.g., rhinoplasty, canthoplasty, cranioplasty, genioplasty, orthognathic surgery) [7]. These are important procedures because satisfaction with appearance has been identified as a central factor for psychological well-being and emotional health for individuals with craniofacial conditions [9]. Yet there are adolescents who decide that they are not interested in these final procedures. Some parents may be reluctant to accept the adolescent's position because they fear that the adolescent will come to regret this decision in the future. Other parents feel strongly that all procedures recommended by the adolescent's surgeon should be completed because parents feel an obligation to make sure 'everything possible' is done for their child. When faced with these types of disagreements, there is no 'right' solution. Rather, surgeon, parents, and adolescent need to come to a decision that is as comfortable as possible for all participants.

The team psychologist can play a valuable role in helping to resolve this type of situation. The psychologist first needs to ensure that both parents and adolescent are able to articulate the surgical plan including the goals of the procedure as well as the risks related to the procedure. Then parents and adolescent need to fully understand what influences their own positions. A useful paradigm for assisting families with this process is what we have called the *Self-Understanding Model* (*SUM*) [10–12]. This model encourages both caregivers and adolescents to identify the feelings, thoughts, physiologic reactions, and behaviors that are associated with the recommendation for surgery. A satisfying solution can often be found by talking about and working through the different reactions of caregivers and adolescents.

Adolescents may state that they are satisfied with their current appearance and not desirous of further changes. The reasons for this lack of interest vary but may include "surgery fatigue", after many procedures throughout childhood, the teen has just had enough. Teens may also be reluctant to cope with readjusting to a new appearance after surgery or unwilling to cope with questions/comments from peers that might be reactivated by a change in appearance [13]. Others express the more philosophical ideas that they have worked hard to accept their appearance and don't see the need to change it, for example, they've been told appearance is not as important as internal characteristics, so they wonder why the adults (parents, surgeons) are now advocating for more external changes [14]. The thoughts associated with these scenarios range from "I just can't handle another surgery" to "I don't want another change in appearance—I've had enough changes". Emotions can range from sadness to anger while physiological reactions may include stomach pain, headaches, or a feeling of tension throughout the body. The adolescent may react by lashing out at caregivers or even the surgeon or they may withdraw in depression. By working with the adolescent, the team psychologist is able to help the patient articulate their thoughts and feelings and subsequently modulate their physiological and behavioral reactions. That doesn't mean that every adolescent will agree to the recommended procedure, but it will help the adolescent and family understand what is driving the decision. The team psychologist assists the adolescent in understanding, articulating, accepting, and eventually coping with their emotional turmoil. Interventions to equip the patient with coping skills necessary to manage the anxiety and stress associated with another surgery are essential for supporting positive psychological and medical outcomes.

Parents can go through a similar process when faced with a decision about additional surgery. When an adolescent is refusing additional procedures, parents' reactions also range from sadness to anger. By helping parents articulate their own thoughts and emotional reactions to the situation, the team psychologist is able to facilitate more open communication between the adolescent and parents. Other strategies such as those recommended by Foster and Robin [15] and Dishion and Stormshak [16] can be implemented as needed to foster open communication and respect between parents and adolescent. The tools of the SUM model can help parents understand and cope with their emotions and stressors as well as increase their understanding of the stresses their child faces. When surgery is advisable, motivational interviewing strategies can empathically assist the family in coming to terms with the challenges and ambivalence of medical decision-making [12].

26.3 Fostering Child Social, Emotional, and Behavioral Adjustment

Children with craniofacial conditions, including craniosynostosis, are at risk for social, emotional, and behavioral problems. Van der Vlugt et al. [17] reported Child Behavior Checklist scores on 115 children between the ages of 5 and 16 who had either single suture ($N = 62$) or syndromic ($N = 53$) craniosynostosis. There were no significantly different rates of psychological risk between the two craniosynostosis groups. Overall, 23% of the children were at risk for internalizing problems (depression, anxiety, withdrawal, somatic complaints), 21% were at risk for externalizing problems (aggression, conduct problems), and 30% fell in the at-risk range on the total problems scale (includes internalizing and externalizing problems as well as social problems, thought problems, and attention problems). When rates of risk were examined based on Full Scale IQ scores, frequencies of risk for children who had scores ≥85 were similar to the normative data. In contrast, the children with Full Scale IQs < 85 were significantly more likely to fall in the high-risk range particularly for Internalizing and Total Problems (Internalizing = 40%, Externalizing, 19%, and Total Problems, 50%). In their studies of metopic and sagittal craniosynostosis, Osborn and colleagues [18–20] reported that behavior problems were more common in children with operated metopic craniosynostosis with prevalence rates ranging from 27% based on objective report to 37% when examining parent/teacher reports, for unoperated metopic synostosis, executive functioning problems, and behavior problems were more prevalent. Results for sagittal craniosynostosis were more variable based on meta-analysis [20]. Speltz et al. [21] found that approximately 1/3 of young elementary age children with single suture craniosynostosis scored above clinical thresholds in one or more areas (internalizing, externalizing, or total problems) compared to 21% of control subjects based on either parent or teacher report. In another study, children (ages 6–13 years) with syndromic craniosynostosis were rated by a parent (generally mother) as at significantly higher risk for internalizing, social, attention, and total problems compared to normative data with moderate to high effect sizes [22]. Similar to Van der Vlugt et al. [17], parents of the children with a measured Full Scale IQ of <85 reported behavior and emotional problems at 2–3.7 times greater frequency than parents of the children whose Full Scale IQ was ≥85 [22].

Due to this increased risk, regular screening for social, emotional, and behavioral problems is an important role for psychologists on craniofacial teams. This screening should include reports from multiple informants when possible [21]. Parent, teacher, and self-reports can be obtained by using appropriate versions of the Child Behavior Checklist [23] or the Strengths and Difficulties Questionnaire [24]. Parent and child-reported outcomes can also be assessed using the patient-reported outcomes measurement information system (PROMIS) developed through the National Institute of Health [25]. PROMIS measures allow psychologists to monitor the physical, mental, and social health of children through age-appropriate parent and self-report. These three groups of measures have been used widely in research involving children with craniofacial conditions but are also appropriate for annual screening during craniofacial team visits.

Early literature on psychological adjustment of children with craniofacial conditions demonstrated that social competence is related to overall adjustment and positive feelings of self-worth [26, 27]. There is also evidence that adolescents whose parents worried less about their friendships and encouraged them to engage with peers displayed greater social competence, while being teased, withdrawn, disliked, or associating with 'bad friends' was correlated with poorer social competence [28]. Peer teasing has also been related to negative social interactions and research shows that teasing or feelings of being discriminated against occur with some frequency for individuals with visible facial differences [29, 30]. Persistence of teasing rather than isolated events may be the more important predictor of later depression and anxiety [31–33]. There is also some evidence to indicate that inconsistent or unpredictable negative responses to facial differences increase negative self-evaluations about appearance as well as anxiety and depression [34]. Finally, studies showed a relationship between social adjustment and self-evaluation of physical appearance for children and adults with craniofacial conditions [13, 30, 35, 36]. Building on these earlier studies, Feragen and Stock [33] postulated that social competence is associated with a positive subjective evaluation of appearance and social acceptance (particularly freedom from teasing).

Satisfaction with appearance is a subjective construct influenced by both internal and external factors as summarized in Fig. 26.1. External factors such as cultural attitudes about appearance and social experiences, both positive or negative, interact with an individual's internal cognitive processes to influence personal judgements about body image. Interventions need to focus on making these internal processes explicit for the individual with a craniofacial condition. The Self-Understanding Model (SUM) described above can be useful in this endeavor [10–12]. The psychologist can help the individual with craniosynostosis identify a situation that one has found particularly stressful with regard to one's appearance. Once a stressful situation is identified, the psychologist can guide the individual as one identifies the thoughts and feelings associated with that situation. The individual should then be directed to consider how one responds to that situation. Are one's thoughts, feelings, and reactions constructive or destructive to one's psychological health? Do their typical responses result in increased satisfaction or dissatisfaction with their appearance? If the interactions of thoughts, feelings, and behavior reactions have a negative impact, the psychologist can help the individuals learn to use cognitive restructuring to change their typical pattern of reaction such that they can reduce appearance concerns and emotional distress while improving positive feelings. Parents can also be taught to help their children with this process so that it can be used at home. Individuals who look different will inevitably face questions, stares, or even negative comments from others in their environment. It is critical to the individuals' mental health that they learn strategies that enable them to cope with these situations in a manner that preserves their self-esteem. The management of these situations can directly affect an individual's attitudes toward one's appearance as self-esteem has been linked to satisfaction with appearance [37].

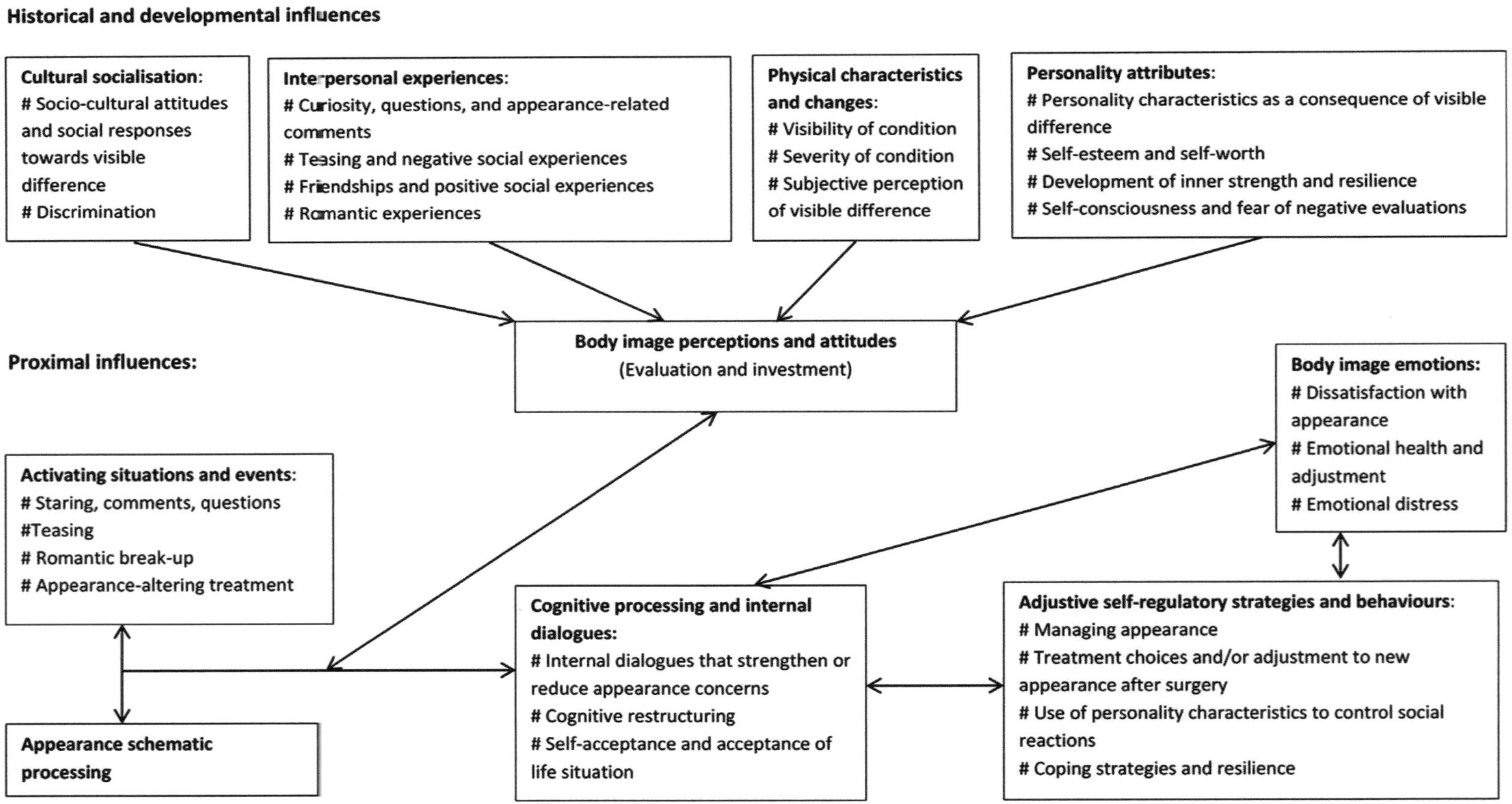

Fig. 26.1 Factors found to affect subjective satisfaction with appearance. (From Feragen and Stock [9]. Used in accordance with Elsevier's permission guidelines)

26.4 Developmental Screening

Knowing that children with craniosynostosis are at increased risk for neuropsychological problems including intellectual ability, gross and fine motor coordination, language, executive functioning, visual-spatial skills, visual-motor coordination, memory, and learning means that it is critical to regularly screen children who are seen in craniosynostosis clinics for these problems [7, 38]. At the youngest ages, this screening should focus on gross and fine motor skills and receptive and expressive language as these are known areas of risk that can be detected at younger ages [39–43]. Parent-reported screening measures such as the Ages and Stages—3 [44] can be used as a first level of screening. The Bayley Scales of Infant Development-4 [45] or similar, but older tests, such as the Mullen Scales of Early Learning [46] can be used to screen infants and toddlers through direct assessments. Early identification of areas of concern along with referral to the appropriate early intervention program can help young children with craniosynostosis develop to their full potential. Developmental screening should occur frequently during the infant to toddler years so that new concerns are not missed.

Once children with craniosynostosis reach the preschool years, screening should focus on a number of pre-academic skills in addition to motor and language skills. These include progress in basic skills such as counting, ABC knowledge, phonological awareness, and paper-pencil control. Children struggling to master rote counting, recitation of ABCs, having difficulty with phonological processing tasks such as rhyming, or identification of initial or ending sounds in words or using a pencil can be referred for more detailed evaluation.

Older children require screening in multiple areas of neuropsychological development including memory, language, executive functioning, visual processing, processing speed, and motor skills as well as problems with academic achievement [47–53]. Screening via direct assessment can be accomplished for older children by selecting subtests from the NEPSY-2 [54] that focus on areas of suspected risk. These subtests can be used individually to screen for neurodevelopmental risk in one or more areas including attention and executive functioning, language, memory and learning, sensorimotor, social perception, and visuospatial processing beginning at age 3. Monitoring of executive functioning skills including attention, organization, and planning can be accomplished via specialized behavior checklists such as the Behavioral Rating Inventory of Executive Function BRIEF [55] beginning by age 5.

As part of the evaluation process, the psychologist should educate parents about services available through their school district. Under the Individuals with Disabilities Education Act of 2004 [56], special educational services are available through public schools beginning at age 3 for children who have documented needs. Disability areas covered by special education law include: autism, deaf-blindness, deafness, an emotional disturbance, a hearing impairment, an intellectual disability (formerly known as "MR"), multiple disabilities, other health impairment (which can include ADHD), an orthopedic impairment, speech/language impairment, a specific leaning disability, traumatic brain injury, or a visual impairment. However, it is not enough to have a diagnosis related to one of those areas; the school district must determine that the disability affects educational performance. School districts will provide diagnostic services evaluating children for global cognitive impairment and learning disorders and will make a determination if the named disability affects education. Schools do not typically perform neuropsychological evaluations and often limit themselves to an educational diagnosis of attention deficit disorder. Children will receive services if they are diagnosed with a cognitive disability. They can also receive speech and language therapy, hearing impaired services, occupational therapy, physical therapy, learning disability services, or interventions for behavior problems. Specialized services for attention problems and other learning challenges are provided through a designation of 'other health impaired'. This designation can be useful if a child does not qualify for services based on other criteria, but is still experiencing learning challenges. The craniofacial team psychologist can help families obtain required services by documenting the child's specialized needs. Indeed, a critical contribution of the psychologist is to assist teachers in understanding the unique needs of their student and to prepare parents to advocate for appropriate supports for their child.

Currently, most school districts in the U.S. strive to provide services for children in what's known as multitiered systems of support (MTSS) [57]. MTSS was developed based on experience with the earlier used Response to Interventions (RTI) [58] and Positive Behavior Interventions and Supports (PBIS) programs [59]. The idea behind all of these programs is that children should receive intervention services before they fail [60, 61]. So rather than waiting for children to fall behind in academic areas, school districts use universal screening of all students early in the school year to identify students in need of services. These services are then offered in three tiered levels of intensity such that children receive services in relationship to their needs. Children who do not respond well to intensified small-group instruction (Tier 2) are the ones who go on to be evaluated for special education interventions (Tier 3). There is ongoing data collection throughout the school year to ensure that services are appropriate and the student is progressing. This program works well for children who have specific needs that can be addressed with less intensive services; however, if improperly applied, the tiered program can delay interventions for children who have greater needs. Many children with craniosynostosis will fall into the latter category and should receive evaluations at the earliest point in their education career as possible. The craniofacial team psychologist plays an important role in ensuring that needed evaluations are completed in a timely fashion.

Psychologists working in countries other than the U.S. need to familiarize themselves with education law and services within their own country.

26.5 Neuropsychological Assessment

Evaluations completed through the school district may not always be detailed enough to identify all areas of cognitive functioning requiring intervention. Psychological and other evaluations completed by the school personal are generally geared to determine if a child qualifies for special education services. These evaluations are not geared to determining if learning or behavior problems experienced by a child are related to underlying brain function or development. For example, a child who struggles to follow instructions in school may be labeled as a behavior problem by the teacher because the teacher sees the child doing something other than the work expected and therefore the first level of intervention may be a behavior plan. However, there are other possible explanations. Executive functioning deficits may be present including the inability to concentrate on the directions or the inability to keep school materials well-enough organized, either of which can look like a behavior problem. In another situation, the child who has a processing speech deficit is not able to complete work in a timely fashion. It's also possible that the child was not able to comprehend the verbal instructions provided and so feels lost as other children begin to work. Or perhaps, the child is not able to remember the instructions provided. A neuropsychological evaluation is most effective in sorting out the etiology of a problem that looks like misbehavior but is really a neuropsychological deficit.

Similarly, reading difficulties can have multiple etiologies. A child may misread words because of impulsivity, suggesting an attention problem. Or a child may misread words due to poor phonological processing abilities suggesting a learning disability. Reading comprehension problems may occur because child speeds through text without concentrating on what is being read, because the child cannot decode unfamiliar words, or because the child doesn't comprehend the information in the text. The etiology of reading comprehension problems can be as disparate as attention problems, problems with phonological processing, or language impairment. Therefore, detailed assessments are needed to sort out learning problems that have similar presentations.

The goal of a neuropsychological evaluation is to better understand how functions such as memory, attention, perception, coordination, language, processing speed ability, or personality characteristics impact learning. The profile of strengths and weaknesses that emerges from the evaluation can help in differential diagnosis. Does the child have ADHD or depression? Is the child's problem with language due to expressive/receptive language delay, difficulty producing speech, shyness, autism, or a cognitive delay? An older child may struggle when expectations for independent work increase. They managed well during early elementary years, but don't succeed when faced with more complicated tasks or multistep projects. The neuropsychological evaluation can identify the underlying causes of a learning problem and help to develop an intervention plan that draws on a child's strengths, builds confidence, and enhances emotional functioning as well as learning. Providing parents with information about the etiology of a child's learning and/or behavior problems and a detailed treatment plan can provide guidance to teachers and ease family tensions around a child's learning struggles.

26.6 Research

A pediatric psychologist on a craniofacial team may be involved in clinical research. Three broad areas of research important to the craniosynostosis field include behavioral, social and emotional adjustment of children, families, and adults; similarities or differences in neurodevelopment within the differing craniosynostosis diagnoses; and finally, the impact of medical treatments on both psychological adjustment and neurodevelopment.

Progress has been made in understanding some of the underpinnings related to psychological adjustment problems, though much more data are needed to develop effective interventions that can be used by craniofacial teams [9, 11, 27, 66]. In particular, studies need to address issues such the validity and generalizability of the constructs to be measured as well as instrumentation or methodology used to measure them, ages to study, and inclusion/exclusion criteria [67, 68]. Multi-site studies that are longitudinal in nature are needed; however, those studies are challenging both from methodological and practical perspectives [69]. Despite the challenges, some studies have examined longitudinal behavioral changes in children with craniosynostosis [21, 63], while other studies have examined correlates of behavioral adjustment [17–20, 22]. Most of the comprehensive work has been done with children who have a cleft lip and palate (e.g., Feragen, Stock [9, 33]). While some of the principal findings may cross-reference to craniosynostosis, additional work is needed to identify the specific factors affecting emotional, social, and behavioral adjustment for individuals born with craniosynostosis.

Considerable progress has been made in identifying neurocognitive patterns in children with nonsyndromic craniosynostosis, primarily, single suture craniosynostosis (SSC). The recent papers on SSC from the Infant and Child Learning Project have demonstrated significant improvements in study design including an improved theoretical basis, a large sample size with a constrained age range, use of a control group, and longitudinal follow-up [21, 38, 41, 42, 49–51, 63–65], while other studies were cross sectional or longitudinal with small sample sizes but used controls (siblings or peers) or applied current neuropsychological theory to their research [4, 18, 20, 66]. There are fewer well-designed studies that investigate neurodevelopment in individuals with syndromic craniosynostosis, likely due to the lower incidence of these disorders, which makes it difficult to acquire a large enough study sample for longitudinal study from one site. Thus, most of the research on craniosynostosis is based on cross sectional designs with small sample sizes, wide age ranges, a single clinic site, and no control group. Recent reviews of the literature on craniosynostosis have highlighted many of the weaknesses in extant studies of these conditions

[2–4, 18, 20, 22, 62]. Even when national samples are available, the number of subjects included per diagnostic group is too small for meaningful comparisons [22]. As recommended by the group developing standards of care for craniosynostosis in the U.S. [7], national data bases are needed in which social, emotional, and behavioral functioning; neuropsychological; medical; and surgical data are systematically collected for all children with craniosynostosis. Psychologists working on craniofacial teams can work together to determine appropriate constructs and instrumentation for the psychological data acquisition.

26.7 Conclusions

Individuals with craniosynostosis may have risks in multiple areas of functioning: social experiences, dissatisfaction with appearance, behavioral difficulties, neurocognitive function, and emotional distress. Risks vary by diagnostic category; however, there is wide variation in functioning among children and adults even within the same diagnostic category of craniosynostosis [62]. A psychologist on a craniofacial team needs to be knowledgeable about risks in each diagnostic category, but more importantly needs to know how to screen for individual risk when an individual presents for evaluation to the craniofacial team.

An individual with craniosynostosis presenting to a craniofacial team will be undergoing multiple evaluations, generally within a single day [7]. It is therefore imperative that the craniofacial psychologist knows how to perform rapid, but effective, screenings within the time frame available. Parent-reported and self-reported screening instruments can be useful strategies to obtain initial information about current concerns. Effective interview techniques can flesh out the information provided by screening instruments. Brief interventions such as using the SUM model to clarify issues related to surgery or social functioning can often be performed within the context of a craniofacial team visit. However, referrals for further evaluation and/or intervention should be made whenever the craniofacial psychologist identifies issues that cannot be easily resolved within the time frame of a team visit. Medical and psychological outcomes of craniosynostosis are intertwined. The team psychologist is an essential support for the patient and families, a resource for educators, and an essential partner and consultant for other members of the multidisciplinary craniofacial team.

References

1. Di Rocco F, Arnaud E, Renier D. Evolution in the frequency of nonsyndromic craniosynostosis. J Neurosurg Pediatr. 2009;4(1):21–5. https://doi.org/10.3171/2009.3.PEDS08355.
2. Speltz ML, Kapp-Simon KA, Cunningham M, Marsh J, Dawson G. Single-suture craniosynostosis: a review of neurobehavioral research and theory. J Pediatr Psychol. 2004;29(8):651–68. https://doi.org/10.1093/jpepsy/jsh068.
3. Kapp-Simon KA, Speltz ML, Cunningham ML, Patel PK, Tomita T. Neurodevelopment of children with single suture craniosynostosis: a review. Childs Nerv Syst. 2007;23(3):269–81. https://doi.org/10.1007/s00381-006-0251-z. Epub 2006 Dec 21.
4. Knight SJ, Anderson VA, Spencer-Smith MM, Da Costa AC. Neurodevelopmental outcomes in infants and children with single-suture craniosynostosis: a systematic review. Dev Neuropsychol. 2014;39(3):159–86. https://doi.org/10.1080/87565641.2014.886690.
5. Tillman KK, Höijer J, Ramklint M, Ekselius L, Nowinski D, Papadopoulos FC. Nonsyndromic craniosynostosis is associated with increased risk for psychiatric disorders. Plast Reconstr Surg. 2020;146(2):355–65. https://doi.org/10.1097/PRS.0000000000007009.
6. Tandon D, Skolnick GB, Naidoo SD, Grames LM, Cradock MM, Smyth MD, Patel KB. Morphologic severity of craniosynostosis: implications for speech and neurodevelopment. Cleft Palate Craniofac J. 2021;58(11):1361–9. https://doi.org/10.1177/1055665620984643. Epub 2021 Jan 20.
7. McCarthy JG, Warren SM, Bernstein J, Burnett W, Cunningham ML, Edmond JC, Figueroa AA, Kapp-Simon KA, Labow BI, Peterson-Falzone SJ, Proctor MR, Rubin MS, Sze RW, Yemen TA, Craniosynostosis Working Group. Parameters of care for craniosynostosis. Cleft Palate Craniofac J. 2012;49(Suppl):1S–24S. https://doi.org/10.1597/11-138. Epub 2011 Aug 17.
8. Kapp-Simon KA, Edwards T, Ruta C, Bellucci CC, Aspirnall CL, Strauss RP, Topolski TD, Rumsey NJ, Patrick DL. Shared surgical decision making and youth resilience correlates of satisfaction with clini-

cal outcomes. J Craniofac Surg. 2015;26(5):1574–80. https://doi.org/10.1097/SCS.0000000000001892.
9. Feragen KB, Stock NM. Factors affecting subjective appearance evaluations among patients with congenital craniofacial conditions: an application of Cash's cognitive-behavioural model of body image development. Body Image. 2018;24:124–36. https://doi.org/10.1016/j.bodyim.2017.12.005. Epub 2018 Feb 3.
10. Kapp-Simon K, Simon D. Meeting the challenge: a social skills training program for adolescents with special needs. Chicago: University of Illinois; 1991.
11. Kapp-Simon KA. Psychological interventions for the adolescent with cleft lip and palate. Cleft Palate Craniofac J. 1995;32(2):104–8. https://doi.org/10.1597/1545-1569_1995_032_0104_piftaw_2.3.co_2.
12. Simon DJ. School-centered interventions: evidence-based strategies for social, emotional, and academic success. Washington, DC: American Psychological Association; 2016. p. 54–68.
13. Stavropoulos D, Hallberg U, Mohlin B, Hagberg C. Living with Crouzon syndrome: how do young adults with Crouzon syndrome handle their life situation? Int J Paediatr Dent. 2011;21(1):35–42. https://doi.org/10.1111/j.1365-263X.2010.01079.x.
14. Searle A, Neville P, Waylen A. Psychological growth and well-being in individuals born with cleft: an application of self-determination theory. Psychol Health. 2017;32(4):459–82. https://doi.org/10.1080/08870446.2016.1275630. Epub 2017 Jan 10.
15. Foster SL, Robin AL. Family conflict and communication in adolescence. In: Mash EJ, Terdal LD, editors. Behavioral assessment of childhood disorders. 2nd ed. New York: The Guilford Press; 1988.
16. Dishion TJ, Stormshak. Intervening in children's lives. Washington, DC: American Psychological Association; 2007.
17. van der Vlugt JJB, van der Meulen JJNM, Creemers HE, Willemse SP, Lequin ML, Okkerse JME. The risk of psychopathology in children with craniosynostosis. Plast Reconstr Surg. 2009;124(6):2054–60. https://doi.org/10.1097/PRS.0b013e3181bcf2dc.
18. Osborn AJ, Roberts RM, Mathias JL, Anderson PJ, Flapper WJ. Cognitive, behavioral and psychological functioning in children with metopic synostosis: a meta-analysis examining the impact of surgical status. Child Neuropsychol. 2019;25(2):263–77. https://doi.org/10.1080/09297049.2018.1441821. Epub 2018 Feb 26.
19. Osborn AJ, Roberts RM, Mathias JL, Anderson PJ, Flapper WJ. Cognitive, behavioral and psychological functioning of children and adults with conservatively managed metopic synostosis. Child Neuropsychol. 2021;27(2):190–208. https://doi.org/10.1080/09297049.2020.1817356. Epub 2020 Sep 8.
20. Osborn AJ, Roberts RM, Dorstyn DS, Grave BG, David DJ. Sagittal synostosis and its association with cognitive, behavioral, and psychological functioning: a meta-analysis. JAMA Netw Open. 2021;4(9):e2121937. https://doi.org/10.1001/jamanetworkopen.2021.21937.
21. Speltz ML, Collett BR, Wallace ER, Kapp-Simon K. Behavioral adjustment of school-age children with and without single-suture craniosynostosis. Plast Reconstr Surg. 2016;138(2):435–45. https://doi.org/10.1097/PRS.0000000000002383.
22. Maliepaard M, Mathijssen IM, Oosterlaan J, Okkerse JM. Intellectual, behavioral, and emotional functioning in children with syndromic craniosynostosis. Pediatrics. 2014;133(6):e1608–15. https://doi.org/10.1542/peds.2013-3077.
23. Achenbach TM. Achenbach system of empirically based assessment. 2021. https://aseba.org/the-achenbach-system-of-empirically-based-assessment/.
24. Goodman R. Strength and difficulties questionnaire. 1998. https://www.sdqinfo.org/a0.html.
25. PROMIS. 2021. https://www.nia.nih.gov/research/resource/patient-reported-outcomes-measurement-information-system-promis.
26. Kapp-Simon KA, Simon DJ, Kristovich S. Self-perception, social skills, adjustment, and inhibition in young adolescents with craniofacial anomalies. Cleft Palate Craniofac J. 1992;29(4):352–6. https://doi.org/10.1597/1545-1569_1992_029_0352_spssaa_2.3.co_2.
27. Endriga MC, Kapp-Simon KA. Psychological issues in craniofacial care: state of the art. Cleft Palate Craniofac J. 1999;36(1):3–11. https://doi.org/10.1597/1545-1569_1999_036_0001_piiccs2.3.co_2.
28. Pope AW, Ward J. Factors associated with peer social competence in preadolescents with craniofacial anomalies. J Pediatr Psychol. 1997;22(4):455–69. https://doi.org/10.1093/jpepsy/22.4.455.
29. Strauss RP, Ramsey BL, Edwards TC, Topolski TD, Kapp-Simon KA, Thomas CR, Fenson C, Patrick DL. Stigma experiences in youth with facial differences: a multi-site study of adolescents and their mothers. Orthod Craniofac Res. 2007;10(2):96–103. https://doi.org/10.1111/j.1601-6343.2007.00383.x.
30. Roberts RM. Discrimination among adults with craniofacial conditions. J Craniofac Surg. 2014;25(1):77–81. https://doi.org/10.1097/SCS.0b013e3182a2e005.
31. Lunde C, Frisén A. On being victimized by peers in the advent of adolescence: prospective relationships to objectified body consciousness. Body Image. 2011;8(4):309–14. https://doi.org/10.1016/j.bodyim.2011.04.010. Epub 2011 Jun 12.
32. McDougall P, Vaillancourt T. Long-term adult outcomes of peer victimization in childhood and adolescence: pathways to adjustment and maladjustment. Am Psychol. 2015;70(4):300–10. https://doi.org/10.1037/a0039174.
33. Feragen KB, Stock NM. A longitudinal study of 340 young people with or without a visible difference: the impact of teasing on self-perceptions of appearance and depressive symptoms. Body Image. 2016;16:133–42. https://doi.org/10.1016/j.bodyim.2016.01.003. Epub 2016 Jan 30.

34. Macgregor FC. Facial disfigurement: problems and management of social interaction and implications for mental health. Aesth Plast Surg. 1990;14(4):249–57. https://doi.org/10.1007/BF01578358.
35. Richman LC. Self-reported social, speech, and facial concerns and personality adjustment of adolescents with cleft lip and palate. Cleft Palate J. 1983;20(2):108–12.
36. Roberts RM, Mathias JL. Psychosocial functioning in adults with congenital craniofacial conditions. Cleft Palate Craniofac J. 2012;49(3):276–85. https://doi.org/10.1597/10-143. Epub 2011 May 2.
37. Bilboul MJ, Pope AW, Snyder HT. Adolescents with craniofacial anomalies: psychosocial adjustment as a function of self-concept. Cleft Palate Craniofac J. 2006;43(4):392–400. https://doi.org/10.1597/05-084.1.
38. Gray KE, Kapp-Simon KA, Starr JR, Collett BR, Wallace ER, Speltz ML. Predicting developmental delay in a longitudinal cohort of preschool children with single-suture craniosynostosis: is neurobehavioral assessment important? Dev Med Child Neurol. 2015;57(5):456–62. https://doi.org/10.1111/dmcn.12643. Epub 2014 Nov 23.
39. Shipster C, Hearst D, Dockrell JE, Kilby E, Hayward R. Speech and language skills and cognitive functioning in children with Apert syndrome: a pilot study. Int J Lang Commun Disord. 2002;37(3):325–43. https://doi.org/10.1080/13682820210138816.
40. Shipster C, Hearst D, Somerville A, Stackhouse J, Hayward R, Wade A. Speech, language, and cognitive development in children with isolated sagittal synostosis. Dev Med Child Neurol. 2003;45(1):34–43.
41. Speltz ML, Kapp-Simon K, Collett B, Keich Y, Gaither R, Cradock MM, Buono L, Cunningham ML. Neurodevelopment of infants with single-suture craniosynostosis: presurgery comparisons with case-matched controls. Plast Reconstr Surg. 2007;119(6):1874–81. https://doi.org/10.1097/01.prs.0000259184.88265.3f.
42. Starr JR, Collett BR, Gaither R, Kapp-Simon KA, Cradock MM, Cunningham ML, Speltz ML. Multicenter study of neurodevelopment in 3-year-old children with and without single-suture craniosynostosis. Arch Pediatr Adolesc Med. 2012;166(6):536–42. https://doi.org/10.1001/archpediatrics.2011.1800.
43. Wilson AT, Den Ottelander BK, Van Veelen MC, Dremmen MH, Persing JA, Vrooman HA, Mathijssen IM, Tasker RC. Cerebral cortex maldevelopment in syndromic craniosynostosis. Dev Med Child Neurol. 2021;64:118. https://doi.org/10.1111/dmcn.14984.
44. Squires J, Bricker D. Ages & stages questionnaires. 3rd ed. Baltimore: Brooks Publishing; 2009.
45. Bayley N, Aylward GP. Bayley scales of infant and toddler development. 4th ed. Bloomington, MN: NCS Pearson; 2019.
46. Mullen EM. Mullen scales of early learning. AGS ed. Circle Pines, MN: American Guidance Service Inc.; 1995.
47. Chieffo D, Tamburrini G, Massimi L, Di Giovanni S, Giansanti C, Caldarelli M, Di Rocco C. Long-term neuropsychological development in single-suture craniosynostosis treated early. J Neurosurg Pediatr. 2010;5(3):232–7. https://doi.org/10.3171/2009.10.PEDS09231.
48. Da Costa AC, Savarirayan R, Wrennall JA, Walters I, Gardiner N, Tucker A, Anderson V, Meara JG. Neuropsychological diversity in Apert syndrome: a comparison of cognitive profiles. Ann Plast Surg. 2005;54(4):450–5. https://doi.org/10.1097/01.sap.0000149387.95212.df.
49. Kapp-Simon KA, Wallace E, Collett BR, Cradock MM, Crerand CE, Speltz ML. Language, learning, and memory in children with and without single-suture craniosynostosis. J Neurosurg Pediatr. 2016;17(5):578–88. https://doi.org/10.3171/2015.9.PEDS15238. Epub 2016 Jan 1.
50. Collett BR, Kapp-Simon KA, Wallace E, Cradock MM, Buono L, Speltz ML. Attention and executive function in children with and without single-suture craniosynostosis. Child Neuropsychol. 2017;23(1):83–98. https://doi.org/10.1080/09297049.2015.1085005. Epub 2015 Sep 18.
51. Wallace ER, Collett BR, Kapp-Simon K, Starr JR, Birgfeld C, Speltz ML. Visuomotor function in school-age children with single-suture craniosynostosis. J Dev Behav Pediatr. 2016;37(6):483–90. https://doi.org/10.1097/DBP.0000000000000319.
52. Speltz ML, Collett BR, Wallace ER, Starr JR, Cradock MM, Buono L, Cunningham M, Kapp-Simon K. Intellectual and academic functioning of school-age children with single-suture craniosynostosis. Pediatrics. 2015;135(3):e615–23. https://doi.org/10.1542/peds.2014-1634.
53. Maximino LP, Ducati LG, Abramides DVM, Corrêa CC, Garcia PF, Fernandes AY. Syndromic craniosynostosis: neuropsycholinguistic abilities and imaging analysis of the central nervous system. Arq Neuropsiquiatr. 2017;75(12):862–8. https://doi.org/10.1590/0004-282X20170171.
54. Korkman M, Kirk U, Kemp S. NEPSY-2nd edition (NEPSY II). San Antonio, TX: Pearson; 2007.
55. Gioia GA, Isquith PK, Guy SC, Kenworthy L. Behavior Rating Inventory of Executive Function®, second edition (BRIEF®2). Lutz, FL: PAR Inc.; 2015.
56. U.S. Department of Education. https://sites.ed.gov/idea/.
57. Stoiber KC. A comprehensive framework for multitiered systems of support in school psychology. In: Thomas A, Harrison P, editors. Best practices in school psychology: data-based and collaborative decision making. Bethesda, MD: National Association of School Psychologists; 2014. p. 41–70.
58. Kovaleski JF, Van Der Heyden AM, Shapiro ES. The RtI approach to evaluating learning disabilities. New York: The Guilford Press; 2013.
59. Sugai G, Homer RR. A promising approach for expanding and sustaining school-wide positive behav-

ior support. Sch Psychol Rev. 2006;35(2):245–59. https://doi.org/10.1080/02796015.2006.12087989.
60. Barrett CA, Burns MK, Maki KE, Clinkscales A, Hajovsky DB, Spear SE. Language used in school psychological evaluation reports as predictors of SLD identification within a response to intervention model. Sch Psychol. 2021;37:107. https://doi.org/10.1037/spq0000485.
61. Fuchs D, Fuchs LS. Rethinking service delivery for students with significant learning problems: developing and implementing intensive instruction. Remedial Spec Educ. 2015;36(2):105–11.
62. Feragen KB, Stock NM. Psychological adjustment to craniofacial conditions (excluding oral clefts): a review of the literature. Psychol Health. 2017;32(3):253–88. https://doi.org/10.1080/08870446.2016.1247838. Epub 2016 Dec 7.
63. Kapp-Simon KA, Collett BR, Barr-Schinzel MA, Cradock MM, Buono LA, Pietila KE, Speltz ML. Behavioral adjustment of toddler and preschool-aged children with single-suture craniosynostosis. Plast Reconstr Surg. 2012;130(3):635–47. https://doi.org/10.1097/PRS.0b013e31825dc18b.
64. Rosenberg JM, Kapp-Simon KA, Starr JR, Cradock MM, Speltz ML. Mothers' and fathers' reports of stress in families of infants with and without single-suture craniosynostosis. Cleft Palate Craniofac J. 2011;48(5):509–18. https://doi.org/10.1597/09-210. Epub 2010 Aug 19.
65. Gray KE, Cradock MM, Kapp-Simon KA, Collett BR, Pullmann LD, Speltz ML. Longitudinal analysis of parenting stress in mothers and fathers of infants with and without single-suture craniosynostosis. Cleft Palate Craniofac J. 2015;52(1):3–11. https://doi.org/10.1597/13-239.
66. Atkinson MJ, Stock NM, Alleva JM, Jankowski GS, Piran N, Riley S, Calogero R, Clarke A, Rumsey N, Slater A, Diedrichs PC, Williamson H. Looking to the future: priorities for translating research to impact in the field of appearance and body image. Body Image. 2020;32:53–61. https://doi.org/10.1016/j.bodyim.2019.10.006. Epub 2019 Nov 29.
67. Stock NM, Feragen KB, Moss TP, Rumsey N. Toward a conceptual and methodological shift in craniofacial research. Cleft Palate Craniofac J. 2018;55(1):105–11. https://doi.org/10.1177/1055665617721925. Epub 2017 Dec 14.
68. Stock NM, Feragen KB. Assessing psychological adjustment to congenital craniofacial anomalies: an illustration of methodological challenges. Cleft Palate Craniofac J. 2019;56(1):64–73. https://doi.org/10.1177/1055665618769661. Epub 2018 Apr 13.
69. Broder HL, Crerand CE, Ruff RR, Peshansky A, Sarwer DB, Sischo L. Challenges in conducting multicentre, multidisciplinary, longitudinal studies in children with chronic conditions. Community Dent Oral Epidemiol. 2017;45(4):317–22. https://doi.org/10.1111/cdoe.12293. Epub 2017 Feb 21.

Part V

Technical Aspects

27 The Role of 3D Technology in the Neurosurgical Management of Craniosynostosis

M. E. L. Nienhuijs, M. Kregel, and H. H. K. Delye

27.1 Introduction

The field of dentistry and maxillofacial surgery has always used 3D models to accurately represent and study 3D structures. Even with very detailed two-dimensional X-ray images or two-dimensional images based on CT or MRI scan, it requires highly trained imaging skills from the physician to combine this information into a mental 3D representation of the structure at hand. The use of physical 3D models enhances the understanding of the surgeon; it helps to study complex cases, to practice procedures, and to teach students and patients [1].

Initially, the use of 3D models concerned an analog workflow with physical plaster models. In the 80s, stereolithography was introduced, which provided insight into the delicate and complex craniofacial anatomy in three dimensions [2]. However, this method has the disadvantage that stereolithographic models are expensive and not reusable once physically printed. Through advances in imaging and visualization techniques, partly driven by the gaming industry, the workflow evolved from plaster models toward virtual 3D models [3]. Compared to physical models, virtual 3D models are faster and less expensive to obtain. In addition, virtual 3D models enable the surgeon to simulate different treatment plans multiple times to determine the best surgical therapy [4]. In contrast to traditional planning, these digital techniques require a specific set of skills to integrate computer technology into the clinical practice. Because of the general growing need to implement different fast developing technologies into the field of medicine, a new training program was developed in the Netherlands in which technical physicians were trained to approach medical problems with a technology-driven solution. These highly skilled technical physicians came into the view of craniofacial surgeons, and their synergy led in our hospital to the creation of the Radboudumc 3D lab. The 3D lab aims to improve clinical practice and patient care by implementing innovative digital technologies. As a result, the technical physician and the surgeon can work closely to offer the best care for patients. In craniosynostosis (CS), a congenital deformity where one or more cranial sutures prematurely fuse, technological advancements enable our multispecialty team to continuously plan, modify, and improve

M. E. L. Nienhuijs (✉)
Department of Oral-, and Maxillofacial Surgery, Radboud University Nijmegen Medical Center, Nijmegen, Netherlands
e-mail: Marloes.Nienhuijs@radboudumc.nl

M. Kregel
Dental School, Radboud University Nijmegen Medical Center, Nijmegen, Netherlands

H. H. K. Delye
Department of Neurosurgery, Radboud University Nijmegen Medical Center, Nijmegen, Netherlands
e-mail: Hans.Delye@radboudumc.nl

F. Di Rocco, J. Kestle (eds.), *Neurosurgical Aspects of Craniosynostosis*,
https://doi.org/10.1007/978-3-031-69386-1_27

treatment modalities, together with the young patient and the parents [5]. In this way, the infant will grow into an adult with a pleasing aesthetic appearance and without functional sequelae.

27.2 Application of 3D Technology

The neurocranium rapidly expands to accommodate the growing brain during infancy and childhood [6]. If premature closure of one or more cranial sutures occurs, compensatory overgrowth ensues at adjacent non-fused sutures, resulting in craniofacial deformity with associated neurodevelopmental and social complications [7, 8]. Treatment of CS primarily aims to halt the developing cranial abnormality and reestablish normal growth [9, 10]. In order to satisfactorily treat CS, it is crucial to assess the cranial abnormality objectively and precisely. Moreover, frequent follow-ups on the infant's head shape and size are needed to evaluate cranial growth before, during, and after treatment [3].

The development of 3D technology and implementation in the treatment strategy for craniosynostosis allows for a huge step forward in the care for CS patients.

The foci for improving the management of CS patients through the implementation of 3D technology encompass the entire length of the treatment process and address the four different phases of surgical and supplemental treatment: the diagnosis, planning, surgery, and evaluation ([11]; Fig. 27.1).

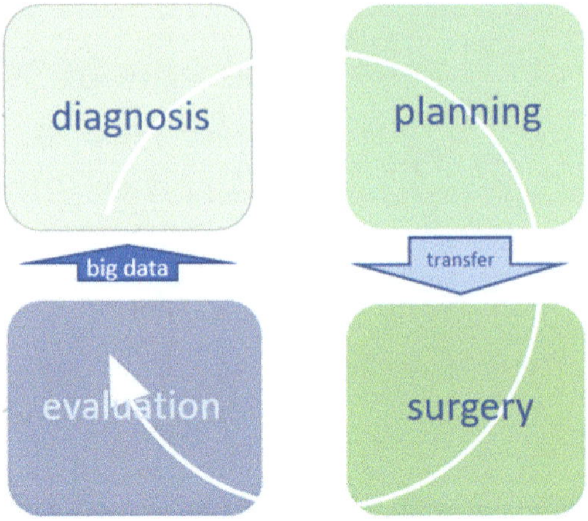

Fig. 27.1 The four different interconnected phases for the treatment of CS and their relationships

- The **diagnosis** of craniosynostosis is critical since the clinical outcome benefits from early and adequate detection. Although diagnosis is based mainly on clinical examination, in selected cases CT scanning or X-ray is still used for diagnosis. However, 3D stereophotogrammetry combined with software algorithms can be implemented to diagnose and classify patients with various types of craniosynostosis without exposure to ionizing radiation [12, 13].
- Preoperative, digital **planning** of CS surgery creates a treatment plan individualized to the patient. This allows for the creation of a patient-specific treatment plan. The use of Virtual Surgical Planning (VSP) has several advantages.. A patient-specific preoperative plan, prepared by the technical physician, provides the surgeon with different treatment options. The surgical plan with the most optimal outcome is selected, finalized, and taken into surgery. The meticulous preoperative planning saves time and discussion in the operation theatre, resulting in less blood loss and shorter postoperative hospital stays [3].
- **Surgery** of CS can be improved using patient-specific guides and templates. When the optimal treatment plan is virtually created, this plan then needs to be accurately transferred to the patient amidst surgery. Patient-specific guides can be virtually designed and fabricated using computer-aided design and manufacturing (CAD/CAM). 3D printed surgical guides and templates assist the surgeon in performing a precise and rapid reconstruction of the cranial vault according to the VSP [3]. The benefits of 3D printed surgical guides have been proved for applications outside craniofacial surgery, such as reconstructive trauma surgery, knee surgery, and spinal surgery [14].

- **Evaluation** of patients during and after treatment is critical for monitoring the patient's well-being. Objective evaluation of surgical outcomes improves the entire treatment process: the diagnosis, planning, surgery, and evaluation wherever possible (Fig. 27.1). The objectification and evaluation of the treatment, i.e. surgery, is Inherent in evaluating the treatment outcomes. Consequently, continuous evaluation of the treatment is the fundamental principle behind the evolution of the surgical and 3D techniques. In turn, this will benefit the treatment of new patients.

It is beyond the scope of this chapter to give a detailed description of all above mentioned steps. The interested reader is referred to the PhD thesis of Meulstee [11].

Nonetheless, we will focus on the application of the most commonly used 3D tools in CS: 3D stereophotogrammetry and virtual planning using CAD/CAM techniques.

27.3 3D Stereophotogrammetry

Conventional imaging modalities that can accurately capture information on cranial morphology are plain radiography, CT, and MRI [12, 15, 16]. In infants, the use of radiation and the need for sedation raise concerns about these traditional imaging techniques [8, 17, 18].

An innovative imaging tool capable of creating 3D photos of a patient in a fraction of a second is 3D stereophotogrammetry [19]. In a setup with five optical pods (Fig. 27.1), it is possible to obtain 3D images of the neurocranium, rendering this imaging modality applicable to the management of CS [19]. The advantages of 3D stereophotogrammetry compared to other imaging modalities are the fast acquisition, high accuracy, and the absence of ionizing radiation [20]. Therefore, this instrument is the preferred method for studying the craniofacial growth of affected newborns and normative controls [3, 6, 19, 21]. In craniofacial surgery, the powerful combination of 3D models with 3D analysis makes it possible to evaluate the cranial shape and size objectively and accurately [19]. Longitudinal datasets of CS patients and healthy references are collected and studied using this non-invasive 3D imaging and analysis combination [13, 22]. Surgery-related outcome measurements also are more easily exchangeable and comparable when the same imaging modality is used. Universal implementation of 3D photogrammetric analysis will make way for the objective comparison of treatment results and help advance the neurosurgical management of CS.

In daily practice, we use 3D stereophotogrammetry mainly for the evaluation and follow-up of craniosynostosis patients treated with endoscopically assisted suturectomy followed by helmet therapy.

The goal of the endoscopic technique is to remove the fused portion of the bone and attempt to recreate normal anatomy as soon as possible. The helmet molding therapy then guides the multidirectional driving force of the expanding brain, without being constrictive, towards the region that was previously restricted in order to compensate for the inability to surgically reconstruct the already existing deformity at time of surgery. The growth of the brain is fastest during the first 3–6 months postpartum, so endoscopic surgery needs to be performed relatively early, preferably around 3 months of age [23].

The day before surgery, a 3D photo is taken as a baseline to compare the growth evolution after surgery. During helmet therapy, which typically starts 2 weeks after surgery, the patient is seen every 3 months at the multidisciplinary craniofacial team. Every time, a 3D photo is taken and compared with the previous photo and the baseline photo. 3D photos are superimposed to measure changes in the head shape and volume and determine the growth of the cranial vault. 3D photogrammetric analysis enables a longitudinal radiation-free follow-up after endoscopically assisted craniosynostosis surgery [24]. Changes in the head volume can be visualized for the parents and clinicians on the spot during the clinical consultation using distance colour mapping (Figs. 27.2 and 27.3). These maps are showing the exact amount of growth at every position of the head that occurred between

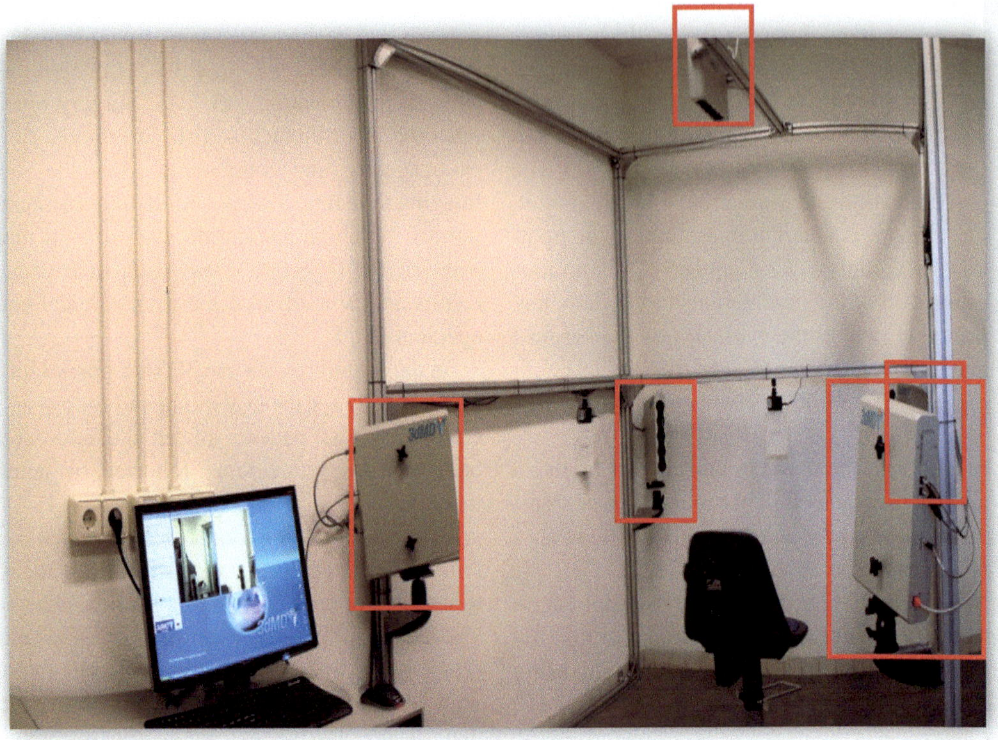

Fig. 27.2 3dMD Cranial System with 5-pod configuration

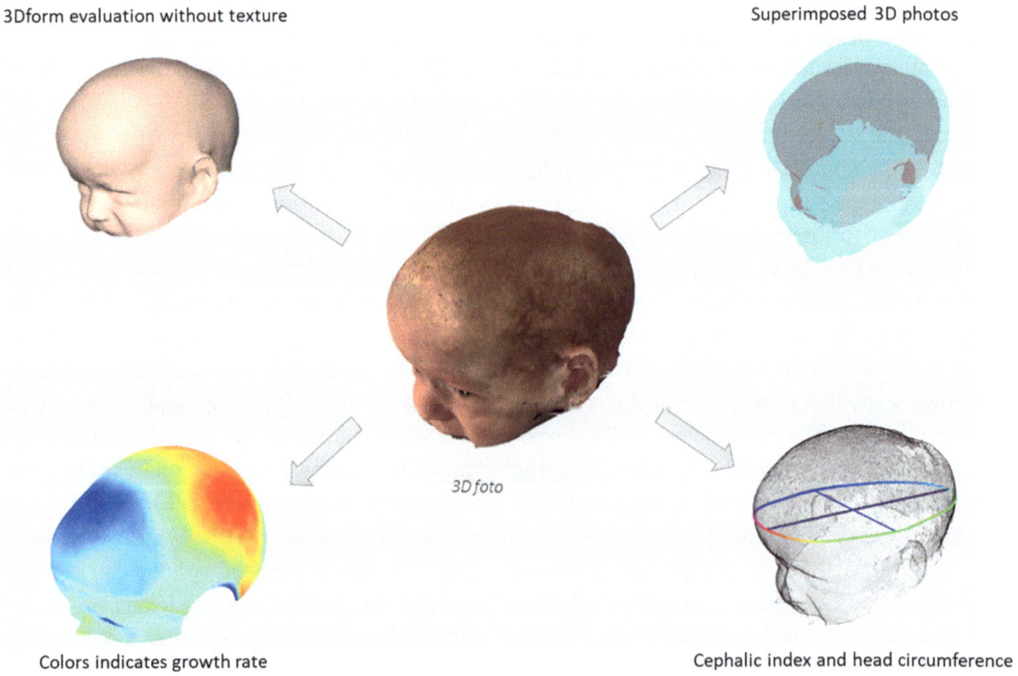

Fig. 27.3 3D analysis of cranial vault using 3D stereophotogrammetry. The 3D photos can be inspected independently using the 3D shape evaluation or superimposed to compare morphological changes and visualize areas of growth. Also, metrices such as the cephalic index and the head circumference can be calculated using the 3D analysis

two photos, expressed in mm. It is our experience that this is greatly appreciated and allows for a better understanding of the treatment protocol by parents. This information is evaluated and aids in the decision of the remaining length of helmet therapy. Typical cephalometric measurements giving an indication of skull growth such as the head circumference and the cephalic index (% skull width/length) are automatically calculated and compared to the preoperative situation (Fig. 27.2).

3D stereophotogrammetry can also be used to evaluate the treatment of larger groups of patients and to objectively compare different treatment modalities, for example, the use of springs or helmets. Although efforts are made to define objective criteria by which 2D photographs and 2D measurements can be used to evaluate the results of CS surgery, still postoperative results are being evaluated by the 'carpenters' eye' and thus biased by subjective evaluation. Using 3D stereophotogrammetry, objective measurements of larger groups of patients can be combined to quantify in an objective manner the actual 3D growth and evolution of the head shape after craniosynostosis surgery for different indications.

Doing this, we evaluated our results of endoscopically treated trigonocephaly patients and objectively showed that this treatment results in flattening of the forehead with a clear flattening and anterior movement of the lateral orbital bar [24].

In addition, the same technology allowed for the recent determination of the normal head growth in infants [13]. By creating this reference data of the normal evolution, we are now capable of not only objectively presenting and evaluating our surgical results, but also of comparing them to the normal growth patterns. This has led to exciting findings considering the postoperative results of endoscopically treated scaphocephaly patients (de Jong et al., in preparation). In general, these reference data of the normal skull development indicate that skull growth patterns in scaphocephalic children tend to normalize 8–11 months after endoscopic treatment.

To conclude, it is very clear that 3D stereophotogrammetry has become indispensable in direct clinical practice as in research to help forward the field of CS treatment.

27.4 Virtual Planning and CAD/CAM Techniques

Endoscopic surgery is only a viable treatment option when the patient is referred before 6 months of age. If a patient presents at an older age, cranial vault remodeling remains the designated therapy. The application of 3D technology in calvarial reconstruction reduces the operative length and intraoperative blood loss, thereby reducing postoperative morbidity and the duration of postoperative hospital stay. The technical physician makes a preoperative (VSP) by simulating different calvarial reconstructions on the 3D CT-scan to improve surgical efficacy. The added value of VSP is demonstrated by three surgical cases below.

27.4.1 Scaphocephaly Case

An age-related average healthy cranial shape is used for reference planning of scaphocephaly. The osteotomy lines are planned and the calvarial segments are studied to determine the optimal reconstructive alignment using the VSP software (Fig. 27.4a). The planned final shape should result in the desired volume increase, reduction of frontal bossing, and widening of the skull. This individualized preoperative plan, made by the technical physician, provides the surgeon with different treatment options. The options are then discussed with the surgeon, and the most optimal plan is chosen (Fig. 27.4b). Marking and reconstructive templates are then designed and printed.

Figure 27.5 demonstrates the intraoperative workflow using 3D VSP. During surgery, the calvaria is exposed, after which the marking template is used to indicate the exact location of the osteotomy lines. The cranial vault is then resected according to the osteotomy lines. The individual bone segments are, thereafter, com-

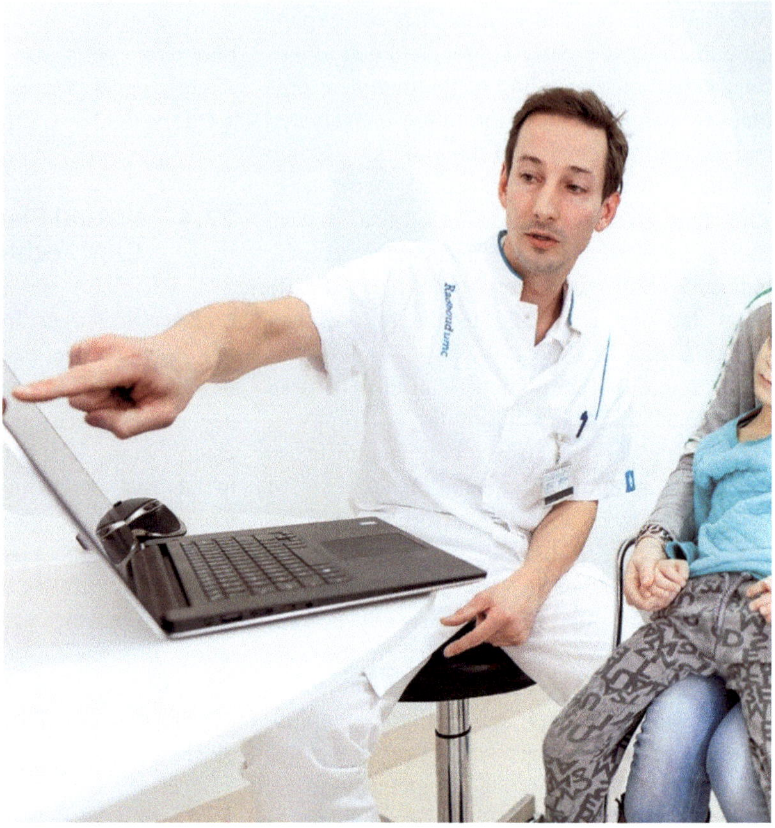

Fig. 27.4 Discussing the treatment progress with the patient's parents using the 3D photo analysis during the postoperative consultation

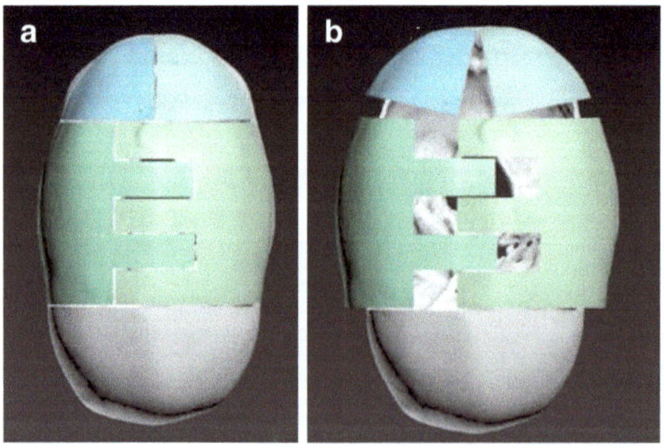

Fig. 27.5 (**a**) Virtual representation of the best reconstructive alignment in order to obtain the desired increase in cranial volume for sagittal suture synostosis where cranial vault remodeling is to be performed. (**b**) Using the VSP software, the exact translational and rotational movements of the individual calvarial segments that result in the desired morphological changes are calculated

bined back together using the reconstruction template via resorbable plates and sutures (Fig. 27.5). The duration of the surgery, blood loss, and comorbidity are all reduced due to the comprehensive preoperative planning performed in the 3D lab.

27.4.2 Plagiocephaly Case

Figure 27.6 shows the preoperative morphology of the patients' skull and the VSP of the cranial reconstruction. In the 3D lab, the existing curvature of the individual frontal bone segments is

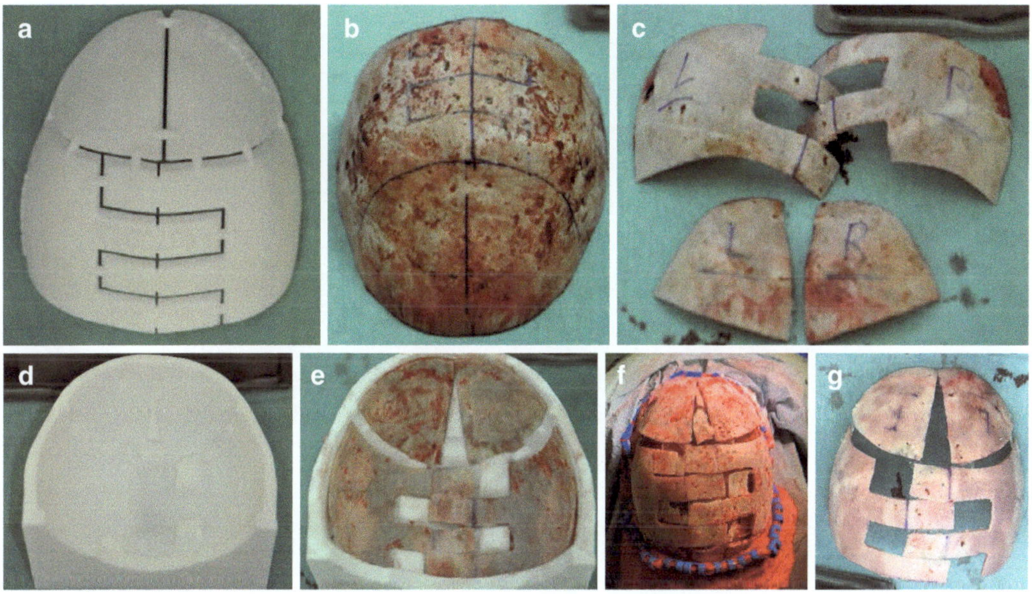

Fig. 27.6 (**a**) The 3D printed marking template is used for transferring the locations of the planned osteotomy lines. (**b**) The resected skull where the planned osteotomy lines have been marked. (**c**) The individual bone segments after completion of the osteotomies. (**d**) The 3D printed reconstruction template is obtained from the VSP. (**e**) The bone segments are positioned in the reconstruction template. (**f**) The bone segments combined together according to the 3D orientation of the reconstruction template. (**g**) The final reconstruction of the cranial vault in situ

studied and used to puzzle together until the final result is as close as possible to the normative reference shape. When the skull is exposed in the operating theatre, the marking template is used to transfer the planned osteotomies onto the skull. The frontal part and the orbital bar are taken out separately. According to the marked osteotomy lines, all parts of the frontal bones are taken out and arranged onto the reconstruction template. The skull elements are then fixed together with resorbable plates. The reconstructed skull is then placed back into the patient (Fig. 27.7). In the case of plagiocephaly, it is important to recreate as much symmetry as possible. The biggest challenge remains optimizing the shape of the orbital bandeau. Using VSP, it is possible to estimate the number and exact placement of the inflection points (Fig. 27.8). This again saves a lot of time and discussion in the OR during the surgery.

27.4.3 Trigonocephaly Case

The fronto-orbital advancement is virtually constructed by the technical physician using reference data of normal, unaffected skulls. The optimal angle of the two orbital segments is again precisely calculated using reference data of healthy individuals (Fig. 27.9). Using VSP, the ideal angle of the orbital segments can be accurately conveyed using the reconstruction template. The frontal bone reconstruction template guides the fixation of the frontal bone segments. The postoperative result shows the absence of the wedge-shaped forehead and the forward displacement of the lateral orbital walls, which gives a more harmonious contour (Fig. 27.10).

In the same way that 3D stereophotogrammetry is used to evaluate the endoscopic approach, the postoperative results of the open reconstruction can also be evaluated. In Fig. 27.11, an example of the growth evaluation of one individual scaphocephaly patient is shown. The red colour shows the preoperative 3D photo, and the blue colour displays the most recent postoperative one. The skull has widened, and the head circumference and the cephalic index have increased. The postoperative heat map shows that skull widening has occurred bilaterally as indicated by the red regions.

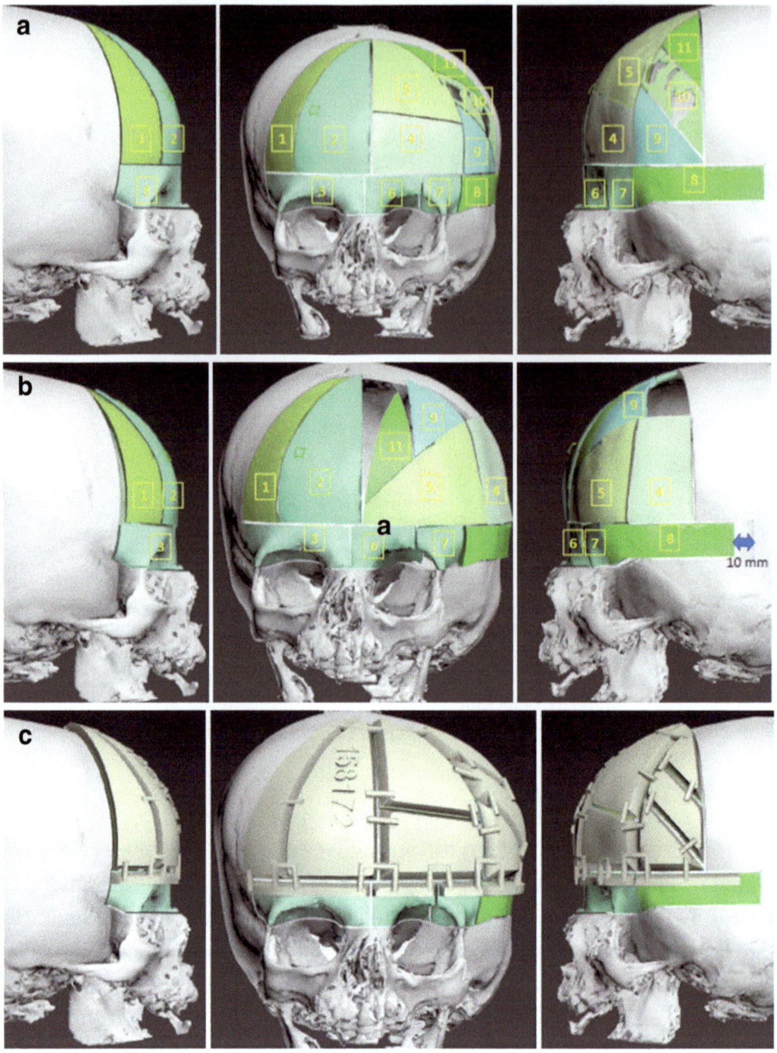

Fig. 27.7 Virtual representation of the patient-specific (**a**) planned osteotomy lines, (**b**) virtual reconstruction in 3D, and (**c**) design of the marking template that will be used to mark the planned osteotomy lines for cranial vault remodeling of plagiocephaly

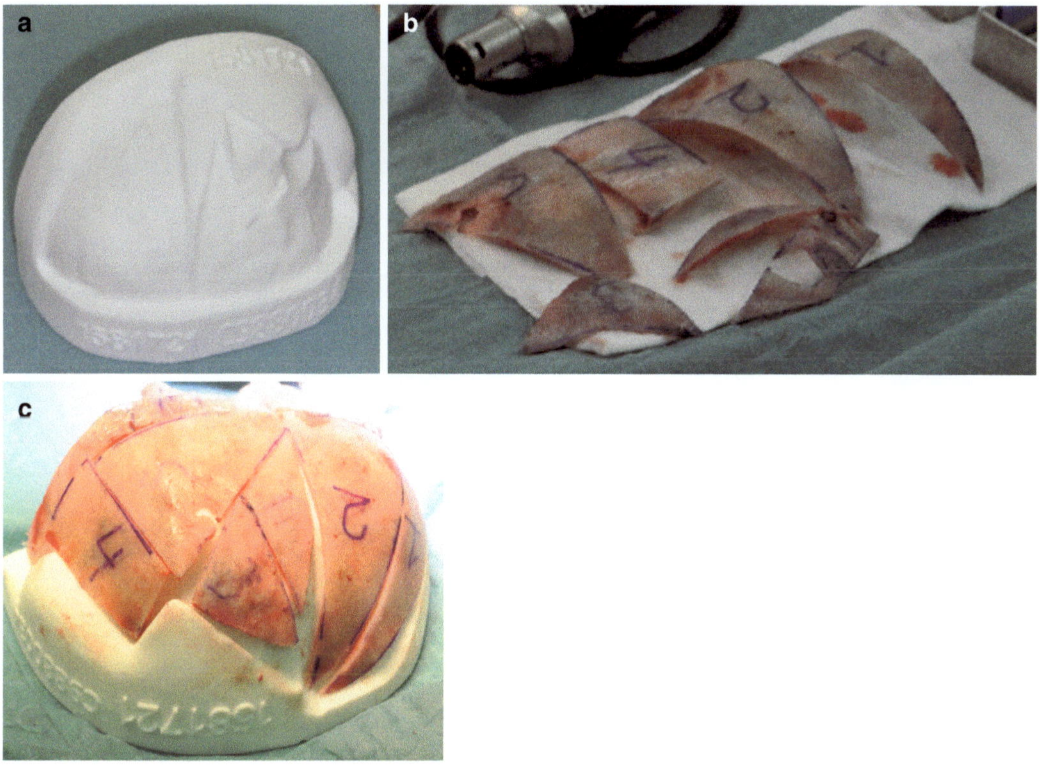

Fig. 27.8 (**a**) 3D printed reconstruction template. (**b**) The individual bone segments after osteotomies. (**c**) The individual bone segments positioned in the reconstruction template according to the planned positioning of the VSP

Fig. 27.9 The virtual surgical plan showing the exact number and placement of inflection points

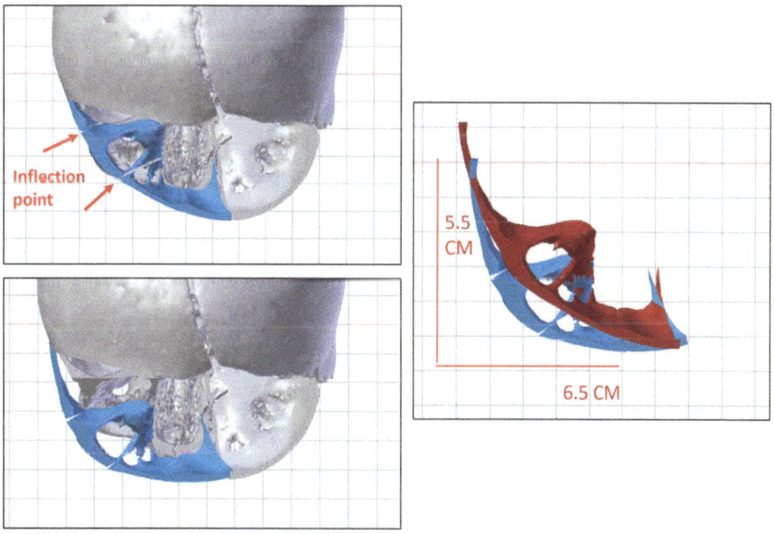

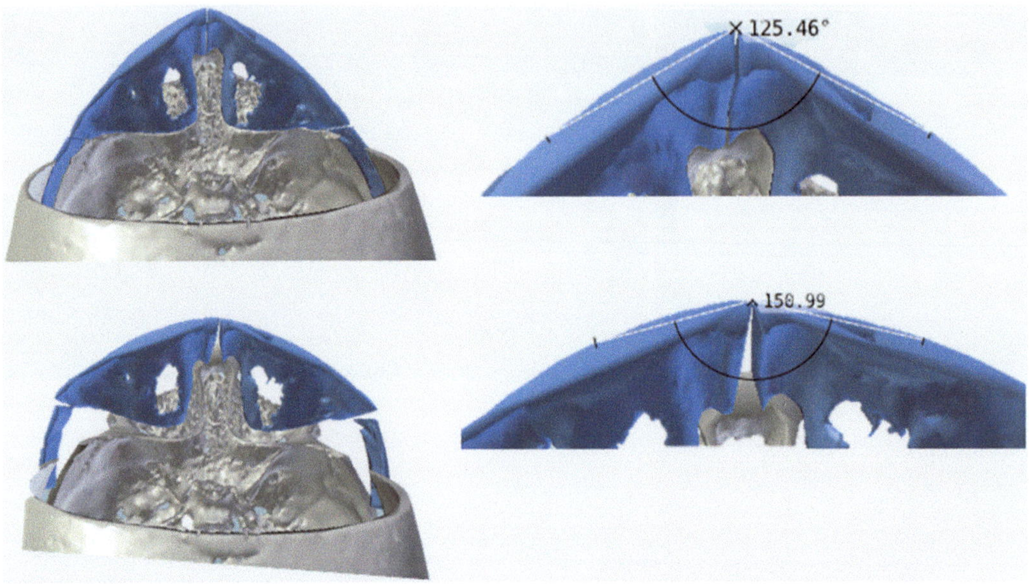

Fig. 27.10 VSP of the planned reconstruction of the two orbital segments with measurements of the angle. The two images above present the preoperative situation of the orbita. The images below show the virtual orbital reconstruction to improve frontal contour

Fig. 27.11 (**a**) Preoperative 3D printed model of a patient with trigonocephaly. (**b**) The 3D printed marking template that will be used intraoperatively to transfer the locations of the osteotomy lines. (**c**) The preoperative situation with the locations of the surgical incisions marked on the patient's cranium. (**d**) Transferring the VSP using the marking template. (**e**) Resected frontal bone segments after osteotomies placed in the reconstruction template. (**f**) The resected orbital bandeau placed in the reconstruction template. (**g**) The reconstructed skull parts are placed back in the patient. (**h**) Immediate postoperative result at the end of the surgery. (**i**) Preoperative frontal view of the trigonocephaly patient showing the characteristic deformity of the forehead. (**j**) Postoperative frontal view of the patient after 6 weeks, showing the improved aesthetic contour

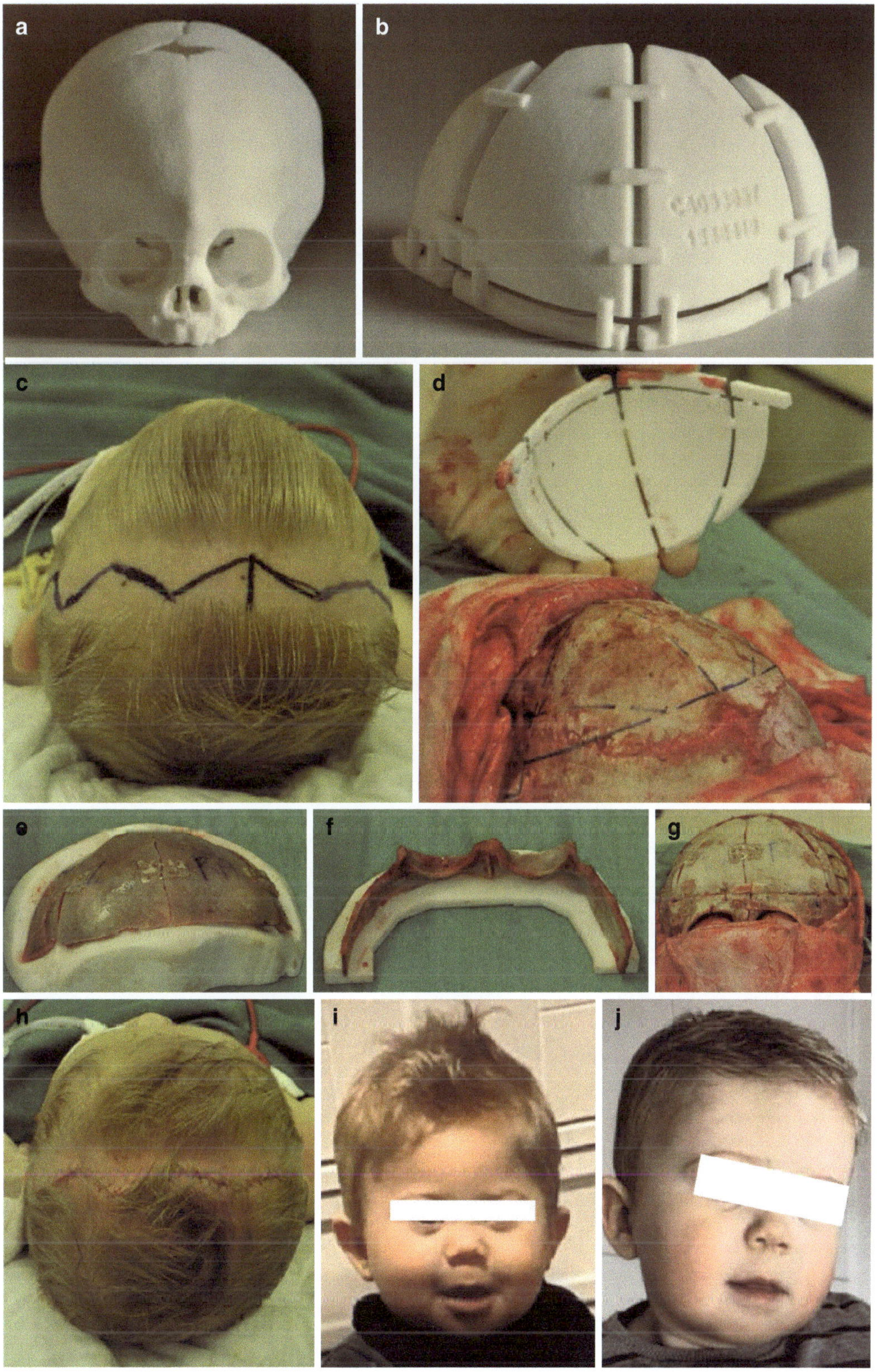
a
b
c
d
e
f
g
h
i
j

27.5 Conclusion

3D stereophotogrammetry enables close monitoring of the cranial development and provides insight into the treatment effect, enabling continuous improvement of the applied surgical techniques. In the case of the endoscopic approach, the postoperative growth is evaluated using superimposed 3D photos which helps clinical decision making, e.g. how long helmet therapy is needed. A 3D preoperative VSP aids in open craniofacial reconstruction because different surgical options are investigated preoperatively, resulting in the most optimal operation plan with a fast and more accurate transfer through operating templates.

27.6 Future Perspectives

As mentioned before, early diagnosis and intervention is important as it often leads to less invasive therapeutic options for the surgeon and more aesthetic outcomes for the patients. In primary and secondary health care sectors, misdiagnosis of CS still occurs due to the lack of expertise. It was recently suggested to combine 3D stereophotogrammetry with the modern machine learning technique called deep learning. Deep learning algorithms can be capable of correctly classifying the head shape of infants on 3D stereophotographs as healthy control or as a CS patient with the subtype scaphoid, trigonal, or anterior plagiocephaly with high accuracy [25]. 3D stereophotogrammetry technology is rapidly evolving, enabling the use of smartphone technology to make accurate 3D photos. This fast and radiation-free modality for capturing the cranial shape can be used in primary healthcare sectors, to make the correct diagnosis quickly. At this time, progress is made on the development of a mobile phone app for this purpose. Another perspective would be that the VSP, which is very labour-intensive, can be automated using artificial intelligence.

Another imaging modality that holds promise is 3D ultrasound. Current ultrasound imaging still has a relatively low detection rate of diagnosing CS [26]. Due to advancements in 3D ultrasound technology, preliminary results show that the detection rate for syndromic CS has improved and is high. Through further improvements, CS could be diagnosed in utero using 3D echoes [27].

One of the difficulties in cranial vault remodeling remains the transfer of the VSP to the skull. That is why marking and reconstruction templates are used nowadays. However, manufacturing such templates is time-consuming and expensive. Therefore, investigations continue to transfer the planning onto the patient using innovative technologies such as augmented reality (AR). Augmented Reality (Fig. 27.12) is the technology of blending virtual objects into the

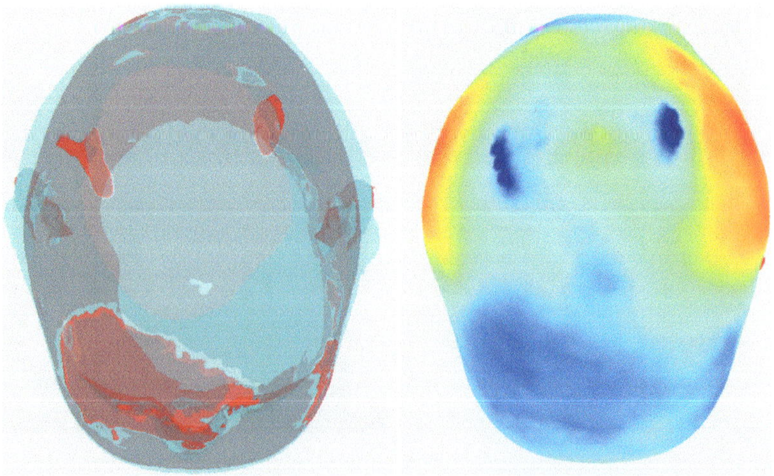

Fig. 27.12 Left: the pre- and postoperative photo of a scaphocephaly case superimposed. Right: distance map where the red color displays where the most volume increase has taken place

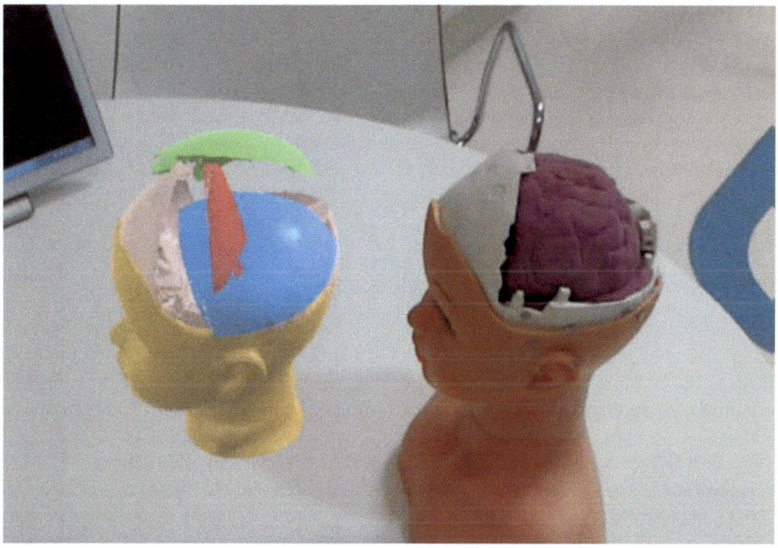

Fig. 27.13 Craniosynostosis planning in the AR-space

real world. AR makes it possible to create a virtual overlay within the surgeon's view. Image data of a patient can be observed directly at the corresponding position on a patient in the operation theatre. With special glasses such as the HoloLens (Microsoft Corporation, Redmond, WA, USA), the VSP could be projected right onto the skull of the patient in the operation theatre, while the surgery is performed [6]. Currently, the implementation of the HoloLens in the surgical field is limited to training and educational purposes.

Like in other specialties, robotics can be of great use in CS surgery. The surgical bots can, more accurately than their human counterpart, transfer the VSP onto the skull of the patient, without the use of a template (Fig. 27.13). One could imagine that this also occurs faster and more accurately. One can even envision that the bots will even perform osteotomies. The use of surgical navigation techniques could become helpful in repositioning the bone segments back into the patient. All these future developments may eventually alter the surgeon's role (Fig. 27.14).

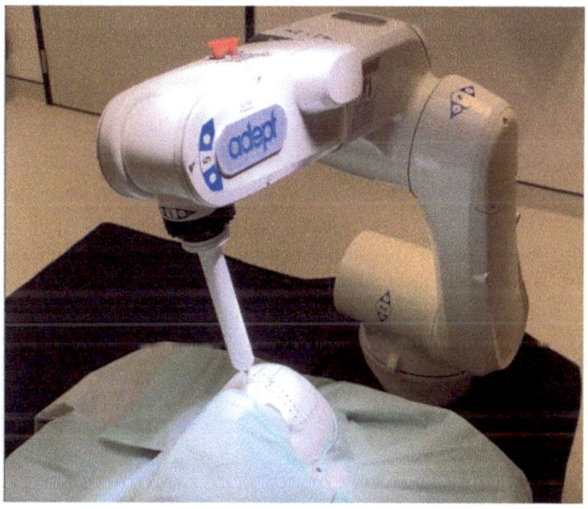

Fig. 27.14 Surgical robot performing craniosynostosis surgery on a dummy to demonstrate the capabilities of surgical robotics

References

1. Tack P, Victor J, Gemmel P, Annemans L. 3D-printing techniques in a medical setting: a systematic literature review. Biomed Eng Online. 2016;15(1):115.
2. Sailer H, Haers P, Zollikofer C, Warnke T, Caris F, Stucki P. The value of stereolithographic models for

preoperative diagnosis of craniofacial deformities and planning of surgical corrections. Int J Oral Maxillofac Surg. 1998;27(5):327–33.
3. García-Mato D, Ochandiano S, García-Sevilla M, Navarro-Cuéllar C, Darriba-Allés J, García-Leal R, et al. Craniosynostosis surgery: workflow based on virtual surgical planning, intraoperative navigation and 3D printed patient-specific guides and templates. Sci Rep. 2019;9(1):17691.
4. Andrew T, Baylan J, Mittermiller P, Cheng H, Johns D, Edwards M, et al. Virtual surgical planning decreases operative time for isolated single suture and multi-suture craniosynostosis repair. Plast Reconstr Surg Glob Open. 2018;6(12):e2038.
5. Chim H, Wetjen N, Mardini S. Virtual surgical planning in craniofacial surgery. Semin Plast Surg. 2014;28(03):150–8.
6. Meulstee J, Nijsink J, Schreurs R, Verhamme L, Xi T, Delye H, et al. Toward holographic-guided surgery. Surg Innov. 2018;26(1):86–94.
7. Proctor M, Meara J. A review of the management of single-suture craniosynostosis, past, present, and future. J Neurosurg Pediatr. 2019;24(6):622–31.
8. Rice H, Frush D, Farmer D, Waldhausen J. Review of radiation risks from computed tomography: essentials for the pediatric surgeon. J Pediatr Surg. 2007;42(4):603–7.
9. Fearon J. Evidence-based medicine. Plast Reconstr Surg. 2014;133(5):1261–75.
10. Hersh D, Bookland M, Hughes C. Diagnosis and management of suture-related concerns of the infant skull. Pediatr Clin N Am. 2021;68(4):727–42.
11. Meulstee J. How augmented reality and 3D visualization techniques can be used in clinical practice and during the treatment of craniosynostosis [dissertation]. Nijmegen, NL: Radboud University; 2021.
12. Kim H, Roh H, Lee I. Craniosynostosis: updates in radiologic diagnosis. J Kor Neurosurg Soc. 2016;59(3):219.
13. Meulstee J, de Jong G, Borstlap W, Koerts G, Maal T, Delye H. The normal evolution of the cranium in three dimensions. Int J Oral Maxillofac Surg. 2020;49(6):739–49.
14. Pugliese L, Marconi S, Negrello E, Mauri V, Peri A, Gallo V, et al. The clinical use of 3D printing in surgery. Updat Surg. 2018;70(3):381–8.
15. Mardini S, Alsubaie S, Cayci C, Chim H, Wetjen N. Three-dimensional preoperative virtual planning and template use for surgical correction of craniosynostosis. J Plast Reconstr Aesthet Surg. 2014;67(3):336–43.
16. Martín-Noguerol T, Paulano-Godino F, Riascos R, Calabia-del-Campo J, Márquez-Rivas J, Luna A. Hybrid computed tomography and magnetic resonance imaging 3D printed models for neurosurgery planning. Ann Transl Med. 2019;7(22):684.
17. Meulepas J, Ronckers C, Smets A, Nievelstein R, Gradowska P, Lee C, et al. Radiation exposure from pediatric CT scans and subsequent cancer risk in The Netherlands. JNCI J Natl Cancer Inst. 2018;111(3):256–63.
18. Artunduaga M, Liu C, Morin C, Serai S, Udayasankar U, Greer M, et al. Safety challenges related to the use of sedation and general anesthesia in pediatric patients undergoing magnetic resonance imaging examinations. Pediatr Radiol. 2021;51(5):724–35.
19. Maal T, Klijn R, Bergé S. 3D imaging for craniomaxillofacial applications in orthognathic and facial surgery planning. Craniomaxillofacial reconstructive and corrective bone. Surgery. 2019:255–81.
20. Brons S, van Beusichem M, Maal T, Plooij J, Bronkhorst E, Bergé S, et al. Development and reproducibility of a 3D stereophotogrammetric reference frame for facial soft tissue growth of babies and young children with and without orofacial clefts. Int J Oral Maxillofac Surg. 2013;42(1):2–8.
21. Meulstee J, Verhamme L, Borstlap W, Van der Heijden F, De Jong G, Xi T, et al. A new method for three-dimensional evaluation of the cranial shape and the automatic identification of craniosynostosis using 3D stereophotogrammetry. Int J Oral Maxillofac Surg. 2017;46(7):819–26.
22. Brons S, Meulstee J, Nada R, Kuijpers M, Bronkhorst E, Bergé S, et al. Uniform 3D meshes to establish normative facial averages of healthy infants during the first year of life. PLoS One. 2019;14(5):e0217267.
23. Delye H, Borstlap W, van Lindert E. Endoscopy assisted craniosynostosis surgery followed by helmet therapy. Surg Neurol Int. 2018;9(1):59.
24. De Jong G, Tolhuisen M, Meulstee J, van der Heijden F, van Lindert E, Borstlap W, et al. Radiation-free 3D head shape and volume evaluation after endoscopically assisted strip craniectomy followed by helmet therapy for trigonocephaly. J Craniofac Surg. 2017;45(5):661–71.
25. De Jong G, Bijlsma E, Meulstee J, Wennen M, van Lindert E, Maal T, et al. Combining deep learning with 3D stereophotogrammetry for craniosynostosis diagnosis. Sci Rep. 2020;10(1):15346.
26. Helfer T, Peixoto A, Tonni G, Araujo Júnior E. Craniosynostosis: prenatal diagnosis by 2D/3D ultrasound, magnetic resonance imaging and computed tomography. Med Ultrason. 2016;18(3):378.
27. Leung K. Applications of advanced ultrasound technology in obstetrics. Diagnostics. 2021;11(7):1217.

3D Models in Craniofacial Surgical Training

28

Giselle Coelho, Stephen Larsen,
Eduardo Varjão Vieira, and Nelci Zanon

28.1 Introduction

Surgeons face the challenge of learning, planning, and performing highly complex surgical procedures. Surgical competence requires technical skills using three-dimensional visualization, and previously it was only possible to train surgeons in real-life situations. Progress in the technologies of three-dimensional (3D) printing and advanced methods in simulation training allow us to design specific training procedures that integrate multiple skills in a safe environment. Given that more than 75% of neurosurgical errors are judged to be avoidable, simulation has a significant role to play in this context [1]. A meta-analysis of McGaghie et al. (2011) has shown that simulation training may influence translational outcomes [1].

The standards for surgical training are shifting from time-based to criterion-based parameters that emphasize obtaining and maintaining competencies [2]. The formation of a surgeon demands significant dedication and effort and considerable time [3]. Currently, well-established methods of surgical training are being challenged as the environment becomes increasingly competitive and litigious with greater scrutiny of patient outcomes [3–8]. In order to increase patient safety and improve treatment outcomes, several strategies including problem-based learning and objective structured clinical examinations have promoted the development of new curricula in surgical education [9–11]. Some of these changes have been driven by events in the 1980s and 1990s, such as medical misconduct and overworked unsupervised resident staff, contributing to patient morbidity and mortality. This has also coincided with a growing medical malpractice crisis.

Concerns arose about the long-established methods of training surgical residents, and solutions were sought to reduce preventable errors and perioperative complications [2, 12]. The airline industry, with the development of flight simulators and pilot coaching methods, proved to be an excellent precedent for innovation in surgical education. Many surgical educators believe such methods are key to accelerating the acquisition of

G. Coelho (✉)
Santa Casa de Misericordia de São Paulo, São Paulo, Brazil

S. Larsen
Harvard University, Cambridge, MA, USA

E. V. Vieira
Bahiana School of Medicine and Public Health, EBMSP, Salvador, Brazil

N. Zanon
Pediatric Neurosurgery Center/CENEPE, São Paulo, Brazil

Discipline of Neurosurgery, Universidade Federal de São Paulo, UNIFESP, São Paulo, Brazil

Hospital Samaritano, Higienópolis, Américas Serviços Médicos, São Paulo, Brazil

F. Di Rocco, J. Kestle (eds.), *Neurosurgical Aspects of Craniosynostosis*,
https://doi.org/10.1007/978-3-031-69386-1_28

fundamental skills and the rate of performance improvement among surgical residents.

Neurosurgical trainees face great challenges in learning to plan and perform increasingly complex procedures in which there is little room for error [15]. The educator's task becomes ever more daunting as the number and complexity of neurosurgical procedures continue to increase in parallel with technological developments. A Yale University study demonstrated that criterion-based simulator training decreased operating time by 30% and operative errors by 85% [13, 14]. The necessity of innovative surgical curriculum development that incorporates safe learning environments and objective skill assessments is obvious and needs to be led by trained surgical educators [16].

Craniosynostosis, first described by Sommerring in 1791, refers to the premature closure of cranial sutures, leading to calvarial deformities [17]. Thus, there is a restriction of skull growth perpendicular to the affected suture, and the continuous increase in brain volume, promoting the compensatory growth of the skull in the other patent sutures, causes progressive deformity typically parallel to the affected suture (Virchow's law) [4]. It is essential to emphasize that the possibilities for hands-on training of surgical techniques to treat craniosynostosis are quite restricted. Training has been performed preferentially on sheep heads, but with many limitations [18]. The sheep head does not present the same pathological condition, and it is not possible to identify the anatomical reference structures. In addition, bone consistency is not adequate to simulate the osteotomy process, impairing the acquisition of physical feedback. Also, emergencies such as bleeding from the superior sagittal sinus are not reproduced.

The limitations of traditional training methods point to the high value of developing new alternative methods. In surgical training generally, and in training for the treatment of craniosynostosis, the educational value of 3D printed models for teaching advanced techniques is derived from their ability to provide the trainee with tactile feedback and to simulate spatial relationships, thus aiding in the memorization of the steps of the surgical procedure.

The first realistic simulator for training surgical techniques for scaphocephaly was published in 2014, presenting a radiological interface and a bleeding effect [19]. As an important complement of the physical simulator, a virtual reality simulator was also developed to emphasize the three-dimensional step by step procedure of craniosynostosis surgical correction [20].

In this chapter, we will describe the available simulators for craniosynostosis surgical training and the current impact of, and future perspectives on, their use in neurosurgical education.

28.2 Craniosynostosis Realistic Simulator

Development authors with a Brazilian institute EDUCSIM (https://educsim.com.br) have worked on creating and improving synthetic models that can provide a reliable model for craniosynostosis training. The first realistic simulator was built with a synthetic thermo-retractile, thermo-sensitive rubber which presents textures, consistencies, and mechanical resistance similar to many human tissues.

Regarding anatomical aspects, the skull shape was based on computerized tomography (CT) in Digital Imaging and Communications in Medicine (DICOM) images of a real patient (6-month-old female). Thin slices were used to enable 3D reconstruction. A special resin, in the shape of the skull, constituted the basic structure of the craniosynostosis module trainer. The module contains the head (the surgical unit, presenting a scaphocephaly type cranial malformation, Fig. 28.1a, b) which is connected to the body by a simulated cervical spine (acrylic composition, Fig. 28.1c). In this way, the head is locked by a simple acrylic connection. With this, training can be performed as if it were a real surgery (Fig. 28.1d). Due to the radiopacity of this simulator, it is possible to perform CT scans (Fig. 28.2) and, consequently, this simulator allows for comparison between pre- and postoperative images.

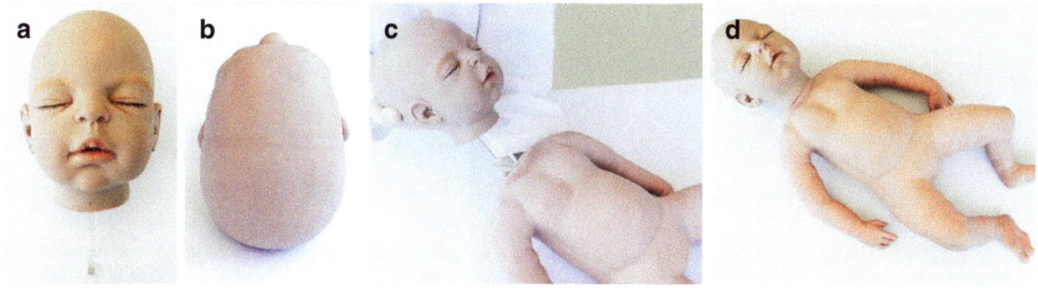

Fig. 28.1 Realistic craniosynostosis simulator. (**a**, **b**) Craniosynostosis Surgical Unit. (**c**) Connection point between the surgical unit (head) and the base of the simulator. (**d**) Anatomical model ready to use

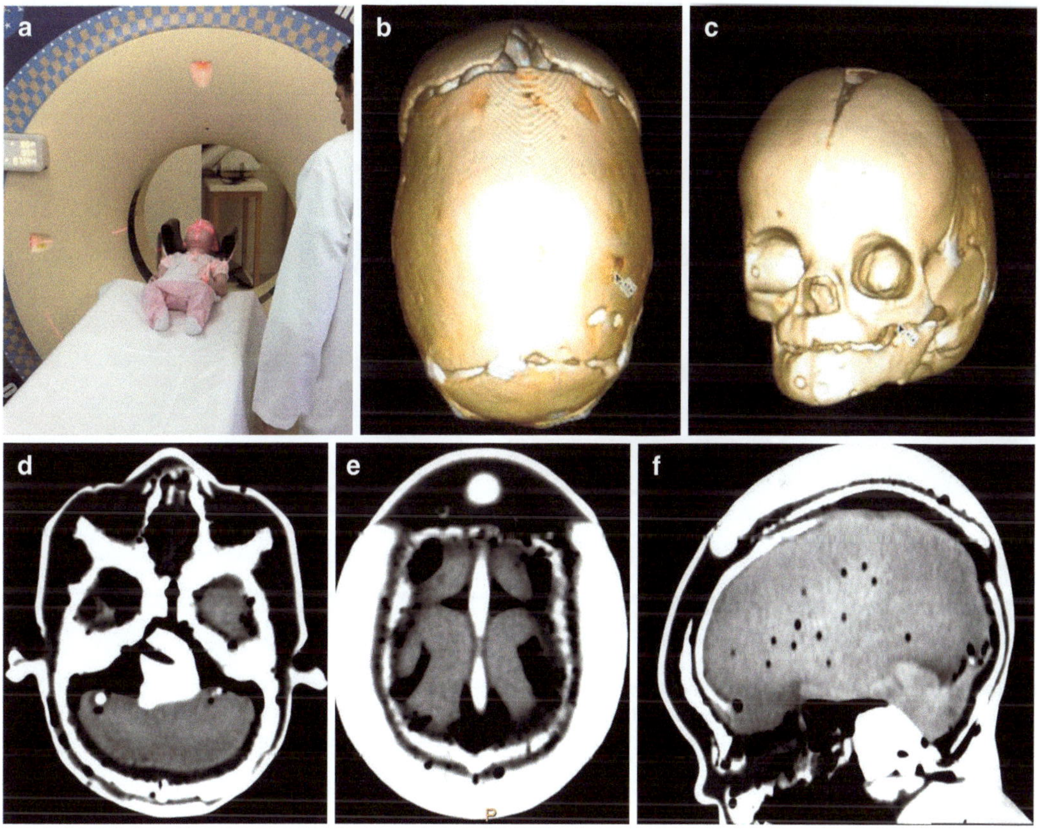

Fig. 28.2 (**a**–**c**) CT images with tridimensional reconstruction. (**d**–**f**) Hyperdensity of superior sagittal sinus (filled with blood simulator)

There are multiple opportunities for practice using this realistic model, including the skin incision, subcutaneous and subperiosteal dissection, osteotomies, and cranial remodeling with absorbable microplates. The presence of superior sagittal and transverse sinuses filled with liquid can simulate emergency situations like bleeding (Fig. 28.3).

This model also can be used to practice endoscopic correction with notable realism [20]. Surgical endoscopic treatment for a case involving both scaphocephaly and trigonocephaly can be performed basing the head model on a combination of real CT images obtained from scaphocephaly and trigonocephaly patients.

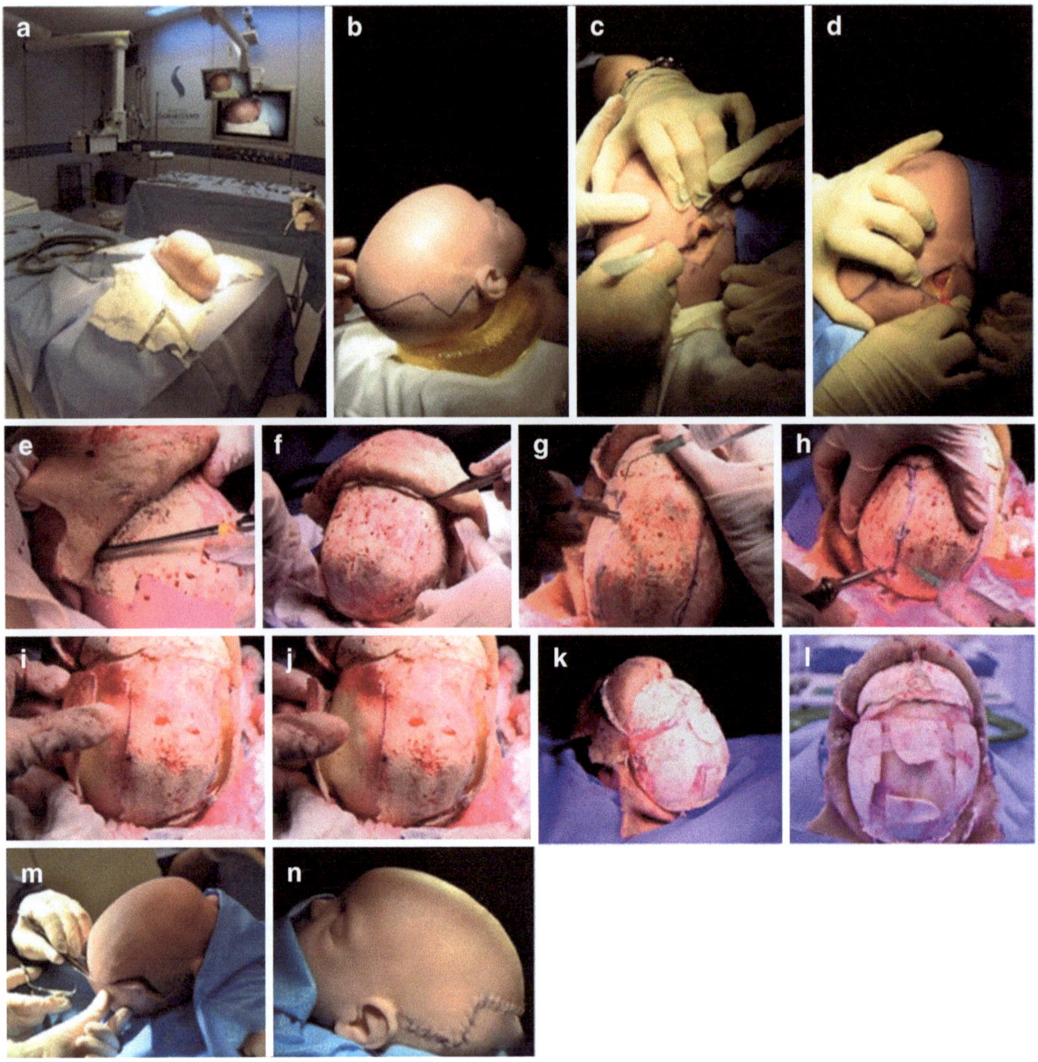

Fig. 28.3 (**a** and **b**) Real simulator in the operating room and delimiting the skin incision. (**c** and **d**) Subcutaneous dissection. (**e** and **f**) Subperiosteal dissection. (**g** and **h**) Delimiting the osteotomy. (**i** and **j**) Green-stick fracture (Renier's "H" technique). (**k** and **l**) Cranial reconstruction (using absorbable plates). (**m** and **n**) Skin closure

28.3 Craniosynostosis Virtual Simulator

The main goal of the virtual simulator is to provide, through virtual simulation, training that mirrors the physical platform. These virtual models don't allow for interaction with the trainee, but they can stimulate the ability to mentally manipulate objects in three dimensions, recreating the intraoperative scenario.

3D videos were developed by a graphic designer and a neurosurgical team using 3DS Max software. They were based on reproduction of the tridimensional anatomy of the skull and real surgical videos [21]. The craniosynostosis virtual modules present the scaphocephaly type and all the stages of the surgical approach by H-Renier technique (Fig. 28.4).

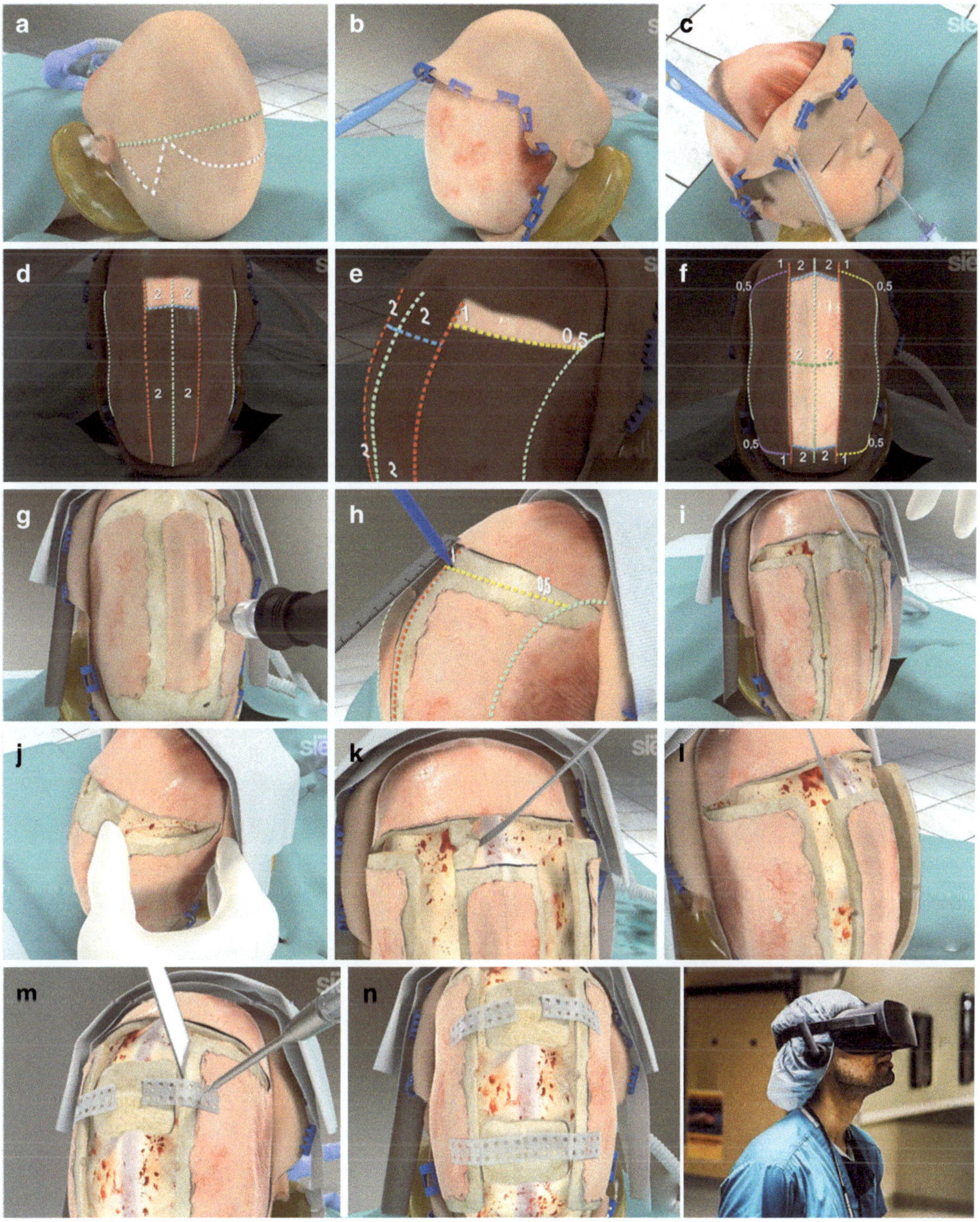

Fig. 28.4 Craniosynostosis virtual simulator. (**a**–**c**) Patient positioning, skin incision, and dissection by plans. (**d**–**i**) Craniotomy area definition—H Renier technique. (**j**) Green stick fracture. (**k** and **l**) Sagittal strip removal. (**m** and **n**) Use of absorbable plates

28.4 Puzzle

A craniosynostosis puzzle was developed to simulate the craniosynostosis correction (scaphocephaly type) using H Renier's technique [22].

The cranial model is created by 1-mm CT scans in the DICOM format. This information is processed using a computing algorithm to generate a 3D printed biomodel in resin. Afterward, planned craniotomies are performed and the skull pieces are fitted with magnets to allow real surgical simulation with the magnetic interface. In this way, it is possible to practice the surgical technique and simulate the cranial reconstruction step by step (Fig. 28.5).

The puzzle is simple to use, portable, and low cost. It can be used many times since it is reusable and recyclable (Fig. 28.5). This is a significant feature, as the number of attempts was proved to be inversely proportional to the number of errors [22].

This tool may be used as a supplementary model to enhance cognitive abilities related to anatomical recognition, allowing a variety of degrees of immersion and realism, establishing a physical reality learning curve, and offering symbolic, geometric, and dynamic information, with 3D visualization.

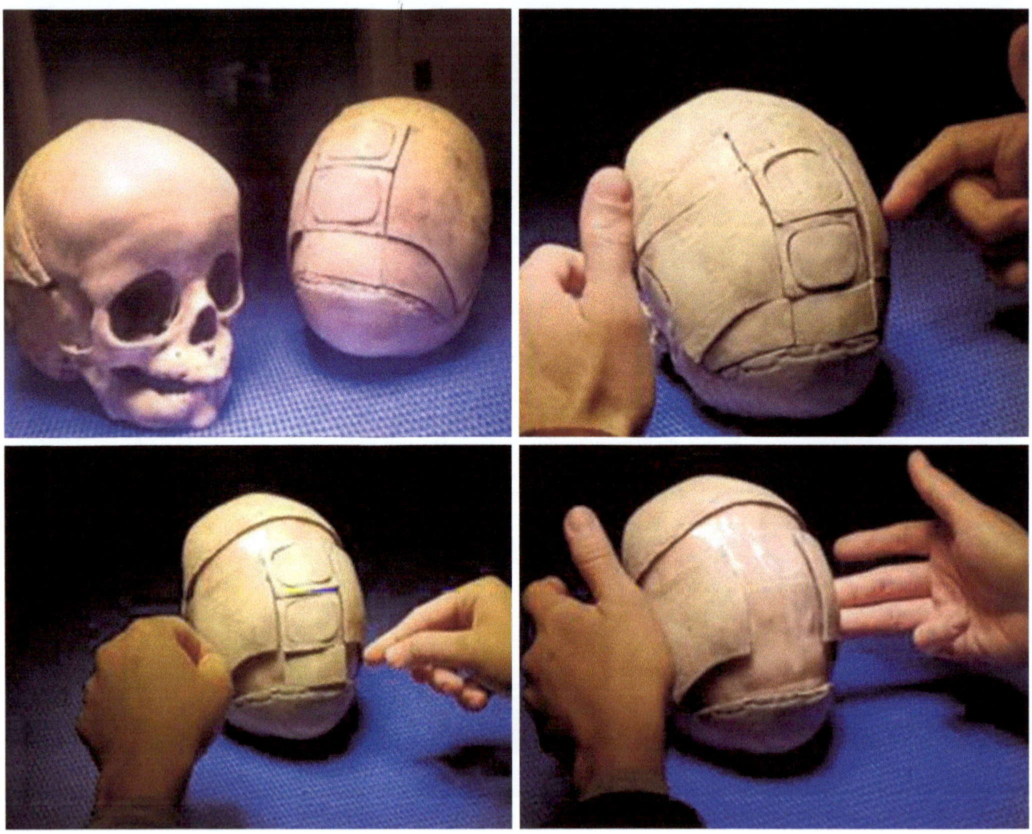

Fig. 28.5 Scaphocephalic skull simulation, with several osteotomies. The magnetic interface of the bone pieces makes possible the "osteotomies" and subsequent posterior cranial remodeling, both correctly and incorrectly

28.5 Patient-Specific Hybrid and Augmented Reality Models

The availability of 3D printing technology has expanded the possibilities for developing life-like models to increase understanding of normal and pathological anatomy [23, 24]. These models combined with augmented reality bring new perspectives to preoperative planning.

Augmented reality (AR) transforms virtual objects into video images in real time, providing specific anatomical information and elaborated metrics [25, 26]. With recent advancements, these systems can be used not only for surgical planning, but also as tools in intraoperative scenarios [25, 27, 28].

An innovative project was developed by Coelho et al. [29] combining a realistic customized model and an augmented reality model for preoperative planning of trigonocephaly correction. In the first step of the development process, a patient-specific hybrid model was created based on the anatomical aspects of the skull. Data were obtained from CT DICOM thin-slice images of a real patient (a 5-month old male infant case patient) which allowed 3D reconstruction (Fig. 28.6). The material was composed of high-performance platinum-cured liquid silicone components used in many applications ranging from creating skin effects to making a variety of different tissues. After the printing process, an artist worked manually to make the model more realistic.

The surgical training using the metopic craniosynostosis model was performed as if it were a real surgery, using surgical instruments. It was possible to simulate the surgical approach step by step with real instruments used to cut the skin (the silicone mimicked the tissue accurately) and to perform the osteotomies and dissection with appropriate tactile feedback (Fig. 28.8). As well, a customized augmented reality model was developed for use with a smartphone app (Fig. 28.7).

The model was considered a fundamental and valuable factor in the multidisciplinary discussion between the neurosurgeons and plastic surgeons. It allowed for a detailed discussion of the aspects of the surgical planning, providing tissues with different tactile and resistance qualities, as well as prediction of the orbit remodeling measurements with excellent precision. The patient operated on in these conditions presented excellent follow-up and an excellent esthetic result [29].

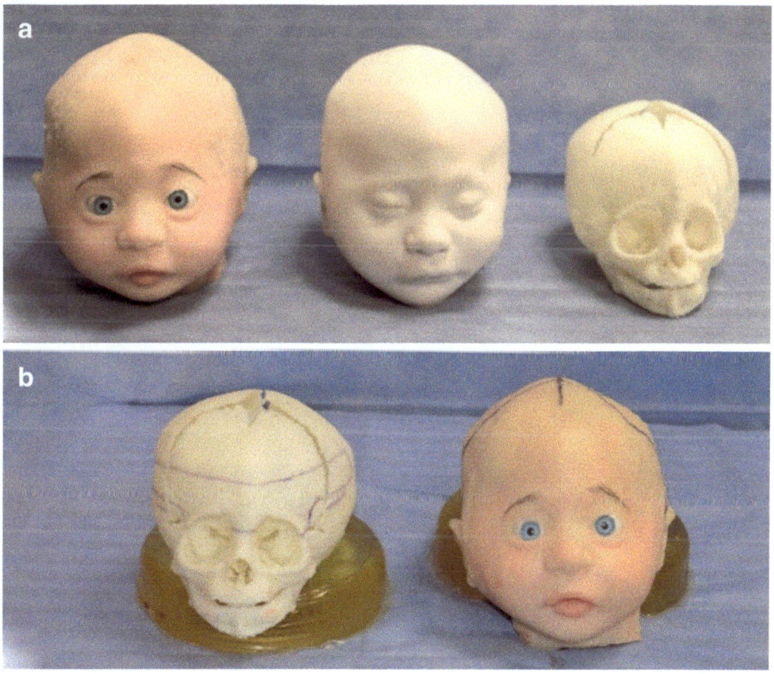

Fig. 28.6 (**a**) Hybrid model and 3D printed models. (**b**) Preoperative planning using the 3D printed and hybrid model

Fig. 28.7 The three layers of visualization in the AR app. (**a**) AR image of patient face in CT scan. (**b**) Whole skull format. (**c**) Possibilities of AR skull creation

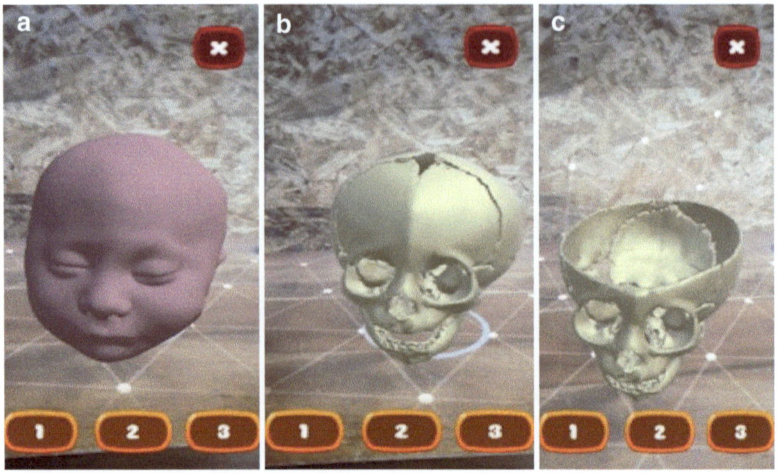

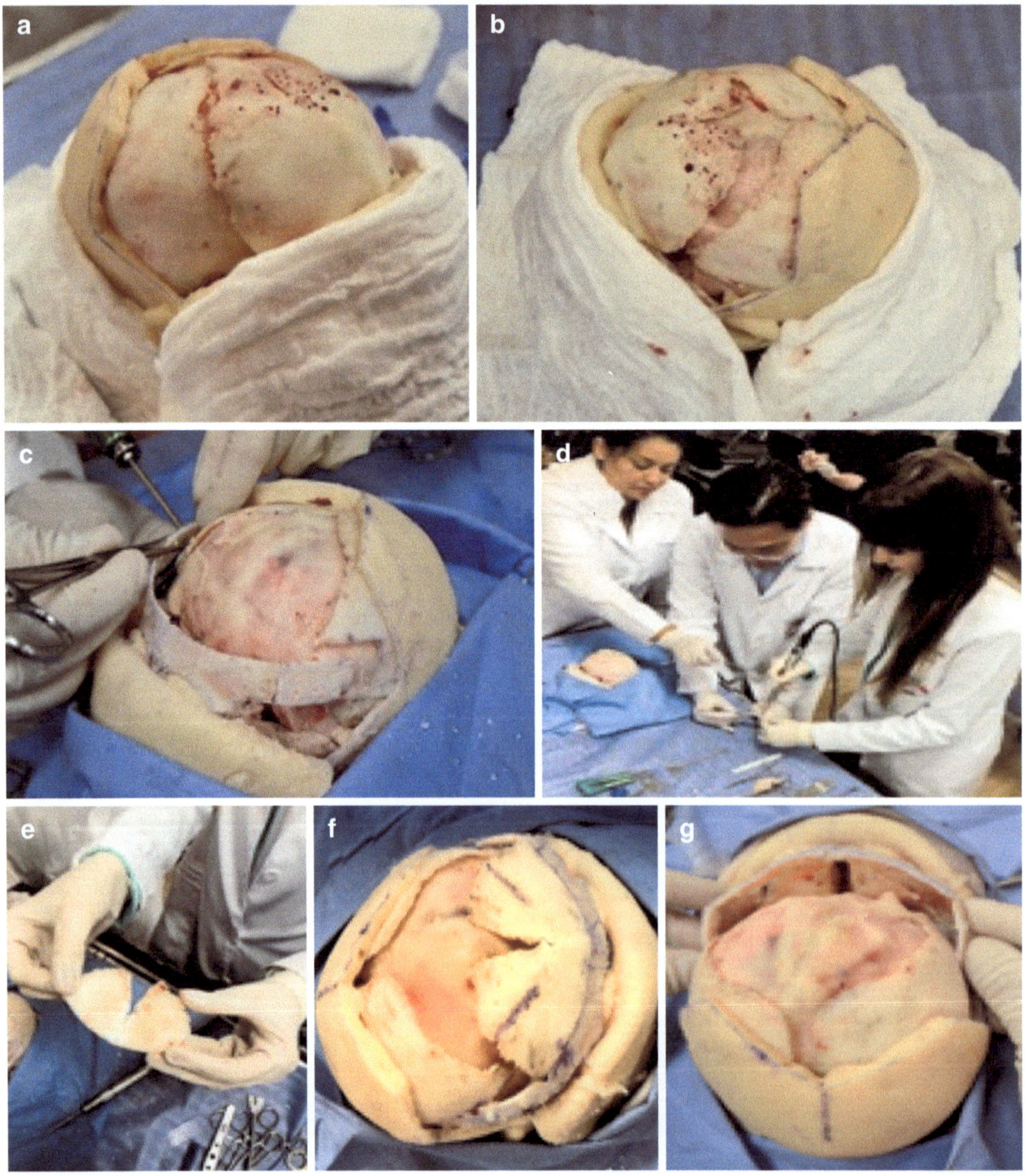

28.6 Discussion

Surgical education in the coming years faces critical challenges, especially in training surgeons to acquire and perfect complex neurosurgical techniques such as those required for successful treatment of craniosynostosis. Disruptions and constraints in both local face-to-face teaching and global mobility inhibit the transfer of knowledge characteristic of the traditional (Halsted) model of surgical apprenticeship and mentorship. Inadequacies in surgical education, whether the effect of exceptional factors like regional or international health crises, prohibitive costs, or political uncertainties, can and must be overcome with advances in teaching technologies and methods, among them the innovative use of highly realistic physical models that simulate the complexities of surgical reality. Such innovations have the further advantage of providing means for supplementary remote training in situations where side-by-side training is impossible or limited in scope, or would benefit from auxiliary methods.

The treatment of craniosynostosis implies extensive surgery and presents a challenge for the surgeon. In this context, training based on surgical simulation is extremely helpful. Multiple meta-analyses have shown that associating simulation with conventional training results in better performance, reduction in surgery time, reduced error rate, and consequently, better patient outcomes [30].

Simulators can be used to facilitate assessment and objectively provide quantifiable measures of learning using multidisciplinary content. Many training models have been created as the initial step in training residents and young neurosurgeons to gain experience with surgical procedures. The majority of these have used animal models, human cadaveric specimens, and occasionally synthetic materials. However, procedures such as craniosynostectomy or cranial vault remodeling can be highly complex to simulate in their entirety. In this respect, the craniosynostosis realistic simulator provides an alternative to the use of animal models and human cadaveric specimens.

Moreover, the realistic simulator presents some notable advantages:

1. material maintenance is convenient
2. the cranium size is appropriate and provides for realistic depth perception
3. the simulator includes all necessary planning steps of the surgery (from positioning to skin closure)
4. real surgical instruments can be used
5. a bleeding effect trains surgeons in the handling of emergency situations
6. there are no ethical or location restrictions to its use

The puzzle can be considered as a complementary tool that allows different degrees of immersion and realism. Also, it enables evaluation of the basic competence of the resident before proceeding to real surgery.

Despite the importance of improving technical skills, operating room conduct, and the interpersonal abilities of those who perform surgical procedures, few studies have examined the use of AR technology in preoperative planning to determine the most favorable surgical approaches [25]. With the development of an AR-based training simulator, surgeons in training can experience realistic simulations of surgical operations comparable to those encountered in actual neurosurgery.

The use of a physical hybrid model and AR in planning the operative technique involved in treating metopic craniosynostosis is particularly noteworthy. The association of physical hybrid model technology with the application of AR can provide a highly effective training environment by facilitating preoperative planning while highlighting important perspectives in medical education. The remarkable realism of this method significantly enhances the teaching of surgical anatomy and operative strategies in the neurosurgical field, especially during residency training, and 3D modeling technology may provide a complementary educational tool in any preoperative surgical planning, enhancing the safety of the

Fig. 28.8 Preoperative planning using the hybrid model. (**a–b**) Skin dissection. (**c**, **d**) Osteotomies. (**e-g**) Cranial reconstruction using absorbable plates. Real surgical tools were used in lll the stages of the preop planning procedure and contributing to a better outcome [29].

Practice with each of these models has particular advantages and disadvantages that are still being elucidated in various validation processes. The choice of the most appropriate training model should be taken into consideration, as well as other qualities such as efficacy, validity, cost-effectiveness, and versatility [31].

Several factors favor the increasing use of surgical simulation in training during medical residency: restrictions on working hours; increased supervision; more formalized educational goals; and rising demand for increased hospital efficiency (with emphasis on the patient and outcomes). The need for new paradigms of training and surgical skills education has led to the development of a variety of simulation methods that refine the technique while objectively assessing the resident's performance.

It is important to emphasize that there is significant evidence demonstrating that technical skills acquired on simulated models directly transfer into performance improvements in the operating room, reinforcing their value in surgical training programs [32, 33]. The ideal simulator has to be realistic in multiple dimensions. Simulation physics, optical properties, haptic feedback, and suitability for the required surgical tasks must be tested to ensure the quality of surgical training.

It is also necessary to validate the ability of the simulation exercise to teach the desired skill set or technique. The identification and measurement of errors permit assessment of the effectiveness of training that is specifically intended to reduce their incidence. Additionally, to be considered a useful tool for training, a simulator should be further evaluated regarding its overall quality. Despite a variety of ways to do it, every simulator should meet three major criteria: validity, reliability, and feasibility [17]. It has been suggested that when adopting a new training paradigm such as a simulator-based curriculum, it is important to utilize the same language and terminology to preserve the standards of assessment [17].

The development of effective surgical simulators is a milestone in the evolution of surgical education. Craniofacial realistic simulators provide a safe and nonthreatening learning context that not only promotes the development of skills, but also allows for objective risk-free testing of a trainee's abilities prior to entering the operating room. Beyond pure technical proficiency, the cognitive skills of anatomical recognition, decision-making, and contingency planning can also be developed. Additionally, these same models can be used in the process of initial certification as well as recertification of existing practitioners similar to performance assessment standards in the airline industry.

28.7 Conclusion

The use of simulation in teaching the operative techniques involved in treating craniosynostosis is particularly noteworthy. The use of realistic simulators can reduce errors, maximize sensitivity in measuring the success of skills transfer, and improve the learning curve prior to undertaking real surgery.

Future studies with accurate learning curve evaluation measurements need to determine whether practice with these described simulators translates into changes in clinical practice, such as reduction of surgical time, complications, and length of hospitalization, with consequent benefits in patient care.

References

1. McGaghie WC, Issenberg SB, Barsuk JH, Wayne DB. A critical review of simulation-based mastery learning with translational outcomes. Med Educ. 2014;48:375–85.
2. Kavic MS. Simulators: a new use for an old paradigm. JSLS. 2006;10(3):281–3.
3. Thomas WEG. The making of a surgeon. Surgery. 2008;26:400–2.
4. Dutta S, Krummel TM. Simulation: a new frontier in surgical education. Adv Surg. 2006;40:249–63.
5. Franzese CB, Stringer SP. The evolution of surgical training: perspectives on educational models

from the past to the future. Otolaryngol Clin N Am. 2007;40:1227–35, vii.
6. Pugh CM, Watson A, Bell RH Jr, Brasel KJ, Jackson GP, Weber SM, Kao LS. Surgical education in the internet era. J Surg Res. 2009;156:177–82.
7. Richardson JD. Training of general surgical residents: what model is appropriate? Am J Surg. 2006;191:296–300.
8. Seymour NE, Gallagher AG, Roman S, O'Brien MK, Bansal VK, Andersen DK, Satava RM. Virtual reality training improves operating roomperformance: results of a randomized, double-blinded study. Ann Surg. 2002;236(4):458–63, discussion 463–4.
9. Dunnington G, Reisner L, Witzke D, Fulginiti J. Structured single-observer methods of evaluation for the assessment of ward performance on the surgical clerkship. Am J Surg. 1990;159:423–6.
10. Sloan DA, Donnelly MB, Johnson SB, Schwartz RW, Strodel WE. Use of an objective structured clinical examination (OSCE) to measure improvement in clinical competence during the surgical internship. Surgery. 1993;114:343–50.
11. Sloan DA, Donnelly MB, Schwartz RW, Strodel WE. The objective structured clinical examination. The new gold standard for evaluating postgraduate clinical performance. Ann Surg. 1995;222:735–42.
12. Committee on Quality of Health Care in America, Kohn LT, Corrigan JM, Donaldson MS. To err is human: building a safer heath system. Washington, DC: National Academy Press; 1999.
13. Satava RM. The future of surgical simulation and surgical robotics. Bull Am Coll Surg. 2007;92(3):13–9.
14. Satava R. Unmanned air vehicles (UAV) for vertical take-off and landing, such as helicopters and ducted-fan air vehicles. Courtesy Satava, Richard, and Public Sources; 2002.
15. Cohen AR, Lohani S, Manjila S, Natsupakpong S, Brown N, Cavusoglu MC. Virtual reality simulation: basic concepts and use in endoscopic neurosurgery training. Childs Nerv Syst. 2013;29(8):1235–44. https://doi.org/10.1007/s00381-013-2139-z.
16. Burt DE. Virtual reality in anaesthesia. Br J Anaesth. 1995;75:472–80.
17. Coelho G, Zanon N, Warf B. The role of simulation in neurosurgery. Childs Nerv Syst. 2014;30:1997–2000.
18. Hicdonmez T, Parsak T, Cobanoglu S. Simulation of surgery for craniosynostosis: a training model in a fresh cadaveric sheep cranium. Technical note. J Neurosurg. 2006;105(2 Suppl):150–2. https://doi.org/10.3171/ped.2006.105.2.150.
19. Coelho G, Warf B, Lyra M, Zanon N. Anatomical pediatric model for craniosynostosis surgical training. Childs Nerv Syst. 2014;30(12):2009–14.
20. Coelho G, Vieira E, Hinojosa J, Delye H. Realistic simulator for craniosynostosis endoscopic approach. Neurosurg Focus Video FOCVID. 2021;4(2).V2. https://thejns.org/video/view/journals/neurosurg-focus-video/4/2/article-pV2.xml. Accessed 29 Jan 2022.
21. Coelho G, Figueiredo EG, Rabelo NN, Teixeira MJ, Zanon N. Development and evaluation of a new pediatric mixed-reality model for neurosurgical training. J Neurosurg Pediatr. 2019;2:1–10.
22. Coelho G, Rabelo NN, Adani LB, Cecilio-Fernandes D, Souza Carvalho FR, Pinto FG, Zanon N, Teixeira MJ, Figueiredo EG. The Craniosynostosis puzzle: new simulation model for neurosurgical training. World Neurosurg. 2020;138:e299–304. https://doi.org/10.1016/j.wneu.2020.02.098. Epub 2020 Feb 25
23. Coelho G, Chaves TMF, Goes AF, Del Massa EC, Moraes O, Yoshida M. Multimaterial 3D printing preoperative planning for frontoethmoidal meningoencephalocele surgery. Childs Nerv Syst. 2018;34:749–56.
24. Wake N, Rosenkrantz AB, Huang R, Park KU, Wysock JS, Taneja SS, et al. Patient-specific 3D printed and augmented reality kidney and prostate cancer models: impact on patient education. 3D Print Med. 2019;5:4.
25. Meola A, Cutolo F, Carbone M, Cagnazzo F, Ferrari M, Ferrari V. Augmented reality in neurosurgery: a systematic review. Neurosurg Rev. 2017;40:537–48.
26. Rice DP. Craniofacial sutures. Development, disease and treatment. Front Oral Biol. 2008;12:xi.
27. Han W, Yang X, Wu S, Fan S, Chen X, Aung ZM, et al. A new method for cranial vault reconstruction: augmented reality in synostotic plagiocephaly surgery. J Craniomaxillofac Surg. 2019;47:1280–4.
28. López Cabrera MV, Valdez García JE. Virtual reality in residents training. Ann Eye Sci. 2019;4:27.
29. Coelho G, Rabelo NN, Vieira E, Mendes K, Zagatto G, Santos de Oliveira R, Raposo-Amaral CE, Yoshida M, de Souza MR, Fagundes CF, Teixeira MJ, Figueiredo EG. Augmented reality and physical hybrid model simulation for preoperative planning of metopic craniosynostosis surgery. Neurosurg Focus. 2020;48(3):E19. https://doi.org/10.3171/2019.12.FOCUS19854.
30. Ferenchick G, Simpson D, Blackman J, DaRosa D, Dunnington G. Strategies for efficient and effective teaching in the ambulatory care setting. Acad Med. 1997;72:277–80.
31. Zymberg ST, Vaz-Guimaraes Filho F, Lyra M. Neuroendoscopic training: presentation of a new real simulator. Minim Invasive Neurosurg. 2010;53:44–6.
32. Lehmann KS, Ritz JP, Maass H, Cakmak HK, Kuehnapfel UG, Germer CT, et al. A prospective randomized study to test the transfer of basic psychomotor skills from virtual reality to physical reality in a comparable training setting. Ann Surg. 2005;241:442–9.
33. Palter VN, Grantcharov T, Harvey A, Macrae HM. Ex vivo technical skills training transfers to the operating room and enhances cognitive learning: a randomized controlled trial. Ann Surg. 2011;253:886–9.

29 Craniosynostosis: Anesthetic Considerations—What the Pediatric Neurosurgeon Should Know

Margaret Ekstein, Jonathan Roth, and Shlomi Constantini

Craniosynostosis is a premature closure of the skull sutures and is categorized as either "single suture synostosis" (SSS) or "multi-suture synostosis" (MSS) [1, 2]. The majority of operated CS are SSS—relating to closure of the sagittal, or metopic sutures. The main effect of SSS is on the appearance of the child with potential secondary psychosocial effects; however, although debatable, some reports have stated long-term neurodevelopmental sequela. Increased intracranial pressure is uncommon in SSS, however it may occur too.

As opposed to SSS, multi-suture synostosis is often associated with syndromes such as Apert, Crouzon, Pfeiffer, and others. MSS impacts the child in many aspects, such as cosmetic and various neurological aspects: increased intracranial pressure is significantly more prevalent compared to SSS, and Chiari malformation and hydrocephalus may occur in about 30%. MSS often involves the skull base sutures, leading to micrognathia and retro-maxilla, affecting the midface and upper airway anatomy. Additionally, MSS may affect the venous outlets of the brain, often leading to large emissary veins and excessively developed and atypical subcutaneous venous pathways [1, 3–6].

Treatment for craniosynostosis is usually performed during the first year of life and sometimes even during the first few months of life [7]. Thus, awareness of the anesthetic—surgical interaction is crucial for ensuring safety during treatment.

29.1 Risk of Anesthesia in the Very Young Patient

Recent studies have found increased risk of complications associated with anesthesia early in life [8, 9]. This risk increases as the age of the child decreases [10]. There has also been a plethora of animal data and some human retrospective studies that suggest the possibility of neurotoxicity of anesthetic agents on the developing brain [11]. Recently, prospective randomized trials have found no negative consequences of general anesthetics on very young infants who received a single short anesthetic [12–14]. Anesthesia for craniosynostosis surgery is neither short nor without its own inherent risks, and we are as yet missing data regarding toxicity of anesthesia for craniosynostosis repair or neurocognitive impact of craniosynostosis itself, repaired or not [15].

M. Ekstein (✉)
Division of Anesthesiology, Intensive Care and Pain Medicine, Tel Aviv Sourasky Medical Center, Tel Aviv, Israel

J. Roth · S. Constantini
Department of Pediatric Neurosurgery, Dana Children's Hospital, Tel Aviv Sourasky Medical Center, Tel Aviv, Israel

F. Di Rocco, J. Kestle (eds.), *Neurosurgical Aspects of Craniosynostosis*,
https://doi.org/10.1007/978-3-031-69386-1_29

29.2 Preparation of the Patient

It is intuitive that preoperative optimization of associated medical conditions of an infant before craniosynostosis surgery will be protective. Surgery for SSS is nearly always elective. Thus, surgery should be postponed in a child with exacerbation of underlying pulmonary disease or a recent upper respiratory tract infection for about 2 weeks to avoid adverse respiratory events perioperatively [16]. Optimization includes pulmonary preparation with inhaled beta agonists and/or steroids or addition of systemic steroids in a child with known chronic lung disease. Since multi-suture synostosis is often part of a multi-organ system syndrome, further workup, including genetic testing, is advised. Syndromes associated with craniosynostosis are reviewed of Meier's recent review [17]. Associated anomalies that should be assessed preoperatively include whether there is midface hypoplasia (Apert's, Crouzon's, Pfeiffer) or whether there is an element of mandibular hypoplasia, or high arched palate with resultant risk of difficult intubation. In addition to anomalous facial features (ptosis, low set ears, hypertelorism, strabismus), there might be associated hearing loss, syndactyly, intellectual deficits in the case of Apert's syndrome; and cardiovascular anomalies, obesity, hypogonadism in the case of Carpenter's syndrome. Preoperative neurologic assessment is necessary for all syndromic patients, and cardiac evaluation is indicated if cardiovascular involvement is suspected. The anesthesiologist should review the full medical history by organ system and include: history of prior anesthetics, allergies, medications, presence of passive smoking, and fasting guidelines. Laboratory examination must include a full blood count, electrolytes including glucose and renal function, coagulation profile, and blood type and cross for transfusion.

29.3 Fasting Guidelines

It is acceptable to fast infants and children prior to general anesthesia or sedation in order to reduce the risk of pulmonary aspiration of gastric contents. The current European Society of Anesthesia and Intensive Care Guidelines recommends a 1-h fast from clear liquids defined as water, tea, juice without pulp, or carbonated drinks; a 3-h fast from breast milk; 4 h from cow's milk, formula and juice with pulp; and 6 h from solid food [18]. Prolonging fasting of clear liquids has negative consequences including risk of hypovolemia and hypoglycemia in small infants, as well as increase in infant irritability and reduced parental satisfaction. In the case of a delay in surgery, it is important to feed the baby sweet clear liquids if a 2-h delay is anticipated, or start intravenous fluid if start time is undetermined.

29.4 Preoperative Anxiety

If surgery involves infants up to 6 months of age, there is high level parental anxiety but not yet significant situational or separation anxiety in the infant. It is important to clearly discuss the procedures and expectations/alternatives of general anesthesia with the parents, answer all questions, and allay their fears. Separate informed consent for general anesthesia including blood transfusion must be obtained. The infant will be able to enter the operating room and undergo inhaled induction with simple distraction techniques to keep them calm. If the child is older than 6 months, it is helpful to administer anxiolysis. The most common anxiolytic agent is midazolam: syrup 0.5 mg–0.7 mg/kg, intranasal 0.2 mg/kg, or intramuscular 0.1 mg/kg. Other agents such as dexmedetomidine, ketamine, and brevital may be given for sedation. Narcotics and nonsteroidal medications can also be given preoperatively for preemptive analgesia [19]. Parental presence during induction of anesthesia is still controversial and depends on the preference of the particular anesthesiologist and individual evaluation of each patient and parent. If a parent is allowed to accompany their child, it is important to prepare the parent as to what to expect and what his/her role is while in the operating room and how he/she will be escorted outside as per the instructions of the anesthesiologist. There must be a staff member dedicated to care for the parent while in the operating room.

29.5 Preparation of the Operating Room

Before arrival to the operating room, the room should be warmed to 24 °C (75 °F), the bed and intravenous fluids should be warmed, and all equipment should be checked. A difficult airway cart should be available, as well as ultrasound for venous and arterial cannulation as needed. Two crossmatched units of packed red blood cells should be checked and available. If blood loss is expected to exceed half of the child's blood volume, fresh frozen plasma and platelets should be ordered from the blood bank and availability of Point of Care analysis of coagulation should be considered.

29.6 Anesthetic Management

29.6.1 Induction and Maintenance of Anesthesia

Standard induction is via inhaled agents: oxygen with or without nitrous oxide and sevoflurane. High concentrations of nitrous oxide are convenient at the start of induction as it is odorless, well tolerated, and promotes a good feeling. It can be used alone for 3 min prior to starting a potent halogenated agent to ease comfort with the mask without causing agitation. During surgery, however, it should be discontinued because of risk of air embolism and N_2O's physical properties which enlarge closed volumes of entrapped air. Once the child is under general anesthesia, intravenous access is obtained and balanced anesthesia follows with both inhaled and intravenous agents, including narcotics and muscle relaxants to ease airway instrumentation and positioning.

29.6.2 Intravenous Access

Two intravenous lines either 22 or 20 gauge comprise our standard practice. Arterial lines are necessary for all open procedures, but can be avoided in minimally invasive procedures in which blood loss is anticipated to be minimal. Ultrasound is often helpful in obtaining access in younger infants or in some in the higher weight percentiles. Central lines are reserved for children with difficult access or in those in whom the necessity of vasoactive agents is anticipated because of underlying cardiac disease [20].

29.6.3 Monitoring

American Society of Anesthesia standard monitoring of ECG, noninvasive blood pressure, pulse oximetry, and temperature is mandatory as well as monitoring of inhaled and exhaled gases. Urinary catheters are not placed routinely. During open craniosynostosis repair, an arterial line is indicated. It is used for beat-to-beat blood pressure assessment as well as for blood sampling; however, its most significant use is its sensitivity to assess fluid responsiveness. The respiratory variations in the arterial waveform, pulse pressure variation across the respiratory cycle, serve as a surrogate to predict the preload's role in augmenting blood pressure in mechanically ventilated patients.

29.6.4 Fluid Management

Goal-directed fluid therapy has evolved from adult intensive care and perioperative fluid management as the ideal way to guide fluid administration. Static variables such as central venous pressure or physical signs are unreliable as predictors of which patients will benefit from a fluid bolus. Dynamic variables based on the heart lung interaction are superior in assessing how fluid will impact stroke volume and cardiac output in ventilated patients [21, 22]. While recent literature supports the use of aortic velocity measurements by ultrasound [22], we use systolic pressure variation during acute hemorrhage occurring in these cases, due to its accessibility intraoperatively, to guide transfusion and crystalloid administration. Blood loss in these small patients is rapid and immediate replacement is necessary to avoid complications of reduced organ perfusion, even if it is transient. Isotonic crystalloids, either lactated ringer's solution or plasmalyte, should be used. Colloid solutions, such as third-generation hydroxyethyl starch (HES 130,000 Daltons) or albumin, may also be used [23]. While HES has been shown to increase risk of renal failure in adults in the intensive care unit, there is no renal dysfunction or effect on perioperative bleeding associated with HES in children at doses up to 20 cc/kg. Administration of HES in this dose has no effect on blood loss or transfusion perioperatively in children and is considered a safe option for restoring blood volume quickly during surgical hemorrhage [24].

29.6.5 Positioning

Proper positioning of the patient for cranial vault surgery is key to safe and effective repair. Sagittal synostosis repairs at early ages (up to about 5–6 months) are best performed in the prone, sphinx position which allows for a full view and access to the margins of craniectomy. Use of a vacuum-stiffened bean bag is standard for these cases [25]; other devices have also been described [26]. The neck is extended and the bed is placed in the reverse-Trendelenburg position. Careful attention must be made to the endotracheal tube (ETT) position as neck extension moves the endotracheal out to a more superficial position in the trachea. If the leak around the ETT increases, or a new leak is heard, repositioning of the ETT to a deeper position is necessary. Careful attention must be paid to the level of the head as compared to the heart, as risk of venous air embolism increases with higher differences between the surgical field and the right atrium. The arms are positioned alongside the body. Legs are positioned flexed with foam, lifting the feet as high as comfortable to promote venous return from the legs (Fig. 29.1). Careful padding with foam should be provided to prevent pressure sores during prolonged surgery. A foam cushion is placed under the buttock and taped to the bed as a slinged hammock to prevent the patient sliding downward in the reverse Trendelenburg position (see Fig. 29.1). Meticulous attention should be paid to eye protection, so no alcohol from the prep solution or debris from the field will touch the eyes. We suggest three layers of protection: first a layer of ophthalmologic ointment or lubricant on the corneas, then watertight dressing on each eye covering the eyebrows, and last a sticky drape which covers the face including the eyes and the tape fixing the ETT. Some surgeons suture the eyelids closed or place corneal protectors, but this is reserved for craniofacial procedures in which there is significant preoperative proptosis typically in syndromic craniosynostosis.

In anterior vault remodeling, the patient is positioned supine, with the head supported by a horseshoe head holder. The head is flexed. Again, careful attention must be paid to ETT position; flexing the neck will advance the ETT deeper into the trachea and might cause a one-lung intubation. Breath sounds must be auscultated in the final position. A foam cushion is placed under the buttock as described above and careful padding of the extremities is necessary. During anterior

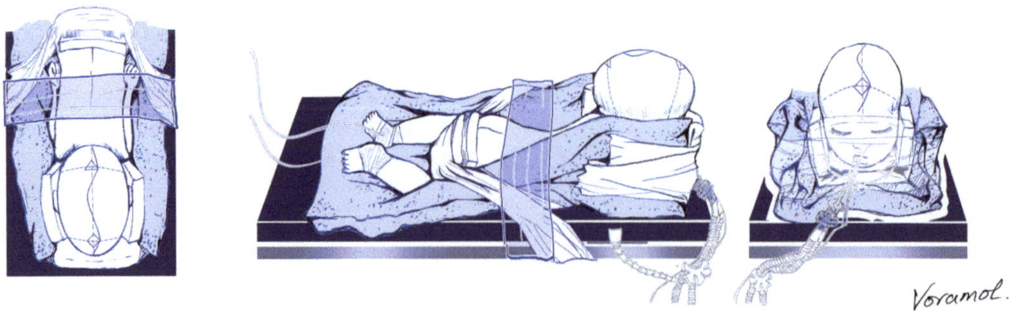

Fig. 29.1 Sketch of patient positioning for repair of saggital craniosynostosis

cranial remodeling, there is risk of extreme neck flexion which can kink the ETT; therefore, we place a foam collar under the neck to prevent exaggerated flexion. Heed the oculo-cardiac reflex during supraorbital bone reconstruction; pressure on the eyes may cause bradycardia which will resolve with cessation of eye pressure; rarely, it is necessary to treat with vagolytic drugs: atropine 0.02 mg/kg.

29.6.6 Venous Air Embolism

A number of factors make the risk of air embolism a particular concern during craniosynostosis surgery, especially when operating on syndromic craniosynostosis, in which emissary veins are more common. Positioning is aimed at reducing blood loss and enhancing surgical exposure to the cranial vault, thus the level of the operative field is often higher than the heart. Bony structures have venous channels (emissary veins) that do not collapse as other veins do. Thus, when exposing and cutting such venous channels, the atmospheric pressure may be higher at the level of the open vein than central venous pressure causing entrainment of air into the right atrium, rather than bleeding in the surgical field. Because of the size of the patient, a small amount of air entrained into the right ventricular outflow tract can cause hemodynamic collapse. Therefore, it is imperative that the surgeons and anesthesiologists monitor for such an event. Monitoring by doppler is most sensitive, but many find it to be overly sensitive, as very small air emboli, present in as much as 82% of craniosynostosis surgeries in one report [27], have no clinical consequence [28]. Large centers have found the incidence of clinically significant air embolism to be less than 5%, which is consistent with our experience, and are detected by acute decrease in end-tidal CO_2, decrease in blood pressure, decrease in oxygen saturation, change in ECG which indicates right ventricular strain, and abrupt increase in CVP after an initial decline.

To mitigate the risk of venous air embolism, it is best to be judicious with positioning, diligent in fluid resuscitation, consider use of positive end expiratory pressure (PEEP) to increase right atrial pressure, and avoid use of nitrous oxide. If venous air embolism is suspected, the surgeon should flood the surgical field with irrigation fluid, search for open venous channels, use bone wax or other hemostatic measures to occlude the entry to the venous system, lower the head of the bed to lower the surgical field to the height of the right atrium, and tilt the bed to the left to protect the right ventricular outflow tract [29]. It is ill-advised to turn the patient to the left lateral position as this might compromise sterility of the surgical field, inhibit effective chest compressions should they be necessary, and there is no evidence that the left lateral position has a protective hemodynamic effect [30]. Blood pressure should be supported with fluid and pressors if needed, increasing inhaled oxygen concentration to improve saturation. Aspiration of air from a central line is theoretically possible, but this author has found this strategy useful only in adults. Aspiration of air includes air with blood, which would worsen hypotension; aspirated blood would have to be returned after air removal which is quite cumbersome in a small child. Sealants should be used with caution as embolism has been described using an aerosolized fibrin sealant; if sealants are used, it's preferable not to deliver with a pressurized delivery device, rather inject sealant using a manual syringe injection [31].

29.7 Blood Transfusion and Conservation Strategies

Open craniosynostosis surgery (as opposed to endoscopic surgery) is associated with significant blood loss. Intraoperative blood loss varies significantly between series and has been reported to be as high as 119 mL/kg [32]. Several factors are associated with increased blood volume loss: length of surgery, young age, lower weight, and the cranial suture related to repair [33, 34]. As a result of the significant intraoperative hemorrhage, transfusion with allogeneic blood products is often necessary during open surgery. According to the pediatric craniofacial surgery perioperative registry, 95% of children younger than 24 months and 79% of older children received transfusions of red blood cells during craniosynostosis surgery. Thirty percent of the younger group received 40 cc/kg of blood, representing 50% of their volume and thus were considered massive transfusion patients [35]. Extent of hemorrhage and transfusion volume is associated with perioperative morbidity. Associated complications include metabolic acidosis, hyperkalemia, hypocalcemia, coagulopathy, hypothermia, hypoxia, and pulmonary complications, venous air embolism, hypotension, bradycardia, and cardiac arrest, as well as longer hospital length of stay [36]. Exposure to allogenic blood is also associated with risks of immunologic and non-immunologic patient reactions, and in the setting of massive blood transfusion, causes coagulopathy and further requirements of blood products transfusion; hence, the stimulus to initiate blood conservation strategies in this population. Minimally invasive endoscopic surgery for craniosynostosis is associated with a significant reduction in blood loss and transfusion [37]. A recent review of 121 endoscopic strip craniectomies (of which 116 were for single suture craniosynostosis) reported intraoperative blood loss to be 5.7 cc/kg; and transfusion rate 21%; intensive care was not needed and hospital stay was a mean of 2.6 days [38]. Analysis of data from the Pediatric Craniofacial Surgery Perioperative Registry of North America compared endoscopic to open craniosynostosis repair. Propensity score matching was used to normalize the inherent age and weight difference in the groups and found that packed red blood cells were given in 26% of endoscopic vs. 81% of open surgeries, coagulation factors in 3% vs. 16%. Adverse events such as hypotension requiring pressors, venous air embolism, hypothermia, and cardiac arrest were not different; however, need for postoperative intubation, intensive care admission, and length of hospital stay were all greater in the open surgery group [39]. Length of surgery was significantly longer, which plays a significant role in blood loss and transfusion volume needed in craniosynostosis surgery [40]. In open procedures, injection of local anesthetic with epinephrine intradermally, use of needle-tip monopolar cautery and Raney clips for skin incision, liberal use of bone wax during osteotomies, and use of appropriate hemostatic agents all minimize surgical bleeding [41]. Other strategies include administration of preoperative oral iron supplements with or without erythropoietin 600–1000 units subcutaneously once a week for 3 weeks prior to surgery to maximize preoperative hemoglobin and hypervolemic hemodilution with infusion of crystalloid solution 20 cc/kg before starting osteotomies [42]. Cell saver may be used but has not been shown to be cost-effective [43]. Landmark randomized prospective trials demonstrated effectiveness of tranexamic acid in reducing blood loss and transfusion during craniosynostosis surgery [32, 44]. Tranexamic acid is an antifibrinolytic agent which depresses the transformation of plasminogen to plasmin, thereby inhibiting binding of plasmin to fibrin clots and reducing clot lysis. The dose of TXA is still debated and ranges from 10 to 20 mg/kg bolus at the beginning of surgery with or without a continuous infusion of 3–10 mg/kg/h [44–46]. Finally, initiation of an institutional protocol using transfusion algorithms has been shown to be effective in reducing blood transfusion during craniosynostosis surgery [41, 47]. Management by a dedicated team of anesthesiologists has also been associated with lower transfusion volume and blood donor exposures [48]. Administration of fresh frozen plasma, platelets, and cryoprecipitate should be guided by laboratory testing as well as thromboelastography (TEG) or other point of care analysis of clot formation [49, 50].

29.8 Postoperative Analgesia

Open craniosynostosis surgery is associated with moderate to severe pain; inadequate pain management is not uncommon in the first 48 h [51]. Multimodal analgesia is recommended [52]. Regional analgesia with a scalp block is an option. This block has been used to blunt response to head pins [53] as well as part of a general anesthetic in children during neurosurgery and other procedures of the head [54]. Local anesthesia, 0.125% levobupivacaine, is infiltrated in multiple sites to target the nerves that innervate the scalp: the supraorbital and supratrochlear nerves as they emerge from the orbit; the auriculotemporal and greater auricular nerves near the ear; the zygomaticotemporal nerve near the zygomatic arch; and the greater, lesser, and third occipital nerves between the inion and the mastoid process posteriorly [53, 54]. The scalp block offers superior pain control in the immediate postoperative period and earlier resumption of feeding compared to morphine alone [54], but not when compared to local anesthesia infiltration [55]. Local anesthesia infiltration with bupivacaine and epinephrine, to reduce scalp bleeding, is our preferred technique. Opioids are necessary for adequate pain control initially. Intravenous morphine is used in boluses of 0.05 mg/kg as needed for the first 24 h, then changed to oral narcotics such as oxycodone 0.2 mg/kg. Adjuvant agents including nonsteroidal anti-inflammatory drugs are given to reduce narcotic requirements and associated adverse events. Ibuprofen 10 mg/kg syrup is given before induction in children older than 3 months and is safe as long as the infant is well-hydrated [56]. Intravenous acetaminophen10-15 mg/kg or dipyrone 10 mg/kg is administered with wound closure [57], and acetaminophen is continued around the clock every 6 h. Intravenous ketorolac 0.5–1 mg/kg every 12 h can also be used and has been shown to have no impact on postoperative bleeding while reducing opioid consumption after cranial vault remodeling [58]. The FLACC pain scale (five categories of Face, Leg movement, Activity, Crying and Consolability each scored between 0 and 2 per for a total score of 0 = no pain to a maximum of 10 = worst pain) is convenient and relevant for the age of craniosynostosis repair, or another pediatric pain scale should be used to guide titration of analgesia. A score of 4 or greater is a trigger for treatment with analgesics.

References

1. Sawh-Martinez R, Steinbacher DM. Syndromic craniosynostosis. Clin Plast Surg. 2019;46(2):141–55.
2. Dempsey RF, Monson LA, Maricevich RS, Truong TA, Olarunnipa S, Lam SK, Dauser RC, Hollier LH, Buchanan EP. Nonsyndromic craniosynostosis. Clin Plast Surg. 2019;46(2):123–39.
3. Frassanito P, Palombi D, Tamburrini G. Craniosynostosis and hydrocephalus: relevance and treatment modalities. Childs Nerv Syst. 2021;37:3465.
4. Coll G, El Ouadih Y, Abed Rabbo F, Gecko V, Sakka L, Di Rocco F. Hydrocephalus and Chiari malformation pathophysiology in FGFR2-related faciocraniosynostosis: a review. Neurochirurgie. 2019;65(5):264–8.
5. Copeland AE, Hoffman CE, Tsitouras V, Jeevan DS, Ho ES, Drake JM, Forrest CR. Clinical significance of venous anomalies in syndromic craniosynostosis. Plast Reconstr Surg - Glob Open. 2018;6(1):1–10.
6. Venkat Raman V, de Beer D. Perioperative airway complications in infants and children with Crouzon and Pfeiffer syndromes: a single-center experience. Paediatr Anaesth. 2021;31:1316–24.
7. Proctor MR, Meara JG. A review of the management of single-suture craniosynostosis, past, present, and future. J Neurosurg Pediatr. 2019;24(6):622–31.
8. Habre W, Disma N, Virag K, Becke K, Hansen TG, Jöhr M, Leva B, Morton NS, Vermeulen PM, Zielinska M, Boda K, Veyckemans F, Klimscha W, Konecny R, Luntzer R, Morawk-Wintersperger U, Neiger F, Rustemeyer L, Breschan C, et al. Incidence of severe critical events in paediatric anaesthesia (APRICOT): a prospective multicentre observational study in 261 hospitals in Europe. Lancet Respir Med. 2017;5(5):412–25.
9. McCann ME, Soriano SG. Does general anesthesia affect neurodevelopment in infants and children? BMJ. 2019;367:1–12.
10. Disma N, Leva B, Dowell J, Veyckemans F, Habre W. Assessing anaesthesia practice in the vulnerable age group: NECTARINE. Eur J Anaesthesiol. 2016;33(4):233–5.
11. Jevtovic-Todorovic V. Exposure of developing brain to general anesthesia: what is the animal evidence? Anesthesiology. 2018;128(4):832–9.
12. Orser BA, Suresh S, Evers AS. SmartTots update regarding anesthetic neurotoxicity in the developing brain. Anesth Analg. 2018;126(4):1393–6.
13. Ing C, Hegarty MK, Perkins JW, Whitehouse AJO, Dimaggio CJ, Sun M, Andrews H, Li G, Sun LS, Von Ungern-Sternberg BS. Duration of general anaesthetic exposure in early childhood and long-term language and cognitive ability. Br J Anaesth. 2017;119(3):532–40.
14. McCann ME, Berde C, Soriano S, Marmor J, Bellinger D, de Graaff JC, de Graaff JC, Dorris L,

Bell G, Morton N, Dorris L, Morton N, Disma N, Giribaldi G, Withington D, Withington D, Grobler A, Stargatt R, Hunt RW, et al. Neurodevelopmental outcome at 5 years of age after general anaesthesia or awake-regional anaesthesia in infancy (GAS): an international, multicentre, randomised, controlled equivalence trial. Lancet. 2019;393(10172):664–77.
15. Speltz ML, Kapp-Simon K, Collett B, Keich Y, Gaither R, Cradock MM, Buono L, Cunningham ML. Neurodevelopment of infants with single-suture craniosynostosis: presurgery comparisons with case-matched controls. Plast Reconstr Surg. 2007;119(6):1874–81.
16. Regli A, Becke K, Von Ungern-Sternberg BS. An update on the perioperative management of children with upper respiratory tract infections. Curr Opin Anaesthesiol. 2017;30(3):362–7.
17. Meier N. Anesthetic considerations for pediatric craniofacial surgery. Anesthesiol Clin. 2021;39(1):53–70.
18. Frykholm P, Disma N, Andersson H, Beck C, Bouvet L, Cercueil E, Elliott E, Hofmann J, Isserman R, Klaucane A, Kuhn F, de Queiroz SM, Rosen D, Rudolph D, Alexander R, Schmidt AS, Stocki D, Sümpelmann R, Stricker PA, Thomas M, Veyckemans F, Afshari A. Pre-operative fasting in children: a guideline from the European Society of Anaesthesiology and Intensive Care. Eur J Anaesthesiol. 2022;39(1):4–25.
19. Cote JC, Jerrold L, Anderson BJ. A practice of pediatric anesthesia for infants and children. 6th ed. Elsevier; 2019. p. 203–24.
20. Bergmans B, Kammeraad JAE, Van Adrichem LNA, Staals LM. Craniosynostosis surgery in an infant with a complex cyanotic cardiac defect. Paediatr Anaesth. 2014;24(7):788–90.
21. Desgranges FP, Desebbe O, Pereira de Souza Neto E, Raphael D, Chassard D. Respiratory variation in aortic blood flow peak velocity to predict fluid responsiveness in mechanically ventilated children: a systematic review and meta-analysis. Paediatr Anaesth. 2016;89:37–47.
22. Morparia KG, Reddy SK, Olivieri LJ, Spaeder MC, Schuette JJ. Respiratory variation in peak aortic velocity accurately predicts fluid responsiveness in children undergoing neurosurgery under general anesthesia. J Clin Monit Comput. 2018;32(2):221–6.
23. Sümpelmann R, Becke K, Zander R, Witt L. Perioperative fluid management in children: can we sum it all up now. Curr Opin Anaesthesiol. 2019;32(3):384–91.
24. Thy M, Montmayeur J, Julien-Marsollier F, Michelet D, Brasher C, Dahmani S, Orliaguet G. Safety and efficacy of peri-operative administration of hydroxyethyl starch in children undergoing surgery. Eur J Anaesthesiol. 2018;35(7):484–95.
25. Park TS, Broaddus WC, Harris M, Persing JA, Jane JA. Vacuum-stiffened beanbag for cranial remodeling procedures in modified prone position. J Neurosurg. 1989;71:623–5.
26. Gander T, Metzler P, Jacobsen C. Simple and safe head positioning device for repair of craniosynostosis with the patient prone. Br J Oral Maxillofac Surg. 2013;51:981–2.
27. Faberowski LW, Black S, Mickle JP. Incidence of venous air embolism during craniectomy for craniosynostosis repair. Anesthesiology. 2000;92(1):20–3.
28. Meyer P, Renier D, Orliaguet G, Blanot S, Carli P. Venous air embolism in craniosynostosis surgery: what do we want to detect? Anesthesiology. 2000;93(4):1157.
29. Adetayo OA, Haider S, Adamo MA, Ehlers MA. Craniosynostosis reconstruction in patients with cyanotic heart defects—risk factors for venous air embolism and overview of preventative strategies. Paediatr Anaesth. 2015;25(7):754–5.
30. Simon G. Management of venous air embolism. Anesth Analg. 2014;119(1):215.
31. Felema GG, Bryskin RB, Heger IM, Saswata R. Venous air embolism from Tisseel use during endoscopic cranial vault remodeling for craniosynostosis repair: a case report. Paediatr Anaesth. 2013;23(8):754–6.
32. Goobie SM, Meier PM, Pereira LM, McGowan FX, Prescilla RP, Scharp LA, Rogers GF, Proctor MR, Meara JG, Soriano SG, Zurakowski D, Sethna NF. Efficacy of tranexamic acid in pediatric craniosynostosis surgery: a double-blind, placebo-controlled trial. Anesthesiology. 2011;114:862.
33. Van Uitert A, Megens JHAM, Breugem CC, Stubenitsky BM, Sen HK, De Graaff JC. Factors influencing blood loss and allogeneic blood transfusion practice in craniosynostosis surgery. Paediatr Anaesth. 2011;21(12):1192–7.
34. Lopez MM, Lee J, Morrison K, Hoffman C, Souweidane M, Ascherman JA. Calculated blood loss and transfusion requirements in primary open repair of craniosynostosis. Plast Reconstr Surg - Glob Open. 2019;7(2):1–5.
35. Stricker PA, Goobie SM, Cladis FP, Haberkern CM, Meier PM, Reddy SK, Nguyen TT, Cai L, Polansky M, Szmuk P. Perioperative outcomes and management in pediatric complex cranial vault reconstruction: a multicenter study from the Pediatric Craniofacial Collaborative Group. Anesthesiology. 2017;126(2):276–87.
36. Stricker PA, Shaw TL, Desouza DG, Hernandez SV, Bartlett SP, Friedman DF, Sesok-Pizzini DA, Jobes DR. Blood loss, replacement, and associated morbidity in infants and children undergoing craniofacial surgery. Paediatr Anaesth. 2010;20(2):150–9.
37. Riordan CP, Zurakowski D, Meier PM, Alexopoulos G, Meara JG, Proctor MR, Goobie SM. Minimally invasive endoscopic surgery for infantile craniosynostosis: a longitudinal cohort study. J Pediatr. 2020;216:142–149.e2.
38. Arts S, Delye H, van Lindert EJ, Blok L, Borstlap W, Driessen J. Evaluation of anesthesia in endoscopic strip craniectomy: a review of 121 patients. Paediatr Anaesth. 2018;126(3):968–75.
39. Thompson DR, Zurakowski D, Haberkern CM, Stricker PA, Meier PM, Bannister C, Benzon H,

Binstock W, Bosenberg A, Brzenski A, Budac S, Busso V, Capehart S, Chiao F, Cladis F, Collins M, Cusick J, Dabek R, Dalesio N, et al. Endoscopic versus open repair for craniosynostosis in infants using propensity score matching to compare outcomes. Anesth Analg. 2018;126(3):968–75.
40. Hall BR, Barrientos S, Flores LE, Cemaj S, Kugler J, Miller JJ. Perioperative management and factors associated with transfusion in cranial vault reconstruction. J Craniofac Surg. 2019;30:2014.
41. White N, Bayliss S, Moore D. Systematic review of interventions for minimizing perioperative blood transfusion for surgery for craniosynostosis. J Craniofac Surg. 2015;26(1):26–36.
42. Wood RJ, Stewart CN, Liljeberg K, Sylvanus TS, Lim PK. Transfusion-free cranial vault remodeling: a novel, multifaceted approach. Plast Reconstr Surg. 2020;145(1):167–74.
43. Krajewski K, Ashley RK, Pung N, Wald S, Lazareff J, Kawamoto HK, Bradley JP. Successful blood conservation during craniosynostotic correction with dual therapy using procrit and cell saver. J Craniofac Surg. 2008;19(1):101–5.
44. Dadure C, Sauter M, Bringuier S, Bigorre M, Raux O, Rochette A, Canaud N, Capdevila X. Intraoperative tranexamic acid reduces blood transfusion in children undergoing craniosynostosis surgery: a randomized double-blind study. Anesthesiology. 2011;114(4):856–61.
45. Fenger-Eriksen C, D'Amore Lindholm A, Nørholt SE, von Oettingen G, Tarpgaard M, Krogh L, Juul N, Hvas AM, Rasmussen M. Reduced perioperative blood loss in children undergoing craniosynostosis surgery using prolonged tranexamic acid infusion: a randomised trial. Br J Anaesth. 2019;122(6):760–6.
46. Goobie SM, Staffa SJ, Meara JG, Proctor MR, Tumolo M, Cangemi G, Disma N. High-dose versus low-dose tranexamic acid for paediatric craniosynostosis surgery: a double-blind randomised controlled non-inferiority trial. Br J Anaesth. 2020;125:336.
47. Kurlander DE, Ascha M, Marshall DC, Wang D, Ascha MS, Tripi PA, Reeves HM, Downes KA, Ahuja S, Rotta AT, Lakin GE, Tomei KL. Impact of multidisciplinary engagement in a quality improvement blood conservation protocol for craniosynostosis. J Neurosurg Pediatr. 2020;26(4):406–14.
48. Reddy SK, Patel RS, Rogers GF, Gordish-Dressman H, Keating RF, Pestieau SR. Intraoperative management by a craniofacial team anesthesiologist is associated with improved outcomes for children undergoing major craniofacial reconstructive surgery. J Craniofac Surg. 2019;30:418.
49. Haas T, Goobie S, Spielmann N, Weiss M, Schmugge M. Improvements in patient blood management for pediatric craniosynostosis surgery using a ROTEM®-assisted strategy—feasibility and costs. Paediatr Anaesth. 2014;24:774.
50. Nguyen TT, Hill S, Austin TM, Whitney GM, Wellons JC, Lam HV. Use of blood-sparing surgical techniques and transfusion algorithms: association with decreased blood administration in children undergoing primary open craniosynostosis repair. J Neurosurg Pediatr. 2015;16(5):556–63.
51. Kattail D, Macmillan A, Musavi L, Pedreira R, Faateh M, Cho R, Lopez J, Dorafshar AH. Pain management for nonsyndromic craniosynostosis: adequate analgesia in a pediatric cohort? J Craniofac Surg. 2018;29:1148.
52. Brown S, Yao A, Sanati-Mehrizy P, Zackai SP, Taub PJ. Postoperative pain management following craniosynostosis repair: current practices and future directions. J Craniofac Surg. 2019;30:721.
53. Prough DS, Pinosky ML, Fishman RL, Reeves ST, Patel S, Palesch Y, Dorman BH, Harvey SC. Skull block on the hemodynamic. Anesth Analg. 1996;83:1256–61.
54. Festa R, Tosi F, Pusateri A, Mensi S, Garra R, Mancino A, Frassanito P, Rossi M. The scalp block for postoperative pain control in craniosynostosis surgery: a case control study. Childs Nerv Syst. 2020;36:3063.
55. Cercueil E, Migeon A, Desgranges FP, Chassard D, Bouvet L. Postoperative analgesia for craniosynostosis reconstruction: scalp nerve block or local anesthetic infiltration? Paediatr Anaesth. 2018;28:474
56. Ziesenitz VC, Zutter A, Erb TO, van den Anker JN. Efficacy and safety of ibuprofen in infants aged between 3 and 6 months. Pediatr Drugs. 2017;19:277.
57. Sümpelmann R, Fieler M, Eich C, Becke K, Badelt G, Leimkühler K, Dennhardt N. Metamizole for postoperative pain therapy in infants younger than 1 year. Eur J Pediatr Surg. 2017;27(3):269–73.
58. Tuncer F, Knackstedt R, Murthy A, Patel N. Postoperative ketorolac administration is not associated with hemorrhage in cranial vault remodeling for craniosynostosis. Plast Reconstr Surg - Glob Open. 2019;7:e2401.

Hemostasis and Transfusion in Craniosynostoses Surgery

30

Martina Messing-Jünger

Craniosynostosis correction is associated with a high risk of significant perioperative blood loss, which is responsible for the majority of complications. Most of the patients are young infants with small blood volume and physiological anemia, e.g., in preterm babies [1]. Several strategies to minimize blood loss are available and a variety of clinical protocols for the reduction of transfusion rates exist. Beside patient age and body volume, the extent of the surgical approach and the operative time are important factors influencing blood loss and transfusion rate [2, 3]. Significant blood loss also causes coagulopathy, which must be avoided as well [4]. In the following chapter, techniques and strategies to reduce blood loss in craniofacial surgery are discussed.

30.1 Preoperative Measures

A child's preoperative hemoglobin and coagulation parameters play an important role for the entire perioperative course in craniosynostosis surgery. In former times, a prophylactic blood transfusion with or without plasma substitution was often the only strategy to reduce severe complications following significant blood loss in this patient group with physiologically low hematocrit and hemoglobin values. In these cases, preoperative erythropoietin (EPO) and/or ferrous sulfate [5–8] administration elevates hematocrit and hemoglobin values and reduces the blood transfusion rate. Abnormal coagulation parameters must be corrected before surgery in any elective craniosynostosis repair.

30.2 Surgical Technique

The surgical technique plays an important role for the prevention of excessive blood loss. Skin and galea are well vascularized and local administration of a lidocain/epinephrine-solution (up to 20 mL of 0.25% lidocaine with 1:400,000) at the incision site can reduce uncontrolled oozing from skin edges [8]. Skin incision with a Colorado needle tip may also help to control unnecessary bleeding. The application of Raney clips is not advisable due to the thin and soft skin in infants. Small curved clamps can also be used for a temporary hemostasis of the galea.

Subperiostal dissection is performed in most craniofacial surgeries, but sometimes causes excessive bleeding from bony perforator vessels. Subgaleal dissection can help to reduce blood loss, e.g., in fronto-orbital advancement [9].

The deflected galea flap may be covered by hydrogen peroxide-soaked gauzes, which control blood ooze from the tissue during exposure.

M. Messing-Jünger (✉)
Pediatric Neurosurgery Department, Asklepios Children's Hospital, Sankt Augustin, Germany
e-mail: m.messing@asklepios.com

F. Di Rocco, J. Kestle (eds.), *Neurosurgical Aspects of Craniosynostosis*,
https://doi.org/10.1007/978-3-031-69386-1_30

The infantile skull bone, although very thin, is an important site of hematopoiesis and very well perfused. The blood loss from bone edges can be significant and sealing is important. Bone wax should not be used since it causes bone defects and bears the risk of late infections. Gel foam is a good hemostatic material and facilitates bone regeneration.

Oozing from dural sinuses is frequent as well and it is advisable to cover them with gel foam or oxidized regenerated cellulose (ORC). Gel foam and ORC are well-established hemostyptic agents in neurosurgery. Both materials will be fully resorbed and rarely cause late effects. A variety of new hemostyptic products are available, but a careful consideration of possible complications is recommended.

One of the most important blood saving factors is a short operative time [2]. Craniofacial procedures should be performed by an experienced team only in order to keep the exposure time as short as possible. Minimal invasive procedures can reduce the need for blood transfusion significantly, not only due to less soft tissue and bone manipulation, but also due to a short operative time and should be offered to patients as often as feasible. In their prospective observational study, Shah et al. (2011) compared open vault reconstruction with endoscopic strip craniectomy in sagittal synostosis. The mean operating time for the endoscopic procedure was 88 min versus 179 min for the open surgery and mean blood loss 29 mL versus 218 mL, respectively. Only 6.4% endoscopy cases underwent transfusion, whereas all patients with open procedures needed transfusion [10].

The use of specific bone cutting tools does not seem to influence the amount of blood loss. The time of the bone incision and the subsequent sealing of the bleeding edges or the adjacent tissues is of importance [11].

The benefit of wound drainages in craniofacial surgery is unclear. On one side, they may reduce postoperative swelling, on the other side increased postoperative blood loss and infections are possible associated complications [12].

30.3 Anesthesia Management

The anesthesia management is decisive for a good outcome in any craniosynostosis surgery. The most important task is the prevention of a potentially life threatening hypovolemia and anemia and to avoid coagulopathy and a high expertise is an important prerequisite.

Several protocols to prevent hypovolemia and reduce blood transfusion exist. In a systematic review, White et al. (2015) evaluated 18 studies; 14 were case series with controls and only four randomized controlled trials. Several relevant aspects remained unaddressed in the available studies. The use of erythropoietin and tranexamic acid is well studied. Less evidence exists regarding cell saver, acute normovolemic hemodilution, and aprotinin. Preoperative autologous donation and ε-aminocaproic acid were not investigated. The administration of tranexamic acid is clinically effective in reducing allogeneic blood transfusion. Also, cell saver use and EPO show a clinical effect [13].

The Children's Hospital of Richmond protocol includes preoperative administration of recombinant EPO until a preoperative hemoglobin of 15 g/dL was reached, intraoperative autologous blood recycling using small bowls of 30 or 55 mL and accepting a transfusion trigger of ≤7 g/dL hemoglobin. These measures significantly decreased the transfusion rate ($p < 0.001$) [14].

The Vancouver group published their 10-year experience of all consecutive cases during this period. The acceptance of a transfusion threshold of 6 g/dL hemoglobin in hemodynamically stable patients led to an overall low transfusion rate of 24% (28% in redo cases). Seventy five percent of transfusions occurred intraoperatively, 21% postoperatively, and 4% intra- and postoperatively [15].

The Pediatric Craniofacial Collaborative Group (PCCG) analyzed 935 children ≤24 months of age with craniosynostosis and found that the likelihood of a perioperative transfusion was 95%. The mean volume of erythrocyte containing blood products transfused intraoperatively for infants was 37.3 ± 26.2 mL/

kg, and the mean volume transfused postoperatively was 16.7 ± 9.3 mL/kg [16]. Beethe et al. (2020) started a quality improvement initiative for reducing the transfusion rate in craniosynostosis patients below 2 years of age and were able to reduce a 100% into a final overall allogeneic transfusion rate of 22.7% at their institution. The following precautions were part of the protocol: Before skin incision, a 20 mL/kg bolus of crystalloid and a tranexamic acid (TXA) bolus of 12.5 mg/kg were administered. Skin incision was performed after administration of up to 20 mL of 0.25% lidocaine with 1:400,000 epinephrine. A close communication between anesthetists, surgeons, and nurses guaranteed permanent information on bleeding status, laboratory values, and vital parameters and ensured timely measures. In order to maintain normovolemic conditions, a total crystalloid administration of 30 up to 100 mL/kg was necessary. Cell saver was used for all patients with a minimum of 25 mL returning to the patient. Perioperative hypothermia has been avoided using air warmers or warm blankets and increasing the operating room temperature up to 22 °C. The intra- and postoperative transfusion threshold was set at 7 g/dL under stable hemodynamics [8].

Escher et al. (2021) compared 21 patients without preoperative EPO and iron administration and perioperative TXA with 15 patients who received both treatments (study group). There were no significant differences between groups in demographics, operative time, intraoperative crystalloid volume, craniofacial syndromes, or sutures affected. Preoperative Hb (13.9 ± 1.0 vs. 12.6 ± 0.8 g/dL, $p < 0.001$) was higher and intraoperative Hb nadir (7.4 ± 1.8 vs. 9.2 ± 1.2 g/dL) lower in the study group. The intraoperative transfusion rate dropped to 66.7% compared to 100% in the control group ($p = 0.008$). The postoperative transfusion rate was 0% versus 28.6% in the control group ($p = 0.03$). The amount of packed red blood cells units dropped as well (0.7 ± 0.6 vs. 1.5 ± 0.9 units) [5].

A randomised trial investigated the usefulness of prolonged TXA administration in craniosynostosis surgery [17]. The children received either TXA (bolus dose of 10 mL kg^{1} injected before surgical incision, followed by 8 h continuous infusion of 3 mL kg^{1} h^{1}). Total blood loss dropped from a mean of 52 mL kg^{1} to 28 mL kg^{1} ($P < 0.001$). Intraoperative red blood cell (RBC) were reduced in the treatment group from 14.0 mL kg^{1} to 8.2 mL kg^{1} and FFP from 13.0 mL kg^{1} to 7.8 mL kg^{1} [17].

In a retrospective international multicenter study, the Pediatric Craniofacial Collaborative Group (PCCG) analyzed a total of 6583 patients, who had open craniofacial surgery either without antifibrinolytic treatment or with TXA or ε-aminocaproic acid and compared seizure rates. The overall seizure rate was 0.24%, with 0.20% in the no antifibrinolytic group, 0.22% in the TXA-group, and 0.44% in the ε-aminocaproic acid group. These results prove the safety of TXA [18].

Krajewski et al. (2008) investigated the benefit of a blood conserving therapy with preoperative Procrit (eopoetin alpha) together with an intraoperative cell saver and found a significant reduction of transfusion rates. In the study group, transfusion rates were 5% versus 100% in the control group. The volumes transfused were lower as well (0.05 versus 1.74 pediatric units). The study group received recombinant human erythropoietin at 3 weeks, 2 weeks, and 1 week preoperatively resulting in a preoperative hematocrit of 36.2%. Eighty percent of patients in the study group received cell saver blood [19].

Aprotinin, a pancreatic trypsin inhibitor with antifibrinolytic activity, has also been tested in craniofacial surgery. Blood loss was lower under aprotinin treatment with 3.9% of circulating blood volume versus 22.0% resulting in a transfusion rate of 0% versus 21.1%. No allergic or other possible aprotinin-specific complications were observed [20].

Another study addressed the administration of fresh frozen plasma (FFP). Prophylactic versus reactive FFP transfusion has been compared. The prophylactic group received a significantly greater average volume of FFP compared to the reactive group (29.7 mL kg^{1} versus 16.1 mL kg^{1}; $p < 0.001$). Coagulation parameters improved similarly; however, there was no difference in blood transfusion requirements or blood loss between the two groups [21].

Excessive packed red blood cells (PRBC) transfusion to maintain target hematocrit can result in coagulopathy from coagulation factor depletion when hemorrhage approaches 1.5 times estimated blood volume. Perioperative monitoring of coagulation parameters is as important as hemoglobin and hematocrit assessment [4].

Substitution of human fibrinogen concentrate is also able to improve blood coagulation in craniofacial surgery in the case of massive blood loss and necessary intravascular volume therapy avoiding the need for FFP or platelets transfusion. However, no comparative or controlled studies exist so far [22].

30.4 Postoperative Care

During the postoperative surveillance, regular hemoglobin, hematocrit, platelet, and coagulation parameter controls are indispensable, since postoperative blood count and coagulation changes are often seen after craniofacial surgery. In general, a transfusion threshold of ≤7 g/mL hemoglobin under stable hemodynamics is recommended, although lower hemoglobin values may be tolerated in selected and well-controlled patients [15]. Thorough wound and eventual drainage controls by the surgeon are important as well in order to detect any postoperative bleeding complications.

30.5 Summary

Craniosynostosis surgery is associated with a high risk of excessive blood loss and meticulous hemostasis during surgery as well as a variety of precautions already starting before hospital admission can help to minimize the need for blood transfusion. The usefulness of protocols or standard operating procedures (SOP) with the aim to reduce blood loss and transfusion rates has been proven in several studies and the implementation of such a protocol in any institution treating children with craniosynostoses is strongly recommended.

References

1. Widness JA. Pathophysiology of anemia during the neonatal period, including anemia of prematurity. NeoReviews. 2008;9(11):e520–5.
2. Chocron Y, Azzi AJ, Galli R, Alnaif N, Atkinson J, Dudley R, u. a. Operative time as the predominant risk factor for transfusion requirements in nonsyndromic Craniosynostosis repair. Plast Reconstr Surg - Glob Open. 2020;8(1):e2592.
3. Barone CM, Jimenez DF. Endoscopic craniectomy for early correction of craniosynostosis. Plast Reconstr Surg. 1999;104(7):1965–73.
4. Williams GD, Ellenbogen RG, Gruss JS. Abnormal coagulation during pediatric craniofacial surgery. Pediatr Neurosurg. 2001;35(1):5–12.
5. Escher PJ, Tu AD, Kearney SL, Linabery AM, Petronio JA, Kebriaei MA, u. a. A protocol of situation-dependent transfusion, erythropoietin and tranexamic acid reduces transfusion in fronto- orbital advancement for metopic and coronal craniosynostosis. Childs Nerv Syst. 2021;37(1):269–76.
6. Escher PJ, Tu A, Kearney S, Wheelwright M, Petronio J, Kebriaei M, et al. Minimizing transfusion in sagittal craniosynostosis surgery: the Children's Hospital of Minnesota Protocol. Childs Nerv Syst. 2019;35(8):1357–62.
7. Aljaaly HA, Aldekhayel SA, Diaz-Abele J, Karunanayka M, Gilardino MS. Effect of erythropoietin on transfusion requirements for craniosynostosis surgery in children. J Craniofac Surg. 2017;28(5):1315–9.
8. Beethe AB, Spitznagel RA, Kugler JA, Goeller JK, Franzen MH, Hamlin RJ, u. a. The road to transfusion-free craniosynostosis repair in children less than 24 months old: a quality improvement initiative. Pediatr Qual Saf. 2020;5(4):e331.
9. Hönig JF, Merten HA, Ludwig H, Bebnke-Mursch J. Subgaleal versus subperiosteal dissection in fronto-orbital advancement procedures. J Craniofac Surg. 2001;12(3):287–91.
10. Shah MN, Kane AA, Petersen JD, Woo AS, Naidoo SD, Smyth MD. Endoscopically assisted versus open repair of sagittal craniosynostosis: the St. Louis Children's Hospital experience: clinical article. J Neurosurg Pediatr. 2011;8(2):165–70.
11. Martini M, Röhrig A, Reich RH, Messing-Jünger M. Comparison between piezosurgery and conventional osteotomy in cranioplasty with fronto-orbital advancement. J Craniofac Surg. 2017;45(3):395–400.
12. Vasudevan K, Oh A, Tubbs RS, Garcia D, Reisner A, Chern JJ. Jackson-Pratt drainage in pediatric craniofacial reconstructive surgery: is it helping or hurting? J Neurosurg Pediatr. 2017;20(4):341–6.
13. White N, Bayliss S, Moore D. Systematic review of interventions for minimizing perioperative blood transfusion for surgery for craniosynostosis. J Craniofac Surg. 2015;26(1):26–36.

14. Vega RA, Lyon C, Kierce JF, Tye GW, Ritter AM, Rhodes JL. Minimizing transfusion requirements for children undergoing craniosynostosis repair: the CHoR protocol. J Neurosurg Pediatr. 2014;14(2):190–5.
15. Bonfield CM, Sharma J, Cochrane DD, Singhal A, Steinbok P. Minimizing blood transfusions in the surgical correction of craniosynostosis: a 10-year single-center experience. Childs Nerv Syst. 2016;32(1):143–51.
16. Stricker PA, Goobie SM, Cladis FP, Haberkern CM, Meier PM, Reddy SK, u. a. Perioperative outcomes and management in pediatric complex cranial vault reconstruction. Anesthesiology. 2017;126(2):276–87.
17. Fenger-Eriksen C, D'Amore Lindholm A, Nørholt SE, von Oettingen G, Tarpgaard M, Krogh L, u. a. Reduced perioperative blood loss in children undergoing craniosynostosis surgery using prolonged tranexamic acid infusion: a randomised trial. Br J Anaesth. 2019;122(6):760–6.
18. King MR, Staffa SJ, Stricker PA, Pérez-Pradilla C, Nelson O, Benzon HA, u. a. Safety of antifibrinolytics in 6583 pediatric patients having craniosynostosis surgery: a decade of data reported from the multicenter Pediatric Craniofacial Collaborative Group. Pediatr Anesth. 2022;32(12):1339–46.
19. Krajewski K, Ashley RK, Pung N, Wald S, Lazareff J, Kawamoto HK, u. a. Successful blood conservation during craniosynostotic correction with dual therapy using Procrit and cell saver. J Craniofac Surg. 2008;19(1):101–5.
20. Gunnarsson I, Hlynsson BÖ, Rosmundsson T, Thorsteinsson A. Haemostatic effect of aprotinin during craniosynostotic surgery in children: aprotinin and craniosynostotic surgery. Acta Anaesthesiol Scand. 2011;55(8):1010–4.
21. Pieters BJ, Conley L, Weiford J, Hamilton M, Wicklund B, Booser A, et al. Prophylactic versus reactive transfusion of thawed plasma in patients undergoing surgical repair of craniosynostosis: a randomized clinical trial. Pediatr Anesth. 2015;25(3):279–87.
22. Haas T, Fries D, Velik-Salchner C, Oswald E, Innerhofer P. Fibrinogen in craniosynostosis surgery. Anesth Analg. 2008;106(3):725–31.

Principles and Techniques of Endoscopic Management

31

Joshua D. Bernstock, Neil Klinger, and Mark R. Proctor

31.1 Principles of Endoscopic Surgery

31.1.1 Evolution of Surgical Treatment for Craniosynostosis

Understanding the role of endoscopic approaches in contemporary therapy requires some understanding of the history of craniosynostosis operations and how surgical practice has changed over time. As is true for the breadth of neurosurgery, treatment for craniosynostosis historically carried high morbidity and mortality. The first reported case of suture release for presumed sagittal synostosis was published in 1890. Two years later, the first report of craniosynostosis treated with the so-called 'linear craniectomy' or 'strip craniectomy' was published, though the child died only hours after the operation (attributed to the alcohol, chloroform, and ether anesthetic used) [1]. In 1893, Abraham Jacobi, regarded as "the Father of American Pediatrics", detailed a series of 33 patients treated with linear craniectomy for microcephalus at the International Congress of Medicine in Rome. He had compiled the data from 6 American surgeons, which had resulted in 14 deaths (42%). Only 3 patients demonstrated "some" or "much" improvement as a result of surgery [2]. As such, the operation fell out of favor for several decades. These poor initial results were likely obtained due to improper patient selection and the state of surgical and anesthetic techniques at the time. It is likely that many of these early surgeries were performed on patients with nonsynostotic microcephaly—strip craniectomy would later be recounted as "…mistakenly used in the treatment of anencephalic microcephaly and other incurable forms of idiocy" [3]. In addition, the surgery was frequently performed far too late in childhood after skull growth was largely completed.

There would be a call to revive linear craniectomy in 1924, but this time as a way to prevent the late sequelae of synostosis. With improved surgical techniques and proper patient selection, this next wave of treatment was far more successful and led to the modern field. In particular, it was cited as a preventative measure for vision loss and not as a treatment for microcephalus [4]. It also became clear that the procedure should be performed as early in childhood as was deemed safe to do so to have the greatest impact. This was advocated for within the first 6 months of life [3], and in 1943, was suggested to be optimal during the first 1–3 months of life during periods of rapid skull and brain growth [5]. This technique, with or without additional osteotomies, was prac-

J. D. Bernstock · N. Klinger · M. R. Proctor (✉)
Department of Neurosurgery, Boston Children's Hospital, Boston, MA, USA
e-mail: jbernstock@bwh.harvard.edu; nklinger@bwh.harvard.edu; mark.proctor@childrens.harvard.edu

F. Di Rocco, J. Kestle (eds.), *Neurosurgical Aspects of Craniosynostosis*,
https://doi.org/10.1007/978-3-031-69386-1_31

ticed for several decades. One major limitation of the operation was suture re-ossification within several months, leading to inadequate corrections. In attempts to combat this, many synthetic and caustic substances were applied to bone edges [6–8], while other surgeons advocated for removal of more extensive amounts of bone [9]. In 1968, Shillito and Matson reviewed an impressive 519 patients treated for craniosynostosis that aided in quelling much of the criticism of the technique's safety (0.58% patients with lasting undesirable sequela) and efficacy (only 2% of patients with adequate follow-up failed to show cosmetic improvement) [10]. Other criticisms of the strip craniectomy (as originally described) include leaving an "unprotected" area over the vertex, and that removing a single suture will not alter the compensatory growth at other sutures (a discovery important to the understanding of skull growth and craniosynostosis [11]), making it less likely to provide a satisfactory cosmetic outcome. As an alternative to strip craniectomy, John Jane introduced an open cranial remodeling procedure in 1978 [12]. This so-called 'pi procedure' was named for the 'π'-shaped piece of calvarium removed for the treatment of sagittal synostosis. Numerous variations of this procedure have since been described, and it is significant for ushering in the era of immediate surgical correction, as opposed to release of the pathological suture with the hope for normalized growth over time [13]. Around the same time, complex craniofacial reconstruction was also being pioneered for the correction of craniofacial dysostoses (familial craniosynostosis, generally affecting the cranial vault, base, and midfacial skeleton). Paul Tessier described the foundations upon which current practice is derived throughout the 1960s and 1970s [14, 15]. However, despite the remarkable innovations introduced by these larger corrections, they also came with significant drawbacks. First, the magnitude of surgery is quite significant, and performing these large operations on young infants could be a daunting task. Perhaps more importantly, creating an ideal skull shape at surgery did not always lead to ideal long-term results, as growth patterns over time are not normal after such major disruption of the skull and soft tissues. This led to high frequency of revision surgery for issues including poor cosmesis and skull defects. Due to some of the drawbacks of large open reconstructions, we have now evolved to an era where both reconstructive and release techniques have a role, and it is incumbent on the craniofacial team to understand the nuances. Indeed, modern craniofacial centers should be able to offer both techniques based on factors including the age of the patient, severity of the condition, and family preference (Fig. 31.1).

With several important modifications, strip craniectomy was reintroduced as a treatment for craniosynostosis in the 1990s. Pioneering work from Barone (plastic surgery) and Jimenez (pediatric neurosurgery) improved upon the traditional open procedure by introducing the minimally invasive endoscopic strip craniectomy (ESC) with postoperative adjuvant therapy. Using an endoscope to aid with visualization, they combined smaller skin incisions, boney removal akin to that of the open linear craniectomy, and the concept of so-called 'directed growth' as a way to achieve the desired cosmetic result over time. Their aim was to achieve similar outcomes as its open counterpart, while mitigating the perioperative morbidity as well as improving the long-term outcomes. Using these techniques, surgeons can avoid the need for extensive removal and reshaping of bone at the time of surgery, thereby shortening the length of the procedure and decreasing blood loss. With directed growth, restoration of skull shape is achieved over time by minimizing skull growth in the overcompensated regions and promoting it in the undercompensated regions. Current options by which directed growth is achieved is with postoperative helmet orthoses, implanted springs, or implanted distractors (discussed in techniques section below).

Current and historic literature regarding surgical therapies for synostosis has been plagued by a lack of standardized nomenclature with which techniques are described [16]. To begin, labelling the modern variant of these procedures as 'endoscopic', in truth, is a mischaracterization. Rather, the procedure is more appropriately described as an endoscope-assisted minimally invasive strip

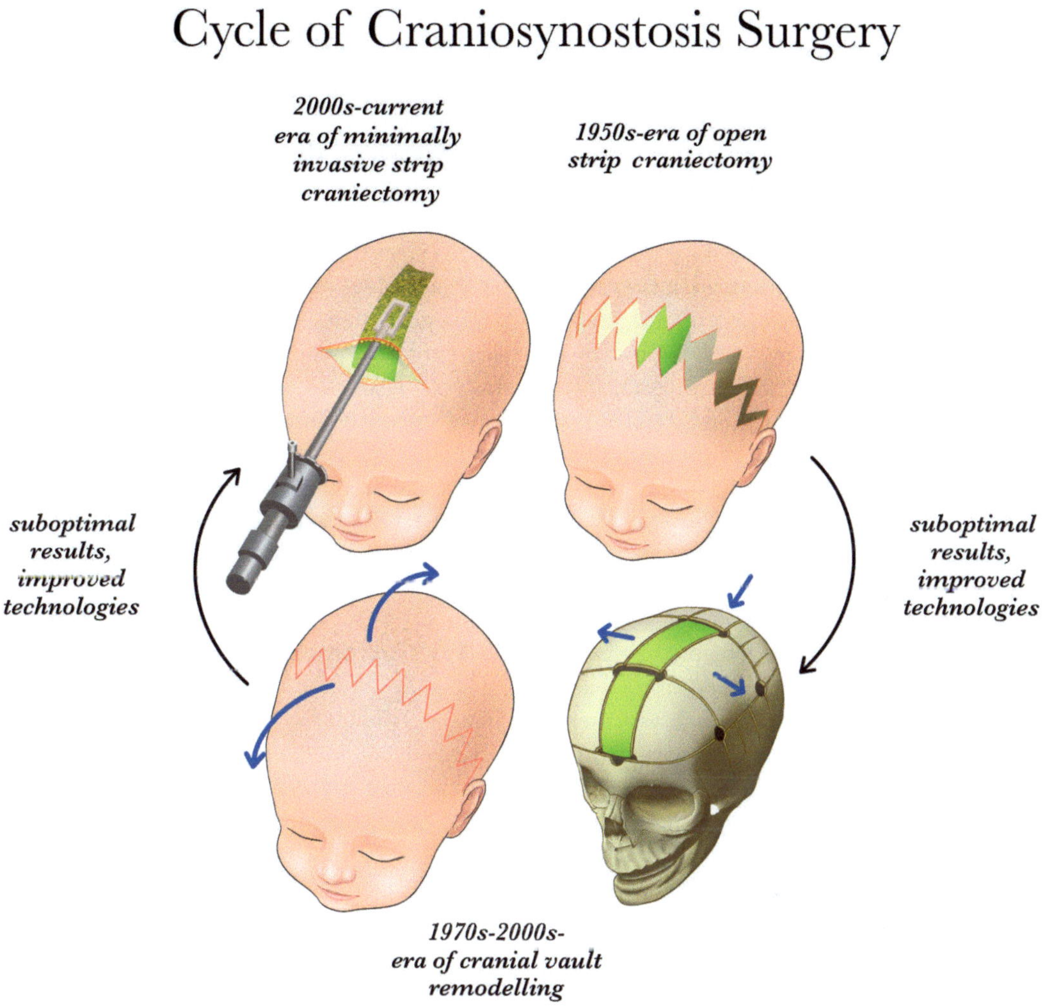

Fig. 31.1 Cycle of craniosynostosis surgery. This pictorial demonstrates the evolution of surgery for the treatment of craniosynostisis, beginning with the open strip (or 'linear') craniectomy. Innovation for these early procedures plateaued around the 1950s. Open strip craniectomy had a number of shortcomings, not the least of which was the relative infrequency with which a satisfactory outcome was achieved. This was primarily owed to premature suture re-ossification before optimal correction was achieved. This, along with the need to treat the more complex craniofacial syndromes, drove innovation in calvarial vault remodeling (CVR) procedures in the 1970s. While these techniques allowed for powerful immediate correction, they also were fraught with high blood loss, transfusion requirements, and prolonged hospital stays, and the results were not always durable over time. The need to minimize perioperative morbidity combined with innovative use of endoscopic visualization allowed Barone and Jimenez to reinvent the strip craniectomy. Their procedure used much smaller incisions, had fewer perioperative complications, and achieved satisfactory outcomes in patients who maintained compliance with helmet therapy after surgery. The minimally invasive strip craniectomy is currently the procedure of choice for appropriate candidates

craniectomy. The primary use of the endoscope for these operations is in helping to visualize along the length of the suture that is being removed, and ensuring the dura is free prior to removal. This allows for the use of smaller skin incisions (and hence 'minimally invasive'), while maintaining adequate visualization to assess hemostasis and adequacy of the surgical procedure. Variations in surgical technique have also led to variations in terminology used to describe those techniques, further clouding the literature and the ability to compare the conditions being treated and the efficacy of the procedures. The type and quantity of primary osteotomy (e.g., sagittal versus bilateral parasagittal) and adjunct osteotomies performed can vary widely, as can the size of strip craniectomy performed (so-called 'extensive strip craniectomy' or 'wide vertex craniectomy'), if/how many 'barrel staves' are used, if/how many wedge osteotomies are performed, and even terminology pertaining to removal of the ossified suture (linear craniectomy versus strip craniectomy versus suturectomy versus synostectomy). This variance in terminology and surgical technique further complicates higher-order data examination such as meta-analyses.

ESC has evolved to optimally treat its own niche of patients. To say that it is a competing therapy with open approaches is denying patients a holistic approach to the problem. A more contemporary view would place endoscopic surgery as a mature procedure (i.e., standard practice), with its own appropriate subset of patients that is complementary to open procedures. In general, ESC should be considered over open reconstruction when patients are younger, have fewer sutures involved, and are not syndromic, although these techniques also play a role in syndromic patients, often as a first stage in a treatment algorithm. Recent systematic reviews and meta-analyses have helped us to understand the relative advantages and disadvantages of one procedure over the other based on factors such as age and complexity.

31.1.2 Surgical Goals

The desired clinical outcome for any craniosynostosis procedure is the same—restoration of the cranium to a more normal configuration with potential for normal brain growth over time. However, the intraoperative goals and the methods by which these outcomes are achieved are vastly different between open remodeling and endoscopic procedures. In general, the goal of ESC is to perform a limited craniectomy through a small skin incision to allow mobility between the prematurely fused bones. This will allow normal growth to occur in the previously restricted direction. The intraoperative goal is not immediate correction of the deformity. With restoration of mobility at the suture location, brain and directed bone growth will lead to the desired cranial morphology. The minimal disruption of both surrounding bone and soft tissues also allows for relatively normal growth patterns over time and the oft detected formation of a 'neosuture', essentially a suture indistinguishable from a non-pathological suture that occurs at the affected suture after endoscopic release [17, 18]. This contrasts the goals of open remodeling procedures, where surgery establishes the desired outcome at the time of the operation, but it is more difficult to predict and account for future growth. Since its inception, ESC has also been adapted for application to multi-suture release and syndromic cases.

31.1.3 Outcomes

Since its introduction by Barone and Jimenez, a large body of literature on endoscope-assisted strip craniectomy has reported cosmetic outcomes substantially equivalent to open procedures. Smaller incisions, unsurprisingly, have yielded smaller scars and less pruritis. Importantly, studies that examine a variety of photographic, radiographic, and anthropomorphic measurements also confirm equivalent cosmetic outcomes following these procedures [19–22]. At this point in time, the outcomes of endoscopic procedures have been fairly rigorously scrutinized and comprise one of the most studies aspects of craniosynostosis surgery. As such, it will be important going forward to look at other outcome measures.

Since the cosmetic outcomes are well established, going forward it will be important to consider neurodevelopmental outcomes among these patients and discovering if avoidance of any potential untoward effects imposed by premature suture closure is possible. Unfortunately, the entire field of synostosis remains somewhat immature in this regard, both with regard to the baseline concerns and the effects of treatment. Data from single-suture synostosis suggest low levels of cognitive disability including developmental delays. Early on, these tend to manifest as psychomotor issues. Among the few studies to include older children, some data suggest impaired neuropsychological functions such as attention, language skills, visual spatial skills, and processing speed [23]. While randomized trials do not exist (and likely never will), some studies have been performed that demonstrate a beneficial effect conferred by operative intervention. Patel et al. found that surgery, either whole-vault cranioplasty or strip craniectomy, before 6 months of age improved long-term neurologic outcomes (higher scores in IQ, reading and comprehension, spelling, and math) [24]. Other reports do not demonstrate this benefit [25]. More rigorous studies are needed to determine any causative factors for adverse neurodevelopmental outcomes, and which, if any, treatment option would most successfully avoid them.

Safety outcomes are important to consider when determining surgical approaches. It is now widely recognized that endoscopic procedures have lower complication rates, less transfusion requirements, lower EBL, shorter operative times, and shorter length of stay [26–28]. As expected, many retrospective series demonstrate that endoscopic surgeries are being performed on patients who are younger than open surgeries. Those amenable to endoscopic correction are done so at a much earlier age, and those who require an open reconstruction are either captured at a later age or done so electively when their physiology better tolerates the more demanding operation. Of course, any surgical intervention carries risk. Many series have been published that detail complication rates around 5–10%, with durotomies and surgical site infections listed as the most frequent occurrences [29–31]. When examining the National Inpatient Sample database, Abraham et al. report risk factors for the development of postoperative complications in patients undergoing surgery (by any technique) for craniosynostosis ($n = 6010$) as advanced age (13–36 months vs. 7–12 months vs. 0–6 months; OR = 1.32), syndromic patients (OR = 1.92), and requiring intraoperative transfusion (OR = 1.60) [32], all of which are known to be mitigated by endoscopic procedures.

In contemporary medicine, additional emphasis is being placed on healthcare costs. To evaluate the economic burden of craniosynostosis, it is important to consider the cost of procedure itself, the hospital stay, any postoperative travel incurred, future visitation to the surgeon or multidisciplinary team, postoperative orthoses (when applicable), and potentially follow-up procedures (such as the case for removal of implanted springs). Factoring in all costs, multiple studies have demonstrated that endoscopic correction is substantially less economically burdensome than open cranial vault remodeling, owing to a much shorter initial hospital stay and less ICU requirements [33–36].

One drawback to endoscopic procedures is its reliance on brain and skull growth to achieve correction, necessitating surgery at an earlier age. This requires patients to have their condition recognized and referred to the appropriate practitioners for treatment expeditiously. For the surgery to be effective, the patient also needs to be treated postoperatively using molding orthoses or with an additional operation for removal of implanted springs or distractors. In addition, an important disadvantage to consider is the lack of immediate correction. This becomes important when considering appropriate surgical candidates for endoscopic procedures and should be discussed with the family.

31.1.4 Patient Selection and Preoperative Evaluation

Proper patient selection is critical to achieve satisfactory results with ESC. Several important factors must be considered, both in the patient and the family. Patients selected to undergo endoscopic strip craniectomy should ideally be less than 6 months of age; preferably around 3 months. Compliance with orthosis is also important to maximize the likelihood of achieving a good outcome. The patient and family need to be able to tolerate wearing it for approximately 23 h/day, for at least 6 months to 1 year. It should be well understood by the family that a good outcome is tied to compliance with this therapy, even if opti-

Table 31.1 Multidisciplinary care team for patients with craniosynostoses, especially those with craniofacial syndromes

Medical/surgical teams	Ancillary support
Pediatrics	Audiology
Genetics	Family counselor
Psychology	PT/OT
Otolaryngology	SLP
Neurosurgery	Social work
Plastic and reconstructive	Nutrition
Ophthalmology	Researchers
Anesthesia	Respiratory care
Dentistry	Care coordinator

mal duration of therapy is not well understood. To this end, they must also understand that correction is achieved over time and not immediately.

Apart from routine preoperative workup, centers that treat craniosynostosis should have a well-established multidisciplinary care team [37, 38]. This is especially true when craniofacial syndromes are present. These patients and their families often benefit from having a craniofacial care coordinator. This coordinator is responsible for liaising between the various specialties and helping the family to receive appropriate, specialized, timely care for the various issues caused by their syndrome. Table 31.1 is an example of some of the patient care teams responsible for intervening and rigorously monitoring their progress during development. Anesthesia care for patients with craniosynostosis or craniofacial syndromes is a challenging field, and it has been established that an OR and anesthesia team experienced in the care of these patients leads to better outcomes [39].

31.2 Techniques of Endoscopic Management

31.2.1 Intraoperative Management

Surgical techniques specific to each suture are reviewed in detail in subsequent chapters. As a broad overview, the following framework derived from the authors' institutional practices can be used to inform endoscopic management with helmet therapy.

31.2.1.1 Anesthesia

It is important to partner with anesthesia teams experienced in treating these patients. Nonetheless, several points of intraoperative management are important for the neurosurgeon to understand while performing endoscopic craniosynostosis procedures. Beyond standard anesthetic monitoring techniques (electrocardiography, noninvasive blood pressure monitoring, pulse oximetry, and temperature monitoring), patients should have precordial doppler ultrasonography whenever working near the dural venous sinuses. Perioperative dosing of prophylactic antibiotics and pain regimens differ by institution, but it is our practice to use a single intravenous dose of a broad-spectrum antibiotic (cefazolin 30 mg/kg). Inhaled sevoflurane with oxygen and nitrous oxide is typically used for induction of general anesthesia, and muscle relaxation accomplished with rocuronium at a dose of 600 mg/kg. Special attention will be needed for airways of patients with compromised facial or laryngeal structures, and oxygenation techniques modified accordingly. For example, Apert syndrome is known to cause difficult mask ventilation due to midface hypoplasia, proptosis, small nares, and choanal stenosis [40]. Ophthalmological ointment is applied for every case.

31.2.1.2 Positioning

Ideal positioning will vary depending on intended surgical target(s). For metopic and coronal sutures, patients will be supine on a cerebellar headrest, whereas prone positioning may be preferred for sagittal and lambdoid sutures. Midline, neutral to slightly flexed position is used for bicoronal, or metopic synostoses. We prefer modified prone (sphinx) positioning during correction of sagittal synostosis to ensure adequate anterior-posterior access to the sagittal suture. The surgical bed will be rotated with the head between 90° or 180° from anesthesia, giving the surgeon the most ergonomic access. To facilitate operative efficiency, we have our scrub tech setup on the surgeons right when possible (right-handed surgeon) and have the endoscopic tower opposite the surgeon's gaze.

31.2.1.3 Incisions

Most endoscopic operations require one or two small (~2 cm) skin incisions perpendicular to the fused suture that will be removed. Skin incisions are typically made using a #15 blade scalpel to gain access to the stenosed suture. Monopolar electrocautery (needle tip) at 15W is then used to develop the bloodless plane in the loose areolar space between the galea and pericranium. This is then scored and stripped with the monopolar to facilitate osseous removal.

31.2.1.4 Craniectomies

We access the intracranial space using a pediatric perforator to create a bur hole at each incision, generally centered directly on the fused suture, which is then enlarged with Kerrison rongeurs. A 4-mm rigid 0° endoscope is then introduced into the epidural space. Endoscopic visualization is crucial for safe dissection of the dura mater from the overlying bone, typically in a bimanual fashion with the use of a Penfield #1 or suction. The type of endoscope employed is a matter of preference to the surgeon, though in its original description, an 0° rigid endoscope was used during the scalp dissection, and 30° rigid scope during dural inspection/separation. Once the dura has been freed and hemostasis ensured, the osteotomy is enlarged longitudinally along the axis of the suture with a combination of angled Kerrison rongeurs, bone (pituitary type) rongeurs, and bone cutting scissors. The intended craniectomy width used in our group is approximately 1–2 cm for any suture involved. Osseous hemostasis is achieved with careful monopolar cautery under direct visualization, and we leave gelfoam lining the bone gap. The incisions are then closed with 4-0 monocryl in a simple running fashion. As with all surgery, meticulous hemostasis should be sought, and thoughtful communication with anesthesia should occur throughout the case. Blood loss is usually minimal, but failure to prepare for unanticipated losses is inadvisable.

31.2.2 Postoperative Treatment

Immediate perioperative pain is treated with administration of intravenous morphine. The patient is started and maintained on acetaminophen, which is often used post discharge for 2–3 days. Typical LOS is one night. We do not routinely give postoperative antibiotic prophylaxis.

Based on historical data, we know that suture removal by itself often does not result in a good outcome. Unchecked compensatory growth at the unfused sutures will continue, and the cut bone margins may rapidly refuse, resulting in failure to obtain a corrected shape. This was recognized when the linear craniectomy was being developed [41] and drove subsequent advances in the field. It is now understood that bone growth needs to be promoted in the direction that was previously restricted. Growth should also be limited, but not prevented, in the previously overcompensated direction. Several methods have been studied to direct growth: use of molding orthoses, implanted spring distractors, and standard implanted distractors.

31.2.2.1 Molding Orthoses

The use of molding helmets for postoperative-directed growth for the treatment of craniosynostosis after endoscopic suturectomy was popularized by Barone and Jimenez [42–45]. The concept of molding an infant's head was not new at that time. Molding helmet use after craniofacial surgery was described in 1986, though evidence suggests that the practice of changing the shape of an infant's head with external pressure has been there since at least the Bronze age [46]. Helmet therapy has several advantages to the other described techniques. They can be modified over time to alter restrictions/freedoms to dynamically achieve a desired result without any additional procedures. They can also mold in 3 dimensions, whereas springs and distractors only work in a single plane. Finally, there will be no need for additional surgery to remove the device. Of course, the family needs to be compliant with the treatment, and the helmet requires periodic adjustment, necessitating additional travel to and from the treating facility. In addition to an ill-fitting orthotic, complications include reports of skin irritation and soft tissue infection, generally at the onset of therapy [47, 48]. Some groups report not having these issues [22, 49].

In our practice, patients are admitted to the inpatient (floor) unit for observation overnight and discharged the following morning after ESC. They then undergo laser scan on 3–4 days after surgery to obtain baseline anthropometric measurements. A custom-made ethylene copolymer helmet is then manufactured and fitted to the child within 7–10 days after surgery. Some children will gain correction with a single helmet, but it is possible to need a second, and rarely a third helmet as the child's head grows and changes shape. Helmet therapy lasts on average 7 months, and in our practice, we always discontinue the helmet by the child's birthday. Patients are then followed on an annual basis until at least 6 years of age.

31.2.2.2 Spring Distractor Osteogenesis

Spring therapy is a relatively newer technique adapted for use with craniosynostosis. The technique of implantable spring (nickel-chromium-iron alloy) for craniofacial reshaping was first introduced by Claes Lauritzen in 1998 [50]. They were manufactured by hand from wire and adjusted with a pressure gauge to ensure appropriate force is applied. Subsequent analysis of the first 100 patients treated this way confirmed the safety and efficacy of the technique [51]. They can be deployed either in open or endoscopic cases. One substantial benefit to spring distraction over helmet therapy is that it does not rely on the rapid periods of brain and skull growth. Therefore, the use of spring distraction extends the age for which endoscopic management can be offered. An obvious downside to their use is that it necessitates a second operation for removal of the device. Compared to standard distraction osteogenesis, there is also no control over the force or rate of force applied after implantation. Complications include spring shifting leading to suboptimal or undesirable bone movement, dislodgement, or wound issues [51].

31.2.2.3 Distraction Osteogenesis

Distraction osteogenesis is a cranial remodeling technique whereby distractors are surgically implanted and affixed to the bones after separation. This technique requires a portion of the device to exit through the skin to allow for subsequent adjustment. The screw is turned daily to expand the distractor at a rate of approximately 1 mm/day. Compared to spring-assisted distraction osteogenesis for the treatment of sagittal synostosis, operative times are longer (216 min versus 104 min), blood loss is greater (250 mL versus 82.5 mL), and hospital stay is longer (16.9 days versus 5.5 days) [52]. Overall complication rates are estimated to be 23%, with the majority of complications being due to infection, scalp/wound dehiscence, and traction pin loosening [52]. Systematic review does not demonstrate statistically significant differences in these parameters as compared to open cranial remodeling surgery [52]. Its use is generally reserved for cases of advanced age where helmeted treatment will not be effective, those with craniofacial deformities, or cases where spring therapy would be deemed ineffective.

31.3 Summary

Endoscopic surgery for the treatment of synostosis has become a well-established treatment paradigm. It should be considered a complementary treatment to open procedure, and one that any modern craniofacial center should have competency in. As compared to open procedures, the operation is performed at a younger age, and the treatment is followed by a postoperative adjuvant, most commonly a helmet, although springs or distractors can also be used. The cosmetic and safety components of this operation are well established and compare quite favorably to open surgery. Future investigation comparing the neurocognitive outcomes of open versus endoscopic surgery is a field that requires additional study.

References

1. Lane LC. Pioneer craniectomy for relief of mental imbecility due to premature sutural closure and microcephalus. J Am Med Assoc. 1892;XVIII:49–50. https://doi.org/10.1001/jama.1892.02411060019001f.
2. Jacobi A. Non nocere. Med Rec A Wkly J Med Surg. 1894;45:609–18.
3. Faber HK, Towne EB. Early Craniectomy as a preventive measure in oxycephaly and allied conditions. Am J Med Sci. 1927;173:701–11. http://content.wkhealth.com/linkback/openurl?sid=WKPTLP:landingpage&an=00000441-192705000-00012.
4. Faber HK. The importance of early diagnosis in oxycephaly and allied cranial deformities, with reference to the prevention of blindness and other sequelae. Cal West Med. 1924;22:542–5. http://www.ncbi.nlm.nih.gov/pubmed/18739466.
5. Faber HK, Towne EB. Early operation in premature cranial synostosisfor the prevention of blindness and other sequelae. J Pediatr. 1943;22:286–307. https://linkinghub.elsevier.com/retrieve/pii/S0022347643801682.
6. Anderson FM, Johnson FL. Craniosynostosis; a modification in surgical treatment. Surgery. 1956;40:961–70. http://www.ncbi.nlm.nih.gov/pubmed/13371461.
7. Ingraham FD, Matson DD, Alexander E. Experimental observations in the treatment of craniosynostosis. Surgery. 1948;23:252–68. http://www.ncbi.nlm.nih.gov/pubmed/18901014.
8. Simmons DR, Peyton WT. Premature closure of the cranial sutures. J Pediatr. 1947;31:528–47. https://linkinghub.elsevier.com/retrieve/pii/S0022347647801428.
9. Magge SN, Bartolozzi AR, Almeida ND, Tsering D, Myseros JS, Oluigbo CO, et al. A comparison of endoscopic strip craniectomy and pi craniectomy for treatment of sagittal craniosynostosis. J Neurosurg Pediatr. 2019;23:708–14. https://thejns.org/view/journals/j-neurosurg-pediatr/23/6/article-p708.xml.
10. Shillito J, Matson DD. Craniosynostosis: a review of 519 surgical patients. Pediatrics. 1968;41:829–53. http://www.ncbi.nlm.nih.gov/pubmed/5643989.
11. Delashaw JB, Persing JA, Broaddus WC, Jane JA. Cranial vault growth in craniosynostosis. J Neurosurg. 1989;70:159–65. https://thejns.org/view/journals/j-neurosurg/70/2/article-p159.xml.
12. Jane JA, Edgerton MT, Futrell JW, Park TS. Immediate correction of sagittal synostosis. J Neurosurg. 1978;49:705–10. https://thejns.org/view/journals/j--neurosurg/49/5/article-p705.xml.
13. Boulos PT, Lin KYK, Jane JA, Jane JA. Correction of sagittal synostosis using a modified Π method. Clin Plast Surg. 2004;31:489–98. https://linkinghub.elsevier.com/retrieve/pii/S0094129804000148.
14. Tessier P. Ostéotomies totales de la face. Syndrome de Crouzon, syndrme d'Apert: oxycéphalies, scaphocéphalies, turricéphalies. Ann Chir Plast. 1967;12:273–86. http://www.ncbi.nlm.nih.gov/pubmed/5622570.
15. Tessier P. The definitive plastic surgical treatment of the severe facial deformities of craniofacial dysostosis: Crouzon's and Apert's diseases. Plast Reconstr Surg. 1971;48:419–42. http://journals.lww.com/00006534-197111000-00002.
16. Garland CB, Camison L, Dong SM, Mai RS, Losee JE, Goldstein JA. Variability in minimally invasive surgery for sagittal craniosynostosis. J Craniofac Surg. 2018;29:14–20. https://journals.lww.com/00001665-201801000-00007.
17. Salehi A, Ott K, Skolnick GB, Nguyen DC, Naidoo SD, Kane AA, et al. Neosuture formation after endoscope assisted craniosynostosis repair. J Neurosurg Pediatr. 2016;18:196–200. https://thejns.org/view/journals/j-neurosurg-pediatr/18/2/article-p196.xml.
18. Sauerhammer TM, Seruya M, Ropper AE, Oh AK, Proctor MR, Rogers GF. Craniectomy gap patency and neosuture formation following endoscopic suturectomy for unilateral coronal craniosynostosis. Plast Reconstr Surg. 2014;134:81e–91e. http://journals.lww.com/00006534-201407000-00022.
19. Farber SJ, Nguyen DC, Skolnick GB, Naidoo SD, Smyth MD, Patel KB. Anthropometric outcome measures in patients with metopic craniosynostosis. J Craniofac Surg. 2017;28:713–6. http://journals.lww.com/00001665-201705000-00032.
20. Le MB, Patel K, Skolnick G, Naidoo S, Smyth M, Kane A, et al. Assessing long-term outcomes of open and endoscopic sagittal synostosis reconstruction using three-dimensional photography. J Craniofac Surg. 2014;25:573–6. http://journals.lww.com/00001665-201403000-00067.
21. Nguyen DC, Patel KB, Skolnick GB, Naidoo SD, Huang AH, Smyth MD, et al. Are endoscopic and open treatments of metopic synostosis equivalent in treating trigonocephaly and hypotelorism? J Craniofac Surg. 2015;26:129–34. https://journals.lww.com/00001665-201501000-00027.
22. Shah MN, Kane AA, Petersen JD, Woo AS, Naidoo SD, Smyth MD. Endoscopically assisted versus open repair of sagittal craniosynostosis: the St. Louis Children's Hospital experience—clinical article. J Neurosurg Pediatr. 2011;8:165–70. https://thejns.org/view/journals/j-neurosurg-pediatr/8/2/article-p165.xml.
23. Kapp-Simon KA, Speltz ML, Cunningham ML, Patel PK, Tomita T. Neurodevelopment of children with single suture craniosynostosis: a review. Childs Nerv Syst. 2007;23:269–81. https://doi.org/10.1007/s00381-006-0251-z.
24. Patel A, Yang JF, Hashim PW, Travieso R, Terner J, Mayes LC, et al. The impact of age at surgery on long-term neuropsychological outcomes in sagittal craniosynostosis. Plast Reconstr Surg. 2014;134:608e–17e. http://journals.lww.com/00006534-201410000-00031.

25. Collett BR, Kapp-Simon KA, Wallace E, Cradock MM, Buono L, Speltz ML. Attention and executive function in children with and without single-suture craniosynostosis. Child Neuropsychol. 2017;23:83–98. https://doi.org/10.1080/09297049.2015.1085005.
26. Goyal A, Lu VM, Yolcu YU, Elminawy M, Daniels DJ. Endoscopic versus open approach in craniosynostosis repair: a systematic review and meta-analysis of perioperative outcomes. Childs Nerv Syst. 2018;34:1627–37. https://doi.org/10.1007/s00381-018-3852-4.
27. Yan H, Abel TJ, Alotaibi NM, Anderson M, Niazi TN, Weil AG, et al. A systematic review and meta-analysis of endoscopic versus open treatment of craniosynostosis. Part 1: the sagittal suture. J Neurosurg Pediatr. 2018;22:352–60. https://thejns.org/view/journals/j--neurosurg-pediatr/22/4/article-p352.xml.
28. Yan H, Abel TJ, Alotaibi NM, Anderson M, Niazi TN, Weil AG, et al. A systematic review of endoscopic versus open treatment of craniosynostosis. Part 2: the nonsagittal single sutures. J Neurosurg Pediatr. 2018;22:361–8. https://thejns.org/view/journals/j--neurosurg-pediatr/22/4/article-p361.xml.
29. Arts S, Delye H, van Lindert EJ. Intraoperative and postoperative complications in the surgical treatment of craniosynostosis: minimally invasive versus open surgical procedures. J Neurosurg Pediatr. 2018;21:112–8. https://thejns.org/view/journals/j--neurosurg-pediatr/21/2/article-p112.xml.
30. Esparza J, Hinojosa J. Complications in the surgical treatment of craniosynostosis and craniofacial syndromes: apropos of 306 transcranial procedures. Childs Nerv Syst. 2008;24:1421–30. https://doi.org/10.1007/s00381-008-0691-8.
31. Han RH, Nguyen DC, Bruck BS, Skolnick GB, Yarbrough CK, Naidoo SD, et al. Characterization of complications associated with open and endoscopic craniosynostosis surgery at a single institution. J Neurosurg Pediatr. 2016;17:361–70. https://thejns.org/view/journals/j-neurosurg-pediatr/17/3/article-p361.xml.
32. Abraham P, Brandel MG, Dalle Ore CL, Reid CM, Kpaduwa CS, Lance S, et al. Predictors of postoperative complications of craniosynostosis repair in the National Inpatient Sample. Ann Plast Surg. 2018;80:S261–6. https://journals.lww.com/00000637-201805005-00007.
33. Chan JWH, Stewart CL, Stalder MW, St. Hilaire H, McBride L, Moses MH. Endoscope-assisted versus open repair of craniosynostosis: a comparison of perioperative cost and risk. J Craniofac Surg. 2013;24:170–4. http://journals.lww.com/00001665-201301000-00040.
34. Garber ST, Karsy M, Kestle JRW, Siddiqi F, Spanos SP, Riva-Cambrin J. Comparing outcomes and cost of 3 surgical treatments for sagittal synostosis: a retrospective study including procedure-related cost analysis. Neurosurgery. 2017. https://academic.oup.com/neurosurgery/article-lookup/doi/10.1093/neuros/nyx209.
35. Vogel TW, Woo AS, Kane AA, Patel KB, Naidoo SD, Smyth MD. A comparison of costs associated with endoscope-assisted craniectomy versus open cranial vault repair for infants with sagittal synostosis. J Neurosurg Pediatr. 2014;13:324–31. https://thejns.org/view/journals/j-neurosurg-pediatr/13/3/article-p324.xml.
36. Zubovic E, Lapidus JB, Skolnick GB, Naidoo SD, Smyth MD, Patel KB. Cost comparison of surgical management of nonsagittal synostosis: traditional open versus endoscope-assisted techniques. J Neurosurg Pediatr. 2020;25:351–60. https://thejns.org/view/journals/j-neurosurg-pediatr/25/4/article-p351.xml.
37. Buchanan EP, Xue Y, Xue AS, Olshinka A, Lam S. Multidisciplinary care of craniosynostosis. J Multidiscip Healthc. 2017;10:263–70. https://www.dovepress.com/multidisciplinary-care-of-craniosynostosis-peer-reviewed-article-JMDH.
38. McCarthy JG, Warren SM, Bernstein J, Burnett W, Cunningham ML, Edmond JC, et al. Parameters of care for craniosynostosis. Cleft Palate-Craniofacial J. 2012;49:1–24. https://doi.org/10.1597/11-138.
39. Reddy SK, Patel RS, Rogers GF, Gordish-Dressman H, Keating RF, Pestieau SR. Intraoperative management by a craniofacial team anesthesiologist is associated with improved outcomes for children undergoing major craniofacial reconstructive surgery. J Craniofac Surg. 2019;30:418–23. http://www.ncbi.nlm.nih.gov/pubmed/30614991.
40. Thomas K, Hughes C, Johnson D, Das S. Anesthesia for surgery related to craniosynostosis: a review. Part 1. Pediatr Anesth. 2012;22:1033–41. https://doi.org/10.1111/j.1460-9592.2012.03927.x.
41. Ingraham FD, Alexander E, Matson DD. Clinical studies in craniosynostosis analysis of 50 cases and description of a method of surgical treatment. Surgery. 1948;24:518–41. http://www.ncbi.nlm.nih.gov/pubmed/18884128.
42. Barone CM, Jimenez DF. Endoscopic craniectomy for early correction of craniosynostosis. Plast Reconstr Surg. 1999;104:1965–73. http://journals.lww.com/00006534-199912000-00003.
43. Jimenez DF, Barone CM. Endoscopy-assisted wide-vertex craniectomy, "barrel-stave" osteotomies, and postoperative helmet molding therapy in the early management of sagittal suture craniosynostosis. Neurosurg Focus. 2000;9:1–6. https://thejns.org/view/journals/neurosurg-focus/9/3/foc.2000.9.3.3.xml.
44. Jimenez DF, Barone CM. Endoscopic craniectomy for early surgical correction of sagittal craniosynostosis. J Neurosurg. 1998;88:77–81. https://thejns.org/view/journals/j-neurosurg/88/1/article-p77.xml.
45. Jimenez DF, Barone CM, Cartwright CC, Baker L. Early management of craniosynostosis using endoscopic-assisted strip craniectomies and cranial orthotic molding therapy. Pediatrics.

2002;110:97–104. https://doi.org/10.1542/peds.110.1.97.
46. Persing JA, Nichter LS, Jane JA, Edgerton MT. External cranial vault molding after craniofacial surgery. Ann Plast Surg. 1986;17:274–83. http://journals.lww.com/00000637-198610000-00002.
47. Freudlsperger C, Bodem JP, Kargus S, Castrillon-Oberndorfer G, Hoffman J, Engel M. The incidence of complications associated with molding helmet therapy. J Craniofac Surg. 2015;26:e299–302. https://journals.lww.com/00001665-201506000-00137.
48. Wilbrand J-F, Wilbrand M, Malik CY, Howaldt H-P, Streckbein P, Schaaf H, et al. Complications in helmet therapy. J Cranio-Maxillofacial Surg. 2012;40:341–6. https://linkinghub.elsevier.com/retrieve/pii/S101051821100120X.
49. Jimenez DF, Barone CM, McGee ME, Cartwright CC, Baker CL. Endoscopy-assisted wide-vertex craniectomy, barrel stave osteotomies, and postoperative helmet molding therapy in the management of sagittal suture craniosynostosis. J Neurosurg Pediatr. 2004;100:407–17. https://doi.org/10.3171/ped.2004.100.5.0407.
50. Lauritzen C, Sugawara Y, Kocabalkan O, Olsson R. Spring mediated dynamic craniofacial reshaping. Scand J Plast Reconstr Surg Hand Surg. 1998;32:331–8. https://doi.org/10.1080/02844319850158697.
51. Lauritzen CGK, Davis C, Ivarsson A, Sanger C, Hewitt TD. The evolving role of springs in craniofacial surgery: the first 100 clinical cases. Plast Reconstr Surg. 2008;121:545–54. http://journals.lww.com/00006534-200802000-00024.
52. Mundinger GS, Rehim SA, Johnson O, Zhou J, Tong A, Wallner C, et al. Distraction osteogenesis for surgical treatment of Craniosynostosis. Plast Reconstr Surg. 2016;138:657–69. http://journals.lww.com/00006534-201609000-00023.

32 Principles and Technique of Anterior Vault Remodeling

Federico Bianchi and Gianpiero Tamburrini

32.1 Metopic Craniosynostosis

Metopic craniosynostosis is nowadays considered the second most frequent one and its distinctive features are described in detail in another chapter of this book. This chapter will instead address the variety of surgical techniques reported for trigonocephaly treatment.

As previously reported, surgical goal can be so summarized:

1. ICP increase prevention;
2. Cranial morphology normalization;
3. Prevention of neurodevelopmental injury;
4. Prevention of ocular movement disturbances.

All proposed techniques have a step in common, namely the removal of the affected suture while differentiating the dealing of the cranial deformity.

Thus, digging into the problem, trigonocephaly can be treated with open field surgery (fronto-orbital advancement combined with anterior cranial vault reconstruction, FOA), device-assisted procedures (DAP), endoscopy-assisted suturectomy (EAS) followed by postoperative cranial orthotic therapy, or mini invasive microscope-assisted suturectomy (MMAS). Among those options, FOA and EAS can be considered the most used.

FOA is the oldest and more studied technique widely demonstrated as safe and reliable in obtaining surgical goals. Nonetheless, it is burdened by the need for larger incision, longer surgical time, the likely need for blood transfusion, as well as supposed longer hospitalization, increased overall health care costs, and a risk of relapse [1]. FOA user elected this open procedure arguing better reconstruction results obtainable in reasonable surgical times in trained hands as well as highlighting that properly performed incisions can be easily masked [2].

Endoscopic assisted suturectomy (EAS) are surely shorter procedures with lesser blood loss and smaller scars but the need for earlier surgery, postoperative helmet therapy render the result less likely to be predict [3].

Whether the chosen technique mortality is quite low being intravascular disseminated coagulation the major responsible. Surgical results are usually good even though scares literature data are present. This fact is related with long term lack of data as well as the potential disparity between surgeon and family impression on them [3].

F. Bianchi
Pediatric Neurosurgery, Fondazione Policlinico Gemelli IRCCS, Rome, Italy
e-mail: Federico.bianchi@policlinicogemelli.it

G. Tamburrini (✉)
Pediatric Neurosurgery, Fondazione Policlinico Gemelli IRCCS, Rome, Italy

Università Cattolica del Sacro Cuore, Milan, Italy
e-mail: gianpiero.tamburrini@unicatt.it

F. Di Rocco, J. Kestle (eds.), *Neurosurgical Aspects of Craniosynostosis*,
https://doi.org/10.1007/978-3-031-69386-1_32

In the rest of the chapter for each of the previously mentioned surgical techniques will be described what reported in the literature about:

1. Positioning and anesthesia;
2. Exposure;
3. Bony decompression;
4. Reconstruction (FOA) vs device used (DAP) vs molding therapy (EAS and MMAS);
5. Closure.

32.1.1 FOA (Fig. 32.1)

32.1.1.1 Positioning and Anesthesia

The patient is usually anesthetized by a pediatric anesthesiologist, using endotracheal intubation, 2 large-bore intravenous lines and or a central line, and 1 arterial line. Further procedure consists of Foley catheter insertion to monitor urine output. As for the position, the child is supine with the head placed into a support. Some authors advocate the use of a horseshoe headrest to increase head stability [4–7]. Before incision, some authors also recommend local anesthesia with 1:200,000 epinephrine addiction to reduce soft tissue bleeding [4, 5, 8, 9]. Only Seal et al. reported the use of a different dosage using 1:400,000 epinephrine [10].

32.1.1.2 Exposure

FOA approach always starts with a bicoronal incision posterior to the anterior fontanelle whose fashion varies among authors. In fact, some of them prefer a sinusoidal cut [8], while others prefer zig-zag ones [4, 6, 11–15] or double opposing lazy S incision [16], scalloped pattern one [17], lazy W incision [9, 18], and finally straight incision at the vertex with zig-zag pattern on the temporoparietal surface [10, 19]. Independently from the chosen fashion, the cut is customed to reduce esthetic trouble from a wide scar. Most of the authors prefer monopolar diathermy to reduce bleeding with or without previous shallow 15-blade epidermis cut. Manikas et al. also suggest to incise the skin in an oblique fashion to reduce hair follicle damage [20].

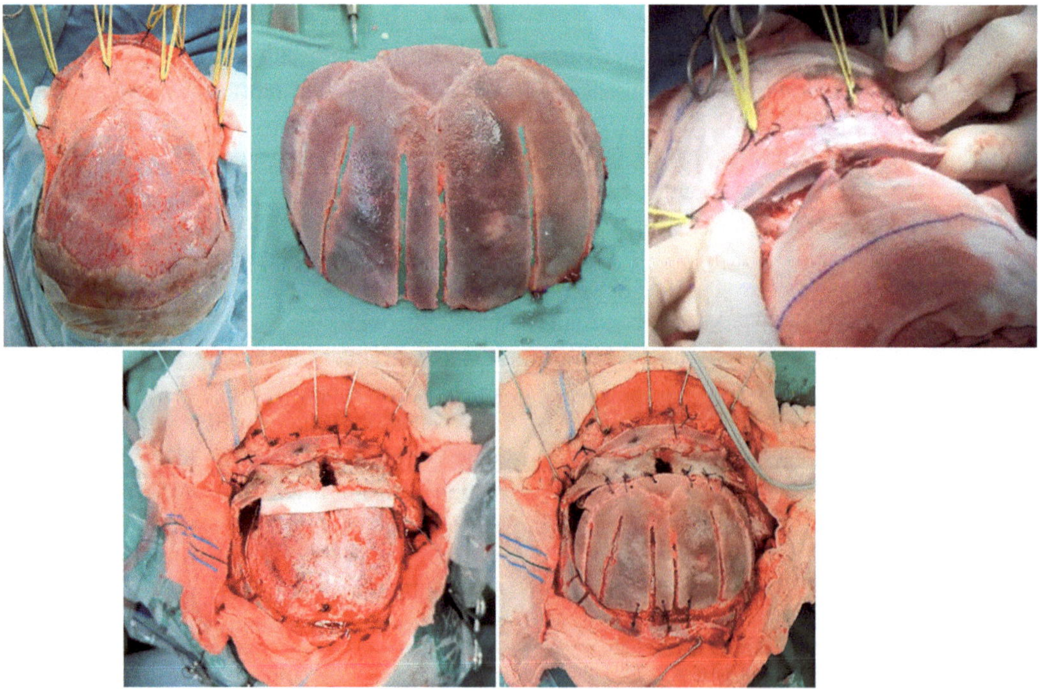

Fig. 32.1 FOA

After incision, exposure proceeds with scalp flap blunt dissection preserving the periosteum in order to create large enough flap to cover the future osteotomies. The aforementioned periosteum flaps extend till 1.5 cm above the superior orbital rims where a different incision, including the external fascia of the temporalis muscle bilaterally, permits the exposure of both the frontal and pterional regions, the lateral margins of the orbits (down to the fronto-zygomatic suture), the superior orbital ridge, and the upper part of the nasal bones, preserving the frontal branches of the supraorbital nerves [5, 6, 8, 10, 12, 17, 20, 21]. Smaller variation of the reported procedures are the ones from Bennet et al. in which the area of periosteum overlaying the metopic suture is removed in order to cancel tissue memory in this region [8] and the ones from Braun et al. (2018) whose technique uses subperiosteal dissection [11].

32.1.1.3 Bone Decompression

Once uncovered the cranial vault and the orbital region, the decompression phase can be started. This phase can be actually divided into two segment, cranial vault decompression and orbital advancement.

While most of the authors concord in the use of a bicoronal craniotomy for vault decompression, many different techniques are reported in the orbital advancement.

Starting with bicoronal craniotomy, it usually extends from posterior the anterior fontanelle till 1.5 cm above the orbital rim to ensure successive orbital advancement. There are a few differences in the bicoronal craniotomy according to the number of flaps collected. In fact, while most of the authors chose to harvest a single bone flap [5, 6, 10, 12], others prefer to divide it into two or more pieces [8].

Some authors also suggest to split the calvarial bone in order to obtain more pieces for reconstruction [8].

As for the orbital bandeau, it is usually created performing osteotomies of the orbital roofs, the medial and lateral orbit walls, and zygomatico-frontal sutures. In removing the bandeau, care must be taken into preserving the supraorbital nerve that might be elevated from its notch or freed from its foramen [4–6, 8, 12, 17]. The aforementioned osteotomies can be carried out completely offering an en-bloc bandeau or trough green-stick fracture according to the surgeon preferences and depending on the severity of the cranial malformation. Surgical instrument useful in performing the orbital bandeau are: the reciprocating saw [8, 18], the piezosurgery scalpel [14, 22, 23], a craniotome or a trephine [24], the chisel [5], and a high-performance ultrasonic aspirator [13].

32.1.1.4 Reconstruction

The reconstruction phase in FOA is definitely the most variable among authors. In fact, either talking about cranial vault reconstruction or orbital bandeau advancement, there are a lot of different opinions.

Starting from the orbital bandeau reconstruction, the supraorbital bar can be remodeled either through green-stick fracture or transecting it and plating it back together in a more anterior position [25]. Complete bandeau advancement supporter argues that, using a free-flap, it is possible to obtain a wider enlargement of the anterior cranial fossa and of the orbits. On the other hand, green-stick fracture supporter states that the central portion of the bandeau is already in the ideal position granting the possibility in trigonocephalic patient to expand only laterally the anterior cranial fossa and the orbits. In addition, bending of the supraorbital bandeau can be added to reach a more spherical contour [8].

Regardless the choice, the new bandeau has to be strongly fixated not to lose the desired correction. Furthermore, most of the authors highlight the importance of hypercorrection in order to compensate for the physiological retrusion of the new construct once the skin flap is closed and to reduce the risk of recurrence.

To obtain such fixation, there are several techniques involving sutures [9], reabsorbable plates [4–6, 20, 21, 24], titanium ones and stainless steel wires [21], and bone grafts [26].

As for cranial vault reconstruction, there are several shapes in which the bone flap can be molded as a way to cover as better as possible the area of craniolacunia. Furthermore, most authors suggest to rotate the bone flap of 180° to use the optimal contour of the parietal bones to reconstruct the forehead. Examples of modeling are the Christmas tree foreheadplasty [16], the shell technique [12], or the cathedral dome procedure [6]. The fixation of the molded flap can be achieved with sutures, reabsorbable plates [10, 20], and stainless steel wires [15, 16, 21]. Some authors also suggest the use of bone particulate and graft to widen even more dural covering [4, 11, 26]. Others also supported the implant of acellular dermal matrix to enhance ossification [27].

32.1.1.5 Closure

In the end, FOA skin flap closure start repositioning the temporalis muscle that has to be advanced to cover for the hollowness left by cranial advancement. Vycril sutures are usually used for the task [4, 8, 28]. Another important step in completing the surgery is the sewing of the periosteum as a lead in future ossification [12, 16]. After that the skin flap is closed in layers using skin suturing reabsorbable stiches, sometimes leaving a subcutaneous drain according to bleeding levels. Nonetheless, some authors still use staples, even though in kids it might be difficult to remove them [9].

32.1.2 Device-Assisted Techniques

Device-assisted techniques resemble FOA in many aspects of the procedures. Positioning, anesthesia, exposure, and closure are practically overlapping, while some differences regard the extent of bony decompression and of course the chosen device. While most of the authors who use this kind of surgery add the device to a standard FOA decompression, others like Bhatti-So¨fteland et al. prefer to carry out barrel stave osteotomies perpendicular to the coronal suture in the anterior parietal region [29]. Fawzy et al., on the other hand, create fronto-orbital osteotomy without separating the bandeau [30]. Finally, some authors prefer to perform a strip craniotomy along the fused suture leaving the distraction to the device [31–33].

Coming to the more commonly implanted devices, it is necessary to distinct among classic distractors [30, 33–35] and springs [29, 31, 32, 36]. Both surgical choices aim to reduce the intraoperative work in exchange for a more prolonged distraction. Supporters of the technique underline the importance of shorter surgical timing and scarring and the possibility of major distraction compared with classical FOA. On the other hand, it is important to remember the added device-related complication as well as the need to remove the device once distraction is completed.

32.1.3 Endoscopic Techniques

Apart from FOA, endoscopic treatment of trigonocephaly represents the second most common surgical procedure. A peculiarity of the technique resides in the need for very malleable bone and, for this very reason, children are usually operated on earlier in comparison with FOA. Most authors refer the age of 3 months as the ideal one for endoscopic treatment. As previously done for FOA, each of the surgical step of the procedure will be covered.

32.1.3.1 Positioning and Anesthesia

Similarly to what happen in FOA, the child is supine with the head located in a cushion or in a pediatric cerebellar head rest [37–40]. Some authors also suggest to infiltrate the skin with a solution of SSF, 25% bupivacaine, and adrenaline 1:1 to reduce bleeding [37, 39].

32.1.3.2 Exposure

Most of the authors perform a small incision, around 3 cm width, behind the hairline posterior to the anterior fontanelle [11, 40, 41], while others prefer to do it anteriorly [37, 42, 43] or over it [38, 44]. In addition to the previously described incisions, some authors add further ones, namely tarsal and periauricular incisions, in order to better reach the lateral orbital aspects, especially in older children [43, 44].

Once completed, the skin opening subgaleal dissection over the metopic ridge is carried above and down from the anterior fontanel to the nasion and frontonasal suture with endoscopic assistance and electrocautery [39, 43].

32.1.3.3 Bone Decompression

Endoscopic bone decompression starts preparing specular burr holes along the midline. Freeing the upper part of the superior sagittal sinuses. The dura is then detached from the intracranial aspect of the suture under 0° straight rigid endoscopic guidance, thus passing onto the suturectomy. Suturectomy can be performed using rongeurs, mayo scissors, piezosurgery, drill, or Leksell [11, 37–39, 42, 43]. Extra care has to be taken in controlling bleeding coming from bridging vein from the superior sagittal sinus, especially in the more nasofrontal portion of the metopic suture. Further osteotomies can be performed transversally to the suturectomy to promote frontal widening [11, 18]. Some authors also change the endoscope optic, preferring a 30° one, to perform osteotomies of the nasofrontal junction [41].

Whenever accessory incisions are performed, bone decompression is also carried out through them. In particular, endoscopic-assisted osteotomies of the orbital roof until anterior cranial fossa, cribriform plate, and lateral orbit walls are reached at the level of pterion and frontomalar union are carried out [43].

32.1.3.4 Molding Therapy

Trigonocephaly endoscopic treatment uses the high malleability of the younger bone together with brain growth to remodel the cranial vault and orbital region. In order to harvest the best result, no endoscopic treatment can be done without planning postsurgical head molding. Children operated on are in fact supposed to wear a helmet for at least 23 h a day for at least 6–9 months after surgery [39, 40, 42, 44]. Such a need represents without a doubt one of the major concerns for surgeons disliking this procedure. The second one resides in the young age needed to successfully perform the technique. Furthermore, it seems more difficult to predict long-term results, also considering the high therapy drop-out rate due to patient discomfort.

32.1.3.5 Microsurgical Mini-invasive Techniques

Finally, a further mini-invasive technique is represented by the microsurgical suturectomy. This technique has a lot in common with the endoscopic resection as it is performed through small incision and requires postsurgical molding therapy. The difference resides in fact in the use of the microscope instead of the endoscope. Truth be told the only to paper regarding such a technique are quite old being from an era in which the endoscopic learning curve was still at its prime for metopic suturectomy [45, 46].

32.1.4 Unicoronal Synostosis

32.1.4.1 Introduction

Unicoronal synostosis (UCS) represents distinct challenges compared with other single-suture craniosynostoses from a surgical point of view. In fact, it represents the form of craniosynostosis in which the cosmetic correction has the highest impact, seen the secondary associated deformation of the orbit and face [47], which is almost invariably progressive in untreated children and destined to have a major psychological impact on the growing child and his family. It is also not negligible the role of surgery in contributing to the correction of ocular movement deficits. In fact, repairing orbital asymmetry contribute in inmproving the impaired ability to fix and follow and visual field defects in these children [48].

Concerning intracranial pressure (ICP), abnormal ICP values have only been seldomly reported in children with unicornal synostosis [49], a finding which is easily explained by the fact that the intracranial volume in UCS overlaps normal volumes of unaffected children up to 18 months of life and that most of the normal ICP recordings which are present in the literature refer to toddlers up to 1 year of age. Conversely, Eley et al. have reported abnormally increased (42%) or borderline ICP values (29%) in unoperated children with mean age of 3.5 years [50]. In spite of the small size of the series (7 cases), results reported by these authors confirm that the risk of increased ICP in unoperated children with craniosynostosis is growing with the child growth. Timing of surgery is a matter of debate. Whereas some author advocate early correction of the deformity (1–4 months) using less invasive techniques, profiting in this case of the malleability of the bone [51], but at the cost of a too early re-ossification and higher intraoperative infectious and hemorrhagic complication rates, other neurosurgeons prefer to operate later on, generally between the fourth and the eighth month of life, to achieve more stable results, but at the cost of an higher rate of bone defects [52].

32.1.4.2 Goals of the Surgery

The goals of the surgical corrections are to restore the shape of the forehead and the orbit, to increase the volume of the ipsilateral anterior cranial fossa and orbit, and to redirect the vectors of growth of the skull, with the final aim of minimizing the facial asymmetry and the neurological and ophthalmological changes. Many techniques are currently available to achieve these goals [6, 16, 53–56].

32.1.5 Surgical Technique: Open Surgery

32.1.5.1 Surgical Steps Specific for Unicoronal Synostosis (Fig. 32.2)

Surgical considerations for anesthesiology and skin incision are similar to what has been reported for metopic synostosis. Similarly, the goal of this step is to expose both the frontal bones (and part of the parietal and the temporal bones), the nasofrontal junction, both the orbits, and the frontozygomatic sutures. The bilateral exposition is

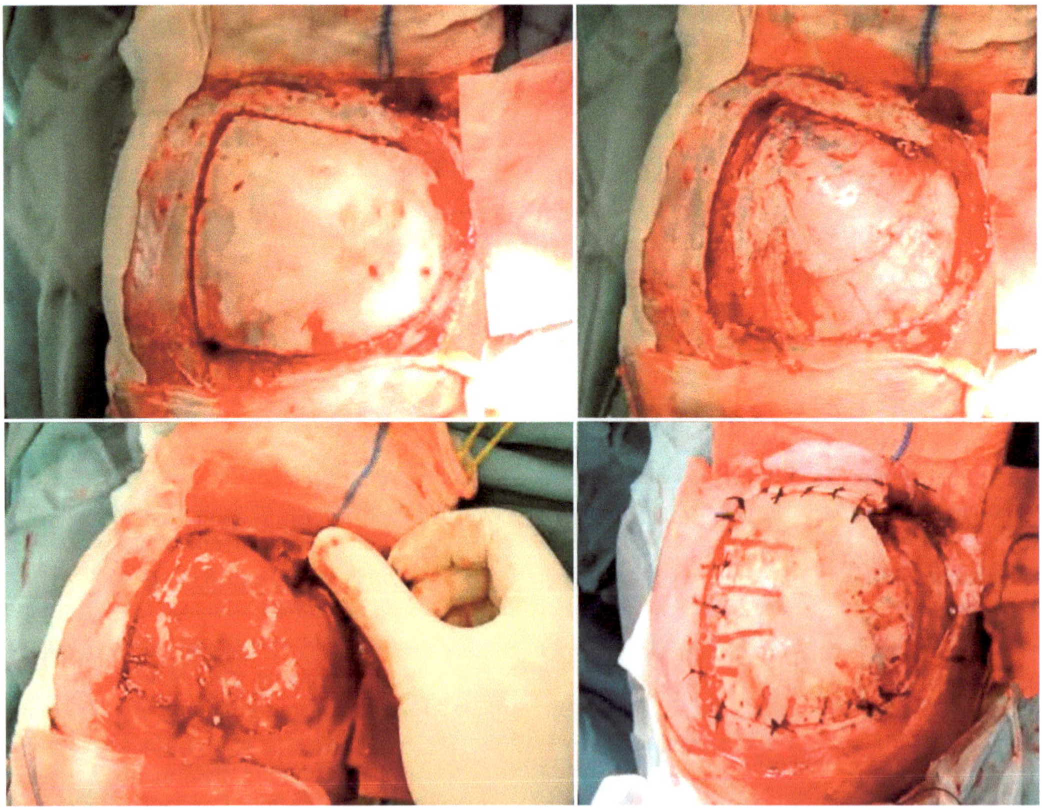

Fig. 32.2 Surgical steps specific for unicoronal synostosis

meant to favor a symmetrical frontal reconstruction, even when the fronto-orbital craniotomy is unilateral. The pericranium is incised parallel to the affected orbit (at least 1½–2 cm above the supraorbital rim to preserve the supraorbital nerve main branch and the vessels), to the metopic and the coronal suture. After a subperiosteal dissection, the pericranium pedunculated on the temporal muscle is overturned toward the ear. In case of a unilateral approach, the dissection of the periosteum, though being substantially unilateral from the affected frontal side, should be extended over the midline for 2 cm; this in order to gain a sufficient amount of tissue to cover the advanced orbital roof. Downward, the dissection is carried out over the supraorbital ridge, extending medially up to the front-nasal junction and, laterally, to the lateral orbital canthus down to the zygomatic body: as a result, the medial, superior, and lateral walls of the orbit are exposed. During this phase of the dissection, the periorbital fascia is separated from the orbital roof taking care to not damage the lacrimal gland. Downward care should be taken to free the supraorbital nerve from its groove or foramen, when closed; in fact, the supraorbital canal is commonly still opened in its inferior border in the great majority of children below 1 year of age. When the canal is closed, sparing of the supraorbital nerve is not always possible, but a spontaneous functional recovery has been observed during the follow-up in the majority of cases [57]. Once this phase is completed, an ipsilateral frontal bone flap is designed according to the frontal flattening and the severity of the retrusion. Templates may be used to better design the flap as well as software designed to preplan the flap using virtual reality or 3D preprinted models are available for this purpose. As a common rule, the bone flap is extended 1 to 3–4 cm beyond the midline which allows to improve remodeling profiting of the contralateral convex frontal bone shape. For a similar purpose, the posterior border of the flap is variably placed a few centimeters behind the affected coronal suture. The anterior limit of the flap is set 1.5–2 cm above the supraorbital rim. The number and location of the burr holes are defined according to the planned craniotomy and the available instrumentation. If the anterior fontanel (AF) is still opened, two burr holes only are needed, the first at the level of the pterional region, the second at the lower medial limit of the frontal bone flap, 1.5-2 cm, above the fronto-nasal-orbital junction. In case of closure of the anterior fontanel, an additional burr hole is placed midline at the frontoparietal junction. Craniotome is used to join the burr holes, substituting it with ultrasonic bone cutting devices (i.e., Piezosurgery®) if available at the inferior border, main advantages being a reduction of the risks of damaging the dura mater as well as a consistent higher possibility to spare bone tissue. The bone flap is elevated after careful dissection from the dura mater and the coronal suture. The thickened pterional bone is removed with rongeur or it is cut with ultrasonic saws along the temporal fossa to unlock the locally restricted regional bone growth.

Bilateral frontal craniotomy, originally proposed by Tessier in 1967, has been alternatively used to unilateral frontal bone flaps. In a bilateral approach, the bilateral frontal flap is realized cutting the bone anteriorly at least 1 cm behind the orbital rim and posteriorly 1 cm behind the coronal suture.

Orbitotomy represents the second step of the surgery. In case of a unilateral approach, the orbitotomy is carried out by cutting the lateral orbital wall at the level of the orbito-zygomatic suture and the roof 1 cm posteriorly and parallel to the superior orbital ridge reaching the upper aspect of its medial wall. Both microdrill and ultrasonic cutting devices may be used for this purpose. The medial wall of the orbit (orbito-nasal surface) is left intact constituting the pivot for the lateral advancement of the superior orbital ridge obtained by means of a green stick fracture at its level. The orbit is recontoured manually, with rongeurs or Tessier bender orbit in a way to make it more arched and more convex anteriorly, mimicking the normal border of the opposite side.

Finally, the orbital ridge is advanced and placed in a hypercorrected position in order to avoid an early postoperative retrusion and it is done both in the sagittal (anteriorly) and in the coronal plane with the objective of overlapping the position of the contralateral orbit; the final position is stabilized with the use of a resorbable plate, fixed on the pterional region proximally and on the lateral border of the orbit distally. Among the several changes that have been proposed, the most common is harvesting a complete (bilateral and in one piece) supraorbital bar [58]. The osteotomies in this case are carried out asymmetrically, ending at the fronto-malar suture on the healthy side and extending to the lateral orbital process of the malar bone on the synostotic side. The bandeau is then contoured to achieve a smooth curved symmetrical contour. One resorbable plate for each side is hence used to fix the orbital bar to the two temporal regions; in order to obtain an adequate correction, the orbital bar is placed obliquely with its higher point in the contralateral side and lower point in the affected side.

Barrel stave osteotomies and greenstick fractures, to weak the bone, and by Tessier bender are used to achieve the right curvature of the frontal bone which is defined case by case based on preoperative imaging, templates, or 3D printed models [10, 59–61].

The bone flap is then replaced, usually rotated by 90 or, less frequently, rotated by 180 or not rotated, according to which rotation assures the best reconstruction [6, 16, 54–56]. The modified frontal bone flap is finally fixed to the advanced orbital bandeau with titanium or biodegradable plates or alternatively sutures.

Concerning sutures, resorbable stitches are preferred to silk for their lower risk to cause granulomatous reactions. In case they're used, the advanced orbit and frontal bone must perfectly fit to maintain their position, in order to reduce the risk of postoperative retrusion. A tip in this case is to buttress a tongue-in-groove bone fragment between the orbit and the sphenoid wing/temporal bone [10].

Titanium miniplates and screws, widely diffused, easy to use, malleable, and relatively cheap, ensure the best rigid fixation and the lower rate of recurrence. However, they are burdened by the higher risk of complications such as disturbance of the growth of the skull, rupture/pull out, skin erosion, and inner migration [62–64]. The inner migration is the main disadvantage of using metallic fixation in craniosynostosis surgery, since a second operation is needed to remove the plates and the screws in cases of their migration, that, due to its relatively high rate of occurrence, is actually suggested for prophylactic purposes to prevent such a complication. Absorbable mini-plates and screws are actually considered to offer the best compromise between reabsorption (Vycril suture) and rigid fixation (titanium). Transient visibility up to their resorption and granulomatous reactions, reported with an incidence of up to 15%, are the main reported complications of these devices [65–67], though their incidence is significantly reduced by the recent improvement in the materials. Actually, in a large multicenter review (1883 patients), device instability rate was as low as 0.3%, the infection rate 0.2%, and the granuloma occurrence rate 0.7% [68]. Actually, the main limitation of absorbable plates is their elevated cost.

Once the bone fixation is ended, the periosteal flap is sutured to cover as much as possible the osteotomies, especially in the orbital region, to drive a good re-ossification.

32.2 Bicoronal Synostosis (Brachycephaly)

Brachycephaly is the definition of the cranial shape that commonly results after premature closure of both sides of the coronal suture. As a consequence of this premature fusion, the anterior fossa adopts a characteristic deformation, broad and short, and there are retruded frontal bones and orbital rims with a vertical, broad, flat forehead and a high bregmatic point. Bicoronal synostosis may appear as an isolated synostosis and has then a favorable prognosis. More often, however, is the clinical manifestation of different syndromic craniosynostoses that share a premature closure of bicoronal sutures and similar phenotype (like Saehtre-Chotzen or Pfeiffer type I syndromes).

Surgical treatment and technique do not differ significantly from what has been previously described for unicoronal synostosis with a bilateral approach. A bilateral skin incision back to the coronal suture and bilateral periosteal flap precede a bilateral frontal craniotomy 2 cm. above the two orbital roofs. A tongue in groove orbital bar is created with similar principles as for the orbital bar, when performed, in unicoronal synostosis. The frontal bone flap is remodeled with radial cuts and reversed more commonly 180° to get the more rounded frontoparietal region to represent the frontal prominences. A recontouring of the orbital bar gaining an adequate curvature follows, with its fixation to the temporal region on the two sides, with special attention to invert the concave curvature as much as possible to make it convex. Suture of the bone flap to the orbital roofs, closure of the periosteal flaps before skin closure, follows the same principles cited above.

32.3 Endoscopic Treatment of Coronal Synostosis (Fig. 32.3)

As for metopic synostosis, endoscopic treatment has been considered as an alternative to open FOA also for coronal synostoses. Indications and limits, including the need of a postoperative helmet, are shared. The technical and directly related points are:

1. 3 cm skin incision 1 cm. back to the coronal suture
2. 1 cm incision lateral 3 cm above the fronto-orbital junction
3. Release of the coronal suture through a 1–1.5 cm. in anteroposterior diameter craniectomy that starts from the midline and it is extended downward and laterally to reach the fronto-orbital junction.

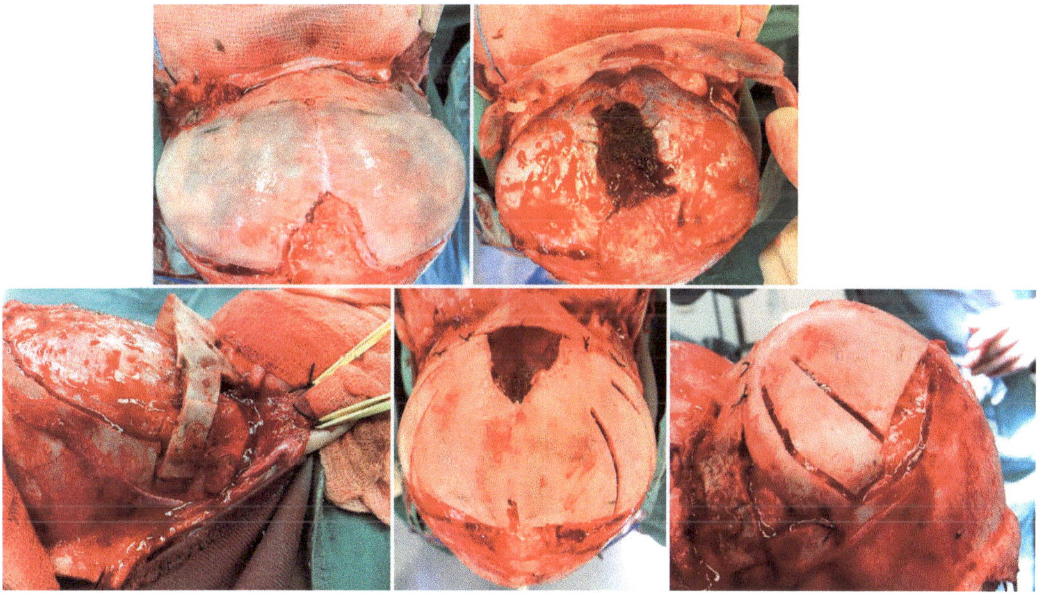

Fig. 32.3 Endoscopic treatment of coronal synostosis

References

1. Chan JWH, Stewart CL, Stalder MW, St Hilaire H, McBride L, Moses MH. Endoscope-assisted versus open repair of craniosynostosis: a comparison of perioperative cost and risk. J Craniofac Surg. 2013;24(1):170–4.
2. Fearon JA, Ruotolo RA, Kolar JC. Single sutural craniosynostoses: surgical outcomes and long-term growth. Plast Reconstr Surg. 2009;123(2):635–42.
3. Jaskolka MS. Current controversies in metopic suture Craniosynostosis. Oral Maxillofac Surg Clin N Am. 2017;29(4):447–63.
4. Guzman R, Looby JF, Schendel SA, Edwards MSB. Fronto-orbital advancement using an en bloc frontal bone craniectomy. Oper Neurosurg Hagerstown Md. 2011;68(suppl_1):68–74.
5. Ozlen F, Kafadar AM, Abuzayed B, Ulu MO, Isler C, Dashti R, et al. Surgical treatment of trigonocephaly: technique and long-term results in 48 cases. J Neurosurg Pediatr. 2011;7(3):300–10.
6. Pang D, Zovickian J, Wong S, Hou YJ, Le HN. Parallel angulated frontal bone slat cuts for treatment of metopic synostosis and other frontal skull deformities: the "cathedral dome procedure". Childs Nerv Syst ChNS. 2013;29(12):2171–82.
7. Robins JMW, Sheikh AJ, Shastin D, Schramm MWJ, Carter P, Russell JL, et al. Fronto-orbital advancement and reconstruction using reverse frontal bone graft without the use of orbital bar: a technical note. Childs Nerv Syst ChNS. 2020;36(6):1295–9.
8. Bennett KG, Liang F, Ranganathan K, Muraszko KM, Vercler CJ, Buchman SR. Surgical hypercorrection of trigonocephaly: evaluation of surgical outcomes. J Craniofac Surg. 2018;29(1):56–61.
9. Hormozi AK, Shahverdiani R, Mohammadi HR, Zali A, Mofrad HRH. Surgical treatment of metopic synostosis. J Craniofac Surg. 2011;22(1):261–5.
10. Seal SKF, Steinbok P, Courtemanche DJ. The cranial orbital buttress technique for nonsyndromic unicoronal and metopic craniosynostosis. Neurosurg Focus. 2015;38(5):E4.
11. Braun TL, Eisemann BS, Olorunnipa O, Buchanan EP, Monson LA. Safety outcomes in endoscopic versus open repair of metopic craniosynostosis. J Craniofac Surg. 2018;29(4):856–60.
12. Di Rocco C, Velardi F, Ferrario A, Marchese E. Metopic synostosis: in favour of a «simplified» surgical treatment. Childs Nerv Syst ChNS. 1996;12(11):654–63.
13. Kampf S, Micko A, Schwartz E, Schopper C, Reinprecht A. Clinical and aesthetic outcome analysis of a case series of trigonocephaly patients after early fronto-orbital advancement. Int J Oral Maxillofac Surg. 2020;49(9):1115–21.
14. Messi M, Consorti G, Lupi E, Girotto R, Valassina D, Balercia P. A new operative open-wings technique to correct the frontoforehead unit in metopic synostosis. J Craniofac Surg. 2015;26(3):902–5.
15. Natghian H, Song M, Jayamohan J, Johnson D, Magdum S, Richards P, et al. Long-term results in isolated metopic synostosis: the Oxford experience over 22 years. Plast Reconstr Surg. 2018;142(4):509e–15e.
16. Britto JA, Gwanmesia I, Leshem D. The Christmas tree foreheadplasty: a novel technique used in combination with a bandeau for fronto-orbital remodelling in craniosynostosis. Childs Nerv Syst ChNS. 2012;28(9):1375–80.
17. Fearon JA, Ditthakasem K, Garcia JC, Herbert M. Abandoning the supraorbital bandeau in anterior craniosynostosis repairs, for a single-segment reconstruction. Plast Reconstr Surg. 2018;142(3):334e–41e.
18. Keshavarzi S, Hayden MG, Ben-Haim S, Meltzer HS, Cohen SR, Levy ML. Variations of endoscopic and open repair of metopic craniosynostosis. J Craniofac Surg. 2009;20(5):1439–44.
19. Paik H, Byeon JH. Anterior two-thirds calvarial remodelling: operative technique for the correction of metopic synostosis in toddlers. J Plast Reconstr Aesthetic Surg JPRAS. 2010;63(1):36–41.
20. Maniskas S, Chandler L, Bruckman K, Pourtaheri N, DiLuna M, Steinbacher DM. Three-dimensional analysis and surgical planning for open correction of trigonocephaly. Plast Reconstr Surg. 2021;147(2):265e–7e.
21. Birgfeld CB, Dufton L, Naumann H, Hopper RA, Gruss JS, Haberkern CM, et al. Safety of open cranial vault surgery for single-suture craniosynostosis: a case for the multidisciplinary team. J Craniofac Surg. 2015;26(7):2052–8.
22. di Rocco F, Gleizal A, Lohkamp L, Szathmari A, Paulus C, Mottolese C. Control of metopic emissary veins in trigonocephaly surgery. Technical note Childs Nerv Syst ChNS. 2018;34(12):2481–4.
23. Massimi L, Rapisarda A, Bianchi F, Frassanito P, Tamburrini G, Pelo S, et al. Piezosurgery in pediatric neurosurgery. World Neurosurg. 2019;126:e625–33.
24. Carter LM, Varley I, Smith IM, Chumas P, Liddington M, Russell JL. Inner table corticectomy of the fronto-orbital bar in correction of metopic and coronal craniosynostoses. J Craniofac Surg. 2013;24(1):195–6.
25. Aryan HE, Jandial R, Ozgur BM, Hughes SA, Meltzer HS, Park MS, et al. Surgical correction of metopic synostosis. Childs Nerv Syst ChNS. 2005;21(5):392–8.
26. Gandolfi BM, Hirji SA, Sobol DL, Allori AC, Marcus JR. Power-assisted particulate bone grafting effectively prevents osseous defects after cranial vault reconstruction. J Craniofac Surg. 2018;29(3):547–52.
27. Madaree A. Use of acellular dermal matrix in craniosynostosis. J Craniofac Surg. 2018;29(1):126–9.
28. Burstein F, Eppley B, Hudgins R, Williams J, Boydston W, Reisner A, et al. Application of the spanning plate concept to frontal orbital advancement: techniques and clinical experience in 60 patients. J Craniofac Surg. 2006;17(2):241–5.
29. Bhatti-Söfteland M, Maltese G, Tarnow P, Hagmarker L, Wikberg E, Bernhardt P, et al. Temporal deformity objectively measured before and after surgery for metopic synostosis: retrusion rather than hollowing. J Craniofac Surg. 2017;28(7):1757–60.

30. Fawzy HH, Choi JW, Ra YS. One-piece fronto-orbital distraction with midline splitting but without bandeau for metopic craniosynostosis: craniometric, volumetric, and morphologic evaluation. Ann Plast Surg. 2019;83(3):285–92.
31. Maltese G, Tarnow P, Lauritzen CG. Spring-assisted correction of hypotelorism in metopic synostosis. Plast Reconstr Surg. 2007;119(3):977–84.
32. Shen W, Cui J, Chen J, Zou J, Ji Y, Chen H, et al. Correction of craniosynostosis using modified spring-assisted surgery. J Craniofac Surg. 2015;26(2):522–5.
33. Sunaga A, Sugawara Y, Kamochi H, Gomi A, Uda H, Sarukawa S, et al. Development of multidirectional cranial distraction osteogenesis for the treatment of craniosynostosis. J Craniofac Surg. 2019;30(1):57–60.
34. Barrientos S, Miller J. Anterior cranial vault reconstruction with distraction for primary and secondary craniosynostosis repair. J Craniofac Surg. 2019;30(2):e109–12.
35. Park DH, Yoon SH. The trans-sutural distraction osteogenesis for 22 cases of craniosynostosis: a new, easy, safe, and efficient method in craniosynostosis surgery. Pediatr Neurosurg. 2011;47(3):167–75.
36. Davis C, Lauritzen CGK. Frontobasal suture distraction corrects hypotelorism in metopic synostosis. J Craniofac Surg. 2009;20(1):121–4.
37. Delgado-Fernández J, Rivero-Garvía M, Márquez-Rivas J. How I do it. 3D endoscopic treatment of metopic craniosynostosis through a single incision. Acta Neurochir (Wien). 2017;159(11):2067–70.
38. Erşahin Y. Endoscope-assisted repair of metopic synostosis. Childs Nerv Syst ChNS. 2013;29(12):2195–9.
39. Jimenez DF, McGinity MJ, Barone CM. Endoscopy-assisted early correction of single-suture metopic craniosynostosis: a 19-year experience. J Neurosurg Pediatr. 2018;23(1):61–74.
40. Lajthia O, Rogers GF, Tsering D, Keating RF, Magge SN. Quantitative outcomes of endoscopic strip craniectomy for metopic craniosynostosis in children with severe trigonocephaly. Childs Nerv Syst ChNS. 2021;37(2):573–9.
41. Gociman B, Agko M, Blagg R, Garlick J, Kestle JRW, Siddiqi F. Endoscopic-assisted correction of metopic synostosis. J Craniofac Surg. 2013;24(3):763–8.
42. Chaichana KL, Jallo GI, Dorafshar AH, Ahn ES. Novel use of an ultrasonic bone-cutting device for endoscopic-assisted craniosynostosis surgery. Childs Nerv Syst ChNS. 2013;29(7):1163–8.
43. Hinojosa J. Endoscopic-assisted treatment of trigonocephaly. Childs Nerv Syst ChNS. 2012;28(9):1381–7.
44. Dalle Ore CL, Dilip M, Brandel MG, McIntyre JK, Hoshide R, Calayag M, et al. Endoscopic surgery for nonsyndromic craniosynostosis: a 16-year single-center experience. J Neurosurg Pediatr. 2018;22(4):335–43.
45. Baumgartner JE, Teichgraeber JF, Waller AL, Grantcherova E, Gateno J, Xia JJ. Microscopic approach to craniosynostosis. J Craniofac Surg. 2005;16(6):997–1005.
46. Teichgraeber JF, Baumgartner JE, Waller AL, Reis SM, Stafford MT, Hollinger LE, et al. Microscopic minimally invasive approach to nonsyndromic craniosynostosis. J Craniofac Surg. 2009;20(5):1492–500.
47. Hankinson TC, Fontana EJ, Anderson RCE, Feldstein NA. Surgical treatment of single-suture craniosynostosis: an argument for quantitative methods to evaluate cosmetic outcomes. J Neurosurg Pediatr. 2010;6(2):193–7.
48. Chieffo D, Tamburrini G, Massimi L, Di Giovanni S, Giansanti C, Caldarelli M, et al. Long-term neuropsychological development in single-suture craniosynostosis treated early. J Neurosurg Pediatr. 2010;5(3):232–7.
49. Tamburrini G, Caldarelli M, Massimi L, Santini P, Di Rocco C. Intracranial pressure monitoring in children with single suture and complex craniosynostosis: a review. Childs Nerv Syst ChNS. 2005;21(10):913–21.
50. Eley KA, Johnson D, Wilkie AOM, Jayamohan J, Richards P, Wall SA. Raised intracranial pressure is frequent in untreated nonsyndromic unicoronal synostosis and does not correlate with severity of phenotypic features. Plast Reconstr Surg. 2012;130(5):690e–7e.
51. Barone CM, Jimenez DF. Endoscopic approach to coronal craniosynostosis. Clin Plast Surg. 2004;31(3):415–22. vi
52. Metzler P, Zemann W, Jacobsen C, Lübbers HT, Grätz KW, Obwegeser JA. Cranial vault growth in multiple-suture nonsyndromic and syndromic craniosynostosis: a postoperative long-term anthropometric follow-up. J Craniofac Surg. 2013;24(3):753–7.
53. Di Rocco C, Paternoster G, Caldarelli M, Massimi L, Tamburrini G. Anterior plagiocephaly: epidemiology, clinical findings,diagnosis, and classification. A review. Childs Nerv Syst ChNS. 2012;28(9):1413–22.
54. Di Rocco C, Frassanito P, Tamburrini G. The shell technique: bilateral fronto-orbital reshaping in trigonocephaly. Childs Nerv Syst ChNS. 2013;29(12):2189–94.
55. Pellerin P, Calibre C, Vinchon M, Dhellemmes P, Wolber A, Guerreschi P. Unicoronal synostotic plagiocephaly: surgical correction: Lille's technique. Childs Nerv Syst ChNS. 2012;28(9):1433–8.
56. Jeyaraj P. A modified approach to surgical correction of anterior plagiocephaly. J Maxillofac Oral Surg. 2012;11(3):358–63.
57. Matushita H, Alonso N, Cardeal DD, de Andrade F. Frontal-orbital advancement for the management of anterior plagiocephaly. Childs Nerv Syst ChNS. 2012;28(9):1423–7.
58. Buchman SR, Muraszko K. Frontoorbital reconstruction. Atlas Oral Maxillofac Surg Clin North Am. 2002;10(1):43–56.
59. Hochfeld M, Lamecker H, Thomale UW, Schulz M, Zachow S, Haberl H. Frame-based cranial reconstruction. J Neurosurg Pediatr. 2014;13(3):319–23.
60. Khechoyan DY, Saber NR, Burge J, Fattah A, Drake J, Forrest CR, et al. Surgical outcomes in craniosynostosis reconstruction: the use of prefabricated tem-

plates in cranial vault remodelling. J Plast Reconstr Aesthetic Surg JPRAS. 2014;67(1):9–16.
61. Pappa H, Richardson D, Webb AAC, May P. Individualized template-guided remodeling of the fronto-orbital bandeau in craniosynostosis corrective surgery. J Craniofac Surg. 2009;20(1):178–9.
62. Courtemanche DJ, Mutimer KL, Holmes AD, Levant BA, Clement JG. Experimental calvarial growth disturbance by micro-plate and screw fixation. Aust N Z J Surg. 1992;62(6):482–8.
63. Duke BJ, Mouchantat RA, Ketch LL, Winston KR. Transcranial migration of microfixation plates and screws. Case report. Pediatr Neurosurg. 1996;25(1):31–4; discussion 35.
64. Panchal J, Uttchin V. Management of craniosynostosis. Plast Reconstr Surg. 2003;111(6):2032–48. quiz 2049
65. Pearson GD, Havlik RJ, Eppley B, Nykiel M, Sadove AM. Craniosynostosis: a single institution's outcome assessment from surgical reconstruction. J Craniofac Surg. 2008;19(1):65–71.
66. Sanger C, Soto A, Mussa F, Sanzo M, Sardo L, Donati PA, et al. Maximizing results in craniofacial surgery with bioresorbable fixation devices. J Craniofac Surg. 2007;18(4):926–30.
67. Goodrich JT, Sandler AL, Tepper O. A review of reconstructive materials for use in craniofacial surgery bone fixation materials, bone substitutes, and distractors. Childs Nerv Syst ChNS. 2012;28(9):1577–88.
68. Eppley BL, Morales L, Wood R, Pensler J, Goldstein J, Havlik RJ, et al. Resorbable PLLA-PGA plate and screw fixation in pediatric craniofacial surgery: clinical experience in 1883 patients. Plast Reconstr Surg. 2004;114(4):850–6; discussion 857.

33 Principles and Techniques of Posterior Vault Remodeling

Claudia Pasquali and Federico Di Rocco

33.1 Principles: Rationale, Indications, and Risks

Posterior cranial deformities can be either asymmetrical (posterior plagiocephaly) or symmetrical (brachy-turricephaly) [1].

Isolated fusion of the lambdoid suture is the rarest form of craniosynostosis: it represents less than 1–5.5% of all cases of craniosynostoses. Its incidence has been considered to be increased up to 8.2% in the last decades because of the "Back to Sleep campaign" of the American Academy of Pediatrics in 1992 to prevent the sudden death of neonates, which has participated actually to increase the incidence of positional calvaria deformations with which the true lambdoid synostosis is misdiagnosed.

True lambdoid craniosynostosis is characterized by the homolateral occipitomastoid bulge with shifting of the ear inferiorly and posteriorly and a contralateral parietal and ipsilateral occipitomastoid bossing which makes the head wider posteriorly than anteriorly, resulting in a trapezoid head shape when viewed from above.

It is estimated that 15% of cases of lambdoid craniosynostosis are bilateral [2]. This condition is characterized by the flattening and widening of the occipital region associated with elongation of the vertex resulting in a brachi-turricephalic aspect of the cranium. The ears are displaced anteriorly and inferiorly.

These aspects can be found in association with synostosis of the sagittal suture in the so-called "Mercedes-Benz syndrome" or be part of a complex, multi-suture syndromic synostosis [3].

The growing brain is the force that guides the neurocranium growing: the calvaria bone is separated and then the osteogenesis process progressively fills the gap [4].

The change in intracranial volume with age is not clearly linear: we can recognize three main period each lasting approximately 5 years (0–5, 5–10, 10–15), characterized by a linear growth of intracranial volume, although the rate of growth differs between these periods.

In 1999, Sgouros et al. showed that in the first few months of life, the intracranial volume is on average 900 cm^3 in boys and 600 cm^3 in girls and that at the age of 2 years it reaches 77% of the volume that il will have at 15 years and at 5 years the 90%. They further demonstrated that patients with craniosynostosis born with a significantly smaller intracranial volume, about 500 cm^3 at the age of 1 month, but at around the age of 6 months the total cranial volume is normalized and since that age they follow the normal head growth pattern. Consequently, any negative constricting effects from craniosynostosis are most likely to

C. Pasquali · F. Di Rocco (✉)
Pediatric Neurosurgery, French Referral Center for Craniosynostosis of Lyon, Hopital Femme Mère Enfant, Université de Lyon, Lyon, France
e-mail: claudia.pasquali@chu-lyon.fr; federico.dirocco@chu-lyon.fr

F. Di Rocco, J. Kestle (eds.), *Neurosurgical Aspects of Craniosynostosis*,
https://doi.org/10.1007/978-3-031-69386-1_33

occur during the first months of life when the difference in intracranial volume between normal and craniosynostosis patients is maximal [5, 6].

An underdeveloped posterior cranial fossa and a consequent craniocerebral disproportion due to the premature fusion of the cranial sutures in children with syndromic or multi-sutural craniosynostosis can be predisposed to a raised intracranial pressure (ICP) with various associations with hydrocephalus or a Chiari type 1 malformation [7, 8].

An incidence of Chiari malformation is described up to 72.2% in children with Crouzon syndrome and between 1.1 and 3% in non-syndromic craniosynostosis [7, 9].

Progressive hydrocephalus has been reported to occur in 9–26% of Crouzon patients and 28–64% of patients with Pfeiffer syndrome. Its origin has to be considered multifactorial, with one of the main recognized mechanisms being crowding in the posterior cranial fossa leading to functional obstruction of cerebrospinal fluid outflow within the cerebral aqueduct [7, 10].

As previously mentioned, the problem of craniocerebral disproportion in craniostenosis, with few exceptions like FGFR2-related craniosynostosis, is maximum in the first month of life, [5, 11] so it cannot be the only mechanism that contributes to increase of intracranial pressure in these patients: airway obstruction [12] and a venous engorgement [13–15] play a non-marginal role in the development of this sequelae which can be considered therefore as a complex and multifactorial pathology (Fig. 33.1) [13].

These patients present a high incidence of anomalies of venous drainage, namely the stenosis of the sigmoid-jugular complex and the transverse sinus agenesis, in particular the one homolateral to the stenosis, associated with various degree of collateral venous collector and in some cases associated with a hypertrophy of the contralateral transvers sinus which can make surgery challenging because of the risk of damage during the dural dissection (Fig. 33.2) [16, 17].

Recent genetic studies speculate on the role of an intrinsic vascular problem associated with the intracranial hypertension. Immunohistochemical examination detected FGFR gene expression products both in synostosic sutures and cranial vascular endothelium: they would stimulate a premature endothelial proliferation resulting in stenosis of these vessels [18]. Loss of expression of the Twist 1 gene seems to have the same implications [19], though clinically Saethre-Choitzen patients do not display the same degree of vascular anomalies than patients with Crouzon or Pfeiffer syndrome.

Venous compression and malformation can also have an impact on surgery: according to the literature, the most exuberant collateral circulation in patients with syndromic craniosynostosis occurs in the posterior fossa, making adequate preoperative planning essential.

Rollins' studies on cerebral venogram find functional stenosis of the jugular foramen in 100% of patients affected with Pfeiffer syndrome, in 62% with Crouzon syndrome, in 50% with Apert syndrome, and in 83% with complex craniosynostosis [20].

Exuberant emissaries are found in 100% of patients with Pfeiffer syndrome, 74% in Crouzon, 36% in Apert, and 33% in Saerthre-Chotzen; occipital and mastoid emissaries are the most common. The persistence of fetal sinus is described in Crouzon and Pfeiffer syndrome, in particular the occipital sinus and the marginal one [21].

The two main objectives of surgery for craniosynostosis are to expand the cranial vault volume to prevent or reduce the raised intracranial pressure and to correct the morphological impact on the anterior cranium [22].

For decades, fronto-orbital advancement (FOA) for cranial vault expansion has been the standard treatment to correct the typical exorbitism, the forehead, and supraorbital bar recession of brachycephaly and to increase the volume of the intracranial cavity.

The high reoperation rate due to the failure in restoring the intracranial pression and the inadequate correction of brachy-turricephaly deformity, described up to 100% in Apert patients, 26% in Crouzon, 38% in Pfeiffer, and 65% in patients with Saethre–Chotzen syndrome, [23] with a reoperation rate of 8.2%, raising to 16.7% in Apert syndrome, even higher if fronto-orbital advancement (FOA) is performed before 6 months of age, stimulates the development of

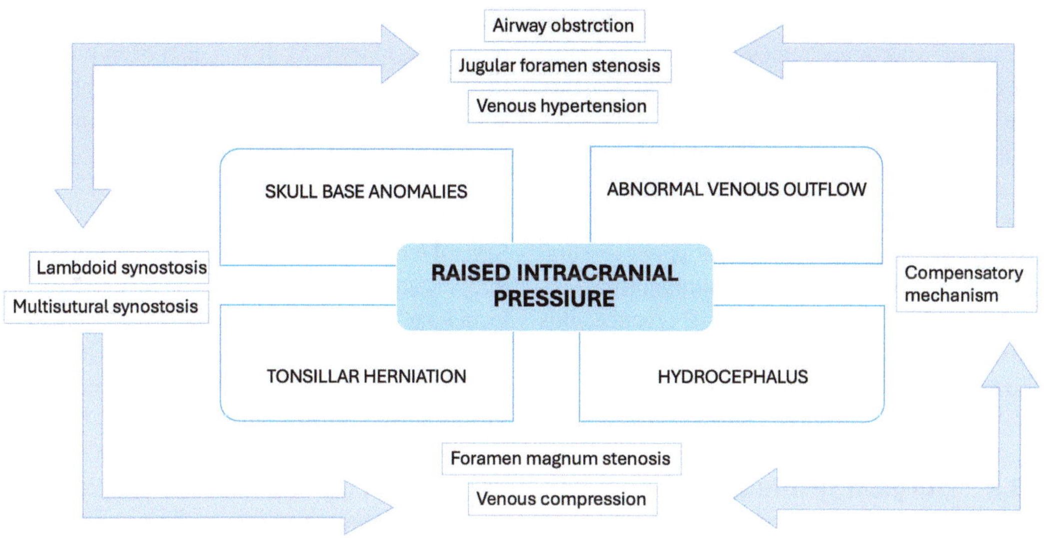

Fig. 33.1 The complex relationship between the factors concurring to a raised intracranial pressure. (Adapted from: Protzenko T et al. Venous anomalies in hypoplastic posterior fossa: unsolved questions. Childs Nerv Syst. 2021;37(10):3177–3187)

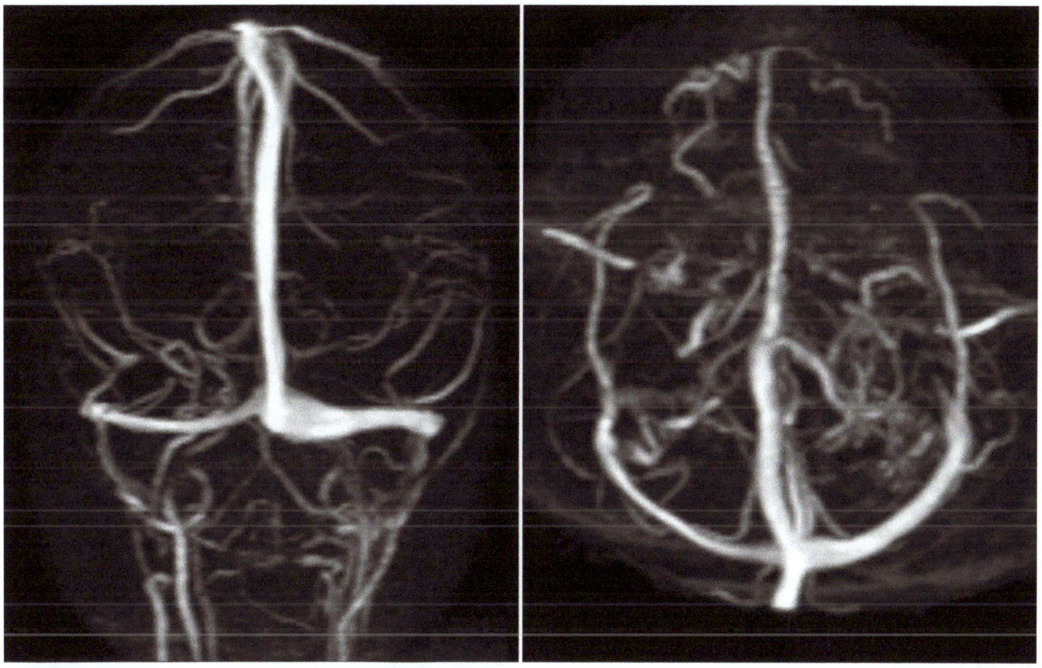

Fig. 33.2 Transversus sinus asymmetry in Crouzon syndrome

surgical procedure for the direct expansion of the posterior cranial vault. Choi's study effectively shows that these procedures can reach intracranial volume expansion approximately 35% greater than anterior cranial vault advancement procedures [24].

The procedure should be made early enough to prevent negative effects on brain development and further progression toward turricephaly, but in case of syndromic craniosynostoses the surgical reconstructions are associated with a higher rate of relapse when performed in very very young children [24]. Thus, the surgical timing is a compromise between developmental stage compatible with safe general anesthesia and surgery and the stage of maximal craniocerebral disproportion to prevent also a supranormal correction of intracranial volume. In practice, this puts the preferred timing between the age of 3 and 6 months [4, 6].

33.2 Surgical Techniques

The posterior cranial vault may be expanded by posterior cranioplasty or by less invasive methods based on gradual posterior cranial vault expansion or distraction [22].

The common goal of all these procedures is to prevent the developing of intracranial hypertension, the progression toward turricephaly, and to reduce any local brain compression within the posterior cranial fossa by increasing the intracranial volume [4].

Posterior skull vault remodeling can either use a single procedure that is necessary in case of pure lambdoid or Mercedes-Benz synostosis or represent the first step of a multistage operative management in cases of complex syndromic craniosynostoses [25].

33.2.1 Fixed Posterior Cranial Vault Expansion (PCVE)

The "conventional" PCVE implies parieto-occipital bon flaps osteotomies, active remodeling, repositioning, rearrangement, reconstruction, advancement, and enlargement plus their fixation, usually elevated from the dura. It is a surgical option suitable for syndromic and non-syndromic unilateral or bilateral lambdoid synostosis, Mercedes-Benz pattern, secondary craniosynostosis due to an over drainage in shunted patients, and correction of scaphocephaly with a severe occipitoparietal narrowing and prominent inion [26]. It has also been proposed in case of severe positional plagiocephaly in which every corrective noninvasive measure applied has failed [27].

33.2.1.1 PCVE Surgical Technique

Several technical nuances are described in literature; [1, 28, 29] here we describe the "Lyonnaise technique" which combines the Tiara-technique, a remodeling procedure described by Goodrich, and the Meander technique, a volume increasing tongue-in-groove procedure.

The patient is in prone position, with the head slightly flexed in a horseshoe headrest. It is very important to pay attention to the positioning of face and eyes to avoid decubitus and pressure damage: a "hellenic helmet" (Fig. 33.3) can be used with this scope [25].

The German group suggests the use of a fixed pediatric headrest system and the spatial registration of patient radiological images with a neuronavigational system to define the position of posterior sagittal and transverse sinuses [1].

A standard ear to ear bicoronal incision is performed. Its location is very important for the further bon exposition: it should be enough anteriorly to permit a large skin flap allowing a resistant coverage of the expanded bone flap and anticipate at the same time the possible need for a secondary frontal surgery.

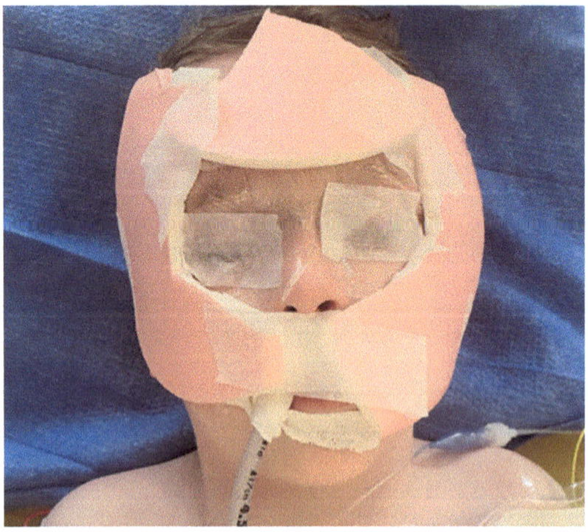

Fig. 33.3 The "hellenic helmet"

A subgaleal flap is then elevated posteriorly until the nuchal line, and a periosteal flap is dissected and elevated down to the insertion of the nuchal muscles: the posterior part of the parietal bones and the superior part of the occipital bone are exposed.

The lateral exposure reaches the posterior part of the temporo-squamosal suture and asterion, while, inferiorly, the dissection reaches the external occipital protuberance.

In case of skull lacunae and potential venous anomalies, care must be taken in order to avoid any dural bleeding and emissary vascular damage. Bone bleeding is controlled with bone wax, if needed.

When the posterior cranial vault is enough exposed, the osteotomy line can be drawn according to the preoperative plan: attention must be taken in case of forehead associated anomalies to spare the temporal region if a secondary distraction surgery of anterior cranial vault could be required.

A carefully dissection of dura mater is made with the help of blunt dissection through the sagittal suture itself or by directly passing through bony lacunas if present. The risk of dural adhesion, and a consequently dural damage, is higher when the lambdoid suture is present and in case of bony spicules that can be embedded extremely deeply within the dura and the parenchyma. Furthermore, particular attention must also be paid because hypertrophic transverse sinuses are described predominantly on the side of the permeable suture [16, 17]. If needed, burr holes are drilled to allow a proper dissection of the epidural plan: a median burr hole on the vertex on the sagittal suture or two paramedian burr holes to protect the sagittal sinus, and a burr hole on the asterion on each side can help a safer dissection.

At this point, in the "Meander technique", four to five tongues with about 2–3 cm of breadth and 10–15 cm of length are created parallel to the sagittal sinus in the technique described by Wagner [29] or perpendicular to the sagittal sinus in the midline in the case of symmetrical brachycephaly or towards the respective side in case of posterior plagiocephaly [1]. The tongues are then elevated from the dura mater and distracted away from the contralateral ones to progressively expanding the convexity of the calvarium and creating additional sub-calvaria, extradural space. The calvaria tongues are then connected in their distracted position [1, 29].

The Lyonnaise technique involves, first, the creation of bony band 1.5 cm width, a "Tiara", from the vertex down to the asterion on both sides that will be used later to enlarge the occipital region, and second, the realization of parietal and occipital osteotomies with the help of craniotome or piezosurgery (Fig. 33.4a).

A better control of potential emissary veins at occipital bone level can be reached with the help of rongeurs instead of craniotome. According to the operative plan, the occipital osteotomies can be carried out up to or even beyond the transverse sinuses.

After completing the dural dissection, the bone flap can then be elevated, the hemostasis controlled, and any eventually dural tear repaired.

At this point, multiple occipitoparietal bone cuts perpendicular to transverse sinus are done with the osteotome or piezosurgery: this maneuver creates occipital bone segments to be bent externally, resulting in a further increase of the skull expansion and intracranial volume increase (Fig. 33.4b) [25].

Finally, the reconstruction step can start. The "parietal-tiara" is placed occipitally and fixed with absorbable plates or absorbable stiches to the skull, creating a dead space allowing the posterior cerebral expansion: normally the bandeau needs a minimal reshaping to achieve a correct morphology, and furthermore, its consistency is hard enough to allow the child to rest on the head subsequently.

The remaining posterior parieto-occipital bone flap is reshaped and replaced over the dura in anatomical position or turned 180° if there is a great asymmetry to correct. Its fixation to the bandeau is usually performed with resorbable stitches. One or several absorbable plates can be used to maintain the posterior expansion and avoiding the bone flap to fall when closing the soft tissues (Fig. 33.4c).

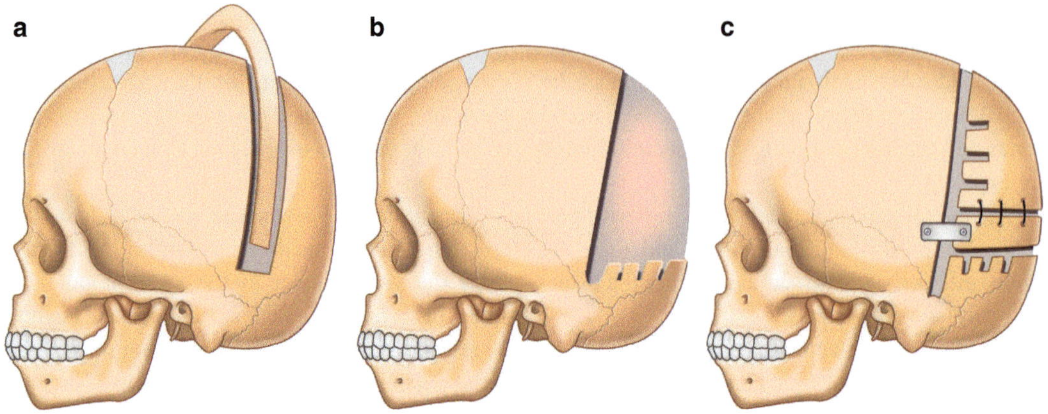

Fig. 33.4 Schematic representation of osteotomies (**a**, **b**) and of the final reconstruction (**c**). (Adapted from: Di Rocco et al. Fixed posterior cranial vault expansion technique. Childs Nerv Syst. 2021;37(10):3137–3141)

Once the bone flap has been fixed, bone powder and bony chips can be added to favor the postoperative ossification [25].

A closure layer by layer is performed; the skin tension can be reduced by an anterior subgaleal undermining.

A subgaleal drain can be placed and removed after 24 h.

Although the infection risk is very small, as there are no external devices, the displaced bone, detached from its blood supplies, acts as a not-vascularized bone graft in the immediate postoperative period time and it could interfere in the medical management of infection because the diffusion of antibiotics in the bone is reduced [25].

33.2.1.2 Advantages and Limits

The fixed posterior vault expansion technique allows an immediate and single-step correction of the deformation and usually permits to reach the exact shape that is planned in the preoperative period. The use of a fixed and rigid occipital bandeau permits the children to rest on the back without modifying or damaging the construct.

Furthermore, in case of raised intracranial pressure, it can offer an immediate control.

The drawback is the impossibility to correct the obtained surgical skull expansion and influence the morphological remodeling in the post operative phase, because of the “fixed” cranial reconstruction.

Perioperative risks are the dural tearing particularly high in case of craniosynostoses associated with severe cranial bone dysplasia and the hemorrhagic risk due both to a large bone osteotomies and remodeling and to a direct damage of emissary veins or of sinuses secondary to a dural tear.

33.2.2 Free Floating Parieto-occipital Cranial Vault Release

The free-floating parieto-occipital cranial vault release exploits brain growth in infants as a driving force for spontaneous and gradual displacement of the free-floating occipital bone flap for posterior cranial vault expansion.

33.2.2.1 Free Floating Parieto-occipital Cranial Vault Release Surgical Technique

The first historical report dates to 1996 with two techniques described, both included in the multi-staged management protocol with the aim of postponing fronto-orbital advancement: the first one consisted in a single bone flap extended 2 cm above the lambdoid sutures with lower limit at the torcula sigmoid sinuses junction (Fig. 33.5a) and the second one in a biparted double bone flap with a midline bone strip craniectomy along the lower third of the sagittal sinus (Fig. 33.5b) [30].

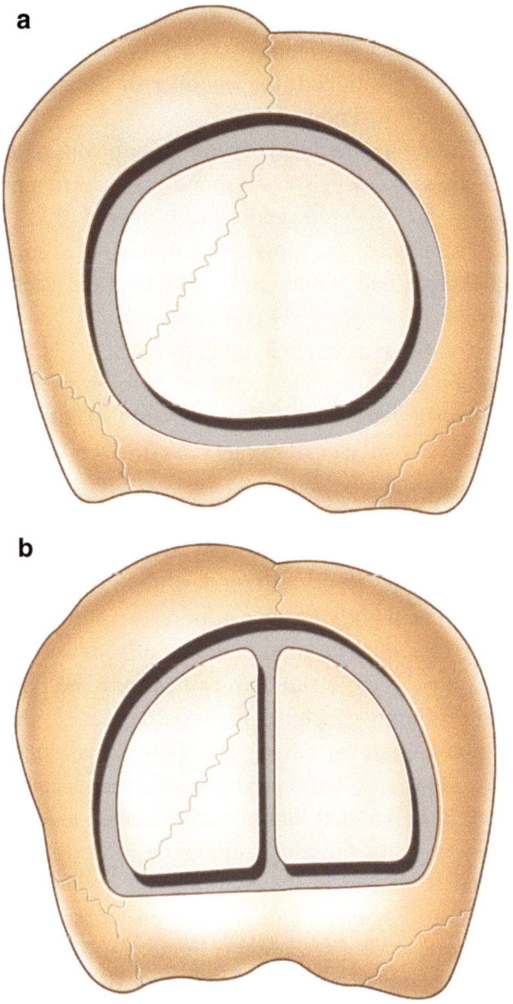

Fig. 33.5 Schematic representation of free-floating craniectomy. (**a**) Single bone flap above the lambdoid sutures. (**b**) Biparted double bone flap with a midline bone strip craniectomy along the lower third of the sagittal sinus. (Adapted from: Sgouros S et al. Posterior skull surgery in craniosynostosis. Childs Nerv Syst. 1996;12(11):727–733)

The procedure can be performed in the prone or semi-sitting position. A posterior bilambdoid [31] or a bicoronaric [4] skin incision is performed to expose the cranial posterior vault in the subgaleal plane to minimize blood loss and avoid injuries to the dura mater protruding through the lacunae. If the coronal suture is involved, the subgaleal dissection can be extended to the bregmatic fontanel and laterally to the pterional region [16, 17].

A carefully dura mater dissection till transverse and sigmoid sinuses is made: in case of children with a honeycomb structure of the bone, the existing holes are used as a pathway to release the bone from the dura dissecting bone limits around the lacunae from the dura by incising the periosteum, while in patients with more compact bone structure, two parietal drill burr holes can be performed 1 cm from the midline and two further burr holes at the level of the lateral third of the transverse sinus [31]. In very young babies, spatula or the cutting edge of the rounded Obwegeser rugine can be used to make the holes [16, 17].

A craniotomy, with craniotome or piezosurgery, is then performed in front of both lambdoid sutures and down to the asterion, and it can be continued caudally under the torcula to the foramen magnum.

The bone is then completely detached from the dural plane except at the level of sagittal sinus, where it is left in place as an anchor point for the bone. If a great venous hypertension is remarked, the flap can be divided into two to protect the sagittal sinus and/or the torcula and reduce the risk of transosseous vein damage [31].

No subcutaneous drain is left in place and a layer-by-layer closure is done. Sometimes an extended subgaleal dissection is needed to have enough tissue for closure [32].

33.2.2.2 Advantages and Limits

Surgical time reduced compared to a conventional PVCE; the minimal blood loss and the immediate relieve of intracranial hypertension make this procedure suitable even for the youngest patients with severe craniostenosis: a recently published series shows safe results of this technique in a cohort of patients aged from 6 days to 6 months [16, 17].

Another advantage is the minimal surgical manipulation which minimizes the risks for dural tears.

Very small babies have great potential of reossification, but the risk of relapse and incomplete ossification is quite high in case of complex craniosynostosis with an "honeycomb" bone-structure.

Its main limitation is related to the mandatory positioning in the postoperative period: alternate lateral positioning is required for a posterior expansion to occur at an age in which there is still a risk of sudden death in the prone position. Indeed, the supine positioning of the infant during the postoperative course could prevent the posterior expansion and could even result in brain compression.

Another limit is the relative ineffectiveness of the technique in correcting the abnormal position of the petrous bone and the deformation of the frontal and facial bones that are present in severe positional plagiocephalies and in all synostotic ones [32].

33.2.3 Spring-Assisted Posterior Vault Expansion (SA-PCVE)

The challenging skin closure using rigid posterior vault expansion incentivized the introduction of gradual and dynamic expansion of posterior vault using devices to support. The use of subcutaneous springs was first described by Lauritzen [33].

The springs can be used alone in case of open lambdoid sutures or in combination with a large osteotomy to obtain a bone flap that will be displaced progressively by the springs in case of closed sutures.

33.2.3.1 Springs Manufacture

The springs are Omega-shaped tools in strainless-free wire introduced in the 1970s for craniofacialsurgery and Lauritzen introduced their use in cranial vault remodeling in late 1990s.

Initially, their wire-form was bent intraoperatively into the desired U shape, and only in 2007, a group of surgeons and engineers of the Great Ormond Street Hospital for Children (GOSH), of London, tried to standardize the device.

Springs are composed by a central loop which extends into two longer arms which end in a footplate that is used to anchor the spring to the bone cuts performed during the surgery. The distance between the tips ("inter-foot distance") is 60 mm at rest and before implantation and the central loop diameter is 10 mm.

When positioned, the opening of the spring narrows its end points.

Three standardized models with different thicknesses, which correspond to a different force, are now currently used: model S10—1.0 mm wire thickness, model S12—1.2 mm thickness, and model S14—1.4 mm thickness [34].

The force at implantation is 11.4 ± 4.3 N for the anterior spring and 11.8 ± 4.1 N for the posterior spring, and studies demonstrate that it takes 10 days from day of surgery for the springs to open completely [35].

33.2.3.2 SA-PCVE Surgical Technique

The patient is positioned prone with the neck in a neutral or slightly flexed position.

A bicoronal incision is done until the subgaleal plane and the skin flap is then reflected posteriorly until reaching the confluence of the lambdoid sutures paying attention to the emissary veins and to the subcutaneous venous anatomy. A pericranial flap is then dissected leaving the temporalis muscle in situ and a subperiosteal plane is created in the retromastoid area at the level of foramen magnum, while the extracranial soft tissue over the torcula is left in situ.

A curved bicoronal osteotomy is done about 5 cm posterior to the skin incision and taken through the soft tissue tunnel towards the foramen magnum (Fig. 33.6a, b).

Along the osteotomy line, burr holes are previously made and the ones in the retromastoid areas are expanded into a small craniotomy to allow visualization of the transverse sinus and to permit the dural dissection towards the foramen magnum under direct vision.

Once the osteotomy is completed, the dura is dissected and stripped from the inner table a few centimeters anteriorly and posteriorly to permit a certain degree of motion of the posterior bone flap: if the flap remains rigid, the osteotomy can be extended towards the torcula and foramen magnum, or the dural dissection can be widened.

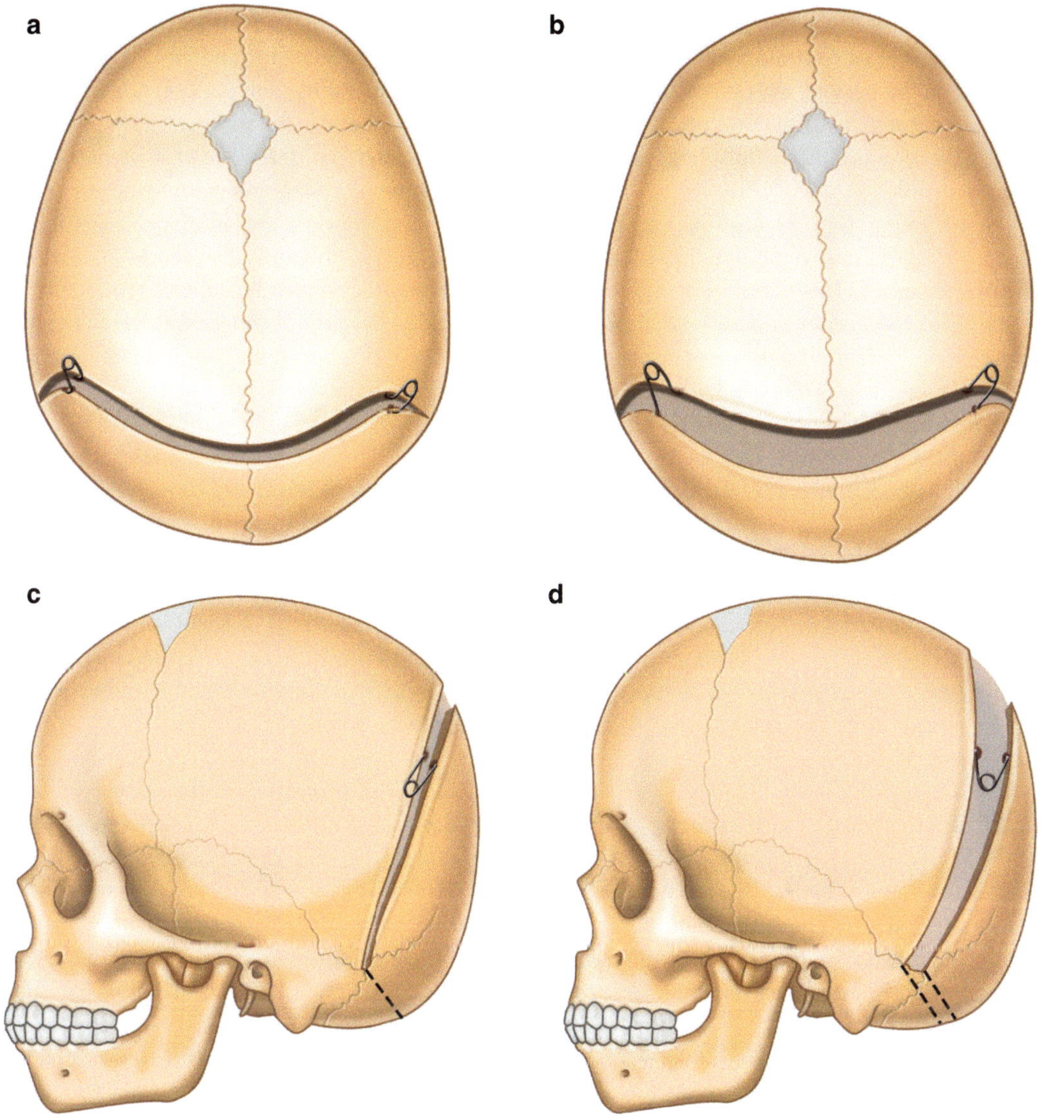

Fig. 33.6 Schematic representation curved osteotomy (**a–c**) and springs placement along the osteotomy line (**b–d**). (Adapted from: Breakey RWF et al. Spring-assisted posterior vault expansion-a single-center experience of 200 cases. Childs Nerv Syst. 2021;37(10):3189–3197)

When the bone mobility is considered sufficient, the springs can be placed across the osteotomy lines (or across the lambdoid sutures when present) [36].

Three different wire diameters are available, resulting in three different spring stiffnesses: normally, younger the child is, the weaker is the spring needed for surgical correction. Two, or occasionally more, springs, if two springs are felt to be insufficient, are placed along the osteotomy line facing each other around 2 cm from either side of the midline into prepared grooves that ensure to lock the spring footplates in position (Fig. 33.6c, d). A resorbable suture is used to anchor the midpoint of the springs to the periosteum to prevent their dislodgement.

The pericranium is closed over the springs. This gives stability to the construct and permits to see how the soft tissues will drape over the springs: any spring protrusion or bony prominence should be overcome at this stage.

The closure of scalp should be done with the compressive help of an assistant, who ensures one hand on the occiput and one on the forehead to avoid compression of the face and eyes.

Once the skin is closed, the springs will begin their expansion.

The treatment time is customized, ranging from some weeks to several months with a mean time of 9 months [37].

Spring removal is done under general anesthesia. The positioning is the same of the insertion and the original scar is reopened. The springs are uncovered using monopolar cautery. Generally, most of the bone gaps have ossified by this time, but careful dissection has to be done to avoid dural tears.

Once the springs are exposed, they are removed with a combination of Mitchel's trimmers, a Tessier periosteal elevator, and a pair of heavy forceps. Care is taken when removing the footplate not to catch any dura in the tip.

The wound is closed layer by layer, and no drain is used [37].

33.2.3.3 Advantages and Limits

SA-PCVE provides a correction of cranial shape based on forces applied to the calvarium rather than on rearrangement of separated bone fragment, reducing the need for multiple osteotomies and thereby the bleeding and surgical time.

The main criticism is the lack of the control over vectors forces and on the degree of bone fragments separation. Furthermore, the largest distraction force is at the beginning, after the force decreases with expansion of the springs: this could cause incomplete ossification, but it appears to be mostly an age-related complication than a technique one [38].

The great ossification capability of the younger has the drawback to make them the group that more likely needs repeat SA-PCVE. The incidence of repeated SA-PCVE is maximum in Apert population, followed by Crouzon-Pfeiffer, and multi-suture craniosynostosis [37]. A study on rabbits shows that 80% of cranial vault expansion is achieved by 2 weeks and 90% by 3 weeks of springs-distraction: at this point of expansion, the residual spring force is 28% of the original one. It shows also that the craniofacial biomechanics modify the expansion curve as the spring force decays; this could explain the relapse if the springs are removed too early, [39] underlying the importance of a close follow-up with serial craniometric studies.

Like all prostheses, they have a non-negligible risk of infection, theoretically reduced by the fact that they are completely subcutaneous (up to 30%, [37]), a risk of dislodgement, skin penetration, LCR leakage, and pressure sores (about 3% in Lauritzen' cohort) [33].

33.2.4 Distractors Osteosynthesis (DO-PCVE)

Transcutaneous distractors' use for cranial vault expansion is based on gradual and controlled separation of bone fragments created by an osteotomy, with a distraction rate that allows a progressive bone formation.

33.2.4.1 Distractors Manufacture

The concept of Distraction Osteogenesis has been directly adopted from orthopedic practice.

The most important characteristics of devices used for distraction osteogenesis are their capacity to transfer distraction forces directly to the bone, and second, the strength to offer the adequate rigidity for osseous consolidation to occur.

The first experimental investigation on cranial osteodistraction was performed in 1957 by Polezhaev and colleagues. Now a variety of plate designs are available to fit your patient's anatomy and your surgical needs.

The main components, all made in lightweight titanium, are the central distractor, the fixation meshes, and the activation arms, which permit the movement of central arm, and so the bone distraction when turned by a screwdriver.

33.2.4.2 DO-PCVE Surgical Technique

The patient is prone-positioned and a bicoronal scalp subgaleal incision is required.

Two types of craniotomies can be used: supratorcular parieto-occipital craniotomy or infratorcular craniotomy below the venous torcular. The choice is determined depending on the crowding of the posterior fossa, presence of tonsillar prolapse, preoperative assessment of the venous anatomy, and perioperative surgical findings [40]. For a maximal volume gain, the vertical part of the osteotomy should be placed at the level of maximal vertical cranial circumference and the horizontal osteotomy as low as possible (Fig. 33.7). The osteotomy is performed with a motor drill or bone rongeur without elevating the cranial bone from the dura matter. Two to four distractors are applied depending on the age of the patient and the vector direction of the bone flap [4, 40].

In the original White's paper, the horizontal osteotomy is placed below the level of the torcula paying attention to the trans-osseous communicating veins to decrease the risk of intraoperative bleeding.

The distractors are positioned and fixated with titanium screws in each temporal region and a superior paramedian to avoid the sagittal sinus [41].

The two types of craniotomies show no significant differences in term of clinical or radiological efficacy. Increasing the number of distractors can enhance construct stability but, at the same time, it increases the risk of wound-related complications and may introduce conflicting vectors. In most cases, two distractors are showed sufficient to allow good expansion [40].

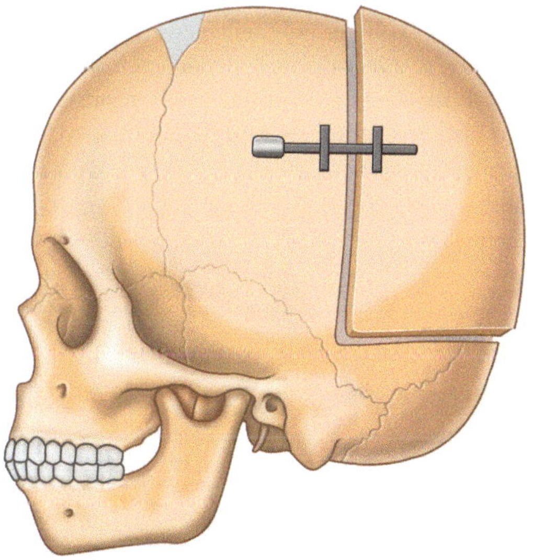

Fig. 33.7 Schematic representation of distractors positioning

It is possible to leave at this early stage few millimeters of distraction, to achieve some degree of distraction.

The direction of the vector will dirige the expansion of the cranial vault: posterior vectors are indicated for cephalo-cranial disproportion with the acceptable overall shape; posteroinferior vectors for turribrachycephaly, bilateral vectors for shunt-related slit ventricle syndrome [42].

Barrel stave osteotomy can be made at inferior occipital segment to expand the cranial vault below the horizontal craniotomy to increase the gain volume [43].

Prior to skin closure, the soft tissues around the activation arms, especially the periosteum, are checked and adapted, if necessary, to avoid pinching them in the rotating parts of the devices during the activation period. The wound is then closed layer by layer, and no drain is used.

After a latency phase of 2–7 days, the distraction phase is characterized by distraction rate of 1 mm/day, divisible once or twice per day. Ong et al. propose a latency period and a distraction rate in function of age: shorter latency period with higher distraction rate for the younger and a longer latency period with smaller distraction rate for the older patients [42].

The distraction is carried out till reaching a slight overcorrection of the preoperative brachycephaly: periodic plain radiographs of the skull are used to monitor the progress of distraction and re-ossification.

Normally, the consolidation period is on average twice as long as the period of activation, but it has to be individualized to each patient [40, 41, 44].

33.2.4.3 Advantages and Limits

Distractors can be used at every age with satisfactory results, but they have to be preferred for infants with a sufficiently thick calvarium.

Goldstein in his cohort of patients aged from 0.3 to 14.1 years documented an overall average volume change of 21% over preoperative intracranial volume measurements, while in patients younger than 12 months the volume increases up to 29%. Furthermore, when the low occiput is included in the distraction segment, it could influence the volume of the posterior cranial base, potentially decompressing a Chiari malformation [44].

Distractors allow a gradual distraction of 0.5–1 mm a day which results in an osteogenetic effect, reducing the risk of severe lacunas [38].

In case of thin bone, the fixation of the distractor may be complex. In order to try and avoid a dislocation while activating the system and reducing the risk of dural tears while positioning the distractor, the use of metallic stainless-steel wires to stabilize the internal distractor has been proposed [45].

Risk related to the device is dislocation or dysfunction; the injury of the underlying dura mater during the placement or fixation of screws and pins in areas of limited bone stock may be up to 10% [4, 40].

Lastly, percutaneous component of the distraction can carry a potential infective risk due to the percutaneous with a tax of infection up to 30% [46].

33.3 Comparison and Conclusions

All these techniques have been proven to permit a satisfying intracranial volume increasing without major significative differences in volume: 13–24% for the free posterior flap, 18–25% for the trans lambdoid springs, 26% for the fixed posterior cranial vault expansion, and 22–29% for the distractors [4, 14, 47].

Not only posterior vault remodeling improves the supratentorial vault volume and skull shape, but posterior cranial vault expansion has shown to permit a complete resolution of Chiari malformation and an accompanying syringomyelia [48].

Internal distractors allow a gradual distraction, resulting in an osteogenetic effect while springs give the largest distraction force in the beginning, and then the force decreases, and this could cause incomplete ossification in older patients because the ossification rate decreases with age [47]. On the other hand, De Jong et al. showed that the spring distraction technique permits larger increase of anteroposterior length in a shorter measurement interval (6.1 versus 8.5 months) when compared to the fixed distraction technique. They concluded that springs permit a larger expansion to the fixed cranial vault expansion, [38] but the fixed cranial vault expansion technique has been shown to have a non-negligible learning curve [47] and it can be a bias in the comparison.

Free floating parieto-occipital cranial vault release could be used in the most unfavorable conditions (tiny honey-comb internal bone structure, severe constriction of intracranial structures) in the very young patient with a reduced surgical time and reduced blood loss. The surgical time is also reduced in all the osteogenic techniques when compared to fixed cranial vault expansion, which has also a higher risk of blood loss [49] and dural tears due to the elevation of the bone flap.

The main drawbacks of springs and distractors are the infectious risk, the device failure, and the need of a second surgery to remove them. Free floating parieto-occipital cranial vault release and spring-assisted expansion share the risk of failure due to the necessity to avoid the dorsal position. On the other hand, fixed posterior cranial vault expansion permits a free posterior postoperative decubitus with the strength and defect of not allowing to adapt the postoperative result.

All the techniques offer good results with good security profile. For the best correction, surgical decision should be based on clinical presentation, age, sutural pattern, and syndromic context.

References

1. Schulz M, Spors B, Haberl H, Thomale UW. Results of posterior cranial vault remodeling for plagiocephaly and brachycephaly by the meander technique. Childs Nerv Syst. 2014;30(9):1517–26. https://doi.org/10.1007/s00381-014-2462-z.
2. Rhodes JL, Tye GW, Fearon JA. Craniosynostosis of the lambdoid suture. Semin Plast Surg. 2014;28(3):138–43. https://doi.org/10.1055/s-0034-1384809.

3. Chivoret N, Arnaud E, Giraudat K, et al. Bilambdoid and sagittal synostosis: report of 39 cases. Surg Neurol Int. 2018;9:206. https://doi.org/10.4103/sni.sni_454_17.
4. Nowinski D, Di Rocco F, Renier D, SainteRose C, Leikola J, Arnaud E. Posterior cranial vault expansion in the treatment of craniosynostosis. Comparison of current techniques. Childs Nerv Syst. 2012;28(9):1537–44. https://doi.org/10.1007/s00381-012-1809-6.
5. Sgouros S, Hockley AD, Goldin JH, Wake MJ, Natarajan K. Intracranial volume change in craniosynostosis. J Neurosurg. 1999;91(4):617–25. https://doi.org/10.3171/jns.1999.91.4.0617.
6. Sgouros S. Skull vault growth in craniosynostosis. Childs Nerv Syst. 2005;21(10):861–70. https://doi.org/10.1007/s00381-004-1112-2.
7. Cinalli G, Spennato P, Sainte-Rose C, et al. Chiari malformation in craniosynostosis. Childs Nerv Syst. 2005;21(10):889–901. https://doi.org/10.1007/s00381-004-1115-z.
8. Marucci DD, Dunaway DJ, Jones BM, Hayward RD. Raised intracranial pressure in Apert syndrome. Plast Reconstr Surg. 2008;122(4):1162–8. https://doi.org/10.1097/PRS.0b013e31818458f0.
9. Engel M, Castrillón-Oberndorfer G, Hoffmann J, et al. Chiari malformation in nonsyndromal single craniosynostosis—much ado about nothing? Acta Neurochir. 2012;154(10):1803–7. https://doi.org/10.1007/s00701-012-1439-5.
10. Collmann H, Sörensen N, Krauss J. Hydrocephalus in craniosynostosis: a review. Childs Nerv Syst. 2005;21(10):902–12. https://doi.org/10.1007/s00381-004-1116-y.
11. Coll G, Abed Rabbo F, Jecko V, Sakka L, Di Rocco F, Delion M. The growth of the posterior cranial fossa in FGFR2-induced faciocraniosynostosis: a review. Neurochirurgie. 2019;65(5):221–7. https://doi.org/10.1016/j.neuchi.2019.09.005.
12. Lo LJ, Chen YR. Airway obstruction in severe syndromic craniosynostosis. Ann Plast Surg. 1999;43(3):258–64. https://doi.org/10.1097/00000637-199909000-00006.
13. Protzenko T, Bellas A, Ribeiro CMC, Gonzalez SMC, Horovitz DDG. Venous anomalies in hypoplastic posterior fossa: unsolved questions. Childs Nerv Syst. 2021;37(10):3177–87. https://doi.org/10.1007/s00381-021-05315-4.
14. Taylor JA, Derderian CA, Bartlett SP, Fiadjoe JE, Sussman EM, Stricker PA. Perioperative morbidity in posterior cranial vault expansion: distraction osteogenesis versus conventional osteotomy. Plast Reconstr Surg. 2012;129(4):674e–80e. https://doi.org/10.1097/PRS.0b013e3182443164.
15. Taylor WJ, Hayward RD, Lasjaunias P, et al. Enigma of raised intracranial pressure in patients with complex craniosynostosis: the role of abnormal intracranial venous drainage. J Neurosurg. 2001;94(3):377–85. https://doi.org/10.3171/jns.2001.94.3.0377.
16. Vinchon M, Guerreschi P, Karnoub MA, Wolber A. Linear craniectomy for early posterior decompression in craniosynostoses: technique and results. Childs Nerv Syst. 2021a;37(10):3113–8. https://doi.org/10.1007/s00381-021-05117-8.
17. Vinchon M, Guerreschi P, Karnoub MA, Wolber A. Synostosis of the lambdoid suture: a spectrum. Childs Nerv Syst. 2021b;37(6):1991–2000. https://doi.org/10.1007/s00381-020-05003-9.
18. Ignelzi MA Jr, Wang W, Young AT. Fibroblast growth factors lead to increased Msx2 expression and fusion in calvarial sutures. J Bone Miner Res. 2003;18(4):751–9. https://doi.org/10.1359/jbmr.2003.18.4.751.
19. Tischfield MA, Robson CD, Gilette NM, et al. Cerebral vein malformations result from loss of Twist1 expression and BMP signaling from skull progenitor cells and dura. Dev Cell. 2017;42(5):445–461.e5. https://doi.org/10.1016/j.devcel.2017.07.027.
20. Rollins N, Booth T, Shapiro K. MR venography in children with complex craniosynostosis. Pediatr Neurosurg. 2000;32(6):308–15. https://doi.org/10.1159/000028959.
21. Copeland AE, Hoffman CE, Tsitouras V, et al. Clinical significance of venous anomalies in syndromic craniosynostosis. Plast Reconstr Surg Glob Open. 2018;6(1):e1613. https://doi.org/10.1097/GOX.0000000000001613.
22. Di Rocco F. Introduction to the focus session on posterior vault surgery in craniosynostosis. Childs Nerv Syst. 2021;37(10):3091–2. https://doi.org/10.1007/s00381-021-05323-4.
23. Wong GB, Kakulis EG, Mulliken JB. Analysis of fronto-orbital advancement for Apert, Crouzon, Pfeiffer, and Saethre-Chotzen syndromes. Plast Reconstr Surg. 2000;105(7):2314–23. https://doi.org/10.1097/00006534-200006000-00002.
24. Choi M, Flores RL, Havlik RJ. Volumetric analysis of anterior versus posterior cranial vault expansion in patients with syndromic craniosynostosis. J Craniofac Surg. 2012;23(2):455–8. https://doi.org/10.1097/SCS.0b013e318240ff49.
25. Di Rocco F, Licci M, Paasche A, Szathmari A, Beuriat PA, Mottolese C. Fixed posterior cranial vault expansion technique. Childs Nerv Syst. 2021;37(10):3137–41. https://doi.org/10.1007/s00381-021-05270-0.
26. Ros B, Iglesias S, Selfa A, Ruiz F, Arráez MÁ. Conventional posterior cranial vault expansion: indications and results-review of the literature. Childs Nerv Syst. 2021;37(10):3149–75. https://doi.org/10.1007/s00381-021-05318-1.
27. Muakkassa KF, Hoffman HJ, Hinton DR, Hendrick EB, Humphreys RP, Ash J, Lambdoid synostosis. Part 2: review of cases managed at the Hospital for Sick Children, 1972-1982. J Neurosurg. 1984;61(2):340–7. https://doi.org/10.3171/jns.1984.61.2.0340.
28. Goodrich JT, Argamaso R. Lambdoid stenosis (posterior plagiocephaly) and craniofacial asymmetry: long-

term outcomes. Childs Nerv Syst. 1996;12(11):720–6. https://doi.org/10.1007/BF00366157.
29. Wagner W, Schwandt E, Huthmann A, Vulcu S, Tschan C. Posterior calvarial augmentation in premature craniosynostosis: a technique avoiding foreign implants or free bone flaps. Childs Nerv Syst. 2010;26(11):1549–53. https://doi.org/10.1007/s00381-010-1158-2.
30. Sgouros S, Goldin JH, Hockley AD, Wake MJ. Posterior skull surgery in craniosynostosis. Childs Nerv Syst. 1996;12(11):727–33. https://doi.org/10.1007/BF00366158.
31. Tamburrini G, Offi M, Massimi L, Frassanito P, Bianchi F. Posterior vault "free-floating" bone flap: indications, technique, advantages, and drawbacks. Childs Nerv Syst. 2021;37(10):3143–7. https://doi.org/10.1007/s00381-021-05281-x.
32. Di Rocco F, Marchac A, Duracher C, et al. Posterior remodeling flap for posterior plagiocephaly. Childs Nerv Syst. 2012;28(9):1395–7. https://doi.org/10.1007/s00381-012-1842-5.
33. Lauritzen CGK, Davis C, Ivarsson A, Sanger C, Hewitt TD. The evolving role of springs in craniofacial surgery: the first 100 clinical cases. Plast Reconstr Surg. 2008;121(2):545–54. https://doi.org/10.1097/01.prs.0000297638.76602.de.
34. Jeelani NUO, Borghi A, Florez NR, Bozkurt S, Dunaway D, Schievano S. The science behind the springs: using biomechanics and finite element modeling to predict outcomes in spring-assisted sagittal synostosis surgery. J Craniofac Surg. 2020;31(7):2074–8. https://doi.org/10.1097/SCS.0000000000006865.
35. Borghi A, Schievano S, Rodriguez Florez N, et al. Assessment of spring cranioplasty biomechanics in sagittal craniosynostosis patients. J Neurosurg Pediatr. 2017;20(5):400–9. https://doi.org/10.3171/2017.1.PEDS16475.
36. Arnaud E, Marchac A, Jeblaoui Y, Renier D, Di Rocco F. Spring-assisted posterior skull expansion without osteotomies. Childs Nerv Syst. 2012;28(9):1545–9. https://doi.org/10.1007/s00381-012-1843-4.
37. Breakey RWF, van de Lande LS, Sidpra J, et al. Spring-assisted posterior vault expansion-a single-centre experience of 200 cases. Childs Nerv Syst. 2021;37(10):3189–97. https://doi.org/10.1007/s00381-021-05330-5.
38. de Jong T, van Veelen ML, Mathijssen IM. Spring-assisted posterior vault expansion in multisuture craniosynostosis. Childs Nerv Syst. 2013;29(5):815–20. https://doi.org/10.1007/s00381-013-2033-8.
39. Davis C, Windh P, Lauritzen CG. Spring expansion is influenced by cranial biomechanics. J Craniofac Surg. 2010;21(3):843–6. https://doi.org/10.1097/SCS.0b013e3181d7a803.
40. Di Rocco F, Usami K, Protzenko T, Collet C, Giraudat K, Arnaud E. Results and limits of posterior cranial vault expansion by osteotomy and internal distractors [published correction appears in Surg Neurol Int. 2019 Feb 13;10:19. Rocco, Federico Di [corrected to Di Rocco, Federico]]. Surg Neurol Int. 2018;9:217. https://doi.org/10.4103/sni.sni_465_17.
41. White N, Evans M, Dover MS, Noons P, Solanki G, Nishikawa H. Posterior calvarial vault expansion using distraction osteogenesis. Childs Nerv Syst. 2009;25(2):231–6. https://doi.org/10.1007/s00381-008-0758-6.
42. Ong J, Harshbarger RJ 3rd, Kelley P, George T. Posterior cranial vault distraction osteogenesis: evolution of technique. Semin Plast Surg. 2014;28(4):163–78. https://doi.org/10.1055/s-0034-1390169.
43. Steinbacher DM, Skirpan J, Puchała J, Bartlett SP. Expansion of the posterior cranial vault using distraction osteogenesis. Plast Reconstr Surg. 2011;127(2):792–801. https://doi.org/10.1097/PRS.0b013e318200ab83.
44. Goldstein JA, Paliga JT, Wink JD, Low DW, Bartlett SP, Taylor JA. A craniometric analysis of posterior cranial vault distraction osteogenesis. Plast Reconstr Surg. 2013;131(6):1367–75. https://doi.org/10.1097/PRS.0b013e31828bd541.
45. Di Rocco F, Szathmari A, Mottolese C. Wire fixation of internal distractor for cranial vault remodeling. Childs Nerv Syst. 2016;32(6):1131–3. https://doi.org/10.1007/s00381-016-3031-4.
46. Komuro Y, Shimizu A, Shimoji K, Miyajima M, Arai H. Posterior cranial vault distraction osteogenesis with barrel stave osteotomy in the treatment of craniosynostosis. Neurol Med Chir (Tokyo). 2015;55(8):617–23. https://doi.org/10.2176/nmc.ra.2014-0401.
47. Pennacchietti V, Schulz M, Tietze A, Schwarz K, Thomale UW. Extended experience in parieto-occipital expansion surgery by meander technique-clinical and radiological evaluation. Childs Nerv Syst. 2021;37(10):3199–207. https://doi.org/10.1007/s00381-021-05355-w.
48. Levitt MR, Niazi TN, Hopper RA, Ellenbogen RG, Ojemann JG. Resolution of syndromic craniosynostosis-associated Chiari malformation type I without suboccipital decompression after posterior cranial vault release. J Neurosurg Pediatr. 2012;9(2):111–5. https://doi.org/10.3171/2011.11.PEDS11268.
49. Kim SW, Shim KW, Plesnila N, Kim YO, Choi JU, Kim DS. Distraction vs remodeling surgery for craniosynostosis. Childs Nerv Syst. 2007;23(2):201–6. https://doi.org/10.1007/s00381-006-0209-1.

34 Technical Tips for Surgery in Older Children

Nirali Patel, Kelsi M. Chesney, Gregory Keating, Gary F. Rogers, Hasan R. Syed, and Robert F. Keating

34.1 Introduction

Most children with craniosynostosis are identified and managed in infancy. There is, however, a subset of patients in whom the diagnosis of craniosynostosis is delayed, either through a lack of recognition or because they lack some or all of the sentinel cranial shape changes. In addition, revision surgery may be required in some patients to address persistent or recurrent issues of cranial shape and/or volume. Nevertheless, the indications for surgical correction remain the same as for the younger cohort: cranial shape/appearance and the possibility of intracranial hypertension. Surgical assessment and intervention in older patients present a unique set of challenges when compared to the treatment of younger patients. The epidemiology, pathophysiology, and key treatment considerations are the subject of this chapter.

N. Patel · K. M. Chesney · G. Keating
Department of Neurosurgery, Children's National Hospital, Washington, DC, USA

Department of Neurosurgery, MedStar Georgetown University Hospital, Washington, DC, USA
e-mail: Nirali.P.Patel@gunet.georgetown.edu; gfk9@georgetown.edu

G. F. Rogers
Department of Plastic Surgery, Children's National Hospital, Washington, DC, USA
e-mail: Grogers@childrensnational.org

H. R. Syed · R. F. Keating (✉)
Department of Neurosurgery, Children's National Hospital, Washington, DC, USA

Department of Neurosurgery, George Washington University, Washington, DC, USA
e-mail: hsyed@childrensnational.org; RKeating@childrensnational.org

34.2 Epidemiology and Pathophysiology

The incidence of nonsyndromic craniosynostosis, defined as abnormal or premature fusion of one or more cranial sutures, is 1 in 2000 live births. Craniosynostosis typically results in characteristic changes in cranial form and volume that herald the presence of the condition, and these changes may lead to adverse effects on cerebral growth and function. Most studies support early intervention to help mitigate these undesirable outcomes, but only 75% of affected patients will be referred to neurosurgery and receive treatment within the first year of life [1, 2]. The underlying causes for delayed treatment are multifactorial and include failure to diagnose or refer in a timely fashion, impaired access to care, or more rarely, development of latent suture fusions [3–6]. The latter category is rare but can result from postnatal environmental influences including: metabolic bone diseases such as rickets, hypophosphatasia, pseudohypoparathyroidism, osteopetrosis, and mucopolysaccharidosis [7]; mechanical forces [8]; or natural population

F. Di Rocco, J. Kestle (eds.), *Neurosurgical Aspects of Craniosynostosis*,
https://doi.org/10.1007/978-3-031-69386-1_34

variability in suture closure patterns [9]. Children with rickets have an increased incidence of craniosynostosis (both single and multiple sutures) and are more likely to suffer from increased ICP when compared to other patients with craniosynostosis [10]. Cerebrospinal fluid (CSF) shunts have also been associated in certain studies with development of secondary craniosynostosis in nearly 50% of patients [8]. Furthermore, recent studies of children evaluated for head trauma demonstrate that approximately 7% of normal infants with otherwise normal head shape will have developed fusion of the sagittal suture before the age of two [9]. While the effect of these latent forms of craniosynostosis on cranial shape and volume can be minor or negligible, increased intracranial pressure has been reported and careful clinical oversight is necessary [11].

Revision surgery is also more likely to be performed in older patients. The indications for revision surgery are esthetic concerns or elevated intracranial pressure, which can occur due to inadequate primary surgery or insufficient cranial growth after an adequate reconstruction. Risk factors include a syndromic diagnosis, surgery before age 6 months, and the number and type of suture fusions (sagittal highest of single suture fusions) [12–16]. Revision surgery may involve longer operating times, greater overall blood loss, and more intraoperative complications related to existing bone defects, scarring of the dura, or elevated intracranial pressure.

34.3 Clinical Presentation

The clinical presentation of patients who present with craniosynostosis later in life varies significantly depending on the reason for the delay. Patients with latent fusion (postnatal) may have little or none of the characteristic changes in cranial shape. These patients can be nearly impossible to identify clinically and are often detected only by fortuitous imaging or other findings. Patients with characteristic cranial shape changes in whom diagnosis was made later in life tend to have more pronounced craniofacial abnormalities, especially at the cranial base, secondary to compensatory calvarial growth, and appear to have an increased risk of increased intracranial pressure (ICP) and developmental delay [11, 12, 17, 18]. Typical signs and symptoms of elevated intracranial pressure such as headaches, nausea/vomiting, and/or vision changes/papilledema are often absent in older children with craniosynostosis [12]. Workup should include a detailed history and physical exam which includes the trajectory of head circumference growth since birth, a fundoscopic examination, and a low threshold for radiographic evaluation (CT, MRI) to assess subtle changes consistent with increased pressure. ICP monitoring may be indicated for patients who manifest minor changes to cranial shape or in whom the decision to proceed with surgical correction is predicated on the presence or absence of intracranial hypertension (e.g., older with reasonable head shape and volume, or parental uncertainty).

The presence of elevated intracranial pressure is an absolute indication for cranial vault expansion, but the beneficial effect of surgery on long-term neurocognitive outcomes is less clear. Developmental delay and neurocognitive deficits have been well demonstrated in older children with untreated synostosis by several groups; up to a three to fivefold increase in risk in some studies [17–21], but a few studies have documented that surgical intervention improves these parameters, especially in older children. A study by Starr et al. also demonstrated significant delay both before and after surgery in patients with isolated single-suture synostosis [22]. Even when these patients have normal IQ scores, they tend to have significant learning disabilities secondary to impairments in executive dysfunction [20]. Functional imaging studies have confirmed altered neural connectivity in patients with sagittal synostosis [23] and surgical intervention prior to 6 months of age has been shown to improve longitudinal outcomes in these kids and has led many to recommend correction at an early age [24]. However, a small prospective study by Fontana et al. has shown developmental improvement even in older patients undergoing cranial vault remodeling encouraging craniosynostosis repair in this cohort [17].

34.4 Surgical Considerations

Treatment of craniosynostosis addresses two concerns: cranial shape and intracranial volume. The choice and timing of treatment depend on many variables including patient age and comorbidities, the number and type of fused sutures, prior cranial vault procedures, presence or absence of intracranial pressure, and others.

1. *Blood Loss*

   The increased thickness of the scalp and bone in an older child may increase the risk of bleeding. Use of meticulous surgical technique, perioperative tranexamic acid (TXA) or aminocaproic acid, and a well-coordinated team effort to minimize operative time can mitigate the need for blood transfusion. This is especially important in revision surgery. Through these measures, our transfusion rate for patients over 2 years of age undergoing cranial reconstruction has been less than 50%. Although rarely used in our center, preoperative use of virtual surgical planning (VSP) can also aid in optimizing the final calvarial shape and reduce surgical time with the help of printed 2D templates to guide osteotomies [25, 26].
2. *Bone Contouring and Stabilization*

   Bone of older children is thicker and more brittle than in infants and often requires more releasing cuts to permit remodeling or shape changes. This can result in bone edges that may be visible or palpable postoperatively, and smoothing of any rough or prominent bone edges with a burr is recommended. We typically use resorbable plates on the endocortical surface to maintain the new bony contour and to stabilize any bony advancement. Although titanium plates are a reasonable option in older children, we prefer resorbable hardware if possible. There are less issues in the long run with prominent plates, etc.
3. *Bone Defects*

   After the age of 18–24 months, the chance of spontaneous healing of significant residual cranial defects decreases dramatically [19, 27]. We routinely cover all areas of exposed dura with autologous particulate graft and this practice has reduced the rate of residual bone defects and need for secondary cranioplasty at our center to nearly zero. The technique has been well-described and uses a Hudson brace and D'Errico bit to obtain the bone graft from the endocortical surface of any removed bone segments or the ectocortical surface of the intact calvaria (Figs. 34.1a–c and 34.2).
4. *Hydrocephalus*

   It is important to assess any degree of cerebral ventriculomegaly and the possibility of hydrocephalus. While ventriculomegaly can contribute to an increase in the ICP, draining the ventricles with a shunt may reduce cerebral growth and internal support for the bony reconstruction, and potential lead to fusion of other cranial sutures. A shunt or CSF diversion should be reserved for the patient with clearly demonstrable hydrocephalus. A progressive Chiari malformation or the presence of syringomyelia may offer potential clues in this regard. One of the most helpful tools is evaluating changes in head circumference percentile. Patients with restricted calvarial growth (due to craniosynostosis) will usually manifest a decreasing percentile over time, whereas the patient with hydrocephalus demonstrates the opposite with an increasing or stable head circumference percentile.
5. *Infection*

   The risk of infection is also increased in these patients. This increase is mainly twofold: due to increased exposure and longer operative times required for the more extensive surgery, but also due to the potential pneumatization of the frontal sinus in the older patient. In a study looking at over 8000 children undergoing craniosynostosis repair at multiple locations, Bruce et al. demonstrated an increased risk of all complications, including bleeding and infection in children undergoing a repair after 12 months of age. The conclusions held true even after they control for procedure type and presence of comorbidities [2].
6. *Relapse*

   Multiple studies have confirmed that surgical correction of craniosynostosis in very

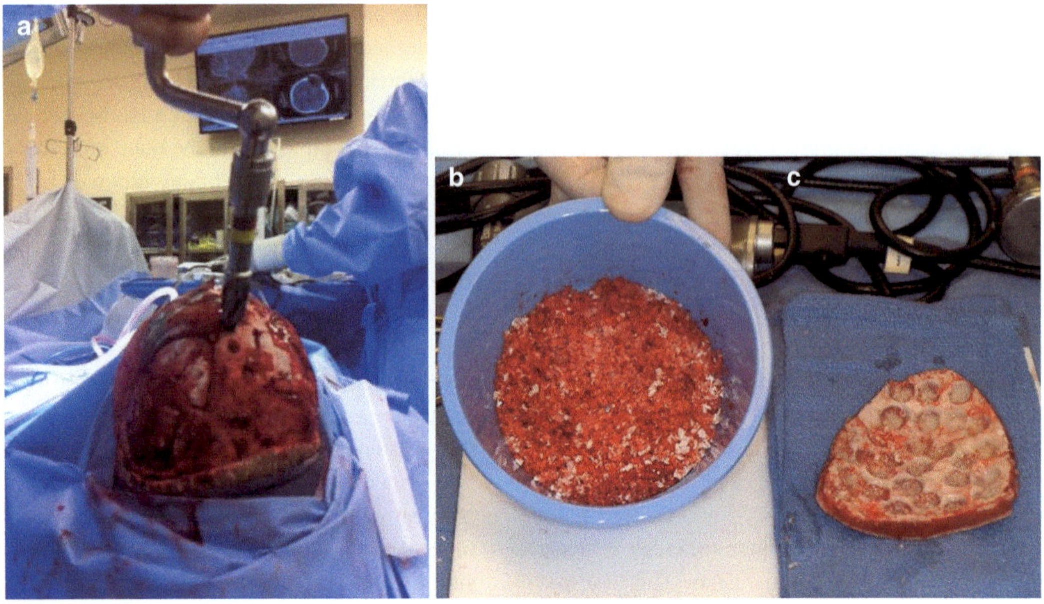

Fig. 34.1 (**a**) A Hudson brace being used on the extracranial surface to harvest cortex and intradiploic bone fragments which will be used for bone particulate cranioplasty material. (**b**) A relatively large amount of particulate bone graft may be harvested from the extra/intracranial surface of the skull. (**c**) Harvesting bone particulate cranioplasty material from the inner surface of a bone flap

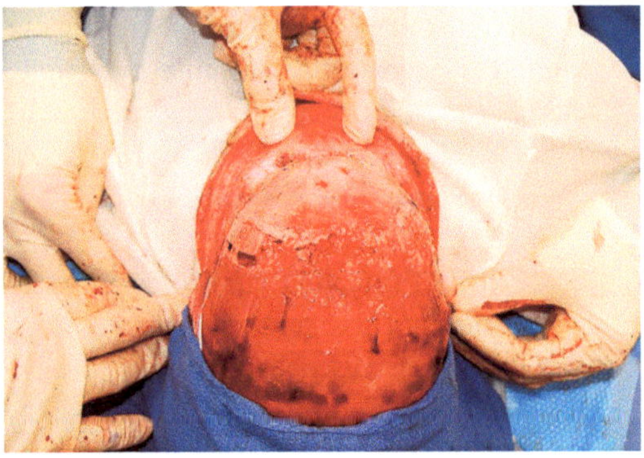

Fig. 34.2 Placing the bone particulate cranioplasty material into residual calvarial defects with fibrin glue (Tisseal TM) as a binding matrix

young infants (i.e., <6 months of age) or in patients with certain craniosynostosis syndromes results in a higher likelihood of relapse and need for revision surgery [16]. Most surgeons compensate for this by overcorrecting the bone movements during the cranial reconstruction. Since older children are further along in their cranial growth, the need for overcorrection and likelihood of relapse of the deformity are much smaller. The surgeon should consider the amount of cerebral growth remaining in determining how much to increase the intracranial volume or advance the bone segments. This is especially important in fronto-orbital advancement surgery where overcorrection of an older patient can lead to a disfiguring or stigmatizing result as well as difficulty in closing the surgical flap and increasing the likelihood of wound breakdown or infection.

34.5 Reconstructive Techniques for Common Forms of Craniosynostosis

While there are multiple approaches in dealing with the older patient with craniosynostosis, ranging from simple radial osteotomies to external distraction, general principles of positioning, anesthetic considerations, minimizing morbidity/blood loss, and ultimately having a defined and cogent reconstructive plan are critical components to a successful surgery. At the outset, one must decide on the principal indication for surgery: cosmesis or increased intracranial pressure, or the frequent presentation of both. Patients presenting at an older time frame often have significant calvarial distortions as well as evidence for increased ICP (thinned calvarium, papilledema, decelerating head circumference percentile, headache, or cognitive decline). Thus, the goal of reducing ICP by increasing skull volume is often intertwined with a desire for an improved morphological appearance. It doesn't take a significant increase in calvarial volume to markedly reduce the patient's ICP and the extent of volumetric expansion will be dictated by the patient's age. Patients approaching 5–6 years of age are unlikely (but still seen on rare occasions) to need additional volumetric expansion for purposes of intracranial pressure, whereas the younger patients (2–4 years) will need to be followed closely, especially in the setting of multi-suture synostosis. For the younger patient, every attempt is made to maximize the increase in volume (e.g., frontal advancement for bifronto-orbital conditions), but this is often limited by the ability of the scalp to accommodate >2 cm frontal advancement.

For reasons that remain unclear, older patients most often present with scaphocephaly and may be at the highest risk for increased ICP for single-suture craniosynostosis. Bilateral coronal synostosis is the second most frequently seen condition, whereas single coronal suture or even metopic suture synostosis usually presents earlier due to the significant calvarial asymmetry seen at an early age. While both types may require a need to increase the calvarial volume, methods to do so vary markedly and ultimately offer different esthetic considerations.

34.5.1 Fronto-orbital Advancement: Metopic Synostosis

While the presence of increased ICP may be less common in the delayed presentation of metopic or coronal synostosis and cosmetic considerations may be paramount, an adequate advancement of the fronto-orbital bar will usually accomplish both goals of improving appearance while simultaneously increasing intracranial volume if there are any concerns about pressure. Fronto-orbital advancement is the most predictable surgical option in older patients with trigonocephaly. This method has predictably good outcomes in older children if done correctly. With the patient in the supine position, the frontal bones and orbital bandeau are removed.

The greatest challenge in these kids may be the presence of a frontal sinus, although this usually develops after 7–8 years of age. In the event that the frontal (or ethmoidal sinus) is encountered, then it is critical to adequately remove all sinus mucosa (exenteration) and seal off this extracranial compartment from the intracranial cavity. This may be accomplished by using bone fragments harvested during the craniotomy and small pieces of temporalis muscle to plug the nasofrontal duct (or adjacent bony defects) and subsequently using fibrin glue to hold the matrix in place. It is often prudent to leave the pericranium intact during the exposure, to potentially use this as a vascularized pedicle to overlie the area (Fig. 34.3). This will help promote healing of this graft and lead to a true sequestration of the extra from intracranial compartments. The additional time and morbidity are minimal compared to the added potential of a well-healed site (Fig. 34.4a–d).

The V-shaped bandeau is expanded, and if necessary, the flat lateral segments are contoured to increase the convexity. In severe cases, the expanded bandeau may require a midline separation and leveling of each half. If this creates a gap, it can be filled with a trapezoidal or triangular bone. The nasal process of each frontal bone is long and should be shortened. The bandeau is intentionally overcorrected in the temporal areas and fixed with resorbable plates. The coronal gap can be filled with a rectangular piece of bone harvested from the vertex to stabilize the bandeau, provide bony continuity, and prevent any possibility of collapse. While the frontal elements are off, a particulate bone graft can be harvested from the inner table and stored in a blood-filled container on the back table (see Fig. 34.1). This

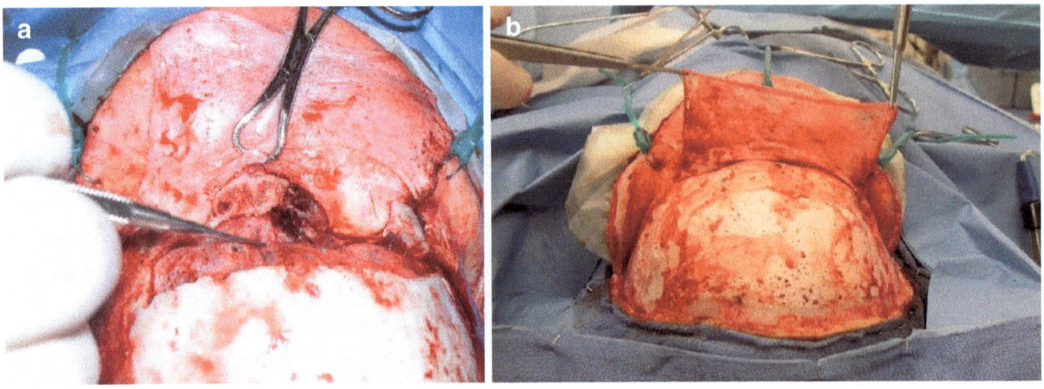

Fig. 34.3 (**a**, **b**) Exposure of the frontonasal duct and ethmoid sinuses via a recently aerated frontal sinus. A portion of pericranium has been preserved to be used as a vascularized pedicle covering the exposed sinus which has been cleared of all mucosa and walled off from the extracranial compartments (with bone fragments)

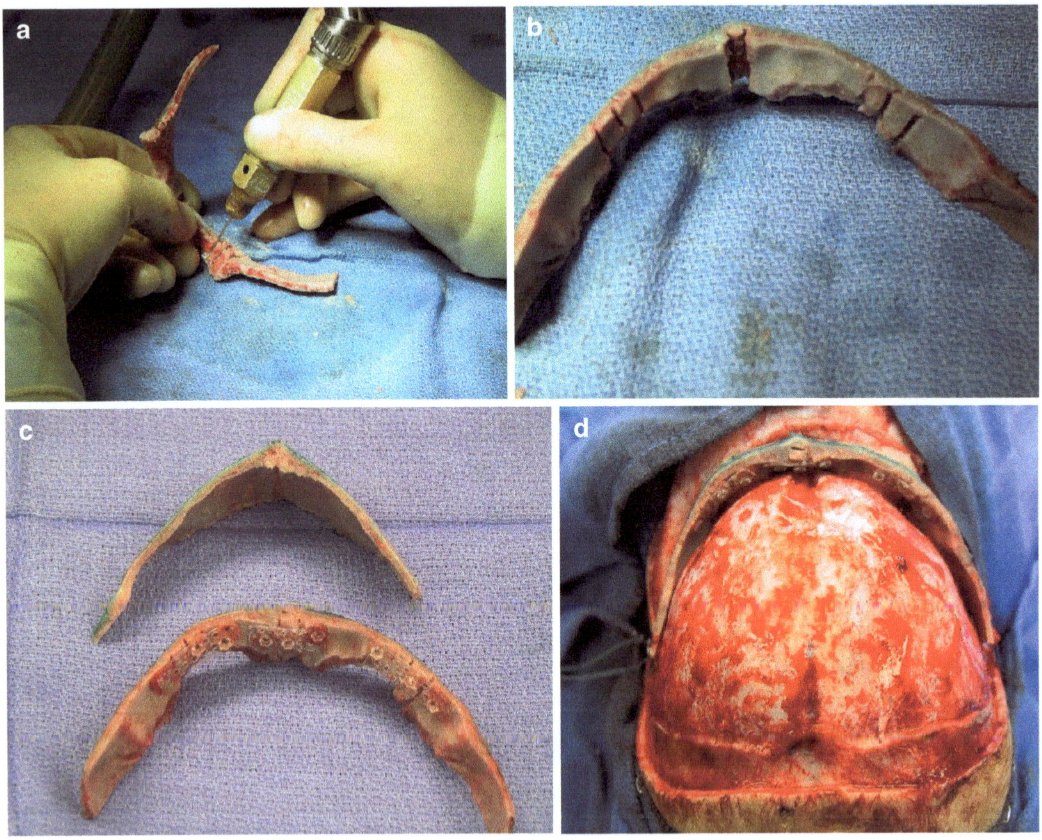

Fig. 34.4 (**a**–**d**) After the frontal bandeau is removed, its shape may be reconfigured by performing osteotomies to facilitate bending the lateral structures as well as the midline. Absorbable plates are used on the endocortical surface to maintain the desired new configuration. When the newly shaped frontal orbital bandeau is returned to its original position, one can appreciate the significant change in the new position (and shape) relative to the preexisting frontal lobes

will provide bone graft to repair any defects created by the advancement or harvest of full-thickness bone graft. Each frontal bone is then remodeled with a shaping burr or radial osteotomies and then orthotopically or heterotopically affixed to the bandeau. The frontoparietal segments can be affixed to the bandeau with resorbable plates or secured with wires or sutures. To create a smooth transition with the widened frontal segments, the parietal bones laterally should be out-fractured using horizontal barrel staves and stabilized to the frontal elements with absorbable plates. Although the lateral bone gaps between the frontal and parietal segments could be left to heal spontaneously, repair with full-thickness cortical bone harvested from the vertex provides bone continuity and reduces the likelihood of depression (temporal hollow) in this area. The temporalis muscle should be advanced anteriorly and resuspended. If the soft tissue closure is tight, the galea can be scored to reduce tension on the repair. This should not induce alopecia if done properly—the scoring must not enter the fat layer where the hair follicles reside.

The older patient often has many areas of calvarial deficiencies after any frontal advancement or bilateral parietal expansion. It is best to ensure that the frontal and other areas of cosmetic priority have adequate bony reconstruction in these regions. Additional bone may be harvested by using split-calvarial cranioplasty as well as using particulate bony matrix harvested from the inner table using a Hudson brace [28]. This technique affords a considerable amount of graft material which when mixed with fibrin glue (Tisseel) will fill in many leftover defects and provides a solid fusion construct most of the time.

Other challenges unique to the added fronto-orbital length include the frequent difficulty of closing an older and less compliant scalp over a greater volume (especially when advancing more than 2 cm). A number of techniques can be employed to facilitate this often late in the course of surgery challenge. The simplest is to use a through and through heavy duty stitch at three to five locations through the scalp to approximate the skin edges as best as possible and then to use a smaller subcutaneous suture to gradually bring the edges together much like a zipper before using a final and superficial skin closure with 3-0 monocryl (absorbable) or nylon suture. This will usually work for most significant advancements if done gradually and carefully. However, one must be cognizant of the amount of tension on the skin edges and the possibility of wound breakdown contributing to a greater chance of infection as well as development of a hypertrophic scar. If this is unsuccessful or if the skin edge tension appears problematic, another approach is to score the galea on the inner surface of the flap, being careful not to extend this too close to the surface or to compromise the dermal vascular layer of the flap. This will also offer greater relaxation of the flap and potentially minimize any later healing problems.

Subgaleal drains are universally used with a catheter on each side of the head (in case one falls out) and have been seen to reduce postop pain and swelling and decrease the length of stay. It is also important to use generous postoperative intravenous steroids to minimize any fronto-orbital swelling that is not only uncomfortable, but can also compromise healing of a flap under tension. We usually start the steroids at the time of induction and use the steroids for 3 days with a diminishing dose each day. To date, we have not seen any added morbidity from a short course of modest steroids, but have seen significant improvement in pain as well as universal discharges to home by postop day #3.

34.5.2 Fronto-orbital Advancement: Unilateral Coronal Synostosis

After the removal of the frontal bones and bandeau, each is remodeled. The frontal bone is remodeled using radial osteotomies, or selective fractures are performed to achieve the desired form. The bandeau is contoured to increase the convexity of the flattened side. A resorbable plate placed on the endocortical surface is excellent for maintaining the bandeau shape. There is a tendency for the correction to relapse in younger children who are still growing, so many surgeons advocate recontouring and sagittal overcorrection of the bandeau and frontal bone on the side of the fusion. Some authors have recommended using an onlay bone graft over the orbital rim on the ipsilateral side to help accentuate the sagittal projection, but it is the authors' experience that onlay grafts resorb. The bandeau repositioned with ipsilateral over-advancement and affixed to each temporal fossa with resorbable plates is, in our opinion, a better option. A full-thickness rectangular bone graft behind the bandeau will help prevent postoperative collapse and ensure bony healing. The frontal bone plates are reattached to the orbital bandeau with resorbable plates. The frontal bones should be attached to the parietal segments with absorbable plates to prevent collapse during the redraping of the coronal flaps. Full-thickness bone grafts harvested from the vertex can be used to fill the lateral coronal gap, especially on the more advanced side. Particulate cranial bone graft harvested from the endocortex of the frontal elements, or ectocortex of the parietal bones, can easily cover all remaining bone defects. The asymmetry of the palpebral fissure can be corrected with a lateral canthopexy on the side of the fusion.

34.5.3 Total Cranial Vault Remodeling: Sagittal

Surgical correction for delayed recognition of scaphocephaly more often may be undertaken for concerns regarding increased ICP, although morphological constraints may also be significant contributor as an indication (Fig. 34.5).

Thus, this approach needs to adequately increase the intracranial volume while concomitantly improving the cephalic index. Many of the usual principles for a safe and effective cranial reconfiguration will apply here, but there are a few concerns to consider differently in this cohort. With careful dissection during the bicoronal incision (leaving the periosteum intact on the bone), in addition to controlled systemic hypotension (55–60 mmHg) as well as preoperative administration by anesthesia of TXA/Amicar, one should be able to minimize bleeding during the opening to less than 50 cc. Starting off with a minimal blood loss during the opening increases the likelihood of not needing any transfusion for these cases and our transfusion rate routinely runs between 25–40% for the older patient. The most important factor is performing a meticulous dissection and watching for the innocuous slow oozing occurring under the towels or in a pocket of the flap. One can lose a large amount of blood over an extended period of time without truly appreciating the loss due to the slow and unimpressive volume at the outset.

In the older child, the degree of anterior-posterior shortening that is safe is considerably less than in a young infant and it is usually not necessary to do any frontal advancement. One may leave the fronto-orbital bar intact, which greatly facilitates the operation as well as reduces postoperative morbidity. The primary goal is to increase the intracranial volume while expanding the biparietal diameter. This is best facilitated by performing a "sunrise" series of frontal osteoto-

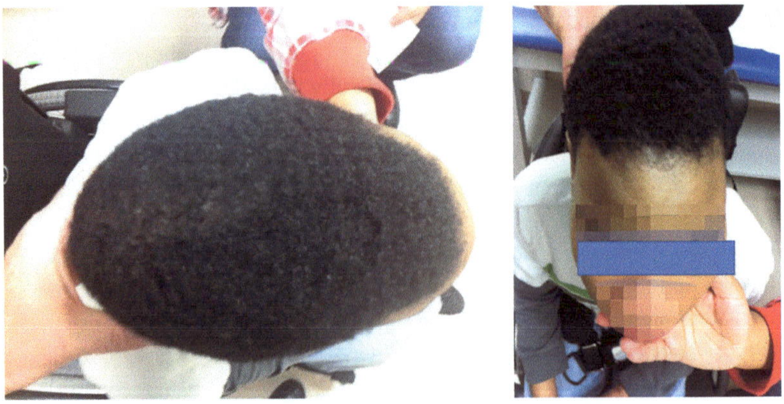

Fig. 34.5 Five year-old male with untreated scaphocephaly referred because of teasing in school. Note the significant skull base changes as well as the narrow face

mies leaving the fronto-orbital base predominantly intact but expanding the lateral and posterior portions of the frontal bone while expanding both parietal bones hinged off the intact and midline sagittal strut (Fig. 34.6a, b).

Total vault remodeling for sagittal synostosis requires exposure from the glabella anteriorly to the posterior cranial base. Supine positioning on a cerebellar head holder is the senior author's preferred position for addressing all types of craniosynostosis as it permits full exposure of the entire cranium and eliminates some potential complications with prone positioning. The entire occiput is easily accessed by simply turning the head to one side or the other. Frontal bossing has been shown to correct naturally with growth and, thus, does not require setback or manipulation. Low temporal and parietal regions barrel stave osteotomies are performed, and the segments are out-fractured. This expands the parietal width and provides a complete release. The cone-shaped occiput is remodeled with radial osteotomies and bending to give a more gradual convex curvature. The bifrontal fragment is radially osteotomized and similarly reshaped. Shortening the anteroposterior length is not usually required. However, this can be accomplished by resecting a portion of the frontal and parietal bones at the midline. The remaining parietal bone fragments are remodeled to increase the lateral convexity. Once the bone fragments are remodeled satisfactorily, they are secured in a more lateralized position with absorbable plates. The exposed dura is covered with particulate bone graft that can be harvested from the endocortical surface of the parietal bones. Plate stabilization assures that the expansion and shape correction achieved intraoperatively will not relapse or collapse postoperatively (Fig. 34.7a–c).

34.5.4 Cranial Vault Distraction

The distraction of the cranium is a newer technique that has shown promise for certain types of craniosynostosis (e.g., bicoronal craniosynostosis), but is used more liberally by some surgeons for all types of craniosynostosis. Distraction can be used for patients of all ages and allows large movements of cranial bone that would be difficult, if not impossible, to achieve with minimally invasive or open cranial remodeling procedures. Because this is a gradual process, ossification of the bone gaps is quite good. But this procedure does require a significant open dissection comparable to a conventional open vault operation to perform the craniotomy and place the distractors. It requires a second procedure to remove the

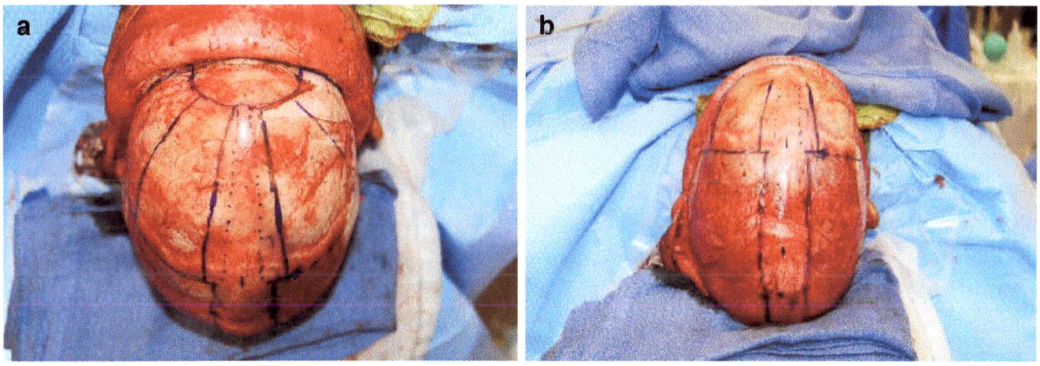

Fig. 34.6 (a, b) Sunrise technique for calvarial vault reconfiguration in the setting of delayed presentation of sagittal synostosis. The frontal bone is left in place, but the lateral and posterior components are opened up by radial osteotomies to expand the width of the frontal bone. Partial thickness osteotomies are represented by the dotted lines, whereas the full thickness osteotomies are planned along the solid lines. The midline bone overlying the sagittal sinus is left in place to protect the sinus as well as being used as a scaffold for fixation of the new calvarial bone flaps

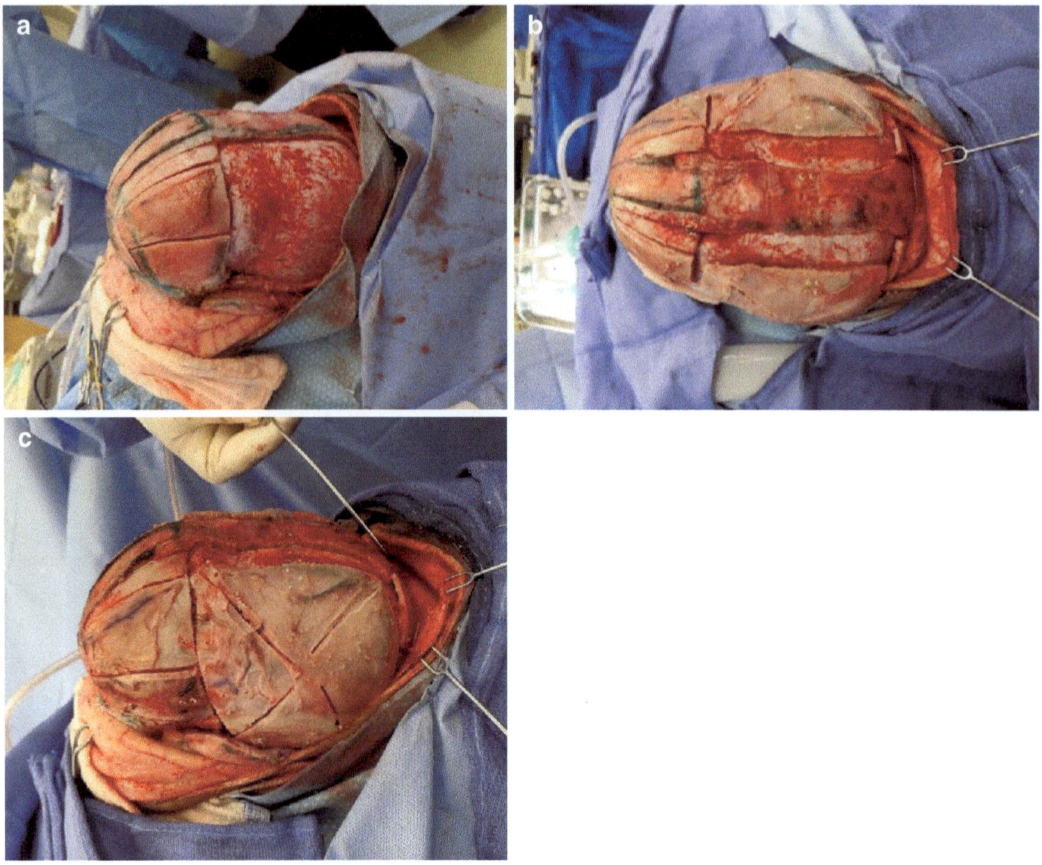

Fig. 34.7 (**a**–**c**) After the frontal osteotomies, the expanded frontal width is now configured to the newly expanded biparietal flaps (also with radial osteotomies) to increase the total width of the head as well as offer greater intracranial volume. The construct is maintained using absorbable plates

device. The greatest limitation for distraction in single suture fusions is that each distractor moves the bone segment in one direction and there is no capacity for bone remodeling or complex three-dimensional shape changes. Thus, its utility and benefits for most types of single-suture craniosynostosis are dubious at best. In the case of bilateral coronal craniosynostosis, some centers have begun to emphasize early posterior expansion, often using distraction and a later staged anterior procedure to improve frontal shape. Advocates suggest that this approach provides the neurocognitive benefits of early decompression, avoids the development of compensational turribrachycephaly, and permits a later anterior reconstruction (presumably less relapse). The disadvantage of this algorithm is that it requires three procedures early in life, including a relatively large procedure to create the posterior osteotomies and place the distractors, another minor procedure to remove the distractors, and the frontal procedure at some time in the future. The procedure also results in the closure of the normal lambdoid sutures—the effect of this is unknown.

34.6 Conclusions

Most children with non-syndromic craniosynostosis present to neurosurgical attention in early infancy and undergo surgical repair prior to 1 year of age. However, a subset of patients may present in a delayed fashion due to several factors and often present unique challenges for the craniofacial team. These children are at risk for presenting with increased ICPs and may manifest developmental delay from the growth restriction placed on the skull and brain in infancy. They also tend to have more craniofacial abnormalities and require more extensive surgery with an increased risk of potential complications. However, with detailed preoperative planning and a few key considerations, these patients can safely undergo repair for both aesthetic purposes and alleviation of any increased ICP as well as potential improvement in any cognitive deficits.

Pearls and Pitfalls

- One must look carefully for any possible sign of increased ICP in the older patient, even those of a single suture synostosis. This entails a detailed history and exam (the HC trajectory is a critical piece of information) as well as radiographic evaluation (CT, MRI) and funduscopic evaluation to look for subtle changes consistent with increased pressure. It may also be necessary to place an ICP monitor for those patients who remain less than clear with respect to their ICP.
- The use of TXA or Amicar at the time of induction (before surgery has started) in addition to keeping the mean systolic BP between 55–60 mmHg has been shown to significantly reduce the need for perioperative transfusion and has allowed our transfusion rates to be <50% in the older kids. Unpublished data from our institution comparing both agents have demonstrated equal efficacy between the two agents.
- For the patient with cerebral ventriculomegaly or suspected hydrocephalus, a shunt or CSF diversion should be reserved only for the patient with clear-cut hydrocephalus (over time); with a progressive Chiari malformation (can also be seen with pansynostosis) or syringomyelia as potential clues.
- The older patient often has many areas of calvarial deficiencies after any frontal advancement or bilateral parietal expansion. It is best to ensure that the frontal and other areas of cosmetic priority have adequate bony reconstruction in these regions. Additional bone may be harvested by using split-calvarial cranioplasty as well as using particulate bony matrix harvested from the inner table using a Hudson brace. This technique affords a considerable amount of graft material which when mixed with fibrin glue (Tissel) will fill in many left over defects and provides a solid fusion construct the majority of the time.
- It doesn't take a significant increase in calvarial volume to markedly reduce the patient's ICP and the extent of volumetric expansion will be dictated by the patient's age. Patients approaching 5–6 years of age are unlikely (but still seen on rare occasions) to need additional volumetric expansion for purposes of intracranial pressure, whereas the younger patients (2–4 years) will need to be followed closely, especially in the setting of multi-suture synostosis.
- Subgaleal drains are universally used with a catheter on each side of the head (in case one falls out) and have been seen to reduce postop pain and swelling and decrease the length of stay.
- In the event of a challenging effort to reapproximate bicoronal skin flaps after a significant frontal advancement, one may score the galea on the inner surface of the flap, being careful not to extend this too close to the surface or to compromise the dermal vascular layer of the flap. This will offer greater relaxation of the flap and potentially minimize any later healing problems.

References

1. Bruce DA. Difficult questions facing the craniofacial team. Oral Maxillofac Surg Clin North Am. 2004;16:429–38.
2. Bruce WJ, Chang V, Joyce CJ, Cobb AN, et al. Age at time of craniosynostosis repair predicts increased complication rate. Cleft Palate Craniofac J. 2018;55(5):649–54.
3. Gandolfi BM, Sobol DL, Farjat AE, Allori AC, Muh CR, Marcus JR. Risk factors for delayed referral to a craniofacial specialist for treatment of craniosynostosis. J Pediatr. 2017;186:165–71.
4. Lin Y, Pan IW, Harris DA, Luerssen TG, Lam S. The impact of insurance, race, and ethnic-

ity on age at surgical intervention among children with nonsyndromic craniosynostosis. J Pediatr. 2015;166(5):1289–96.
5. Mozaffari MA, Hauc SC, Junn AH, Junn A, et al. Socioeconomic disparities in the surgical management of craniosynostosis. J Craniofac Surg. 2022;33(1):294–7.
6. Hoffman C, Valenti AB, et al. Impact of health disparities on treatment for single-suture craniosynostosis in an era of multimodal care. Neurosurg Focus. 2021;50(4):E13.
7. Blessing M, Gallagher ER. Epidemiology, genetics, and pathophysiology of craniosynostosis. Oral Maxillofac Surg Clin North Am. 2022;34(3):341–52. https://doi.org/10.1016/j.coms.2022.02.001. Epub 2022 Jul 2.
8. Bryant JR, Mantilla-Rivas E, Keating RF, Rana MS, Manrique M, Oh AK, Magge SN, Murnick J, Oluigbo CO, Myseros JS, Rogers GF. Craniosynostosis develops in half of infants treated for hydrocephalus with a ventriculoperitoneal shunt. Plast Reconstr Surg. 2021;147(6):1390–9.
9. Manrique M, Mantilla-Rivas E, Rana MS, Crowder H, Oh N, Oh AK, Keating RF, Rogers GF. Normocephalic sagittal craniosynostosis in young children is common and unrecognized. Childs Nerv Syst. 2022;38(8):1549–56.
10. Vega RA, Opala C, Harshbarger RJ, et al. Hypophosphatemic rickets and craniosynostosis: a multicenter case series. J Neurosurg Pediatr. 2016;17:694–700.
11. Wall SA, Thomas GPL, Johnson D, Byren JC, et al. The preoperative incidence of raised intracranial pressure in nonsyndromic sagittal craniosynostosis is underestimated in the literature. J Neurosurg Pediatr. 2014;14(6):674–81.
12. Seruya M, Oh AK, Boyajian MJ, Posnick JC, Myseros JS, Yaun AL, Keating RF. Long-term outcomes of primary craniofacial reconstruction for craniosynostosis: a 12-year experience. Plast Reconstr Surg. 2011;127(6):2397–406.
13. Parikh RP, Farber SJ, Nguyen D, Skolnick GB, Patel K, Woo AS. Risk factors for postoperative complications after surgical correction of craniosynostosis: a nationwide analysis of 1357 intracranial procedures. Plast Reconstr Surg. 2015;136(4S):40.
14. Moore MH, Chaisrisawadisuk S, Prasad V, Santoreneos S, Molloy CJ. Secondary raised intracranial pressure after cranial vault remodeling for isolated sagittal craniosynostosis. J Craniofac Surg. 2021;32(8):2651–5.
15. Thomas GP, Johnson D, Byren JC, Judge AD, Jayamohan J, Magdum SA, Richards PG, Wall SA. The incidence of raised intracranial pressure in nonsyndromic sagittal craniosynostosis following primary surgery. J Neurosurg Pediatr. 2015;15(4):350–60.
16. Utria AF, Lopez J, Cho RS, Mundinger GS, Jallo GI, Ahn ES, Kolk CV, Dorafshar AH. Timing of cranial vault remodeling in nonsyndromic craniosynostosis: a single-institution 30-year experience. J Neurosurg Pediatr. 2016;18(5):629–34.
17. Fontana SC, Belinger S, Daniels D, Tuttle M, et al. Longitudinal assessment of development outcomes in infants undergoing late craniosynostosis repair. J Craniofac Surg. 2018;29:25–8.
18. Renier D, Lajeunie E, Arnaud E, et al. Management of craniosynostoses. Childs Nerv Syst. 2000;16:645–58.
19. Iyengar RJ, Klinge PM, Chen WS, Boxerman JL, et al. Management of craniosynostosis at an advanced age: controversies, clinical findings, and surgical treatment. J Craniofac Surg. 2016;27:e435–41.
20. Becker DB, Petersen JD, Kane AA, Cradock MM, Pilgram TK, Marsh JL. Speech, cognitive, and behavioral outcomes in nonsyndromic craniosynostosis. Plast Reconstr Surg. 2005;116:400–7.
21. Spetzl ML, Kapp-Simon KA, Cunnigham M, et al. Single-suture craniosynostosis: a review of neurobehavioral research and theory. J Peditr Psychol. 2004;29:651–68.
22. Starr JR, Kapp-Simon KA, Cloonan YK, et al. Presurgical and postsurgical assessment of the neurodevelopment of infants with single-suture craniosynostosis: comparison with controls. J Neurosurg. 2007;107(2 suppl):103–10.
23. Beckett JS, Brooks ED, Lacadie C, Vander Wyk B, Jou RJ, Steinbacher DM, Constable RT, Pelphrey KA, Persing JA. Altered brain connectivity in sagittal craniosynostosis. J Neurosurg Pediatr. 2014;13(6):690–8. https://doi.org/10.3171/2014.3.PEDS13516. Epub 2014 Apr 18.
24. Patel A, Yang JF, Hashim PW, et al. The impact of age at surgery on long-term neuropsychological outcomes in sagittal craniosynostosis. Plast Reconstr Surg. 2014;134:608e–17e.
25. Chim H, Wetjen N, Mardini S. Virtual surgical planning in craniofacial surgery. Semin Plast Surg. 2014;28(3):150–8.
26. Garcia-Mato D, Ochandiano S, Garcia-Sevilla M, et al. Craniosynostosis surgery: workflow based on vritual surgical planning, intraoperative navigation and 3D printed patient-specific guides and templates. Sci Rep. 2019;9:17691.
27. Rottgers SA, Kim PD, Kumar AR, et al. Cranial vault remodeling for sagittal craniosynostosis in older children. Neurosurg Focus. 2011;31:E3.
28. Oh AK, Greene AK, Mulliken JB, Rogers GF. Prevention of temporal depression that follows fronto-orbital advancement for craniosynostosis. J Craniofac Surg. 2006;17(5):980–5. https://doi.org/10.1097/01.scs.0000230015.16401.1d.

Hydrocephalus and Craniosynostosis

35

Matthias Schulz and Ulrich-Wilhelm Thomale

35.1 Aetiology

The impaired growth capacity of the cranial vault due to craniosynostosis—especially in the event of multiple fused cranial sutures—results in a situation termed "cephalo-cranial disproportion" which is characterized by insufficient intracranial volume increment for the developing brain and subsequently chronic elevation in intracranial pressure (ICP) [1, 2]. In the case of insufficient volume development of the posterior fossa, this disproportion may further adversely impact the CSF circulation and contribute to a developing hydrocephalus. Tonsillar herniation (Chiari malformation) is a further known manifestation of the cephalo-cranial disproportion affecting the posterior part of the cranial vault and the posterior fossa. In one large series about 8% of the children with craniosynostosis (29/329) presented with Chiari Malformation. The incidence was highest for children with multiple/syndromic craniosynostosis with 35% (14/40) and with isolated lambdoid synostosis (56%, 6/9). The average area of the foramen magnum has been demonstrated to be smaller in children affected by syndromic craniosynostosis and a correlation between the area of the foramen and the size of the ventricular system has be shown by Rijken et al. [3]. In accordance with Coll et al., a correlation between smaller size of the foramen magnum and hydrocephalus as well as an association of hydrocephalus and tonsillar herniation was observed [4].

Several factors contribute to a disturbed circulation of the cerebro-spinal fluid (CSF) resulting in a hydrocephalic condition [5]. In craniosynostosis, relevant factors are restricted skull growth with possible secondary displacement of intracranial structures and impaired venous outflow, which may result in CSF resorption impairment as a possible contributing factor for CSF circulation disturbance. Anatomical displacement will more often be seen in multiple synostosis conditions most likely due to decreased volume of the posterior fossa. This may lead to major CSF pathway occlusion at locations such as the Sylvian aqueduct or the outlets of the fourth ventricle. Secondary tonsillar herniations may obstruct the foramen magnum, which might reduce the transmission of CSF pulsation between the intracranial and the spinal compartment in which the dura is imbedded in epidural fat tissue. This spinal dural elasticity normally enables to balance the pulsatile ICP wave which is impaired in condition of tonsilar herniation. In addition, impaired absorption capacity of the CSF back into the venous system secondary to intracranial venous hypertension is caused by altered skull base growth and compression of venous sinuses within the posterior fossa—both leading to increased

M. Schulz · U.-W. Thomale (✉)
Pediatric Neurosurgery, Campus Virchow Klinikum, Charité Universitätsmedizin Berlin, Berlin, Germany
e-mail: matthias.schulz@charite.de; Ulrich-Wilhelm.Thomale@charite.de

F. Di Rocco, J. Kestle (eds.), *Neurosurgical Aspects of Craniosynostosis*,
https://doi.org/10.1007/978-3-031-69386-1_35

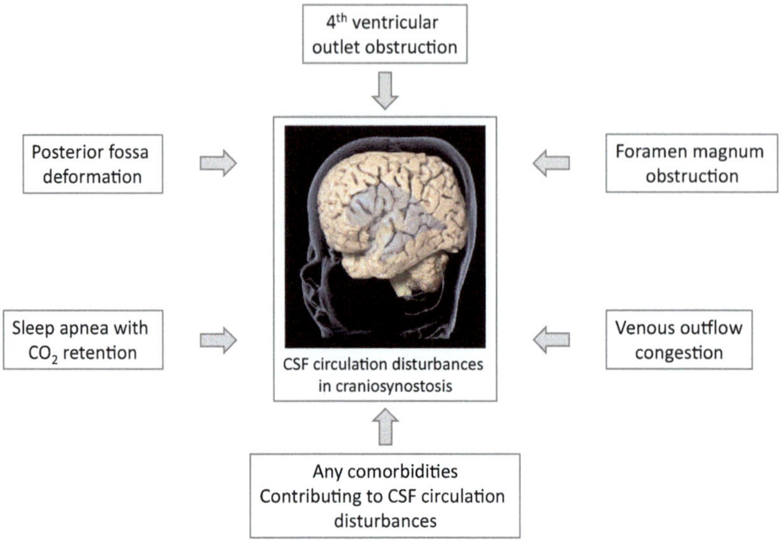

Fig. 35.1 The ventricular system as well as the external CSF spaces may show disbalance in circulation more often in the context of multiple craniosynostosis affecting the posterior fossa growth. Possible contributing factors for CSF circulation disturbances may be major CSF pathway obstruction at the outlets of the fourth ventricle or the foramen magnum, venous outflow disturbances, and CO_2 retention due to sleep apnea or comorbidities contributing to hydrocephalus development

venous outflow resistance [6, 7]. Possible obstructive sleep apnea (OSA) secondary to impaired midfacial growth or brainstem compression causing CO_2 retention and thereby increased intracranial blood volume has been furthermore discussed as a contributing factor for ICP elevation [8–10] (Fig. 35.1).

35.2 Epidemiology

The prevalence of hydrocephalus in children with craniosynostosis depends on the underlying aetiology of craniosynostosis. In non-syndromic children with single suture craniosynostosis, the prevalence is reported to be rare—between 0.28 and 1.8% (4/1447—5/275) [11, 12]. Some of the reported children in those series were furthermore affected by concurring comorbidities known to predispose hydrocephalus (e.g. previous haemorrhage, myelomeningocele). Thus, primary CSF circulation disturbances due to single suture synostosis alone may even be less frequent. On the contrary, the incidence of hydrocephalus in children with multiple or syndromic craniosynostosis is reported to be significantly higher and will certainly dependent also on the underlying genetic precondition. Although inconsistently discussed in the literature, several authors differentiate between hydrocephalus requiring surgical treatment and non-progressive ventriculo- or subarachnomegaly (Fig. 35.1).

The prospectively collected data of the Hydrocephalus Clinical Research Network confirm the disparity of the incidence of hydrocephalus between non-syndromic and syndromic children—in this cohort of children who were treated for hydrocephalus ($n = 6152$), only 42 children were affected by craniosynostosis. Of those, 79% (33/42) presented with multiple craniosynostosis and the remaining 21% (9/42) with single-suture craniosynostosis (3 with unilateral coronal, 3 with sagittal, and 2 with lambdoid suture craniosynostosis). For the majority of children (90%, 38/42), an underlying craniofacial syndrome was identified (the largest share being Crouzon Syndrome in 42% (16/38)) [13].

For children with Crouzon syndrome, the rates of hydrocephalus are reported to be 15.9% (10/63) and of ventriculomegaly to be 35% according to Collmann et al. [11], 16.6.% for hydrocephalus and 33.3% for ventriculomegaly according to Noetzel et al. [14], and 29% (4/14) for hydrocephalus according to Coll et al. [4]. For children with Pfeiffer Syndrome, even higher rates are reported—60% (9/15) with hydrocephalus and further 15% (3/15) with ventriculomegaly according to Collmann et al., 40% (2/5) according to Noetzel et al., and 33% (2/6) according to

Coll et al. On the contrary, the rates of hydrocephalus are low in children with Apert Syndrome—between 0 and 8.3%. Nevertheless, the rate of ventriculomegaly without the necessity for a surgical intervention is reported to be substantial at 43–100% [4, 11, 14, 15]. For children with a combination of bilateral lambdoid and sagittal suture synostosis ("Mercedes-Benz-Pattern"), a 5.1% rate of concomitant hydrocephalus and 28.8.% rate of ventriculomegaly have been reported [16]. For other craniofacial syndromes, the incidence of hydrocephalus seems to be negligible—none of the children affected by Muenke-Syndrome ($n = 24$) of Saethre-Chotzen-Syndrome ($n = 37$) demonstrated features of hydrocephalus [11].

35.3 Diagnostics

For children with syndromic craniosynostosis, a correlation between occipito-frontal head circumference and intracranial volume has been documented and underlines the value of repetitive head circumference measurements to detect insufficient growth [17]. In infants, the open fontanelle allows an indirect but easy assessment of the ICP and by means of transfontanellar ultrasound, the imaging and repetitive monitoring of the dimensions of the ventricular system and Doppler sonography for "resistance index" evaluation, which may indicate an increased ICP via decreased end-diastolic flow.

However, the higher quality imaging modes for the evaluation of the intracranial compartment are CT and MRI. Although both methods allow assessment of the dimensions of the ventricular system, the repetitive utilization of CT should be deferred in favour of MRI because of the documented increased life-time risk for smaller children to develop a malignancy after exposure to ionizing radiation [18, 19]. Furthermore, the MRI offers the better soft-tissue differentiation and the possibility of dynamic CSF circulation studies including T2-sequences in three dimensions, venous MR angiography and sagittal midline CISS sequence for evaluation of the cisternal and intraventricular membranes and superior evaluation of a possible tonsillar herniation and thus may be considered as diagnostic measure of choice [20].

35.4 Treatment Options

(a) Craniofacial Treatment Options

Children with craniosynostosis and concomitant hydrocephalus constitute a difficult and complex situation, because utilized treatment steps may favourably or adversely impact various aspects of the primary pathology. Clinical outcome and consecutive treatment. As a basic rule, both aetiology and pathophysiology of the existent hydrocephalus as direct result of intracranial volume reduction should be taken into consideration to establish the appropriate order of treatment steps. If ever possible, treatment should attempt to reverse the underlying aetiology of hydrocephalus. In this regard, one of the first questions to answer is whether the development of the intracranial volume so far has been and will presumably remain sufficient. In a child with obvious cephalo-cranial disproportion with cranial restriction and hydrocephalus, an expansive cranioplasty to enlarge the intracranial volume should be performed at first step if clinically feasible. That will always be preferable to any CSF diverting measures, since a shunt system constitutes a risk of overdrainage and may even further diminish calvarial growth or compromise previous expansion results.

Posterior calvarial expansion may play a relevant role to influence CSF circulation since it seems to more effectively increase intracranial volume (by 35%) than anterior calvarial vault expansion—as demonstrated for three simulated translational and similar distances of advancement [21]. Furthermore, posterior cranial vault expansion addresses the part of the calvarium in anatomical relation to the disturbed CSF circulation such as the foramen magnum, tonsillar herniation, draining veins and sinuses, and the compressed fourth ventricle. Therefore, the suggested order of cranial vault enlargement in cephalo-cranial disproportion with secondary signs of increased ICP is a posterior vault cranioplasty at the age of 3–6 months followed by later anterior advancement (e.g. by fronto-orbital advancement) at 10–12 months [22, 23].

Several techniques of posterior cranial vault remodeling (PCVR) have been published, allowing increase of the intracranial volume between 13 and 29% [24–27]. As an advantage, a PCVR procedure allows the treatment of a Chiari Malformation—a possible contributing factor for hydrocephalus—by a suboccipital craniectomy (and laminectomy C1, if necessary) [28, 29]. One published series compared the influence of the applied cranioplasty technique: regarding the rate of hydrocephalus, no difference was demonstrated between posterior vault distraction osteogenesis (PVDO, $n = 49$) without however involving the foramen magnum and calvarial vault remodeling (CVR, $n = 23$). The rate of developing tonsillar herniation was significantly lower after PVOD compared to CVR, possibly due to the larger achievable expansion distance after PVDO [30]. In a series of 41 patients receiving posterior cranial vault expansion, five hydrocephalus surgeries were done before the expansion surgery including four VP shunt implantation. During mean follow-up of 18 months (3–72), none of the patients needed any VP shunt implantation while only 2 had additional ETV surgeries [27] (Fig. 35.2).

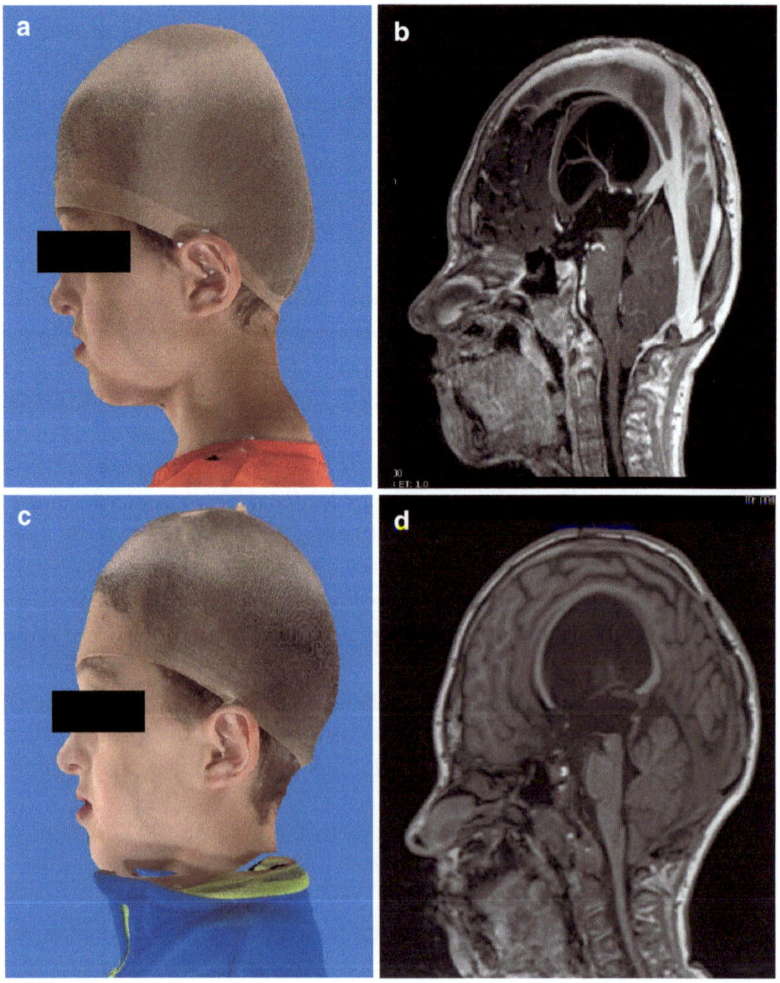

Fig. 35.2 9.5 year old boy with pansynsotosis who received early total calvarial vault remodeling externally with secondary pansynositosis, brachycephaly, and severe headaches (**a**, **b**). Parieto-occipital expansion was performed, which enhanced the posterior cranial vault curvature (**c**). In follow-up MRI, the relief of posterior fossa and establishment of CSF flow anterior to the tonsils can be appreciated (**d**), which resolved the headaches

The recommendation to consider and perform a cranial vault expansion prior to the insertion of a CSF diverting shunt is based on the obvious risk that a CSF diversion may further adversely affect cranial growth and may aggravate cephalo-cranial disproportion. In a series by Nilsson et al., significantly smaller head circumferences were observed in children (age 2–3 years) who underwent a shunt insertion during their first year of life compared to children without a shunt. Furthermore, chronic shunt-induced overdrainage has been reported to induce secondary craniosynostosis. Especially in the setting of tonsillar herniation and pre-existing cephalo-cranial disproportion, a shunt insertion may have deleterious effects [31–33].

(b) CSF Diverting Treatment Options

In addition to the discussed specific cranial expansion treatment options, all possible established CSF diverting treatment options remain available for children affected by craniosynostosis and concomitant hydrocephalus if necessary.

Depending on the underlying pathophysiology, the primary treatment option may be the endoscopic third ventriculo-cisternostomy (ETV) to establishing an alternative intracranial CSF pathway in the setting of a non-communicating hydrocephalus. Extracranial CSF diverting shunt implantation remains appropriate for communicating hydrocephalus if alternative options are not available.

For both treatment options for hydrocephalus, a substantial amount of data in children without craniosynostosis have been published. The reported revision-free survival after ETV in a pediatric cohort of 336 children with hydrocephalus of all causes (median age of 6.9 years, IQR 1.7–12.6 years) was 64.8%, 61.7%, and 57.8% after respective 6 months, 1 year, and 2 years [34]. After shunt implantation in a large cohort of 1036 children (mean age of 131 ± 228 weeks, among them 56% less than 6 months old), a revision rate of 33% and an infection rate of 7.6% after a median follow-up of 264 days were documented [35]. The treatment of hydrocephalus in the context of craniosynostosis was evaluated by data of the prospective registry of the Hydrocephalus Clinical Research Network [13]. The median age of the 42 treated children was 0.6 years (IQR 0.3–1.7 years) at the time of the first craniosynostosis surgery and 1.2 years (IQR 0.5–2.5 years) at the first hydrocephalus surgery—thereby underlining the suggested order of antecedent craniosynostosis intervention before hydrocephalus surgery. Only 28% of the treated children underwent hydrocephalus treatment prior to craniosynostosis intervention. Hydrocephalus treatment was performed via shunt insertion in 2/3 of the patients (28/42); the remaining third underwent endoscopic third ventriculostomy (ETV). After 12 months, in total 34% of the children (14/42) required revision surgery—8 (28.6%) after shunt insertion and 6 (42.9%) after ETV. After a follow-up of 5.2 years (range 0.1–9.7 years), in total 50% of the patients (21/42) required an operative revision—there was no significant difference between the success rate of shunt insertion and ETV which supports the author's statement that ETV must be considered as a relevant alternative to shunting in this group of patients. This is in accordance with prior reports of success rates of ETV of 63.6% (7/11) children in children with craniofacial syndromes [36] (Fig. 35.3).

The choice of ETV over extracranial CSF diversion is especially supported by the typical signs of an existing pressure gradient between the internal CSF spaces and the external CSF spaces—including outward bulging membranes of the third ventricle such as the floor of the third ventricle, the lamina terminalis, and the pineal recess on sagittal midline MRI. In the absence of those signs and if cranial vault expansion is not necessary because of sufficient intracranial overall volume, extracranial CSF diversion may become unavoidable. In these situations, the shunt system and its valve should be chosen with the possibility to avoid overdrainage at all measures. A recent review has more precisely defined the possible signs of

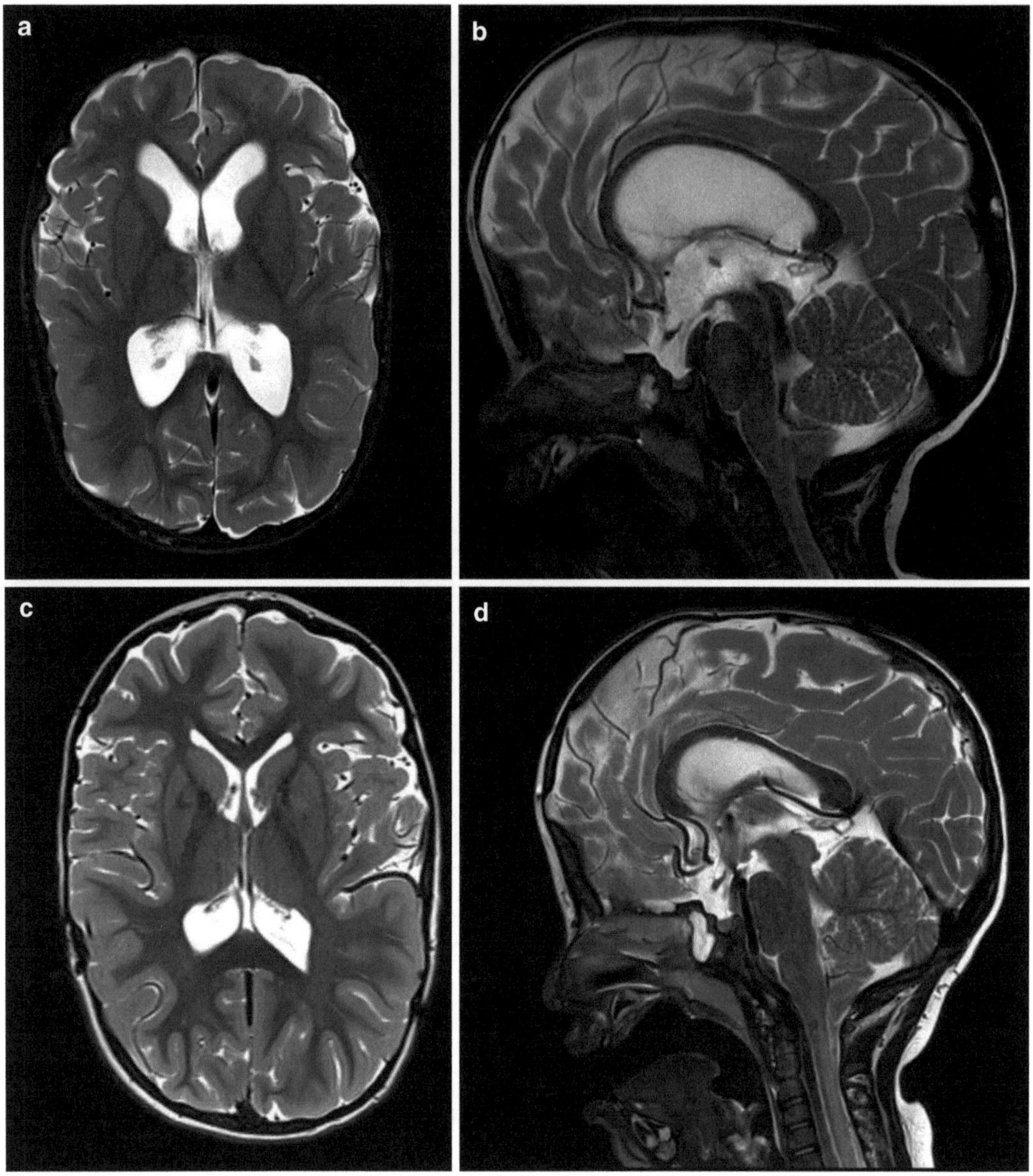

Fig. 35.3 1 year 4 months old patient with Crouzon syndrome showing ventricular enlargement and Chiari malformation while cranial expansion surgeries were already accomplished (**a**, **b**). An endoscopic third ventriculostomy was performed in condition of relative ventricular enlargement. MRI at 2 years follow-up (age: 3 year 4 months) showed decreased ventricular size and a patent ETV stoma due to stabilized CSF circulation disturbances (**c**, **d**)

CSF overdrainage such as postural dependent headache, vomiting and mood change/irritability, sunken fontanelle (if present), decreasing head circumference, and/or radiological signs as slim ventricles/complete ventricular collapse, subdural hygroma/haematoma, and overriding or fused cranial sutures [37]. In order to avoid these conditions, we strongly recommend the use of any overdrainage protecting units such as anti-gravitational units or any alternative effectively counteracting the hydrostatic effect in standing position. In addition, the adjustability of the valve resistance furthermore will allow patient-specific adaptation of valve drainage without the need for surgical shunt revision in a situation of overdrainage. The resistance in the entire valve system should be adjusted principally at a higher level compared to other hydrocephalus entities since the expected amount of required CSF diversion will be relatively low.

In infants with adjustable valves implanted within the first year of life, the option to adapt the setting of the valve was utilized in 31% and 42% of the children after 1 and 2 years and in a majority of 61% of the children by the time of the latest follow-up [38]. Concordantly, in older children (n = 53, mean age of 7.3 years), 35.8% underwent adaptation of valve settings after shunt insertion within a mean observation period of 15.2 month [39] which could be supported in subsequent reports with the same shunt system [40, 41]. Alternatively to adjustable valves with anti-siphoning units, flow-regulated valves demonstrated low primary overdrainage situations [42] (Fig. 35.4). Regarding the entry point of the ventricular catheter—the parietal entry offers the advantage that it might interfere less with later fronto-facial advancements and the necessary internal or external distraction devices. However, in the author's experience with exclusively frontally inserted ventricular catheters, no significant problems secondary to catheter location have been encountered. The site of the catheter entry is usually not

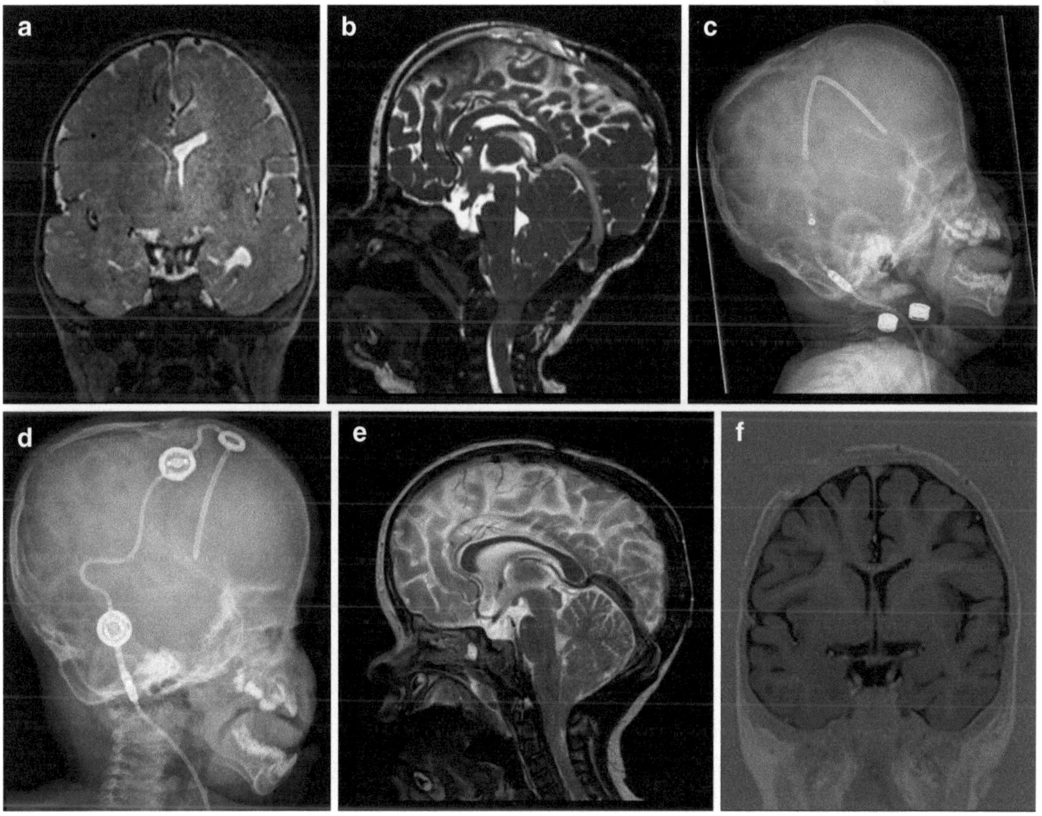

Fig. 35.4 One year old girl with Crouzon syndrome, received fronto-orbital advancement at an external center including VP shunt insertion (Codman hakim valve plus shunt assistant (SA) at 3/+20 = 3/23 cmH_2O with overdrainage showing the SA not in strict vertical position (**a**–**c**)). A craniocervical decompression and shunt valve exchange with higher valve resistance (proV and proGAV: 20 + 10/+30 – 30/60 cmH_2O) were performed followed by occipital expansion and later cranio cervical decompression establishing a better harmony in head shape and ventricular appearance

incorporated in the advanced part of the forehead and meticulous dissection as well as anti-infective measures ensures that secondary damage or infection of the shunt system is avoided.

It remains essential that in any child after treatment of hydrocephalus, close clinical and radiological follow-up with 3D photography, head circumference measures, and serial MRIs are mandatory to observe long-term effects to the ventricular system and the related anatomical structures.

Bullet Points

- Different pathophysiological mechanisms contribute to disturbed CSF circulation in craniosynostosis patients such as venous outflow impairment and major pathway obstruction, especially in volume-deficient posterior fossa anatomy mainly in children with multiple suture craniosynostosis.
- Avoid primary extracranial CSF diversion, if ever possible and clinically acceptable. Consider cranial expansion and/or foramen magnum decompression prior to any extracranial CSF diversion.
- Posterior cranial vault remodeling possibly has a more advantageous effects on disturbed CSF circulation than anterior advancement. The staged combination of both will effectively increase the intracranial volume with beneficial effects on CSF circulation and venous outflow.
- Consider ETV as appropriate first choice before any extracranial CSF diverting shunt especially in enlarged ventricles and posterior fossa crowding.
- If shunt implantation becomes unavoidable, consider the selection of relative high differential pressure settings in combination with counteracting the hydrostatic effect in upright position by the use of antihydrostatic units (gravitational/anti-siphoning units) to reduce the risk of overdrainage.
- Consider the use of adjustable valves to establish the option to alter valve resistance if clinical or radiographic signs of overdrainage are observed during follow-up.
- Maintain close clinical follow-up to assure sufficient shunt function and to identify possible overdrainage at early stages.

References

1. Hoffman HJ, Tucker WS. Cephalocranial disproportion. A complication of the treatment of hydrocephalus in children. Childs. Brain. 1976;2(3):167–76.
2. Di Rocco C, Frassanito P, Massimi L, Peraio S. Hydrocephalus and Chiari type I malformation. Childs Nerv Syst. 2011;27(10):1653–64.
3. Rijken BF, Lequin MH, Van Veelen ML, de Rooi J, Mathijssen IM. The formation of the foramen magnum and its role in developing ventriculomegaly and Chiari I malformation in children with craniosynostosis syndromes. J Craniomaxillofac Surg. 2015;43(7):1042–8.
4. Coll G, Arnaud E, Collet C, Brunelle F, Sainte-Rose C, Di Rocco F. Skull base morphology in fibroblast growth factor receptor type 2-related faciocraniosynostosis: a descriptive analysis. Neurosurgery. 2015;76(5):571–83; discussion 83.
5. Thomale UW. Integrated understanding of hydrocephalus—a practical approach for a complex disease. Childs Nerv Syst. 2021;37(11):3313–24.
6. Copeland AE, Hoffman CE, Tsitouras V, et al. Clinical significance of venous anomalies in syndromic craniosynostosis. Plast Reconstr Surg Glob Open. 2018;6(1):e1613.
7. Ghali GZ, Zaki Ghali MG, Ghali EZ, et al. Intracranial venous hypertension in craniosynostosis: mechanistic underpinnings and therapeutic implications. World Neurosurg. 2019;127:549–58.
8. Gonsalez S, Hayward R, Jones B, Lane R. Upper airway obstruction and raised intracranial pressure in children with craniosynostosis. Eur Respir J. 1997;10(2):367–75.
9. Hayward R, Gonsalez S. How low can you go? Intracranial pressure, cerebral perfusion pressure, and respiratory obstruction in children with complex craniosynostosis. J Neurosurg Pediatr. 2005;102(1):16–22.
10. Marucci DD, Dunaway DJ, Jones BM, Hayward RD. Raised intracranial pressure in apert syndrome. Plast Reconstr Surg. 2008;122(4):1162–8.
11. Collmann H, Sörensen N, Krauß J. Hydrocephalus in craniosynostosis: a review. Childs Nerv Syst. 2005;21(10):902–12.
12. Cinalli G, Sainte-Rose C, Kollar EM, et al. Hydrocephalus and craniosynostosis. J Neurosurg. 1998;88(2):209–14.
13. Bonfield CM, Shannon CN, Reeder RW, et al. Hydrocephalus treatment in patients with craniosynostosis: an analysis from the hydrocephalus clinical research network prospective registry. Neurosurg Focus. 2021;50(4):E11.

14. Noetzel MJ, Marsh JL, Palkes H, Gado M. Hydrocephalus and mental retardation in craniosynostosis. J Pediatr. 1985;107(6):885–92.
15. Renier D, Arnaud E, Cinalli G, Sebag G, Zerah M, Marchac D. Prognosis for mental function in Apert's syndrome. J Neurosurg. 1996;85(1):66–72.
16. Balestrino A, Secci F, Piatelli G, et al. Pure bilateral lambdoid and posterior sagittal synostosis (Mercedes-Benz syndrome): case report and literature review. World Neurosurg. 2019;128:77–82.
17. Rijken BFM, den Ottelander BK, van Veelen M-LC, Lequin MH, Mathijssen IMJ. The occipitofrontal circumference: reliable prediction of the intracranial volume in children with syndromic and complex craniosynostosis. Neurosurg Focus. 2015;38(5):E9.
18. Pearce MS, Salotti JA, Little MP, et al. Radiation exposure from CT scans in childhood and subsequent risk of leukaemia and brain tumours: a retrospective cohort study. Lancet. 2012;380(9840):499–505.
19. Miglioretti DL, Johnson E, Williams A, et al. The use of computed tomography in pediatrics and the associated radiation exposure and estimated cancer risk. JAMA Pediatr. 2013;167(8):700–7.
20. Robson CD, MacDougall RD, Madsen JR, Warf BC, Robertson RL. Neuroimaging of children with surgically treated hydrocephalus: a practical approach. AJR Am J Roentgenol. 2017;208(2):413–9.
21. Choi M, Flores RL, Havlik RJ. Volumetric analysis of anterior versus posterior cranial vault expansion in patients with syndromic craniosynostosis. J Craniofac Surg. 2012;23(2):455–8.
22. Swanson JW, Samra F, Bauder A, Mitchell BT, Taylor JA, Bartlett SP. An algorithm for managing syndromic craniosynostosis using posterior vault distraction osteogenesis. Plast Reconstr Surg. 2016;137(5):829e–41e.
23. Carlson AR, Taylor JA. Posterior vault distraction osteogenesis: indications and expectations. Childs Nerv Syst. 2021;37(10):3119–25.
24. Schulz M, Spors B, Haberl H, Thomale UW. Results of posterior cranial vault remodeling for plagiocephaly and brachycephaly by the meander technique. Childs Nerv Syst. 2014;30.1517.
25. Nowinski D, Di Rocco F, Renier D, SainteRose C, Leikola J, Arnaud E. Posterior cranial vault expansion in the treatment of craniosynostosis. Comparison of current techniques. Childs Nerv Syst. 2012;28(9):1537–44.
26. Goldstein JA, Paliga JT, Wink JD, Low DW, Bartlett SP, Taylor JA. A craniometric analysis of posterior cranial vault distraction osteogenesis. Plast Reconstr Surg. 2013;131(6):1367–75.
27. Pennacchietti V, Schulz M, Tietze A, Schwarz K, Thomale UW. Extended experience in parieto-occipital expansion surgery by meander technique-clinical and radiological evaluation. Childs Nerv Syst. 2021;37(10):3199–207.
28. Cinalli G, Chumas P, Arnaud E, Sainte-Rose C, Renier D. Occipital remodeling and suboccipital decompression in severe craniosynostosis associated with tonsillar herniation. Neurosurgery. 1998;42(1):66–72.
29. Scott WW, Fearon JA, Swift DM, Sacco DJ. Suboccipital decompression during posterior cranial vault remodeling for selected cases of Chiari malformations associated with craniosynostosis. J Neurosurg Pediatr. 2013;12(2):166–70.
30. Lin LO, Zhang RS, Hoppe IC, et al. Onset and resolution of Chiari malformations and hydrocephalus in syndromic craniosynostosis following posterior vault distraction. Plast Reconstr Surg. 2019;144(4):932–40.
31. Weinzweig J, Bartlett SP, Chen JC, et al. Cranial vault expansion in the management of postshunt craniosynostosis and slit ventricle syndrome. Plast Reconstr Surg. 2008;122(4):1171–80.
32. Bhadkamkar MA, Albright SB, Wolfswinkel EM, Bollo R, Buchanan EP. Posterior cranial vault distraction in the treatment of shunt-induced craniosynostosis. J Craniofac Surg. 2015;26(1):e70–2.
33. Nilsson D, Svensson J, Korkmaz BA, Nelvig H, Tisell M. Decreased head circumference in shunt-treated compared with healthy children. J Neurosurg Pediatr. 2013;12(5):483–90.
34. Kulkarni AV, Riva-Cambrin J, Holubkov R, et al. Endoscopic third ventriculostomy in children: prospective, multicenter results from the hydrocephalus clinical research network. J Neurosurg Pediatr. 2016;18(4):423–9.
35. Riva-Cambrin J, Kestle JR, Holubkov R, et al. Risk factors for shunt malfunction in pediatric hydrocephalus: a multicenter prospective cohort study. J Neurosurg Pediatr. 2016;17(4):382–90.
36. Di Rocco F, Jucá CE, Arnaud E, Renier D, Sainte-Rose C. The role of endoscopic third ventriculostomy in the treatment of hydrocephalus associated with faciocraniosynostosis. J Neurosurg Pediatr. 2010;6(1):17–22.
37. Pedersen SH, Prein TH, Ammar A, et al. How to define CSF overdrainage: a systematic literature review. Acta Neurochir. 2023;165(2):429–41.
38. Bock HC, von Philipp G, Ludwig HC. An adjustable gravitational valve for initial VP-shunt treatment in hydrocephalic preterm neonates and infants below 1 year of age. Childs Nerv Syst. 2021;37(11):3497–507.
39. Rohde V, Haberl EJ, Ludwig H, Thomale UW. First experiences with an adjustable gravitational valve in childhood hydrocephalus. J Neurosurg Pediatr. 2009;3(2):90–3.
40. Thomale UW, Gebert AF, Haberl H, Schulz M. Shunt survival rates by using the adjustable differential pressure valve combined with a gravitational unit (proGAV) in pediatric neurosurgery. Childs Nerv Syst. 2013;29(3):425–31.
41. Gebert AF, Schulz M, Schwarz K, Thomale UW. Long-term survival rates of gravity-assisted, adjustable differential pressure valves in infants with hydrocephalus. J Neurosurg Pediatr. 2016;17(5):544–51.
42. Henderson D, Budu A, Zaki H, et al. A comparison between flow-regulated and adjustable valves used in hydrocephalus during infancy. Childs Nerv Syst. 2020;36(9):2013–9.

Management of Hydrocephalus in Patients with Craniosynostosis

36

Eduardo Jucá
and Carolina Carmona Pinheiro Machado

36.1 Contextualization and Epidemiology

Interest in the challenges posed by the association between craniostenosis and hydrocephalus dates back to the 1970s and 1980s, coinciding with a period of exponential progress in the understanding and development of operative techniques for the management of craniostenosis. In fact, as they represent two of the most important diseases faced by pediatric neurosurgeons and both have the risk of intracranial hypertension leading to neurodevelopmental delay and cognitive impairment, the two entities entail particularities and specific challenges in their treatment when combined [1, 2].

More specifically, while the incidence of hydrocephalus seems to be fortuitous and anecdotal in nonsyndromic craniostenosis involving early closure of one or more cranial sutures, most cases of association affect children with syndromic craniostenosis in all reported series.

Back in 1985, in a study that actively researched hydrocephalus and cognitive impairment in cases of craniostenosis, Noetzel et al. found no cases of hydrocephalus in 27 cases of nonsyndromic craniostenosis, but identified 5 occurrences in 23 cases of syndromic craniostenosis, including cases of Crouzon syndrome, Pfeiffer syndrome, and cloverleaf deformity [2].

Golabi et al. also reported in 1987 a series of 10 patients with hydrocephalus in a total of 250 patients treated for craniostenosis in 5 consecutive years. Of these, four had Pfeiffer's syndrome, three had Crouzon's syndrome, two had syndromic features but without a defined syndrome, and only one patient had a single suture craniostenosis, a case of scaphocephaly due to sagittal suture closure. The origin of hydrocephalus in the latter case was associated with prematurity; therefore, there was no causal association between the two entities [1].

In 2010, Di Rocco et al. described a series of 2194 cases conducted at the craniofacial surgery unit of the Necker Hospital in Paris between 1995 and 2008, with the identification of 293 patients with syndromic craniosynostosis and 46 of these cases (15.69%) with progressive hydrocephalus in need of surgical treatment [3].

Overall, the incidence of hydrocephalus was estimated at 12.1% of cases of syndromic craniostenosis and 0.3% of cases of isolated craniostenosis by Cinalli et al. in a study in 1998. In this large survey involving 1727 patients, the authors advanced in order to suggest which syndromes present a higher risk of developing hydrocephalus among affected patients. According to the report, patients with cloverleaf deformity have hydrocephalus as a typical feature, whereas patients with Crouzon syndrome have a higher

E. Jucá (✉) · C. C. P. Machado
University of Fortaleza, Fortaleza, Brazil

F. Di Rocco, J. Kestle (eds.), *Neurosurgical Aspects of Craniosynostosis*,
https://doi.org/10.1007/978-3-031-69386-1_36

risk of hydrocephalus than patients with other syndromes, and patients with Appert syndrome have overall increased ventricular dimensions, but without progressive character and with less need for surgical treatment [4].

All this background in the literature and the questions still to be answered regarding the best way to manage cases of association between craniostenosis and hydrocephalus demonstrate the need for additional studies that elucidate the contribution of each pathological entity in the clinical picture of affected children, so that the better treatment for controlling intracranial hypertension and preserving the cognitive development potential is achieved.

36.2 Pathophysiology

The pathophysiological mechanisms that lead a patient with craniostenosis to develop progressive hydrocephalus are unclear. Understanding these factors is very important for therapeutic planning. There are some clues to the marked predominance in cases of syndromic craniostenosis and also to the greater risk in certain syndromes over others. Although the literature on the subject is not very extensive, several hypotheses have already been raised to explain the development of hydrocephalus in patients with craniostenosis.

Certainly, a distortion of the anatomy manifested in different ways in a syndromic cases leads to obstruction of the cerebrospinal fluid flow. In this context, a tight posterior fossa that causes herniation of the cerebellar tonsils through the foramen magnum with obliteration of the fourth ventricle outflow ways, compression of the aqueduct of Sylvius, and venous return difficulties based mainly on the narrowing of the jugular foramina seem to play a key role [3].

Among these structural alterations, impaction or even herniation of the cerebellar tonsils in the foramen magnum seems to be of special importance, obliterating the outflow ways of the fourth ventricle through the foramina of Luschka and Magendie. In fact, Chiari type I alteration is present in most cases of syndromic craniostenoses (Fig. 36.1). An additional argument in favor of this pathophysiological mechanism in the development of hydrocephalus is the fact that the surgical treatment of space restriction in the posterior fossa, either in the classic way with suboccipital median craniectomy, or with posterior cranial enlargement through implantation of distractors, is capable, in many cases, of controlling the progression of ventricular dilation and avoiding the indication of ventricular shunting. On the other hand, Chiari type I malformation is present in 90% of children with hydrocephalus and syndromic craniostenosis, as highlighted by Frassanito et al. Synergistically, hydrocephalus and Chiari I could be part of a cyclical mechanism in which one entity could worsen the evolution of the other: the impaction of the tonsils impairing the flow of cerebrospinal fluid and hydrocephalus functioning as a downward force promoting the passage of tonsils through the foramen magnum [5].

Compression of the cerebral aqueduct can also be included in the general picture of conflict between continent and content in the posterior fossa, reproducing obstructive hydrocephalus

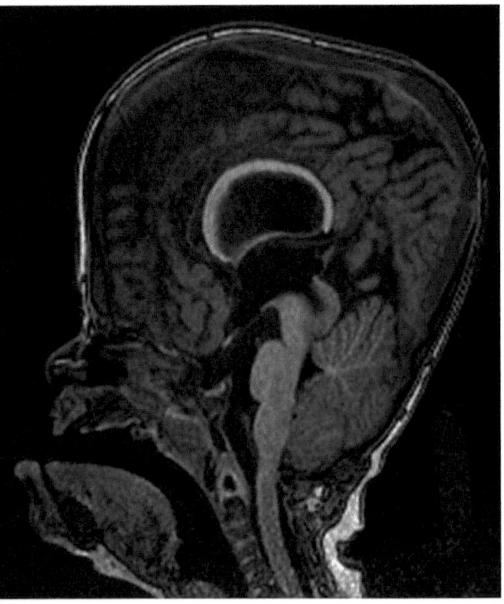

Fig. 36.1 Magnetic resonance imaging of a child with Crouzon syndrome showing herniation of the cerebellar tonsils through the foramen magnum (Chiari I) and supratentorial ventricular dilatation

with the possibility of treatment by endoscopic third ventriculostomy. Although it is currently difficult to define the exact topography of the obstruction to cerebrospinal fluid flow, the possibility of improving this topographic localization in the future may serve as a basis for improving the choice of therapeutic modality.

In addition to structural abnormalities and anatomical distortions with mechanical consequences, there is evidence of functional elements that contribute to the blockade of CSF absorption with consequent progressive ventricular dilation. Among these factors is the difficult passage of CSF through hypoplastic subarachnoid spaces in syndromic craniostenosis and also the difficulty in venous return due to the alteration of the venous sinuses anatomy and the characteristic narrowing of the jugular foramina in these patients. Thus, one of the causal factors for the appearance of hydrocephalus would be the impairment of the full return of CSF to the venous compartments due to the slowing of the venous return flow [3, 5].

In practice, all these possibilities may be combined in the genesis of hydrocephalus related to syndromic craniostenosis. In fact, a possible common origin for most of these pathophysiological processes would be the early fusion of the basiooccipital and lambdoid sutures, leading, at the same time, to the narrowing of the jugular foramina with overlying venous hypertension and to hypoplasia of the posterior fossa leading to mechanical constriction of the cerebrospinal fluid flow. An important argument in favor of this theory is the higher incidence of hydrocephalus in FGFR-2 gene-related craniostenosis, reaching 88% of cases in Pfeiffer syndrome. Furthermore, a difference in the osteogenic action of the FGFR-2 gene in the early fusion of intraoccipital synchondrosis in Crouzon and Appert syndromes could explain the higher incidence of hydrocephalus in patients with Crouzon syndrome [5].

Indeed, in Appert syndrome, it is common to find ventriculomegaly without evidence of progression or intracranial hypertension that requires surgical treatment with shunt. This situation can also occur with other forms of syndromic and even nonsyndromic craniostenosis, since a child with isolated suture fusion is also subject to factors such as prematurity or the coexistence of other causes of hydrocephalus such as aqueductal stenosis.

Another way in which a disturbance of CSF circulation can occur in patients with craniostenosis, in addition to hydrocephalus, is the identification of subdural collections, also known as pericerebral effusions. This topic was addressed by Usami and colleagues in a very focused study in 2021 with patients diagnosed with scaphocephaly. In this survey of 63 children, 57% had pericerebral effusions greater than expected for their age, 57% had ventriculomegaly according to the Evans index greater than 0.3 criterion, and 46% had both conditions. The main hypothesis raised for this increased risk of subdural collections in patients with scaphocephaly was venous hypertension caused by compression of the superior sagittal sinus by the synostotic sagittal suture. Supporting this possibility is the fact that most patients had regression of measurements of both the subdural space and the ventricular dimensions after surgical correction, which included sagittal suturectomy in the technique with release of the superior sagittal sinus from eventual compression. This postulation makes the surgical indication even stronger in isolated craniostenosis, in addition to the aesthetic, structural, and control of intracranial hypertension aspects [6]. Although the aforementioned study focused only on patients with scaphocephaly, this situation can potentially be reproduced with other types of nonsyndromic craniostenosis involving the superior sagittal sinus, such as brachycephaly or trigonocephaly, as shown in Fig. 36.2.

Finally, a specific situation of combined hydrocephalus and craniosynostosis that may require the attention of the pediatric neurosurgeon is craniosynostosis secondary to treatment of hydrocephalus with a ventricular shunt. In this case, the pathophysiological sequence is inverted and the drainage of the cerebrospinal fluid for the treatment of hydrocephalus is the cause of the fusion of one or more cranial sutures. The mechanism underlying this phenomenon would be a decrease in intracranial pressure leading to loss of stimulus for skull expansion, which is based

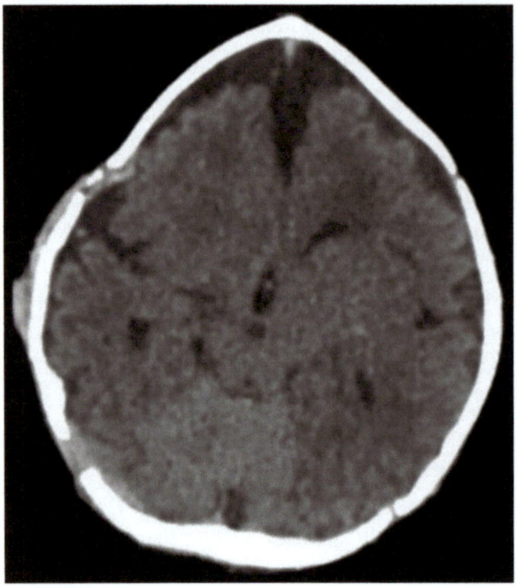

Fig. 36.2 Computed tomography scan of the skull of a 3-month-old child showing trigonocephaly and frontal pericerebral effusion

on osteogenic proliferation mainly on the cranial sutures [7, 8].

In a 2021 study, Bryant and colleagues studied with computed tomography (CT) and 3D reconstruction a population of 125 children treated for hydrocephalus with a ventriculoperitoneal shunt. Almost half of the patients presented fusion of one or more sutures in exams performed on average 26 months after shunt surgery. The influence of these image findings on cranial growth and the development of intracranial hypertension, however, was unclear [7].

In fact, it is necessary to identify early cases in which a secondary craniosynostosis may represent only an image finding and situations in which there is cranial deformity or worsening intracranial hypertension as consequences. Golinko et al. described a series of 13 patients with ventricular shunt-induced craniostenosis in which surgical skull remodeling was performed. The criteria adopted for the indication of cranial remodeling in this series were the existence of cranial deformity, clinical or radiological evidence of intracranial hypertension, evidence of suture fusion in image studies, and absence of shunt malfunction signs [8].

Knowledge about all these pathophysiological variables is very important for adequate guidance during patient assessment and for adequate therapeutic decision-making. The management options in the face of the association between hydrocephalus and craniosynostosis can range from ventricular shunt to endoscopic third ventriculostomy, including or not skull remodeling procedures. Understanding the mechanisms underlying the clinical picture and the structural changes should contribute to the best choice for the management of each individual case.

36.3 Assessment

The assessment, both clinically and by neuroimaging, of cases involving the association of hydrocephalus and craniostenosis imposes difficulties related to the manifestations of each entity and the specific contribution to the clinical presentation of each patient.

In the case of nonsyndromic craniosynostosis involving fusion of one or more sutures, incidental cases of hydrocephalus can be identified based on the usual clinical presentation of the disease in infants, which includes increased head circumference outside the expected curve for age, fontanelle bulging, and neurodevelopmental delay. CT or MRI shows increased ventricular dimensions with occasional indirect signs of intracranial hypertension, such as ependymal transudation and effacement of sulci and cisterns. Special attention must be paid to these clinical and radiological signs in cases of risk factors for hydrocephalus, such as prematurity.

In cases of syndromic craniostenosis, given the considerable percentage of patients who develop hydrocephalus, it is necessary to actively seek clinical and radiological manifestations, since one in eight patients will need surgical treatment for hydrocephalus. Thus, from the diagnosis of craniostenosis and the related syndrome, it is necessary to look for clinical manifestations of intracranial hypertension and for radiological signs of progressive ventricular dilatation. The initial assessment is performed by means of CT of the skull, and the same exam used to study the sutures and cranial conformation already allows the observation of ventricular dimensions and signs of hydrocephalus. However, the need for more detail and the search for causal factors in each specific case should lead to obtaining a brain MRI.

In addition to assessing the size of the ventricles and the use of objective criteria such as the Evans index, it is necessary to observe other factors on MRI, potentially related to the origin of hydrocephalus: descent of the tonsils through the foramen magnum, size of the fourth ventricle, tight appearance of the posterior fossa, compression of the aqueduct of Sylvius, distortion of the position of the floor of the third ventricle, and alteration in the anatomy of the venous sinuses [3].

In a complementary way, obtaining a CT angiography, especially when planning a surgical approach to craniostenosis with anterior or posterior remodeling and distractions, can help in the planning of osteotomies in order to respect and preserve venous drainage, preventing possible damage to the venous network that could cause an additional increase in intracranial pressure by impairing venous return.

Although all the mentioned clinical manifestations and radiological findings are important in the global assessment of children with craniostenosis at risk of developing hydrocephalus, it must be recognized that the main question to be answered is whether there is intracranial hypertension that leads to the indication of a specific treatment for hydrocephalus. Some initiatives have already taken place to directly assess intracranial pressure in patients with craniostenosis through the intracranial implantation of specific catheters for this purpose, both preoperatively and intraoperatively [9, 10]. Thompsom and colleagues found intracranial hypertension in 28 out of 53 cases of syndromic craniostenosis, but also in 20 out of 83 cases of nonsyndromic cases [9]. Although direct measurement is the most reliable method, this can be invasive and costly, even requiring the child to be hospitalized for a few days for an adequate study to be carried out.

To make the estimation of intracranial pressure more practical, without the need for hospitalization, less invasive methods have been developed. An assessment technique that has gained prominence is the measurement of pulse waves by a sensor fitted close to the skull (Fig. 36.3). This method quantitatively evaluates the relationship between the various components of pulse waves and suggests that there is a loss of intracranial compliance caused by hypertension

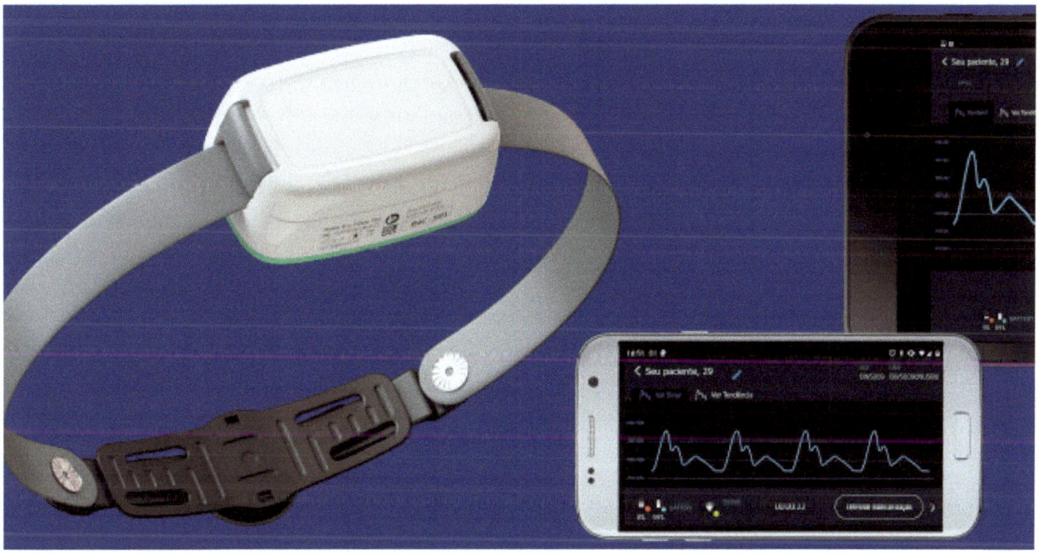

Fig. 36.3 Monitoring screen and sensor used to assess intracranial compliance by measuring pulse waves and the P1/P2 ratio

when there is an increase in the P2 component in relation to the P1 component, with a P2/P1 ratio predominantly above 0.8. The strategy has already proved to be useful in cases of hydrocephalus not associated with craniostenosis and could be applied with a view to decision-making in cases of association between the two diseases [11].

All assessment strategies described, including clinical, imaging, or functional phenomena, must be globally taken into account to support the choice of the best management in cases of hydrocephalus associated with craniostenosis. Since there is no repetition of a single pattern between cases, all information needs to be collected, so that the best decisions are reached.

36.4 Treatment

Clinical evaluation of active hydrocephalus in the craniostenosis context is difficult, the patient may present with nonspecific symptoms and the condition may be masked by the craniostenosis deformity. In addition, ventricular dilation is often only identified after decompression surgery [12]. Because of the complexity and multifactorial aspect of the etiology of hydrocephalus, there is still discussion about which would be the best treatment choice [5].

Craniosynostosis is treated with combinations of techniques that involve suturectomy, decompressive craniectomy, and bone remodeling. The procedure itself can stabilize and improve intracranial pressure and ventricular dilation by providing space for the brain to expand. Even so, patients with syndromic craniosynostosis, who have a higher incidence of progressive hydrocephalus, may develop ventricular dilatation after surgery, threatening the life of these patients and requiring immediate resolution [2].

The pathophysiology of hydrocephalus in syndromic craniostenosis is still under study; however, it is known that jugular stenosis and posterior fossa constriction are important factors. According to Frassanito et al., there are three scenarios for the occurrence of hydrocephalus such as (1) ventricular dilation begins to progressively worsen before surgery, and then, there is surgical intervention to reduce intracranial hypertension. (2) Hydrocephalus is only apparent after decompression surgery as a complication of CSF leakage. (3) Patients with stable ventricular dilatation and/or nonspecific signs of intracranial hypertension who improve with decompressive surgery [5].

The current recommendation is: if there is no accurate and confirmed diagnosis of active hydrocephalus, surgery to correct craniostenosis should be chosen as a first step, observing ventricular development and monitoring intracranial pressure afterwards. If hydrocephalus is evident prior to decompressive surgery, primary resolution of hydrocephalus should be chosen, as the patient's condition may worsen with increased intracranial pressure after craniostenosis surgery [13].

Figure 36.4 illustrates the management of a personal case of the author of this chapter, in which a 14-month-old boy, 29 weeks' gestation premature, presented with increased head circumference and ventricular dilatation, while he had a craniofacial deformity compatible with left anterior plagiocephaly. An option was made for initial correction of craniostenosis and cranial decompression was sufficient to contain the progression of hydrocephalus and to stabilize the growth of the head circumference in the curve (Fig. 36.4).

Over the past 70 years, the ventriculoperitoneal shunt has been the method of choice for the treatment of hydrocephalus due to its effectiveness, cost and clinical benefit. However, the technique has been questioned due to frequent complications. Device-related morbidity is higher in syndromic craniosynostosis, and the risks of hemorrhage, infection, and device dysfunction are some of the related factors. The ventriculoperitoneal shunt may also impair skull growth by excessively decreasing pressure from the inside to the outside and may excessively drain the CSF, causing hypotension and impairing bone remodeling (secondary synostosis), especially in patients with multiple suture craniosynostosis. In addition, an increase in epidural dead space may occur, which increases the risk of infections.

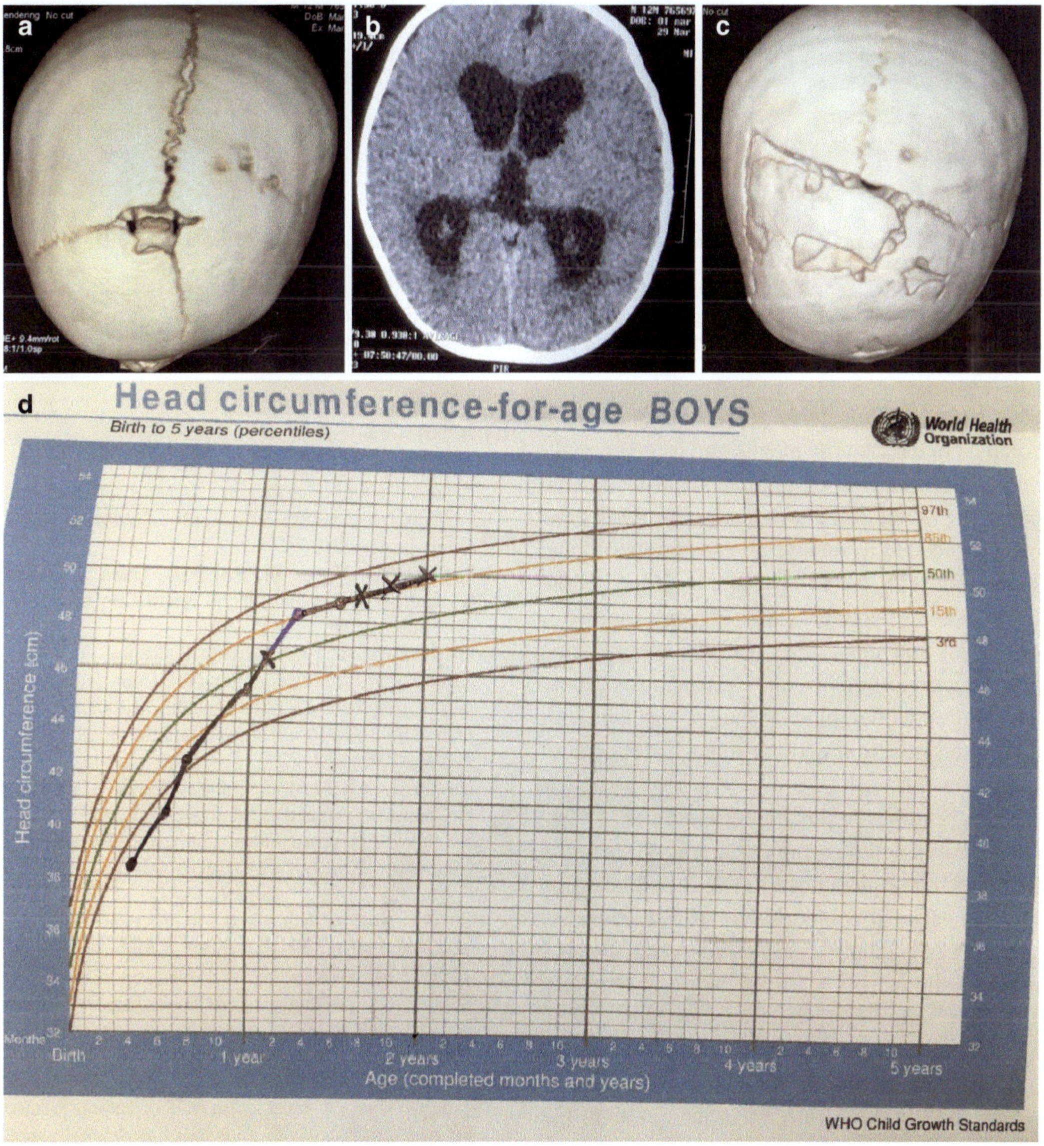

Fig. 36.4 Preoperative image of a child with anterior plagiocephaly showing significant cranial asymmetry (**a**) and ventricular dilatation (**b**). 3D tomography after surgical correction of craniostenosis (**c**). Reversal of disproportionate growth of head circumference after correction of craniostenosis

Bonfield, in a 2021 article, points out that 50% of patients with a shunt for hydrocephalus and craniostenosis need shunt revision, especially those with syndromic craniosynostosis, because of their more challenging anatomy, which can lead to infections, dysfunctions, and failures. The same study reports similarity of results between ventricular shunt and third ventriculostomy, making the use of the endoscopic method advantageous [14].

ETV can minimize risks by maintaining intracranial CSF flow and preventing hypotension, in addition to being effective in cases of obstructive hydrocephalus due to anatomical variations or Chiari malformations.

In a 2010 study, DiRocco et al. described a series of 11 cases of syndromic craniosynostosis with hydrocephalus treated with ETV (Fig. 36.5). All cases presented features such as aqueduct

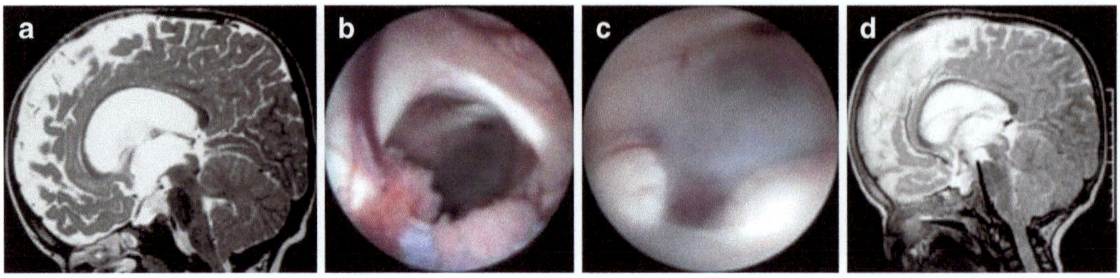

Fig. 36.5 Preoperative image (**a**), view of intraoperative anatomy (**b**, **c**) and postoperative image with flow sign through the floor of the third ventricle (**d**) of a patient with Crouzon Syndrome and hydrocephalus treated with endoscopic third ventriculostomy. (From di Rocco et al., 2010, with permission from the authors)

obstruction, tight posterior fossa, and mechanical conflicts in the cisterna magna and foramen magnum. The presence of jugular stenosis in nine patients was not a contraindication for ETV. Four patients needed to receive a ventriculoperitoneal shunt after ETV failure. In eight patients, endoscopy was effective with disappearance of symptoms and signs of intracranial hypertension and reduction of ventricular dimensions. Among the children with implanted shunts, one had shunt associated infection and the other had mechanical dysfunction [3].

Thus, endoscopic treatment would be preferable in cases with favorable anatomy. Even when there is a subsequent need for shunt implantation in some cases, it is possible to spare a considerable part of patients from the definitive installation of a shunt.

When ventricular shunt cannot be avoided, systems including adjustable valves and antisiphoning devices should be preferred in order to reduce the risk of excess CSF drainage. If, during cranial reconstruction surgery, there is a complication with the development of active hydrocephalus, an external shunt can be put in place for primary containment of the problem and subsequent assessment of the need for a shunt.

Finally, for both nonsyndromic and syndromic craniosynostosis, the decision-making regarding the primary treatment or not of hydrocephalus must be carefully planned, individualizing each case with their particularities and issues such as age, general condition of the patient, severity of craniosynostosis, and neurological impairment.

References

1. Golabi M, Edwards M, Ousterhout D. Craniosynostosis and hydrocephalus. Neurosurgery. 1987;21:63–7.
2. Noetzel MJ, Marsh JL, Palkes H, Gado M, Louis S. Hydrocephalus and mental retardation in craniosynostosis. 1985.
3. Di Rocco F, Jucá CE, Arnaud E, Renier D, Sainte-Rose C. The role of endoscopic third ventriculostomy in the treatment of hydrocephalus associated with faciocraniosynostosis: clinical article. J Neurosurg Pediatr. 2010;6:17–22.
4. Cinalli G, Saint-Rose C, Kollar E, Zerah M, Brunelle F, Chumas P, Arnaud E, Marchac D, Pierre-Kahn A, Renier D. Hydrocephalus and craniosynostosis. J Neurosurg. 1998;88:209–2014.
5. Frassanito P, Palombi D, Tamburrini G. Craniosynostosis and hydrocephalus: relevance and treatment modalities. Childs Nerv Syst. 2021;37:3465–73.
6. Usami K, Nicolini F, Arnaud E, Di Rocco F. Cerebrospinal fluid collections in sagittal suture synostosis. Childs Nerv Syst. 2016;32:519–25.
7. Bryant JR, Mantilla-Rivas E, Keating RF, et al. Craniosynostosis develops in half of infants treated for hydrocephalus with a ventriculoperitoneal shunt. Plast Reconstr Surg. 2021;147:1390. https://doi.org/10.1097/PRS.0000000000007988.
8. Golinko MS, Atwood DN, Ocal E. Surgical management of craniosynostosis in the setting of a ventricular shunt: a case series and treatment algorithm. Childs Nerv Syst. 2018;34:517–25.
9. Thompson DNP, Harkness W, Jones B, Gonsalez S, Andar U, Hayward R. Subdural intracranial pressure monitoring in craniosynostosis: its role in surgical management. Childs Nerv Syst. 1995;11:269. https://doi.org/10.1007/BF00301758.
10. Judy BF, Swanson JW, Yang W, Storm PB, Bartlett SP, Taylor JA, Heuer GG, Lang SS. Intraoperative intracranial pressure monitoring in the pediatric craniosynostosis population. J Neurosurg Pediatr. 2018;22:475. https://doi.org/10.3171/2018.5.PEDS1876.

11. Ballestero MFM, Frigieri G, Cabella BCT, de Oliveira SM, de Oliveira RS. Prediction of intracranial hypertension through noninvasive intracranial pressure waveform analysis in pediatric hydrocephalus. Childs Nerv Syst. 2017;33:1517–24.
12. Collmann H, Sörensen N, Krauß J. Hydrocephalus in craniosynostosis: a review. Childs Nerv Syst. 2005;21:902–12.
13. Tcherbbis Testa V, Jaimovich S, Argañaraz R, Mantese B. Management of ventriculomegaly in pediatric patients with syndromic craniosynostosis: a single center experience. Acta Neurochir. 2021;163:3083–91.
14. Bonfield CM, Shannon CN, Reeder RW, et al. Hydrocephalus treatment in patients with craniosynostosis: an analysis from the hydrocephalus clinical research network prospective registry. Neurosurg Focus. 2021;50:E11. https://doi.org/10.3171/2021.1.FOCUS20979.

Postoperative Management and Long-Term Follow-Up After Surgery for Craniosynostosis

37

Elena Kurudza and John R. W. Kestle

37.1 Introduction

The postoperative management of children after craniosynostosis surgeries depends predominantly on the surgical technique used. This chapter will discuss general early and late postoperative management, as well as specific variations in management associated with each surgical technique.

37.2 Early Postoperative Management

Regardless of the surgical technique, the immediate postoperative management should be geared towards early identification of potential immediate postoperative complications. Typically, this should include monitoring of neurologic status, hemodynamics, feeding, and pain control. Although the following complications are rare, a high clinical suspicion should always be maintained for hematoma, seizure, and cerebrospinal fluid (CSF) leak in the immediate postoperative setting [1]. A patient's length of stay, level of care, need for blood transfusion, and drain management, among other factors, depend on surgical technique and will be discussed further below.

E. Kurudza . J. R. W. Kestle (✉)
Department of Neurosurgery, University of Utah, Salt Lake City, UT, USA
e-mail: neuropub@hsc.utah.edu

37.3 Technique-Specific Postoperative Management

37.3.1 Endoscopic-Assisted Craniectomy

37.3.1.1 Length of Stay and Level of Care

Children treated with endoscopic-assisted craniectomy usually do not have syndromes or significant systemic illness. Their postoperative care is therefore less complicated, and most do not require admission to an intensive care unit (ICU). Length of stay is typically shorter in endoscopic-assisted craniectomies when compared with cranial vault remodeling. Centers have reported a mean length of stay of 1–2 days and the majority of patients were managed on the surgical ward postoperatively [2–4]. For example, in a retrospective study of 225 patients by Dalle Ore et al. [5], the median length of stay for endoscopic-assisted craniectomy was 1 day, with 216 (96%) patients admitted directly to the surgical ward postoperatively. Of the 8 patients that were admitted to the ICU postoperatively, 7 had preexisting medical conditions that the team had identified preoperatively as necessitating a planned ICU admission.

F. Di Rocco, J. Kestle (eds.), *Neurosurgical Aspects of Craniosynostosis*,
https://doi.org/10.1007/978-3-031-69386-1_37

37.3.1.2 Special Postoperative Considerations

The main considerations in the postoperative setting for endoscopic-assisted craniectomy include monitoring for blood loss, pain control, and adequate oral intake. As noted above, most patients are able to meet discharge criteria within 1–2 days postoperatively. Typically, subgaleal drain placement is not necessary; however, postoperative day 1 hemoglobin and hematocrit levels are routinely checked. Although transfusion threshold varies, multiple studies have reported significantly lower rates of transfusion after endoscopic-assisted craniectomy, ranging from 6.4 to 26% [2, 4, 6], when compared with cranial vault remodeling.

Pain management varies depending on which suture has been treated. Children who undergo endoscopic-assisted craniectomy on the sagittal suture usually experience more discomfort than those whose treatment addresses the metopic or coronal sutures, and they often require oral or intravenous (IV) narcotics overnight. Most of them feel much better the next day and are comfortable on over-the-counter oral pain medications such as acetaminophen. Patients are usually able to tolerate oral intake within a few hours of surgery. Overall, discharge readiness is determined by postoperative hemoglobin and hematocrit levels, pain control on oral medications, and ability to tolerate oral intake. Imaging is not routinely obtained for these patients, but specific instances will be discussed further below.

37.3.2 Cranial Vault Remodeling

37.3.2.1 Length of Stay and Level of Care

Compared with endoscopic approaches, open cranial vault approaches are associated with a longer hospital stay, with reported averages of approximately 4 days [2, 4]. Although practice varies by institution, in a multicenter study, 24 out of 29 institutions routinely admitted patients undergoing open cranial vault procedures to the ICU, with a median length of ICU stay of 2 days [4]. Despite these findings, there is recent literature that demonstrates that routine ICU admission may not be necessary in the majority of cases [7].

37.3.2.2 Special Postoperative Considerations

As with endoscopic approaches, the postoperative management for open cranial vault surgeries involves monitoring neurologic status, need for postoperative transfusion, and pain control; however, in addition to the aforementioned discharge readiness requirements, special considerations for open cranial vault surgeries include drain management, postoperative antibiotics, postoperative imaging, and hemodynamic monitoring.

Open cranial vault surgeries are associated with a higher rate of blood transfusion when compared with endoscopic approaches, with reported rates of intraoperative transfusion in 81% of cases and postoperative transfusion in 25.1% of cases, according to one multicenter study [4]. In addition, 16% of patients received coagulation blood products (defined as platelets, fresh frozen plasma, or cryoprecipitate) [4]. Other studies report an even higher frequency of postoperative blood transfusion [2].

When it comes to pain control, multimodal analgesia remains the mainstay; however, in contrast to endoscopic approaches where patients' pain is routinely controlled on oral medications, open cranial vault surgeries are associated with more frequent use of IV analgesics, including IV acetaminophen and IV opioids [8, 9]. In a recent review, Brown et al. [8] proposed an increasing role for dexmedetomidine to minimize IV opioid use.

Unique postoperative considerations for open cranial vault surgeries include drain management, antibiotic use, hemodynamic monitoring, and postoperative imaging. Again, while practice varies per institution, it is common practice at our institution to leave a subgaleal drain in place postoperatively. In a survey of 19 American craniofacial teams, 63% reported using a drain [9]. The timing of removal as well as indications for removal are not well established in the literature, but in our practice, drains are commonly in place for 2 to 3 nights unless drainage is minimal before that. In the same survey, 75% of teams reported routine use of arterial lines for postoperative hemodynamic monitoring in the ICU setting and 75% reported using prophylactic antibiotics postoperatively [9]. Finally, there is additional variation between institutions regarding postoperative imaging. Shah et al. [2] reported that nearly all patients that underwent open cranial vaults in their prospective study had a computed tomography (CT) scan before discharge, but Binning et al. [10] reported no significant association with postoperative events, including seizures, prolonged ICU stay, or reoperation in patients without shunts who underwent CT, although there was an increased rate of identifying shunt malfunction in patients with shunts. Thus, at our institution, we only obtain CTs as clinically indicated.

Discharge readiness is determined by stable hemoglobin and hematocrit levels, ability to tolerate oral intake, and pain controlled on oral medications. Discharge typically requires at least twice the number of hospital days on average to meet this in comparison with endoscopic surgeries. At our institution, patients usually spend 3 to 4 nights in the hospital before discharge.

37.3.3 Distraction Osteogenesis

37.3.3.1 Length of Stay and Level of Care

Overall, standard distraction osteogenesis is considered a less invasive option compared with cranial vault reconstruction and is thought to be associated with shorter operating times and less blood loss when compared with cranial vault remodeling, although this difference was not statistically significant in a systematic review including 181 cases [11]. Additionally, the use of distraction osteogenesis rather than cranial vault remodeling does not translate to a significant difference in postoperative management, as the two procedures have similar transfusion rates, postoperative ICU length of stay, and overall hospital length of stay [11–13]. Additionally, like patients who undergo cranial vault remodeling, most patients who undergo distraction osteogenesis require IV medication for pain management.

37.3.3.2 Special Postoperative Considerations

Unique considerations in the postoperative setting for distraction osteogenesis include the importance of caregiver education in regard to operating the distractor. Distractors are also associated with higher rates of dural tears intraoperatively [12, 14]. As such, special attention should be paid to early detection of CSF leak in the postoperative setting. Distractors are also associated with higher rates of infection, wound dehiscence, and device failure, so there should be routine monitoring in place for these complications [14]. At follow-up, it is also common practice for the patient to undergo routine three-dimensional CT imaging as often as every 1–3 weeks to monitor progress after activation [15]. Finally, it is important to consider that unlike endoscopic strip craniectomies and cranial vault reconstructions, distractor osteogenesis requires the patient to return for a second surgery for removal.

37.3.4 Spring-Assisted Cranioplasty

37.3.4.1 Length of Stay and Level of Care

Breakey et al. [16] performed a retrospective review of 200 cases at their institution and found that the median length of hospital stay for spring-assisted cranioplasty was three nights; however, there remains variability among institutions regarding the level of postoperative care for patients undergoing spring-assisted cranioplasty. As with open vault surgeries, most patients are admitted to the ICU postoperatively, but in a single-center retrospective study, the average length of stay in the ICU was 30.9 h, which is shorter than that of patients who have been treated with open cranial vault procedures [17]. In addition, Malmqvist et al. [18] performed a small observational study during which they used a simplified protocol for postoperative pain management. They found that there was no significant difference in the number of patients with FLACC (Face, Legs, Activity, Cry, Consolability) pain scores >4 with intermittent injections of morphine and clonidine rather than a morphine infusion [18]. This made it possible for their patients to avoid an ICU admission, which many centers are starting to avoid.

37.3.4.2 Special Postoperative Considerations

Monitoring hemoglobin and hematocrit levels is crucial because transfusion is common in the postoperative setting in spring-assisted craniectomy [17]. In their study, Breakley et al. [16] found that the most common complications were related to infection, so special attention should be paid to wound healing at follow-up. Finally, as with distractors, this technique requires that the patient return for a second operation for removal, usually between 4 and 6 months later.

37.3.5 Imaging

There are undefined postoperative imaging protocols for craniosynostosis surgery, and practice varies widely by institution. In a retrospective study of 1150 patients who underwent cranial vault reconstructions across the United States, 28.4% of patients underwent routine postoperative CTs. Of those that underwent a CT, only 7.1% were found to have an associated intracranial hemorrhage [19]. At our institution, we do not routinely obtain immediate postoperative imaging.

During long-term follow-up, the majority of patients who underwent cranial vault reconstructions underwent a CT within 1 year of surgery and 95% had undergone a head CT for follow-up within 6 years [19].

37.4 Long-Term Follow-Up

Special consideration for follow-up must occur in the cases of helmet therapy associated with endoscopic-assisted craniectomy as well as spring-assisted craniectomy. In the case of endoscopic-assisted craniectomies, most patients are fitted for a helmet within 4–5 days postoperatively and begin wearing the helmet about 2 weeks postoperatively. They are then followed by the orthotist every 2–3 weeks over the first 3–6 months to monitor growth and to have helmet adjustments. The surgical team also sees them when they first get the helmet (about 2 weeks postoperatively), then 3, 6, 9, and 12 months after surgery, and then yearly to 5 years of age. It has been demonstrated that peak cephalic index is reached at 7–9 months. Prolonged helmet therapy beyond this did not demonstrate any clear benefit [20, 21], but longer follow-up is recommended to monitor head growth, development, and the rare occurrence of symptoms of raised intracranial pressure.

Distractors typically are used beginning 3–5 days postoperatively and are turned one to two times daily for 2–3 weeks. Caregivers are instructed on how to operate the device before discharge, and patients are seen in the clinic with skull X-rays each week. Patients typically return for a second surgery at 3 months for removal of the distractors.

For patients who undergo open cranial vault procedures, the time to first follow-up varies based on institution. At our institution, we typically schedule an initial postoperative follow-up appointment for 4–6 weeks after discharge.

At follow-up visits for all procedures, special attention is paid to head shape, cranial index, signs of high intracranial pressure, and signs of infection/wound breakdown and bony defects. The mean length for follow-up is reported to be just over 2 years [21]; however, Ridgway et al. [21] proposed follow-up should last until at least 6 years of age to allow for completion of intracranial growth.

In our practice, regardless of the surgical technique, we continue annual clinical follow-up for a minimum of 5 years. Patients are evaluated for symptoms, particularly problematic headache, cranial shape, and or defects. We also monitor patients' developmental progress. We do not routinely obtain imaging of patients unless they present with problematic headache, flattening of the head circumference percentile, or a new deformity that would suggest delayed fusion of previously untreated sutures. In those patients, we would have an ophthalmology evaluation of their fundi, a new three-dimensional CT scan, and, in those with a developmental concern, a formal developmental assessment. Nonsyndromic children who have no issues after 5 years of follow-up are then seen on an as-needed basis, but syndromic children and those with issues described above are monitored and treated as appropriate. In rare situations where the symptoms are out of proportion to the other findings, we have used intracranial pressure monitoring to assess these children.

One report describes very long follow-up of isolated sagittal synostosis patients [22]. At a mean of 26.5 years' postoperative follow-up, these patients were as happy with their facial appearance as were age- and gender-matched controls. Socioeconomic situation and general health were also similar to those of controls.

As with so many other aspects of pediatric neurosurgery, craniosynostosis has lifelong implications, and adequate follow-up and availability of pediatric neurosurgical care are essential.

References

1. Jubbal KT, Agrawal N, Hollier LH Jr. Analysis of morbidity, readmission, and reoperation after craniosynostosis repair in children. J Craniofac Surg. 2017;28(2):401–5.
2. Shah MN, Kane AA, Petersen JD, Woo AS, Naidoo SD, Smyth MD. Endoscopically assisted versus open repair of sagittal craniosynostosis: the St. Louis Children's Hospital experience: clinical article. J Neurosurg Pediatr. 2011;8(2):165–70.
3. Riordan CP, Zurakowski D, Meier PM, Alexopoulos G, Meara JG, Proctor MR, et al. Minimally invasive endoscopic surgery for infantile craniosynostosis: a longitudinal cohort study. J Pediatr. 2020;216:142–9.e2.
4. Thompson DR, Zurakowski D, Haberkern CM, Stricker PA, Meier PM, Bannister C, et al. Endoscopic versus open repair for craniosynostosis in infants using propensity score matching to compare outcomes: a multicenter study from the Pediatric Craniofacial Collaborative Group. Anesth Analg. 2018;126(3):968–75.
5. Dalle Ore CL, Dilip M, Brandel MG, McIntyre JK, Hoshide R, Calayag M, et al. Endoscopic surgery for nonsyndromic craniosynostosis: a 16-year single-center experience. J Neurosurg Pediatr. 2018;22(4):335–43.
6. Cartwright CC, Jimenez DF, Barone CM, Baker L. Endoscopic strip craniectomy: a minimally invasive treatment for early correction of craniosynostosis. J Neurosci Nurs. 2003;35(3):130–8.
7. Chocron Y, Azzi A, Galli R, Alnaif N, Atkinson J, Dudley R, et al. Routine postoperative admission to the intensive care unit following repair of nonsyndromic craniosynostosis: is it necessary? J Craniofac Surg. 2019;30(6):1631–4.
8. Brown S, Yao A, Sanati-Mehrizy P, Zackai SP, Taub PJ. Postoperative pain management following craniosynostosis repair: current practices and future directions. J Craniofac Surg. 2019;30(3):721–9.
9. Srivatsa S, Heiman AJ, Gray MC, Carpenter C, Patel A. Variations in postoperative management of pediatric open-vault craniosynostosis. J Craniofac Surg. 2021;32(1):305–9.
10. Binning M, Ragel B, Brockmeyer DL, Walker ML, Kestle JR. Evaluation of the necessity of postoperative imaging after craniosynostosis surgery. J Neurosurg. 2007;107(1 Suppl):43–5.
11. Mundinger GS, Rehim SA, Johnson O 3rd, Zhou J, Tong A, Wallner C, et al. Distraction osteogenesis for surgical treatment of craniosynostosis: a systematic review. Plast Reconstr Surg. 2016;138(3):657–69.
12. Kamel GN, Wong A, Segal RM, Carbulido MK, Hornacek M, Ewing E, et al. A single-center retrospective review of perioperative complications and reoperation rates between open cranial vault remodeling and distraction osteogenesis for unilateral coronal craniosynostosis. J Craniofac Surg. 2021;32(7):2373–8.
13. Taylor JA, Derderian CA, Bartlett SP, Fiadjoe JE, Sussman EM, Stricker PA. Perioperative morbidity in posterior cranial vault expansion: distraction osteogenesis versus conventional osteotomy. Plast Reconstr Surg. 2012;129(4):674e–80e.
14. Greives MR, Ware BW, Tian AG, Taylor JA, Pollack IF, Losee JE. Complications in posterior cranial vault distraction. Ann Plast Surg. 2016;76(2):211–5.
15. Park DH, Yoon SH. Transsutural distraction osteogenesis for 285 children with craniosynostosis: a single-institution experience. J Neurosurg Pediatr. 2016;17(2):230–9.
16. Breakey RWF, van de Lande LS, Sidpra J, Knoops PM, Borghi A, O'Hara J, et al. Spring-assisted posterior vault expansion-a single-centre experience of 200 cases. Childs Nerv Syst. 2021;37(10):3189–97.

17. Jones VM, Thomas SG, Siska R, Massary D, David LR, Dillingham CS, et al. Spring-assisted surgery for treatment of sagittal craniosynostosis. J Craniofac Surg. 2021;32(1):164–7.
18. Malmqvist C, Paganini A, Johansson L, Maltese G, Tarnow P, Olsson R, et al. Simplified postoperative care after spring-assisted strip craniotomy for sagittal synostosis: a prospective before-and-after study. J Craniofac Surg. 2021;32(4):1507–10.
19. Makar KG, Gunaseelan V, Waljee J, Vercler CJ, Buchman SR. Variation in the utilization of postoperative computed tomography for patients with nonsyndromic craniosynostosis: a national claims analysis. Cleft Palate Craniofac J. 2020;57(3):288–95.
20. Iyer RR, Ye X, Jin Q, Lu Y, Liyanage L, Ahn ES. Optimal duration of postoperative helmet therapy following endoscopic strip craniectomy for sagittal craniosynostosis. J Neurosurg Pediatr. 2018;22(6):610–5.
21. Ridgway EB, Berry-Candelario J, Grondin RT, Rogers GF, Proctor MR. The management of sagittal synostosis using endoscopic suturectomy and postoperative helmet therapy. J Neurosurg Pediatr. 2011;7(6):620–6.
22. Salokorpi N, Savolainen T, Sinikumpu J-J, Ylikontiola L, Sándor GK, Pirttiniemi P, et al. Outcomes of 40 nonsyndromic sagittal craniosynostosis patients as adults: a case-control study with 26 years of postoperative follow-up. Oper Neurosurg. 2019;16(1):1–8.

Part VI

Surgical Atlas: How I Do It (Sagittal, Metopic, Coronal, Lambdoid)

38 Sagittal Suture Synostosis: Endoscopic Approach, Key Points for the Neurosurgeons

Nikita Alexiades and John R. W. Kestle

38.1 Introduction

Since its introduction by Jimenez and Barone in 1998, the endoscopic minimally invasive approach to sagittal suture synostosis has gained wide acceptance [1]. It has proven to be a safe and effective technique that minimizes operative time, blood loss, transfusion rates, cost, and the length of hospital stays while resulting in excellent and durable surgical results compared with open cranial vault remodeling when done in patients under 6 months of age [2–7]. This approach, called the strip craniectomy, entails a craniectomy encompassing the entire length of the fused sagittal suture with or without wedge osteotomies, followed by the postoperative use of a custom-made cranial molding helmet. This approach can be broken down into two subtypes, a wide (4- to 6-cm) strip craniectomy with parietal wedge osteotomies as described by Jimenez and Barone or a narrow (2-cm) strip craniectomy without additional osteotomies. The wide approach pioneered by Jimenez and Barone has a more robust body of the literature supporting it, but a number of studies have demonstrated similar outcomes with the narrow strip approach [8–10].

In a recent retrospective multicenter study of outcomes, open cranial vault remodeling and strip craniectomies showed satisfactory postoperative cephalic indices, but wide strips were associated with a greater improvement in the cephalic index (CI) than narrow strips [10]. It is our practice to perform the wide strip approach with small biparietal wedge osteotomies. Our operative approach is detailed below and can be modified easily to a narrow strip approach by planning a smaller craniectomy and forgoing wedge osteotomies.

38.2 Preoperative Planning

It is our practice to perform low-dose computed tomography (CT) scans with three-dimensional reconstruction on all patients as part of our preoperative evaluation. Special attention should be paid both to bony defects within the planned dissection area and the bony anatomy of the suture overlying the sinus, particularly at its posterior extent. A preoperative hematocrit value should be obtained to guide decision-making regarding the

N. Alexiades
Department of Neurosurgery, University of Utah, Salt Lake City, UT, USA

Department of Neurosurgery, University of Arizona College of Medicine – Phoenix, Phoenix, AZ, USA

J. R. W. Kestle (✉)
Department of Neurosurgery, University of Utah, Salt Lake City, UT, USA
e-mail: neuropub@hsc.utah.edu

F. Di Rocco, J. Kestle (eds.), *Neurosurgical Aspects of Craniosynostosis*,
https://doi.org/10.1007/978-3-031-69386-1_38

need for intraoperative or postoperative transfusions. A blood type and cross match should also be performed, and blood should be readily available even though it is often not needed with this approach.

38.3 Anesthetic Considerations and Positioning

Proper positioning coupled with excellent communication between the surgical team and anesthesiologist are vital to surgical success. Adequate intravenous access should be obtained prior to positioning as it is essential in the event of significant blood loss and the need for fluid resuscitation. We employ the sphinx position to provide sufficient access to the entirety of the sagittal suture. To facilitate airway management in this position, nasotracheal intubation is performed and the tube is secured using a silk purse string suture through the nasal septum. It is essential to confirm that all bony prominences, including the chin, are well padded to prevent pressure necrosis and ensure that the neck remains supple in extension. We use gel bolsters under the chest along with a beanbag wrapping under and around the neck and shoulders. The patient is then taped securely in place using silk surgical tape.

38.4 Operative Procedure

After the patient is appropriately positioned, the skull is palpated to identify the anterior fontanelle, sagittal suture, and lambda. Two 4- to 5-cm transverse incisions are marked, one anteriorly several centimeters behind the anterior fontanelle and one posteriorly several centimeters in front of the lambda, each centered on the midline. Each incision is infiltrated with an appropriate amount of local anesthetic for the patient's weight, and sterile prepping and draping is completed. An incision is made with a 15 blade through the dermis and into the subcutaneous fat. A monopolar cautery is used to further dissect through the galea and then to widely dissect subgaleally in the loose areolar tissue. It is important to leave the periosteum in place to minimize unnecessary blood loss from diploic venous channels. Once the subgaleal dissection is adequate and the incisions are in communication, the craniectomy is planned. We prefer a rectangular craniectomy 5 cm in width spanning the anterior fontanelle to the lambdoid sutures. The monopolar cautery is used to mark planned burr hole sites 2.5 cm lateral to the midline bilaterally in line with both the anterior and posterior incisions. We then mark oblique, medially oriented cuts on either side from the anterior burr holes to the anterior fontanelle. Posteriorly, our cuts are marked bilaterally from the burr holes to the lambdoid sutures. Figure 38.1 demonstrates the planned craniectomy and osteotomies.

The craniectomy is begun by making the anterior burr holes using a 7-mm perforator bit, bony edges are waxed, and a Penfield 3 dissector is used to strip the dura first anteriorly towards the fontanelle and then gently across the midline. The craniotome is then used to make the anteriorly directed cuts and then to cross the midline and connect the two burr holes. At this point, the bone fragment will still adhere via fibrous tissue to the anterior fontanelle. The bone is hinged forward under gentle traction and then cut at its attachment using Mayo scissors. Hemostasis from bone edges is achieved using the monopolar cautery with cotton patties to protect the dura along with bone wax as needed. The bipolar cautery is used to gently coagulate any dural vessels and the fibrous tissue at the anterior fontanelle. Next, in a similar fashion, burr holes are made at the posterior incision and stripped with a Penfield 3 dissector, and the craniotome is used to make the posteriorly directed cuts towards the lambdoid sutures and then a cut connecting the burr holes. Care must be taken in stripping the dura in the midline here because it can be densely adherent or overgrown with bone (Figs. 38.2 and 38.3). If needed, we will perform small bilateral craniectomies here to allow for direct visualization of the midline dural dissection. Once all posterior cuts are made, the bone is reflected and hinged at the lambdoid sutures and cut with Mayo scissors. Dural bleeders are then coagulated with bipolar cautery, and bony hemostasis

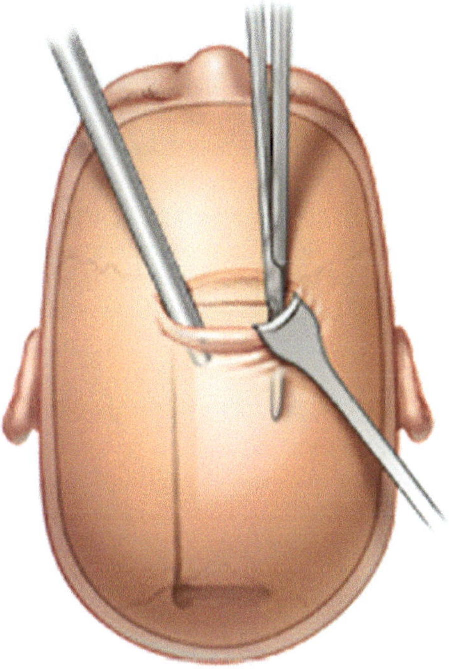

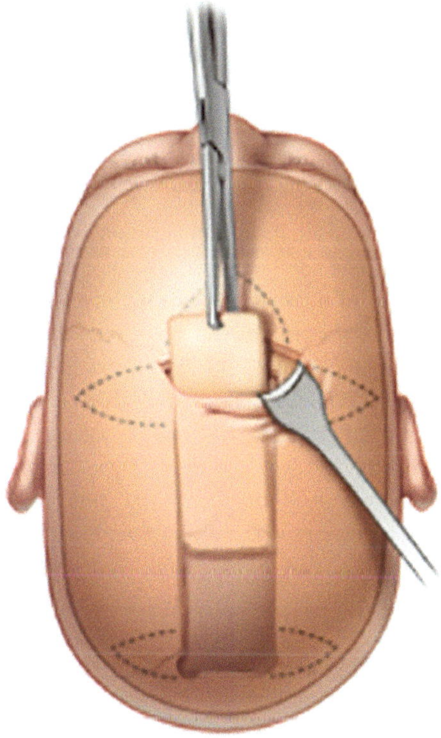

Fig. 38.1 Illustration of the planned craniectomy and wedge osteotomies along with the locations of planning incisions

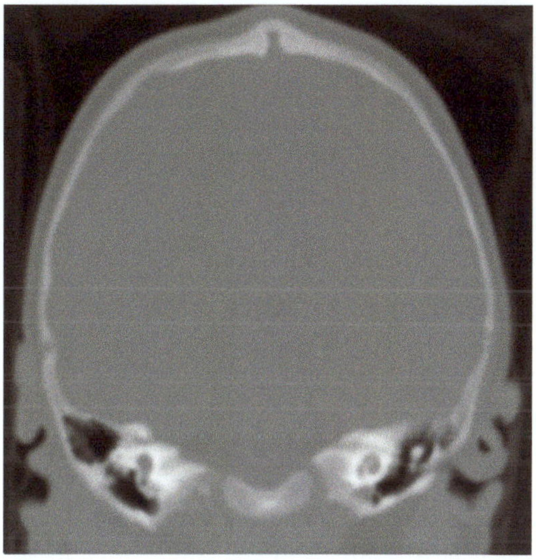

Fig. 38.2 Coronal bone windowed CT scan demonstrating bony overgrowth with investment of the posterior sagittal sinus within it

is achieved with monopolar cautery and bone wax as needed.

Once the anterior and posterior bone windows have been created, we next perform an endoscopic dissection along the remaining bone flap. The surgeon is seated for this portion of the procedure. A 2-mm rigid 30° endoscope is advanced lateral to the midline from the anterior incision to the posterior bony opening. A suction device is used in the surgeon's other hand and advanced just in front of the endoscope to maintain visualization and provide gentle downward pressure to strip the dura. With the room lights lowered, the progress of the endoscope can be tracked via transillumination through the skull and skin. Once the posterior bony opening is reached, the endoscope is retracted and gently swept laterally to provide additional dissection for wedge osteotomies. The same maneuver is then repeated on the contralateral side, and the endoscope is angled medially to visualize the full dissected epidural space overlying the sagittal sinus. Curved Mayo scissors are then used to fashion the lateral bony cuts. Our preferred maneuver is to place the nondominant hand at the corner of the posterior opening and gently advance the Mayo scissors with the concavity directed medially towards the posterior opening. The cut is

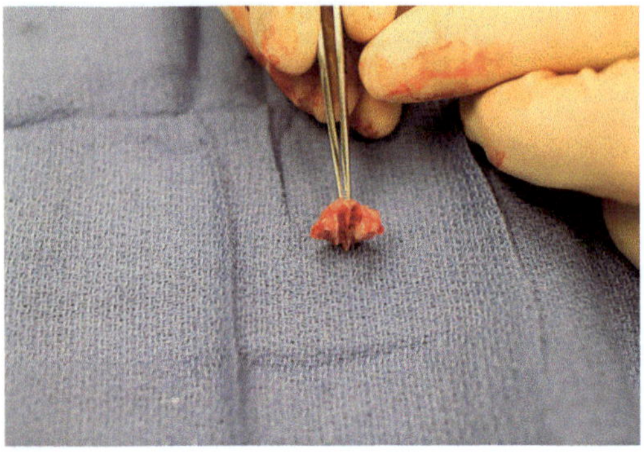

Fig. 38.3 Operative photo of bone that was overlying the posterior sagittal sinus showing evidence of ingrowth

repeated on the contralateral side, and the bone fragment is gently removed; care is taken to not allow the posterior margin to drive into the exposed dura in the process. A lighted retractor is then used to retract the scalp, and any bleeding dural vessels are coagulated with the bipolar cautery. Bone edge hemostasis is achieved by using the monopolar cautery with cotton patty protection and bone wax as needed.

Our plastic surgery colleagues then perform two sets of parietal wedge osteotomies just behind the coronal suture and just in front of the lambdoid suture. Once these are completed and bony hemostasis is assured, a large piece of dry compressed Gelfoam is cut to size and placed in the epidural space. The incisions are then closed by using inverted, interrupted 4-0 monocryl sutures in the galea and a running, nonlocking 5-0 Rapide suture in the skin. The incisions are cleaned, and dry sterile dressings are placed. The patient is then carefully removed from the sphinx position, and care is returned to anesthesia for extubation.

38.5 Complications

Complication avoidance begins with good positioning and anesthesia preparation. Adequate intravenous access is critical in the event of significant blood loss, as is the ready availability of cross-matched blood. Communication with the anesthesia team is critical as soon as any significant bleeding is encountered. Injury to the sagittal sinus is a real risk, and the low circulating blood volume in these patients can rapidly lead to hemorrhagic shock. The modified sphinx position and extensive bone work puts these patients at risk for venous air emboli. If encountered, the field must be immediately flooded with saline, and the head of bed lowered. If needed, the patient must be rapidly turned supine and flat. We limit the use of irrigation during our bony opening to readily identify any dural tears. If cerebrospinal leakage is identified, any tears should be promptly closed to prevent the development of large pseudomeningoceles, given the extensive dead space under the scalp.

38.6 Postoperative

Patients are monitored in the hospital overnight. We check a repeat hematocrit level the morning after surgery. Patients are discharged once they are feeding normally and pain is controlled with only oral pain medications.

Key Points

- The modified sphinx position requires meticulous attention to detail. We employ nasal intubation secured via suture, given the lack of easy access to the oropharynx once positioned. Particular attention should be paid to the degree of neck extension and appropriate padding of the chin in addition to the more commonly addressed bony prominences.
- We obtain preoperative a low-dose CT scan on all patients. In some instances, varying degrees of bony overgrowth around the posterior sagittal sinus may be observed. In such cases, piecemeal removal of the bone to obtain adequate visualization for sinus dissection is key. We will occasionally leave an island of bone on the sinus if needed, with our craniectomy extending to the lambdoid suture on either side of the midline.
- Awareness of the starting hematocrit level and careful attention to hemostasis will decrease the need for intraoperative and postoperative transfusions.

- During initial dissection, leaving the periosteum in place aside from planned bony cuts will limit unnecessary blood loss from diploic veins.
- Care should be taken to not cross the midline initially when performing epidural dissection using the endoscope. Transillumination of the scope through the skin can guide the dissection.
- In some older children with thicker bone, Mayo scissors may be insufficient to make the lateral bony cuts. We have occasionally used sternotomy scissors to accomplish this.
- The large bone fragment must be removed gently without levering it into the underlying dura and brain. If necessary, it should be removed in pieces.
- A handheld lighted retractor can be particularly helpful once the bone is removed to evaluate the craniectomy and obtain hemostasis.
- There are often midline veins emerging from the sinus at its posterior extent that require gentle bipolar cautery to obtain hemostasis.

References

1. Jimenez DF, Barone CM. Endoscopic craniectomy for early surgical correction of sagittal craniosynostosis. J Neurosurg. 1998;88(1):77–81.
2. Jimenez D, Barone C, Cartwright C, Baker L. Early management of craniosynostosis using endoscopic-assisted strip craniectomies and cranial orthotic molding therapy. Pediatrics. 2002;110:97–104.
3. Jimenez D, Barone C. Endoscopic technique for sagittal synostosis. Childs Nerv Syst. 2012;28:1333–9.
4. Jimenez D, Barone C. Endoscopy-assisted wide-vertex craniectomy, "barrel-stave" osteotomies, and postoperative helmet molding therapy in the early management of sagittal suture craniosynostosis. Neurosurg Focus. 2000;9(3):e2.
5. Vogel T, Woo A, Kane A, Patel K, Naidoo S, Smyth M. A comparison of costs associated with endoscope-assisted craniectomy versus open cranial vault repair for infants with sagittal synostosis. J Neurosurg Pediatr. 2014;13:324–31.
6. Ridgway E, Berry-Candelario J, Grondin R, Rogers G, Proctor M. The management of sagittal synostosis using endoscopic suturectomy and postoperative helmet therapy. J Neurosurg Pediatr. 2011;7:620–6.
7. Shah M, Kane A, Petersen J, Woo A, Naidoo S, Smyth M. Endoscopically assisted versus open repair of sagittal craniosynostosis: the St. Louis Children's Hospital experience. J Neurosurg Pediatr. 2011;8:165–70.
8. Wood BC, Ahn ES, Wang JY, Oh AK, Keating RF, Rogers GF, et al. Less is more: does the addition of barrel staves improve results in endoscopic strip craniectomy for sagittal craniosynostosis? J Neurosurg Pediatr. 2017;20(1):86–90.
9. Dlouhy BJ, Nguyen DC, Patel KB, Hoben GM, Skolnick GB, Naidoo SD, et al. Endoscope-assisted management of sagittal synostosis: wide vertex suturectomy and barrel stave osteotomies versus narrow vertex suturectomy. J Neurosurg Pediatr. 2016;18(6):674–8.
10. Baker CM, Ravindra VM, Gociman B, Siddiqi FA, Goldstein JA, Smyth MD, et al. Management of sagittal synostosis in the Synostosis Research Group: baseline data and early outcomes. Neurosurg Focus. 2021;50(4):E3.

39 Sagittal Suture Synostosis: Open Vault Surgery in Young Children, Key Points for Neurosurgeons

Kelsi M. Chesney, Gregory Keating, Nirali Patel, Hasan R. Syed, and Robert F. Keating

39.1 Introduction

39.1.1 Background

Sagittal craniosynostosis is an anatomical condition resulting from premature fusion of the sagittal suture that causes abnormal calvarial formation and potential limitation of underlying brain growth. Of all the cranial sutures, sagittal synostosis is the most commonly affected by early fusion, comprising more than half of patients with nonsyndromic synostosis and 2:1 ratio for males:females [1]. Over the past few decades, several different surgical approaches have been employed to treat this condition. The two principal treatments are strip craniectomy and cranial vault reconstruction with each procedure having multiple technical variations. Endoscopic strip craniectomy is most effective in children under 4–6 months of age while open cranial vault reconstruction has historically been the standard of care and an alternative approach employed when the patients are older or there are multiple sutures involved. Open vault surgery is characterized by an open craniotomy with strategic osteotomies to expand the cranial vault, reduce intracranial pressure (ICP), and improve calvarial symmetry as well as cosmesis. In this chapter, we will review the preoperative planning objectives, surgical techniques, postoperative care, and complications associated with open vault surgery in the pediatric population.

K. M. Chesney · G. Keating · N. Patel
Department of Neurosurgery, Children's National Hospital, Washington, DC, USA

Department of Neurosurgery, MedStar Georgetown University Hospital, Washington, DC, USA
e-mail: gfk9@georgetown.edu; Nirali.P.Patel@gunet.georgetown.edu

H. R. Syed · R. F. Keating (✉)
Department of Neurosurgery, Children's National Hospital, Washington, DC, USA

Department of Neurosurgery, George Washington University, Washington, DC, USA
e-mail: hsyed@childrensnational.org; Rkeating@childrensnational.org

39.2 Clinical Presentation

Infants (age < 12 months) presenting with craniosynostosis are most often referred for abnormal head shape. Sagittal synostosis may be identified by a scaphocephalic head shape such that the biparietal diameter is narrowed compared to an elongated occipitofrontal diameter. This ratio is defined as the *cephalic index*. Normal cephalic indices fall between 75 and 80. Values less than 75 are predictive of sagittal synostosis. Additional characteristics may include ridging of the sagittal suture as well as prominent bulging of the frontal and occipital regions (Fig. 39.1).

Of note, breech positioning in utero may mimic a scaphocephalic head shape with overlap-

F. Di Rocco, J. Kestle (eds.), *Neurosurgical Aspects of Craniosynostosis*, https://doi.org/10.1007/978-3-031-69386-1_39

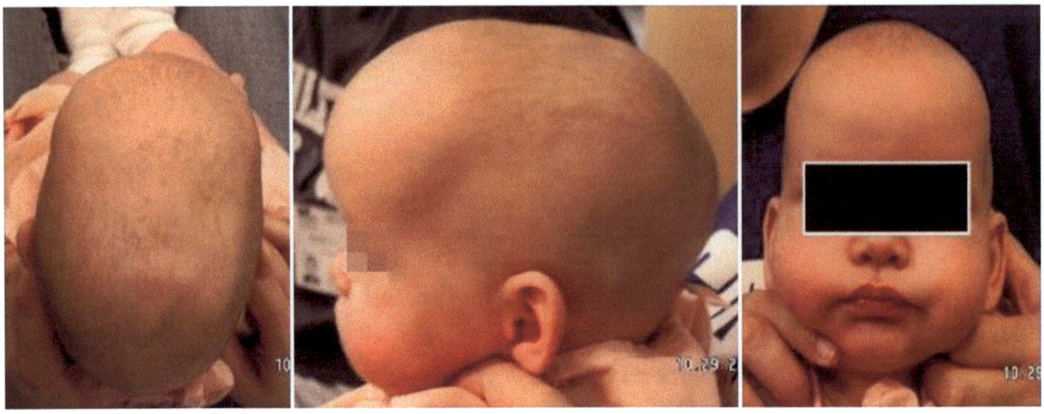

Fig. 39.1 An infant with sagittal synostosis characterized by a scaphocephalic head shape with frontal and occipital bossing

ping parietal bones being mistaken for a ridge. This condition will typically resolve within a few days of birth compared to sagittal synostosis that will persist and/or worsen with time. Another mimic of scaphocephaly includes persistence of the mendosal suture that produces a bathrocephalic head shape in addition to an occipital protuberance. This condition has no effect on brain growth and should not undergo surgical treatment [2]. One also has to consider secondary scaphocephaly related to prematurity or lack of overall brain growth. In this setting, the scaphocephaly is not related to premature fusion of the sagittal suture but rather to biparietal brain growth.

Older children tend to present with more subtle calvarial abnormalities and may manifest mild neurocognitive difficulties. While IQ scores tend to fall within a normal range, up to 50% of patients with single-suture sagittal synostosis may have learning disabilities secondary to impairments in executive functioning [3]. Functional imaging studies have confirmed altered neural connectivity in patients with sagittal synostosis [4]. The etiology behind these deficits has not yet been elucidated, though restricted brain growth due to an abnormal skull shape has been proposed to play a role. For the same reason, older patients may also present with symptoms of elevated ICP, such as headache, nausea/vomiting, and vision changes. Unlike coronal and metopic synostosis, ophthalmic dysfunction is less common in sagittal synostosis; however, routine preoperative ophthalmologic evaluation may be helpful in identifying elevated ICP [5].

39.3 Pathophysiology

Regarding factors that contribute to the act of bony fusion, there are both intrinsic and extrinsic conditions that may occur in utero, with primary craniosynostosis, or postnatal, with secondary synostosis. It is critical that the treating physician appreciate these factors and determine whether the craniosynostosis is primary versus secondary. Environmental exposures such as parental age as well as a mother's smoking status, medications, and vitamin consumption carry variable risks across all types of craniosynostosis [6]. Regarding sagittal synostosis, thyroid dysfunction during pregnancy and the action of thyroid hormone on osteogenesis in utero has been observed with a positive association. Postnatal, metabolic bone disorders such as, rickets, hypophosphatasia, pseudohypoparathyroidism, osteopetrosis, and mucopolysaccharidosis, may also play a role in sagittal synostosis [6].

Genetic factors have been more clearly identified in syndromic craniosynostosis, which in turn have a higher likelihood of increased ICP as well as greater chance of needing additional surgery in the long run. Alpert's, Pfeiffer's, and Crouzon's have all been strongly linked to fibroblast growth factor genes. With respect to single-suture craniosynostosis, Clark et al. identified causative genetic factors in just 15% of 391 patients presenting with single suture synostosis [7]. In an even smaller percentage of patients (3.8%), sagittal synostosis suggests familial inheritance [8]. The increased incidence of sagittal suture synostosis in males supports a genetic component. Despite these observations, there are no enough data to warrant genetic testing in this population unless there is concern for an underlying syndrome.

39.4 Diagnosis and Treatment

(a) **Diagnostic imaging**
(b) **Surgical management**

Physical exam, as described previously, has been shown to accurately diagnose sagittal craniosynostosis alone [9]. However, it is a typical practice to obtain radiographic confirmation in patients with strong suggestive features. Computed tomography (CT) will show a fused sagittal suture in addition to other anatomical features that are helpful for preoperative planning. In 3–5% of patients, an additional fused suture may be identified on imaging that ultimately affects management [10–12]. Once confirmed, the family should be counseled on their treatment options.

Prior studies focused on the natural history of sagittal synostosis indicate that the skull deformity is likely to worsen without intervention [13]. Although still controversial, there are some data to support that patients with neurocognitive deficits may demonstrate improvement with surgical intervention [14]. If the patient is less than 4–6 months of age, an endoscopic strip craniectomy may be offered. If the patient is older than 4–6 months or there are barriers to complying with helmet therapy, other surgical options, including open cranial vault surgery, may be offered (discussed below).

39.5 Preoperative Planning

Surgical treatment aims to provide an optimal long-term aesthetic and neurocognitive outcome. As sagittal synostosis often presents with a wide variety of deformities (frontal vs occipital bossing, scaphocephaly), the surgical approach will be tailored to correct the most salient deformity. The specific technique will also differ based on anatomical features such as bone quality, volumetric analysis, and venous anatomy, particularly in the occipital region.

Three-dimensional, computer-aided planning with CT may assist with surgical planning. The placement of osteotomies and repositioning of bone flaps can be strategically planned for the safest desired outcome as well as to decrease operative time and morbidity. Experimental growth models have also been studied to predict skull morphology based on planned surgical technique [15–17]. A majority of patients require remodeling of the anterior 2/3 of the cranium. Some patients also require posterior cranial remodeling of the occiput. Recontouring of the occipital region increases the element of morbidity especially in the vicinity of the transverse sinus and often addressing the anterior 2/3 of the calvarium improves the aesthetic appearance adequately to obviate the need for a posterior operation. If needed (rarely) this can be addressed by a later operation. Calvarial growth over time often self-corrects this issue. Other variations of cranial vault reconstruction that are used less often but have efficacious value are the pi and reverse pi procedures.

Patient age and comorbidities should also be considered prior to surgical intervention. The ideal timing of surgery has been debated. Studies focused on neuropsychological outcomes advocate for surgical correction prior to 6 months of age [18]. While surgery performed at a younger age minimizes growth restriction of the developing brain, there is a higher likelihood of postoperative bony growth requiring reoperation. Open cranial vault surgery is also associated with longer operative times and higher estimated blood loss than endoscopic approaches. The effects of anesthetic and blood loss may be significant in a young patient population. Preoperative volume status should be optimized. Administration of erythropoietin (EPO) 7–10 days before surgery or tranexamic acid (TXA) or aminocaproic acid (Amicar) at the start of surgery should be considered to decrease intraoperative blood loss with significant literature supporting its efficacy [19, 20]. The patient should also be type and crossed and blood products made available for administration intraoperatively with donor-designated blood as an option.

39.6 Operative Technique

(a) **General principles**
(b) **Π and modified Π procedures**
(c) **Foreshortening and lateral expansion of the cranium activated by gravity (FLAG)**
(d) **Open cranial vault remodeling**

An observational study by Baker et al. demonstrated that operative techniques for the treatment of single suture sagittal synostosis vary widely and additional studies are necessary to determine best outcomes [10]. The goal of this section is to describe the most commonly adopted principles, including the modified Π procedure, foreshortening and lateral expansion of the cranium activated by gravity (FLAG), and current approaches to open cranial vault remodeling techniques.

In most cases, the patient is typically positioned in a supine or prone position to achieve exposure of the calvarium that extends from the forehead to the lambdoid suture. A bicoronal incision is planned to mitigate and obscure resultant scarring and hair loss [21]. Subgaleal dissection is carried out both anteriorly and posteriorly with preservation of the periosteum (this helps to minimize bleeding). Exposure typically extends anteriorly to the orbital rims and posteriorly to the occiput, depending upon the preop planning. Careful attention should be paid to preserving the superior temporal artery during exposure and preservation of the supraorbital vessels and nerves if possible.

The extent of bony removal is dependent on the degree of deformity. Great care should be taken separating the bone from its underlying dura so as not to inadvertently injure underlying brain or vascular sinus, if exposed. Any opportunity to stay clear of the sinus should be undertaken. Hemostasis is periodically achieved from bleeding points on the dura using bipolar electrocautery or bone edges using bone wax. The craniotomy and reconstruction are then performed based upon the surgical technique employed. During closure, deep galeal and epidermal sutures are placed in a standard fashion. If skin closure is under significant tension due to significant cranial expansion, galeal scoring may assist with approximation as well as additional subaleal dissection. A surgical site drain is used at the discretion of the surgeon and absorbable sutures are used at the surface.

The Pi (Π) procedure was first proposed by Jane et al. [22, 23] as a total cranial value reconstruction for the treatment of sagittal synostosis and typically performed between 6 and 9 months of age. The technique was named because of the shape of the bone removal to address the primary stenosis as well as the resultant deformity of the cranial vault (Fig. 39.2). In this technique, the patient is placed in a prone position and the bone is removed with a craniotome roughly outlining the Greek letter pi (Π). The parietal bone removal is made anterior to the lambdoid and posterior to the coronal sutures and down as far as possible towards the squamosal sutures in the temporal region. Minimizing any interruption of the coronal or lambdoid sutures may help in avoiding delayed craniosynostosis of these sutures in the future. The bone can be removed in one piece or as two pieces, as in the letter "L," to avoid dissection of the anterior sagittal suture. The anterior-posterior (AP) diameter is then shortened using two Neurolon sutures from the frontal bone and remaining overlying piece of bone over the sagittal sinus. Leaving the stenosis sagittal suture in place does not jeopardize normalization of the calvarial growth. Care is taken not to tighten this gap too much (~1 cm), to avoid any potential compression of the underlying sagittal sinus. When the remaining sagittal strip is brought forward (~1 cm), the lateral pieces of parietal bone often move in more lateral direction and often

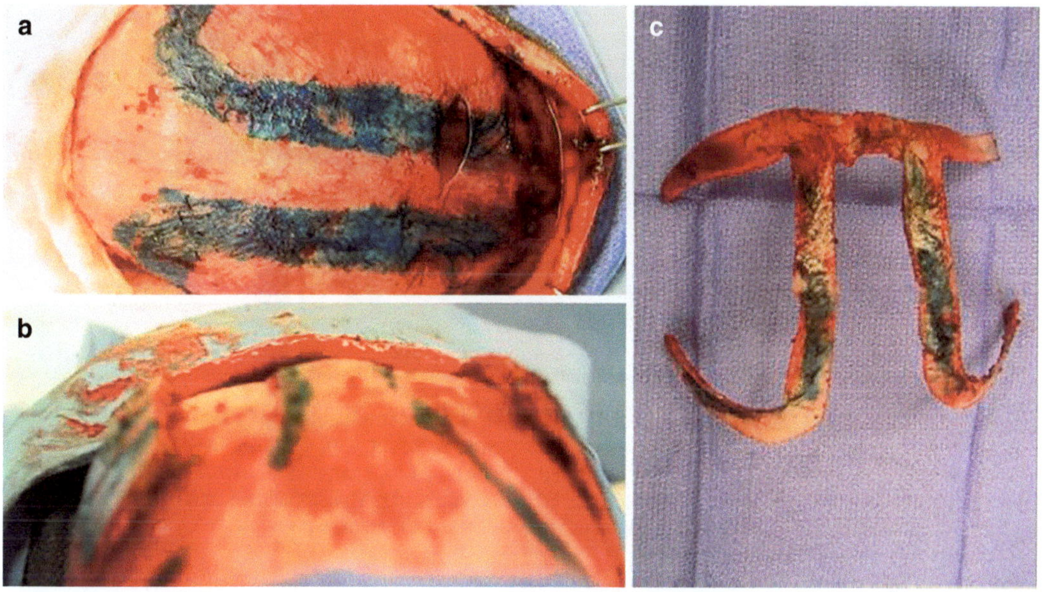

Fig. 39.2 Intraoperative photographs of a Π procedure. (**a**) An axial view of the planned bony removal with anterior and posterior boundaries. (**b**) A close-up view of the remaining sagittal suture that is left in place following the previously outlined cuts and biparietal widening. (**c**) An image of the bone flap removed with a distinct shape for which the procedure is named

requires the parasagittal osteomy to made wider than the frontal and occipital cuts, to facilitate skin closure due to the newly expanded parietal bones. The parietal bone removal is made anterior to the lambdoid and posterior to the coronal sutures and down as far as possible towards the squamosal sutures in the temporal region.

The Pi procedure has undergone many variations and modifications over time. The modified Π procedure was described by Jane et al. to address the variations in phenotypical patterns seen in sagittal synostosis and typically performed in children older than 3 months of age [22]. In this technique, sagittal, bilateral coronal, and lambdoid sutures are first removed, and the parietal bones are out-fractured to increase the biparietal diameter. The sagittal suture is then cut and used as strut grafts to maintain the outward position. Depending on the phenotypic variation, frontal bossing is corrected by performing a bifrontal craniotomy and radial barrel staves for contouring. Similar craniotomy and radial barrel staves are performed in the occipital bone for occipital bossing with careful attention to dissecting where the dural sinuses are located. The additional osteotomies add to the complexity and morbidity of the surgery and the long-term outcomes remain lacking.

The FLAG procedure was first described by Amm et al. as a technique for sagittal synostosis correction that *avoids* the use of hardware in infants between 6 and 12 months of age [24]. In this procedure, the patient is positioned prone in order to expose the occipital bullet. A bicoronal incision is performed, and subperiosteal dissection exposes the fused sagittal suture and the occipital prominence. A 3-cm parietal craniectomy is performed encompassing the sagittal suture (Fig. 39.3). Closing wedge osteotomies are resected posteriorly over the lambdoid sutures. Lateral barrel stave osteotomies are then performed behind the coronal sutures, out-fracturing the parietal bones to allow for a widened biparietal diameter. A trough is then drilled to thin the lower aspect of the occipital bone and allow it to hinge anteriorly with digital pressure. The parents are instructed to keep the infants strictly supine for 3 weeks during recumbence to allow flattening of the occipital prominence.

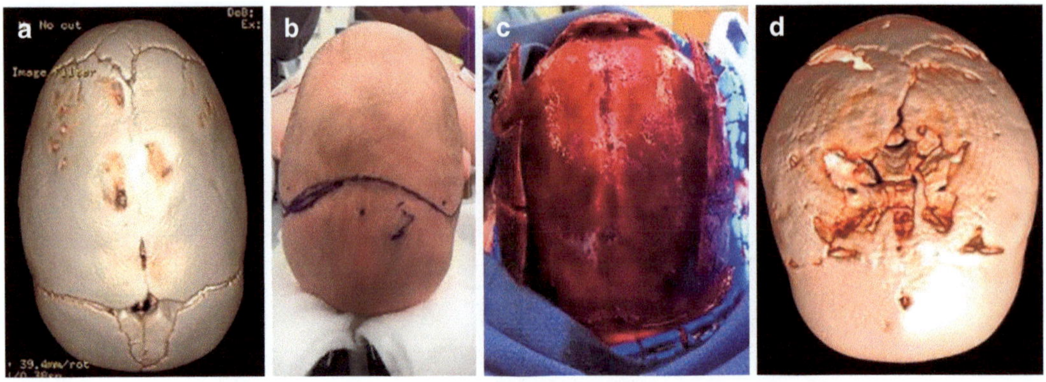

Fig. 39.3 Example of the FLAG procedure in a 5-month old child. (**a**) Preoperative axial CT diagnosing sagittal synostosis with a fused sagittal suture and an elongated frontooccipital length. (**b**) Preoperative photograph of patient in prone position with planned cranial incision. (**c**) An intraoperative photograph showing biparietal craniectomy including with posterior wedge osteotomies and bilateral parietal barrel stave osteotomies. No hardware is necessary. (**d**) A postoperative axial CT demonstrating improved CI without restenosis

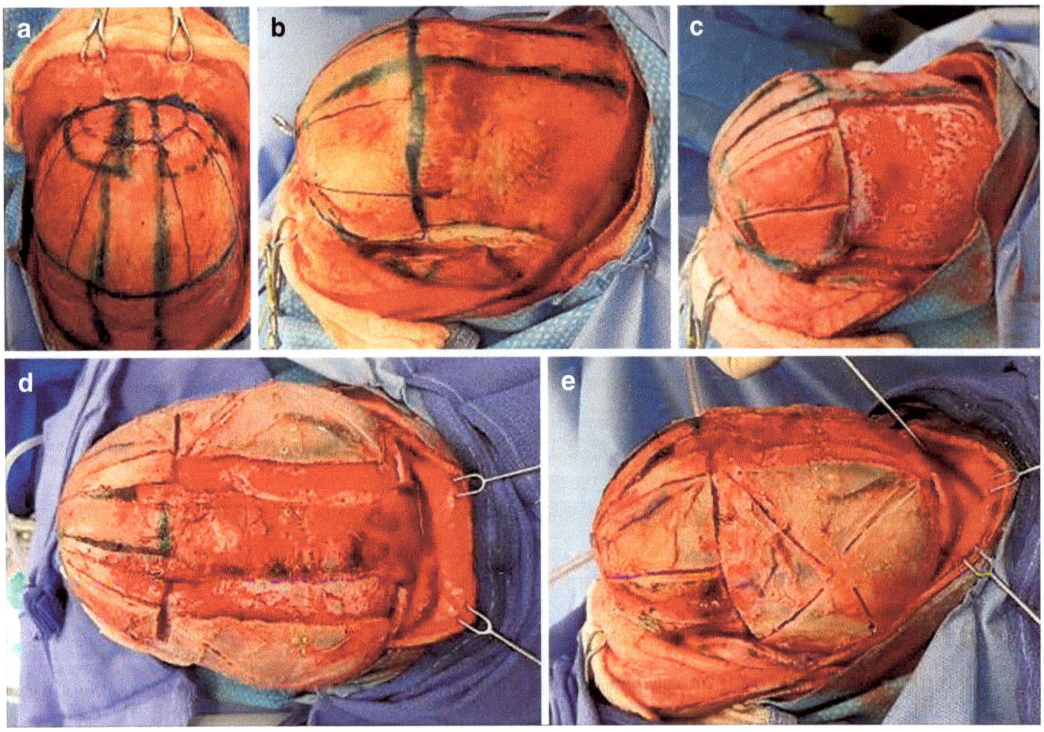

Fig. 39.4 An example of open cranial vault remodeling surgery. (**a**, **b**) Axial and sagittal views of the planned cuts to include parietal craniectomies and radial barrel stave osteotomies (**c**) Image following parietal craniectomies and posterior barrel stave osteotomies. Note that the sagittal suture is left in place. (**d**) Photo showing replacement of the parietal bone flaps in a position that increases biparietal diameter. The flaps are anchored to the sagittal suture and native occipital bone with absorbable plates and screws. (**e**) Native bone and particulate bone graft are used to fill the gaps created by widening the skull

At Children's National Hospital, variations of the open cranial vault remodeling surgery are employed; more specifically, cranial vault remodeling for sagittal synostosis diagnosed beyond 4–6 months of age (Fig. 39.4).

In these cases, calvarial remodeling is initiated with burr holes just lateral to the fused sagittal suture. Parietal bone flaps are removed, and lateral osteotomies are performed above the squamosal sutures to increase the biparietal diameter. A sagittal bar is maintained over midline as an anchoring point for reconstruction, while minimizing the risk to the sagittal sinus. Radial barrel staves are performed in both anterior and posterior directions to promote greater frontal and occipital width. Finally, the parietal bone flaps are affixed to the native skull as well as the intact midline bone over the sagittal sinus and positioned in a configuration to increase the biparietal diameter. The cranial bones are secured using absorbable hardware. Endocortical particulate bone graft is harvested using the Hudson brace from the parietal bone flaps, and any bony gaps or larger deficits are subsequently filled with this bone material affixed by fibrin glue over the area of defects.

39.7 Postoperative Care

Those patients who have had Pi or FLAG procedures are generally monitored in a skilled postop nursing unit and are usually ready for discharge to home the next day after their drains are removed and their hemacrit/hemaglobin is stable. Antibiotics and routine analgesia is given in the postoperative period.

Patients having undergone open vault reconstruction for sagittal craniosynostosis should receive routine postoperative monitoring in a pediatric intensive care unit with neurological monitoring for 24 h. While it has been demonstrated that intensive therapy is generally not needed in a healthy, nonsyndromic patient [25], it is still important to perform frequent neurologic exams to assess for potential intracranial complications. In the event of a neurologic change, imaging should be obtained. Given the risk of significant blood loss, hemoglobin and hematocrit should be trended in the postoperative period and blood products transfused as needed. Drains are removed when the hematocrit is stable and output from the drains is less than 30 cc over 8 h. Antibiotics are given for 24 h (until the subcutaneous drains are removed) and routine analgesia is provided. Patients are discharged home when they have established neurological and hemodynamic stability, have adequate pain control and demonstrate stability of any anticipated postop edema. The mean length of hospital stay in patients undergoing cranial vault reconstruction is 3 days [10].

39.8 Complications/Outcomes

Overall, cranial vault surgery for sagittal synostosis has a low complication rate [20, 26]. However, when complications occur, they can have devastating consequences and attention to technique should be paid to avoid these outcomes. Blood loss may occur from multiple cuts through cancellous bone. Hemodynamic monitoring along with adequate intravascular volume replacement and meticulous hemostasis should be employed to avoid significant blood loss, especially in younger children. Although uncommon, blood transfusion reactions may also occur. In addition, osteotomies in the bone increase risk for venous air embolism and this should always be considered, especially if there is a sudden change in blood pressure or in end-tidal CO2. Patients should have an optimized circulating volume prior to surgery and systolic blood pressure should be well-controlled during osteotomies. A precordial doppler may be placed and carbon dioxide monitoring should be employed throughout the operation in order to detect an intraoperative venous air embolism but the practice of placing a central line is seldom done due to the rarity of such an event. Venous sinus injury is a rare but potentially severe complication and always should be kept in mind. Major venous structures should be identified on preoperative imaging and the steps of bony removal incorporated to avoid injury. Wound infection rate ranges from 2.5 to 12.1% [27] and increases with patient age and lower weight [28]. Pneumonia is an additional postoperative complication found to occur more often in patients >12 months [26].

Patients are followed over the long term (till 10 years) for morphological and developmental progress and monitored for delayed complications. The symmetry of the calvarium and cranial index are trended clinically as well as the head circumference percentile. While the utility of cranial index as a measure of surgical success has been debated, it is still widely used to assess deformity correction. Any time the head circumference percentile decreases or the cephalic index deteriorates, it is reasonable to check for any potential increased ICP by utilizing a head CT (to evaluate the calvarial bone) as well as an ophthalmological exam of the fundus to rule out papilledema. Cranial vault reconstruction tends to result in more dramatic CI changes from baseline compared to strip craniectomy with an average associated improvement of 0.11 [10]. Long-term complications include restenosis and delayed intracranial hypertension. When an open approach is indicated for sagittal synostosis, the rate of reoperation ranges 5.2–16.7% [29–31]. Alternatively, some patients require reoperation for cranioplasty to address persistent cranial defects [32], although we have found this issue to be uncommon in our practice. There is ongoing research investigating long-term neurocognitive outcomes with some data that favors cranial vault reconstruction to alternative methods for improvement in cognitive function [33, 34].

39.9 Conclusion

(a) **Summary of key points, important considerations**
(b) **Future directions for research and treatment**

Open cranial vault reconstruction for the treatment of nonsyndromic single suture sagittal craniosynostosis is an important tool with various techniques to suit a patient's particular deformity. For older patients and those with significant deformity, it may be the most effective treatment available. Given the extensive nature of this operation, it is important to consider the operative time and expected blood loss in a younger patient population. Complication rates are low but special attention should be paid to preoperative anatomy to avoid any devastating vascular sinus injury. Long-term follow-up (10 years) should be undertaken to monitor for recurrent cranial deformities and possible intracranial hypertension. Research that explores genetic contributions and neurocognitive outcomes may aid in surgical selection and timing. The utilization of advanced imaging techniques and predicted growth models will also contribute to optimized surgical outcomes.

Pearls and Pitfalls

- It is important to differentiate between primary and secondary scaphocephaly. A CT scan will demonstrate fusion of the sagittal suture in the setting of normal appearing brain. Whereas secondary scaphocephaly will show an underlying element of lack of cerebral development.
- Recontouring of the occipital region increases the element of morbidity especially in the vicinity of the transverse sinus and often addressing the anterior 2/3 of the calvarium improves the aesthetic appearance adequately to obviate the need for a posterior operation. If needed (rarely), this can be addressed by a later operation. Calvarial growth over time often self-corrects this issue.
- For the Pi procedure, the parietal bone removal includes up anterior to the lambdoid and posterior to the coronal sutures and down as far as possible towards the squamosal sutures in the temporal region. Minimizing any interruption of the coronal or lambdoid sutures may help in avoiding delayed craniosynostosis of these sutures in the future.

References

1. Schraw JM, Woodhouse JP, Langlois PH, et al. Risk factors and time trends for isolated craniosynostosis. Birth Defects Res. 2021;113(1):43–54. https://doi.org/10.1002/bdr2.1824.
2. Gallagher ER, Evans KN, Hing AV, Cunningham ML. Bathrocephaly: a head shape associated with a persistent mendosal suture. Cleft Palate Craniofac J. 2013;50(1):104–8. https://doi.org/10.1597/11-153.
3. Becker DB, Petersen JD, Kane AA, Cradock MM, Pilgram TK, Marsh JL. Speech, cognitive, and behavioral outcomes in nonsyndromic craniosynostosis. Plast Reconstr Surg. 2005;116(2):400–7. https://doi.org/10.1097/01.prs.0000172763.71043.b8.

4. Beckett JS, Brooks ED, Lacadie C, et al. Altered brain connectivity in sagittal craniosynostosis. J Neurosurg Pediatr. 2014;13(6):690–8. https://doi.org/10.3171/2014.3.PEDS13516.
5. Ntoula E, Nowinski D, Holmstrom G, Larsson E. Ophthalmological findings in children with non-syndromic craniosynostosis: preoperatively and postoperatively up to 12 months after surgery. BMJ Open Ophthalmol. 2021;6(1):e000677. https://doi.org/10.1136/bmjophth-2020-000677.
6. Blessing M, Gallagher ER. Epidemiology, genetics, and pathophysiology of craniosynostosis. Oral Maxillofac Surg Clin North Am. 2022;34(3):341–52. https://doi.org/10.1016/j.coms.2022.02.001.
7. Clarke CM, Fok VT, Gustafson JA, et al. Single suture craniosynostosis: identification of rare variants in genes associated with syndromic forms. Am J Med Genet A. 2018 Feb;176(2):290–300. Am J Med Genet A. 2018;176(11):2522. https://doi.org/10.1002/ajmg.a.38846.
8. Greenwood J, Flodman P, Osann K, Boyadjiev SA, Kimonis V. Familial incidence and associated symptoms in a population of individuals with nonsyndromic craniosynostosis. Genet Med. 2014;16(4):302–10. https://doi.org/10.1038/gim.2013.134.
9. Fearon JA, Singh DJ, Beals SP, Yu JC. The diagnosis and treatment of single-sutural synostoses: are computed tomographic scans necessary? Plast Reconstr Surg. 2007;120(5):1327–31. https://doi.org/10.1097/01.prs.0000279477.56044.55.
10. Baker CM, Ravindra VM, Gociman B, et al. Management of sagittal synostosis in the Synostosis Research Group: baseline data and early outcomes. Neurosurg Focus. 2021;50(4):E3. https://doi.org/10.3171/2021.1.FOCUS201029.
11. Jimenez DF, Barone CM, McGee ME, Cartwright CC, Baker CL. Endoscopy-assisted wide-vertex craniectomy, barrel stave osteotomies, and postoperative helmet molding therapy in the management of sagittal suture craniosynostosis. J Neurosurg. 2004;100(5 Suppl Pediatrics):407–17. https://doi.org/10.3171/ped.2004.100.5.0407.
12. Magge KT, Magge SN, Keating RF, et al. Incidental findings on preoperative computed tomography for nonsyndromic single suture craniosynostosis. J Craniofac Surg. 2014;25(4):1327–30. https://doi.org/10.1097/SCS.0000000000000797.
13. Persing J, Babler W, Winn HR, Jane J, Rodeheaver G. Age as a critical factor in the success of surgical correction of craniosynostosis. J Neurosurg. 1981;54(5):601–6. https://doi.org/10.3171/jns.1981.54.5.0601.
14. Chieffo D, Tamburrini G, Massimi L, et al. Long-term neuropsychological development in single-suture craniosynostosis treated early. J Neurosurg Pediatr. 2010;5(3):232–7. https://doi.org/10.3171/2009.10.PEDS09231.
15. Cross C, Khonsari RH, Larysz D, Johnson D, Kölby L, Moazen M. Predicting and comparing three corrective techniques for sagittal craniosynostosis. Sci Rep. 2021;11(1):21216. https://doi.org/10.1038/s41598-021-00642-7.
16. Tu L, Porras AR, Oh A, et al. Radiation-free quantification of head malformations in craniosynostosis patients from 3D photography. Proc SPIE Int Soc Opt Eng. 2018;10575:105751U. https://doi.org/10.1117/12.2295374.
17. Porras AR, Tu L, Tsering D, et al. Quantification of head shape from three-dimensional photography for presurgical and postsurgical evaluation of craniosynostosis. Plast Reconstr Surg. 2019;144(6):1051e–60e. https://doi.org/10.1097/PRS.0000000000006260.
18. Patel A, Yang JF, Hashim PW, et al. The impact of age at surgery on long-term neuropsychological outcomes in sagittal craniosynostosis. Plast Reconstr Surg. 2014;134(4):608e 17e. https://doi.org/10.1097/PRS.0000000000000511.
19. Eustache G, Nardi N, Rousseau C, et al. Importance of tranexamic acid in pediatric monosutural craniosynostosis surgery. J Neurosurg Pediatr. 2022;29(4):412–8. https://doi.org/10.3171/2021.10.PEDS21438.
20. Reddy SK, Patel RS, Rogers GF, Gordish-Dressman H, Keating RF, Pestieau SR. Intraoperative management by a craniofacial team anesthesiologist is associated with improved outcomes for children undergoing major craniofacial reconstructive surgery. J Craniofac Surg. 2019;30(2):418–23. https://doi.org/10.1097/SCS.0000000000005086.
21. Munro IR, Fearon JA. The coronal incision revisited. Plast Reconstr Surg. 1994;93(1):185–7. https://doi.org/10.1097/00006534-199401000-00031.
22. Boulos PT, Lin KY, Jane JA. Correction of sagittal synostosis using a modified Pi method. Clin Plast Surg. 2004;31(3):489–98, vii. https://doi.org/10.1016/j.cps.2004.03.011.
23. Jane JA, Edgerton MT, Futrell JW, Park TS. Immediate correction of sagittal synostosis. J Neurosurg. 1978;49(5):705–10. https://doi.org/10.3171/jns.1978.49.5.0705.
24. Amm CA, Denny AD. Correction of sagittal synostosis using foreshortening and lateral expansion of the cranium activated by gravity: surgical technique and postoperative evolution. Plast Reconstr Surg. 2005;116(3):723–35. https://doi.org/10.1097/01.prs.0000176897.76579.7c.
25. Seruya M, Sauerhammer TM, Basci D, et al. Analysis of routine intensive care unit admission following fronto-orbital advancement for craniosynostosis. Plast Reconstr Surg. 2013;131(4):582e–8e. https://doi.org/10.1097/PRS.0b013e3182818e94.
26. Puthumana JS, Lopez CD, Lake IV, Yang R. Evaluation of complications and outcomes in Craniosynostosis by age of operation: analysis of the National Surgical Quality Improvement Program-Pediatric. J Craniofac Surg. 2023;34(1):29–33. https://doi.org/10.1097/SCS.0000000000008872.
27. Fearon JA, Yu J, Bartlett SP, Munro IR, Chir B, Whitaker L. Infections in craniofacial surgery: a combined report of 567 procedures from two centers.

Plast Reconstr Surg. 1997;100(4):862–8. https://doi.org/10.1097/00006534-199709001-00006.

28. Reilly FOF, Clinton S, Dillon P, et al. Examining the relationship between wound complications and the use of resorbable plates in cranial vault reconstruction. J Craniofac Surg. 2021;32(7):2310–3. https://doi.org/10.1097/SCS.0000000000007663.
29. Baykal D, Balçın RN, Taşkapılıoğlu M. Amount of reoperation following surgical repair of non-syndromic craniosynostosis at a single center. Turk J Med Sci. 2022;52(4):1235–40. https://doi.org/10.55730/1300-0144.5428.
30. Agrawal D, Steinbok P, Cochrane DD. Reformation of the sagittal suture following surgery for isolated sagittal craniosynostosis. J Neurosurg. 2006;105(2 Suppl):115–7. https://doi.org/10.3171/ped.2006.105.2.115.
31. Seruya M, Oh AK, Boyajian MJ, et al. Long-term outcomes of primary craniofacial reconstruction for craniosynostosis: a 12-year experience. Plast Reconstr Surg. 2011;127(6):2397–406. https://doi.org/10.1097/PRS.0b013e318213a178.
32. Flores CA, French BM, Alexander AL, et al. Vascularized Pericranial flap as a method to prevent persistent skull defects after craniectomy for sagittal synostosis. J Craniofac Surg. 2021;32(8):2744–8. https://doi.org/10.1097/SCS.0000000000007851.
33. Alperovich M, Runyan CM, Gabrick KS, et al. Long-term neurocognitive outcomes of spring-assisted surgery versus cranial vault remodeling for sagittal synostosis. Plast Reconstr Surg. 2021;147(3):661–71. https://doi.org/10.1097/PRS.0000000000007640.
34. Hashim PW, Patel A, Yang JF, et al. The effects of whole-vault cranioplasty versus strip craniectomy on long-term neuropsychological outcomes in sagittal craniosynostosis. Plast Reconstr Surg. 2014;134(3):491–501. https://doi.org/10.1097/PRS.0000000000000420.

Sagittal Suture Synostosis: Distraction Osteogenesis, Key Points for the Neurosurgeons

40

Kyu Won Shim and Eun Kyung Park

40.1 Introduction

Sagittal synostosis is the most common form of craniosynostosis. Dolichocephalic cranial morphology is a distinguishable characteristic that allows a clear diagnosis of sagittal synostosis [1]. The surgical treatment is inevitable, and various techniques (total skull remodeling, pi-plasty or modified pi-plasty, endoscopic suturectomy, and distraction osteogenesis) have been used [2–5]. In younger patients (4–6 months) with the innate capability of early reossification, corrective methods include removing the pathologic sagittal suture and waiting for natural reformation following brain growth [6]. Cranial molding helmets have also been used to support realignment [4].

The brain volumetric growth will transmit the tensile strains to the sutures and stimulate the bone deposition at the cranial vault suture [7]. The functional matrix theory insists that the functional enlargement or development of an organ system is the primary force in changing its overall shape and determining its final form. Brain enlargement is clearly the engine of skull remodeling and the vault suture plays a critical role in the development of the skull pathology associated with craniosynostosis [8].

Sagittal craniosynostosis can notably distort and deform the cranial vault and the underlying brain parenchyma. Intracranial pressure (ICP) and neurocognitive impairment are reasonably assumed that there is a probable linear relationship with skull deformation or distortion. Neuroanatomical changes resulting from the interaction between the growing skull and the developing brain can extend beyond the region directly beneath the fused suture [9]. The development of the brain and skull is quite independent and follow different trajectories. The growth of brain does not correlate with the morphology of skull. The deformational stress on the cerebral cortex affects subcortical structures and also affects the overall spread throughout the brain [10, 11]. Sagittal craniosynostosis usually shows cognitive impairment, and there have been several studies suggesting that the occurrence of cognitive impairment is directly due to cranial deformation [12]. Skull growth is regionally restricted [13], but the brain volume in these cases is usually within [14, 15] or exceeding [15]

K. W. Shim (✉) · E. K. Park
Department of Pediatric Neurosurgery, Severance Children's Hospital, Yonsei University College of Medicine, Seoul, South Korea
e-mail: shimkyuwon@yuhs.ac; estherpark@yuhs.ac

F. Di Rocco, J. Kestle (eds.), *Neurosurgical Aspects of Craniosynostosis*,
https://doi.org/10.1007/978-3-031-69386-1_40

normal limits. Our recent data are consistent with these findings regarding the intracranial volume. A smaller preoperative intracranial volume might suggest a low developmental score compared to the normal volume, although in most cases, the volume is not smaller than the age-matched average [16].

At school age, learning disabilities or related problems associated with neurocognitive impairment do become apparent, because of the fact that children are positioned into more intellectually demanding surroundings, combined with higher expectancies of social interaction [17]. A comprehensive and team-based close follow-up should be needed.

40.2 Positioning

All procedures are performed by plastic and neurosurgery professionals [16]. In each instance, "a baseline circumferential osteotomy" is performed starting 5 mm above the supraorbital rim and connecting the near inion. Midsagittal and horizontal bicoronal osteotomy lines are variably implemented (Fig. 40.1).

For this basic surgical scheme, the supine position has been used at our institute (Fig. 40.2). To address both anterior and posterior aspects of the skull without the need for repositioning, modified prone position is recommended [18]. This modified prone position has been used for whole

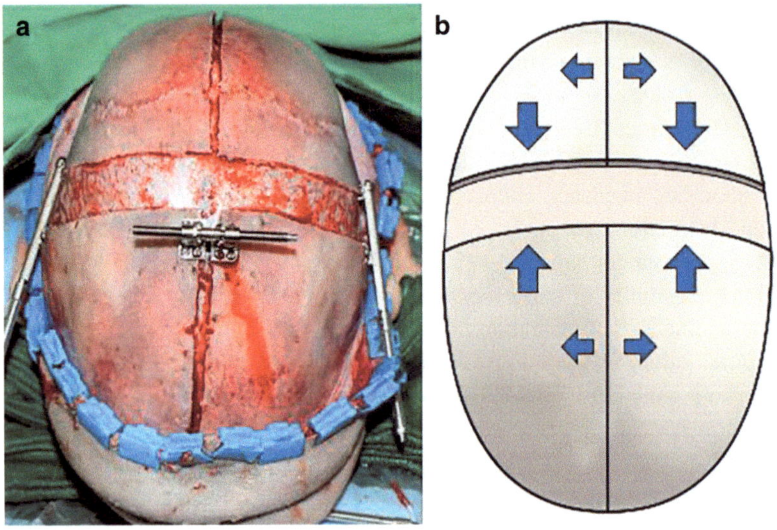

Fig. 40.1 Intraoperative photo (**a**) and schematic diagram (**b**) of anteroposterior compression with the bitemporal expansion technique. Craniotomy lines are shown (frontal-vertex-occipital and bitemporal-vertex), dividing the hemisphere into quadrants. An additional hairband-shaped craniectomy line (bitemporal vertex) is made for anteroposterior compression as needed

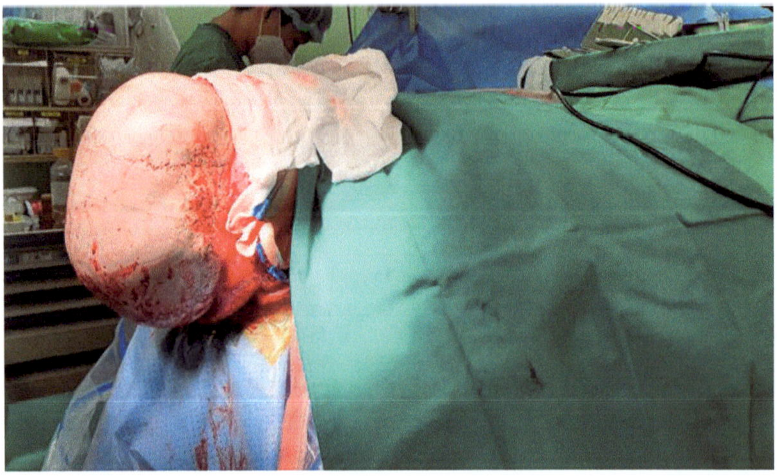

Fig. 40.2 Supine position. A small gap or space between surgical table or head rest/horse shoe and patient's head will be enough to be passed by electrical craniotome to make a craniotomy line

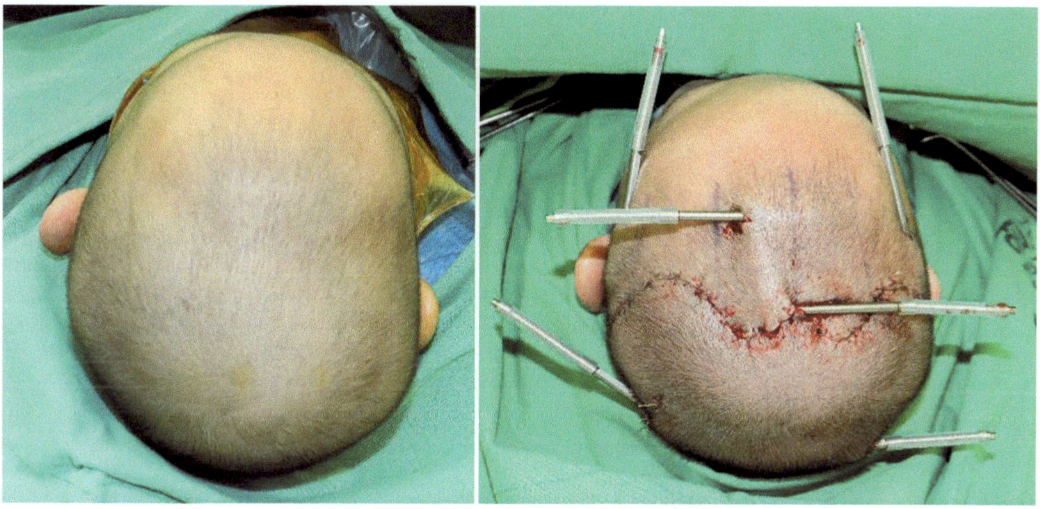

Fig. 40.3 Sagittal craniosynostosis with moderate plagiocephaly. An incision is curvilinear wave pattern along to coronal line and multiple additional incision for exit of internal distractors. Only internal distractors were used for this case. This case used three internal devices for midline distraction

cranial vault remodeling surgery. However, our circumferential craniotomy technique does not require "the easy access to the area of inion and posterior inferior part of cranium." Our technique needs only a small gap or space between surgical table or head rest/horse shoe and patient's head to be passed by electrical craniotome to make a craniotomy line. This standard supine position is very comfortable for patients as well as anesthesiologist to access the patients, but it may be uncomfortable to surgeons (Fig. 40.2). In case of emergency situation like a hypovolemic shock, supine position will be tremendously beneficial for patient's safety. When an operator is making craniotomy line at posterior parietal bone and occipital bone which is very dependent position and narrow access to the field reverse, the Trendelenburg position of 15–30° will give a better approach angle toward the surgical field.

40.3 Incision

Main skin incision is curvilinear wave pattern along to the coronal line to minimize the visualization of scar. Curvilinear wave pattern incision will be covered and a scar exposure will be minimized by hair growth. Small multiple additional incisions for the outlet of distractors are needed. The author's institute uses two types of distractors, which are internal and external type. Small additional incision for their outlet will be adjusted according to the position and type of distractors. For the external distractor, additional skin incision for outlet will not be necessary. However, the internal distractor usually has another outlet, so additional skin incision is necessary. As you can see in Fig. 40.4, the shape of the internal distractor distal half of distractor is flexible and long tailed. When the fixation of distractor, the outlet and direction of that should be considered to minimize the additional incision and scar (Fig. 40.3).

40.4 Instrumentation

Distraction devices [19] are developed by plastic surgeon of the author's institute. The internal and external distractors are shown in Fig. 40.4. The internal device consists of two parts, proximal rigid which has two foot plates for fixation on craniotomy edges with eight holes for screw and distal flexible parts covered by silicon sheath (Fig. 40.4a). This distal flexible part is useful for exiting skin through additional incision and hiding inside dressing. This internal device can be used

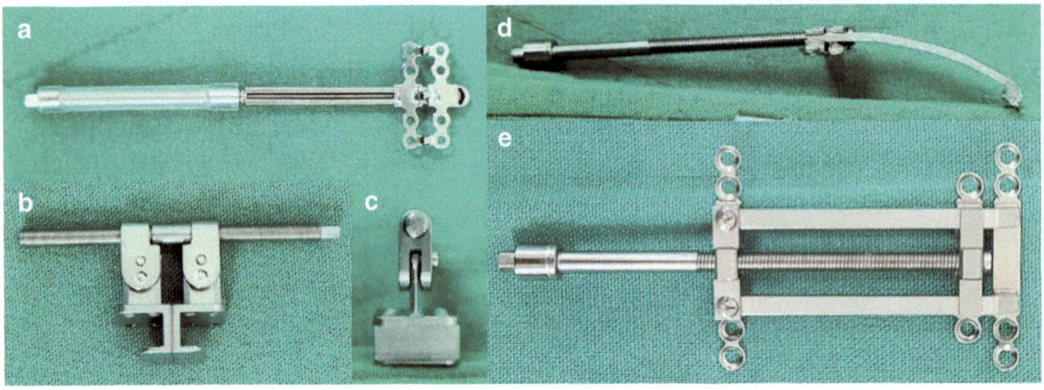

Fig. 40.4 Distraction devices which the authors developed. (**a**) Internal device, (**b**, **c**) external devices, and (**d**, **e**) malleable distractor

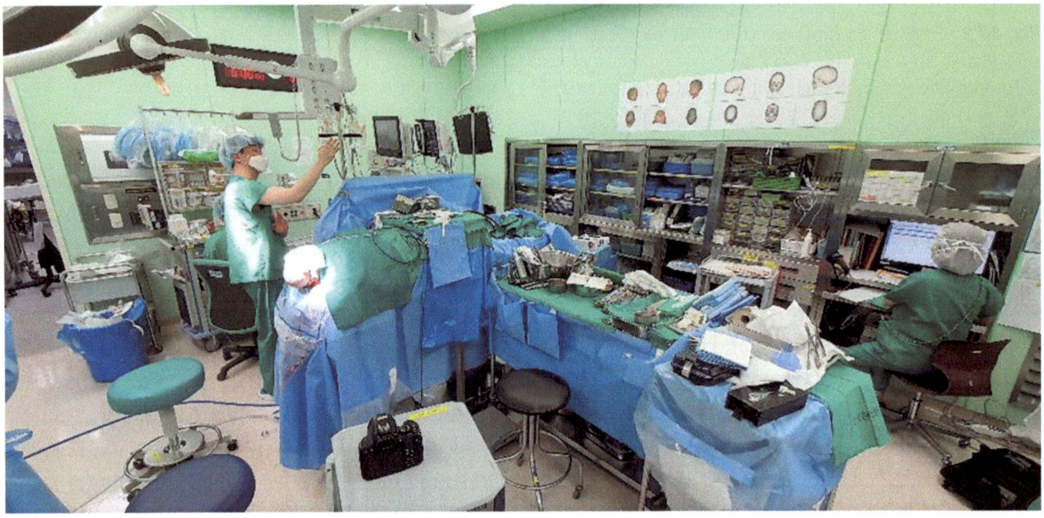

Fig. 40.5 The panoramic view of the operating theater. Anesthesiologist is usually on the left side of patient, i.e., deep inside of the operating room. Green chair at the left lower corner is for surgeon. Surgical instruments are positioned at the right side of patient's foot. The black round chair is for scrub nurse

for distracting and compressing. The internal device is not so tough to withstand hard distraction or compression, so an external device is useful for hard distraction. Hard distraction shall be applied to distract two big bone flaps in the middle of two parietal bones. Our institute uses three external devices for distracting midline bones of sagittal craniosynostosis because the distracting line is too long for single distractor. An external device is strong enough to hold and distract thick and large bone flaps (Fig. 40.4b, c). It has large profile and is heavier than the internal device, but no additional incision is needed. Both distraction devices can distract or compress by a linear vector. There is another one for curved vector distraction (Fig. 40.4d, e). The main body of this distractor is malleable so that the operator can adjust the curvature of the distractor, as shown in Fig. 40.4d.

40.5 Position of Surgical Team

Surgical procedures are performed by engaging a team of professionals (i.e., plastic surgeon, neurosurgeon, anesthesiologist, geneticist, and pediatric psychologist). Figure 40.5 clearly shows operating theater and the position of surgical team. The anesthesiologist team dedicated to pediatric craniofacial surgery is prepared all about anesthesia inside of the room. As shown in Fig. 40.5, the patient is positioned supine next to the anesthesiologist. The area of patient's head is freely open for surgeons to ensure full access to the whole area of the calvarial bone. Surgical instruments are kept ready which are perpendicular to the surgical table. Scrub nurse can access surgical instruments and assist surgeons simultaneously at the corner of the patient's and instrument table.

40.6 Intraoperative Monitoring

The author's institute has not done with any type of intraoperative ICP monitoring. The reason is the main purpose of the surgical correction of craniosynostosis is not ICP control. And also, we did a study of preoperative measurement of ICP through a lumbar puncture while the patients are on the general anesthesia and ophthalmologic exam for papilledema (unpublished). There has been no clear evidence for those parameters that could be essential for patients to be decided for surgical treatment or surgical extent so far. Elevated ICP may be one of the considerations for decision-making although the normal variation of ICP with age is not well delineated. And only small portion of single-suture craniosynostosis patients show elevated ICP [19]. Recently, Brendan et al. [20] did an intraoperative ICP monitoring before and after craniectomy or craniotomy using a flexible ICP fiberoptic probe. They reported that in the mean precraniectomy ICP, there was no significant difference between syndromic and nonsyndromic patients (17.68 vs. 15.58 mmHg, $p = 0.239$). In regard to postcraniectomy ICP, there was no significant difference between syndromic and nonsyndromic patients (8.68 vs. 8.96 mmHg, $p = 0.820$) [20].

Distraction osteogenesis shows statistically significant decreased blood loss and reduced amount of blood transfusion [21]. However, the absolute amount of blood loss is still large for infant. In the author's institute, a standardized anesthesia protocol has been used and bleeding monitoring was published, which was developed by an anesthesiology team [22]. At the author's institute, the following standardized general anesthesia protocol is used: induction with 2 mg/kg propofol and 1 μg/kg fentanyl, neuromuscular blockade with 0.6 mg/kg rocuronium bromide, maintenance with desflurane or sevoflurane in an oxygen-air mixture (fraction of inspired oxygen, 0.5), and administration of intermittent bolus doses of fentanyl and rocuronium. A central venous catheter is placed in the femoral or internal jugular vein, whereas an arterial catheter is placed in the radial artery. Urine output is monitored using a urinary catheter. Rectal temperature is measured and maintained at normothermic levels with a forced-air blanket throughout the surgery. Due to the inaccuracy in estimating blood loss during surgery, blood loss is calculated by the anesthesiologist using a previously adopted formula for this patient population [23–25]: estimated red cell volume $(ERCV)_{lost} = ERCV_{preoperative} + ERCV_{transfused} - ERCV_{postoperative}$ where ERCV is estimated blood volume (EBV) × Hct/100. EBV is 80 mL/kg for infants younger than 12 months and 75 mL/kg for children older than 12 months. $ERCV_{transfused}$ is calculated as follows: $ERCV_{transfused}$ = transfused volume of packed RBC (mL) × Hct of packed RBC/100 Hct of packed RBC is estimated to be approximately 60% by the local blood bank. Therefore, EBV_{lost} is calculated as follows: EBV_{lost} (mL/kg) = $ERCV_{lost}$ (mL)/[Weight (kg) × $Hct_{preoperative}$/100]. Routine fluid management during surgery consisted of continuous administration of balanced crystalloid with additional SD 1:4 solution (0.2% NaCl with dextrose). The amount of fluid administered is determined based on preoperative fasting time, intraoperative deficits, and basal fluid maintenance. Colloid (hydroxyethyl starch (6%, 130/0.4) in a balanced electrolyte solution, Volulyte; Fresenius Kabi, Schelle, Belgium) up to 20 mL/kg/day is administered in case of acute and massive perioperative blood loss prior to the initiation of blood product preparation and transfusion. Controlled hypotension is not performed during surgery.

TXA-induced hemostasis involves the inhibition of plasminogen-plasmin interactions on the surface of fibrin, thereby preventing fibrin degradation [26]. The antifibrinolytic activity of TXA resulted in reduced transfusion requirement until postoperative day 2 in our institute [22].

40.7 Hemostasis Control

Tranexamic acid (TXA) is effective for reducing blood loss and the need for transfusions during surgeries [22, 26]. TXA is administered as an intravenous loading dose of 10 mg/kg over 15 min, followed by continuous intravenous infusion at 5 mg/kg/h from the beginning of the surgery until skin closure [22, 27].

The initial skin incision starts when blood transfusion is ready. A local infiltration of local anesthetics along the incision is commonly used to minimize bleeding. Small size scalp clip for pediatric patient is applied to reduce the bleeding from the open scalp wound during operation.

There are many active possible bleeding points while performing craniotomy. Supraorbital bony sinus or bone marrow, pterional meningeal artery, and bone bleeding around the anterior fontanelle are main sites of bleeding. Bleeding along the coronal craniotomy site is frequently encountered as well as from sagittal venous sinus. There are many commercially available hemostatic materials with various application techniques such as Bone wax, absorbable hemostat (Surgicel® fibrillar), microfibrillar collagen hemostat (Avitene®), fibrin sealant patch (Tachosil®), and hemostatic matrix (Floseal®), etc. These materials are unique feature of hemostatic mechanisms, so surgeons can choose several of them according to the nature of bleeding and oozing.

40.8 Bone Opening

Under general anesthesia, the patient is placed in the supine position on a horse-shoe head rest. A curvilinear wave pattern incision is made along the scalp as a bicoronal line. Subperiosteal dissection is done to the supraorbital rim anteriorly and below the inion posteriorly. In each instance, a baseline circumferential osteotomy is carried out, starting at a point 5 mm above the supraorbital rim and connecting the near inion. Two additional straight osteotomy lines are variably implemented as needed; the first is a mid-sagittal line, and the second is a horizontal bicoronal line. Furthermore, bicoronal strip ostectomy (width, 10–20 mm) is performed along the bicoronal osteotomy line. Once removed, internal distraction devices are applied for fronto-occipital compression, incorporating vectors of frontal bossing. Along the mid-sagittal osteotomy, two or three distraction devices are then applied for bitemporal expansion (Fig. 40.6) [12].

For safe and efficient craniotomy, initial burr hole should be carefully made at critical point along the designed craniotomy line. At the age of 1 year, the sutures are tight and ligamentous nature, so they are not easy to directly cross with craniotomy burr. For effective correction of sagittal craniosynostosis, circumferential craniotomy to detach calvarial bone from the skull base should be made. Coronal sutures, pterion, squamosal suture, and lambdoid sutures are crossed for basal circumferential craniotomy. If a suture is too tough to directly cross, dissecting burr can be helpful to cross the suture and also the removal of tight ligamentous tissues. However, the pterion crossing the internal bony ridge is problematic and craniotome is used to be stuck. A gentle "to and fro" maneuver of craniotome may cross the internal ridge, otherwise dissecting burr should be used carefully to remove the internal bony ridge. Frontal base craniotomy is little challenging because usually there is an internal sharp bony ridge. And also, there is long and tough midline ridge underneath the midline of the frontal bone. For a patient who has prominent frontal bossing, this midline frontal craniotomy is needed. Most of the midline internal ridge is not so high to be removed by simple craniotomy. A gentle "to and fro" maneuver of craniotome and feeling the "grinding out of the ridge" will help to overcome this ridge. Posterior 2/3 of the midline is quite challenging due to the position of the patient and very tight dura around the lambdoid

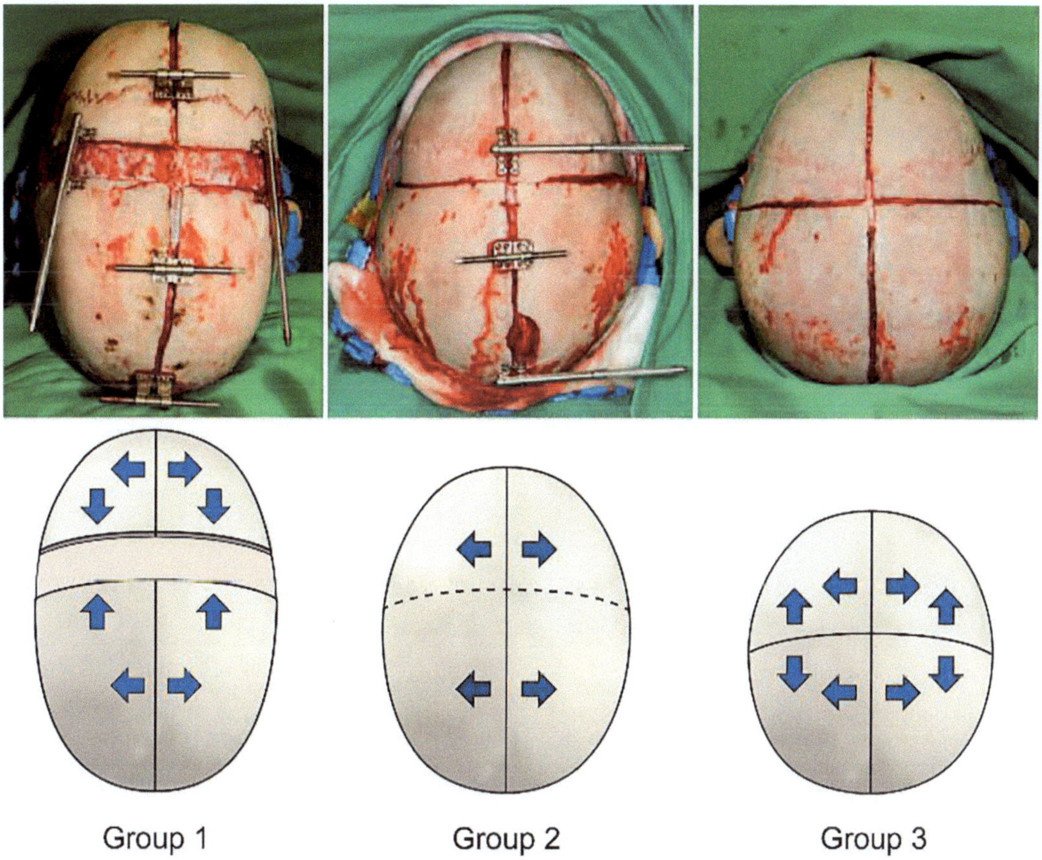

Fig. 40.6 Intraoperative photographs and schematic diagrams of surgical techniques for each therapeutic group. The arrows indicate the distraction direction, and the shaded area represents the cranial segment removed. The dotted line in the bitemporal distraction procedure denotes the craniotomy line, which was performed when anterior and posterior cranium expansions differed. Group 1, anteroposterior compression with bitemporal expansion (left); group 2, bitemporal expansion (center), and group 3, anteroposterior expansion with bitemporal expansion (right) [12]

suture. Similar principle can be applied. A gentle "to and fro" maneuver of craniotome and feeling the "grinding out of the bone" will help. For tight lambdoid suture, dissecting burr should be used not to injure the sagittal sinus. Craniotomy for occipital bone is very difficult for the surgeon because patients are supine and craniotomy line is in dependent position.

In group 1, a bicoronal strip ostectomy (width, 10–20 mm) is performed along the bicoronal osteotomy line. Once removed, distraction devices are applied for antero-occipital compression, considering frontal bossing vectors. Two or three distraction devices are then applied along the midsagittal osteotomy for bitemporal expansion (Fig. 40.7) [12].

In group 2, a midsagittal osteotomy is performed, and two or three distraction devices are applied along the midsagittal osteotomy for bitemporal expansion. A bicoronal osteotomy was performed to correct disparate front-to-back width, applying distraction devices to each flap (Fig. 40.8) [12].

In group 3, midsagittal and bicoronal osteotomies are performed, and distraction devices are placed along osteotomy lines to expand in the bitemporal and antero-occipital directions (Fig. 40.9) [12].

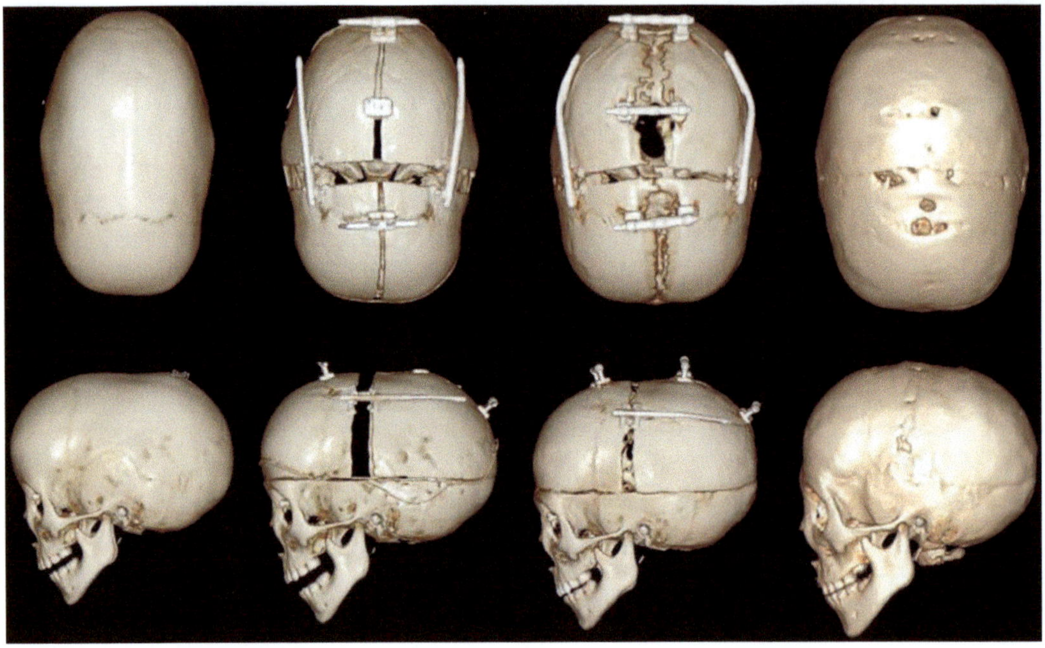

Fig. 40.7 Anteroposterior compression procedure for distraction osteogenesis in dolichocephalic sagittal synostosis. Sagittal synostosis noted preoperatively with intact coronal and lambdoid sutures (left). Devices were applied at craniotomy sites for anteroposterior compression and bitemporal expansion to perform distraction in distinguishable vectors (second from left and second from right). Correction of scaphoid cranial shape and excessive frontal bossing were confirmed, and newly generated calvarial bone was verified at the sagittal suture point (right)

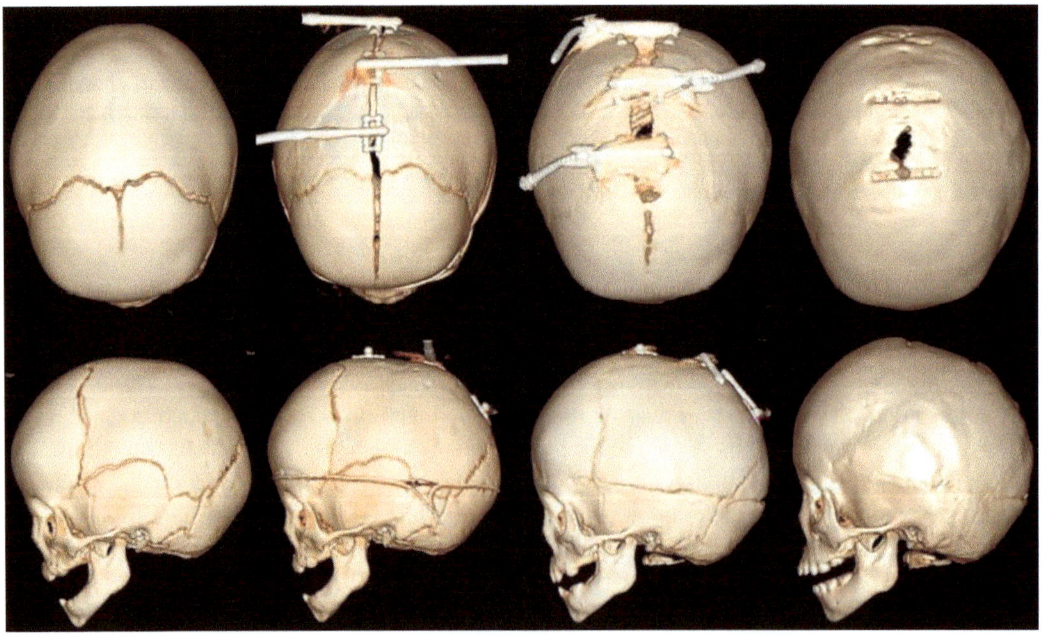

Fig. 40.8 Bitemporal expansion procedure for distraction osteogenesis in sagittal synostosis, with a cranial index of 75–80. Sagittal synostosis was noted preoperatively, with intact coronal and lambdoid sutures (left). Devices were applied at craniotomy sites for bitemporal expansion to perform distraction (second from left and second from right). Correction of constricted cranial growth at midline was confirmed. Newly generated calvarial bone was verified at the area of the former sagittal suture (right)

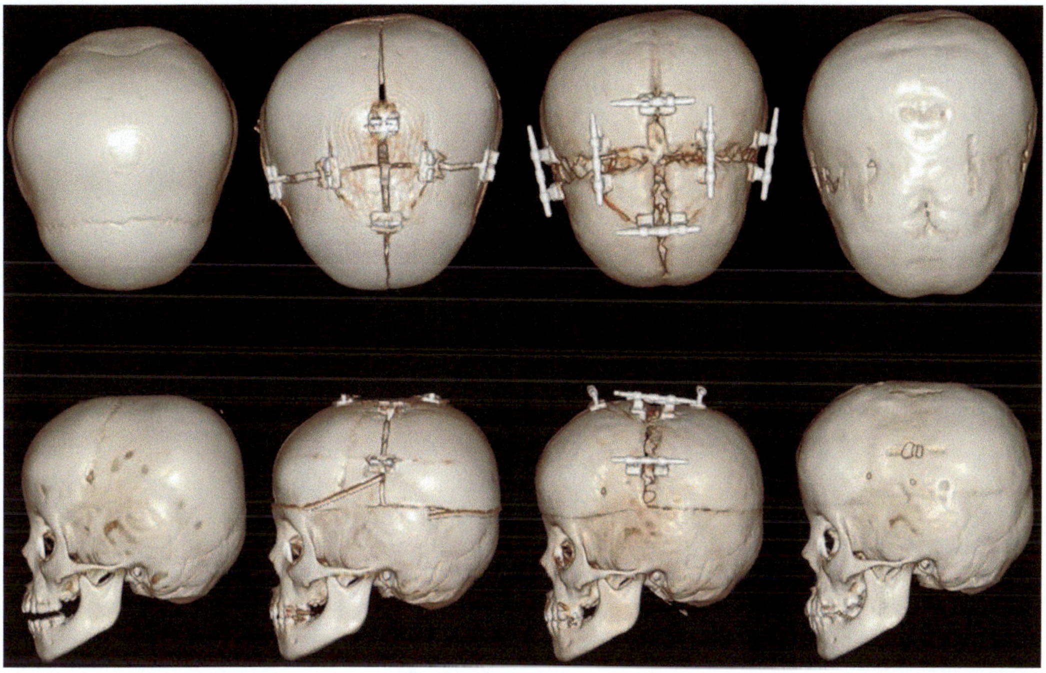

Fig. 40.9 Anteroposterior and bitemporal expansion procedure for distraction osteogenesis in nondolichocephalic sagittal synostosis. Sagittal synostosis was noted preoperatively, with intact coronal and lambdoid sutures (left). Devices were applied at craniotomy sites for anteroposterior and bitemporal expansion, and distraction was performed in the expansile vector (second from left and second from right). Correction of nondolichocephalic cranial shape was confirmed, and newly generated calvarial bone was verified at the distraction site (right)

40.9 Postoperative Drain

The scalp is closed with resorbable sutures, and a compressive dressing is applied. Whole calvarial bone is usually exposed, so two silicone vacuum drainage bags are inserted anteriorly and posteriorly. While patients are monitored in the neurosurgical intensive care unit for 1–2 days, the drains are monitored hourly. Usually, the drainages are maintained for 3–4 days postoperatively. Removal of drainage depends on the amount of drainage.

40.10 Postoperative Dressing and Surveillance

The patients are monitored at recovery room immediately after operation until patient's vital signs and general condition are considered stable. In most of the patients, chest X-rays are taken at the recovery room to monitor the volume status, because the infused fluids including blood products are plenty. The anesthesiologist and neurosurgeon decide to transfer the patient to the neurosurgical care unit. A 3D head CT is usually performed if the patient's condition permits, while the patient is being transferred to the neurosurgical care unit.

40.11 Postoperative Intensive Care at Neurosurgical Care Unit

Patients are monitored in the neurosurgical intensive care unit for 1–2 days. Heart rate with electrocardiography, respiration rate, blood pressure with arterial line and oxygen saturation. After patients are stabilized at the neurosurgical care unit, a dressing is changed to inspect the undetected hematomas collection and active bleeding from distractor exit sites, usually 6 h after the end of operation. One hour before midnight, a dressing is inspected by the plastic surgeon and neurosurgeon to check bleeding or oozing. Complete blood counts and coagulation profiles are checked. Other routine chemistries are also checked. Additional infusion of volume expander or transfusion of blood is decided according to the results of laboratory test and the amount of drainage.

The next day after the operation, most of the patients are sent to the general ward to proceed the rest of the postoperative care and take an instruction for distraction and wound care at home.

40.12 Outpatient Clinic Follow-Up

Five days after the procedure, distraction is initiated at a rate of 0.5–1.0 mm/day and continued until the shape of the skull is satisfactory by appearance and on radiographic images. Overall perioperative management adhered to critical pathways of the institute for craniosynostosis patients. Seven days after admission, guardians may make adjustments to distraction on an outpatient basis. In outpatient clinic, the status is checked at 1–2 week interval with skull X-ray and visual inspection until they reach the planed shape of expansion and compression. Usually, 3–4 weeks are enough for distraction and compression.

40.13 Removal of Instrumentation

After completion of distraction or compression, a consolidation period is given for 8–12 weeks according to the status of the skull and patient's age. The devices are removed under general anesthesia after consolidation. Absorbable plates are placed on each expansion site to maintain distracted gaps, which help retain stability and overcome adjacent soft-tissue pressure until complete reossification is achieved.

40.14 Postop Helmet

As shown in Figs. 40.7, 40.8, and 40.9, cranial indices are much improved. But there are usually certain amount of bone gaps/defects and skull growth is still taking place after the completion of distraction. Helmet orthosis can assist symmetrical growth of skull and provide a guidance for proper filling of the bone defect. The duration of helmet assist depends on the postoperative status of patients.

40.15 Neurosurgeon's Perspectives

Dolichocephalic sagittal craniosynostosis can be treated effectively by circumferential cranial reformation, strategically using distraction osteogenesis for maximal benefits. Sagittal craniosynostosis with a normal intracranial volume is corrected through distraction osteogenesis in combination with antero-posterior compression and bitemporal expansion. These procedures resulted in neurodevelopmental improvement, demonstrating the validity of expansion linked with a compression technique [12, 16]. Most of nondolichocephalic sagittal craniosynostosis showed subnormal intracranial volume. The preoperative psychomotor developmental index is mostly lower than dolichocephalic sagittal craniosynostosis [12]. Table 40.1 shows the assessment results of neurodevelopmental outcomes

Table 40.1 Age-dependent neurodevelopmental assessment results

	Age at operation <1 year ($n = 48$)		Age at operation >1 year ($n = 17$)	
	MDI	PDI	MDI	PDI
Preoperative	86.75 ± 10.12	88.13 ± 18.79	81.83 ± 17.53	80 ± 12.18
Postoperative	100.23 ± 12.34	101.98 ± 13.68	88.92 ± 17.43	84.92 ± 13.27
p	0.001*	0.004*	0.073	0.052

MDI mental developmental index; *PDI* psychomotor developmental index
* $p < 0.05$

(unpublished data). The "Golden Time" for surgical correction is 4–6 months old [28]. According to studies of patients with sagittal synostosis, early surgery (i.e., <6 months of age) with a more comprehensive approach yielded a better neurological outcome than strip craniectomy (endoscopic or otherwise) before 3 months of age [29, 30]. Distraction osteogenesis has advantages of larger volume expansion and effective correction of the vault shape [21].

References

1. Persing JA. MOC-PS(SM) CME article: management considerations in the treatment of craniosynostosis. Plast Reconstr Surg. 2008;121(4 Suppl):1–11.
2. Nakajima H, Sakamoto Y, Tamada I, Ohara H, Kishi K. Dynamic total skull remodeling by a combination of morcellation craniotomy with distraction osteogenesis: the MoD procedure. J Craniofac Surg. 2011;22(4):1240–6.
3. Guimaraes-Ferreira J, Gewalli F, David L, Darvann TA, Hermann NV, Kreiborg S, et al. Sagittal synostosis: II. Cranial morphology and growth after the modified pi-plasty. Scand J Plast Reconstr Surg Hand Surg. 2006;40(4):200–9.
4. Ridgway EB, Berry-Candelario J, Grondin RT, Rogers GF, Proctor MR. The management of sagittal synostosis using endoscopic suturectomy and postoperative helmet therapy. J Neurosurg Pediatr. 2011;7(6):620–6.
5. Derderian CA, Bastidas N, Bartlett SP. Posterior cranial vault expansion using distraction osteogenesis. Childs Nerv Syst. 2012;28(9):1551–6.
6. Massimi L, Di Rocco C. Mini-invasive surgical technique for sagittal craniosynostosis. Childs Nerv Syst. 2012;28(9):1341–5.
7. Moss ML. Functional anatomy of cranial synostosis. Childs Brain. 1975;1(1):22–33.
8. Moss ML. Growth of the calvaria in the rat; the determination of osseous morphology. Am J Anat. 1954;94(3):333–61.
9. Aldridge K, Kane AA, Marsh JL, Panchal J, Boyadjiev SA, Yan P, et al. Brain morphology in nonsyndromic unicoronal craniosynostosis. Anat Rec A Discov Mol Cell Evol Biol. 2005;285(2):690–8.
10. Aldridge K, Marsh JL, Govier D, Richtsmeier JT. Central nervous system phenotypes in craniosynostosis. J Anat. 2002;201(1):31–9.
11. Munakata Y, Casey BJ, Diamond A. Developmental cognitive neuroscience: progress and potential. Trends Cogn Sci. 2004;8(3):122–8.
12. Lee MC, Shim KW, Yun IS, Park EK, Kim YO. Correction of sagittal craniosynostosis using distraction osteogenesis based on strategic categorization. Plast Reconstr Surg. 2017;139(1):157–69.
13. Camfield PRCC, Cohen MM. Neurologic aspects of craniosynostosis. In: Cohen MMMR, editor. Craniosynostosis: diagnosis, evaluation, and management. New York: Oxford Press; 2000. p. 177–83.
14. Polley JW, Charbel FT, Kim D, MaFee MF. Nonsyndromal craniosynostosis: longitudinal outcome following cranio-orbital reconstruction in infancy. Plast Reconstr Surg. 1998;102(3):619–28; discussion 29–32.
15. Posnick JC, Armstrong D, Bite U. Metopic and sagittal synostosis: intracranial volume measurements prior to and after cranio-orbital reshaping in childhood. Plast Reconstr Surg. 1995;96(2):299–309; discussion 10–5.
16. Lee MC, Shim KW, Park EK, Yun IS, Kim DS, Kim YO. Expansion and compression distraction osteogenesis based on volumetric and neurodevelopmental analysis in sagittal craniosynostosis. Childs Nerv Syst. 2015;31(11):2081–9.
17. Kapp-Simon KA. Mental development and learning disorders in children with single suture craniosynostosis. Cleft Palate Craniofac J. 1998;35(3):197–203.
18. Heller JB, Heller MM, Knoll B, Gabbay JS, Duncan C, Persing JA. Intracranial volume and cephalic index outcomes for total calvarial reconstruction among nonsyndromic sagittal synostosis patients. Plast Reconstr Surg. 2008;121(1):187–95.
19. Thompson DN, Harkness W, Jones B, Gonsalez S, Andar U, Hayward R. Subdural intracranial pressure monitoring in craniosynostosis: its role in surgical management. Childs Nerv Syst. 1995;11(5):269–75.
20. Judy BF, Swanson JW, Yang W, Storm PB, Bartlett SP, Taylor JA, et al. Intraoperative intracranial pressure monitoring in the pediatric craniosynostosis population. J Neurosurg Pediatr. 2018;22(5):475–80.
21. Kim SW, Shim KW, Plesnila N, Kim YO, Choi JU, Kim DS. Distraction vs remodeling surgery for craniosynostosis. Childs Nerv Syst. 2007;23(2):201–6.
22. Kim EJ, Kim YO, Shim KW, Ko BW, Lee JW, Koo BN. Effects of tranexamic acid based on its population pharmacokinetics in pediatric patients undergoing distraction osteogenesis for craniosynostosis: rotational thromboelastometry (ROTEM(TM)) analysis. Int J Med Sci. 2018;15(8):788–95.
23. Goobie SM, Meier PM, Pereira LM, McGowan FX, Prescilla RP, Scharp LA, et al. Efficacy of tranexamic acid in pediatric craniosynostosis surgery: a double-blind, placebo-controlled trial. Anesthesiology. 2011;114(4):862–71.
24. Stricker PA, Shaw TL, Desouza DG, Hernandez SV, Bartlett SP, Friedman DF, et al. Blood loss, replacement, and associated morbidity in infants and children undergoing craniofacial surgery. Paediatr Anaesth. 2010;20(2):150–9.
25. Kearney RA, Rosales JK, Howes WJ. Craniosynostosis: an assessment of blood loss and transfusion practices. Can J Anaesth. 1989;36(4):473–7.

26. Dunn CJ, Goa KL. Tranexamic acid: a review of its use in surgery and other indications. Drugs. 1999;57(6):1005–32.
27. Goobie SM, Meier PM, Sethna NF, Soriano SG, Zurakowski D, Samant S, et al. Population pharmacokinetics of tranexamic acid in paediatric patients undergoing craniosynostosis surgery. Clin Pharmacokinet. 2013;52(4):267–76.
28. Marchac D, Renier D, Broumand S. Timing of treatment for craniosynostosis and facio-craniosynostosis: a 20-year experience. Br J Plast Surg. 1994;47(4):211–22.
29. Patel A, Yang JF, Hashim PW, Travieso R, Terner J, Mayes LC, et al. The impact of age at surgery on long-term neuropsychological outcomes in sagittal craniosynostosis. Plast Reconstr Surg. 2014;134(4):608e–17e.
30. Hashim PW, Patel A, Yang JF, Travieso R, Terner J, Losee JE, et al. The effects of whole-vault cranioplasty versus strip craniectomy on long-term neuropsychological outcomes in sagittal craniosynostosis. Plast Reconstr Surg. 2014;134(3):491–501.

41 Spring-Mediated Cranioplasty for Treatment of Sagittal Synostosis

Michael R. Bykowski, Michael M. McDowell, John T. Smetona, Jesse A. Goldstein, and Ian F. Pollack

41.1 Introduction

Nonsyndromic sagittal craniosynostosis (SCS) causes an abnormally long and narrow head shape. Surgical management for SCS can be classified into two general approaches such as (1) traditional open cranial vault remodeling (CVR) and (2) early management with less-invasive techniques. While these approaches are vastly different, they share the same fundamental goals such as (1) to restore normal cranial appearance and (2) to prevent future neurocognitive impairment. CVR techniques are performed around after 6 months of age through an open bicoronal approach, whereby the affected skull is removed and reshaped into a normal form at the time of surgery. While CVR enables immediate and consistent outcomes, the benefits are negatively weighted by the risk of intraoperative blood loss, larger scar burden, need for postoperative critical care, and length of stay in the hospital. To overcome these limitations, less-invasive alternatives were developed wherein the sagittal suture is surgically "released," followed by postoperative reshaping with either an external cranial orthosis or, more recently, internal stainless-steel springs.

In 1998, Jimenez and Barone pioneered endoscopic-assisted strip craniectomy (ESC) for early treatment of SCS around 3–6 months of age [1]. Unlike CVR, cranial shape is not corrected at the time of ESC. Instead, head shape is passively molded by rapid infantile brain growth and an external cranial orthosis. The cranial orthosis is worn 23.5 h daily for 6–9 months. Noncompliance with the intense, prolonged treatment course leads to less predictable outcomes.

In 2008, spring-mediated cranioplasty (SMC) was popularized in the literature by Lauritzen and colleagues after reporting the results of the first 100 cases [2]. Strip craniectomy is performed; however, in lieu of postoperative helmet therapy, correction is achieved with internal stainless-steel springs. Like ESC, head shape is not corrected at the time of surgery. Parietal bone widening occurs over the course of several weeks as expansile and resistive forces reach equilibrium. Springs are removed in 3–4 months after bone consolidation. The primary challenges of SMC are (1) understanding the nuanced interplay between spring attributes and the viscoelastic properties of the pediatric skull and (2) how can we apply this knowledge for guiding surgical decision-making to achieve consistent results

Supplementary Information The online version contains supplementary material available at https://doi.org/10.1007/978-3-031-69386-1_41.

M. R. Bykowski · J. T. Smetona · J. A. Goldstein
Departments of Plastic Surgery, UPMC Children's Hospital of Pittsburgh, University of Pittsburgh School of Medicine, Pittsburgh, PA, USA

M. M. McDowell · I. F. Pollack (✉)
Departments of Neurological Surgery, UPMC Children's Hospital of Pittsburgh, University of Pittsburgh School of Medicine, Pittsburgh, PA, USA

F. Di Rocco, J. Kestle (eds.), *Neurosurgical Aspects of Craniosynostosis*,
https://doi.org/10.1007/978-3-031-69386-1_41

across the phenotypic spectrum of SCS. As such, there is a learning curve when first incorporating SMC into practice.

Over the last 25 years, more and more craniofacial treatment centers have adopted less-invasive techniques to treat patients with sagittal craniosynostosis. The growing body of the literature demonstrates that ESC and SMC are effective alternatives to CVR. The more favorable perioperative risk profiles have led some to prefer ESC and SMC as first-line treatments. Despite the growing popularity of SMC, however, there is wide variability in technique and other factors important to surgical decision-making [3]. These issues are addressed in the following sections describing preoperative evaluation, patient selection, surgical planning, and technique variations with respect to incisions, spring implantation, and strip craniectomy.

In this chapter, we define which patients are appropriate candidates for SMC, highlight factors important for surgical decision-making, and illustrate SMC with detailed step-by-step notes.

41.2 Eligible Surgical Candidates

SMC is indicated for infants with isolated SCS prior to 6 months of age. Surgery is typically performed between 3 and 6 months of age. Children younger than 3 months are less tolerant to surgical blood loss due to the physiologic nadir of hematocrit [4]. Their relatively thin skull also makes spring use unfavorable. Surgical timing should consider gestational age; SMC is delayed for children born preterm until they are 3–6 months from the term date. Patients with contraindications at a young age (major comorbidities) or those older than 6 months of age at the time of presentation are monitored and later treated with CVR.

41.3 Patient Evaluation

Infants with suspected SCS undergo a detailed craniofacial assessment. The degree of scaphocephaly, frontal bossing, biparietal narrowing, and occipital bulleting is noted. Ridging of the sagittal suture is often present. The cephalic index is measured with calipers. It is important to perform a full history and physical examination to identify extracranial comorbidities or syndromic manifestations. Preoperative three-dimensional (3D) photographs serve as a useful baseline assessment of morphologic shape allowing for objective analysis of future cranial growth. A low-dose 3D CT scan is performed to confirm SCS, evaluate patency of other cranial sutures, evaluate bone thickness, and rule out any intracranial abnormalities.

Comprehensive evaluation should be performed by a multidisciplinary team consisting of plastic surgery, neurosurgery, ophthalmology, and genetics. Dilated ophthalmologic exam, visual-evoked potential (VEP) and/or optical coherence tomography are performed to assess for signs of elevated intracranial pressure, which are rare in infants, but provide a useful baseline for future comparisons. Routine preoperative laboratory assessment includes a complete blood cell count, electrolyte panel, type and cross-match, and prothrombin time to screen for bleeding disorders.

Parietal bone thickness of 0.5–1.5 cm from the suture line, along the strip craniectomy site, may predict perioperative outcomes. Thicker bone, but not patient age, has been reported to be associated with increased surgical blood loss, need for transfusion, and hospital length of stay [5], although this may vary based on technique.

41.4 Surgical Decision-Making

The long term goals of SMC are to (1) restore normal cranial appearance and (2) prevent future neurocognitive impairment. The technical goals are to implant springs sufficient to slowly widen the parietal bones such that cephalic index is normalized over the subsequent weeks following surgery. Surgical outcomes ultimately relate to a combination of patient age, phenotypic severity, spring characteristics, and surgical technique. While our understanding of these factors is still incomplete, we discuss considerations for surgical decision-making.

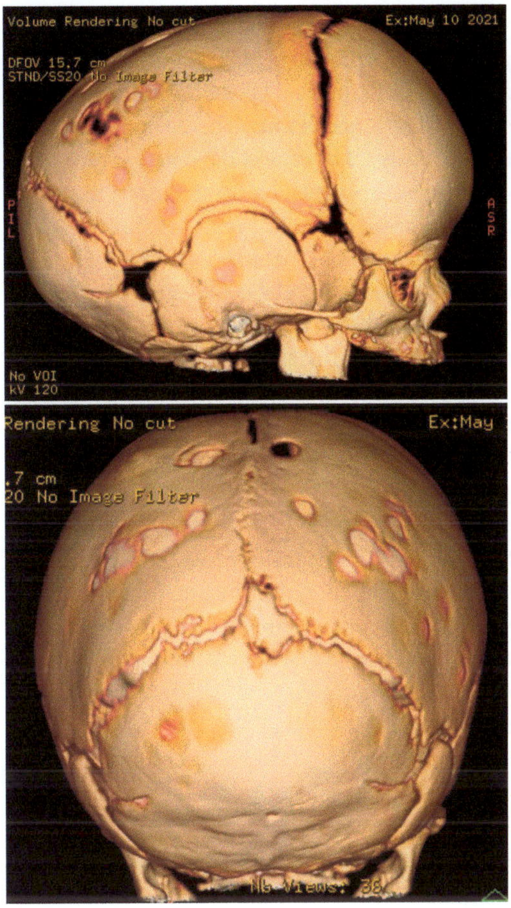

Fig. 41.1 Sagittal (**upper**) and coronal (**lower**) computerized tomography 3D bony reconstructions, highlighting both the sagittal synostosis and the bony thinning that may warrant consideration for spring placement versus postoperative helmeting

41.5 Patient Age

Many techniques typically describe performing surgery between 3 and 6 months, because treatment efficacy wanes with older age. One retrospective study reported that for every month increase in age, the change in the cephalic index decreased by 1.3 [6]. Bone thickness increases and viscoelastic compliance of the skull decreases during this time, which counterbalances the expansile forces of the springs. Implanted springs stop expanding once force equilibrium is reached against resistive forces of the skull. Patients presenting for surgery closer to 6 months of age benefit from technique modifications to increase force exerted across the craniectomy.

The most dramatic changes to the cranial shape occur over the first several weeks as the skull is actively expanded transversely. However, postoperative improvements to forehead and occiput aesthetics are observed over subsequent months, even after the springs have been removed. Bearing in mind that SMC primarily addresses the midvault in the transverse dimension, changes to the forehead and occiput rely on postoperative brain growth after brain matter is restored to its normal distribution within the transversely expanded vault. As such, it may be prudent to treat children with severe phenotypes around 3 months of age to maximize the secondary molding benefit of the brain. However, a limiting factor is that bone in younger patients is thinner, more fragile, and at risk for fracturing under the pressure from springs. Spring force should be adjusted accordingly. If preoperative CT images demonstrate especially thin bone (Fig. 41.1), the treatment team may consider postponing surgery or alternative treatment with ESC and postoperative cranial orthosis. During the informed consent process, regardless of bone thickness, parents should be informed of the possibility of intraoperative bone fracture and the need to switch to ESC with postoperative helmeting.

41.6 Spring Design

Generally, two or three U-shaped stainless steel springs are used [7–10]. Standardized, prefabricated springs are commercially available (OsteoMed SmartFlex, Acumed; Fig. 41.2). Springs exert expansile forces across the craniectomy site to slowly widen the parietal bones and, thereby, normalize cephalic index. The two most important factors for increasing CI are spring expansile force and spring excursion [10]. Indeed, while there is some minimum spring force that is required to overcome the intrinsic resistive forces of the bone and scalp, maximizing spring force may counterintuitively decrease total skull expansion. With commercially available springs, spring force is inversely proportional to arm length. Higher force springs have shorter arms and, consequently, less excursion potential when compared to lower force springs. Additionally, high-force springs increase bone contact point-

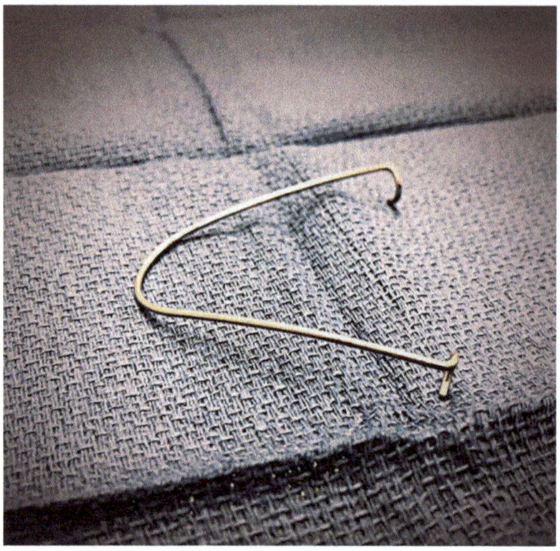

Fig. 41.2 The appearance of a typical spring. Arm length and force dynamics are factors that can be modified to fit the procedure, as discussed in the text

force and may erode through the bone rather than pushing the bone, decreasing total biparietal expansion.

Custom-made springs can be fabricated by the surgical team to modify spring characteristics. However, the biomechanical relationship between springs and cranial expansion is complex, still poorly understood, and requires further systematic clinical investigation. Nonetheless, there are several modifiable spring characteristics that impact the cumulative force translated to the parietal bones, including number of springs used, opening angle, wire thickness, spring compression, and arm length.

Generally, 2–3 springs have been used with intrinsic forces of each ranging between 5 newtons (N) and 10 N [7–10]. Posterior bone is thicker and often fitted with a larger force spring. Use of three springs enables a larger total force to be applied compared to two springs by distributing the force more gradually and reducing point-force along bone contact points. While reducing the risk of bone erosion, implanting additional springs can also be problematic due to spring overcrowding, interlocking, spring dislodgement, and undue soft tissue tension. The intrinsic force of the springs can also be modified as desired. A wider "U" bend generates greater distracting force versus a narrower bend independent of spring length. Heavier gauge wire generates even greater distracting force when compared to alterations in the spring "U" bend independent of spring length and width. The strip craniectomy can be designed to exploit the inherent properties of springs. Springs compressed to a narrower defect width (e.g., 10 versus 40 mm) exert a greater distracting force: per Hooke's law, the distraction force correlates to degree of compression at the time of implantation across the suturectomy width. Maintaining a narrow strip craniectomy is, therefore, advantageous to maximizing spring-mediated skull expansion, and we recommend keeping this width to no more than 10–15 mm.

Finally, biparietal widening can be maximized using long-arm springs because the length of the spring arm dictates the maximal spring excursion. Longer arm springs exert a slower, more uniform expansion with less initial distracting force when compared to shorter arm springs (e.g., 60 versus 40 mm), which exert an accelerated expansion initially but reach their maximal opening earlier. Thus, there is less relative expansion immediately after placement of longer springs but greater expansion in the longer term [10]. Because spring length is inversely related to force, longer springs are less likely to fracture the skull. Taking these caveats together, the greatest amount of distraction is typically achieved when utilizing multiple wide, thick, long-armed springs, and a narrow strip craniectomy width.

41.7 Operative Technique: *Spring-Mediated Cranioplasty*

41.7.1 Overview

We find that a simple, standardized approach to patient selection, strip craniectomy, and spring selection reliably corrects cephalic index by 0.1–0.15. Most children who present with a cephalic index ranging from 0.6 to 0.7 benefit from the approach described below without major modifications. Surgical timing, spring force, and spring arm length may be modified for patients with CI outside of this range.

41.7.2 Surgical Timing

Surgical timing for spring meditated cranioplasty must weigh the benefits of rapid head growth early in infancy with increasing bone integrity, and thus spring function, with age. Although SMC has been described in patients ranging from 3 to 6 months of age, in our experience, the ideal time for spring placement is 4 months of age (corrected for any prematurity). At this age, the brain growth trajectory is still rapid, but skull thickness has increased enough that springs can be placed with low concern for footplate-induced bone fractures.

41.7.3 Implants and Instrumentation

Two prefabricated 0.051″ thick stainless steel U-shaped cranial springs are selected (OsteoMed SmartFlex, Acumed). Instruments are shown in Fig. 41.3. The 30° endoscope is used with the optical dissector (Karl Storz, Germany). The fenestrated spatula at the distal end of the optical dissector retracts the scalp and prevents blood from obscuring the camera.

41.7.4 Anesthesia Considerations

Anesthesia is delivered by experienced anesthesiologists well-versed in craniofacial surgery. Two intravenous (IV) catheters are placed. One catheter delivers IV fluids and medications while the other delivers tranexamic acid (loading dose: 10 mg/kg; continuous infusion: 5 mg/kg/h) to reduce blood loss and need for transfusion [11]. Unlike more invasive open CVR procedures, early aggressive fluid resuscitation is unnecessary with meticulous hemostasis. For this reason, SMC can be safely performed without an arterial line or Foley catheter [12]. Precordial Doppler monitoring is not routinely used. Weight-based IV prophylactic antibiotics are administered. Cross-matched blood is immediately available in the operating room.

41.7.5 Patient Positioning and Preparation

The operative table is turned 180° away from the anesthesia team. While SMC can be performed with the patient positioned supine, prone positioning facilitates more efficient access to the

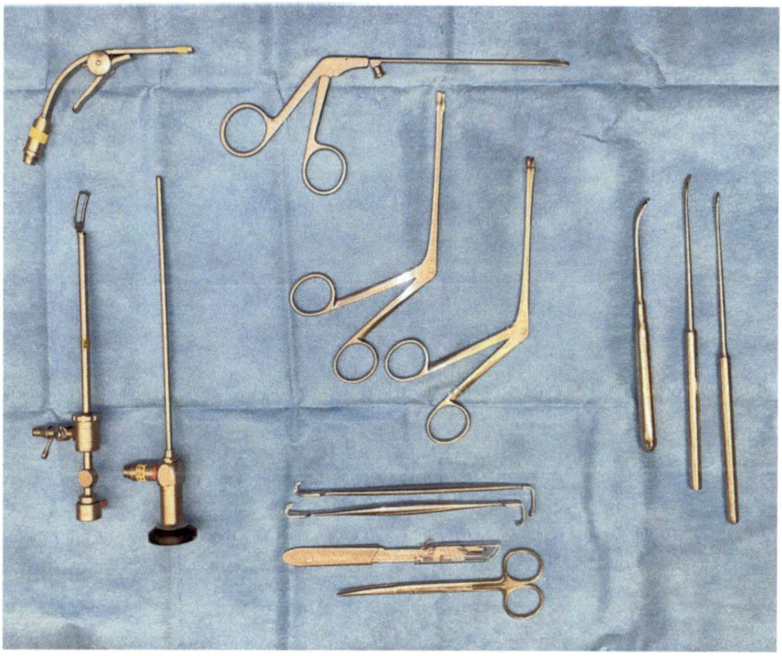

Fig. 41.3 Typical instrumentation used during the SMC procedure

mid- and posterior vault, especially in cases of severe scaphocephaly. The forehead and cheeks are padded with Reston foam to prevent pressure-indued injury of the face and orbits. The scalp is shaved, scrubbed with a chlorhexidine brush, and then infiltrated with local anesthesia (0.25% bupivacaine with epinephrine 1:200,000). The surgical field is sterilely prepped with povidone-iodine solution and draped with a craniotomy drape.

41.7.6 Scalp Incision

The anterior fontanelle and lambda are demarcated on the skin with a marking pen. A midline 2–3 cm incision is marked slightly dependent to the midpoint between the prior markings (Fig. 41.4). The scalp is incised with a #15 blade 10 min after local anesthetic injection allowing the epinephrine hemostatic effect to develop. The galea is bluntly separated from the pericranium with Metzenbaum scissors. The sagittal suture is exposed with minimal undermining creating a subgaleal tunnel between the anterior fontanel and the lambdoid sutures. A 1-cm wide strip craniectomy is demarcated by scoring the periosteum (centered on the midline) with electrocautery.

An alternative skin incision commonly used involves two transverse incisions near the anterior fontanelle and lambdoid sutures. We prefer a single vertex incision as described above to minimize scar visibility, especially in the case of males due to the possibility of a receding hairline with aging. The trade-off, however, is that endoscopic-assisted surgery can be technically more challenging. In our early experience, we found the endoscope to be unwieldy when performing the anterior strip craniectomy. The operating surgeon is forced to operate in the opposite direction of the camera (i.e., reverse alignment "mirror image" visualization). We found that by placing the 2–3 cm incision in a slightly dependent manner, we can avoid this situation without lengthening the scar or compromising surgical efficiency. The anterior bone is removed comfortably and expeditiously under direct visualization using a lighted retractor. The endoscope is often only used when performing the posterior strip craniectomy, which is straightforward because the camera faces in the same direction as the operating surgeon. For severe cases that require extensive anterior and posterior visualization, we use endoscope monitors at both the head and foot of the patient to allow normal viewing orientation in both directions.

41.7.7 Strip Craniectomy

A parasagittal burr hole is drilled while carefully avoiding the sagittal sinus. Dura is dissected free from adjacent bone with a modified Penfield 4. The craniectomy is initiated at the burr hole with a Kerrison rongeur and proceeds in the dependent direction to avoid pooling of blood in the operative field. If the patient is prone, the anterior strip craniectomy is performed first with a small rongeur and lighted retractor. Sequential dural dissection is performed as the craniectomy continues anteriorly until it is continuous with the anterior fontanelle. In cases of severe scaphocephaly, a straight Blakesley Thru-Cut forceps is used to complete the distal craniectomy.

The strip craniectomy proceeds posteriorly in similar fashion with a small rongeur and a lighted retractor until it becomes ergonomically unfavorable. The lighted retractor is exchanged for a 30° endoscope with optical dissector and attached irrigation syringe. A short-angled drill attachment (Stryker, Kalamazoo, MI) and a 4-mm coarse diamond round drill bit is used to obliterate the outer cortex (Video 41.1). The coarse diamond bit simultaneously cauterizes bone controlling hemostasis, which is particularly helpful if there is a thick midline ridge, which is common posteriorly (Fig. 41.5). A suction tip is used to protect the dura while simultaneously clearing irrigation. The inner cortex is removed with Thru-Cut forceps extending to the lambdoid sutures while also ensuring that the craniectomy width is minimal. Once the entire fused suture is removed, the parietal bones will be "unlocked" and independently mobile. Adequate mobility is confirmed by alternating manual depression of the scalp over the parietal and occipital bones

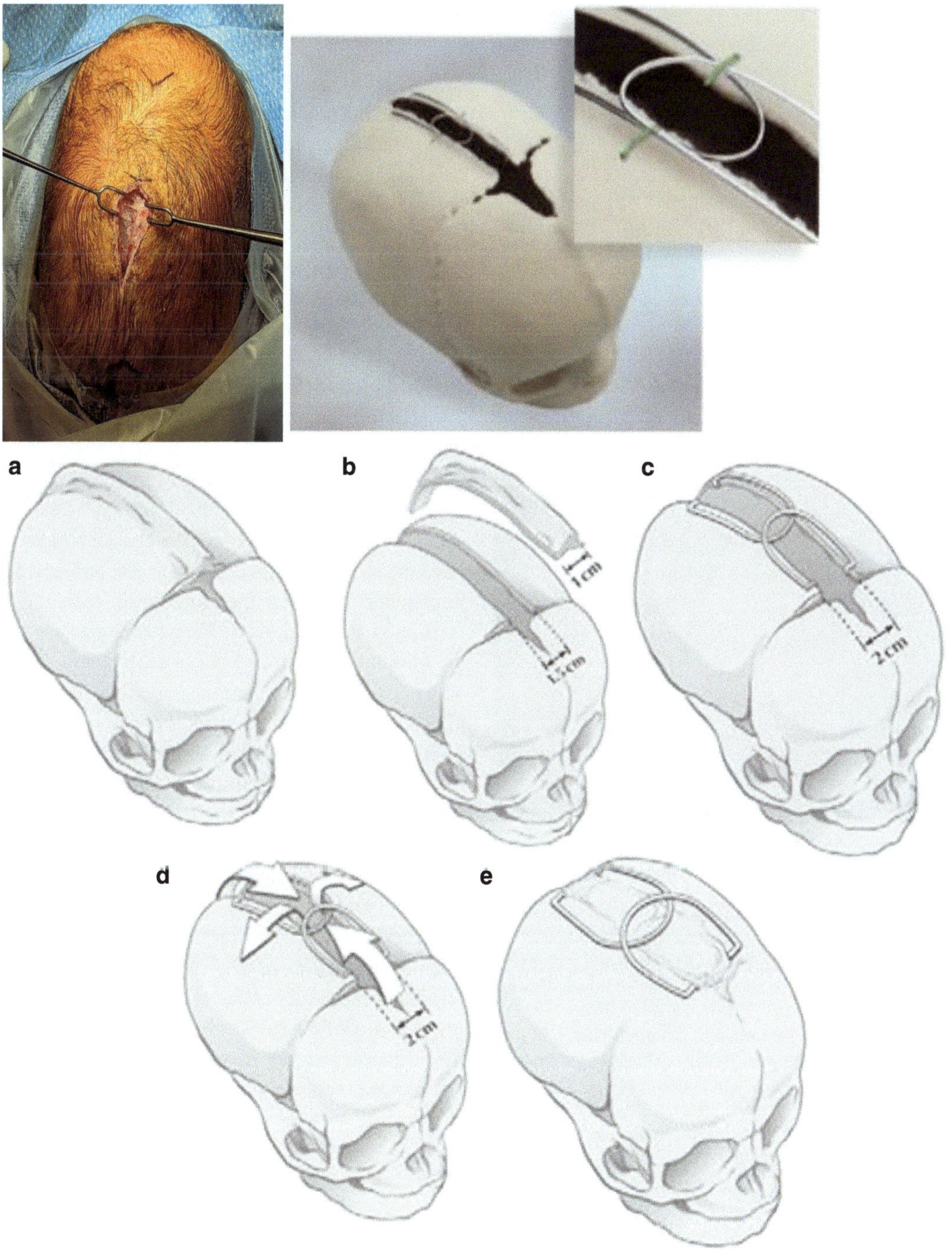

Fig. 41.4 **Upper:** The skin incision and schematic of the intended spring placement on typical procedure. **Lower:** Multistep schematic of the various steps in bone removal and spring placement and the resultant remodeling dynamics that contribute to the ultimate cranial reshaping

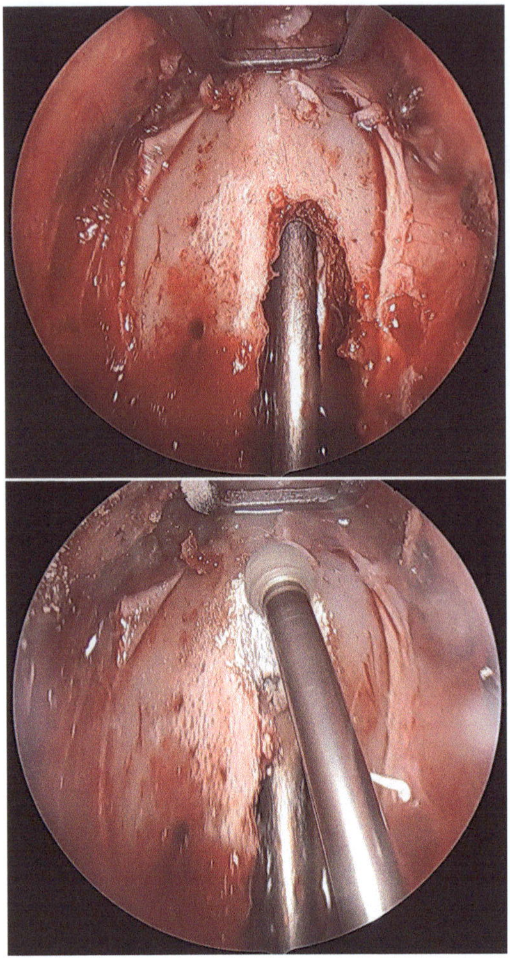

Fig. 41.5 **Upper:** Endoscopic view, showing the periosteal incision and endoscope-mediated visualization of the posterior sagittal suture. The dura is protected with a suction in preparation for additional bone removal. **Lower:** The thick midline keel is thinned down using a short-angled drill and a 4-mm coarse diamond burr, and then removed with a Thru-Cut forceps. This step is repeated until the lambdoid suture junction is reached. Right- and left-angled forceps are sometimes used to remove bone at the sagittal/lambdoid junction to obtain free mobility of posterior parietal bone plates

while simultaneously visualizing the lambdoid suture with the endoscope. If the bony plates do not move independently across the lambdoid suture, dura is dissected from the proximal lambdoid sutures and additional bone is removed until mobility is satisfactory. Hemostasis at the bone margins and the dura are obtained.

41.7.8 Spring Insertion

Two stainless steel U-shaped springs with hooked footplates are selected (0.051-inch wire diameter; OsteoMed SmartFlex, Acumed). Matched osteotomy notches are made using a 1-mm Kerrison rongeur along each margin of the strip craniectomy where the footplates will engage, approximately 1–2 cm posterior to the coronal sutures and 1–2 cm anterior to the lambdoid sutures. Springs are then prepared for implantation. For the majority of 4-month-old patients who fall within the 0.6–0.7 range of cephalic index, 7 or 7.5 Newton Smartflex springs are chosen. First, the spring opening angle is manually widened to increase the distance between the footplates to 70–75 mm from the "out-of-package" resting state of 55–65 mm. This step is critical to maximize the potential skull expansion. Second, spring implantation through the small scalp incision is facilitated by using a 4–0 Vicryl suture to secure the footplates to within 1 cm of each other (Video 41.1). The spring is positioned such that the footplates engage with the osteotomy notches and, while the dura is protected with a wide malleable, the suture is cut with scissors releasing the spring. At this point, it is important to confirm that the (1) long axis of the spring is parallel to the strip craniectomy to ensure symmetric transverse expansion of parietal bones; (2) springs are not interlocking such that one spring prevents full opening excursion of the other; and (3) spring footplates are firmly engaged with bone to prevent migration. Generally, we like to see widening of the strip craniectomy by up to 1 cm at this point. Springs are then secured to the periosteum with a 4–0 Vicryl suture on each side where springs overlap.

41.7.9 Incision Closure

The skin is closed in two layers. The galea and dermis are captured in a single pass using 3–0 Vicryl suture. Skin edges are approximated with a running subcuticular 4–0 Monocryl suture. Subgaleal drains are not used. The incision is covered with bacitracin and xeroform, and a craniofacial head wrap is placed.

41.7.10 Postoperative Monitoring

Patients are monitored for one night on a regular inpatient surgical floor. Surveillance in the intensive care unit is not necessary unless otherwise warranted by patient comorbidities. In the rare instance that a blood transfusion was required, a Complete Blood Count is collected the following morning. Four-view skull X-rays are obtained prior to discharge (Fig. 41.6). The head wrap is removed on postoperative day two at home.

The degree of cranial expansion observed 1-month postoperatively serves as a gross clinical endpoint of expansion. If long-arm springs are used, expansion may take longer (up to 2–3 months). Ongoing remodeling of frontal bossing or occipital bulleting can be clinically observed for several months, even after springs are removed.

41.8 Operative Technique: *Spring Removal*

41.8.1 Overview

Springs are removed 4 months after implantation to allow consolidation of bone. X-ray is performed to document expansion width and evaluate interpositional bone formation.

41.8.2 Patient Positioning

The surgical table is turned 180° away from the anesthesia team. The patient is positioned supine with a Mayfield head rest. The scalp is with scrubbed a chlorhexidine brush, and then infil-

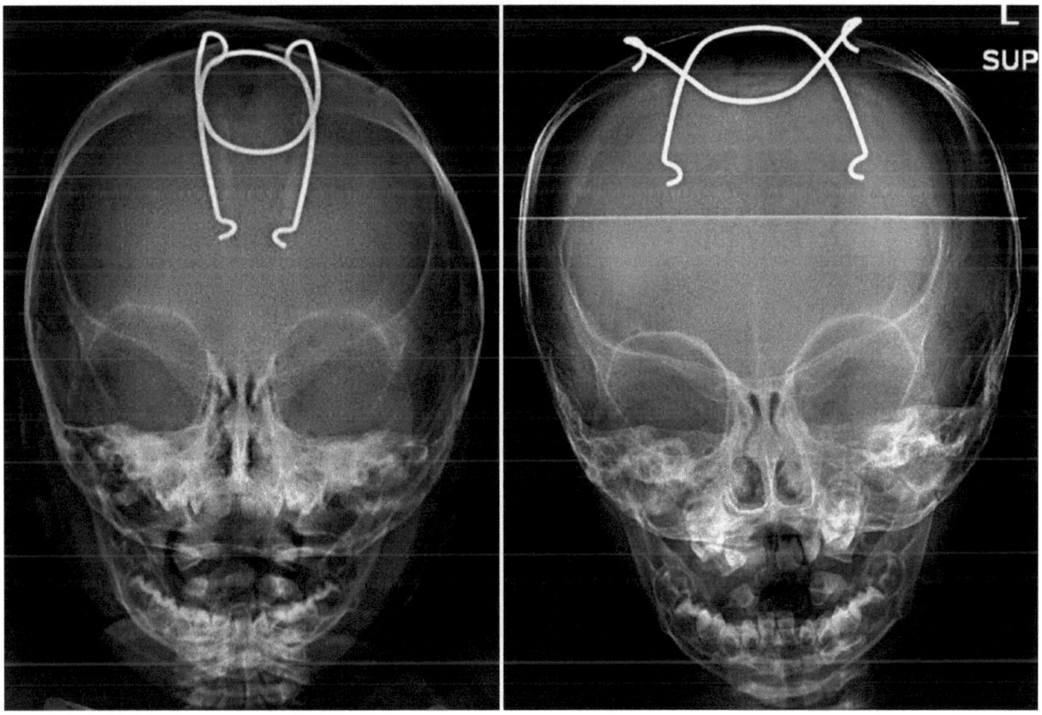

Fig. 41.6 Immediate postoperative (**left**) and 3-month follow-up (**right**) x-rays in a child who was 5-months of age at the time of surgery, illustrating the degree of spring expansion and resultant cranial expansion that can be achieved. CI has normalized from 0.69 to 0.82 during this interval

trated with local anesthesia (0.25% bupivacaine with epinephrine 1:200,000). The surgical field is sterilely prepped with povidone-iodine solution and draped with a craniotomy drape.

41.8.3 Spring Removal

The existing scalp scar has often widened due to the transverse spring forces on the soft tissues during distraction. As such, the scar is revised with full-thickness incision. Cranial springs are easily accessed through this incision. Metzenbaum scissors are used to bluntly separate the galea from the springs. The springs are freed from adherent soft tissues with an elevator. A Kirschner wire cutter is used to divide both springs at their apex. At this point, spring segments should be easily manipulated with minimal resistance from adherent soft tissues. Each segment is removed separately with a simple two-step maneuver. First, a heavy needle driver is used to rotate the spring segment in the axial plane away from midline so that the footplate is retracted from its subcranial position. Second, the spring is rotated in the coronal plane away from the midline and then removed. These steps are repeated for each leg. The incision is closed in the same manner as the initial operation. Patients are discharged home the same day.

41.9 Complications and Pitfalls

SMC is a relatively safe procedure when performed by experienced craniofacial surgeons. Nonetheless, there are potential serious complications, particularly during the midline strip craniectomy. Life-threatening bleeding is the most serious complication. Sizable bridging veins between the dura and bone may be encountered and should be addressed in controlled fashion. Wax is applied as bone is sequentially removed to minimize bleeding and the risk of air embolism. Caution must be exercised to avoid tearing as the dura is separated from overlying bone without excessive traction.

The most common complications are minor, including delayed wound healing and surgical site infection. Hardware removal or additional surgical intervention are rarely necessary. There are several potential pitfalls to avoid during spring placement. The number of springs should be minimized to avoid overcrowding, spring interlocking, undue soft tissue tension, and skin erosion. Generally, only two springs are necessary to adequately widen the skull. In severe cases, the surgeon can use longer, higher force springs and a narrower strip craniectomy to maximize expansion without adding a third spring. A third spring also increases the probability of spring dislodgement and interlocking, both of which can result in inadequate expansion. Springs should be secured to the periosteum with suture while ensuring the planes of expansion do not overlap. Spring footplates are positioned such that the long axis of the spring is parallel to the strip craniectomy defect; otherwise, asymmetric cranial expansion will occur. Finally, thin bone is less tolerant to the point-force of springs and can result in erosion of the spring through parietal bone. When excessively thin bone is noted intraoperatively, surgery is converted to strip craniectomy only followed postoperative helmet molding.

References

1. Jimenez DF, Barone CM. Endoscopic craniectomy for early surgical correction of sagittal craniosynostosis. J Neurosurg. 1998;88(1):77–81.
2. Lauritzen CGK, Davis C, Ivarsson A, Sanger C, Hewitt TD. The evolving role of springs in craniofacial surgery: the first 100 clinical cases. Plast Reconstr Surg. 2008;121(2):545–54.
3. Garland CB, Camison L, Dong SM, Mai RS, Losee JE, Goldstein JA. Variability in minimally invasive surgery for sagittal craniosynostosis. J Craniofac Surg. 2018;29(1):14–20.
4. Kates EH, Kates JS. Anemia and polycythemia in the newborn. Pediatr Rev. 2007;28(1):33–4.
5. Villavisanis DF, Cho DY, Shakir S, Kalmar CL, Wagner CS, Cheung L, et al. Parietal bone thickness for predicting operative transfusion and blood loss in patients undergoing spring-mediated cranioplasty for nonsyndromic sagittal craniosynostosis. J Neurosurg Pediatr. 2022;29(4):419–26.

6. Sun J, Ter Maaten NS, Mazzaferro DM, Wes AM, Naran S, Bartlett SP, et al. Spring-mediated cranioplasty in sagittal synostosis: does age at placement affect expansion? J Craniofac Surg. 2018;29(3):632–5.
7. David LR, Plikaitis CM, Couture D, Glazier SS, Argenta LC. Outcome analysis of our first 75 spring-assisted surgeries for scaphocephaly. J Craniofac Surg. 2010;21(1):3–9.
8. Pyle J, Glazier S, Couture D, Sanger C, Gordon S, David L. Spring-assisted surgery-a surgeon's manual for the manufacture and utilization of springs in craniofacial surgery. J Craniofac Surg. 2009;20(6):1962–8.
9. Taylor JA, Maugans TA. Comparison of spring-mediated cranioplasty to minimally invasive strip craniectomy and barrel staving for early treatment of sagittal craniosynostosis. J Craniofac Surg. 2011;22(4):1225–9.
10. Shakir S, Humphries LS, Lanni MA, Kalmar CL, Vu G, Heuer G, et al. What is the role of force in correcting scaphocephaly through spring-mediated cranial vault expansion for sagittal craniosynostosis? J Craniofac Surg. 2021;32(8):2615–20.
11. Goobie SM, Staffa SJ, Meara JG, Proctor MR, Tumolo M, Cangemi G, et al. High-dose versus low-dose tranexamic acid for paediatric craniosynostosis surgery: a double-blind randomised controlled non-inferiority trial. Br J Anaesth. 2020;125(3):336–45.
12. Ririe DG, Smith TE, Wood BC, Glazier SS, Couture DE, Argenta LC, et al. Time-dependent perioperative anesthetic management and outcomes of the first 100 consecutive cases of spring-assisted surgery for sagittal craniosynostosis. Paediatr Anaesth. 2011;21(10):1015–9.

Sagittal Suture Synostosis: Surgical Technique in Older Children

42

Scott Boop, Srinivas Susarla, Amy Lee, Hannah E. Goldstein, and Craig Birgfeld

42.1 Introduction

Sagittal craniosynostosis (SCS) is the most common type of premature cranial suture fusion, occurring in approximately 1 in 2000 people [1]. Historically, a wide variety of techniques have been used for surgical correction of this malformation, with varying degrees of success and risk to the patient depending on surgical timing, team composition and experience, and technique [2–7]. Initial correction of craniosynostosis was first described by Lane in 1892, but surgery for this fell out of favor for a time due to high complication and mortality rates owing to long surgeries and high blood loss early on. A more minimally invasive technique was developed in the form of strip craniectomy, which removed the affected suture, but frequently led to inadequate correction. In the 1960s, Paul Tessier established the first multidisciplinary craniofacial team in Paris, and was able to demonstrate effective and safe open cranial vault remodeling procedures [7].

Since this time, improvements in the surgical technique and anesthetic management have made what was once a difficult surgery with high risk into a relatively routine procedure at high-volume craniofacial centers. At Seattle Children's Hospital, the management of craniosynostosis is provided by a multidisciplinary team, with patients placed in a treatment pathway that sees them through initial consultation to eventual discharge following surgical correction [8–10]. Corrective techniques are tailored to the age and affected suture(s) of each patient [11]. For sagittal synostosis, patients younger than 9 months old are treated via a modified pi procedure; for those diagnosed after 9 months old, total cranial vault expansion is the preferred method of surgical correction.

42.2 Preoperative Evaluation

Initial diagnosis of isolated sagittal synostosis or multisuture synostosis involving the sagittal suture involves a multidisciplinary team at our institution. This team includes a pediatrician trained in craniofacial deformity and syndromes, craniofacial plastic surgeon, and pediatric neurosurgeon. When patients present with multisuture synostosis or concern for an underlying syndromic cause, the team is expanded to include geneticists, otolaryngologists, dentists, ophthalmologists, and other needed specialties.

S. Boop · S. Susarla · A. Lee (✉) · H. E. Goldstein · C. Birgfeld
Seattle Children's Hospital, University of Washington, Seattle, WA, USA
e-mail: sboop92@uw.edu; Srinivas.Susarla@seattlechildrens.org; Amy.Lee@seattlechildrens.org; hannah.goldstein@seattlechildrens.org; craig.birgfeld@seattlechildrens.org

F. Di Rocco, J. Kestle (eds.), *Neurosurgical Aspects of Craniosynostosis*, https://doi.org/10.1007/978-3-031-69386-1_42

Diagnosis is typically made by physical examination by the primary craniofacial team and confirmed by preoperative CT scan with 3D reconstructions. This aids in diagnosis as well as in reconstruction planning, and serves as a baseline to assess morphologic calvarial change longitudinally. Preoperatively, consultation with an experienced anesthesia team is of utmost importance. During this consultation, the team reviews family and medical history, physical exam, and a thorough preop laboratory workup is performed as well as discussion of anesthetic risks. Critical preoperative lab workup includes CBC, CMP, analysis of coagulation status, and preoperative type and screen for transfusion planning.

42.3 Intraoperative Considerations

Operating room set up is an important consideration for streamlining these surgeries. The OR team consists of a pediatric anesthesiologist who is a member of the craniofacial group, typically a fellow, resident, or CNA under their supervision, a craniofacial plastic surgeon and pediatric neurosurgeon and their respective assistants, a surgical scrub nurse with experience in these procedures, and one to two circulator nurses. Patients are brought in under the care of the pediatric anesthesia team. After induction, IV access is obtained with two large bore peripheral catheters as well as an arterial line for continuous BP monitoring. An endotracheal tube is placed (in those patients with syndromic conditions and other craniofacial anomalies, often via fiberoptic intubation) and secured with a silk circum-mandibular suture. A continuous end tidal CO2 monitor is placed as well as a precordial Doppler to monitor for air embolism during the case. All pressure points are padded. Appropriate preoperative antibiotics are infused and redosed at appropriate intervals throughout the case. For cases of isolated sagittal synostosis, patients are typically positioned prone with the head resting on a Mayfield horseshoe headrest in order to facilitate middle and posterior vault expansion. However, depending on which other sutures are affected and based on the preoperative plan made by the reconstructive team, supine positioning may be necessary (i.e., if patients also require fronto-orbital advancement or another form of anterior/middle vault expansion). Padding around the face and eyes is placed, and a precordial Doppler is secured in place and padded prior to flipping the patient over.

The head of the bed is turned 90 degrees with the surgical team at the head, anesthesia and scrub technician on either side of the bed, and bulky equipment (suction towers, etc.) at the foot. Hyperventilation is typically initiated to reduce intracranial pressure prior to the start of the case. Cross-matched packed red blood cells and fresh frozen plasma are available in the room prior to incision. Unless otherwise indicated, transfusion of the first units of pRBCs and FFP is initiated around the time the first burr hole is placed for intracranial access. Further blood product administration is based on the anesthesia team's careful monitoring of vital signs, serial hematocrits, and other indicated labs. Intraoperative autotransfusion is typically not utilized at our institution given prior studies showing minimal benefit [12]. Intraoperative steroids are typically used for nausea control by the anesthesia team but are typically not required for specific intracranial effects. Tranexamic acid is routinely used at our institution for open cranial vault remodeling.

The head is fully shaved prior to positioning and corneal protectors placed. A coronal incision is marked out in a zig zag pattern in order to reduce tension on the scalp wound and camouflage the future scar (Fig. 42.1). The incision is infiltrated with local anesthetic. The patient is prepped and draped in sterile fashion with the entire head, face, and ears visible. The scalp is reflected in the subperiosteal plane using a combination of monopolar cautery and blunt/sharp dissection. The anterior flap includes the temporalis muscle, the posterior flap is dissected laterally past the squamosal sutures (Fig. 42.2a). Following exposure, the outline of the craniec-

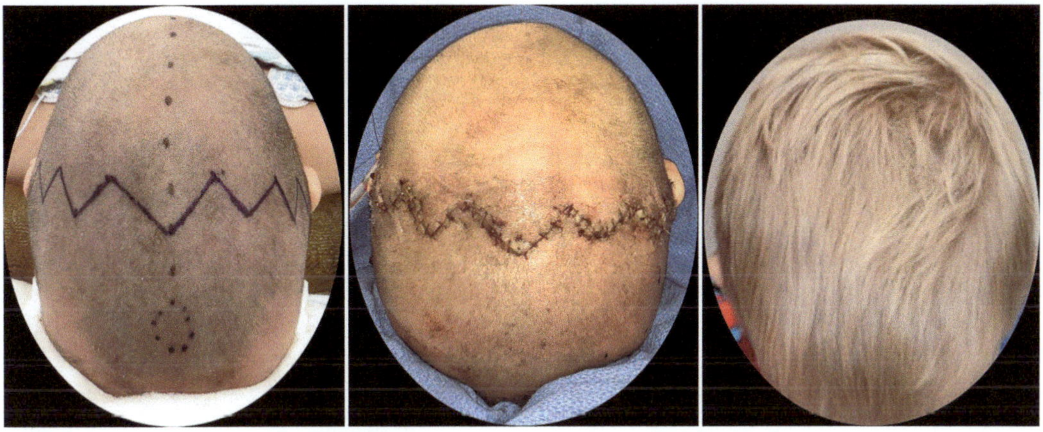

Fig. 42.1 A zig-zag coronal incision is our preferred approach for exposure (left). The zig zag incision facilitates easy closure (middle image) results in a less conspicuous scar after healing (right)

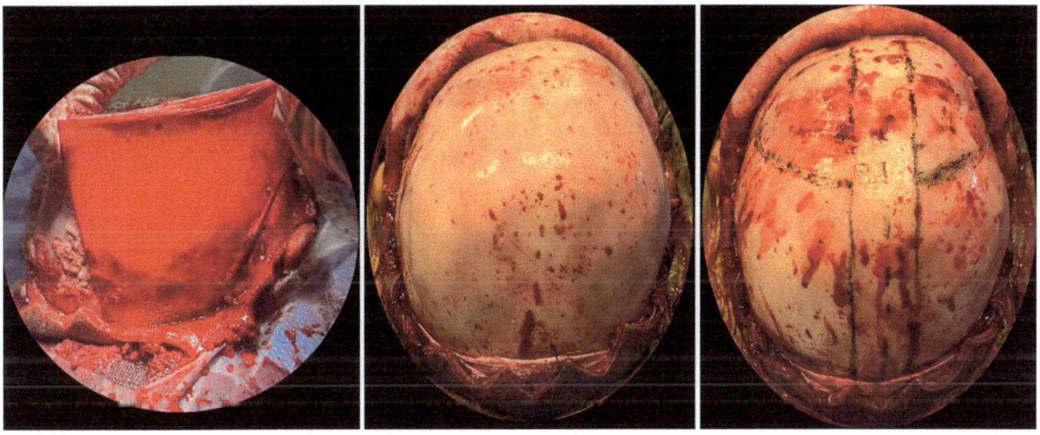

Fig. 42.2 Initial exposure is completed in the subpericranial plane. A pericranial flap (left) can be developed as a separate layer if needed (e.g., to cover shunt hardware). The skull exposure is completed 2 cm anterior to the coronal sutures, just past the squamosal sutures laterally, and just past the external occipital protuberance posteriorly (middle). Once the exposure is completed, the craniotomies are marked using a sterile pencil (right). The craniotomy patterns are based upon the morphology to be treated, but typically include parietal and occipital cuts, as well as liberation of the central strip containing the fused sagittal suture

tomies is drawn onto the bone using pencil (Fig. 42.2b). The neurosurgery team then undertakes burr hole craniotomy for intracranial access.

Burr holes are placed with an acorn drill bit parasagittally along the marked strip of bone, typically three per side. These are then widened with a Kerrison rongeur until a Penfield #3 can be used for epidural dissection. Two additional burr holes are made on each side laterally in the parietal bones. Following this, the acorn is swapped for a craniotome drill bit to complete the parasagittal cuts along the marked lines. Throughout this portion, the dura is protected under direct visualization. The dura is stripped from the lambdoid sutures bilaterally as well as the occipital bones. Wing osteotomies are made to remove the occipital bones and the prior marked cuts are used to remove the parietal bones bilaterally as well. Careful dissection is used to free the midline sagittal strip of bone from the underlying dura, taking care to protect the sagittal sinus underneath. Depending on the degree of correction needed, the sagittal bone strip is either removed as well or can be reshaped in situ using a Tessier rib bender. The dura is thoroughly checked for any defects that might require repair, and these are addressed in the appropriate fashion (Fig. 42.3a). At this point, the craniofacial plastic surgery team proceeds with the reconstruction.

Reconstruction is achieved primarily off the surgical field on a back table. The removed segments of the skull are reshaped using a combination of radial osteotomies with a reciprocating saw for aggressive out-fracturing or the Tessier rib bender for more gradual correction. Prior to reshaping them, a particulate bone is harvested from the endocranial surface with a cortical bone scraper. The ultimate goal of recontouring is to achieve satisfactory biparietal widening, occipital flattening, increase in vertex height, and shortening of AP dimension. Once this is complete, the bone is secured in situ using a combination of resorbable plates (KLS Martin SonicWeld®, Jacksonville, FL) laterally and 3–0 PDS suture medially (Fig. 42.4). After thorough irrigation, the harvested cortical bone particulates are mixed with fibrin sealant and interposed in the gaps created by the expansion. Throughout the procedure, hemostasis is achieved using a combi-

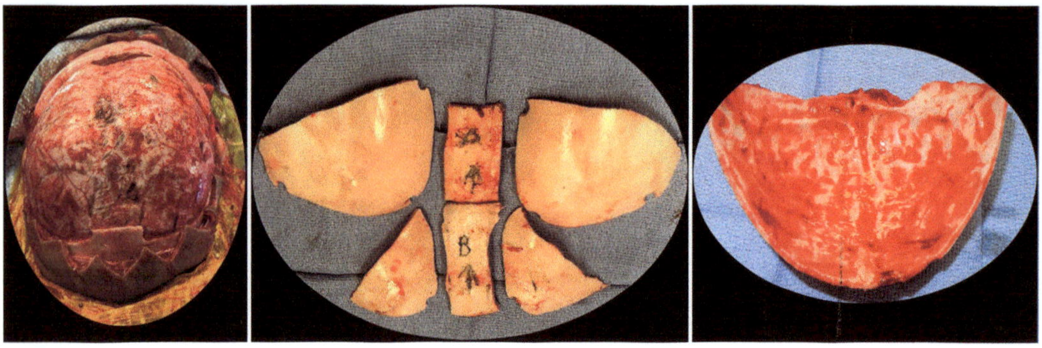

Fig. 42.3 Bur holes are drilled and a complete epidural dissection is completed. The craniotomies are then completed and the bone flaps removed. The dura is then inspected to verify its integrity (left). The bone flaps (middle) are then taken to the back table for contouring. It is not uncommon to see evidence of intracranial hypertension, such as thumbprinting of the bone flaps (right)

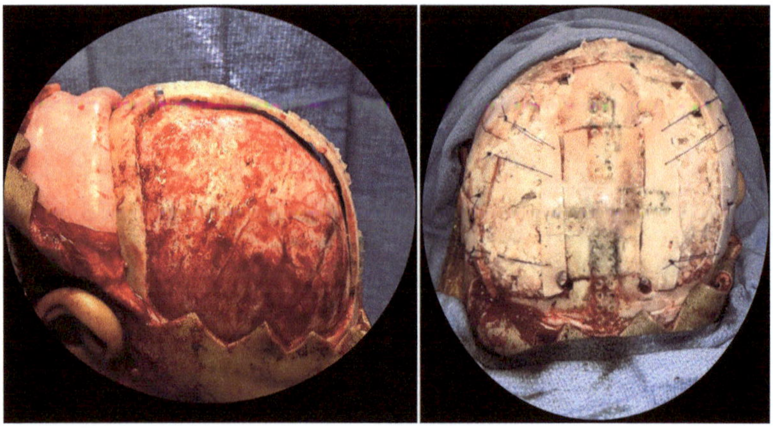

Fig. 42.4 (Left) Central strip recontouring to achieve appropriate vertex position and height, (right) parietal and occipital bone flaps are contoured by creating radial osteotomies and bending the done using rib benders. They are then affixed using resorbable plates and sutures. The interpositional gaps created by the expansion are filled with cortical and particulate bone graft mixed with fibrin sealant. No exposed dura should remain following grafting

nation of bone wax (particularly important during the initial scalp flap advancement to stop bleeding from the calvarium), gel foam and sponges soaked in thrombin, and liquid gel foam (applied liberally to the dura to prevent microhemorrhages).

Once reconstruction is complete, hemostasis is again verified and a drain is placed. Typically, a single flat Jackson Pratt drain is placed subgaleally in the posterior aspect of the wound bed and tunneled out behind the ear and secured with suture. The team then turns their attention to closure, with a typical layered scalp closure that reapproximates the galea in interrupted fashion and then the skin with running absorbable suture (Fig. 42.1b). Following this, the scalp is examined to ensure adequate vascularization. Should excessive tension on the scalp be a concern, regular slashes in the galea can be made in order to provide scalp advancement, which may be more of a concern in older children. The skin is cleaned and dried and antibiotic ointment liberally applied to the incision . The patient is the carefully repositioned supine and turned over to the anesthesia team for extubation following removal of the suture securing the ET tube. Occasionally, at the discretion of the anesthesia team depending on procedure length and patient anesthetic tolerance, extubation may be deferred immediately postop.

42.4 Postoperative Care

Following extubation, the patient is taken by the anesthesia and surgical teams for an immediate postoperative head CT (Fig. 42.5), again with 3D reconstructions included. This serves the dual purpose of ensuring that there are no immediate postoperative concerns regarding hematoma formation or intradural injury and serves as a new baseline for longitudinal assessment of calvarial remodeling. The patient

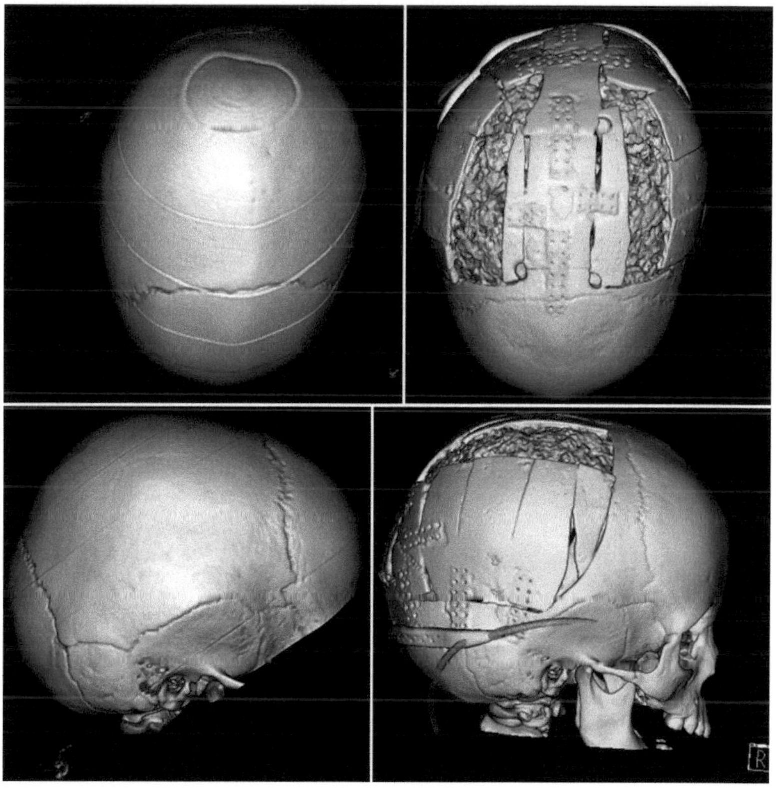

Fig. 42.5 (Left) Preoperative imaging demonstrating sagittal craniosynostosis with biparietal narrowing and occipital constriction. (Right) Postoperative appearance after open cranial vault expansion with parietal and occipital craniotomies, reshaping using radial osteotomies, central strip recontouring to achieve appropriate vertex height, and placement of calvarial bone graft into interpositional defects

is then transferred to the pediatric ICU for close monitoring and further resuscitation if needed.

There exists at our institution as part of the surgical pathway for craniosynostosis patients a standardized postoperative order set [10]. This includes immediate postoperative CBC, INR, PT, PTT, fibrinogen level, and electrolyte panel. Patients with hematocrits less than 25 postoperatively receive further blood products in the unit. CBC is further checked following additional transfusion and the morning of POD 1. JP drain output is carefully monitored, and the surgical team is alerted for outputs greater than 50 cc/h for the first 2 h, then 100 cc/h following this initial interval, which may indicate an active bleeding process that may require surgical intervention. Continuous pulse oximetry is performed while in the PICU, which may help to detect rare delayed venous sinus embolism. Continuous isotonic IV fluids are administered until the patient can tolerate sufficient PO intake, which is encouraged as soon as possible following the operation. The head of bed is adjusted initially to 30 degrees to promote resolution of postoperative facial and scalp edema. Perioperative antibiotics are continued for 24 h postop, and pain is closely monitored and controlled using IV and PO medications. NSAIDs are typically avoided within the first 24-h postoperatively, and a scheduled postoperative bowel medication regimen is implemented.

Following 24 h of ICU monitoring, as long as there are no contraindications, the patients are transferred to an acute care surgical ward. Patients remain in the hospital until their JP drains are removed (typically once outputs at <20 cc per day), their pain is controlled on a PO regimen and they are tolerating feeds without bowel/bladder issues, and their postoperative periorbital edema has improved to the point where they are able to open one or more eyes. Typical length of stay is usually 3–4 days in uncomplicated cases. Antibiotic ointment is applied to the incision twice a day for a total of 7 days postoperatively. No helmets are provided either for protection or remodeling in cases of total vault reconstruction.

Longer term, the patients return for a 2–4-week postoperative wound check. If no immediate issues are identified, they will then follow-up at a 1-year interval with a repeat 3D reconstructed CT scan at 2-years postoperatively (Fig. 42.6). At this point, several issues are evaluated, including skull shape and contour, presence of large (>3 × 3 cm) calvarial defects, issues with scar formation/healing, and any other concerns for an underlying syndromic cause that might require further genetic testing if not already performed. Assuming that there are no issues identified that might require surgical revision, patients then have further follow-up with serial imaging at 2-years postop, and at 5–6 years of age [10].

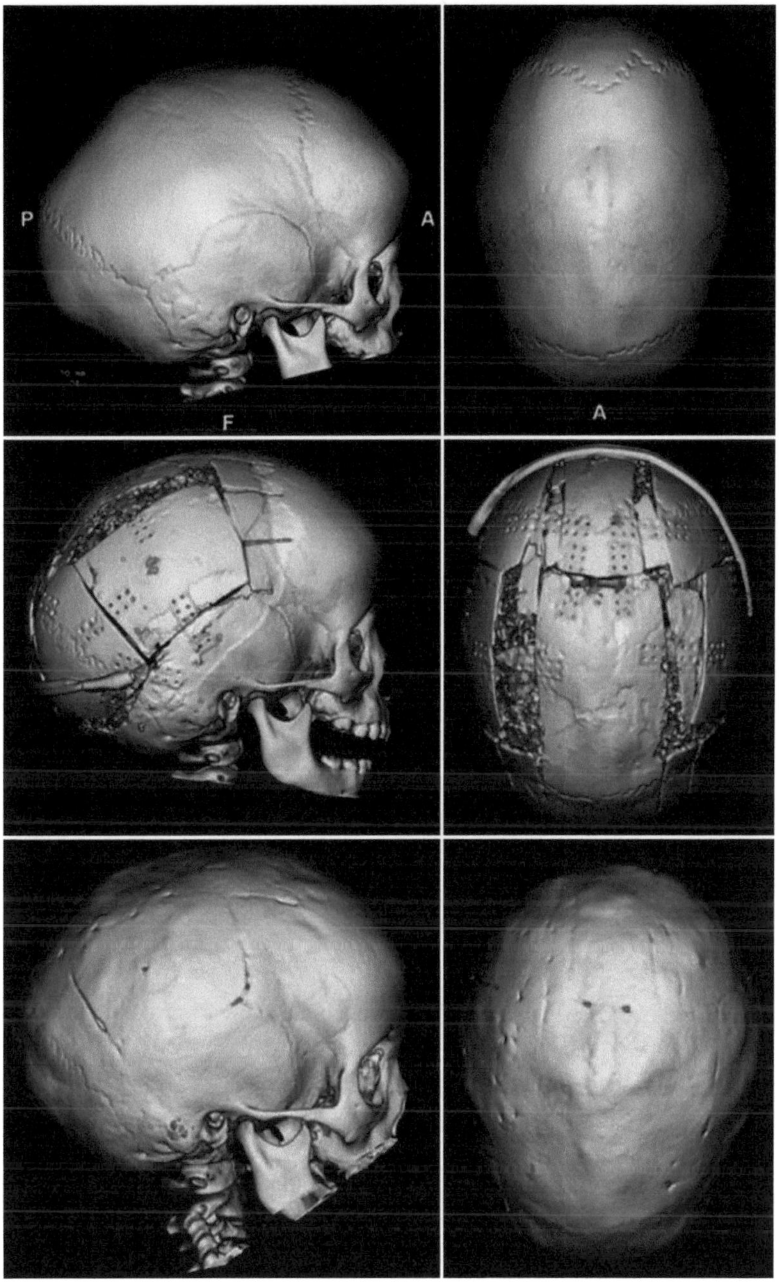

Fig. 42.6 Preoperative (top), immediate postoperative (middle) and 2-years postoperative (bottom) three-dimensional computed tomographic images for a patient treated at 2 years of age for sagittal craniosynostosis

References

1. Baker CM, Ravindra VM, Gociman B, Siddiqi FA, Goldstein JA, Smyth MD, Lee A, Anderson RCE, Patel KB, Birgfeld C, Pollack IF, Imahiyerobo T, Kestle JRW, for the Synostosis Research Group. Management of sagittal synostosis in the synostosis research group: baseline data and early outcomes. Neurosurg Focus. 2021;50(4):E3.
2. Maugans TA, McComb JG, Levy ML. Surgical management of sagittal synostosis: a comparative analysis of strip craniectomy and calvarial vault remodeling. Pediatr Neurosurg. 1997;27(3):137–48. https://doi.org/10.1159/000121241.
3. Dlouhy BJ, Nguyen DC, Patel KB, Hoben GM, Skolnick GB, Naidoo SD, Woo AS, Smyth MD. Endoscope-assisted management of sagittal synostosis: wide vertex suturectomy and barrel stave osteotomies versus narrow vertex suturectomy. J Neurosurg Pediatr. 2016;25(6):674–8. https://doi.org/10.3171/2016.6.PEDS1623. Epub 2016 Sep 9. PMID: 27611899; PMCID: PMC5333556
4. Smyth MD, Tenenbaum MJ, Kaufman CB, Kane AA. The "clamshell" craniotomy technique in treating sagittal craniosynostosis in older children. J Neurosurg. 2006;105(4 Suppl):245–51. https://doi.org/10.3171/ped.2006.105.4.245.
5. McComb JG. Occipital reduction-biparietal widening technique for correction of sagittal synostosis. Pediatr Neurosurg. 1994;20(1):99–106. https://doi.org/10.1159/000120772.
6. Mackenzie KA, Davis C, Yang A, MacFarlane MR. Evolution of surgery for sagittal synostosis: the role of new technologies. J Craniofac Surg. 2009;20(1):129–33. https://doi.org/10.1097/SCS.0b013e318190e1cf.
7. Kyutoku S, Inagaki T. Review of past reports and current concepts of surgical management for craniosynostosis. Neurol Med Chir (Tokyo). 2017;57(5):217–24. https://doi.org/10.2176/nmc.ra.2017-0006.
8. Forrest CR, Hopper RA. Craniofacial syndromes and surgery. Plastic Reconstr Surg. 2013;131(1):86e–109e. https://doi.org/10.1097/PRS.0b013e318272c12b.
9. Birgfeld CB, Dufton L, Naumann H, et al. Safety of open cranial vault surgery for single-suture craniosynostosis: a case for the multidisciplinary team. J Craniofac Surg. 2015;26(7):2052–8. https://doi.org/10.1097/SCS.0000000000001940.
10. Seattle Children's Hospital, Birgfeld C, Heike C, Herrman A, Popalisky J, Turner A. Craniosynostosis Pathway. March 2019. http://www.seattlechildrens.org/pdf/craniosynostosis-pathway.pdf.
11. Weinzweig J, Baker SB, Whitaker LA, Sutton LN, Bartlett SP. Delayed cranial vault reconstruction for sagittal synostosis in older children: an algorithm for tailoring the reconstructive approach to the craniofacial deformity. Plast Reconstr Surg. 2002;110(2):397–408. https://doi.org/10.1097/00006534-200208000-00003.
12. Deva AK, Hopper RA, Landecker A, Flores R, Weiner H, McCarthy JG. The use of intraoperative autotransfusion during cranial vault remodeling for craniosynostosis. Plast Reconstr Surg. 2002;109(1):58–63. https://doi.org/10.1097/00006534-200201000-00010.

Metopic Suture Synostosis: Endoscopic Approach, Key Points for the Neurosurgeons

43

Yusuke S. Hori and Mark R. Proctor

43.1 Background

Children with pathologic metopic craniosynostosis present with a characteristic head shape known as trigonocephaly. This needs to be distinguished from normal early closure of the metopic suture, as it closes in many normal babies by 3 months of age, with either no sequelae or just a simple ridge associated with a normal forehead shape, which does not require treatment. To date, studies have not shown a clear association between severity of trigonocephaly and cognitive development [1], although several reports have shown that patients with metopic synostosis and associated trigonocephaly may develop cognitive impairment and behavioral disturbances [2, 3]. As a definitive treatment, surgical correction is recommended not only to improve appearance, but also because it has the potential to improve the neurodevelopmental outcomes, although the data on this latter point remains unclear [4].

The mainstay of the surgical treatment has been open surgery near the maturation of skull shape development in the range of 8–12 months, at which point, trigonocephaly correction requires a fairly extensive and invasive procedure [5]. Endoscope-assisted repair was introduced in the early 2000s, and studies have shown its safety and effectiveness [6–8]. Jimenez et al. have reported the largest case series with the mean estimated blood loss of 35 mL, mean operative time of 56 minutes, and the total transfusion rate of 4.3% [7]. Lajthia et al. have reported the effectiveness of this procedure in patients with severe trigonocephaly [8]. Furthermore, several studies have shown the comparative results of open vs. endoscope-assisted repair [9–11]. The results have demonstrated that endoscopic repair had significant better perioperative outcomes including estimated blood loss, transfusion rate, operative time, and hospital LOS [9, 10], while maintaining comparable postoperative morphological results [11].

43.2 Institutional Experience at Boston Children's Hospital

In our institution, we introduced endoscope-assisted metopic craniosynostosis repair in 2006, and since then, over 130 cases have been treated with this minimally invasive technique. The cumulative results have shown its effectiveness in both safety and cosmetic outcome. As a brief summary, our institutional data showed the mean age was 14 weeks at the time of treatment with the mean weight of 6 kg. Approximately 80% of the patients were male and 20% were female, similar to other large series [7]. Perioperatively,

Y. S. Hori · M. R. Proctor (✉)
Department of Neurological Surgery, Boston Children's Hospital, Harvard Medical School, Boston, MA, USA
e-mail: Yusuke.Hori@childrens.harvard.edu; Mark.Proctor@childrens.harvard.edu

F. Di Rocco, J. Kestle (eds.), *Neurosurgical Aspects of Craniosynostosis*,
https://doi.org/10.1007/978-3-031-69386-1_43

the transfusion rate for the last 10 years was 6.7%, also comparable to the previously reported rate [7]. Postoperatively, no patients experienced recurrence of metopic synostosis requiring operative repair, with one minor revision for a bony prominence that was drilled down for cosmetic reasons.

43.3 Procedure

Our preferred age for treatment is 10–12 weeks, with a minimum weight of 5 kg. We do not routinely obtain preoperative imaging, although many patients present to our clinic with a CT scan, and on rare occasions, we obtain one if there is question of a syndromic diagnosis. The patient is taken to the operating room and two intravenous (IV) lines and routine cardiorespiratory monitors are placed. General endotracheal anesthesia is employed. We do not routinely use an a-line, but often employ tranexamic acid to aid with hemostasis. Precordial doppler to monitor for air embolism is routinely employed. A baseline blood specimen is obtained to assess the hematocrit and hemoglobin, which is repeated at the end of the case to assess the blood loss. The patient is placed in a spine position, and the fused metopic suture is confirmed by palpation for surgical planning. The incision is outlined, directly at the hairline, and then, hair is clipped (Fig. 43.1a). Sterile prep is performed with betadine scrub and paint. Standard surgical drapes are applied (Fig. 43.1b). A single dose of antibiotics is administered 30 min prior to the incision, and cefazolin is our preferred antibiotic.

After surgical time-out, local injection is performed using bupivacaine with epinephrine (Fig. 43.2a). A small 5-mm incision is placed at the edge of the preplanned incision site with a 15 blade surgical scalpel (Fig. 43.2b). The incision is extended with a platinum tipped microdissection needle to open in a bloodless fashion while minimizing skin injury (Fig. 43.2c). The deeper layer is then explored while preserving as much periosteum as possible (Fig. 43.2d), as it seems helpful to minimize soft tissue disruption. The planned burr hole site is cauterized at the midline, with further dissection performed under the periosteum, which is elevated with a retractor. A small midline burr hole is carefully created using the high-speed drill (Fig. 43.3a and b), and then expanded with curettes and Kerrison rongeurs until an approximately 1 cm gap is achieved.

At this point, suture removal is directed towards the anterior fontanelle using the rongeur, and a dissector is used to strip the perios-

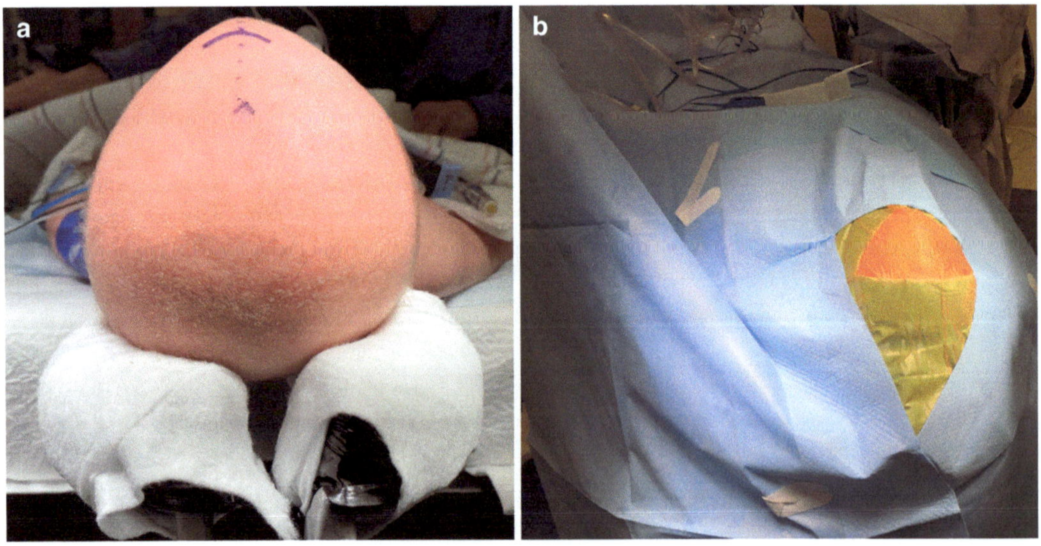

Fig. 43.1 Presurgical preparation. Incision is outlined (**a**) and standard surgical drapes are applied (**b**)

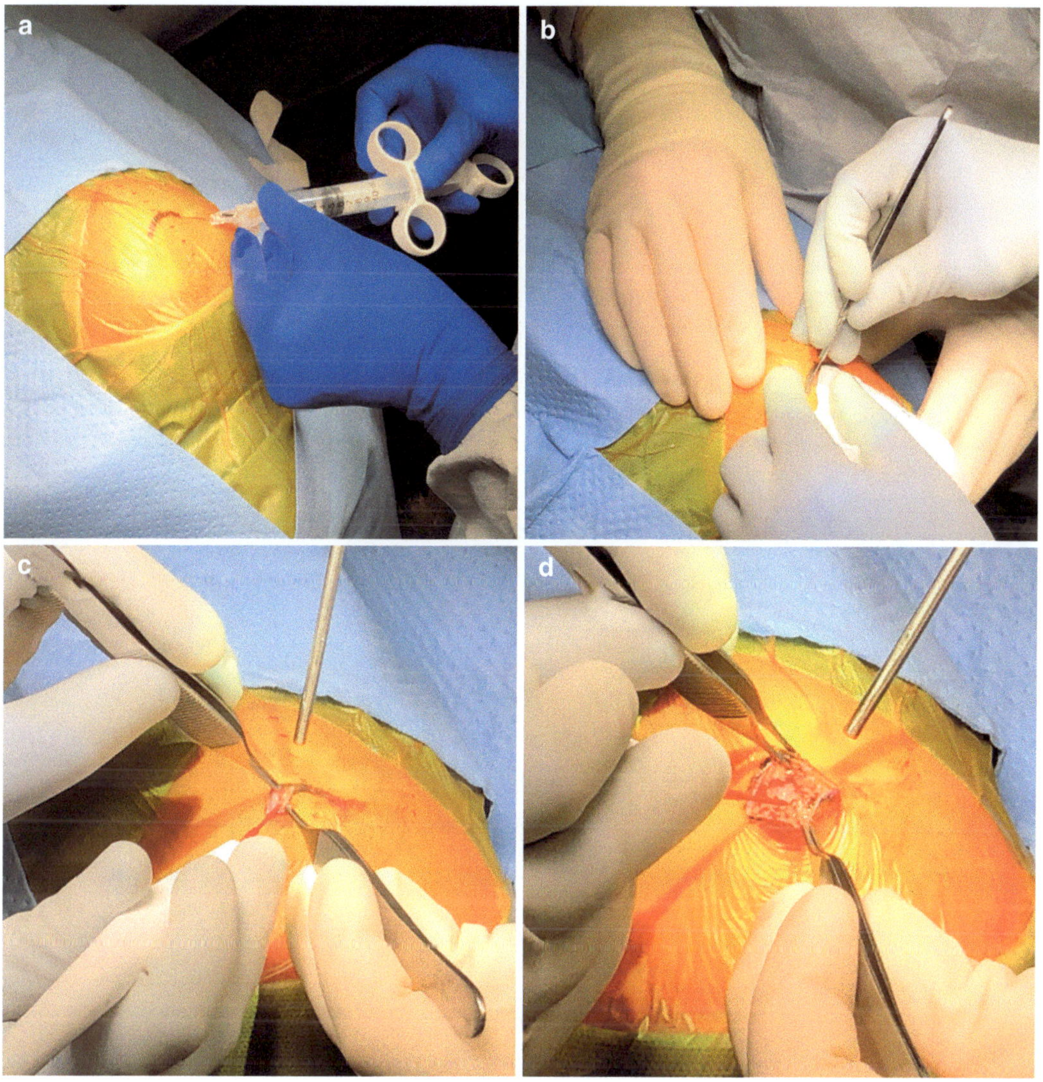

Fig. 43.2 Local injection with bupivacaine with epinephrine (**a**). A 5-mm incision is placed (**b**) extended with a platinum tipped microdissection needle (**c**). Deeper layer is then explored while preserving periosteum (**d**)

teum off the external surface of the bone to the fontanelle (Fig. 43.4a). A zero-degree endoscope is introduced to help dissect the dura off the undersurface of the bone (Fig. 43.4b). After confirming that we have reached the anterior fontanelle and the dura is sufficiently stripped, bone-cutting scissors are used to complete the strip craniectomy extending to the fontanelle (Fig. 43.4c–e).

Once the superior portion of the bone is removed, the suture removal is next directed towards the inferior portion. Similar to the superior site, the periosteum and dura are stripped off the undersurface of the bone with a Penfield 1 dissector. Bone is initially removed with a Kerrison rongeur, but as one dissects inferiorly the bone rapidly becomes quite thickened (Fig. 43.5a) in most children and is not easily amenable to cut-

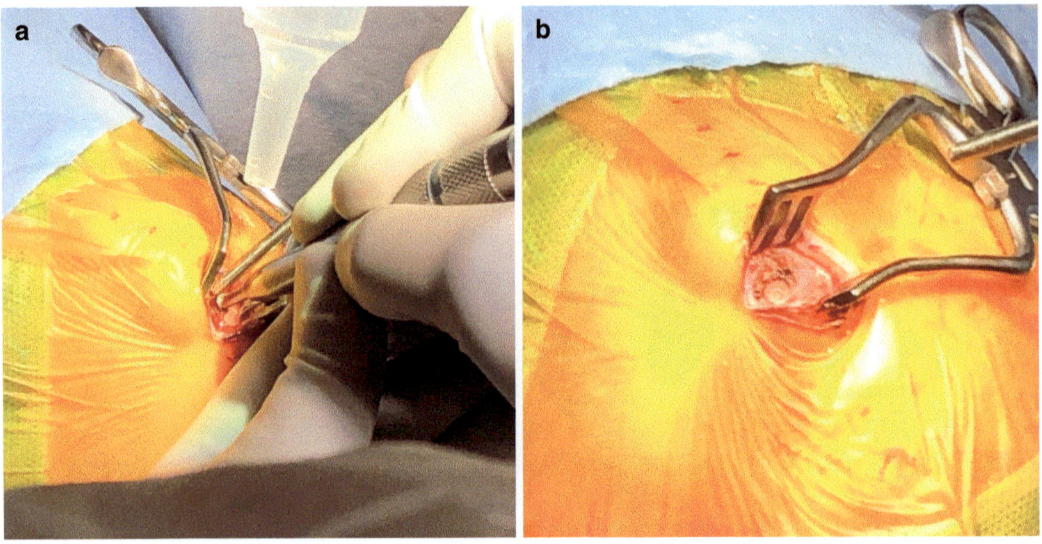

Fig. 43.3 A small burr hole is created using the high-speed drill (**a**). A tiny dural exposure is observed at the center of the hole (**b**)

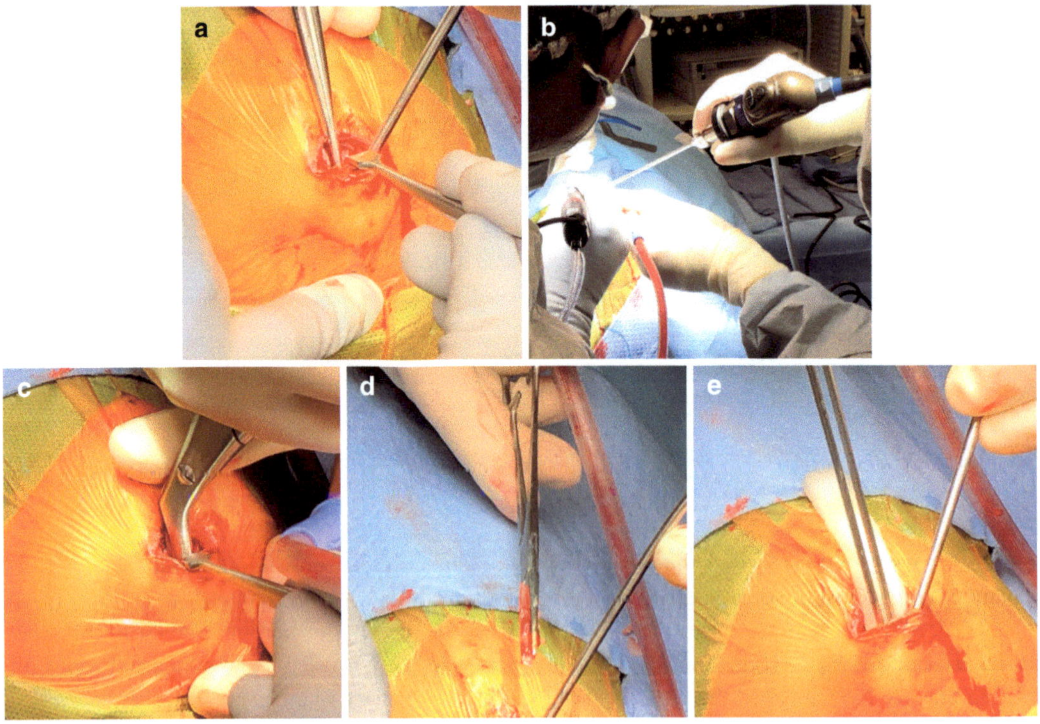

Fig. 43.4 Stripping the periosteum off the external surface of the bone using dissector (**a**). A zero-degree endoscope is introduced to help dissect the dura (**b**). Bone-cutting scissors (**c**) are used to complete the strip craniectomy (**d**). Absorbable gelatin sponges are placed along the removed suture (**e**)

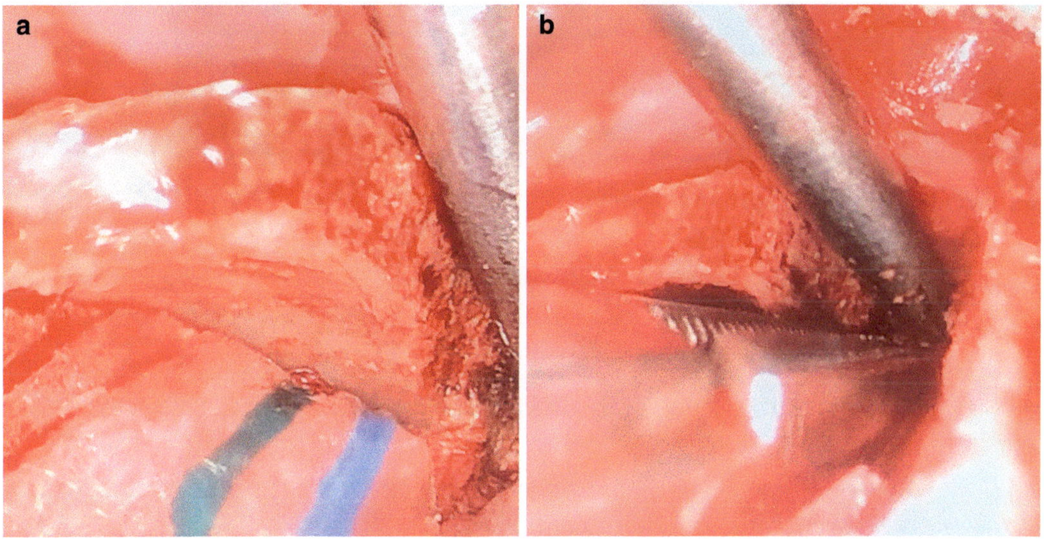

Fig. 43.5 Thickened bone is typically observed inferiorly (**a**) and an endoscope-assisted ultrasonic bone aspirator is used to dissolve the bone all the way down to the nasofrontal junction (**b**)

ting with scissors. After careful dissection and coagulation of the midline emissary views, usually one on either side of center, an ultrasonic bone aspirator is used to dissolve the bone all the way down to the nasofrontal junction (Fig. 43.5b). At the completion, the surgeon should confirm that the two frontal bones are completely disconnected by physically moving them and being sure they move independently (Fig. 43.6a). At the completion, a gap between the frontal bones is observed with a width of approximately 1 cm.

Absorbable gelatin sponges are placed along the removed suture to help hemostasis. The wound is meticulously irrigated with bacitracin or betadine, along with saline (Fig. 43.6b). After confirming hemostasis, the incision is closed in subcutaneous (Fig. 43.6c) and skin (Fig. 43.6d) layers with absorbable sutures. A sterile dressing and a pressure wrap are applied. The patient is transferred to the anesthesia recovery room.

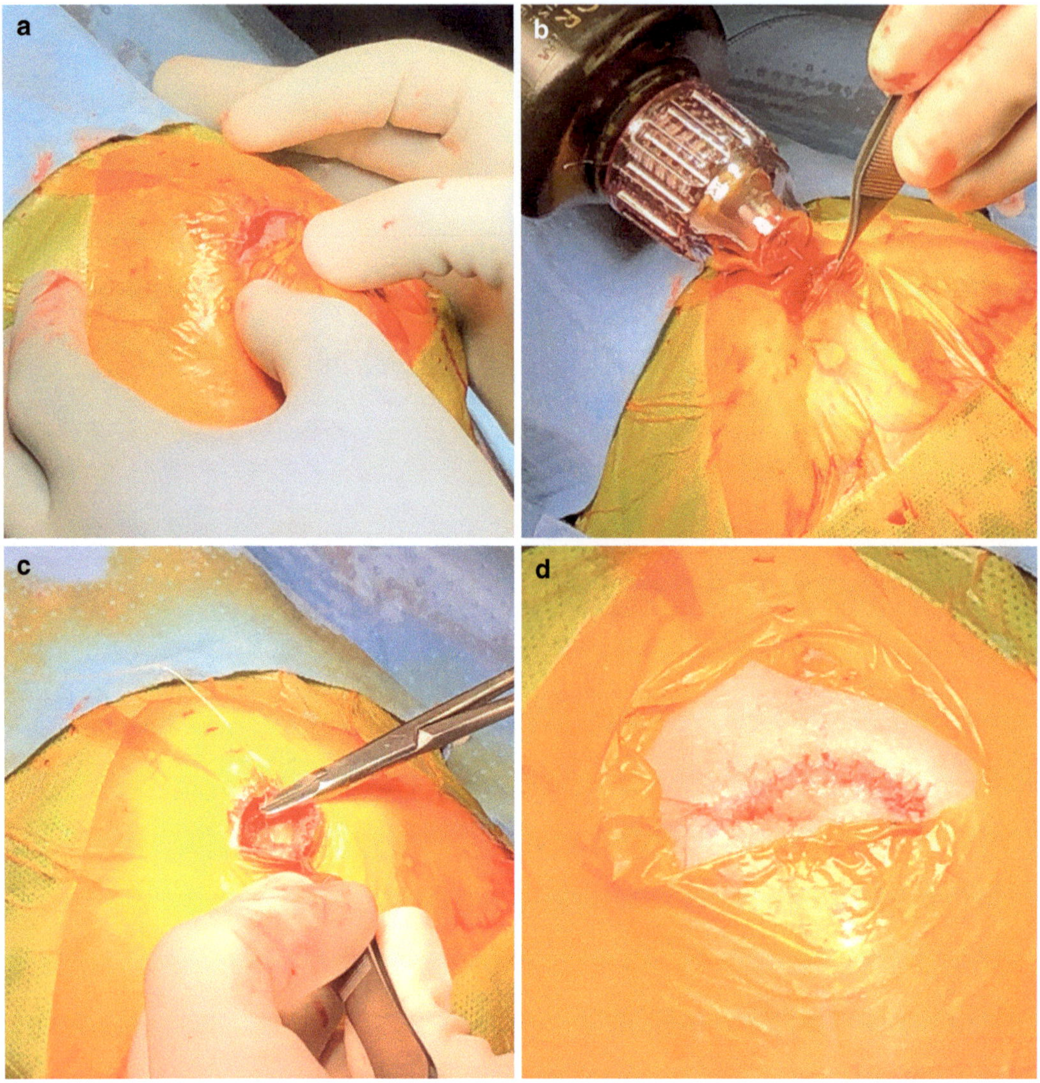

Fig. 43.6 Confirming that the two frontal bones are completely disconnected by physically moving them (**a**). Wound irrigation with betadine (**b**). Subcutaneous (**c**) and skin (**d**) layers are closed with absorbable sutures

43.4 Postoperative Course

A hemoglobin and hematocrit is sent at the completion of the case, with a typical hematocrit decrease of 7% comparing pre- vs. postoperative specimens. A very low percentage of infants require transfusion as described in our institutional experience section. The patient is observed overnight on the neurosurgical floor. Pain control might require a dose or two of narcotic, with IV morphine 0.1 mg/kg being our preferred drug, but with rapid transition to acetaminophen, which is the only discharge medication. The vast majority of patients are discharged on postoperative day 1 after confirming that pain is well controlled and oral intake is sufficient. Helmet fitting is performed 2–4 days after surgery, with a goal of instituting helmet therapy by day 7. The patient is followed up at the outpatient clinic in 1 month. The family is informed that helmet therapy may continue until 1 year of age, but the typical duration of the helmet therapy is less than 7 months.

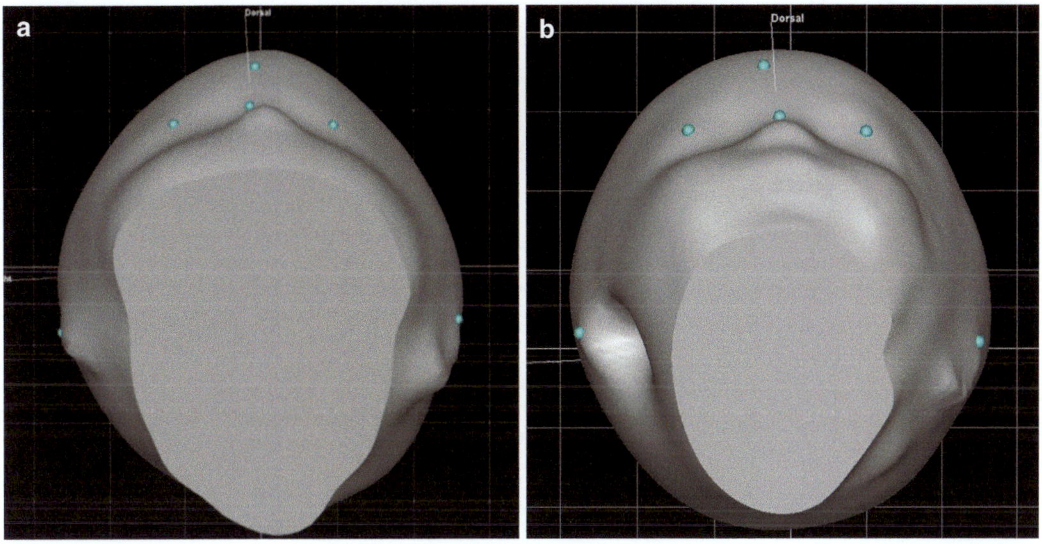

Fig. 43.7 Representative laser scan images demonstrating significant improvement of trigonocephaly. Immediate postoperative (**a**, 3 days after the procedure) and 6-month follow-up (**b**)

Completion of helmet therapy is not a specified duration but based on response.

As for any patient with synostosis, it is important that these children be followed for at least 5 years. This corresponds to the essential completion of brain growth, as brain weight and size reach maturity at 5–6 years [12]. Routine follow-up should always include annual head circumference measurement, and routine eye exams to rule out papilledema. Although the reoperation rates for metopic synostosis are exceedingly low, any child with synostosis is at risk for refusion of the original suture, or other sutures, prior to full brain maturity. Specific to metopic synostosis, the family and surgeon will notice an indentation where the prominence had been over the first year or two. The goal of the therapy in the first year is to achieve lateral frontal growth and a normalized forehead shape (Fig. 43.7). It will still appear slightly indented in the midline and have some slight angularity at the release site at 1 year of age. This improves over the next few years as the bone gap completely fills in and the surrounding frontal bones thicken.

It is our experience that children with metopics synostosis tend to have a slightly narrower forehead than the average population after treatment, which this is true with both endoscopic and open operations. This is why some surgeons have advocated for extreme hypercorrection when they do a frontal orbital advancement [13]. That said, children with this condition have slightly narrow facial features, so that if you overly widen the forehead it actually appears to be a mismatch between the forehead and frontal region, and in our view, this is not advised.

For some forms of synostosis repair, it is the opinion of the authors that the endoscopic outcomes are actually superior to the open cranial reconstructions due to minimization of scar and excellent skull morphology. Although the literature often notes very comparable anthropometric outcomes for open and endoscopic procedures metopic synostosis, and in our experience patient and family satisfaction rates have been very high, we do believe that the open operations often achieves a slightly wider forehead configuration. With that caveat, in the authors' experience, a family has never requested a repeat operation after endoscopic metopic suture release, and they have been very happy that they chose the minimally invasive technique.

43.5 Conclusion

Endoscope-assisted repair is a safe and effective treatment for metopic synostosis. The estimated blood loss is much less and the operative time is significantly shorter when compared with open procedures. This procedure rarely require intra- or postoperative transfusion. The cosmetic outcome of the treatment is comparable to open repair with very high rates of family satisfaction. This chapter details the actual procedure as a reference for those considering endoscope-assisted metopic suture repair, which should be part of the treatment algorithm for a complex craniofacial center.

References

1. Starr JR, Lin HJ, Ruiz-Correa S, Cunningham ML, Ellenbogen RG, Collett BR, Kapp-Simon KA, Speltz ML. Little evidence of association between severity of trigonocephaly and cognitive development in infants with single-suture metopic synostosis. Neurosurgery. 2010;67(2):408–15.
2. Sidoti EJ Jr, Marsh JL, Marty-Grames L, Noetzel MJ. Share. Long-term studies of metopic synostosis: frequency of cognitive impairment and behavioral disturbances. Plast Reconstr Surg. 1996;97(2):276–81.
3. van der Vlugt JJB, van der Meulen JJNM, Creemers HE, Verhulst FC, Hovius SER, Okkerse JME. Cognitive and behavioral functioning in 82 patients with trigonocephaly. Plast Reconstr Surg. 2012;130(4):885–93.
4. Kunz M, Lehner M, Heger A, Armbruster L, Weigand H, Mast G, Peraud A. Neurodevelopmental and esthetic results in children after surgical correction of metopic suture synostosis: a single institutional experience. Childs Nerv Syst. 2014;30(6):1075–82.
5. Delashaw JB, Persing JA, Park TS, Jane JA. Surgical approaches for the correction of metopic synostosis. Neurosurgery. 1986;19(2):228–34.
6. Gociman B, Agko M, Blagg R, Garlick J, Kestle JR, Siddiqi F. Share. Endoscopic-assisted correction of metopic synostosis. J Craniofac Surg. 2013;24(3):763–8.
7. Jimenez DF, McGinity MJ, Barone CM. Endoscopy-assisted early correction of single-suture metopic craniosynostosis: a 19-year experience. J Neurosurg Pediatr. 2018;23(1):61–74.
8. Lajthia O, Rogers GF, Tsering D, Keating RF, Magge SN. Quantitative outcomes of endoscopic strip craniectomy for metopic craniosynostosis in children with severe trigonocephaly. Childs Nerv Syst. 2021;37(2):573–9.
9. Braun TL, Eisemann BS, Olorunnipa O, Buchanan EP, Monson LA. Safety outcomes in endoscopic versus open repair of metopic craniosynostosis. J Craniofac Surg. 2018;29(4):856–60.
10. Ha AY, Skolnick GB, Chi D, Nguyen DC, Naidoo SD, Smyth MD, Patel KB. School-aged anthropometric outcomes after endoscopic or open repair of metopic synostosis. Pediatrics. 2020;146(3):e20200238.
11. Nguyen DC, Patel KB, Skolnick GB, Naidoo SD, Huang AH, Smyth MD, Woo AS. Are endoscopic and open treatments of metopic synostosis equivalent in treating trigonocephaly and hypotelorism? J Craniofac Surg. 2015;26(1):129–34.
12. Dekaban AS. Changes in brain weights during the span of human life: relation of brain weights to body heights and body weights. Ann Neurol. 1978;4(4):345–56.
13. Bennett KG, Liang F, Ranganathan K, Muraszko KM, Vercler CJ, Buchman SR. Surgical hypercorrection of trigonocephaly: evaluation of surgical outcomes. J Craniofac Surg. 2018;29(1):56–61.

44 Metopic Suture Synostosis: Open Vault Surgery: Key Points for the Neurosurgeon

Vijay M. Ravindra, Barbu Gociman, and John R. W. Kestle

44.1 Introduction

Premature closure of the metopic suture accounts for about 15% of all single-suture fusion cases [1–8]; it occurs in 1 in 2500 to 1 in 70,000 live births in the U.S [9, 10].Typically, closure of the metopic suture occurs by 9 months of age, although the suture may remain patent until 2 years of age, which allows for growth of the frontal bones [11]. In some cases, however, physiologic closure may occur by 3 months. Premature fusion of the metopic suture results in restriction of the normal growth of the frontal bones. When clinically significant fusion is present, it is theorized to occur during intrauterine development, although some fusion may occur after birth [12, 13]. Most diagnosed cases of metopic synostosis are single-suture conditions without syndromic involvement, although syndromic cases may appear in conjunction with Opitz C syndrome, Say-Meyer syndrome, or Frydman syndrome [10, 14, 15]. Most cases of metopic synostosis occur in males, who make up 65–85% of cases [4, 16, 17].

The clinical presentation of metopic synostosis includes trigonocephaly—a wedge-shaped frontal region with significant ridging (Fig. 44.1), hypotelorism, and temporal narrowing [18]. It is important to realize that not all patients who experience premature closure will develop trigonocephaly. The wedge-shaped frontal bones also result in prominence of the lateral supraorbital rims. With metopic synostosis, the orbits are medialized in position, which results in hypotelorism. In addition to the cosmetic effects of premature metopic suture fusion, there is the possibility of cognitive deficits or elevated intracranial pressure (ICP) [2, 19], and there are often intracranial abnormalities, such as congenital anomalies, extra-axial fluid collections, and so-called "copper beaten" skull [20].

V. M. Ravindra
Department of Neurosurgery, University of Utah, Salt Lake City, UT, USA

Department of Neurosurgery, University of California San Diego, San Diego, CA, USA

Department of Neurosurgery, Naval Medical Center San Diego, San Diego, CA, USA

B. Gociman
Division of Plastic Surgery, Primary Children's Hospital, University of Utah, Salt Lake City, UT, USA

J. R. W. Kestle (✉)
Department of Neurosurgery, University of Utah, Salt Lake City, UT, USA
e-mail: neuropub@hsc.utah.edu

F. Di Rocco, J. Kestle (eds.), *Neurosurgical Aspects of Craniosynostosis*,
https://doi.org/10.1007/978-3-031-69386-1_44

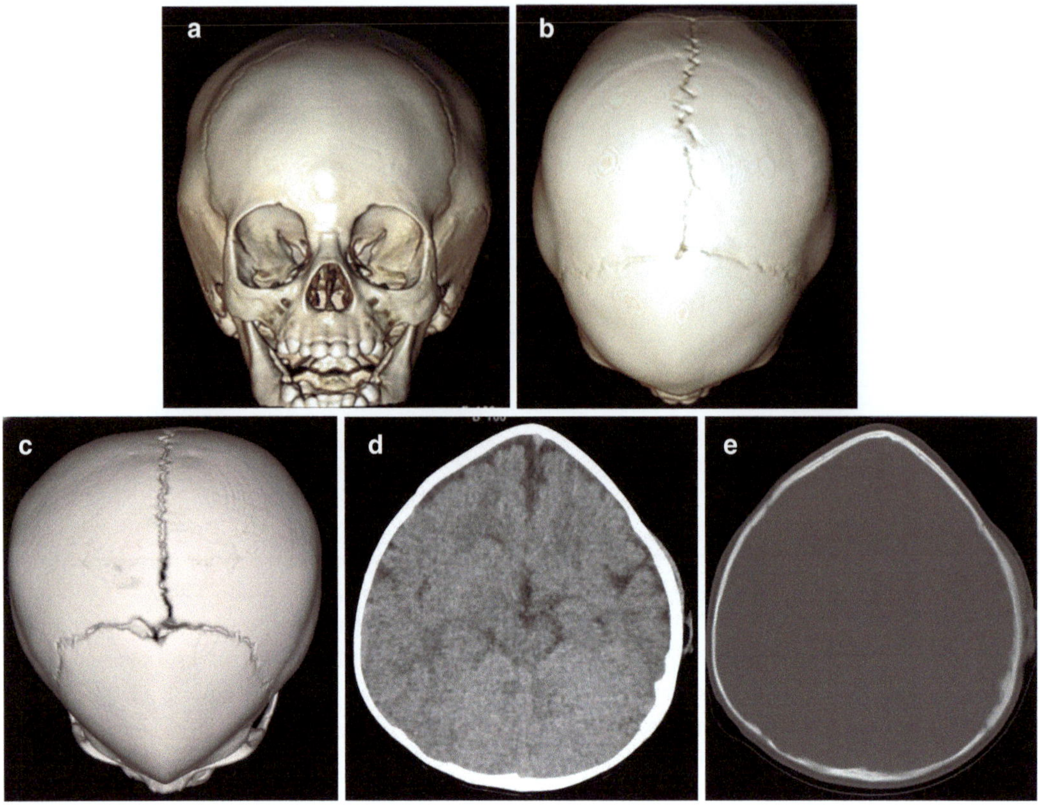

Fig. 44.1 (**a**, **b**) Three-dimensional computed tomography (CT) reconstruction (left anterior view, right superior view) demonstrating a mild metopic ridge with no significant narrowing of the anterior cranial fossa; a child with this type of deformity does not require surgery. (**c**) In contrast, a 3D CT reconstruction of a child with significant metopic synostosis and trigonocephaly and axial brain (**d**) and bone (**e**) window images demonstrate an example of a narrow anterior cranial fossa in metopic synostosis

44.2 Choice of Surgical Procedure/Goal of Surgery

The two main indications for surgical treatment of craniosynostosis are to correct the skull shape for both cosmetic and psychosocial considerations and to ensure there is adequate room for normal brain growth and development. As with any craniosynostosis correction, the goal is to achieve the most durable and best cosmetic result possible while keeping the risk profile low. For mild cases, observation alone may be warranted. Otherwise, when choosing the type of surgical correction, the age of the patient is the most important factor. For infants younger than 3 months of age, endoscopic correction with subsequent prolonged helmet therapy may be applied. For older children, open vault surgery is necessary. In this chapter, we focus on the key aspects of open vault surgery, but knowledge of additional treatment options is important.

44.3 Preoperative Evaluation/Surgical Planning

The diagnosis of metopic synostosis is most often made during a clinical examination. Preoperative computed tomography with three-dimensional (3D) reconstruction of the skull can be useful for identification of additional suture involvement or preoperative planning, but this imaging is not necessary for diagnosis and rarely alters surgical plans [20]. Surgical planning is often performed in conjunction with craniofacial surgeons as part of a multidisciplinary team.

The decision to operate on affected children is based on the degree of deformity of the forehead and anterior fossa and also on the risk of raised ICP. At one extreme on the spectrum of severity of deformity, there are children with a virtually normal forehead contour with a simple ridge superimposed on the metopic suture. These children do not need intervention (Fig. 44.1a and b). At the other extreme are patients with severe trigonocephaly with reduced anterior fossa volume (Fig. 44.1c–e) who clearly need corrective surgery. Between these two scenarios, there are various degress of deformity, and surgeons vary in their threshold for suggesting corrective surgery. Surgery for mild deformity has been advocated [21, 22] but is controversial [23, 24]. Birgfeld et al. [25] proposed some criteria to differentiate between true metopic synostosis and a simple metopic ridge. They suggested that the relationship between the lateral frontal bone and lateral orbit is helpful in distinguishing the two and that CT can be helpful not to confirm suture closure but rather to investigate other characteristics of metopic craniosynostosis including upsloping of the superior orbital rim, absence of pulled anterior fontanelle, position and shape of lateral frontal bone, frontal bone tangent to midline, and orbital/intraorbital narrowing.

Generally, patients with single-suture synostosis demonstrate a low rate of elevated ICP, and the mean ICP for children with metopic craniosynostosis in a study by Kalmar et al. [26] was 12.5 mmHg, significantly lower than in their unicoronal or sagittal counterparts; in addition, no children had an ICP measurement of ≥20 mmHg. In this study, including children with single and multisuture synostosis with syndromic and nonsyndromic disease, the authors found that syndromic status, older age at intervention, and multiple suture involvement were associated with elevated ICP. Although the relationship among bony abnormality, ICP, and neurocognitive outcome has been questioned [27], Starr et al. [28] found that children with metopic synostosis had neurodevelopmental scores 0.9–4.5 points worse than those of children with sagittal synostosis. Similarly, Baird et al. [29] found that children with metopic suture have the highest rate of cognitive impairment among the single-suture synostoses. For further detailed discussion of these issues and the indications, see Chap. 8.

If there is no concern for high ICP and the child presents outside the window for endoscopic release, then open vault surgery is typically delayed until the child reaches at least 6–12 months of age. This allows the circulating blood volume in the child to increase and enables the child to deal better with the stress of a cranial vault operation [30]. All children undergoing cranial vault remodeling should be prepared for blood transfusion; family is given the option to donate before surgery in most cases.

44.4 Positioning

For open cranial vault remodeling surgery, the patient is placed supine on a horseshoe headrest with even pressure distributed through the scalp (Fig. 44.2). A bicoronal incision, which can be

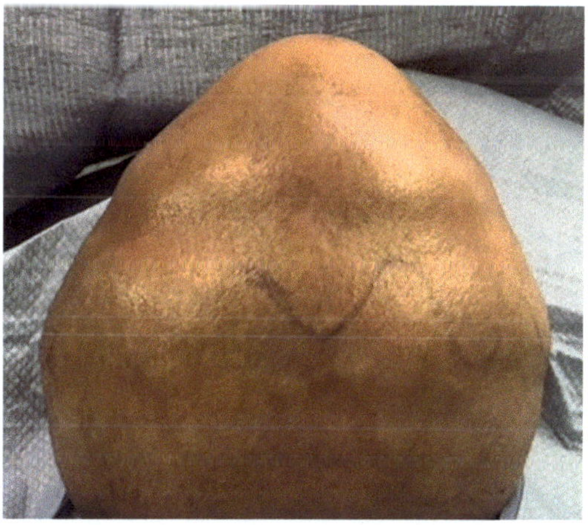

Fig. 44.2 Photograph (superior view) of a child with trigonocephaly. Characteristic findings include a frontal keel, bitemporal narrowing, coronal sutures displaced anteriorly (not pictured), compensatory bulging of the parieto-occipital region, bizygomatic narrowing, and posterior displacement of the superolateral orbital rim (not pictured)

linear, wavy, or zigzag, is planned. Skin preparation is undertaken well behind the coronal incision posteriorly and anteriorly/inferiorly to the eyebrow and to the skin of the upper eyelids. The use of 5% povidone-iodine *ophthalmic* ophthalmic solution allows prepping near the eyebrows with corneal guards. Extending the prep inferiorly helps post-correction visualization of the fronto-orbital, supraorbital advancement by allowing full view of the structures from an anterior, lateral, and superior view after reconstruction is completed [30].

44.5 Blood Loss

Standard measures should be taken to minimize blood loss during cranial vault surgery. Adequate intravenous access with accurate monitoring of blood loss is essential to safe reconstruction. The use of central venous access and precordial Doppler ultrasound placement is at the discretion of the pediatric anesthesia provider and surgical team.

Significant bleeding may occur during scalp incision and osteotomies. Meticulous attention to hemostasis is important to minimize the need for transfusion. A needle tip Bovie electrocautery can be used to complete the scalp incision and elevate the scalp flap to prevent blood loss. The use of tranexamic acid can decrease the rate of transfusion in cranial vault remodeling [31].

44.6 Bifrontal Craniotomy

The scalp is elevated in the subgaleal plane as an anterior flap and a posterior flap. The anterior flap dissection is carried on to approximately 2 cm from the brow. A large anteriorly based pericranial flap can then be elevated based on the supraorbital and supratroclear arterial blood supply. The flap is elevated past the brow, into the orbits. At the end of surgery, this flap will help to cover the entire reconstructed anterior cranial vault and provide good blood supply to promote bony healing (Fig. 44.3). The bony portion of the procedure begins with the neurosurgical team performing a bifrontal craniotomy. The posterior margin is just behind the coronal sutures. Anteriorly, the craniotomy cut goes across the inferior frontal region, leaving a supraorbital bar at least 1 cm in width attached to the orbits (Fig. 44.4). Burr holes are placed at the temporal regions bilaterally, and in the midline posterior to the coronal suture and adjacent to the midline anteriorly, just above the orbital bar. The burr holes should be placed so that the orbital bar is spared in its entirety to facilitate the reconstruction. Dural separation is then carefully performed through these burr holes using Penfield dissectors. The dura may be quite adherent under the normal coronal sutures, and if dissection from one direction is difficult, another burr hole and approach to the adherent area should be attempted. In addition, there is frequently in-folding and invagination of the dura into the metopic ridge and a midline ridge on the inner table of the skull just above the orbital bar. All of these should be carefully dissected. It is very common to find a pair of large diploic veins low down, near the orbital bar on either side of the midline. If these bleed, the area should be packed with surgical foam while the craniotomy is opened. Finally, great care

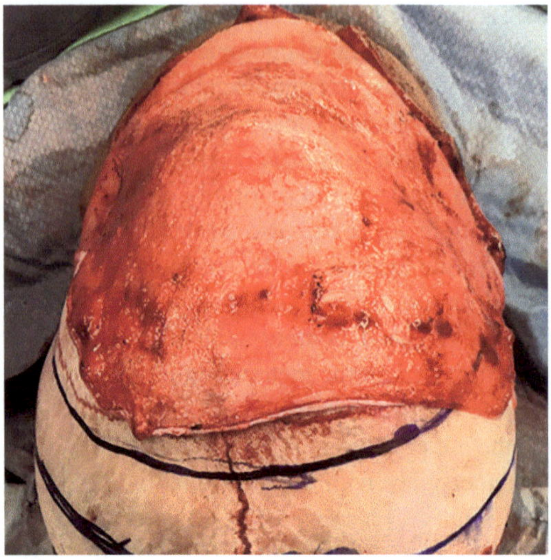

Fig. 44.3 Dissected pericranial flap (superior view). This flap can be useful to cover the entire reconstructed anterior cranial vault and provide good blood supply to promote bony healing

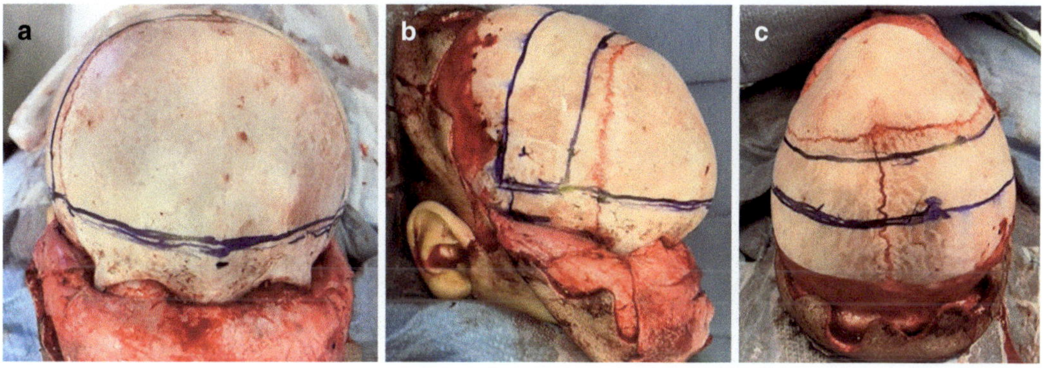

Fig. 44.4 Intraoperative photographs after reflection of the scalp demonstrating the margins of cranial bone removal. (**a**) Anteriorly, the craniotomy cut goes across the inferior frontal region (marked line indicating the delineation between the frontal bone and supraorbital bar). (**b**) A supraorbital bar about 1 cm in width attached to the orbits (lateral view). (**c**) Superior view demonstrating the posterior aspect of the craniotomy well behind the coronal suture and parietal bone to facilitate reconstruction and remodeling (marked line delineating the posterior aspect of the bone removal)

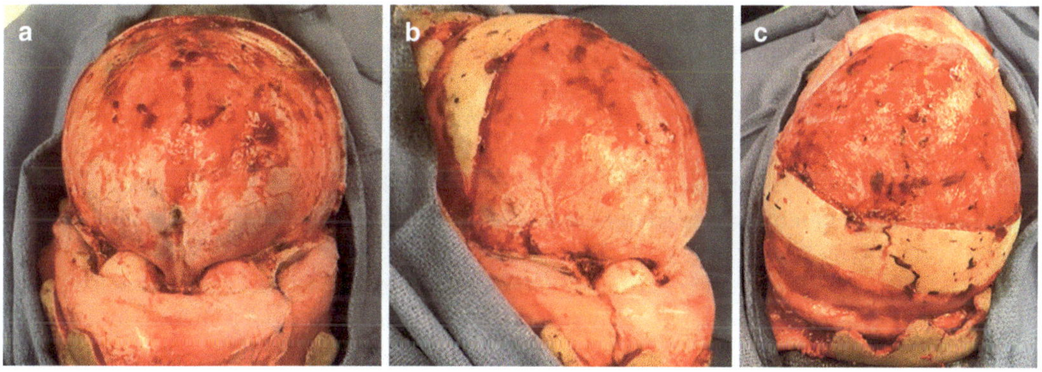

Fig. 44.5 (**a**) Intraoperative photograph (anterior view) demonstrating exposure of the dura to the level of the nasofrontal suture and orbital contents after removal of the frontal bone bilaterally and the orbital bandeau. (**b**) Lateral photograph demonstrating the inferior aspect of the bone removal as well as clear exposure of the orbital contents indicating the amount of bone removal needed for full mobilization of the orbital bandeau and bone removal well behind the coronal suture over the parietal dura. (**c**) Superior view showing the entire extent of frontal and parietal craniotomies

should be taken in dissecting the dura and sinus from the bone at the posterior margin of the craniotomy. Two burr holes, one on either side of the midline, may be needed to do this safely. Once the dura is clear, the craniotomy is cut circumferentially and elevated from posterior to anterior. As it is elevated, the dura should be visualized and bleeding points coagulated. An approximately 5-cm-wide parietal craniotomy is then made. This allows for complete reshaping of the anterior vault and provides ample bone graft for the reconstruction. In the unlikely event of a dural tear, primary closure can usually be done with an absorbable 4–0 suture.

The dura is then dissected from the floor of the anterior fossa and the anterior aspect of the middle fossa bilaterally. In the midline, the dura should be elevated down to the nasofrontal suture (Fig. 44.5). Dissection of the periorbita of the supraorbital rim is carried out and extended at least 1–1.5 cm off the orbital roof bilaterally. Next, a sagittal saw or a piezoelectric bone cutter is used to create an osteotomy in the orbital roof from medial to lateral. Very gen-

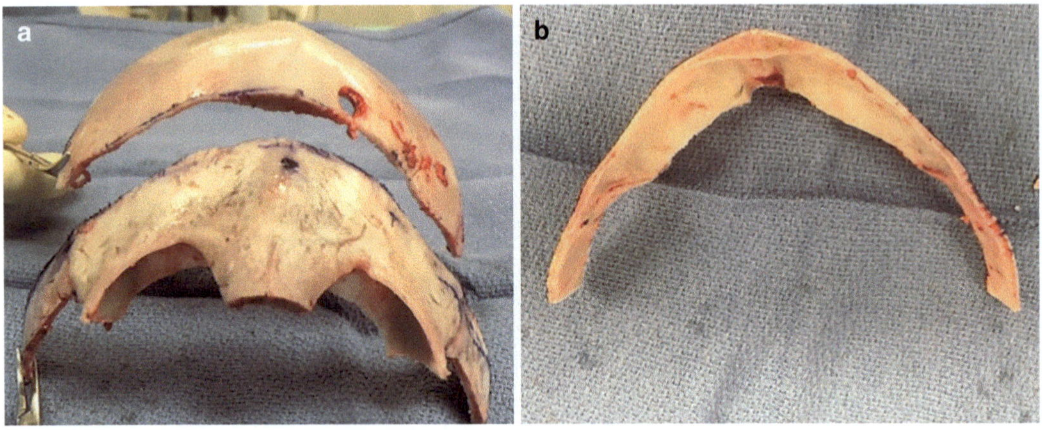

Fig. 44.6 Intraoperative photographs demonstrating the removed bony segments from the frontal bone and orbital bandeau (**a**, front view) and supraorbital bar/orbital bandeau (**b**, superior view)

tle retraction is placed on the frontal lobe dura and periorbita. Typically, no augmentation for ICP is needed or recommended at this point. The osteotomy is extended laterally to the greater wing of the sphenoid bone. In the midline, the osteotomy is completed anterior to the foramen cecum with a small osteotome or the piezoelectric bone cutter, and the orbital bar is removed (Fig. 44.6).

44.7 Reconstruction

44.7.1 Fronto-Orbital Advancement Technique

The goals of the reconstruction are to increase the volume of the anterior cranial fossa by advancing and widening the forehead and to reshape the orbits. This is achieved by straightening and widening the orbital bar. To straighten the bar, the inner table is removed just lateral to the level of the lateral orbital wall, which makes the bone more malleable and allows for reshaping. The supraorbital bar can be split at the midline and then reshaped and widened with an interposition bone graft to correct the hypotelorism. The orbits are burred as needed to achieve a harmonious and symmetrical shape (Fig. 44.7). Prior to reattachment of the reconstructed orbital bar, barrel staving of the temporal bone bilaterally is done to further enlarge the anterior cranial fossa in the transverse dimension. The staves are made approximately 2 cm in width and 4 cm in length and greenstick out-fractured to preserve their viability (Fig. 44.8). The supraorbital bar is advanced approximately 1–2 cm anteriorly from its original position and secured to the temporal bone and the lateral orbital walls at the level of the frontozygomatic sutures using a resorbable plating system. Any gaps present at the level of the bar fixation points are filled with well-fitted bone grafts to prevent dislodgement. No plating is done at the level of the nasal bone. The bar is placed over the nasal bone for a overlap distance of approximately 2 mm in the vertical dimension. The inner table of the bar is removed with a burr at the level of the overlap to prevent any significant prominence (Figs. 44.8 and 44.9).

The frontal and parietal bone flaps are typically split down the middle. Each half of the frontal bone flap is rotated to obtain a broader contour of the forehead. The contour of the frontal bone can often be achieved with a bone bender in younger patients, but if the bone is too rigid then radial osteotomies can be performed. To enlarge the anterior cranial vault, the parietal bone flaps are split at the level of the diploic

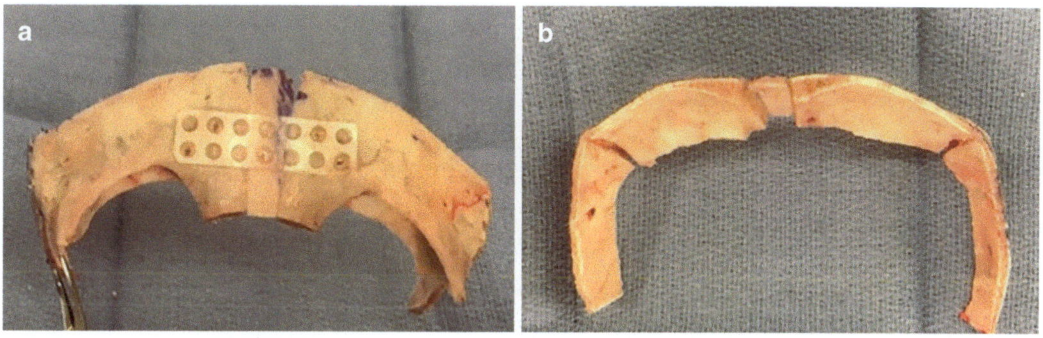

Fig. 44.7 Intraoperative photographs (**a**, front view; **b**, superior view) demonstrating the technique of splitting supraorbital bar at the midline and reshaping and widening it with an interposition bone graft to correct the hypotelorism

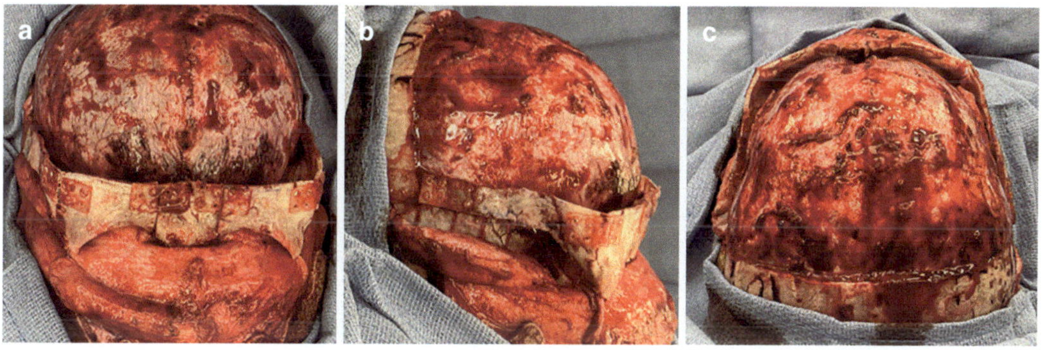

Fig. 44.8 Inset of the supraorbital bar showing the increase in volume at the level of the anterior cranial fossa (**a**, anterior view; **b**, lateral view; **c**, superior view). The bar is advanced approximately 1–2 cm anteriorly and secured using a resorbable plating system to the temporal bone and the lateral orbital walls at the level of the at the frontozygomatic sutures. Any gaps present at the level of the bar fixation points are filled with well-fitted bone grafts to prevent dislodgement. No plating is done at the level of the nasal bone. In **b**, the barrel staving technique of the temporal bone bilaterally is done to further enlarge the anterior cranial fossa in transverse dimension. The staves are approximately 2 cm in width and 4 cm in length and greenstick out-fractured to preserve their viability

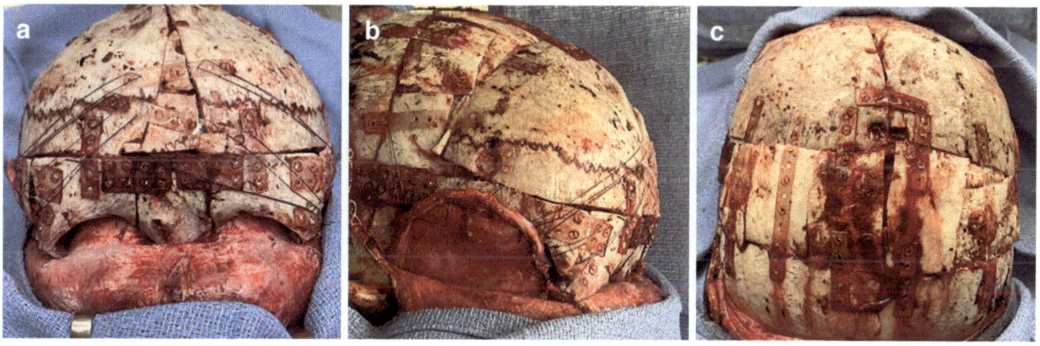

Fig. 44.9 Intraoperative photographs of case 1 (**a**, anterior view; **b**, lateral view; **c**, superior view) demonstrating the technique of splitting the frontal bone flap and rotating the halves to obtain a broader contour of the forehead. The contour of the frontal bone can be achieved with a bone bender or radial osteotomies (if the bone is too rigid). To enlarge the anterior cranial vault, the parietal bone flaps are split at the level of the diploic space using osteotomes. The resulting bony pieces are used to reconstruct the anterior cranial vault by enlarging it and giving it a well-proportioned shape. All of the pieces are secured using resorbable plates and screws, and no defects are left ungrafted

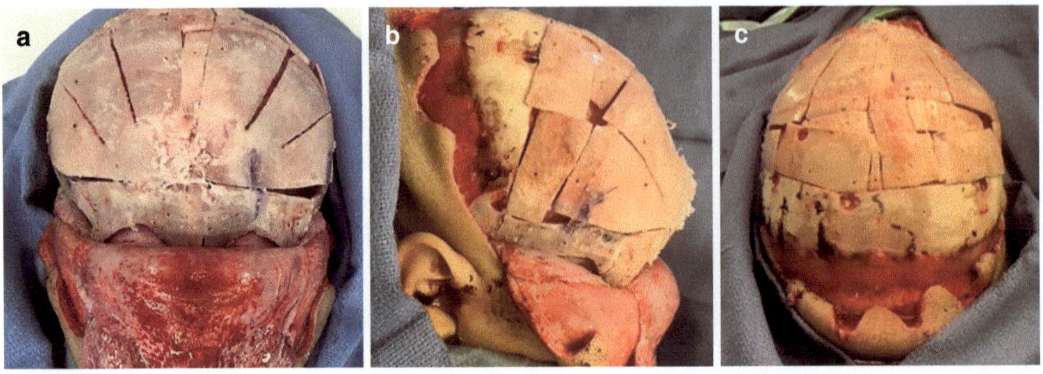

Fig. 44.10 Intraoperative photographs of case 2 (**a**, anterior view; **b**, lateral view; **c**, superior view) demonstrating the potential reconstruction based on the malleability of the bone flaps and the size and quality of the split calvarial bone grafts

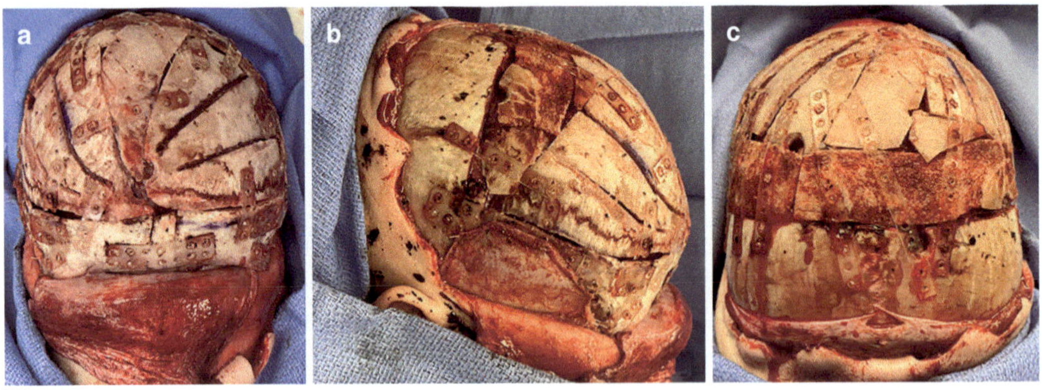

Fig. 44.11 Intraoperative photographs of case 3 (**a**, anterior view; **b**, lateral view; **c**, superior view) demonstrating another unique reconstruction based on the malleability of the bone flaps and the size and quality of the split calvarial bone grafts

space using osteotomes. The resulting bony pieces are used to reconstruct the anterior cranial vault by enlarging it and giving it a well-proportioned shape. All of the pieces are secured using resorbable plates and screws, and no defects are left ungrafted. Every reconstruction is unique based on the malleability or rigidity of the bone flaps and the size and quality of the split calvarial bone grafts, as illustrated by the three different cases presented (Figs. 44.9, 44.10, and 44.11). An alternative to split calvarial bone grafting is filling of the bony defects with inner table bone shavings obtained by using a burr or a bone scraper. It is imperative to reflect the scalp over the correction intermittently to ensure the desired cosmetic result is

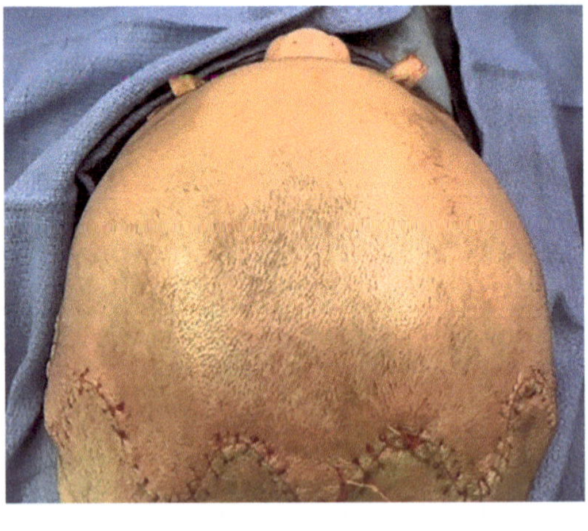

Fig. 44.12 Intraoperative photograph demonstrating skin closure over the newly contoured bone structure of the frontal bones and orbital bandeau

being achieved, specifically at the end of the correction (Fig. 44.12).

44.7.2 Single-Segment Reconstruction

Fearon et al. [32] described an alternative method of remodeling the frontal bone using a single-segment bone flap (Fig. 44.13). The reconstruction method involves harvesting an appropriately sized biparietal bone flap after measurement of the nonhair-bearing forehead skin to correctly size the repair.

The exposure reaches the level of the supraorbital rims, but no intraorbital dissection is necessary. Once the scalp is reflected using a coronal incision, further donor-site inspection is required to harvest the most appropriately shaped bone graft that will match the curvature for reconstructing the forehead as a single unit. On the basis of their experience, Fearon et al. [32] noted that this often comes from the posterior half of the parietal bone.

A frontal craniotomy is performed, and the low supraorbital region is excised to the level of the floor of the anterior fossa; the orbital roof is left undisturbed. All bone removed is then split on the back table, and forehead reconstruction proceeds with fixation of the biparietal bone flap (Fig. 44.12), which is often rotated 180 degrees, so the posterior aspect of the harvested flap becomes the most inferior portion of the supraorbital/frontal bone. The flap is secured in the midline with a U-shaped suture that is secured through two holes in the glabella, and the lateral outer aspects of the donor flap are advanced on either side. The single-piece reconstruction replaces the bandeau and frontal bone with the most anterior inferior aspect, giving rise to the new supraorbit. After the new frontal bone has been secured in place, removal of bone in the temporal region is undertaken, which permits bone-to-bone inset of the posterolateral aspects of the new frontal bone, similar to the traditional fronto-orbital advancement procedure described above.

Once the contour and reconstruction are cosmetically suitable, the posterior parietal bone donor site is reconstructed with the former frontal bones, supraorbital bone, and split calvarial grafts. The outcomes for this method are comparable with the traditional supraorbital ban-

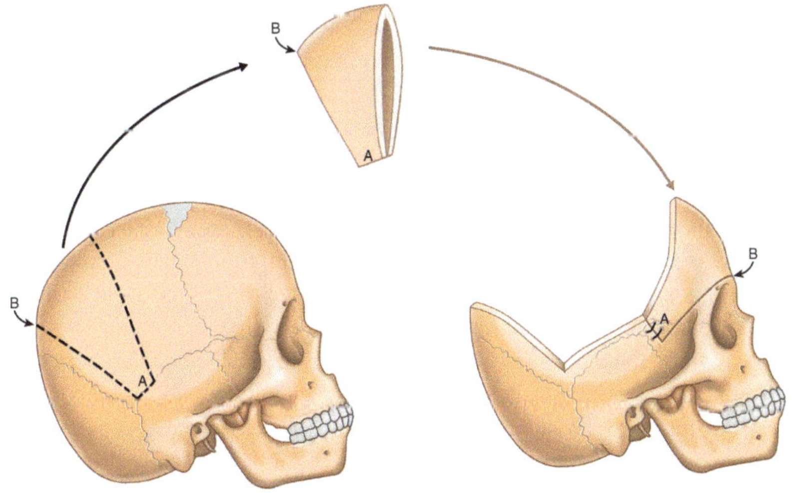

Fig. 44.13 Image demonstrating single-piece reconstruction using a biparietal harvested bone flap for recreating the supraorbital bandeau and frontal bone. The technique described by Fearon et al. [32] involves rotation of the harvested parietal flap 180 degrees, so the posterior aspect of the flap becomes the inferior aspect of the supraorbital/frontal bone. (From Fearon JA, Ditthakasem K, Castro García J, Herbert M. Abandoning the Supraorbital Bandeau in Anterior Craniosynostosis Repairs, for a Single-Segment Reconstruction. Plast Reconstr Surg. 2018 Sep;142 (3):334e-41e)

deau method with respect to surgical time, blood loss, and complication rates, and there is some evidence of lower reoperation rates (0 vs. 2.7%) and improved aesthetic outcomes [32].

44.8 Postoperative Care

The most immediate concern after surgery is acute blood loss anemia. Serum hemoglobin is usually drawn 4–6 h postoperatively and the next morning. Transfusion thresholds may vary, but a hemoglobin level less than 8 g/dL should trigger consideration of transfusion. The presence of significant periorbital edema is normal between postoperative days 1 and 3 and is often accompanied with emesis and fever. The most common postoperative complication is fever [33], and this is usually self limiting.

When absorbable cranial plating systems are used, there can be painless scalp swelling approximately 9–12 months after surgery that coincides with plate resorption [34]. Reassurance should be provided to the family during this time.

44.9 Complications

44.9.1 Intraoperative Sagittal Sinus Injury

Injury to the superior sagittal sinus should be extremely rare if dural dissection and craniotomy cuts are done carefully. Bleeding from the sinus can be mitigated with gentle pressure and often closed primarily with a suture. Care should be taken while doing this to avoid air embolus, so the head should be flat, and the assistant should provide irrigation while the suture is placed. More severe bleeding may require placement of a dural patch, or in extreme circumstances, sacrifice of the sinus. Ligation of up to one third of the anterior sagittal sinus can be performed with low risk of venous infarction but should be reserved for the extremely rare severe sinus injury that cannot be controlled by other means.

44.9.2 Postoperative Infection

Infection is an uncommon complication after craniosynostosis surgery, with mean infection rates reported to be 2% [33], but should be identified and dealt with in a similar manner as other post-craniotomy infections. Superficial or incisional infections may be treated with local wound care and antibiotic therapy, but deep infection may require open debridement. If there is concern for or evidence of osteomyelitis, then removal of the flap is required with prolonged antibiotic therapy. Although bone flap removal is not ideal, a period of observation is a reasonable option before planning any secondary flap replacement or reconstruction because bone gaps may fill in on their own in very young children.

44.9.3 Poor Postoperative Cosmetic Outcome

The long-term success with open reconstruction is more than 90% in patient with nonsyndromic metopic synostosis [16, 35–39]. The cosmetic outcomes are highly dependent on the severity of the preoperative deformity. Overall, rates of new metopic ridging or progression are very low, although reoperation may be necessary [40]. An additional source for potential reoperation arises from temporal hollowing, which can occur in 15% of patients [41].

Decisions to intervene or reoperate should be made with the knowledge that each additional surgery carries an increased risk of dural injury, vascular injury, bleeding, and potential for no appreciable improvement in cosmetic deformity. Ideally, a shared, multidisciplinary decision-making approach should occur.

As mentioned above, the use of a single-segment bone flap has been described with similar results to conventional fronto-orbital advancement [32, 42]. At present, the selection of the method for reconstruction should be based on surgeon experience and outcomes because further head-to-head study is needed to compare these techniques.

44.10 Conclusion

Premature closure of the metopic suture is usually a single-suture pathology but rarely can be seen in the setting of syndromic conditions. Open vault surgery is typically performed after 6 months of age with the goal of correcting the associated trigonocephaly, hypotelorism, and temporal narrowing with abnormal shape of the supraorbital rim. Open surgical treatment usually includes a 1-cm fronto-orbital advancement with recontouring of the frontal bones and widening of the orbital rim. An alternative single-segment reconstruction has been proposed. Correction should be tailored to the nature of the deformity. Careful neurosurgical dissection of the dura and hemostasis will avoid many of the potential complications that might otherwise occur.

Author Disclaimer The views expressed in this article are those of the author and do not necessarily reflect the official policy or position of the Department of the Navy, Department of Defense, nor the U.S. Government.

References

1. Anderson FM, Geiger L. Craniosynostosis: a survey of 204 cases. J Neurosurg. 1965;22:229–40.
2. Anderson FM, Gwinn JL, Todt JC. Trigonocephaly. Identity and surgical treatment. J Neurosurg. 1962;19:723–30.
3. Bottero L, Lajeunie E, Arnaud E, Marchac D, Renier D. Functional outcome after surgery for trigonocephaly. Plast Reconstr Surg. 1998;102(4):952–8; discussion 9–60
4. Genitori L, Cavalheiro S, Lena G, Dollo C, Choux M. Skull base in trigonocephaly. Pediatr Neurosurg. 1991;17(4):175–81.
5. Sadove AM, Kalsbeck JE, Eppley BL, Javed T. Modifications in the surgical correction of trigonocephaly. Plast Reconstr Surg. 1990;85(6):853–8.
6. Shillito J Jr, Matson DD. Craniosynostosis: a review of 519 surgical patients. Pediatrics. 1968;41(4):829–53.
7. Sloan GM, Wells KC, Raffel C, McComb JG. Surgical treatment of craniosynostosis: outcome analysis of 250 consecutive patients. Pediatrics. 1997;100(1):E2.
8. Collmann H, Sorensen N, Krauss J. Consensus: trigonocephaly. Childs Nerv Syst. 1996;12(11):664–8.
9. Alderman BW, Fernbach SK, Greene C, Mangione EJ, Ferguson SW. Diagnostic practice and the estimated prevalence of craniosynostosis in Colorado. Arch Pediatr Adolesc Med. 1997;151(2):159–64.
10. Cohen M. Syndromes with craniosynostosis. In: Cohen M, editor. Craniosynostosis: diagnosis, evaluation, and management. New York, NY: Raven; 1986. p. 413–590.
11. Currarino G, Silverman FN. Orbital hypotelorism, arhinencephaly, and trigonocephaly. Radiology. 1960;74:206–17.
12. Azimi C, Kennedy SJ, Chitayat D, Chakraborty P, Clarke JT, Forrest C, et al. Clinical and genetic aspects of trigonocephaly: a study of 25 cases. Am J Med Genet A. 2003;117A(2):127–35.
13. Scarfo GB, Tomaccini D. Trigonocephaly: some clinical and surgical features. Acta Neurol Belg. 1980;80(3):137–43.
14. Sargent C, Burn J, Baraitser M, Pembrey ME. Trigonocephaly and the Opitz C syndrome. J Med Genet. 1985;22(1):39–45.
15. Schaap C, Schrander-Stumpel CT, Fryns JP. Opitz-C syndrome: on the nosology of mental retardation and trigonocephaly. Genet Couns. 1992;3(4):209–15.
16. Dhellemmes P, Pellerin P, Lejeune JP, Lepoutre F. Surgical treatment of trigonocephaly. Experience with 30 cases. Childs Nerv Syst. 1986;2(5):228–32.
17. Marsh J, Schwartz H. The surgical correction of coronal and metopic craniosynostosis. J Neurosurg. 1983;59:245–51.
18. Aryan HE, Jandial R, Ozgur BM, Hughes SA, Meltzer HS, Park MS, et al. Surgical correction of metopic synostosis. Childs Nerv Syst. 2005;21(5):392–8.
19. Paige KT, Cohen SR, Simms C, Burstein FD, Hudgins R, Boydston W. Predicting the risk of reoperation in metopic synostosis: a quantitative CT scan analysis. Ann Plast Surg. 2003;51(2):167–72.
20. Ravindra VM, Awad AW, Baker CM, Lee A, Anderson RCE, Gociman B, et al. Preoperative imaging patterns and intracranial findings in single-suture craniosynostosis: a study from the synostosis research group. J Neurosurg Pediatr. 2021;28(3):344–50.
21. Shimoji T, Shimabukuro S, Sugama S, Ochiai Y. Mild trigonocephaly with clinical symptoms: analysis of surgical results in 65 patients. Childs Nerv Syst. 2002;18(5):215–24.
22. Shimoji T, Tominaga D, Shimoji K, Miyajima M, Tasato K. Analysis of pre- and post-operative symptoms of patients with mild trigonocephaly using several developmental and psychological tests. Childs Nerv Syst. 2015;31(3):433–40.
23. Ijichi S, Ijichi N. Mild trigonocephaly with clinical symptoms. Childs Nerv Syst. 2002;18(12):659–60. author reply 61–2

24. Ijichi S, Ijichi N, Ishida A, Yotsumoto M, Nagata J, Tanuma R, et al. Ethical fallacies, tricky ambiguities, and the misinterpretation of the outcomes in the cranioplasty for mild trigonocephaly. Childs Nerv Syst. 2015;31(7):1009–12.
25. Birgfeld CB, Saltzman BS, Hing AV, Heike CL, Khanna PC, Gruss JS, et al. Making the diagnosis: metopic ridge versus metopic craniosynostosis. J Craniofac Surg. 2013;24(1):178–85.
26. Kalmar CL, Zapatero ZD, Kosyk MS, Carlson AR, Bartlett SP, Heuer GG, et al. Elevated intracranial pressure with craniosynostosis: a multivariate model of age, syndromic status, and number of involved cranial sutures. J Neurosurg Pediatr. 2021;28:716–23.
27. Hayward R, Britto J, Dunaway D, Jeelani O. Connecting raised intracranial pressure and cognitive delay in craniosynostosis: many assumptions, little evidence. J Neurosurg Pediatr. 2016;18(2):242–50.
28. Starr JR, Collett BR, Gaither R, Kapp-Simon KA, Cradock MM, Cunningham ML, et al. Multicenter study of neurodevelopment in 3-year-old children with and without single-suture craniosynostosis. Arch Pediatr Adolesc Med. 2012;166(6):536–42.
29. Baird L, Proctor MR. Craniosynostosis. In: Albright A, Pollack IF, Adelson P, editors. Principles and practice of pediatric neurosurgery. 3rd ed. New York, NY: Thieme; 2014.
30. Aldana P, Ranalli N. The surgical repair of metopic synostosis. In: Cohen A, editor. Pediatric neurosurgery: tricks of the trade. New York, NY: Thieme; 2015. p. 138–40.
31. Goobie SM, Meier PM, Pereira LM, McGowan FX, Prescilla RP, Scharp LA, et al. Efficacy of tranexamic acid in pediatric craniosynostosis surgery: a double-blind, placebo-controlled trial. Anesthesiology. 2011;114(4):862–71.
32. Fearon JA, Ditthakasem K, Garcia JC, Herbert M. Abandoning the supraorbital bandeau in anterior craniosynostosis repairs, for a single-segment reconstruction. Plast Reconstr Surg. 2018;142(3):334e–41e.
33. Esparza J, Hinojosa J. Complications in the surgical treatment of craniosynostosis and craniofacial syndromes: apropos of 306 transcranial procedures. Childs Nerv Syst. 2008;24(12):1421–30.
34. Aldana PR, Wieder K, Postlethwait RA, James HE, Steinberg B. Ultrasound-aided fixation of biodegradable implants in pediatric craniofacial surgery. Pediatr Neurosurg. 2011;47(5):349–53.
35. Albin RE, Hendee RW Jr, O'Donnell RS, Majure JA. Trigonocephaly: refinements in reconstruction. Experience with 33 patients. Plast Reconstr Surg. 1985;76(2):202–11.
36. Cohen SR, Maher H, Wagner JD, Dauser RC, Newman MH, Muraszko KM. Metopic synostosis: evaluation of aesthetic results. Plast Reconstr Surg. 1994;94(6):759–67.
37. Di Rocco C, Velardi F, Ferrario A, Marchese E. Metopic synostosis: in favour of a "simplified" surgical treatment. Childs Nerv Syst. 1996;12(11):654–63.
38. Posnick JC, Lin KY, Chen P, Armstrong D. Metopic synostosis: quantitative assessment of presenting deformity and surgical results based on CT scans. Plast Reconstr Surg. 1994;93(1):16–24.
39. Schneider EN, Bogdanow A, Goodrich JT, Marion RW, Cohen MM Jr. Fronto-ocular syndrome: newly recognized trigonocephaly syndrome. Am J Med Genet. 2000;93(2):89–93.
40. Wall SA, Goldin JH, Hockley AD, Wake MJ, Poole MD, Briggs M. Fronto-orbital re-operation in craniosynostosis. Br J Plast Surg. 1994;47(3):180–4.
41. van der Meulen J. Metopic synostosis. Childs Nerv Syst. 2012;28(9):1359–67.
42. Zapatero ZD, Zimmerman CE, Kosyk MS, Kalmar CL, Carlson AR, Humphries LS, et al. Single segment neo-bandeau fronto-orbital advancement in children with craniosynostosis: technique adaptation and craniometric analysis. J Craniofac Surg. 2021;32(7):2393–6.

Unicoronal Suture Synostosis: Endoscopic Approach for the Neurosurgeons

45

David F. Jimenez

45.1 Introduction

Premature closure of the coronal suture leads to a number of significant deformations of the facial and cranial skeleton. The phenotypic clinical presentation includes the following findings:

1. Disorbitism in the primary form of vertical dystopia.
2. Strabismus.
3. Ipsilateral frontal plagiocephaly.
4. Nasal tip deviation to the contralateral side.
5. Ipsilateral proptosis.
6. Cranial scoliosis and sagittal cranial and facial imbalance.

Altogether, these findings present the neurosurgeon and his/her craniofacial team with a major treatment challenge. The classical and common way of treating this condition is with an orbitofrontal advancement, which is typically done between the ages of 9 and 12 months. The problem with this approach, in my view, is that the cranial-facial skeleton settles in the specific level of deformity and correction of the aforementioned issues become extremely difficult. For example, repositioning of the entire orbital osseous complex to correct the vertical dystopia becomes an impossibility. Simply moving forward the supraorbital rim and forehead does not address the sagittal imbalance, nasal deviation, or vertical dystopia. On the contrary, releasing the stenosed suture at an early age allows the brain to correct all of these complex deformities, as will be shown in this chapter.

D. F. Jimenez (✉)
Department of Neurosciences, Pediatric Neurosurgery, El Paso Children's Hospital, El Paso, TX, USA

Neurosurgery Department, University Medical Center, El Paso, TX, USA

45.2 Procedure

Given the simple and uncomplicated nature of the endoscopic release of the stenosed coronal suture, minimal preoperative preparation is needed. The diagnosis is simply a clinical one and no CT scan, X-rays, or unnecessary radiation exposure to the patient is needed if the patient has the classical phenotype presentation. The only laboratory value to obtain is a hemoglobin/hematocrit level after the patient is placed under anesthesia. No arterial or central venous lines are placed. No Foley is used, and only one or two peripheral intravenous lines are inserted. The table is rotated 180° from the anesthesiologist and the head is placed on a cerebellar horseshoe headrest. Lubricated corneal shield protectors are placed under the eyelids. A precordial Doppler is placed over the heart to auscultate for possible venous air emboli during the procedure. The head is slightly rotated to the contralateral side in order to expose the entire affected suture (Fig. 45.1). A small strip of hair is shaved at the proposed

F. Di Rocco, J. Kestle (eds.), *Neurosurgical Aspects of Craniosynostosis*,
https://doi.org/10.1007/978-3-031-69386-1_45

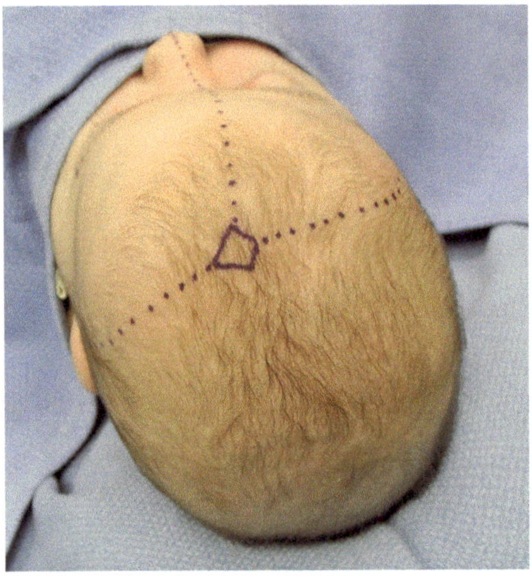

Fig. 45.1 A patient with right coronal synostosis is placed on the cerebellar horseshoe headrest with the head slightly rotated to the left side for improved surgical access

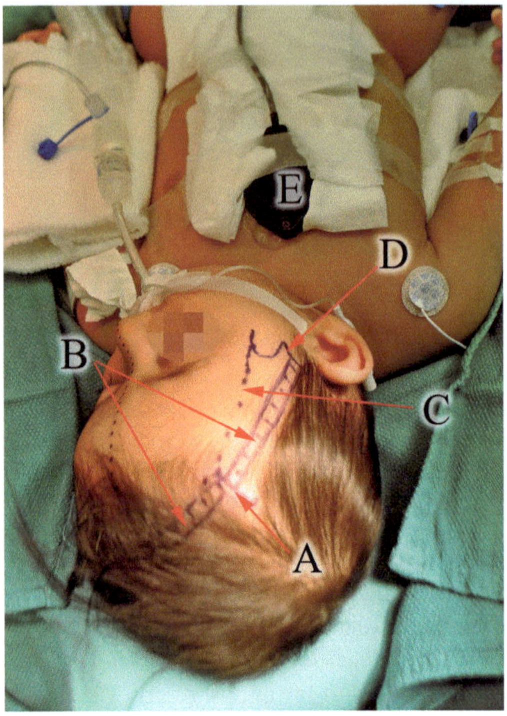

Fig. 45.2 The location of the incision is placed midway between anterior fontanel and pterion. (**a**) The stenosed coronal suture (**c**) is denoted by the dotted line. A strip of bone (4 mm width) shown and marked (**b**), is located behind the stenosed suture and must reach the squamosal suture (**d**). (**e**) Denotes the precordial Doppler

incision site. The incision is made half way between the anterior fontanelle and the squamosal suture immediately in front of the ear (Fig. 45.2). The head and face are prepped with povidone-iodine solution, and a single dose of antibiotics is given 30 min prior to skin incision.

The incision (≈2 cm) is made with the monopolar electrocautery unit using the needle tip set at 10 W on the cut mode. Once the dermis is opened, the rest of the opening through the galea is done using the coagulation mode at 20 W of energy. A rhinoplasty hand held lighted retractor is used to elevate the galea and develop the subgaleal plane towards the anterior fontanelle. A zero-degree rigid endoscope can also be used to perform this dissection. A craniotome with a 7 mm perforator is used to create a burr hole at the incision. A Woodson elevator is used to dissect the dura around the burr hole. A 4 mm Kerrison rongeur is used to remove bone towards the fontanelle for about a centimeter. This maneuver allows the introduction of a 30° rigid endoscope with the angled end aimed at the bone. A small, 7 French suction is inserted and advanced in tandem with the endoscope, developing the epidural plane until reaching the fibers of the anterior fontanelle (Fig. 45.3). Using bone biting pituitary-like rongeurs, a 4 mm osteotomy is created by removing the bone, in a piece-meal fashion under visualization. Once the frontal bone is released from the parietal bone, the diploë is cauterized with suction coagulator. Gentle manipulation of the frontal and parietal bones will demonstrate release and disconnection of these bones (Fig. 45.4).

Once the medial release has been done, attention is directed towards the greater wing of the sphenoid bone and pterion. The subgaleal plane is developed above the temporalis muscle with blunt dissection using a dissector (Fig. 45.5). The endoscope is inserted under the bone and advanced toward the greater wing of the sphenoid (Fig. 45.6), pterion, and the open squamosal suture is identified (Fig. 45.7). The temporalis muscle can be elevated and mobilized from the temporal and parietal bones using the #1 Penfield

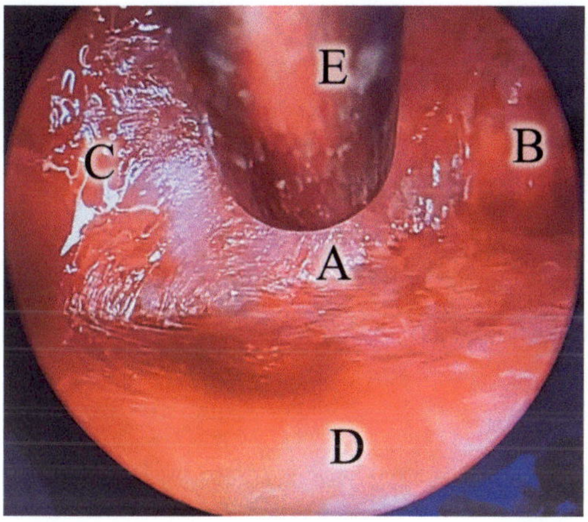

Fig. 45.3 Endoscopic view of the anterior fontanelle (**a**). After dissecting the epidural plane medially. The frontal bone (**b**) and parietal bone (**c**) are visualized. The dura (**d**) and the section-dissector (**e**) are also seen

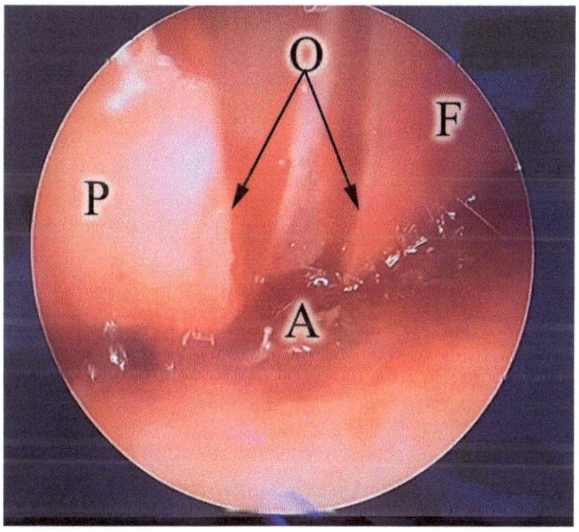

Fig. 45.4 The osteotomy/craniectomy (O) has been extended all the way to the anterior fontanelle. The arrows denote the edges of the osteotomy. The frontal bone (F) has been fully detached from the parietal bone (P) medially

dissector. The bone biting rongeur is used to create a 4 mm osteotomy all the way down past the squamosal suture (Fig. 45.8). This completes the separation of the fronto-orbital complex from the parietal bone (Fig. 45.9). The diploic space is coagulated using suction electrocautery in order to obtain full homeostasis. Surgiflo is sprayed along the osteotomy. The galea is closed with 4.0 monocryl suture. The skin is sealed with Mastisol and Steri-strips, which are removed 6 days later.

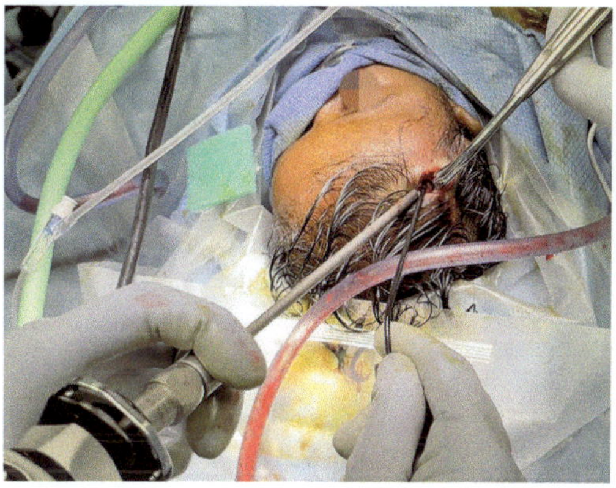

Fig. 45.5 Having completed the osteotomy medially from the fontanelle, attention is directed towards the pterion. A right endoscope is on the surgeon's left hand, and a dissector is used to develop the epidural space with the right hand. The assistant elevates the scalp with a lighted retractor

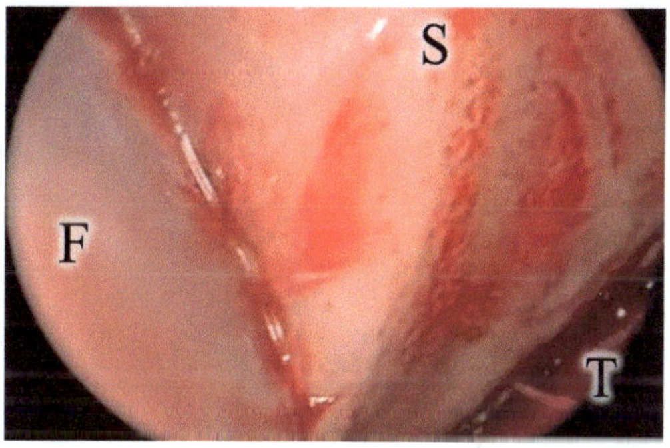

Fig. 45.6 Endoscopic view of the greater wing of the sphenoid (S), the dura of the frontal lobe (F) and temporal lobe (L). The sphenoid wing must be first identified as a primary landmark prior to moving the endoscope posteriorly to look for the squamosal suture

The patient is admitted to the hospital for a 23-h observation period and discharged the next morning. Pain is controlled with alternating doses of acetaminophen and ibuprofen every 3 h for 3 days. On postop day 4, the patient is scanned for a postoperative cranial orthosis, which is manufactured the same day and fitted on the following day. The patient wears the cranial orthosis until correction of the vertical dystopia, advancement of the ipsilateral supraorbital rim, and nasal deviation corrects, usually 6–9 months. The last to correct is the frontal plagiocephaly, which may take several years to fully correct.

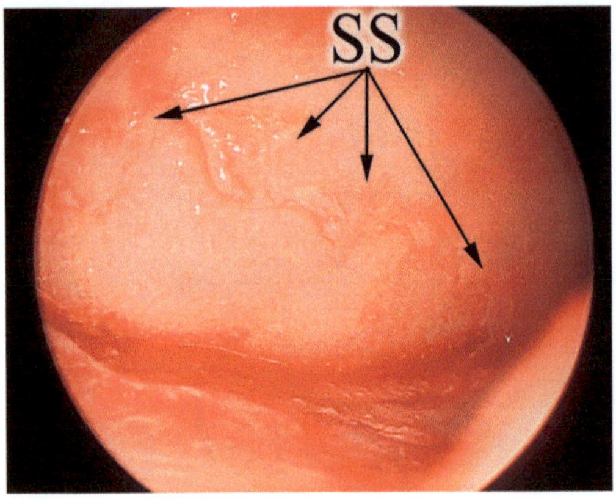

Fig. 45.7 The endoscope has moved posteriorly and inferiorly. The open squamosal suture (S) is identified as pointed by the arrows

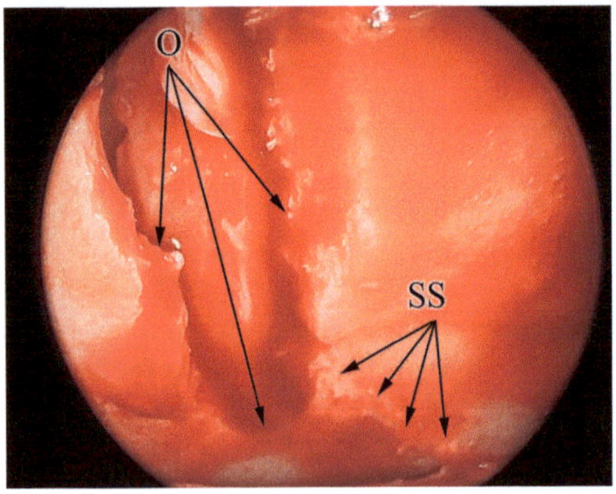

Fig. 45.8 The osteotomy (O) is taken to and past the squamosal suture (SS) to make sure that the frontal and parietal bones have been fully disarticulated

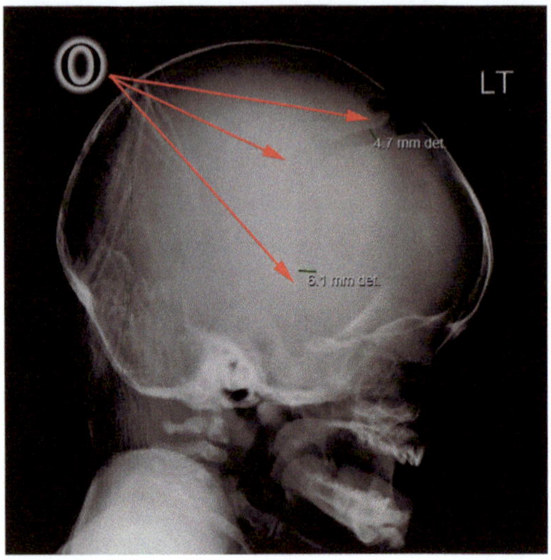

Fig. 45.9 Immediate postoperative lateral skull radiograph shows the 4–6 mm osteotomy (O) extending from the anterior fontanelle to the pterion

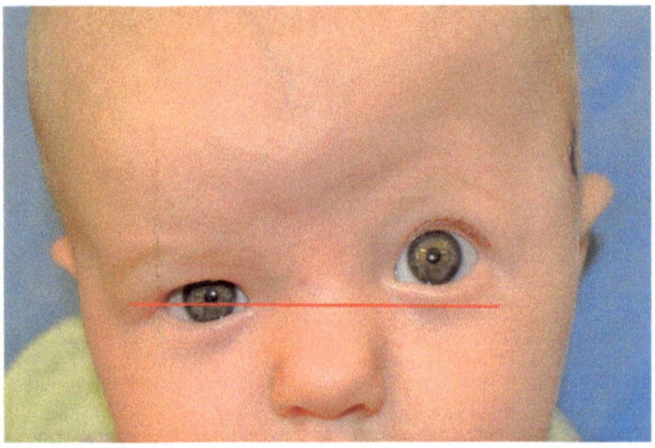

Fig. 45.10 Patient A preoperative photograph of the 3-month-old female with left coronal craniosynostosis and severe vertical dystopia affecting the left eye/orbit

45.3 Outcomes

We have the longest and largest series of unicoronal synostoses treated with endoscopic assisted, minimally invasive techniques. The series expands over 26 years (1996–2023) and comprises a total of 182 patients. There were 112 females (69.3%) and 70 males (30.7%). The median age of the surgery was 4.1 months (0.5–10 months). Median estimated blood loss for the entire cohort was 15 mL. There were no intraoperative blood transfusions and only one patient was transfused postoperative for a 0.7% transfusion rate. The mean surgical time was 43 min. All patients were discharged the morning following the surgery. No patient required the surgery to be converted from endoscopic to an open procedure. Anthropometric analysis with the craniofacial software analysis from the cranial orthosis unit demonstrated marked and significant improvement of the preoperative deformities. Fifty one percent of the patients demonstrated 100% correction of the vertical dystopia and over 2/3 if the patients had over 80% correction of this major deformity (Figs. 45.10, 45.11, 45.12, 45.13, 45.14, 45.15, 45.16, and 45.17). Eighty one percent of the patients presented with sagittal deviation and cra-

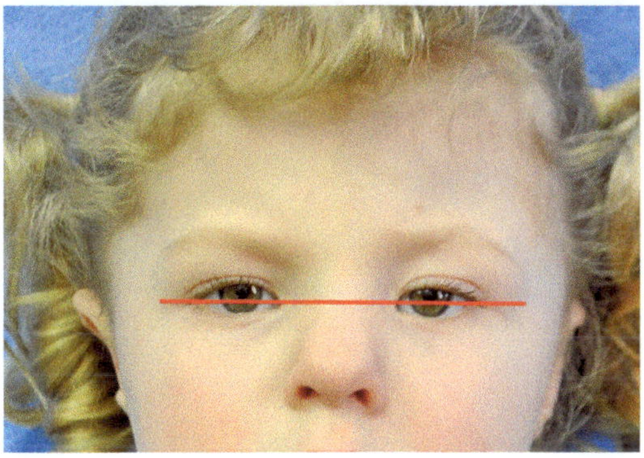

Fig. 45.11 Patient A 2 years postoperatively, the same patient shows that the orbits have realigned along the horizontal exo-endocanthal axis after endoscopic release

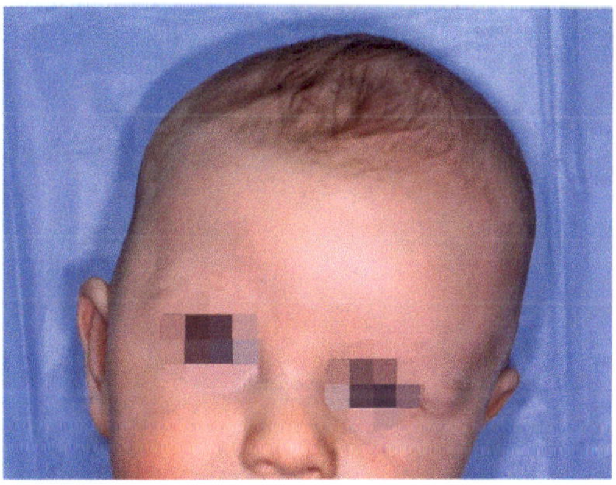

Fig. 45.12 Patient B 4-month-old male with right coronal synostosis and severe vertical dystopia

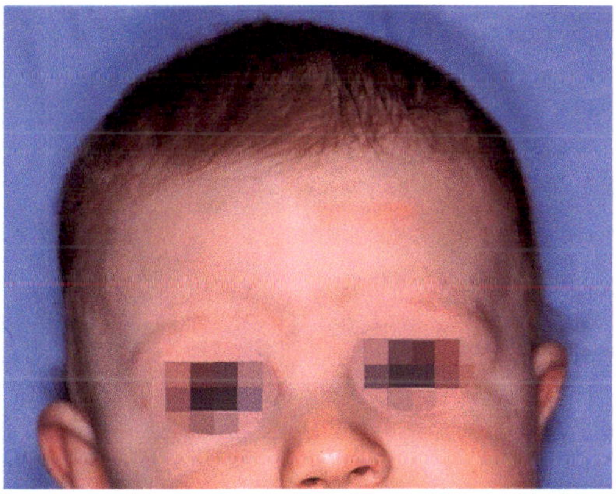

Fig. 45.13 Patient B already at 6 months, he demonstrates significant inferior displacement of the right orbit and improvement of the dystopia

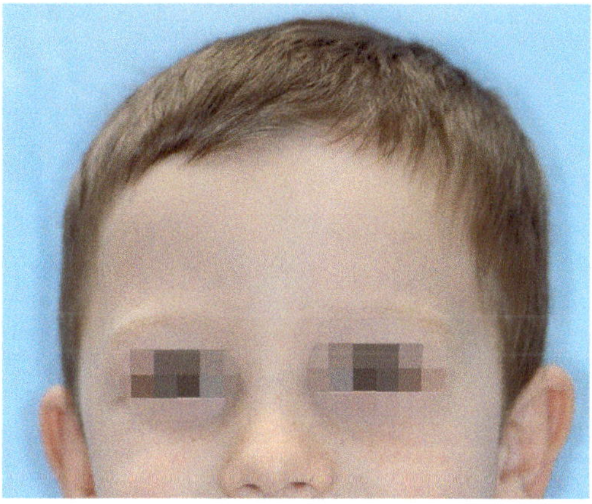

Fig. 45.14 Patient B, 3 years after surgery, the patient demonstrates complete realignment of the eyes along the horizontal axis and no vertical dystopia

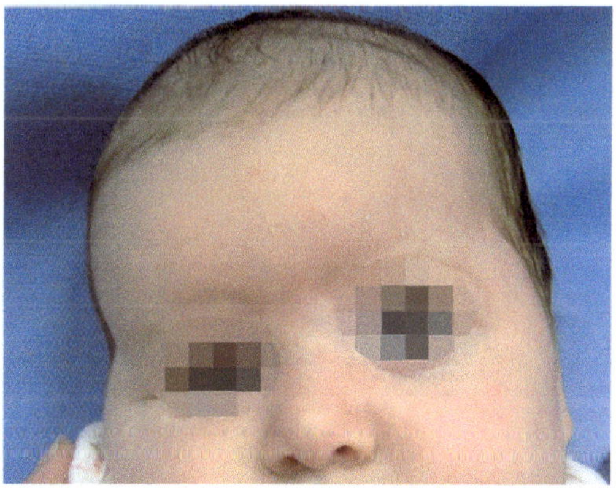

Fig. 45.15 Patient C 2-month-old female with left sided coronal synostosis and vertical dystopia

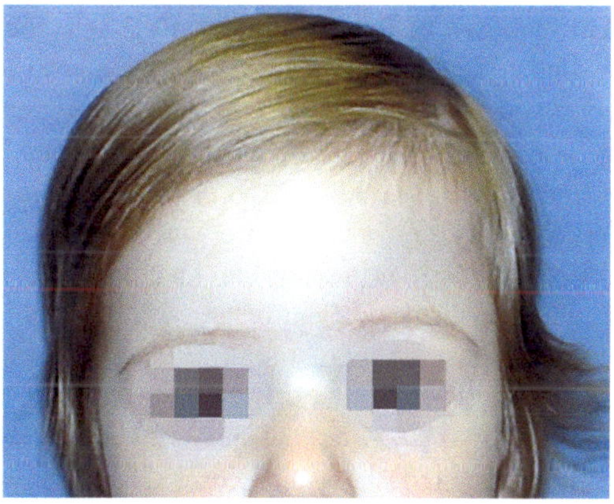

Fig. 45.16 Patients C, 1 year after surgery demonstrates a complete correction of the dystopia

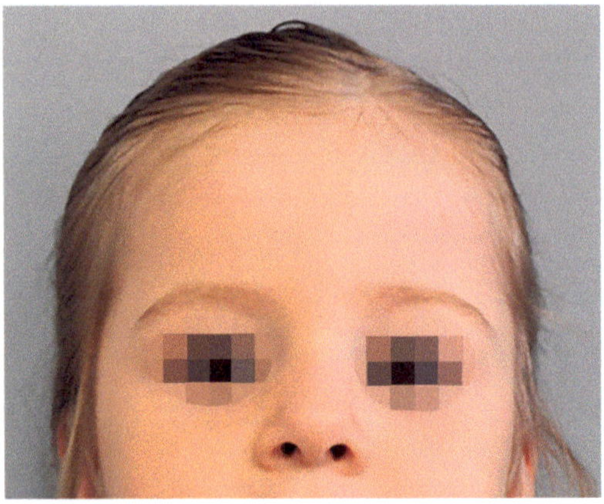

Fig. 45.17 Patient C, 2.5 years after surgery continues to show complete and persistent vertical dystopia correction

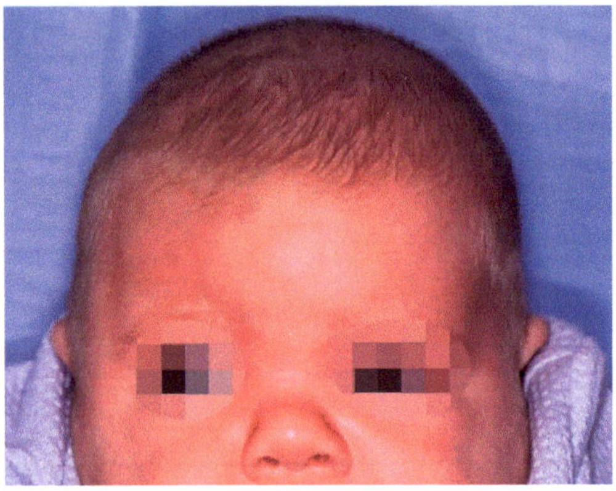

Fig. 45.18 Patient D, 10-week-old male presenting with right coronal craniosynostosis and right eye exotropia

nial scoliosis. Following surgery at a 2-year follow-up, 77% of the patients achieved 100% correction, 4% of the patients achieved correction between 80% and 90%, 8% of the patients achieved 70%, and 12% of the patients achieved less than 70% correction. There were no mortalities. Strabismus is a very common presenting finding and in our patient cohort, 84.3% of the patients presented with strabismus (Figs. 45.18, 45.19, 45.20, 45.21, 45.22, 45.23, 45.24, 45.25, and 45.26). At 3-year follow up, only 3.7% of the patients required strabismus correction surgery. This means that there was an 88.9% correction of the strabismus with a simple craniectomy done at an early age.

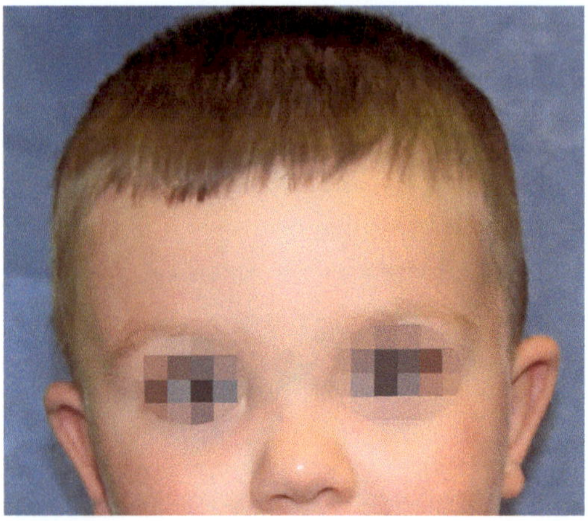

Fig. 45.19 Patient D, 1 year following endoscopic release of the right coronal suture. The strabismus has fully corrected without the need for surgical corrections

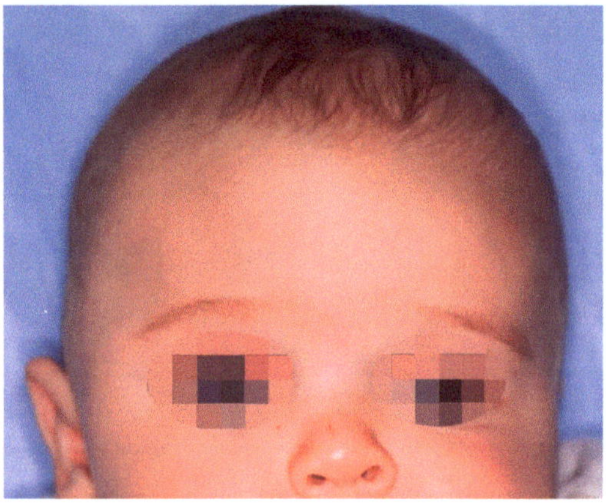

Fig. 45.20 Patient E, 9-week-old male with right coronal synostosis and left exotropia

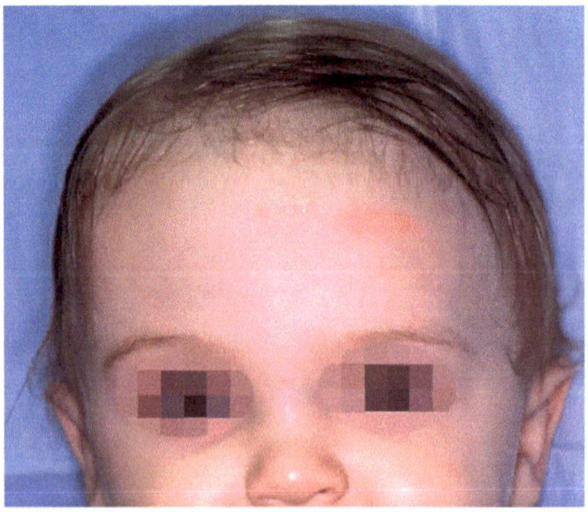

Fig. 45.21 Patient E, 1 year after surgery patient shows complete correction of the strabismus without the need for ocular surgery

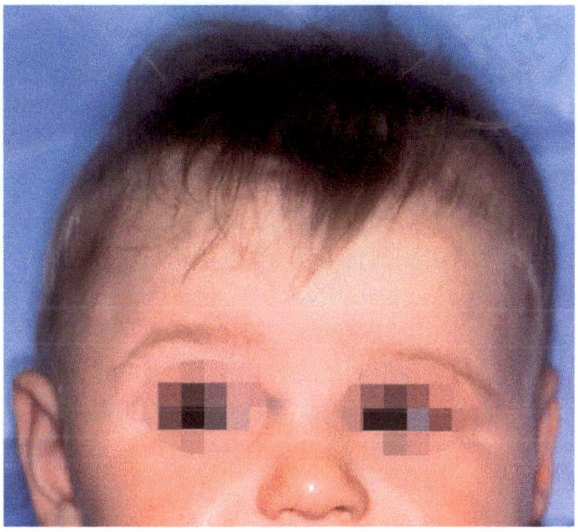

Fig. 45.22 Patient F, 10-week-old male with right coronal synostosis and right exotropia

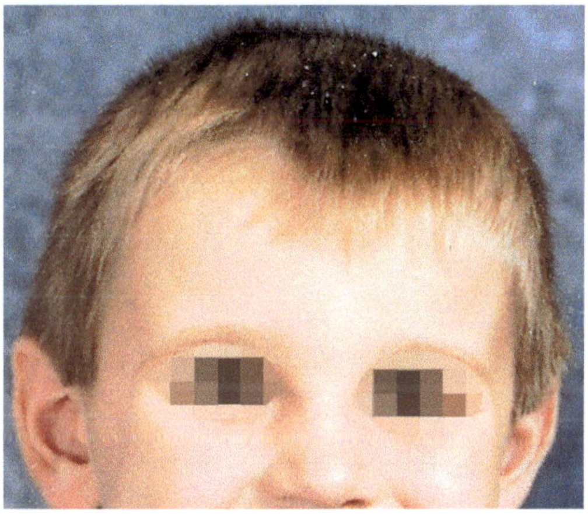

Fig. 45.23 Patient F, 4 years after endoscopic craniectomy, no strabismus, no ocular surgery

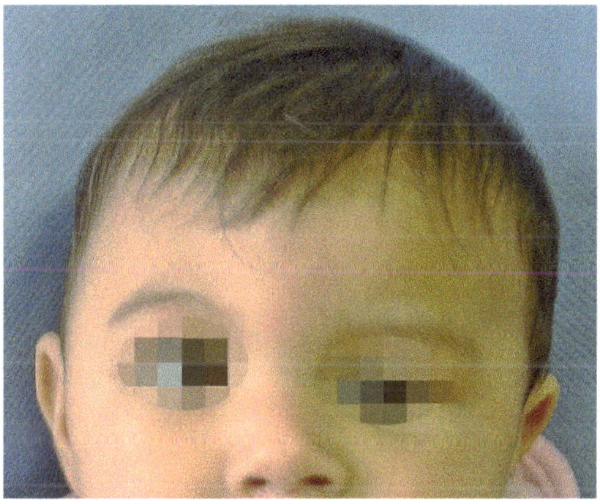

Fig. 45.24 Patient G, 3-month-old male with right coronal synostosis and severe right esotropia

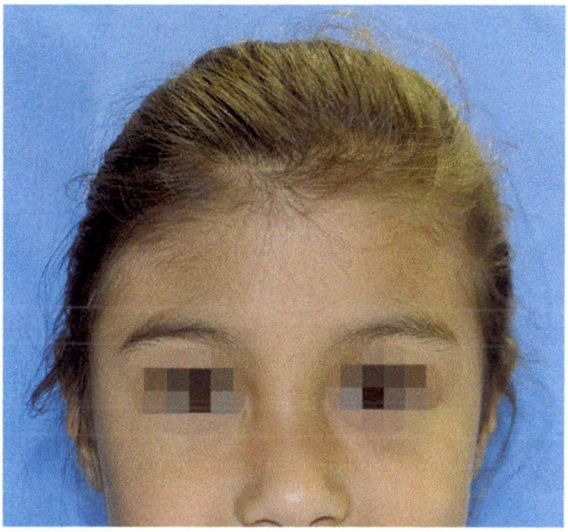

Fig. 45.25 Patient G, 6-years postendoscopic surgery the patient has fully corrected the esotropia without surgery

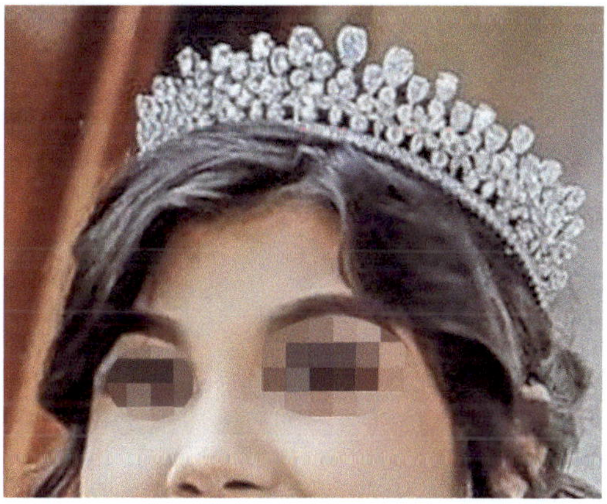

Fig. 45.26 Patient G, 16 years after surgery shows no dystopia, strabismus or midsagittal imbalance correction

45.4 Discussion

Presented in this chapter are the results treating patients with unicoronal craniosynostosis using minimally invasive techniques. This series is the longest (26 years) and the largest (182) reported in the literature. The basic underlying principles supporting this approach are simple. Brain growth doubles in size in the first 6 months. Average brain weight at birth is 400 g, at 6 months the weight doubles to 800 g. This extremely rapid brain growth phase provides an opportunity for the brain to reshape the cranial and facial skeleton once the root cause of the problem is removed by fully releasing the stenosed suture. The results of this series prove that to be the case. Once the suture is released, the ipsilateral frontal lobe, which has been retained in a posterior and superior position in relation to the contralateral lobe, is allowed to resume its normal and preferred position. The brain advances forward and inferiorly. As such, the forehead and supraorbital rim move forward. The orbit moves forward and inferiorly, thereby correcting the sagittal imbalance and cranial scoliosis. The goal of the fronto-orbital advancement surgery is to move the ipsilateral forehead and supraorbital rim about 2–3 cm forward. We have found out that the same can be done with the endoscopic procedure and cranial orthosis without having to do major open surgery (Fig. 45.27a–c).

Furthermore, preliminary unpublished data show there is a mild to moderate elevation of the intracranial pressure which normalizes immediately following the craniectomy. Fundoscopic examination in our patients preoperatively is showing significant abnormalities to include segmental papilledema and retinal vascular abnormalities, which resolve as early as 2 months postoperatively.

Neuropsychological testing done before and after surgery show all of our patients to be average or above average. We have found no underperformers or abnormal patients. We believe that short surgical times (43 min) with minimal exposure to general anesthesia, excellent blood pressure control, and brain perfusion pressures and lack of need for significant blood transfusions (as in calvarial vault surgery) underlie these superb

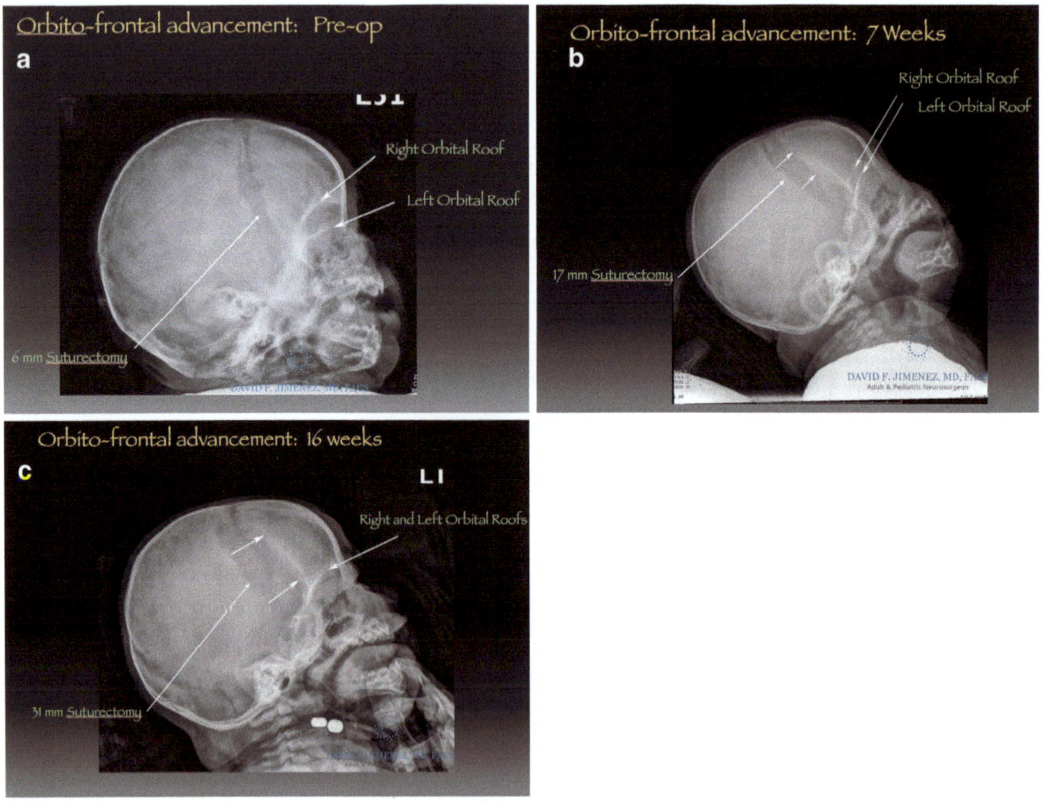

Fig. 45.27 (**a**) Immediate skull ray of a patient with right coronal synostosis who underwent and endoscopic 6 mm craniectomy. Notice the elevation of the right orbital roof in relation to the left. (**b**) 7 weeks post-surgery, the lateral radiograph shows internal fronto-orbital advancement of 11 mm. The right orbital roof has lowered. (**c**) 16 weeks after surgery, the suturectomy has increased to 3.1 cm and both orbital roofs have aligned without the need for a front-orbital advancement

results. Endoscopic treatment of unicoronal craniosynostosis, done at an early age is an excellent option that should be given to all of the parents of those affected children.

References

1. Gencarclli JR, Murphy A, Samargandi OA, Bezuhly M. Ophthalmologic outcomes following fronto-orbital advancement for unicoronal craniosynostosis. J Neurosurg. 1992;76(3):401–6.
2. Sloan GM, Wells KC, Raffel C, McComb JG. Surgical treatment of craniosynostosis: outcome analysis of 250 consecutive. Pediatrics. 1997;100(1):e2.
3. Öwall L, Darvann TA, Larsen P, Hove HD, Hermann W, Bøgeskov L, Kreiborg S. Facial asymmetry in children with unicoronal synostosis who have undergone craniofacial reconstruction in infancy. Cleft Palate Craniofac J. 2016;53(4):385–93.
4. Hansen M, Padwa BL, Scott MR, Stieg PE, Mulliken JB. Synostotic frontal plagiocephaly: anthropometric comparison of three techniques for surgical correction. Plast Reconstr Surge. 1997;100(6):1387–95.
5. McCarthy JG, Glasberg SB, Cutting CB, Epstein FJ, Grayson BH, Ruff G, Thorne CH, Wisoff J, Zide BM. Twenty-year experience with early surge for craniosynostosis: the craniofacial synostosis syndromes and pansynotosis-results and unsolved problems. Plast Reconstr Surg. 1995;96(2):284–95.
6. Barone CM, Jimenez DF. Endoscopic approach to coronal craniosynostosis. Clin Plast Surg. 2004;31(3):415–22.
7. Jimenez DF, Barone CM. Endoscopic technique for coronal craniosynostosis. Childs Nerv Syst. 2012;28(9):1429–32.
8. Jimenez DF, Barone CM. Early treatment of coronal synostosis with endoscopy assisted craniectomy and postoperative cranial orthosis therapy: 16-year experience. J NSurg Pediatr. 2013;12(3):207–19.
9. Jimenez DF, Barone CM. Endoscopic techniques for craniosynostosis. Atlas Oral Maxillofac Surg Clin North Am. 2010;18(2):93–107.
10. Jimenez DF, Barone CM, et al. Early management of craniosynostosis using endoscopic assisted strip craniectomies and cranial orthotic molding therapy. Pediatrics. 2002;110(1):97–104.

Unicoronal Suture Synostosis: Open Vault Surgery, Key Points for the Neurosurgeons

46

Federico Di Rocco

46.1 Introduction

The early fusion of one hemicoronal suture leads to a complex combination of bone anomalies of the cranial basis, the cranial vault, the facies and, in most severe cases, of the upper axis. While the anomalies of the cranial vault and the orbit are satisfactorily corrected by an appropriate surgical treatment those of the face, namely, the deviation of the nasal pyramid and the mandibular asymmetry are faced by the surgeon only when extremely severe and disfiguring. In most cases, they are not addressed due to their limited functional impact (Fig. 46.1).

The anomalies of first vertebra consist of the volumetric combination of the hypotrophy of the lateral mass on the side of the early fused hemicoronal suture and the hypertrophy of the controlateral one. Opposite volumetric changes involve the occipital *condyle*, being hypertrophic the one on the side of the early affected hemicoronal suture and hypotrophic the contralateral one. These "crossed" changes account for the oblique orientation of the craniovertebral junction on the horizontal plane that is responsible of the torticollis which characterizes the most severely affected subjects. The depending functional disturbance is rarely addressed surgically because of the limitations of the techniques currently available. Consequently, when necessary, most of the affected children undergo specific physiotherapic treatments. Also, the peculiar type of strabismus and other abnormalities of ocular movements that can be noticed in many of the infants with anterior plagiocephaly secondary to the alterations in volume and shape of the orbit on the side of the precociously fused hemicoronal suture are rarely treated surgically during infancy [1, 2]. Indeed, the early surgical correction is required only in children with significant functional impairment. Similar considerations can be made for the other bone anomalies that do not cause an evident cosmetic defect or do not bear an important functional impact, e.g., the anterior displacement of the petrous bone in the affected hemicranium or the asymmetry of the mandibula that depends on the anterior displacement of the mandibular articulation on the synostotic side (Fig. 46.1).

On the other hands, some of the osseous anomalies in the coronal-frontosphenoidal, sphenoethmoidal, and frontozygomatic suture associated with the early fusion of the hemicoronal require a prompt surgical correction both to correct the cosmetic defect secondary to the already established bony anomalies and to pre-

F. Di Rocco (✉)
Department of Pediatric Neurosurgery, French Referral Center for Craniosynostosis of Lyon, ERN Cranio, INSERM 1033, Université de Lyon, Hôpital Femme Mère Enfant, Hospices Civils de Lyon, Lyon, France
e-mail: federico.dirocco@chu-lyon.fr

F. Di Rocco, J. Kestle (eds.), *Neurosurgical Aspects of Craniosynostosis*,
https://doi.org/10.1007/978-3-031-69386-1_46

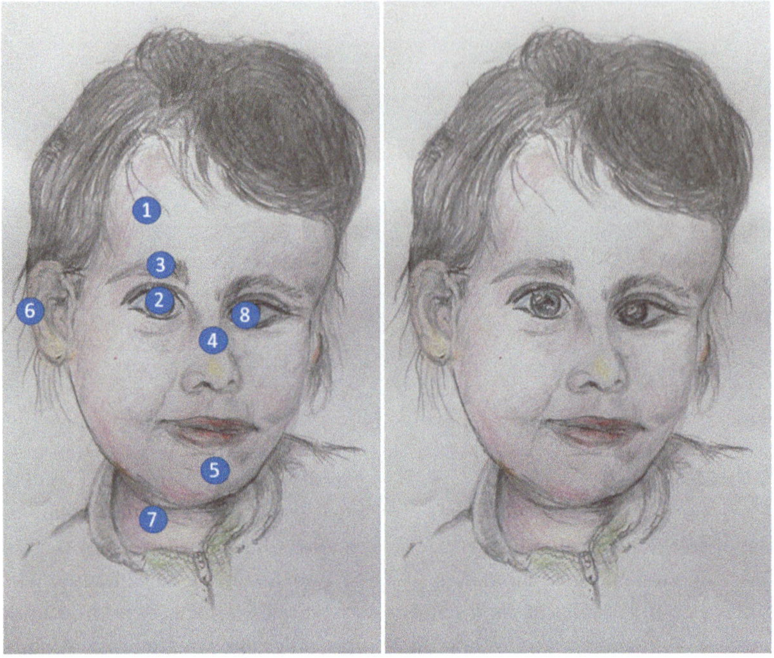

Fig. 46.1 Phenotype of anterior plagiocephaly. The early fusion of the right hemicoronal suture determines several developmental bone anomalies: the flattening and posterior displacement of the right hemifrontal bone (1), the flattening of the orbit with secondary ocular proptosis (2), the flattening and elevation of the right supraorbital ridge (3), the contralateral deviation of the nasal pyramid (4) and mandibula (5), the anterior displacement of the temporal pyramid (6), the volumetric asymmetry of the lateral masses of the first cervical vertebrae associated to an opposite volumetric modification of the occipital condyle resulting in a torticollis (7). Because of the ocular proptosis in the affected side, the normal eye appears smaller. Squint is nearly always associated (8)

vent their further aggravation. This is the case of the hypoplasic and posteriorly displaced hemifrontal bone that may impair the normal growth of the brain and the reduced volume of the abnormally shaped orbit resulting in the typical drop or "harlequin" type deformity and ocular globe proptosis.

Indeed, besides the possible functional abnormalities, the frontal and orbital deformation impact on the facial development of the affected child that might influence the self-perception or social acceptance, so impairing the normal psychomotor development. A similar motivation may encourage the craniofacial surgeon to surgically manage the deviation of the nasal pyramid during adolescence in cases where it aggravates the cosmetic appearance of the C-shaped and twisted face, typical of the condition, already visible in the first months or years of life.

46.2 Surgical Considerations

The surgical management of unilateral coronal synostosis should be modulated, taking into account the degree of severity of the condition in various children. In such a regard, the classification that subdivides the affected population in three main types according to the anomalies of the cranial base as shown by the radiological investigations offers a valid and practical tool both for the surgical indication and the prediction of the surgical outcome (Fig. 46.2).

In *Type I*, the bone anomalies do not involve the anterior skull base. Only the frontal bone on the side of the early fused hemicoronal suture is flattened and displaced posteriorly together with the supraorbital rim. The vomer bone maintains its midline position as well as the nasal pyramid.

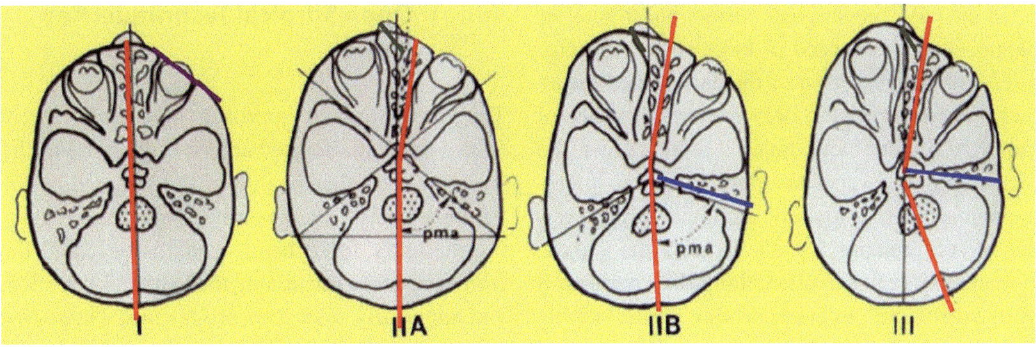

Fig. 46.2 Classification of coronal synostosis according to skull base alterations. (Adapted from Ref. [3])

In *Type II*, the posterior displacement of the hemifrontal bone on the affected side is associated to a deviation of the vomer bone towards the fused suture and to a moderate contralateral deviation of the nasal bones. Type II can be further subdivided into Type II A and Type II B according to the absence or presence of anterior rotation and displacement of the homolateral temporal petrous bone.

Type III is characterized by the obvious anterior displacement of the temporal pyramid, the marked homolateral attraction of the vomer bone towards the affected side and the more pronounced retrocession of the hemifrontal bone, all contributing to a further volumetric reduction of the anterior hemicranial fossa. Also, the contralateral deviation of the nasal pyramid is more obvious. In most severe cases even the occipital fossa is affected with the homolateral deviation of the posterior half of the median basal axis of the skull.

Such a classification is quite useful to anticipate the family's expectations as the surgical result is very satisfactory in Type I and limited in type III. Intermediate results can be expected in Type II anterior plagiocephaly [3, 4].

When planning the surgical management of anterior plagiocephaly synostosis is necessary to take into account the potential underlying genetic condition, e.g., Muenke, TCF12 or Saethre-Chotzen syndromes that are phenotypically expressed as unilateral coronal synostosis in some infants. Indeed, the presence of genetic anomalies is associated to a high risk of recurrence or incomplete cosmetic results that should be anticipated to the parents.

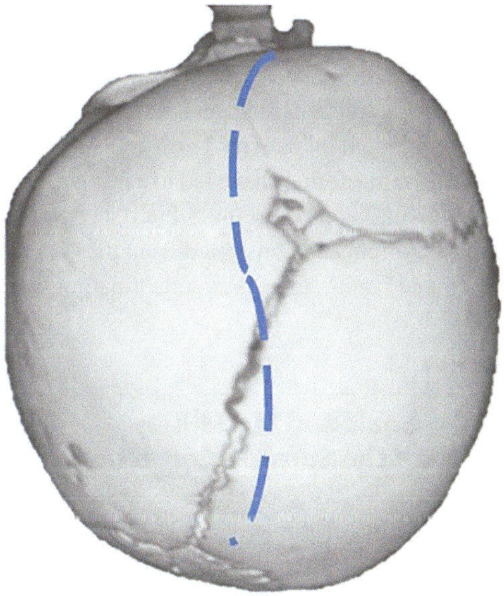

Fig. 46.3 Projection of the superior sagittal sinus position on the skull vault. (Adapted from Ref. [5])

The surgical management starts from a careful analysis of the available imaging in order to anticipate how the vascular structures are displaced. Indeed, the superior sagittal sinus will not be on the midline due to the skull scoliosis (Fig. 46.3). The superior sagittal sinus is usually deviated contralaterally to the closed coronal suture and generally it is deviated contralaterally to the closed coronal suture [5].

In the past, the surgical correction of anterior plagiocephaly consisted of large strip craniectomies with the resection of the early fused suture that proved to provide only a limited release of the frontal bone and failed to counteract the recession of the superior orbital ridge. Strip craniectomies were also associated with a high incidence of relapse, even when the linear craniectomy was extended along the lateral wall of the orbit the inferior orbital fissure in the attempt of addressing the synostosis involving the skull base too [6]. Even the introduction of some technical variations such as the lateral canthal advancement [7] or the apposition of a piece of bone between the surgically advanced lateral canthus and the anterior border of the parietal bone failed to prevent relapse in a significant proportion operated on patients [8]. Surgical failures of linear craniectomies have led to a more aggressive surgical approach, in which a free and advanced forehead is separated from the face and the cranial vault, the so-called "floating forehead" [9, 10].

46.3 Goals and Modalities of the Surgical Correction

The basic aim of the surgical correction of the early fusion of the hemicoronal suture is to advance the anterior cranial vault and the superior orbital rim on the affected side in order to reestablish a normal volume of the anterior cranial fossa and the orbit. To assure a cosmetically rewarding surgical outcome, the advancement of these bone structures is associated to their remodelling to assure a cosmetically rewarding surgical outcome that can be better obtained with an open surgical approach.

The open surgical approach is usually well tolerated by an healthy infant. Nevertheless, the associate blood loss should not be undervalued especially when the operation is carried out in early infancy to profit of the more malleable bone and the pushing of the developing brain, postoperatively.

46.3.1 Open Surgical Technique: Key Points

The open surgical approach allows the direct access to the malformed anterior frontal bone and superior orbit that facilitates the removal of the flattened and retruded hemifrontal bone, containing the early fused hemicoronal suture, and the frontal bandeau containing the flattened, retruded, and superiorly displaced orbital rim. These free bone flaps so obtained are then remodeled prior to their replacement by greenstick fracture of the supraorbital rim to recreate its normal anterior convex shape and by parietal linear bone cuts of the frontoparietal flap to favour the late normalization and possible expansion under the force of the growing brain to compensate for the restricted volume of the anterior cranial fossa.. The remodeled bones are repositioned in a more advanced position to assure sufficient space for the normal cerebral growth (frontoorbital advancement). In most cases, the frontal bone flap is replaced after an appropriate rotation to exploit the curvature of its less flattened superior half in order to create a "normal" frontal bossing similar to that of the contralateral intact hemifrontal bone [6–8]. Spatial overcorrection is often selected by replacing the superior orbital ridge and the frontal bone in a more advanced position as compared to the contralateral intact side to favor a symmetrical aspect in the subsequent late developmental phases and the risk of relapse of the condition [11, 12]. Such a risk is high in cases of syndromic synostosis.

The necessity to count on thick enough but still pliable cranial bones to be remodeled and a stable reconstruction of the anterior skull explains the reason to operate on the affected children between 9 and 12 months of age. However, some authors advocate an earlier correction to fully exploit the action of the developing underlying brain and its ability to mold more compliant bones.

A reliable stabilization of the bone segments utilized for the cranial reconstruction is mandatory to prevent recurrence of the cosmetic defect and, even more important, brain damage related to their postoperative mobility. In the past, metallic screws and plates were utilized for such a purpose. They were abandoned after the demonstration of their migration through the bone in late postoperative radiological controls. Nowadays, biodegradable resorbable plates and screws made from polylactide polymers are commonly utilized, placed whenever possible on the internal face of the bone segment. Resorbable plates and screws provide a rigid fixation for the first 2–3 months up to for 6–9 months before biodegrading around the end of the first postoperative year [13, 14].

The main advantage of the open surgical approach is the immediate correction of the malformation. The main disadvantages are represented by the relative severity of the operation, the perioperative haemorrhagic risk. A further significant disadvantage compared to minimally invasive techniques is the postoperative obvious scar [15–20].

46.3.1.1 Surgical Procedure

The hair is prepared with antiseptic shampooing. The child is then placed supine on the OT, the head resting on a horseshoe headrest. The skin of entire frontoparietal regions and face are prepped with betadine solution, and the head and face are draped up just below the nose. The hair is combed or it might be shaved minimally for a coronal strip, 1 cm in width, from one ear to the other. A zig-zag bilateral coronal incision of the scalp is designed with the end points at 2 cm above the ear of each side. The zig zag incision should be preferred to minimize the risk of enlarging postoperative scar faced by a linear straight incision in case of an excessive tension secondary to the expansion of the frontal lobe. The zig zag incision is thought to better distribute the force vectors in multiple directions. Furthermore, this type of incision is more effectively hidden by the hair even when wet, in children with straight hair too. The scalp incision is then carried out after having infiltrated the subcutaneous tissue and galea with a solution of Lidocaine and Epinephrine in order to reduce blood loss. Hemostasis of the scalp is obtained using the bipolar coagulation, the Colorado needle and/or clips.

A blunt dissection of the galea from the underlying periosteum is then made to reflect the cutaneous flap anteriorly and expose the frontal region. The dissection can also be undertaken directly subperiosteally leaving the periosteum adherent to the skin flap. In all cases, the preservation of the periosteum is important to retain the bone production capacity. The folded frontal flap is reflected anteriorly using elastic bands and protected during the operation by the topic application of wet abdominal pads. Matrix hemostatic sealants might be utilized throughout the operation to favour hemostasis. The periosteum is then incised along the anterior border of the temporal muscle. The muscle is then transected horizontally together with the underlying periosteum at about 1 cm from its proximal insertion on the skull and reflected off the temporal fossa left attached to the scalp flap. The use of electrocautery and accurate hemostasis minimize the blood loss. The incision of the periosteum is then continued inferiorly to expose the lateral orbital rim down to the body of zygomatic bone, approximately at 1 cm posteriorly to the fused hemicoronal suture up to the midline. By contouring the lateral borders of the anterior fontanel the incision is extended anteriorly along the midline ending at 2 cm above the supraorbital ridge to be then continued at this distance parallelly to the inferior border of the frontal bone to reach the periosteal incision in the temporal region. Successively, the frontal incision of the periosteumis extended on the contralateral frontal region to facilitate the anterior reflexion of the membrane above the frontal folded scalp. The nasofrontal suture and the supraorbital notch are exposed. In case when the nerve is running in a groove, it should be made free using a bone scalpel with a delicate manoeuvre meant at preserving its anatomical and functional integrity to avoid postoperative sensorial deficit. The superior surface of the ocular capsule is then detached from the overlaying inferior surface of the orbital roof and the palpebral ligament from the frontozygomatic suture. The intraorbital dissection of the periorbita is extended to the lat-

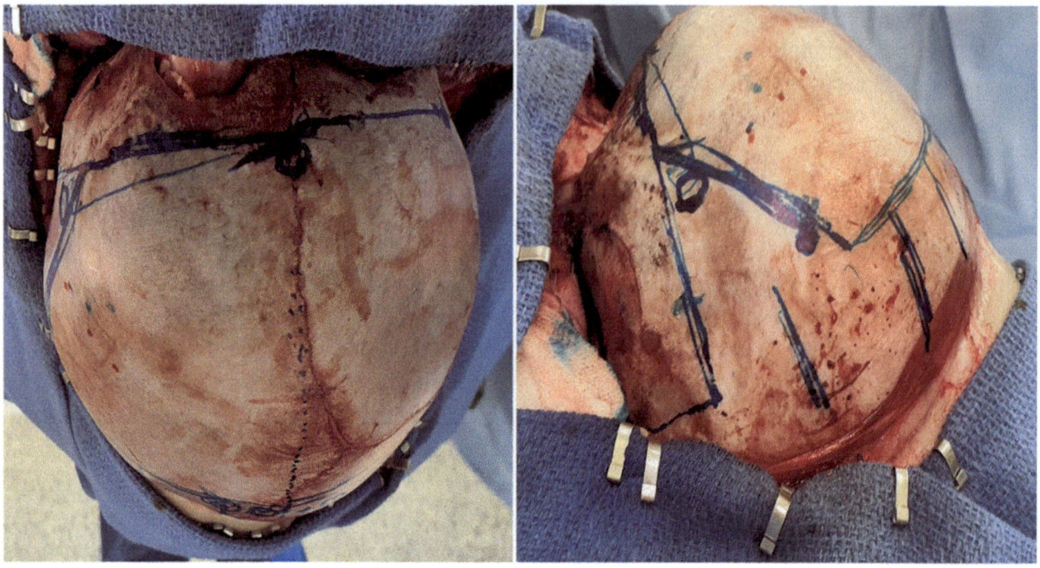

Fig. 46.4 Osteotomy design to correct a left coronal synostosis. Note that the forehead is planned to be tilted inferiorly on the left side in order to correct the asymmetry of the frontal bossing

eral orbital rim and down to the junction of the inferior orbital rim.

The osteotomy design is performed (Fig. 46.4).

The osteotomy plan aims at identifying the orbital bandeau and the future frontal bone. The donor site for the new frontal bone will be adapted to the patient anatomy and degree of deformation. The same forehead might be used after a minor remodeling in case of mild deformation whereas, in case of sever deformation, the forehead must be obtained by a different anatomical region.

The hemifrontal craniotomy is performed after the appropriately blunt dissection of the periosteum along the outlined borders of the osteotomy plan.

One or several burr holes might be performed in order to get an access to the epidural space and separate the dura from the bone that will be cut with a craniotome.

The bone flap can also be obtained using directly an ultrasonic piezosurgery bone scalpel which allows to spare bone and reduces the risk of dural tears or damaging the soft tissues (Fig. 46.5).

A blunt dissector can be the used through the burr holes to detach the dura from the overlying inner cranial surface along the line of the designed craniotomy to facilitate the careful lifting and removal of the frontal bone flap. Care must be taken when dissecting the pterional region in the affected side where the dura can makea fold within the elevated sphenoid ridge. A supraorbital bar is then prepared by removing the inferior border of the frontal bone and the upper part of the nasal bones and cutting the mesial supraorbital ridge anteriorly to the foramen cecum: completely, if the removal of the fronto-orbital bar is planned, or partially in case where only the anterior rotation of the bar is decided by pivoting it on this level after fracturing the residual bone at the mesial superior angle of the orbit. Eventually, the craniotomy can continue laterally and the lateral pillar of the orbit can be included in the bandeau (Fig. 46.6).

The bone cut is then continued across the orbital roof remaining at about 1 cm posteriorly to the superior orbital ridge by retracting the dura mater and the underlying frontal lobe using malleable retractors to protect the brain as well as the capsule of the ocular globe. Laterally the cutting is extended posteriorly and inferiorly, on the lateral wall of the orbit paralleling the zygomatic arch in the region of the frontosphenoidal and frontozygomatic sutures, to create a rectangular "tongue" to be used to advance and lowering the supraorbital bar.

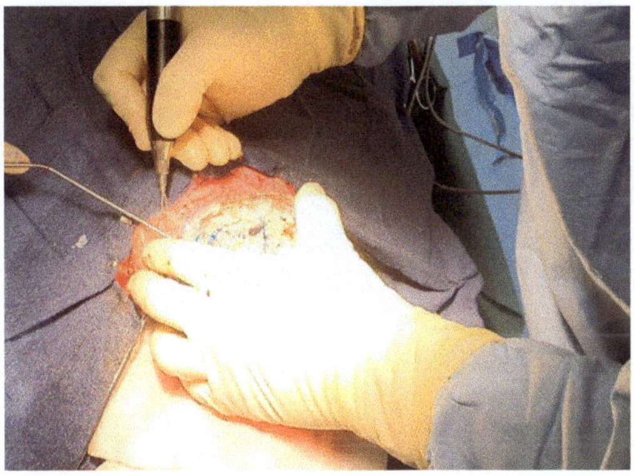

Fig. 46.5 Frontal bone osteotomy using piezoelectric® bone scalpel

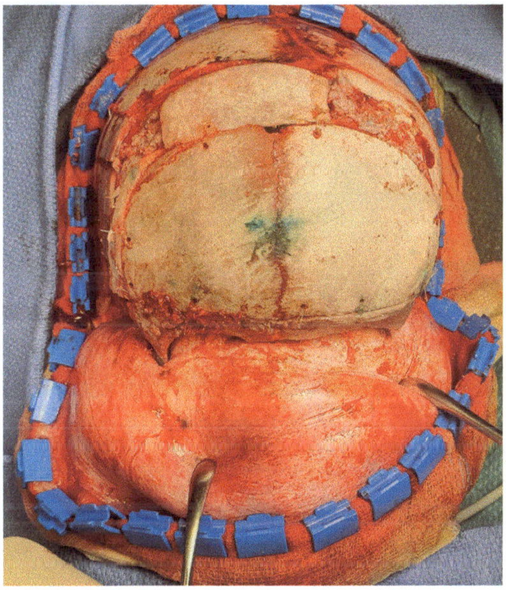

Fig. 46.6 The lateral wall of the right orbit is included in the bandeau advancement. Note that the periosteum is attached to the skin flap

The supraorbital bar is first drilled to obtain symmetrical orbital roofs; then, it is replaced on the skull. It is held in place in the new advanced position with transosseous sutures with PDS or vicryl, and/or bio-resorbable plates and screws. The degree of advancement is related to the severity of the malformation. Usually, the supraorbital bar advancement overcompensates the contralateral side to favour the late outcome [1–12]. The degree of over overcorrection when replacing the supraorbital and the frontal bone is limited by the need of performing a scalp closure without tension. The abnormal superior orbital roof homolateral to the synostosis can be corrected with a greenstick fracture and using a bone bender at this stage.

The supraorbital bar is then replaced, inclined in a ventral direction to correct the usual more vertical and backward slanted development of this structure, so to reestablish the normal angle and assure an immediate better cosmetic reconstruction. The "tongue in groove" portion of the supraorbital bar advanced within the parietal groove assures a stable new position that can be further reinforced by the replacement of the frontal bone flap, appropriately reshaped and rotated (usually by 180°), anchored to the contralateral frontal bone mesially and to the border of the parietal bone superiorly. The reshaping of the frontal bone flap, by means of the bone bending forceps is facilitated by radial cuts that decrease the bone resistance consequently facilitating the action of the instrument. When the anterior portion of the parietal bone is abnormally restricted, it can be enlarged with the same tool after having carried out radial bone cuts.

In case of marked protrusion of the temporal fossa, which is often the case in FGFR3 related plagiocephaly, some remodeling of the temporal bone can also be performed (Fig. 46.7).

Because of the reduced dimensions of the replaced frontal bone, small areas of cranial defects will result from the procedure that increases the volume of the anterior cranial fossa (Fig. 46.8).

The defects reossify spontaneously in nearly all the cases previous the accurate reconstitution of the periosteum and repositioning of the temporal muscle. The elevation of the temporal muscle *en bloc* with the scalp flap and eventually the suturing of its superior end to the periosteum of the parietal bone and/or the replaced frontal bone flap is quite useful to fill the hollow due to the advanced frontal–orbital bone The scalp is sutured in two layers; a subgaleal drainage might be left in place may reduce the volume of postoperative effusions, so allowing a faster and safer healing of the surgical wound.

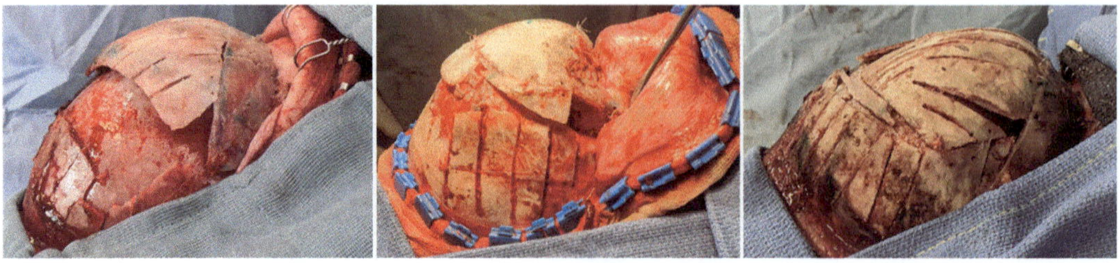

Fig. 46.7 Different types of remodeling of the temporal region

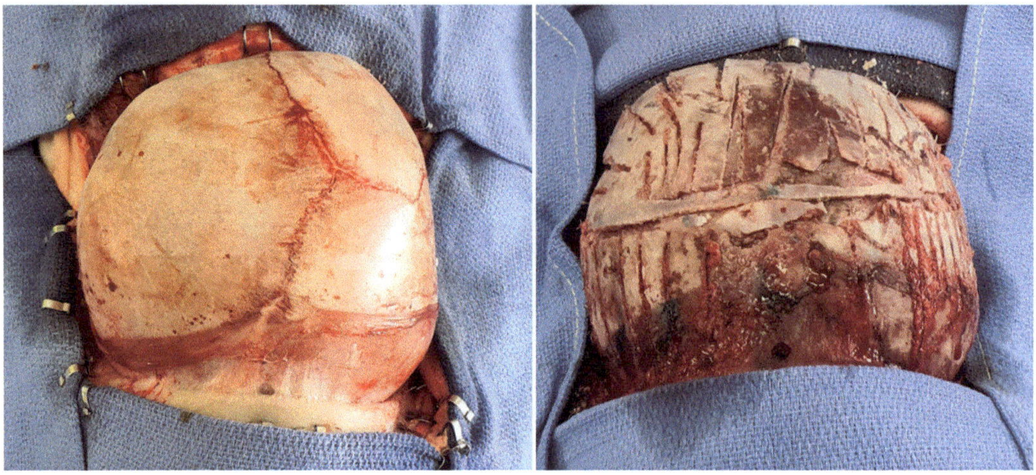

Fig. 46.8 Initial and late intraoperative pictures showing the correction of a left anterior plagiocephaly. Note the overcorrection on the left side

Intraoperative and postoperative (from the postoperative drainage or within the subcutaneous space) surgical losses range between 50 and 400 mL, with a mean value around 200 mL. Intraoperative blood transfusion is required in nearly half of the cases. The operative time commonly range between 2 and 3 h.

After the operation, the child is observed in the pediatric intensive care department for 24 h with monitoring of the hemodynamic and neurological condition. The postoperative hospitalization is about 4–5 days.

Postoperative 3D-CT scan can be used to evaluate the reconstructed skull. However, in most cases, the immediate postoperative result is based on the mere clinical observation to avoid further irradiation.

References

1. Bagolini B, Campos EC, Chiesi C. Plagiocephaly causing superior oblique deficiency and ocular torticollis. A new clinical entity. Arch Ophthalmol. 1982;100(7):1093–6. https://doi.org/10.1001/archopht.1982.01030040071012.
2. Ricci D, Vasco G, Baranello G, Salerni A, Amante R, Tamburrini G, Dickmann A, Di Rocco C, Velardi F, Mercuri E. Visual function in infants with non-syndromic craniosynostosis. Dev Med Child Neurol. 2007;49(8):574–6. https://doi.org/10.1111/j.1469-8749.2007.00574.x.
3. Di Rocco C, Velardi F. Nosographic identification and classification of plagiocephaly. Childs Nerv Syst. 1988;4(1):9–15.
4. Di Rocco C, Paternoster G, Caldarelli M, Massimi L, Tamburrini G. Anterior plagiocephaly: epidemiology, clinical findings, diagnosis, and classification. A review. Childs Nerv Syst. 2012;28(9):1413–22. https://doi.org/10.1007/s00381-012-1845-2.

5. Protzenko Cervante T, Arnaud E, Brunelle F, Di Rocco F. Unilateral coronal synostosis: can we trust the sagittal suture as a landmark for the underlying superior sagittal sinus? J Neurosurg Pediatr. 2016;17(5):589–94.
6. McCarthy JG, Coccaro PJ, Epstein F, Converse JM. Early skeletal release in infant with craniofacial synostosis. The role of the sphenozygomatic suture. Plast Reconstr Surg. 1978;62:335–46.
7. Hoffman HJ, Mohr G. Lateral canthal advancement of the supraorbital margin. A new corrective technique in the treatment of coronal synostosis. J Neurosurg. 1976;45:376–81.
8. Whitaker LA, Schut L, Kerr LP. Early surgery for isolated craniofacial dysostosis. Plast Reconstr Surg. 1977;60:575–81.
9. Tessier P. Osteotomies totales de la face: Syndrome de Crouzon, syndrome d' Apert—oxcephalies, scaphocephalies, turricephalies. Ann Chir Plast. 1967;12:273.
10. Marchac D, Renier D. "Le Front flottant": traitement precocedes facio—craniostenoses. Ann Chir Plast. 1979;24:121.
11. Hilling DE, Mathijssen IMJ, Mulder PGH, Vaandrager JM. Long-term aesthetic results of frontoorbital correction for frontal plagiocephaly. J Neurosurg. 2006;105(1 Suppl Ped):21–5.
12. Mesa JM, Fang F, Murazko KM, Buchman S. Reconstruction of unicoronal plagiocephaly with a hypercorrection surgical technique. Neurosurg Focus. 2011;31:1–8.
13. Surpure SJ, Smith KS, Sullivan SM, et al. The use of resorbable plating system for treatment of craniosynostosis. J Oral Maxillofac Surg. 2001;59:1271. https://doi.org/10.1053/joms.2001.27497.
14. Acosta HL, Stelnicki EJ, Rodriguez L, et al. Use of absorbable poly (d, o) lactic acid plates in cranial vault remodelling: presentation of first case and lessons learned about its use. Cleft Palate Craniofac J. 2005;42:333. https://doi.org/10.1597/03-071.1.
15. Jimenez DF, Constance M. Barone early treatment of anterior calvarial craniosynostosis using endoscopic-assisted minimally invasive techniques. Childs Nerv Syst. 2007;23:1411–9.
16. Satoh K, Mitsukawa N, Hayashi R, Hosaka Y. Hybrid of distraction osteogenesis unilateral frontal distraction and supraorbital reshaping in correction of unilateral coronal synostosis. J Craniofac Surg. 2004;15:953–9.
17. Tellado MG, Lema A. Coronal suturectomy through minimal incisions and distractions osteogenesis are enough without other craniotomies for the treatment of plagiocephaly due to coronal synostosis. J Craniofac Surg. 2009;20:1975–7.
18. Stelniski E, Heger I, Brooks CJ, Ghersi MM, Subbs CB, Bahuleyann B, Paresi R. Endoscopic release of unicoronal craniosynostosis. J Craniofac Surg. 2009;20:93–7.
19. Delye HHK, Borstlap WA, van Lindert EJ. Endoscopy-assisted craniosynostosis surgery followed by helmet therapy. Surg Neurol Int. 2018;9:59.
20. Chong S, Wang K-C, Phi JH, Lee JY, Kim S-K. Minimally invasive suturectomy and postoperative helmet therapy : advantages and limitations. J Korean Neurosurg Soc. 2016;59(3):227–32.

47 Bicoronal Sutures Synostosis

Ricardo Santos de Oliveira and Matheus Ballestero

47.1 Introduction

Bicoronal sutures synostosis is a skull deformity characterized by a shortened anteroposterior skull length and a widened biparietal diameter. This condition may be nonsyndromic, or syndromic. Accurate diagnosis of the type of brachycephaly is paramount in deciding the appropriate treatment options.

The treatment of bilateral coronal synostosis skull deformities is challenging. It is directed at increasing the anteroposterior dimension of the skull, reducing its superior-inferior dimension, releasing the fusion of the coronal sutures, and advancing the supraorbital rims bilaterally. Although helmet therapy is promising [1], surgical intervention is the cornerstone of treatment [2].

Bilateral coronal craniosynostosis gives rise to the so-called brachycephaly, a short and wide head shape due to the fusion of the coronal sutures, restricting anteroposterior growth (Fig. 47.1). The compensatory growth occurs sideways, resulting in upper and midface hypo-

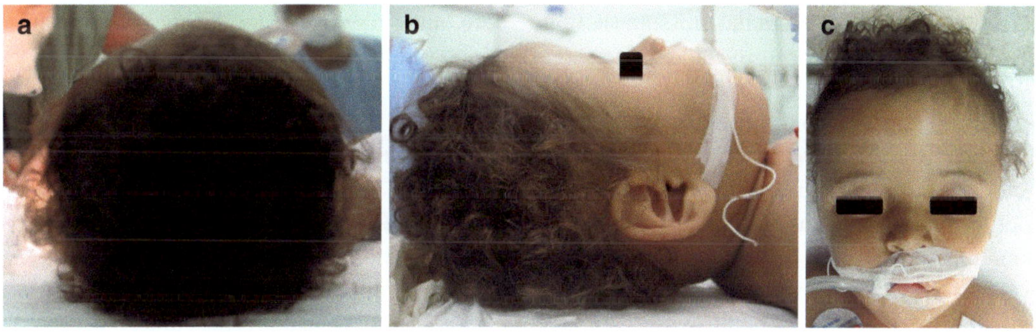

Fig. 47.1 Superior (**a**), lateral (**b**), and frontal (**c**) preoperative view of a brachiocephalic child, showing bilateral coronal synostosis. A typical frontal appearance of brachiocephalic with a short and wide head shape due to the fusion of the coronal sutures, restricting anteroposterior growth

R. S. de Oliveira (✉)
Division of Neurosurgery, School of Medicine of Ribeirão Preto, University of São Paulo, Ribeirão Preto, SP, Brazil

M. Ballestero
Medicine Department, Federal University of São Carlos, São Carlos, SP, Brazil

F. Di Rocco, J. Kestle (eds.), *Neurosurgical Aspects of Craniosynostosis*,
https://doi.org/10.1007/978-3-031-69386-1_47

plasia [3, 4]. Neurosurgeons also must be aware that patients with brachycephaly should be evaluated by a clinical geneticist in order to exclude a syndrome [5].

47.2 Surgical Strategy

47.2.1 Recommendation

Once the diagnosis of craniosynostosis is confirmed, the treatment should be surgical, based on three factors:

47.2.1.1 Brain Compression

The main indication for surgical treatment of craniosynostosis is the risk of chronic intracranial hypertension, and consequent cerebral suffering due to chronic hypoxia, thus leading to cognitive alterations and regression of neuropsychomotor development.

Accelerated brain growth, especially in the first year of life, associated with bone restriction resulting from synostosis, can lead to intracranial hypertension.

In 1982, Renier et al. [6] demonstrated the effects of increased intracranial pressure (ICP) in children with craniosynostosis undergoing surgical correction through pre-and postoperative records. The authors confirmed that even isolated craniosynostosis could present high levels of ICP.

ICP measurement has become an important tool for pre-operative assessment of craniofacial abnormalities prior to calvarial remodelling, as well as postprocedural screening for suspicion of raised ICP in syndromic craniosynostosis. ICP monitoring may also be of value to both the parents and surgeon in cases of mild deformity where there may be doubts as to the need for surgery on a cosmetic basis in addition to concerns about the functional effects of chronic intracranial hypertension [7].

47.2.1.2 Aesthetics/Repair

Psychological studies in patients with nonoperated craniosynostosis in childhood confirm the loss of self-esteem, difficulty in accepting the child by society, by the parents, relatives, and by himself, so the surgical indication should be made in order to repair the installed craniofacial deformity [8].

47.2.1.3 Ophthalmologic Impairment

Orbital alterations are present in some types of nonsyndromic craniosynostosis, such as brachycephaly, oxycephaly, anterior plagiocephaly, and trigonocephaly. Ocular proptosis can lead to corneal exposure, trauma, and consequent visual loss. The involvement of skull base sutures in brachycephaly and oxycephaly (frontoethmoidal and frontosphenoid) may be associated with the appearance of important orbital deformities.

47.2.2 Surgery Time

For the reasons presented, it becomes evident that the surgical indication must be early. In nonsyndromic brachycephaly, surgery is recommended, preferably between 6 and 12 months.

Some factors are essential for the success of the procedure in children under the age of 1 year: the child's weight is sufficient to support a major surgery (>6 kg); neuroanaesthesia, preparation of blood products before the beginning of the procedure and intensive care in the postoperative period (preferably in the pediatric ICU).

47.2.3 Surgical Technique

47.2.3.1 Preparation

The child should preferably be positioned in the supine position, so that the anesthesiologist has easy access to the endotracheal tube, if necessary, during the surgical procedure (Fig. 47.2).

Before starting the surgical procedure, a check must be made regarding:

- Presence of the informed consent for surgery
- Proper and safe patient position
- Eyes closed and protected
- Free access to the endotracheal tube
- Adequate venous access with blood products in the operating room ready for infusion
- Invasive (intraarterial) blood pressure, when possible
- Photographic documentation

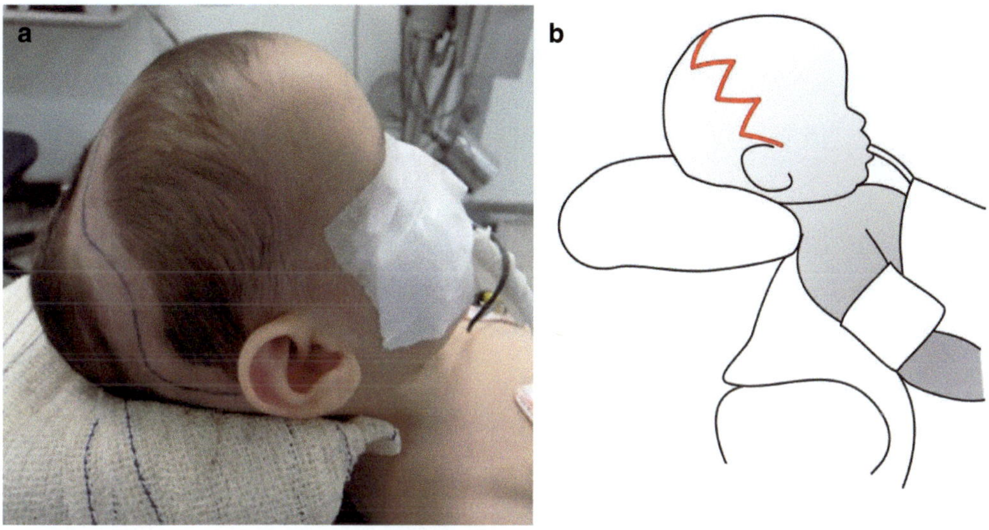

Fig. 47.2 Photography of a brachycephalic child in supine position using horseshoe pad. (**a**) A free and accessible endotracheal tube and cautious protection to the eyes are shown. (**b**) Illustration showed a zig-zag bicoronal scalp incision for cranial-facial surgical correction

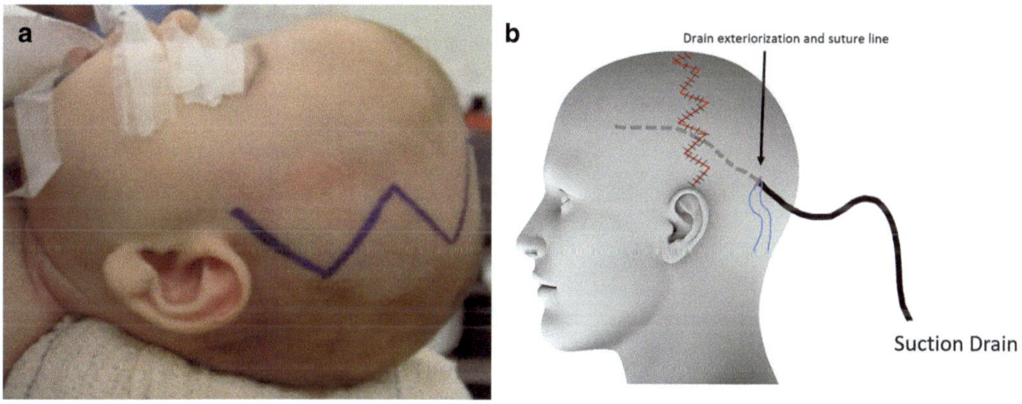

Fig. 47.3 Preoperative photography of a brachicefalic child. (**a**) Lateral view of a bicoronal zig-zag incision. (**b**) Illustration of a suction drain position and exteriorization

47.2.3.2 Incision

In all types of craniosynostosis, a bicoronal zig-zag incision can be made (in a straight or curvilinear way), in order to minimize the effects of late healing. A scalpel with monopolar needle coagulation (Colorado® microdissection) is essential for dissection of superficial planes to minimize blood loss and. Raney clips may also be used, sometimes along with a surgical compress, to make the scalp thicker and archives a more effective compression hemostasis. At the end of the surgery, an aspiration drain is placed to prevent postoperative periorbital hematomas and edema, a suture absorbable line is fixed in the suction drain's exteriorization point, in order to close it with a surgical knot when removing the drain (Fig. 47.3).

47.2.3.3 Cranial Vault Remodeling

The recessed and abnormally wide supraorbital bar is lifted with a bilateral temporal tenon, reshaped and replaced with a bilateral advance-

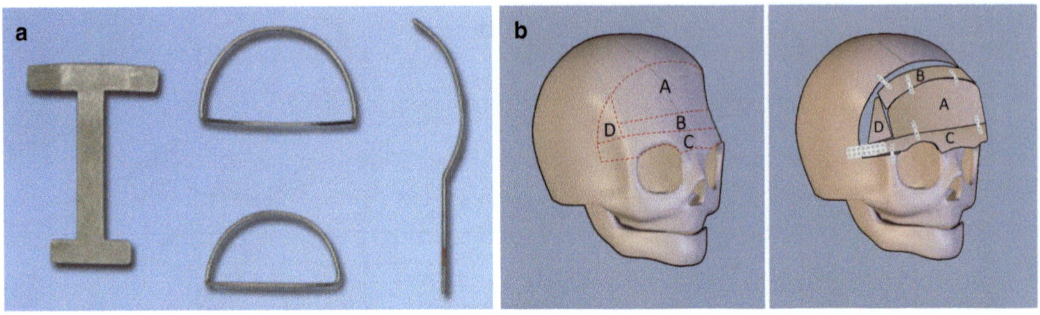

Fig. 47.4 (**a**) Marchac frontal patterns and instruments. From the left to right ruler, frontal model in two sizes and orbital model [11]. (**b**) Surgical planning

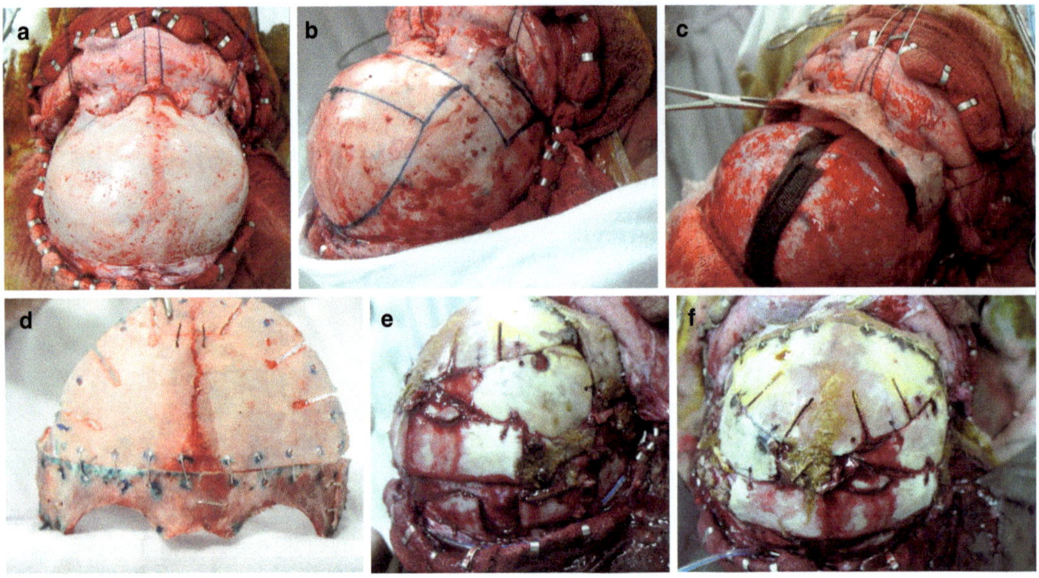

Fig. 47.5 Surgical photographs for brachycephaly deformity correction. Main surgical steps showing a cranial vault remodeling technique. (**a**) Superior view of complete exposition of supraorbital rim and craniofacial bones. (**b**) Craniotomy planning drawn on bone surface. (**c**) Planning of the supraorbital advance. (**d**) Reconstructed and fixed (steel wires) frontal. (**e**) Lateral view of final cranial vault remodeling and bilateral fronto-orbital advancement. (**f**) Superior view of final cranial vault remodeling

ment. The upper forehead is usually constructed from the existing forehead (Fig. 47.4), which is fixed back onto the supraorbital bar in its new position. The bulging of the temporal fossae is corrected by lifting a small bone flap and putting it back with the concavity outward. In infants younger than 6 months, the forehead is fixed in the advanced position only at the root of the nose and lateral orbital walls, without any fixation to the posterior cranial vault. This allows the brain to push freely on the forehead, realizing what we have called the "floating forehead" [9, 10]. Bony defects should be filled in by bone grafts fixed with fibrin glue (Fig. 47.5).

The fixation of the frontal and the supraorbital bar can be obtained with absorbable plates, when available, or through steel wires (Aciflex®) (Fig. 47.6). Currently, the preference to stabilize the fronto-orbital bar and the new frontal are the absorbable plates.

Fronto-orbital advancement allows eye protection in cases where there is marked proptosis,

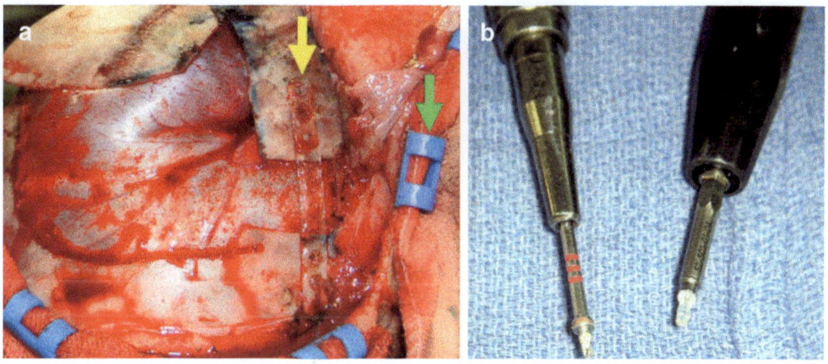

Fig. 47.6 Intraoperative photographs. (**a**) Absorbable plate (yellow arrow) and Raney Clip (green arrow) used for skin hemostasis. (**b**) Screwdrivers and screws used to fixate the absorbable plates (mechanical on the left and ultrasound assisted on the right)

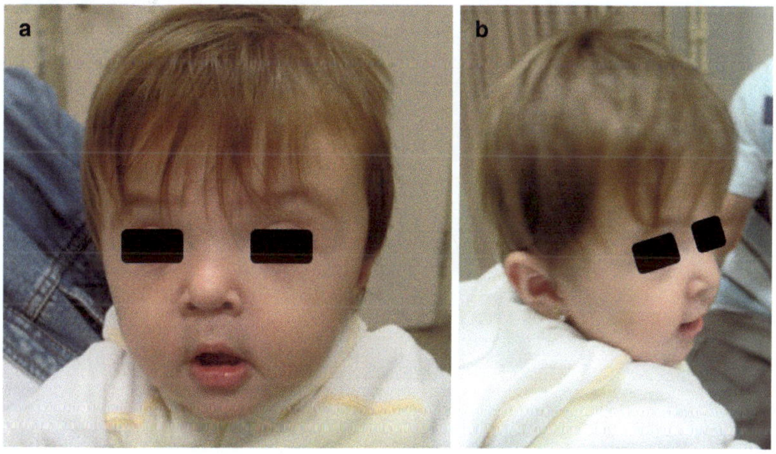

Fig. 47.7 Photography in 4 months follow-up after brachycephaly surgical correction. (**a**) Frontal view. (**b**) Lateral view. There is no visible scar because of zig-zag incision. A gradual normalization of the cranial was observed

in addition to allowing adequate cerebral decompression, minimizing the risk of intracranial hypertension. The bulging of the temporal region is corrected through the inversion of the temporal bone flap.

47.3 Postoperative/Outpatient Follow-Up

At least 24 h of monitoring in the pediatric intensive care unit (UCI) is important to verify the hemodynamic stability, bleeding and to control the hematimetry. On the first or second postoperative, depending on the output, the suction drain must be removed and the exteriorization point sutured. Prescription of intravenous and/or oral analgesia on a regular basis should be recommended.

In general, children remain hospitalized after surgery for a total period of 3 days. After 1 week, the surgical scar should be evaluated on an outpatient basis. The use of absorbable polyglactin 910 4-0 (Vicryl Rapide®) sutures should be encouraged.

A postoperative 3D CT can be performed in selected cases. However, periodic photographic documentation is essential for late assessment of the result (Figs. 47.7 and 47.8).

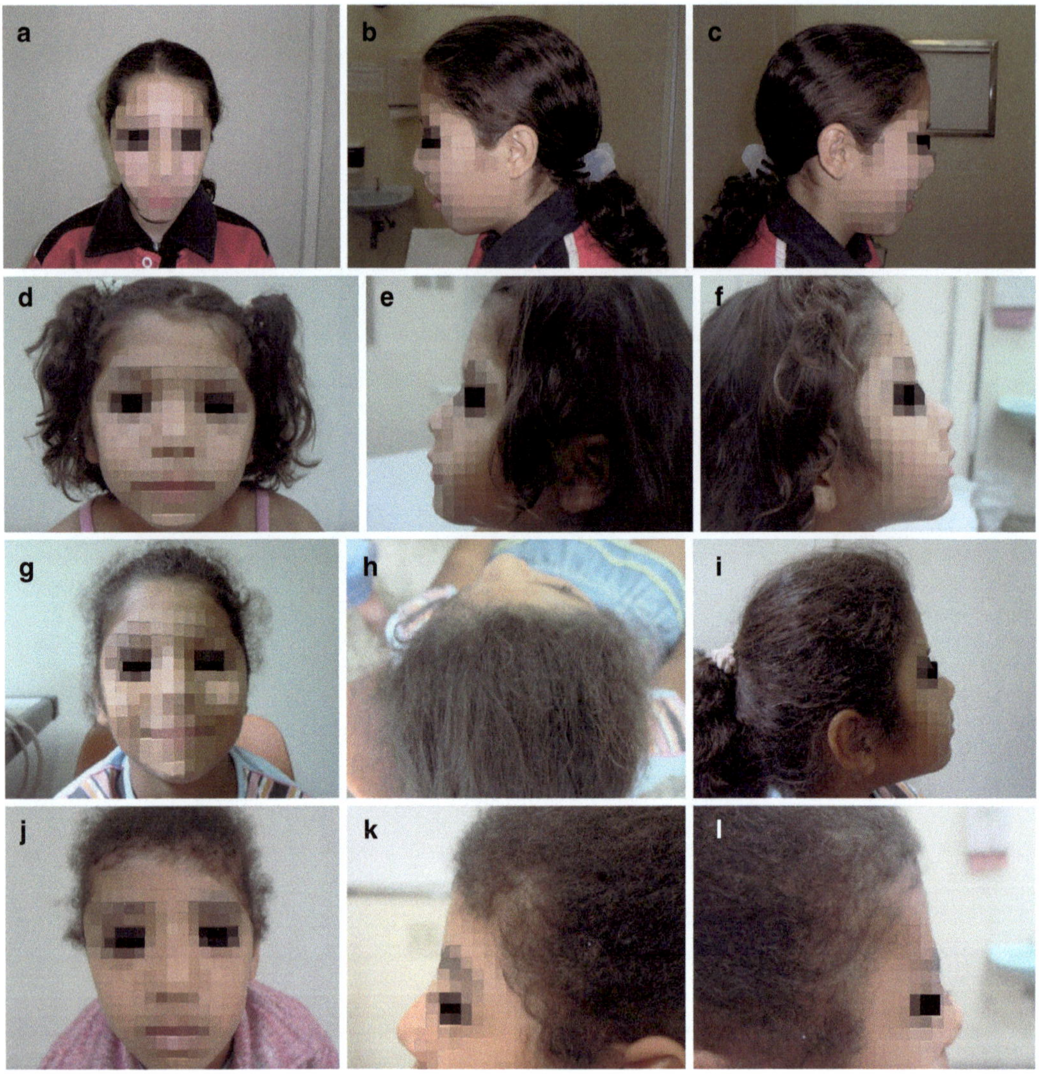

Fig. 47.8 Late postoperative photographs of four children after brachycephaly surgical correction. (**a**, **d**, **g**, **j**) Frontal view. (**b**, **e**, **k**) Left lateral view. (**c**, **f**, **i**, **l**) Left lateral view. (**h**) Superior view

References

1. Choi H, Lim SH, Kim JS, Hong BY. Outcome analysis of the effects of helmet therapy in infants with brachycephaly. J Clin Med Res. 2020;9(4) https://doi.org/10.3390/jcm9041171.
2. Vinchon M, Pellerin P, Baroncini M, Wolber A, Dhellemmes P. Non-syndromic oxycephaly and brachycephaly: a review. Childs Nerv Syst. 2012;28(9):1439–46.
3. Kolar JC. An epidemiological study of nonsyndromal craniosynostoses. J Craniofac Surg. 2011;22(1):47–9.
4. Schmetz A, Amiel J, Wieczorek D. Genetics of craniofacial malformations. Semin Fetal Neonatal Med. 2021;26:101290.
5. Hinojosa J. Syndromic craniosynostosis. In: Textbook of pediatric neurosurgery. Cham: Springer International Publishing; 2018. p. 1–37.
6. Renier D, Sainte-Rose C, Marchac D, Hirsch JF. Intracranial pressure in craniostenosis. J Neurosurg. 1982;57(3):370–7.
7. Wiegand C, Richards P. Measurement of intracranial pressure in children: a critical review of current methods. Dev Med Child Neurol. 2007;49(12):935–41.
8. Renier D, Lajeunie E, Arnaud E, Marchac D. Management of craniosynostoses. Childs Nerv Syst. 2000;16(10–11):645–58.
9. Daniel Marchac DR. Le front flottant, traitement précoce des faciocraniosténoses. Ann Chir Plast. 1979;24:21.
10. Marchac D, Renier D. Cranio-facial surgery for cranio-synostosis. Scand J Plast Reconstr Surg. 1981;15(3):235–43.
11. Marchac D. A frontal pattern for frontocranial remodeling. Ann Plast Surg. 1986;17(3):263–5.

48 Lambdoid Suture Synostosis: Endoscopic Approach, Key Points for Neurosurgeons

David F. Jimenez

48.1 Introduction

Although it is the least common of all craniosynostosis, lambdoid synostosis can be difficult to diagnose and may be easily confused with positional plagiocephaly by many primary care providers unfamiliar with its clinical presentation [1–10]. However, the diagnosis should not be difficult to make for those surgeons and centers that treat craniosynostosis. For the most part, isolated single suture nonsyndromic craniosynostosis is a clinical diagnosis. A well-versed clinician can make the diagnosis by simply observing the patient while doing the physical exam. As such, it is our policy not to obtain CT scans and unnecessarily expose patients to radiation. However, lambdoid synostosis is the exception and as such, we obtain CT scans in all patients suspected of lambdoid synostosis. We do this to rule out positional plagiocephaly and to document the extent of the synostosis. In brief summary, lambdoid craniosynostosis presents clinically as follows: (a) occipital plagiocephaly ipsilateral to the craniosynostosis (Fig. 48.1), (b) inferior displacement of the mastoid process on the affected side (Fig. 48.2), (c) inferior downward displacement of the ipsilateral ear, (d) a bony ridge along the stenosed suture (Fig. 48.3), (e) cranial scoliosis with deviation of the vertex to the contralateral

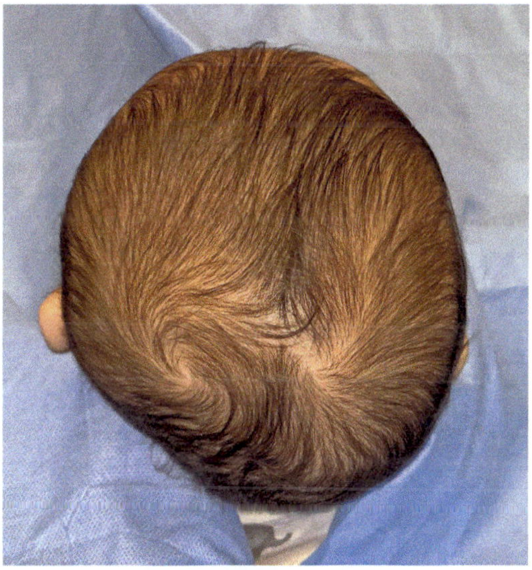

Fig. 48.1 Six-month-old male presenting with left lambdoid synostosis. Significant occipital indentation and plagiocephaly is seen in this view taken from above

D. F. Jimenez (✉)
Department of Neurosciences, El Paso Children's Hospital, El Paso, TX, USA

Pediatric Neurosurgery, El Paso Children's Hospital, El Paso, TX, USA

Neurosurgery Department, University Medical Center, El Paso, TX, USA
e-mail: drj@nexusneurosurgery.com

F. Di Rocco, J. Kestle (eds.), *Neurosurgical Aspects of Craniosynostosis*,
https://doi.org/10.1007/978-3-031-69386-1_48

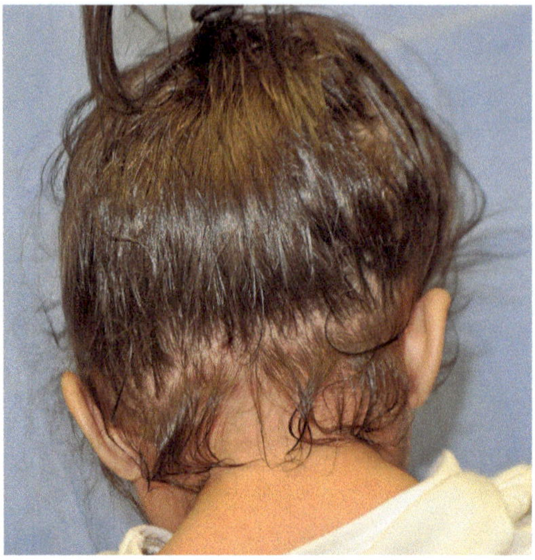

Fig. 48.2 Eight-month-old female with left lambdoid synostosis demonstrates the classic findings of the inferior displacement of the ipsilateral ear and mastoid process

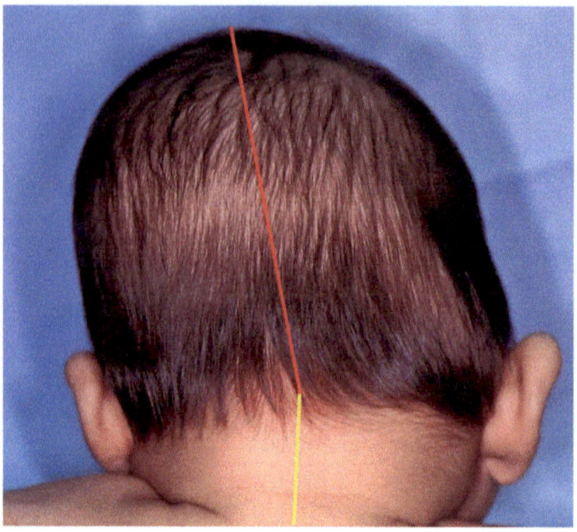

Fig. 48.4 Cranial scoliosis is evident in this patient with right lambdoid synostosis. The yellow line indicates patients midline through the neck and the foramen magnum. Red line indicates midline axis of the cranial vault, which is significantly deviated to the contralateral side

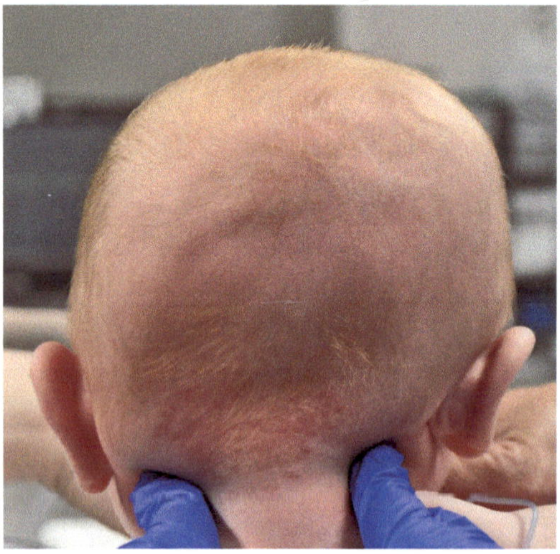

Fig. 48.3 Three-month-old male with left lambdoid synostosis. A bony ridge is seen and can be palpated on the left side along the stenosed lambdoid suture

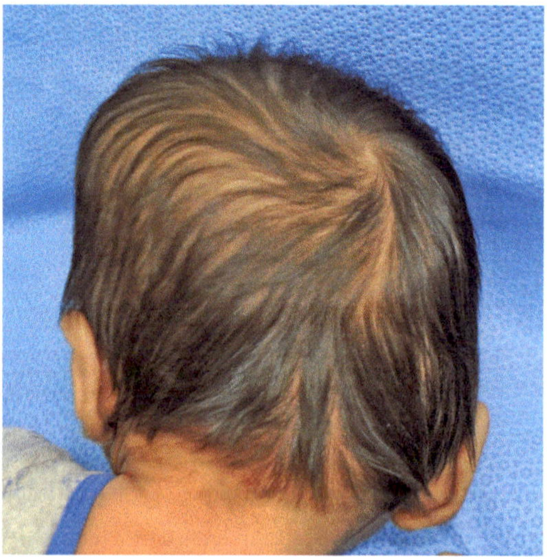

Fig. 48.5 Another classical finding in lambdoid synostosis is the deviation of the vertex of the side contralateral to the stenosis suture, as seen in this patient with right lambdoid stenosis

side (Fig. 48.4), and (f) prominent and protruding parietal eminence of on contralateral side (Fig. 48.5). Contrary with patients with positional plagiocephaly, the forehead tends to be round and symmetrical. When viewed from above, these patients have a "trapezoid" shape (Fig. 48.6) in comparison to the parallelogram shape seen in positional plagiocephaly.

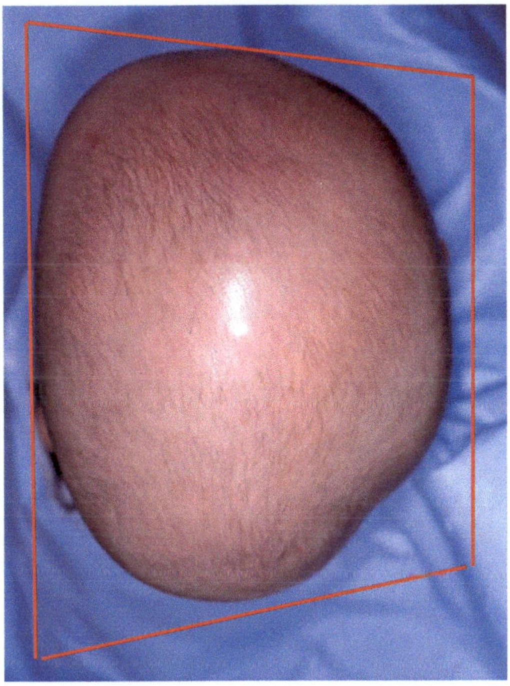

Fig. 48.6 When viewed from above, lambdoid craniosynostosis patients have a "trapezoid" shape (as shown by the red lines) in contrast to the typical parallelogram shape seen in patients with positional plagiocephaly

48.2 Diagnostic Radiology

Plain skull radiographs have high sensitivity and can easily provide the diagnosis, but a Towne's view is necessary. Evident is a sclerotic suture where closure has taken place, as seen in this lateral radiograph (Fig. 48.7). Nevertheless, CT scans are the golden standard for definitive diagnosis. However, 3D reconstructions will clearly show the stenosed suture (Fig. 48.8), and the sagittal view will show if cerebellar tonsillar ectopia is present. Premature suture closure can affect the entire suture or portion of it. The scan will clearly show the location of the stenosis.

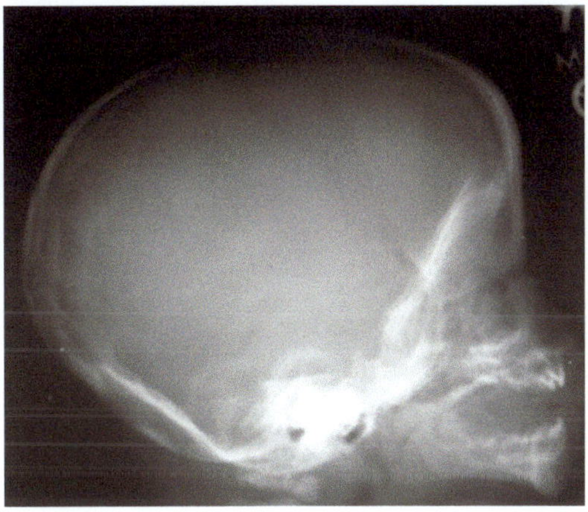

Fig. 48.7 Lateral skull radiograph clearly demonstrates a sclerotic area on the retromastoid region consistent with the stenosed lambdoid suture

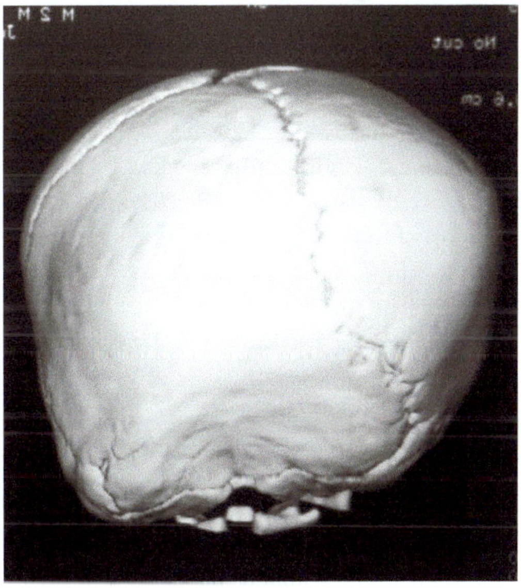

Fig. 48.8 The gold standard for definitive diagnosis is a head CT scan with 3D reconstruction. This CT clearly shows a completely stenosed left lambdoid suture

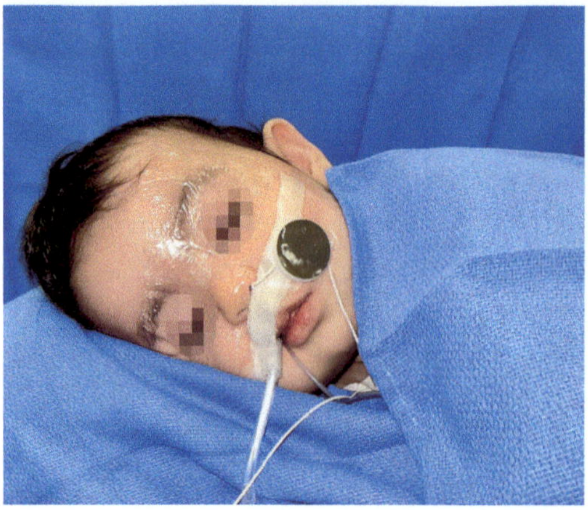

Fig. 48.9 For surgery, the patient is positioned on the lateral decubitus position with the affected suture placed superiorly. This patient, with the left lambdoid synostosis, is resting on a cerebellar horseshoe headrest

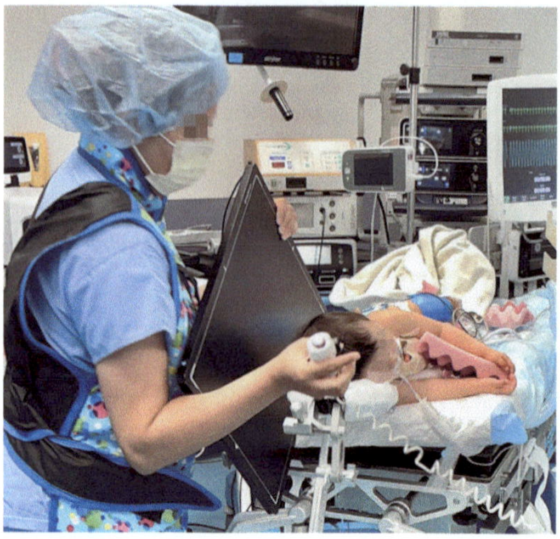

Fig. 48.10 Intraoperative skull X-rays are obtained in order to properly localize lambda and asterion. The tech is seen taking on A-P radiograph trying to localize lambdas

48.3 Patient Positioning

The patient's head is placed on a cerebellar horseshoe headrest. We have tried placing the patient fully prone on the headrest as well as the lateral decubitus position. The latter is our preferred position (Fig. 48.9). All of the standard precautions for placing a patient on the horseshoe headrest are taken, particularly that the contralateral ear is not under pressure.

48.4 Incisions

Proper placement of the incisions is extremely critical when operating on lambdoid synostosis. If not properly placed, the procedure will be very difficult to do. The use of X-rays is critical to localize the lambda and the asterion on the affected side. The radiology technologist takes both A-P, and lateral views (Figs. 48.10 and 48.11). In order to localize lambda, metallic stick-on markers are placed on the estimated location by the surgeon. Oftentimes, the markers need to be relocated and several X-rays taken in

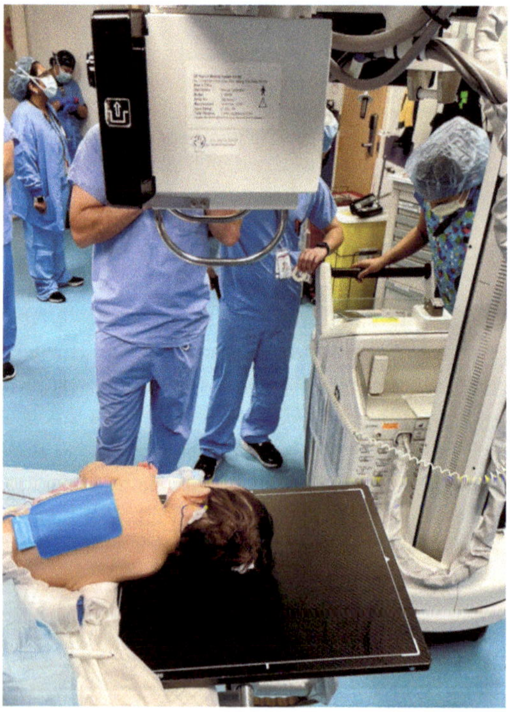

Fig. 48.11 Now the radiology technologist is taken a lateral X-ray for asterion identification

order to localize the proper points (Fig. 48.12). Once the proper location has been selected, a small strip of hair is shaved/clipped for an incision of about 2–2.5 cm. One incision is immediately on top of the lambda and the second immediately medial to the asterion (Fig. 48.13).

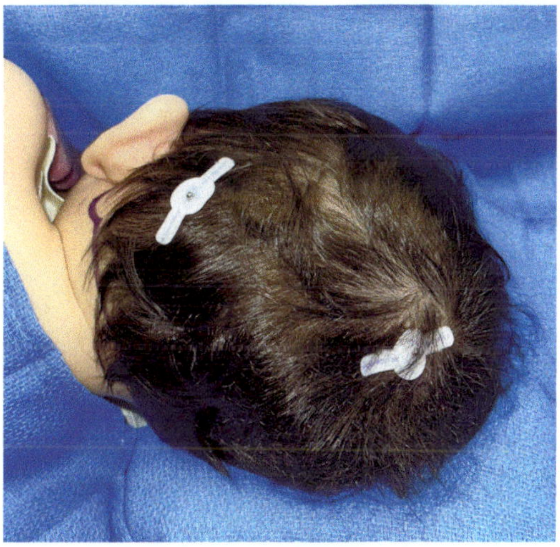

Fig. 48.12 The surgeon places stick-on metallic markers in the approximate location of the lambda and asterion prior to taking intraoperative X-rays

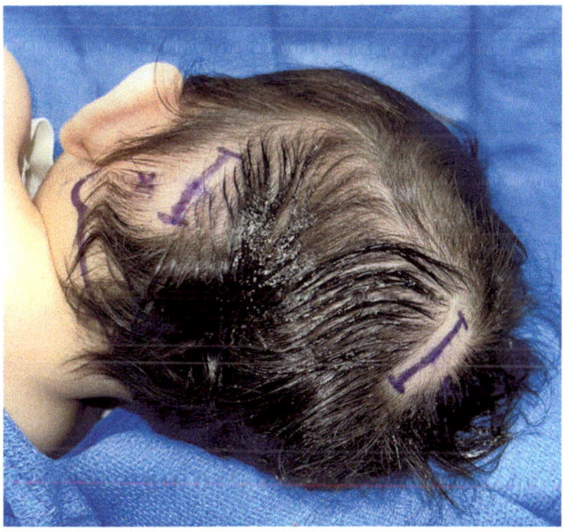

Fig. 48.13 Once the proper location of lambda and asterion is made, a small strip of hair is shaved over the proposed incision sites

48.5 Surgical Procedure

The dermis is open with the monopolar needle tip, and the cautery is set on cut mode at 10 W. This setting causes minimal injury to the dermis, and scars heal superbly and are hardly visible. Both incisions can be opened simultaneously (Fig. 48.14). The next step is to develop the subgaleal plane between the incisions. This can be done with direct endoscopic visualization (Fig. 48.15) using a 0° endoscope. Alternatively, a rhinoplasty lighted retractor and an insulated brain ribbon can be used for the subgaleal dissection (Fig. 48.16). Once the plane is fully developed, a brain ribbon is passed to document complete plane dissection (Fig. 48.17). Identification of lambda is done at the proximal incision using a #1 penfield dissector (Fig. 48.18). Mobilization of the pericranium allows for the identification of the sagittal suture and it's junction with the contralateral opened lambdoid suture. Burr holes are placed at each incision and enlarged (towards each other) with a #4 or 5

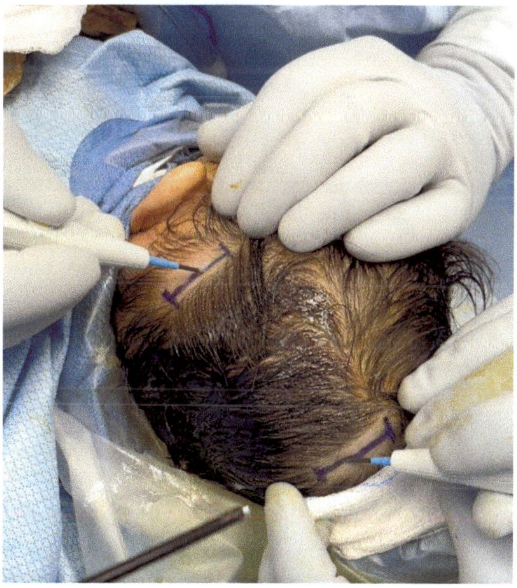

Fig. 48.14 Both incisions are open simultaneously with needle tip Bovie set at 10 W on cut mode

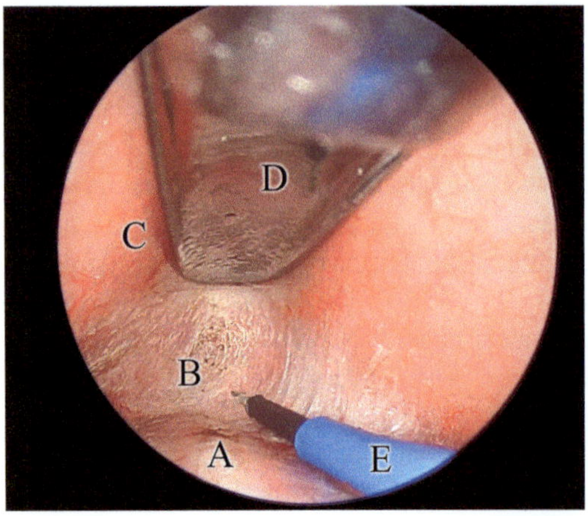

Fig. 48.15 Endoscopic view with a 0° scope, of the loose areolar tissue plane dissection from Lambda to Asterion. (**a**) The stenosed lambdoid suture. (**b**) The loose areolar tissue between the pericranium and galea. (**c**) The galea and the scalp being evaluated by the lighted retractor. (**d**) The Bovie. (**e**) Used for dissecting the plane bloodlessly

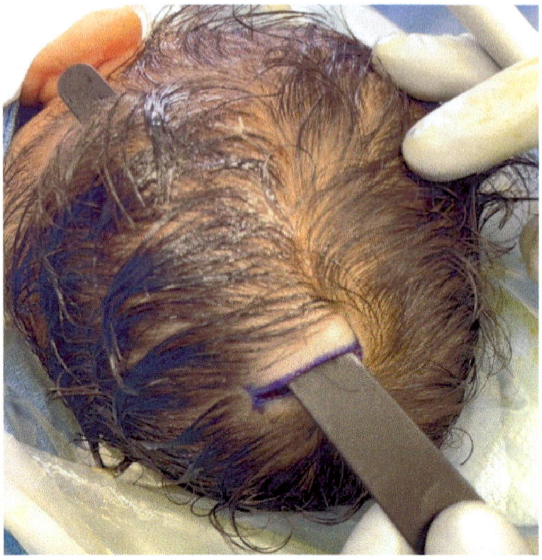

Fig. 48.17 A brain ribbon is placed under the galea between lambda and asterion incisions, indicating complete release

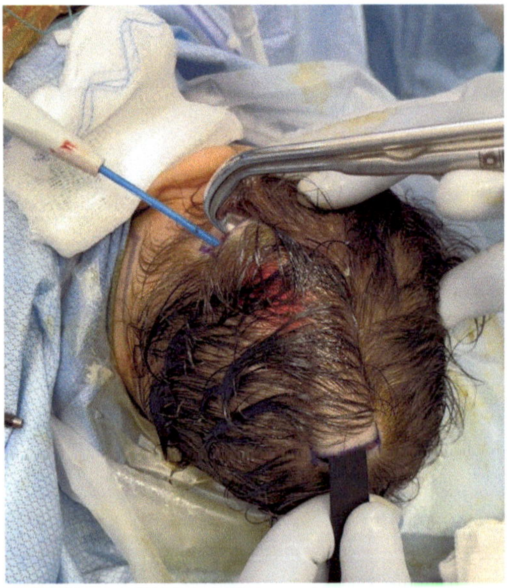

Fig. 48.16 A rhinoplasty lighted retractor can also be used to develop the loose areolar tissue plain under direct visualization

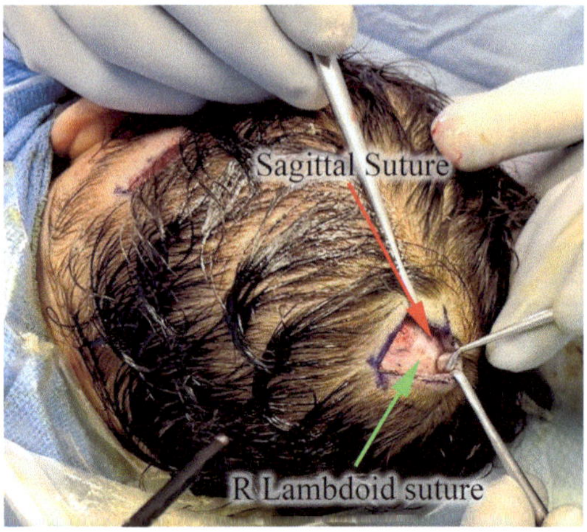

Fig. 48.18 Two Ragnell retractors hold the incision apart. A #1 penfield is used to mobilize the pericranium. The sagittal and open lambdoid sutures are identified

Kerrison rongeurs. Elongation of the burr hole allows for the insertion of a 30° rigid endoscope. With the scope pointing towards the bone, it is advanced and the stenosed suture visualized and followed distally. When coming close to the asterion, the point where the closed suture joins the open asterion is clearly seen (Fig. 48.19). The osteotomy is then created by removing bits of bone in a piece meal fashion using bone cutting rongeurs (Fig. 48.20). The osteotomy is continued until the open suture is found (Fig. 48.21). The osteotomy is fully completed, bone hemostasis is obtained with the Bovie suction coagulator

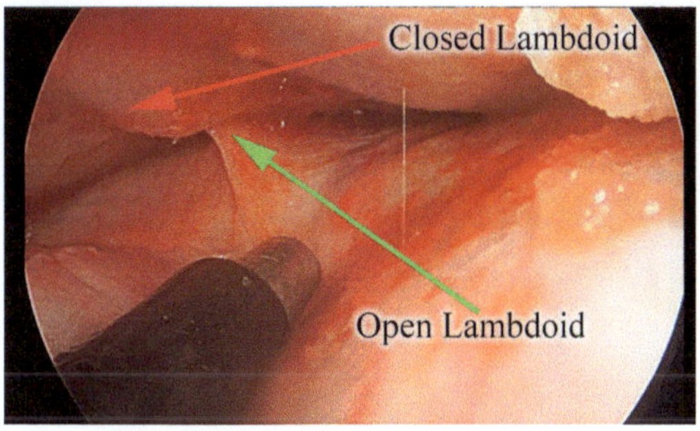

Fig. 48.19 A 30° endoscope is passed under the skull and advanced until the closed lambdoid suture forms the open suture of the asterion

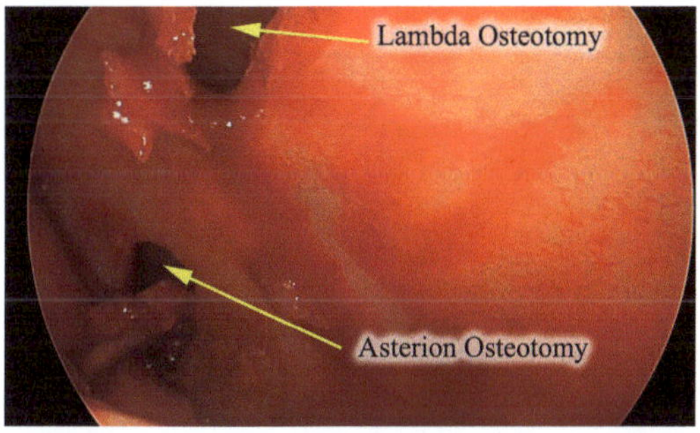

Fig. 48.20 Endoscopic view of the lambda and asterion osteotomies as they are about to unite into a single osteotomy extending between both ends

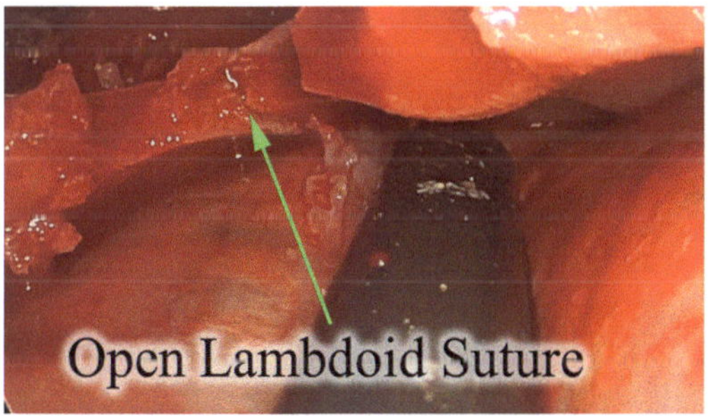

Fig. 48.21 The lambdoid sutures opens as it joins the asterion, as seen in this endoscopic view

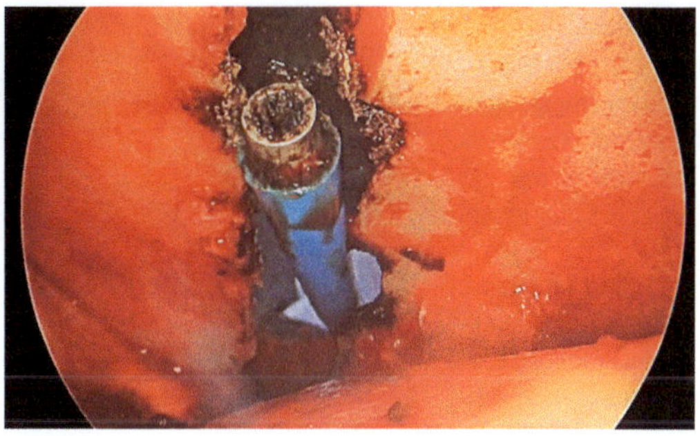

Fig. 48.22 A monopolar suction electrocautery is used to cauterize the osteotomy edges and obtain complete bony hemostasis

set on coagulation mode at 60 W (Fig. 48.22). Hemostasis is completely obtained with Surgiflo® and the incisions closed with absorbable 4-0 galeal suture (Monocryl or vicryl) Mastisol and steri-strips are used to close the dermis.

48.6 Postoperative Management

After extubation, the patient is transferred to the PACU (recovery room) and then moved to the floor for overnight observation. Pain management includes alternating doses of ibuprofen and acetaminophen every 3 h. Intravenous morphine is given as needed for severe breakthrough pain. The patient is discharged the following morning. The patient's head is scanned (infrared) for a cranial orthosis on the postoperative day (POD) #4, and the orthosis filled on (POD) #5. Patient wears the cranial orthosis for 23-h a day for the ensuing 6–10 months (Figs. 48.23, 48.24, 48.25, 48.26, 48.27, and 48.28).

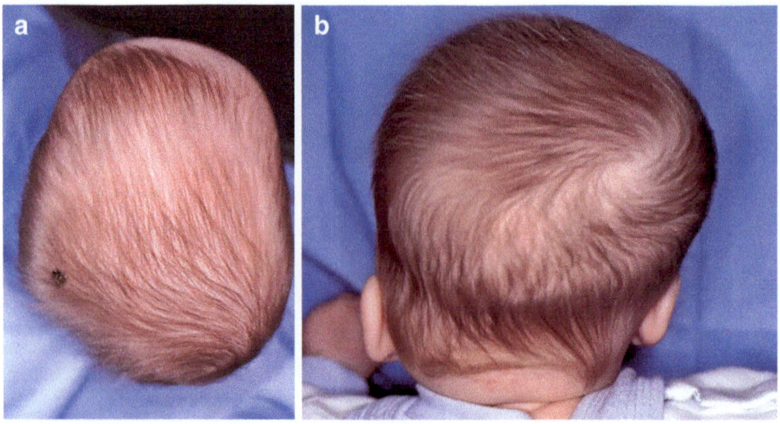

Fig. 48.23 (**a**) Patient A is a 6-month-old female presenting with lambdoid synostosis. Top view shows left-sided plagiocephaly. (**b**) Posterior-anterior (PA) view of same patient shows downward displacement of ear and mastoid as well as contralateral bulging of the parietal eminence

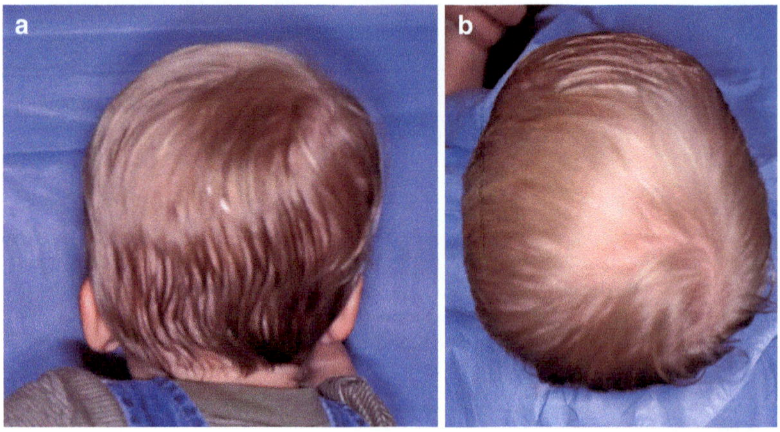

Fig. 48.24 (**a**) Patient A, 9 months after surgery shows improvement of the preoperative findings on PA view. (**b**) Patient A shows complete correction of the left-sided plagiocephaly at 9 months

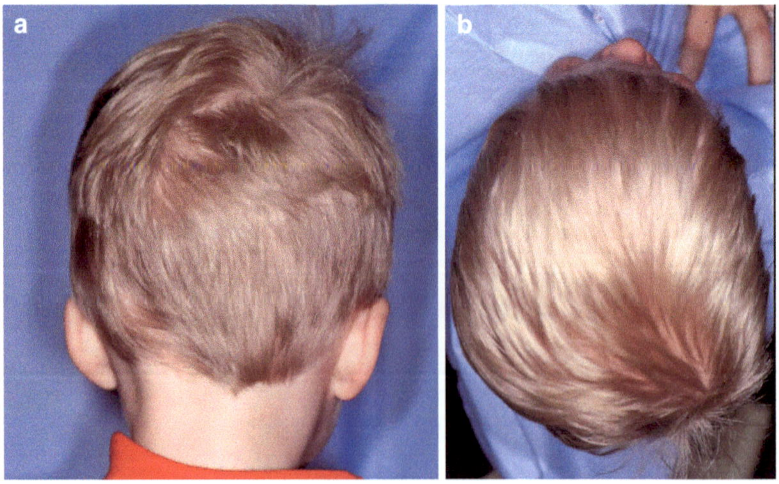

Fig. 48.25 (**a**) Patient A at 2.5 years postop. Notice almost complete correction of the skull base asymmetry as seen by the alignment of the ears along the horizontal plane. (**b**) Patient continues to demonstrate complete correction of plagiocephaly 2.5 years after surgery

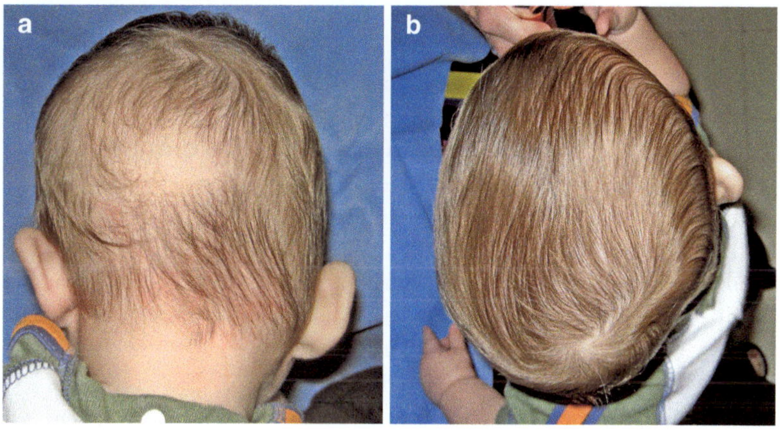

Fig. 48.26 (**a**) Five-month-old male with classical findings on PA view. The right ear significantly displaced inferiorly along with the mastoid suture. (**b**) Top view shows marked indentation posteriorly along the stenosed lambdoid suture

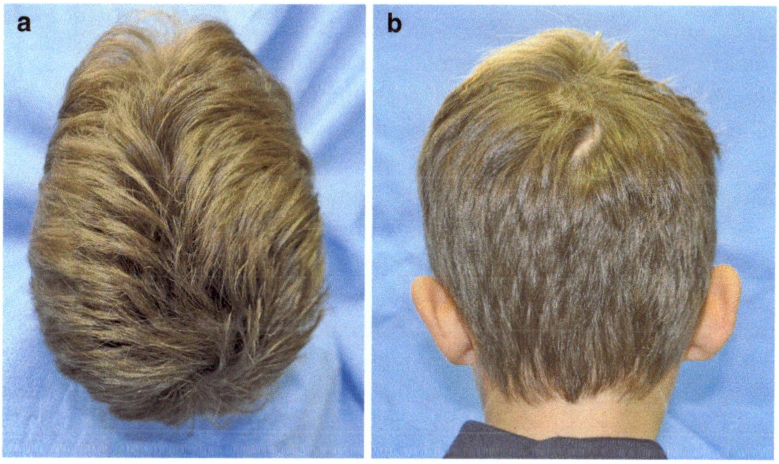

Fig. 48.27 (**a**) Six years after endoscopic release, top view shows normalization of the head. (**b**) Six years after surgery, P-A view shows complete correction of skull based deformity

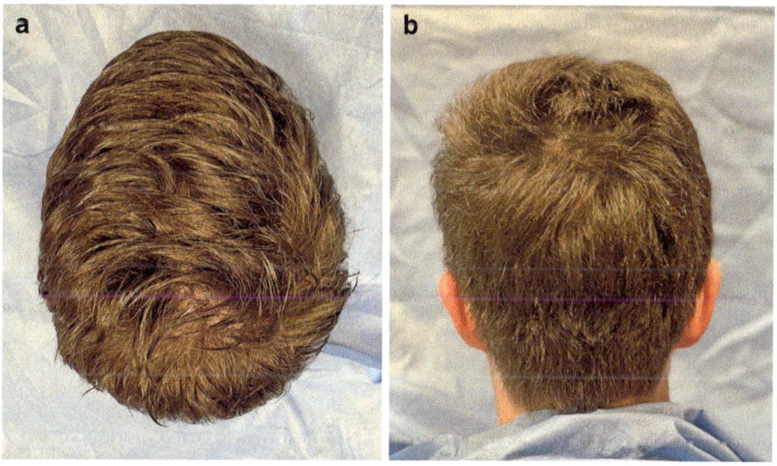

Fig. 48.28 (**a**) Top view of the same patient 11 years after surgery. (**b**) PA view of some patient shows persistent skull based abnormalities and asymmetry correction

48.7 Discussion

Lambdoid craniosynostosis is associated with significant skull-based cranial and in some cases facial deformities. Traditional surgical treatment involves a complete calvarial vault reconstruction of the occipital parietal bones to round the back of the head. Many variations on the theme have been proposed by multiple surgeons and craniofacial centers. Given our immense success with treating the other calvarial sutures using minimally invasive endoscopic techniques, we decided to apply the same principles to the stenosed lambdoid. To our surprise, the patients obtained major and significant correction of their preoperative deformities. The correction is not immediate and requires patience and time. This surgical approach is associated with minimal blood loss. So far, not a single patient has been transfused intra- or postoperatively, there's minimal pain and swelling. Short anesthesia times are one of the extreme benefits to the patient. We strongly believe that the brain is fully responsible for the ultimate shape of the face and entire cranial skeleton to include the skull base. As such, if a stenosed suture is released and the brain allowed to assume its normal morphology, the preoperative cranial and facial deformities will correct as we have clearly shown with other suture synostosis to now include the lambdoid. Endoscopic release is associated with excellent results and is a surgical option that should be given to the parents of children affected with this condition.

References

1. Huang MD, Gruss JS, Clarren SK, et al. The differential diagnosis of posterior plagiocephaly: true lambdoid synostosis versus positional molding. Plast Reconstr Surg. 1996;98(5):765–74.
2. Losee JE, Feldman E, Ketla M, et al. Nonsynostotic occipital plagiocephaly; radiographic diagnosis of the "sticky suture". Plast Reconstr Surg. 2005;116(7):1860–9.
3. Vander Kolk CA, Carson BS. Lambdoid synostosis. Clin Plast Surg. 1994;21(4):575–84.
4. McComb JG. Treatment of functional lambdoid synostosis. Neurosurg Clin N Am. 1991;2(3):665–72.
5. Ortega R. Unkind cut. Wall Street J. 1996: Sect A: 1–5.
6. Nemzek WR, Brodie HA, Hecht ST, et al. CT and plain film imaging of the developing skull base in fetal specimens. AJNR Am J Neuroradiol. 2000;21(9):1699–706.
7. Rhodes JL, Tye GW, Fearon JA. Craniosynostosis of the lambdoid suture. Semin Plast Surg. 2014;28(3):138–43.
8. Zoller JE, Mischkowski RA, Speder B. Preliminary results of standardized occipital advancement in treatment of lambdoid craniosynostosis. J Craniomaxillofac Surg. 2002;30(6):343–8.
9. Goodrich JT, Argamaso R. Lambdoid synostosis (posterior plagiocephaly) and craniofacial asymmetry: long term results. Childs Nerv Syst. 1996;12(11):720–6.
10. Jimenez DF, Barone CM. The sunrise technique: the correction of occipital plagiocephaly using bandeau occipital plate and radial osteotomies. Pediatr Neurosurg. 1995;22:162–5.

49 Lambdoid Suture Synostosis: Open Vault Surgery, Key Points for the Neurosurgeons

Martina Messing-Jünger

Lambdoid suture synostoses are rare. They are found in less than 5% of all cases and diagnosis is often delayed, possibly due to the fact that they are mistaken for positional plagiocephaly. Therefore, open vault remodeling becomes necessary when the patient is older than 4 months of age. Evidence regarding the best surgical management in lambdoid craniosynostosis is sparce, but occasional publications report on similar cosmetic results in endoscopic strip craniectomy versus open vault surgery [1]. Nevertheless, regardless of the applied surgical technique, patients with lambdoid synostosis show persistent asymmetry of the posterior cranial vault and the cranial base [1]. Additional cranial base fusion is not only found in syndromic craniosynostoses, but also in nonsyndromic patients; however, in lambdoid synostosis, no associated cranial base suture fusions could be detected so far [2]. In order to address asymmetry adequately as well as the underlying cause for further deformity progress, it is recommended to perform surgery as soon as possible. Open vault remodeling is best performed at 6 months of age [3, 4].

Growth restriction due to premature lambdoid suture closure can lead to significant volume reduction of the posterior fossa, and it is recommended to perform MRI prior to surgery to rule out secondary Chiari malformation type 1 (Fig. 49.1). This condition can be even more pronounced in bilateral lambdoid fusion (Fig. 49.2). In most cases, the tonsillar displacement will disappear after appropriate cranioplasty, but control MRI is recommended and additional bony foramen magnum decompression should be discussed in persistent Chiari malformation type 1.

Similar to the anterior plagiocephaly caused by coronal suture fusion also, the posterior form leads to complex three-dimensional skull deformity of varying extent. The ipsilateral forehead may be retruded, whereas the contralateral parietal squama is bulging laterally (Fig. 49.3). Both deforming aspects eventually have to be addressed by the remodeling technique [3].

The essentials of open lambdoid suture synostosis correction are the same as in other sutures: to open the fused suture, to expand the restricted cranial volume, and to restore the entire head shape and morphology [5]. It is advisable to communicate with the family prior to the surgery that a complete cosmetic normalization will not be achieved since the already existing displacement of the petrous bone and the mastoid together with the ear position will persist to a certain extend.

In our institution, all craniofacial procedures are managed according to a specific standard operation procedure (SOP) protocol, which includes preoperative hemoglobin elevation in anemic patients, presurgical crystalloid hemodilution, tranexamic acid administration,

M. Messing-Jünger (✉)
Pediatric Neurosurgery Department, Asklepios Children's Hospital, Sankt Augustin, Germany
e-mail: m.messing@asklepios.com

F. Di Rocco, J. Kestle (eds.), *Neurosurgical Aspects of Craniosynostosis*,
https://doi.org/10.1007/978-3-031-69386-1_49

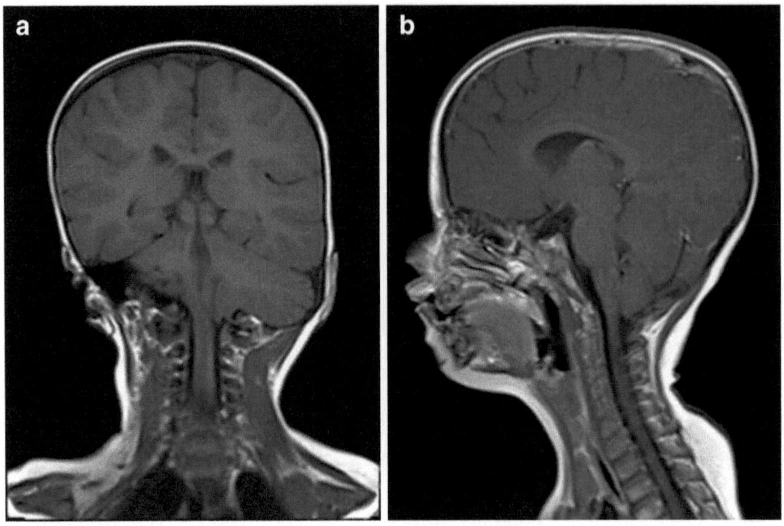

Fig. 49.1 Secondary unilateral tonsillar herniation in left-sided lambdoid craniosynostosis: (**a**) coronal and (**b**) sagittal T1 MRI

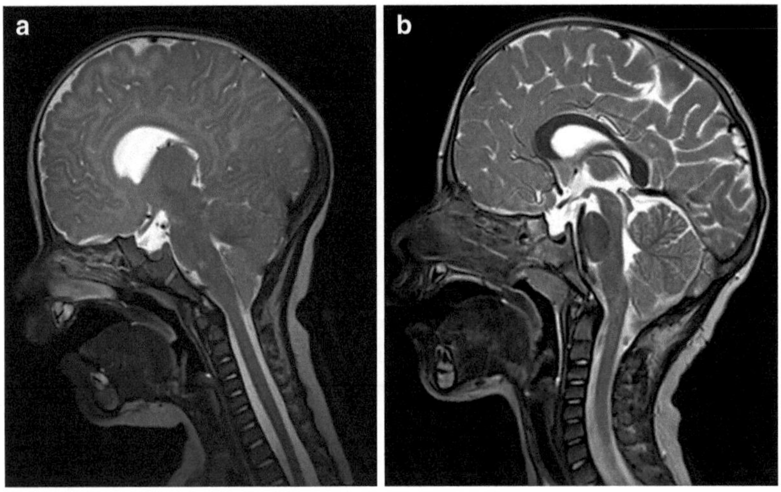

Fig. 49.2 Bilateral lambdoid synostosis with secondary Chiari malformation type 1: (**a**) preoperative and (**b**) postoperative sagittal T2 MRI

positioning on a warming mattress with extremity wrapping, central i.v. line and invasive blood pressure monitoring, and an endotracheal Woodbridge tube. Our technique involves prone positioning on a small size face position cushion (Fig. 49.4) and a curved biparietal skin incision. After preparation of the galeal layer a subperiostal excision of the affected bone structures is performed. We do not follow a strict excision pattern, but adjust the incision lines according to the underlying skull deformity which needs to be corrected. Figure 49.5 demonstrates a left-sided lambdoid craniosynostosis with occipital and additional parietal augmentation. In cases with ipsilateral forehead retrusion, remodeling of the entire calvaria may become necessary. In order to ensure appropriate surgical access, supine position in slight head inclination is advisable in these cases (Fig. 49.6). Bone pieces which are removed en bloc may be contoured ex vivo. Transposition of the parieto-occipital bone flaps is also performed, if the shape allows a good reconstruction. In any case, it is important to completely detach and remove the affected suture from the original site in order to prevent relapse of the deformity. Suture detachment from the underlying dural structures can be difficult, and any injury of the torcular and adjacent sinuses must be avoided. Additional in situ barrel stave osteotomies are added as necessary to create a

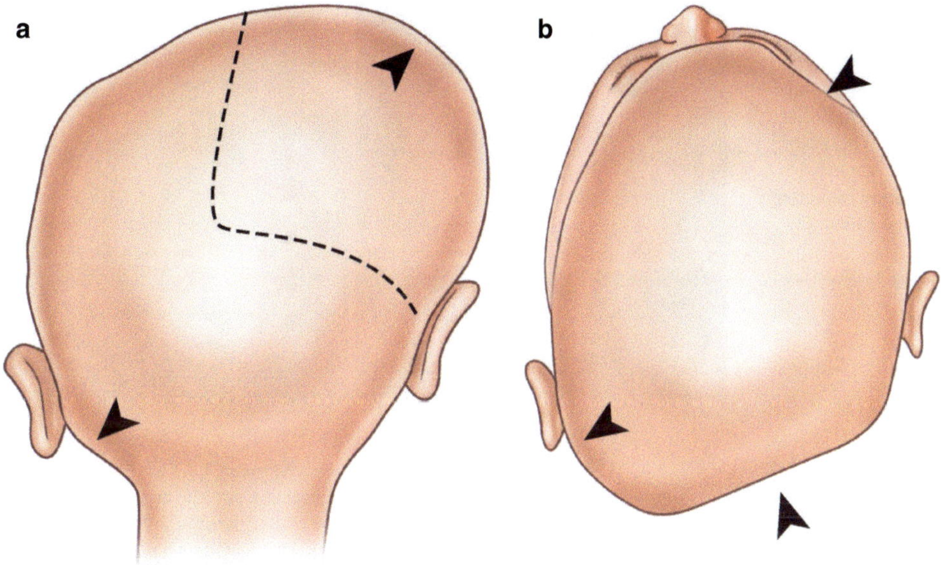

Fig. 49.3 Typical deformity in lambdoid suture synostosis. (**a**) Left-sided fusion with ipsilateral mastoid and contralateral parietal bossing and downward displacement of ipsilateral ear (coronal view). (**b**) Ipsilateral occipital and frontal retrusion with frontal ear displacement and contralateral parietal bossing in right-sided suture fusion (axial view)

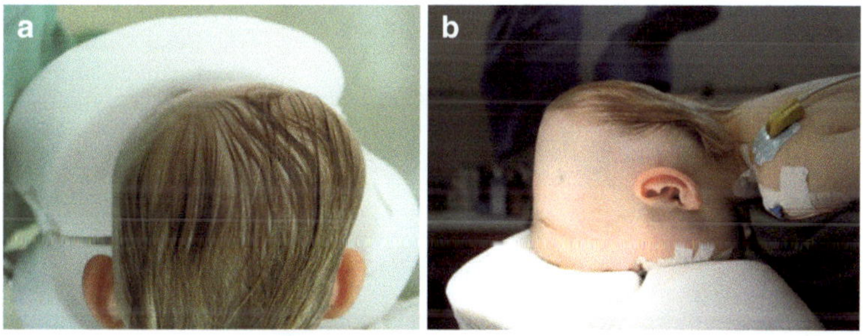

Fig. 49.4 Prone positioning with face position cushion

normal contour. Since the weight of the head during lying position causes significant pressure forces on the osteosynthesis sites, fixation must be as rigid as possible. We therefore still recommend titanium implants, which have to be removed after 3 months in order to prevent them from migration. Alternatively, a postoperative helmet protection must be discussed. We do not have sufficient experience with the use of distraction devices, which are recommended by some authors [6]. Finally, the periosteum is readapted following by a two-layer skin closure with intracutaneous sutures covered by spray dressing and wound cover strips. We are not using suction drains in our institution. Our technique is comparable to the ones published by other groups [4, 5].

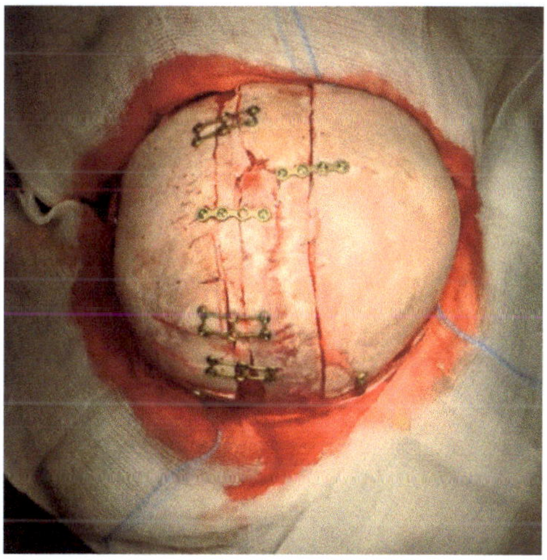

Fig. 49.5 Example of left-sided lambdoid craniosynostosis correction with additional ipsilateral parietal augmentation

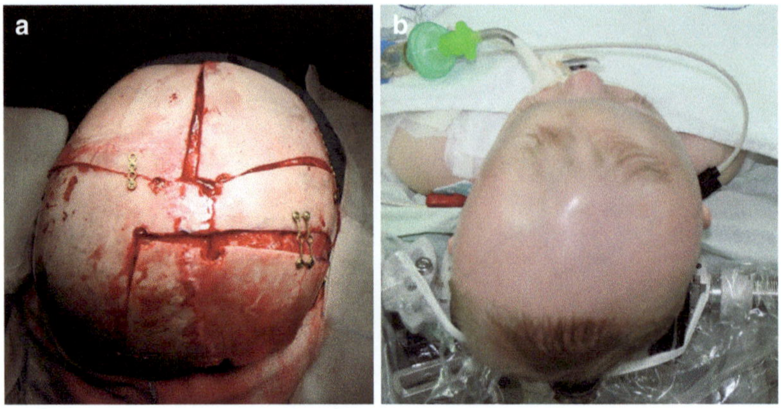

Fig. 49.6 Example of right-sided lambdoid craniosynostosis correction (**a**) in a child with ipsilateral forehead retrusion (**b**). This case was operated on in supine position for better access to the entire calvaria

References

1. Zubovic E, Woo AS, Skolnick GB, Naidoo SD, Smyth MD, Patel KB. Cranial base and posterior cranial vault asymmetry after open and endoscopic repair of isolated lambdoid craniosynostosis. J Craniofac Surg. 2015;26(5):1568–73.
2. Mazzaferro DM, Naran S, Wes AM, Runyan CM, Vossough A, Bartlett SP, et al. Incidence of cranial base suture fusion in infants with craniosynostosis. Plast Reconstr Surg. 2018;141(4):559e–70e.
3. Dempsey RF, Monson LA, Maricevich RS, Truong TA, Olarunnipa S, Lam SK, et al. Nonsyndromic craniosynostosis. Clin Plast Surg. 2019;46(2):123–39.
4. Marbate T, Kedia S, Gupta D. Evaluation and management of nonsyndromic craniosynostosis. J Pediatr Neurosci. 2022;17(5):77.
5. Markiewicz MR, Recker MJ, Reynolds RM. Management of sagittal and lambdoid craniosynostosis. Oral Maxillofac Surg Clin North Am. 2022;34(3):395–419.
6. Kamel GN, McKee RM, Carbulido K, Modi R, Belza C, Ewing E, et al. A posterior rotational flap technique using distraction osteogenesis for unilateral lambdoid craniosynostosis. J Craniofac Surg. 2021;32(4):1365–9.

Foramen Magnum Decompression in Craniosynostosis

50

José Francisco M. Salomão and Tatiana Protzenko

50.1 Introduction

Foramen magnum decompression is performed in some selected cases of craniosynostosis associated with Chiari Deformation Type I (CMI), defined as a cerebellar tonsillar herniation greater than 5 mm below the foramen magnum and also denominated tonsillar herniation (TH) or tonsillar ectopia (TE). These malformations fit on what Raybaud called secondary Chiari deformities on his classification of the Chiari I malformations spectrum [1].

Until the introduction of MRI as a diagnostic method, CMI and craniosynostosis were occasionally reported, usually, as late complications related to hydrocephalus [2–6]. Francis et al. [2] reported a series of patients with Crouzon syndrome in which CMI was found in five out of ten cases. The role of multisutural and syndromic synostosis as a cause of CMI was firstly stressed by the Parisian group in 1995, that reported a high incidence of deformations in 95 patients studied by MRI [7]. Three years later, the same group established the basis of the treatment of this condition [8], and since then, many controversies appeared regarding the best way to manage these conditions. Mutations in the fibroblast growth factor receptors especially the FGFR1 and FGFR2 genes are identified in Pfeiffer and Crouzon and these are identical [9, 10].

50.2 Incidence

CMI was diagnosed in 8% of the craniosynostosis patients treated by Strahle et al. [11] and is rarely seen in a single monosutural craniosynostosis, in which the incidence ranges from 1% to 5% of these cases [12, 13], affecting especially the lambdoid suture [12, 14] and occasionally others [13, 15, 16]. Cinalli et al. [7] stated that the involvement of the lambdoid suture was predictive of tonsillar herniation, both in isolated and multisutural forms. More recently, some authors reported CMI in nearly half of all cases of lambdoid synostosis [11, 17, 18]. It was established that CMI is much more likely in patients with Crouzon–Pfeiffer syndrome than in those with Apert syndrome because in the former the sagittal and lambdoid sutures close significantly earlier and in the last one the posterior fossa attain a normal volume [19].

In complex craniosynostosis, the incidence of CMI ranges from 40% to 75%, being higher in oxycephaly [7, 17]. In syndromic cases, its incidence may reach 82% in Pfeiffer's, 70% in Crouzon's, and 100% in Kleeblattschädel's

J. F. M. Salomão (✉) · T. Protzenko
Division of Pediatric Neurosurgery, Department of Pediatric Surgery, Fernandes Figueira National Institute of Health for Women, Children and Adolescents, Oswaldo Cruz Foundation (IFF-Fiocruz), Rio de Janeiro, Brazil

F. Di Rocco, J. Kestle (eds.), *Neurosurgical Aspects of Craniosynostosis*,
https://doi.org/10.1007/978-3-031-69386-1_50

deformities, being very low in Apert and Sahtre-Schotzen syndromes [7, 11, 13, 14, 20–24].

50.3 Pathophysiology

The pathophysiology of CMI in the sense of craniosynostosis involves several factors such as the reduced posterior fossa volume, the block of the venous outflow through the jugular foramen, and changes in and around the foramen magnum leading to CSF disorders.

The Chiari 1 deformity and the posterior fossa volume: One of the causes of CMI is the disproportionate growth between the hindbrain and the abnormally small posterior fossa. The deformity is acquired and may be progressive over time [25]. The size of the posterior cranial fossa is related not only to the lambdoid suture but also to the early closure of small sutures and synchondroses such as the parieto-squamosal arches [7, 26, 27]. Thompson et al. [28] showed an inverse relationship between the relative size of the posterior fossa and the degree of tonsillar herniation. Consequently, a smaller skull and/or a deformed posterior fossa may result in crowding of its components and tonsillar descent in affected patients, mainly those with lambdoid suture stenosis [8, 14, 19, 22].

It was demonstrated that although patients with craniosynostosis are born with a significantly smaller intracranial volume, by the age of 6 months, most achieve a normal cranial volume [23]. Rijken et al. [29] showed that patients with CMI have similar cerebellar and posterior fossa volume when compared to controls. According to the authors, despite a significantly higher cerebellar volume/posterior fossa ratio, it is not possible to predict which craniosynostosis patients are more prone to developing CMI, and consequently, one should focus on the skull vault and other contributing factors, since the real relationship between them remains obscure.

The foramen magnum: Patients with different types of syndromic or complex CS have a significantly smaller foramen magnum surface area when compared with normal controls [30–32]. Studies have shown that the inner-occipital synchondrosis (IOS) fuses prematurely in patients with Apert, Crouzon, and Pfeiffer [29, 32] and this may be already noted at birth, increasing over time [29]. It is still unclear how much the premature closure of the IOS impairs the development of the FM since it might be influenced by other factors such as hypoplasia of the occipital bones [29]. Dissimilarity in the age of fusion is seen in different series and different types of craniofaciosynostosis, sometimes related to the difficulty to make a clinical diagnosis without routine genetic testing [30].

Venous outflow: Venous outflow impairment is induced by stenosis of the jugular foramen turning difficult CSF absorption and leading to venous hypertension and increased ICP [33]. Abnormalities of cerebral veins in the occipital region were identified in 28% of Strahle's series [11]. According to the literature, the most exuberant collateral circulation in patients with syndromic craniosynostosis occurs in the posterior fossa, being more frequent through the mastoid and condylar emissary veins and seen especially in Crouzon–Pfeiffer syndrome [33–35].

Hydrocephalus and ICP: Hydrocephalus is frequently associated with craniofaciostenosis and is usually multifactorial, including increased CSF pressure due to jugular foramina stenosis, hindbrain herniation, reduced volume of the posterior cranial fossa, and abnormalities at the level of the foramen magnum. The block of the subarachnoid spaces at the FM area increases the pressure in the cranial compartment and consequently dissociation of craniospinal pressure [19, 28, 36]. These children are more prone to have tonsillar herniation than those without hydrocephalus. As ventriculomegaly is frequently observed during the investigation, serial images and clinical follow-up may be necessary to establish or not the diagnosis of active hydrocephalus and intracranial hypertension.

Syringomyelia: Syringomyelia is usually seen when there is tonsillar herniation. In Strahle's series, 10 out of 29 (34%) patients with craniosynostosis also had syringomyelia and all had Crouzon syndrome. Syringomyelia was present in 7 out of 34 patients of Scott's series and among these, 5 had postoperative images available for review.

50.4 Signs and Symptoms

Chiari I malformation may be asymptomatic in syndromic craniosynostosis, and in such cases, the diagnosis is usually established by imaging and MRI is the gold standard. There is a wide range regarding the number of patients that become symptomatic due to TH [14, 19, 37, 38]. Doerga et al. [38] found neurological signs and symptoms in 73% of all patients with syndromic CS, with or without TH, a much higher prevalence than usually reported and that certainly include also mental disabilities and structural brain malformations often seen in patients with Apert syndrome. Phenotypically, syndromic and complex craniosynostosis differ from each other but flattening of the posterior cranium is an important predictor of MCI [7].

The symptoms of CMI are well known, and their detailed description is beyond the scope of this chapter. These may include suboccipital pain, painful torticollis, impaired cerebellar function, motor deficit, coordination disturbances, cranial nerve dysfunction, and other. It is important to emphasize that symptoms may develop rapidly, especially in very young children who may present with breathing problems such as central or obstructive apnea (OSA) or central sleep apnea (CSA) that may lead rapidly to respiratory arrest [14, 20, 38–41].

50.5 Treatment

50.5.1 Hydrocephalus

Hydrocephalus may develop before or after treatment of craniosynostosis. Whenever possible, vault expansion should be done initially but, in some cases, especially those with marked intracranial pressure, hydrocephalus should be treated first [37, 42]. There is no consensus regarding the type of treatment with many authors preferring shunting or third ventriculostomy as the first choice in dealing with hydrocephalus [11, 43].

50.5.2 Surgical Treatment of CMI

Surgical treatment of tonsillar herniation in asymptomatic patients is controversial [8, 44, 45] although the prophylactic decompression premise lacks statistical data and long-term follow-up [14].

Cinalli [8] and the Dallas group [46, 47] proposed an occipital decompression and an in-continuity enlargement of the posterior FM region. This procedure is accepted with some variations by many authors [11, 46, 48]. Figure 50.1 shows an example from the historical series of the authors of a patient with Pfeiffer syndrome, presenting closure of the coronal, sagittal, and lambdoid sutures, cooper beaten sign and "coupe de serpe" sign, which characterizes the interruption of the posterior curvature of the skull due to the hypoplastic posterior fossa. The treatment proposed at the time, as there were no significant associated venous anomalies, consisting of posterior vault remodeling with wide foramen magnum opening and then fronto-orbital advancement. In isolated NSCS, cranial vault remodeling [49] or posterior vault distraction are options to address these conditions [21]. Figure 50.2 shows a case of CMI in a patient with scaphocephaly, where only the remodeling of the skull was enough to correct the clinical-radiological issues of the CMI.

However, even in syndromic forms, in most cases, the posterior vault expansion is sufficient to increase the volume of the posterior fossa. Figure 50.3 demonstrates posterior vault expansion in a patient with Pfeiffer syndrome using springs, with significant improvement in tonsil ectopia and posterior fossa volume. This technique, as well as expansion with external distractors, is an option not only for the large posterior

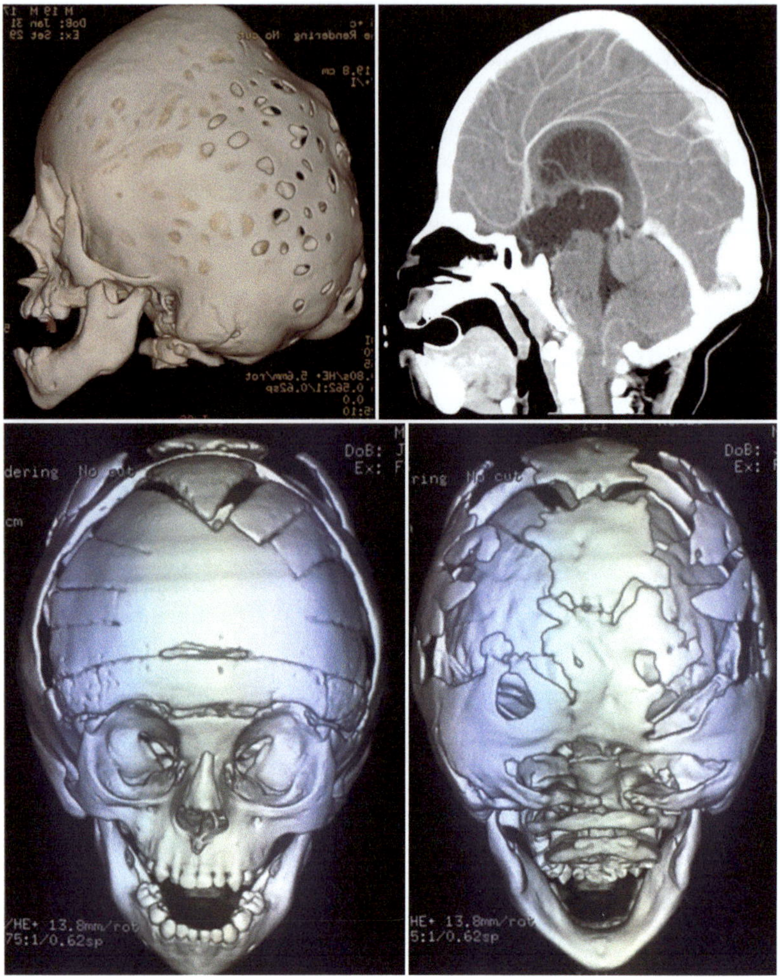

Fig. 50.1 Pfeiffer syndrome patient, presenting pansynostosis and Chiari I malformation. Posterior vault remodeling and wide opening of the foramen magnum is shown

volume acquired, but also to avoid access to the collateral venous circulation commonly found in these patients and which can be life-threatening.

Suboccipital and foramen magnum decompression should be preferable in situations, such as syringomyelia [11], when the correction of the supratentorial deformity and treatment of hydrocephalus are ineffective or if there is a progression of the tonsillar ectopia [11, 24]. Foramen magnum decompression alone has a limited role in the treatment of CMI in the setting of craniosynostosis since the options cited above are usually enough to resolve symptoms in most patients [17].

Considering that a significant number of individuals with syndromic craniosynostosis have intracranial-extracranial venous channels, especially Crouzon-Pfeiffer and Apert, these patients should undergo preoperative CT or MRI venography to identify venous anomalies and avoid excessive bleeding with catastrophic results [33, 34, 38, 45] when approaching the foramen magnum region.

The foramen magnum may be approached through a bicoronal incision when planning the occipital expansion simultaneously or through a midline incision when the isolated treatment is chosen. Some authors recommend excising the posterior arch of C1 [11], but the decompression of the foramen magnum and the adjacent bone of the posterior fossa, as in cases of primary CMI seems to be enough. Irrespective of the extension of the craniotomy, the dura mater is not routinely opened due to the danger of uncontrollable hem-

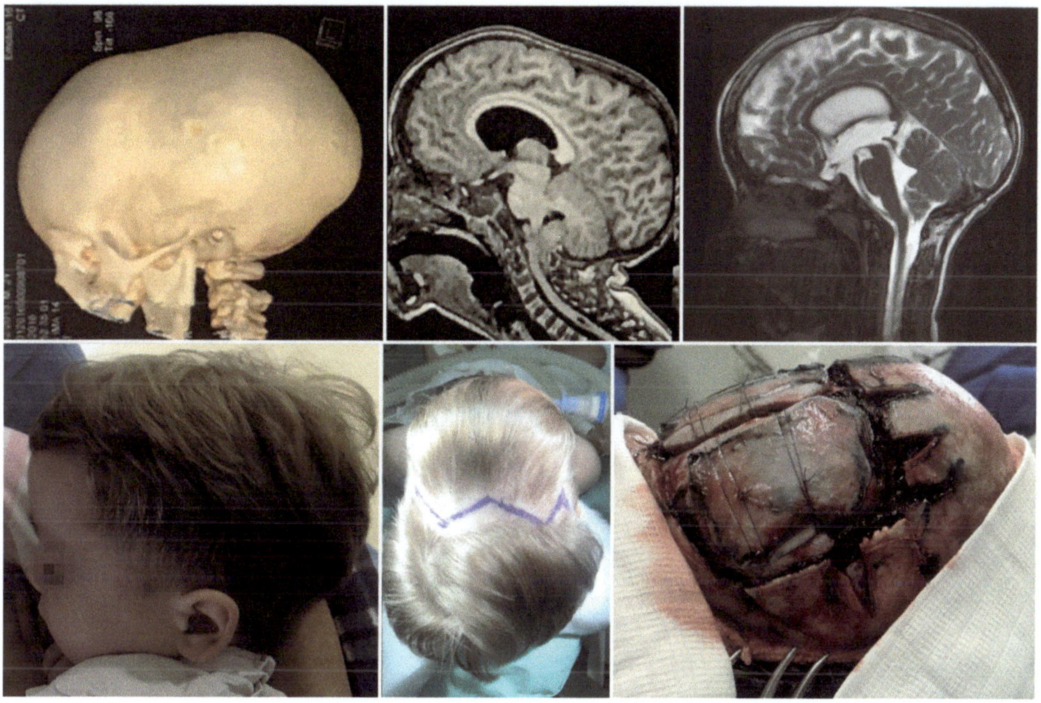

Fig. 50.2 Nonsyndromic scaphocephaly presenting Chiari I malformation treated with cranial vault remodeling. Control MRI shows the resolution of the Chiari I malformation

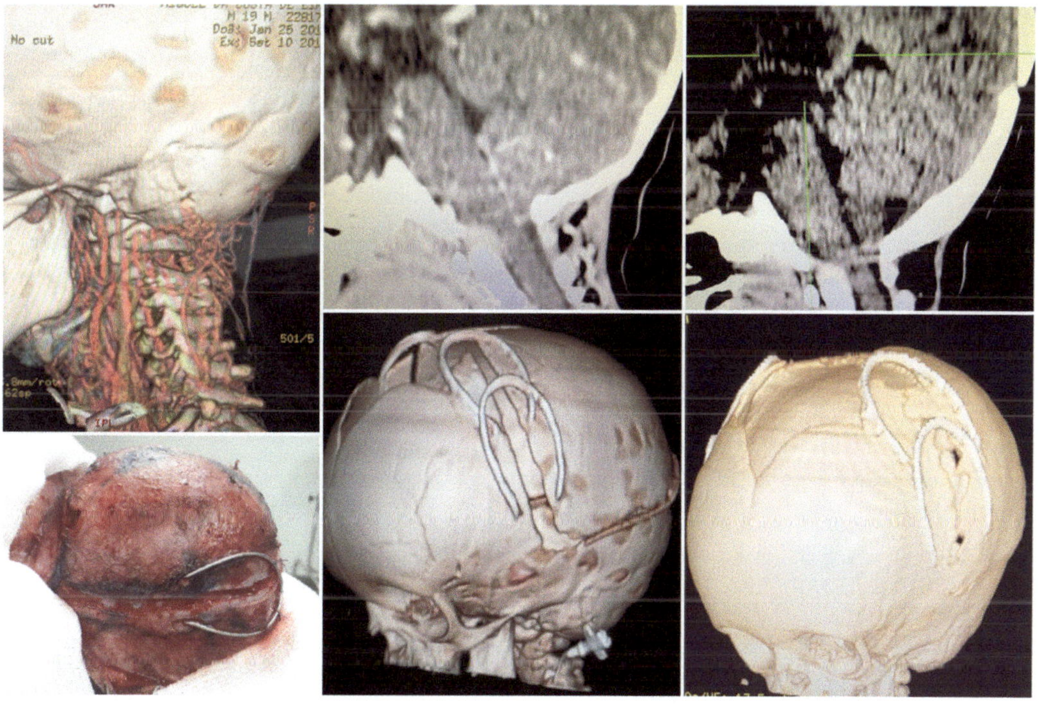

Fig. 50.3 Pfeiffer syndrome patient presenting important venous collateral circulation. Posterior vault expansion was performed with springs. Preop and postop CT scan shows the difference in volume of the posterior fossa

orrhages caused by collateral circulation around the foramen magnum. When the signs and symptoms of CMI appear after correction of craniosynostosis, the decompressive procedure is like that used in other forms of deformity.

50.6 Complications

As stated by Renier [10], the main risk of posterior fossa decompression in CMI/craniosynostosis is hemorrhage. Sandberg [50] reported two cases in which occipital decompression was withheld due to huge venous anomalies noted on imaging studies. Thompson [45] presented the case of a patient with a cloverleaf skull syndrome in whom division of occipital emissary veins during the elevation of the skin flap led to an acute rise in ICP and death of the patient.

50.7 Outcome and Follow-Up

The association of CMI and craniosynostosis is rare, and it is difficult to evaluate the results of FM decompression since the procedure is seldom performed alone, and the treatment of craniosynostosis sensu stricto involves decompression of the brain before or after addressing the foramen magnum. Scott et al. [47] considered that the extent of tonsillar descent and tightness of the foramen magnum are important risk factors, and Addo et al. [20] reported that FM decompression improved CSA in all five patients of their series. Regarding syringomyelia, in all cases of Scott et al. [47], the syrinx was found to be significantly smaller postoperatively. Patients with CMI should have a regular follow-up and screening through MRI. There is no consensus on how long this must be done.

References

1. Raybaud C, Jallo GI. Chiari 1 deformity in children: etiopathogenesis and radiologic diagnosis. In: Manto M, Huisman TAGM, editors. Handbook of clinical neurology, The cerebellum: disorders and treatment, vol. 155. 3rd series. Elsevier; 2018. p. 25–48. https://doi.org/10.1016/B978-0-444-64189-2.00002-0.
2. Francis PM, Beals S, Rekate HL, Pittmann HW, Manwaring K, Reiff J. Chronic tonsillar herniation and Crouzon's syndrome. Pediatr Neurosurg. 1992;18:202–6.
3. Friede RL, Roesmann U. Chronic tonsillar herniation. An attempt at classifying chronic herniation at the foramen magnum. Acta Neuropathol. 1989;34:214–35.
4. Frim DM, Jones D, Goumnerova L. Development of symptomatic Chiari malformation in a child with craniofacial dysmorphism. Pediatr Neurosurg. 1990;16:228–31.
5. Saldino RM, Steinbach HL, Epstein CJ. Familial acrocephalosyndactyly (Pfeiffer syndrome). Am J Roentgenol. 1972;116:609–22.
6. Venes JL. Comment in: Cinalli G, Chumas P, Arnaud E, Sainte-Rose C, Renier D: Occipital remodeling and suboccipital decompression in severe craniosynostosis associated with tonsillar herniation. Neurosurgery. 1998;42:71–2.
7. Cinalli G, Renier D, Sebag G, Sainte-Rose C, Arnaud E, Pierre-Kahn A. Chronic tonsillar herniation in Crouzon and Apert syndrome: the role of the premature synostosis of the lambdoid suture. J Neurosurg. 1995;83:575–82.
8. Cinalli G, Chumas P, Arnaud E, Sainte-Rose C, Renier D. Occipital remodeling and suboccipital decompression in severe craniosynostosis associated with tonsillar herniation. Neurosurgery. 1998;42:66–73.
9. Azoury SC, Reddy S, Shukla V, Deng C-X. Fibroblast growth factor receptor 1 and 2 (FGFR2) mutation related syndromic craniosynostosis. Int J Biol Sci. 2017;13:1479–88. https://doi.org/10.7150/ijbs.22373.
10. Renier D, Lajeunie E, Arnaud E, Marchac D. Management of craniosynostoses. Childs Nerv Syst. 2000;16(10–11):645–58. https://doi.org/10.1007/s003810000320.
11. Strahle J, Muraszko KM, Buchman SR, Kapurch J, Garton HJ, Maher CO. Chiari malformation associated with craniosynostosis. Neurosurg Focus. 2011;31(3):E2. https://doi.org/10.3171/2011.6.FOCUS11107.
12. Engel M, Castrillón-Oberndorfer G, Hoffmann J, Orakcioglu B, Rohde S, Seeberger R, Freudlsperger C. Chiari malformation in nonsyndromal single craniosynostosis—much ado about nothing? Acta Neurochir. 2012;154(10):1803–7. https://doi.org/10.1007/s00701-012-1439-5. Epub 2012 Jul 13.
13. Leikola J, Koljonen V, Valanne L, Hukki J. The incidence of Chiari malformation in nonsyndromic, single suture craniosynostosis. Childs Nerv Syst. 2010;26:771–4.
14. Fearon JA, Swift DM, Bruce DA. New methods for the evaluation and treatment of craniofacial dysostosis-associated cerebellar tonsillar herniation. Plast Reconstr Surg. 2001;108:1855–61.
15. Pouratian N, Sansur CA, Newman SA, Jane JA Jr, Jane JA Sr. Chiari malformations in patients

with uncorrected sagittal synostosis. Surg Neurol. 2007;67:422–8.
16. Valentini LG, Saletti V, Erbetta A, Chiapparini L, Furlanetto M. Chiari 1 malformation and untreated sagittal synostosis: a new subset of complex Chiari? Childs Nerv Syst. 2019;35(10):1741–53. https://doi.org/10.1007/s00381-019-04283-0. Epub 2019 Jul 21.
17. Czerwinski M, Kolar JC, Fearon JA. Complex craniosynostosis. Plast Reconstr Surg. 2011;128(4):955–61. https://doi.org/10.1097/PRS.0b013e3182268ca6.
18. Vinchon M, Guerreschi P, Karnoub MA, Wolber A. Synostosis of the lambdoid suture: a spectrum. Childs Nerv Syst. 2021;37(6):1991–2000. https://doi.org/10.1007/s00381-020-05003-9. Epub 2021 Jan 6.
19. Cinalli G, Spennato P, Sainte-Rose C, Arnaud E, Aliberti F, Brunelle F, et al. Chiari malformation in craniosynostosis. Childs Nerv Syst. 2005;21:889–901.
20. Addo NK, Javadpour S, Kandasamy J, Sillifant P, May P, Sinha A. Central sleep apnea and associated Chiari malformation in children with syndromic craniosynostosis: treatment and outcome data from a supraregional national craniofacial center. J Neurosurg Pediatr. 2013;11(3):296–301. https://doi.org/10.3171/2012.11.PEDS12297. Epub 2012 Dec 14.
21. Feller CN, Jensen JN, Lew SM. Chiari malformation type 1 and syringomyelia in a patient with prior surgically-treated sagittal synostosis effectively treated with posterior cranial vault distraction osteogenesis. J Craniofac Surg. 2021;32(6):2110–3. https://doi.org/10.1097/SCS.0000000000007401.
22. Fiaschi P, Morana G, Anania P, Rossi A, Consales A, Piatelli G, Cama A, Pavanello M. Tonsillar herniation spectrum: more than just Chiari I. Update and controversies on classification and management. Neurosurg Rev. 2020;43(6):1473–92. https://doi.org/10.1007/s10143-019-01198-x. Epub 2019 Nov 10.
23. Sgouros S. Skull vault growth in craniosynostosis. Childs Nerv Syst. 2005;21(10):861–70. https://doi.org/10.1007/s00381-004-1112-2. Epub 2005 Mar 25.
24. Sgulò FG, Spennato P, Aliberti F, Di Martino G, Cascone D, Cinalli G. Contemporary occurrence of hydrocephalus and Chiari I malformation in sagittal craniosynostosis. Case report and review of the literature. Childs Nerv Syst. 2017;33(1):187–92. https://doi.org/10.1007/s00381-016-3189-9. Epub 2016 Jul 22.
25. Venes JL. Arnold-Chiari malformation in an infant with Kleeblattschädel: an acquired malformation? Neurosurgery. 1988;23:360–2.
26. Calandrelli R, D'Apolito G, Gaudino S, Stefanetti M, Massimi L, Di Rocco C, Colosimo C. Radiological assessment of skull base changes in children with syndromic craniosynostosis: role of "minor" sutures. Neuroradiology. 2014;56(10):865–75. https://doi.org/10.1007/s00234-014-1392-5. Epub 2014 Jul 10.
27. Goodrich JT. Skull base growth in craniosynostosis. Childs Nerv Syst. 2005;21:871–9. https://doi.org/10.1007/s00381-004-1113-1.
28. Thompson DN, Harkness W, Jones BM, Hayward RD. Aetiology of herniation of the hindbrain in craniosynostosis. An investigation incorporating intracranial pressure monitoring and magnetic resonance imaging. Pediatr Neurosurg. 1997;26(6):288–95. https://doi.org/10.1159/000121208.
29. Rijken BF, Lequin MH, Van Veelen ML, de Rooi J, Mathijssen IM. The formation of the foramen magnum and its role in developing ventriculomegaly and Chiari I malformation in children with craniosynostosis syndromes. J Craniomaxillofac Surg. 2015;43(7):1042–8. https://doi.org/10.1016/j.jcms.2015.04.025. Epub 2015 May 8. PMID: 26051848
30. Coll G, Sakka L, Botella C, Pham-Dang N, Collet C, Zerah M, Arnaud E, Di Rocco F. Pattern of closure of skull base synchondroses in Crouzon syndrome. World Neurosurg. 2018;109:e460–7. https://doi.org/10.1016/j.wneu.2017.09.208. Epub 2017 Oct 10.
31. Di Rocco F, Dubravova D, Ziyadeh J, Sainte-Rose C, Collet C, Arnaud E. The foramen magnum in isolated and syndromic brachycephaly. Childs Nerv Syst. 2014;30(1):165–72. https://doi.org/10.1007/s00381 013-2245-y. Epub 2013 Oct 18.
32. Rijken BFM, Lequin MH, de Rooi JJ, van Veelen MC, Mathijssen IMJ. Foramen magnum size and involvement of its intraoccipital synchondroses in Crouzon syndrome. Plast Reconstr Surg. 2013;132(6):993e–1000e. https://doi.org/10.1097/PRS.0b013e3182a8077e.
33. Al-Otibi M, Jea A, Kulkarni AV. Detection of important venous collaterals by computed tomography venogram in multisutural synostosis. J Neurosurg Pediatr. 2007;107(6):508–10. https://thejns.org/pediatrics/view/journals/j-neurosurg-pediatr/107/6/article-p508.xml. Accessed 24 Jun 2022.
34. Jeevan DS, Anlsow P, Jayamohan J. Abnormal venous drainage in syndromic craniosynostosis and the role of CT venography. Childs Nerv Syst. 2008;24:1413. https://doi.org/10.1007/s00381-008-0667-8.
35. Protzenko T, Bellas A, Ribeiro CMC, Gonzalez SMC, Horovitz DDG. Venous anomalies in hypoplastic posterior fossa: unsolved questions. Childs Nerv Syst. 2021;37(10):3177–87. https://doi.org/10.1007/s00381-021-05315-4.
36. Coll G, Lemaire JJ, Di Rocco F, Barthélémy I, Garcier JM, De Schlichting E, Sakka L. Human Foramen Magnum Area and Posterior Cranial Fossa Volume Growth in Relation to Cranial Base Synchondrosis Closure in the Course of Child Development. Neurosurgery. 2016;79(5):722–35. https://doi.org/10.1227/NEU.0000000000001309. PMID: 27341342.
37. Mathijssen IM. Guideline for care of patients with the diagnoses of craniosynostosis: Working Group on Craniosynostosis. J Craniofac Surg. 2015;26(6):1735–807. https://doi.org/10.1097/SCS.0000000000002016.
38. Doerga PN, Rijken BFM, Bredero-Boelhouwer H, Joosten KFM, Neuteboom RF, Tasker RC, Dremmen MHG, Lequin MH, van Veelen MLC, Mathijssen

IMJ. Neurological deficits are present in syndromic craniosynostosis patients with and without tonsillar herniation. Eur J Paediatr Neurol. 2020;28:120–5. https://doi.org/10.1016/j.ejpn.2020.06.018. Epub 2020 Jul 21.
39. Strahle J, Spence J, Pasterkamp H, McDonald PJ. Isolated central sleep apnea in type I Chiari malformation: improvement after surgery. Pediatr Pulmonol. 2010;45:1141–4.
40. Tan HL, Kheirandish-Gozal L, Abel F, Gozal D. Craniofacial syndromes and sleep-related breathing disorders. Sleep Med Rev. 2016;27:74–88. https://doi.org/10.1016/j.smrv.2015.05.010. Epub 2015 Jun 6.
41. Tubbs RS, Lyerly MJ, Loukas M, Shoja MM, Oakes WJ. The pediatric Chiari I malformation: a review. Childs Nerv Syst. 2007;23(11):1239–50. https://doi.org/10.1007/s00381-007-0428-0. Epub 2007 Jul 18.
42. Renier D, Arnaud E, Marchac D. [Craniosynostosis: functional and morphologic postoperative results]. Neurochirurgie. 2006;52:302–10.
43. Schulz M, Spors B, Haberl H, et al. Results of posterior cranial vault remodeling for plagiocephaly and brachycephaly by the meander technique. Childs Nerv Syst. 2014;30:1517–26. https://doi.org/10.1007/s00381-014-2462-z.
44. Martinez-Perez D, Vander Woude DL, Barnes PD, et al. Jugular foraminal stenosis in Crouzon syndrome. Pediatr Neurosurg. 1996;25:252–5.
45. Thompson DN, Hayward RD, Harkness WJ, et al. Lessons from a case of kleeblattschädel. Case report. J Neurosurg. 1995;82:1071–4.
46. Fearon JA, Dimas V, Ditthakasem K. Lambdoid craniosynostosis: the relationship with Chiari deformations and an analysis of surgical outcomes. Plast Reconstr Surg. 2016;137(3):946–51. https://doi.org/10.1097/01.prs.0000480014.18541.d8.
47. Scott WW, Fearon JA, Swift DM, Sacco DJ. Suboccipital decompression during posterior cranial vault remodeling for selected cases of Chiari malformations associated with craniosynostosis. J Neurosurg Pediatr. 2013;12(2):166–70. https://doi.org/10.3171/2013.4.PEDS12463. Epub 2013 May 24.
48. Chivoret N, Arnaud E, Giraudat K, et al. Bilambdoid and sagittal synostosis: report of 39 cases. Surg Neurol Int. 2018;9:206. Published 2018 Oct 11. https://doi.org/10.4103/sni.sni_454_17.
49. Leikola J, Haapamäki V, Karppinen A, Koljonen V, Hukki J, Valanne L, Koivikko M. Morphometric comparison of foramen magnum in non-syndromic craniosynostosis patients with or without Chiari I malformation. Acta Neurochir (Wien). 2012;154(10):1809–13. https://doi.org/10.1007/s00701-012-1451-9. Epub 2012 Aug 7. PMID: 22868492.
50. Sandberg DI, Navarro R, Blanch J, Ragheb J. Anomalous venous drainage preventing safe posterior fossa decompression in patients with chiari malformation type I and multisutural craniosynostosis. Report of two cases and review of the literature. J Neurosurg. 2007;106(6 Suppl):490–4. https://doi.org/10.3171/ped.2007.106.6.490.

Part VII

Results and Outcome Analysis

51 Evaluation Tools for Craniosynostosis

Rebecca M. Burke and John R. W. Kestle

51.1 Introduction

Historically, the pre- and postoperative assessment of craniosynostosis was largely subjective and employed the use of imaging modalities such as computed tomography (CT) that resulted in radiation exposure to the developing brain of pediatric patients [1–7]. Consequently, there has been a movement to develop objective and reproducible evaluation tools that do not rely on ionizing radiation to reliably characterize preoperative cranial vault deformity and postoperative correction [8, 9]. Here, we describe the evolution of these assessment tools and their clinical relevance with an emphasis on advancements in the realm of scaphocephaly and trigonocephaly.

R. M. Burke · J. R. W. Kestle (✉)
Department of Neurosurgery, University of Utah, Salt Lake City, UT, USA
e-mail: neuropub@hsc.utah.edu

51.2 Early Attempts at Predicting the Need for Revision Surgery: The Whittaker Classification

One of the earliest attempts to create an assessment tool for postoperative outcomes in craniosynostosis surgery was in 1987 with the development of the Whitaker classification, a 4-point scale that stratifies the degree of revision surgery that would achieve cosmetic normalcy [6, 7]. The classification scheme is as follows: (I) no refinements or surgical revisions considered advisable or necessary by the surgeon or the patient; (II) soft-tissue or lesser bone-contouring revisions desirable, whether performed or not; (III) major alternative osteotomies or bone-grafting procedures needed or performed; and (IV) major procedure duplicating or exceeding in extent the original surgery necessary (Table 51.1). Although this classification has been widely used in the literature, it is limited by the subjective nature of the reporting scheme, which has led to questions about its inter rater reliability demonstrating the need for more objective and reliable assessment tools to properly evaluate the patient with craniosynostosis [6, 10, 11]. In a retrospective analysis by Wes et al. [6], the Whitaker classification demonstrated low interrater reliability and did not successfully predict the need for future operative intervention. The basic premise of this study highlighted the limitations of allowing subjective aesthetic assessments

F. Di Rocco, J. Kestle (eds.), *Neurosurgical Aspects of Craniosynostosis*,
https://doi.org/10.1007/978-3-031-69386-1_51

Table 51.1 Whitaker classification definitions

Classification	Description
I	No refinements or surgical revisions considered advisable or necessary by the surgeon or the patient.
II	Soft-tissue or lesser bone-contouring revisions desirable, whether performed or not.
III	Major alternative osteotomies or bone-grafting procedures needed or performed.
IV	Major procedure duplicating or exceeding in extent the original surgery necessary.

Reproduced with permission from Wes AM, Naran S, Sun J, Mazzaferro D, Xu W, Nguyen P, et al. The Whitaker classification of craniosynostosis outcomes: an assessment of interrater reliability. Plast Reconstr Surg. 2017;140(4):579e–86e

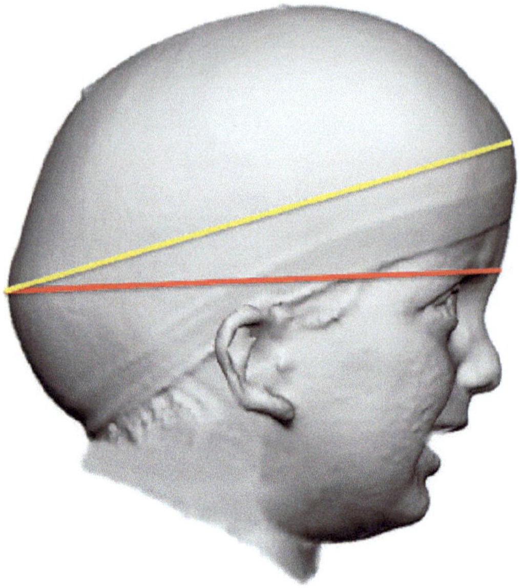

Fig. 51.1 Lateral view of sagittal craniosynostosis with traditional cranial index (red line) and modified cranial index (yellow line). (Reproduced with permission from Al-Shaqsi SZ, Rai A, Forrest C, Phillips J. Standardization of cranial index measurement in sagittal craniosynostosis. J Craniofac Surg. 2019;30:366–9)

to dictate operative decision-making. Although the Whitaker classification laid the groundwork for a system that could guide the need for further intervention, its significant limitations were clear, leading to the development of alternative assessment tools.

51.3 Sagittal Synostosis

51.3.1 Anthropometric Analysis

Because sagittal synostosis represents the most common form of single-suture synostosis, comprising 40–60% of isolated synostoses cases, several parameters have been devised to facilitate its preoperative evaluation and postoperative assessment [11–13]. Historically, the cranial index (CI) has been used as a two-dimensional (2D), linear, quantitative measure of the severity of sagittal synostosis, and its utility has also been observed in outcome assessment [4, 9]. The CI is defined as the ratio of maximum cranial width, which is measured from euryon to euryon, to the maximum cranial length, which is measured from the glabella to the opisthocranion × 100 [4, 14]. Patients with isolated sagittal synostosis (ISS) have an average CI of 60–67%, in contrast to their unaffected counterparts with a CI of 76–78%. Despite the wide utility of the CI in the assessment of ISS, it is not without its limitations, and several studies have called into question its reproducibility [3, 15, 16]. One criticism is the variability in technique used to measure the maximal cranial width and maximal cranial length, which can be further complicated by the variable degrees of frontal and occipital bossing [9, 16]. In fact, the results of a study by Al-Shaqsi et al. [17] indicated that the traditional method of measuring the CI underestimates the severity of scaphocephaly. Instead, they proposed a modified method of measuring the CI, calculated as the ratio of the most anterior point on the cranium to the opisthocranion, to more accurately reflect the severity of scaphocephaly by taking the degree of frontal bossing into consideration (Fig. 51.1). Similarly, in isolation, the CI does not provide information about regional severity [3]. The CI is also generated from 2D measurements to describe a three-dimensional (3D) object and is therefore a descriptive oversimplification [15].

In further recognition of a need for standardized assessment tools in the evaluation of craniosynostosis, Fearon et al. [18] employed the use of anthropometric measurements to evaluate long-term skull growth and surgical outcomes in patients undergoing surgical correction for ISS. Four measurements, including minimum frontal breadth, head circumference, maximum cranial length measured from the glabella to the opisthocranion, and maximal cranial breadth measured from euryon to euryon, were obtained. The anthropometric values obtained were compared with sex- and age-matched controls and converted to standard (*Z*) scores for standardized comparison. The authors demonstrated that the anthropometric measurements normalized 6 weeks postoperatively. However, long-term follow-up revealed a disproportionate restriction in growth in width when compared with length, thus promoting a more scaphocephalic skull morphology over time [18]. Although anthropometric measurements have allowed for significant advances in our understanding of craniosynostosis, they do not provide 3D information, and their use also introduces significant inter- and intraobserver error [3, 9]. Furthermore, obtaining reliable and reproducible anthropometric data from a young, uncooperative pediatric patient can be very challenging [9].

51.3.2 Intracranial Volume Assessment

Early studies relied on the use of CT to evaluate intracranial volume as a mechanism to follow preoperative and postoperative outcomes [19–22]. One study employed thin-cut CT scans, fine-point calipers, a 0.5-mm ruler, and a 1° protractor to evaluate 14 measurements based on bony landmarks to evaluate the morphology of the midface and cranial vault in ISS patients [19]. Another study evaluated scans on a slice-by-slice basis with computerized counting of the number of voxels within the intracranial cavity for the corresponding slice being evaluated [20]. This was repeated for each slice such that the intracranial volume could be extrapolated. Using this methodology, the authors were able to demonstrate that the preoperative intracranial volume and postoperative cranial expansion in patients with ISS was approaching or exceeding that of age-matched controls. David et al. [21] used a 3D laser scan to measure the CI, morphology, and intracranial volume in patients with scaphocephaly pre- and postoperatively (Fig. 51.2). A ratio of anterior to total cra-

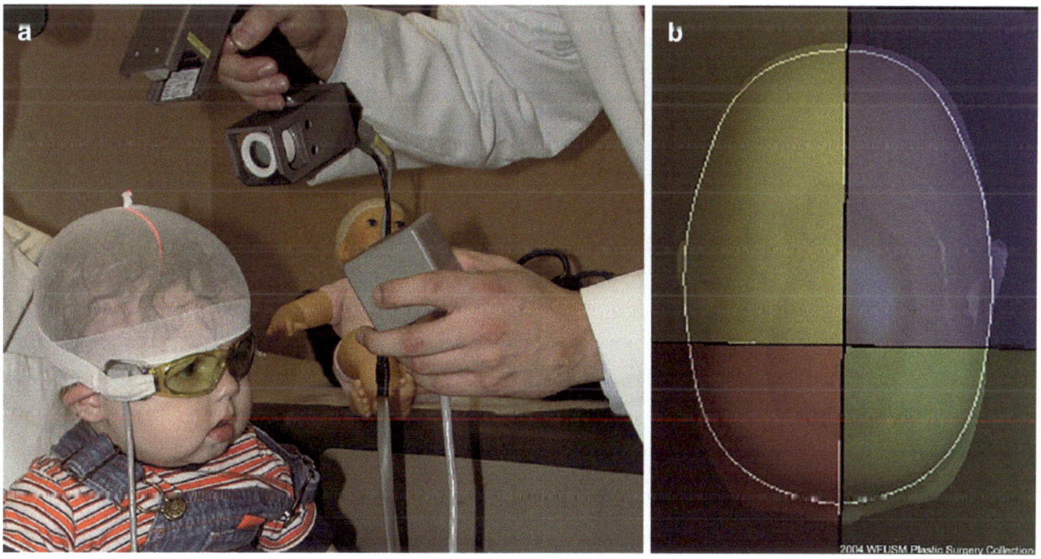

Fig. 51.2 (**a**) Portable laser Doppler scanning device. (**b**) Example of images obtained with volume calculation using Delta Scan Comparison software. (Reproduced with permission from David LR, Plikaitis CM, Couture D, Glazier SS, Argenta LC. Outcome analysis of our first 75 spring-assisted surgeries for scaphocephaly. J Craniofac Surg. 2010;21:3–9)

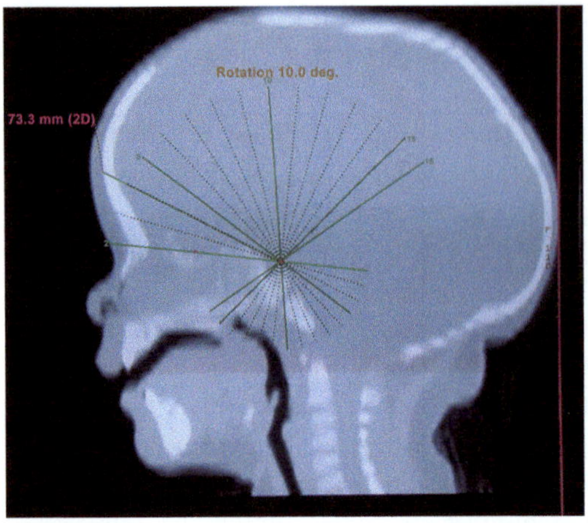

Fig. 51.3 Set of radial vectors at 10° increments are created in radial pattern, emanating from posterior ledge of sella. Measurements are taken to outer table. Analysis is performed pre- and postoperatively to allow qualitative analysis and to provide data suitable for paired statistical analysis. (Reproduced with permission from Marcus JR, Stokes TH, Mukundan S, Forrest CR. Quantitative and qualitative assessment of morphology in sagittal synostosis: mid-sagittal vector analysis. J Craniofac Surg. 2006;17(4):680–6)

nial volume was measured and demonstrated a trend toward normalization after surgery. Although the intracranial volume from a CT can be a useful and objective assessment tool in the analysis of ISS, the radiation exposure required using this modality is not ideal in the developing brain.

51.3.3 CT Vector Analysis

Midsagittal vector analysis has been used to assess pre- and postoperative morphology after cranial vault remodeling [23]. This method uses a radial vector analysis from a single point in the sagittal plane at the level of the sella turcica to assess distances to the cranial surface (Fig. 51.3). Vectors in the frontal, vertex, and occipital regions were calculated pre- and postoperatively from CT scans. Postoperative data demonstrated a reduction in the frontal and occipital prominence, an increase in the height of the vertex, and correction in frontal and occipital bossing [23]. Although this provided a more objective assessment of pre- and postoperative morphology, this technique is limited by its 2D assessment as well as the need for ionizing radiation [9]. Similarly, the decrease in the biparietal diameter in scaphocephaly would not be adequately evaluated using this purely sagittal plane methodology [9].

Ruiz-Correa et al. [16] demonstrated the superiority of scaphocephaly severity indices (SSIs) as compared with the CI in the ability to predict ISS. SSIs were generated by tracing 2D planes defined by several internal anatomical landmarks, including the top of the lateral ventricles, the foramen of Monro, and the maximal dimension of the fourth ventricle, and measuring the ratio of head width and length in each of these planes (Fig. 51.4). It was determined that although CI demonstrates a high level of sensitivity, it lacks specificity in contrast to the SSI, which demonstrates high levels of both sensitivity and specificity [16].

Moreover, CT scan digital analysis has been employed in patients with sagittal synostosis to address whether associated frontal bossing requires direct surgical correction or if there is spontaneous resolution of the frontal bossing over time after posterior cranial vault expansion [24]. In this study, CT scans converted to 3D models were evaluated immediately and 2 years after posterior-middle cranial vault expansion. Quantitative angular and linear measures of frontal bossing were obtained in a standardized fashion in the axial and midsagittal planes and compared with healthy controls. Using CT scan digital analysis, the authors demonstrated that patients with sagittal synostosis who undergo surgery before 1 year of age spontaneously normalize the frontal bossing within a 2-year postoperative window. Thus, using standardized, objective assessment techniques, the authors were able to illustrate that a single-stage operation, if offered within the first year of life, helps avoid forehead contour deformities related to a more extensive procedure as well as multistage procedures that are associated with greater risk of morbidity [24]. Although this addressed some of the limitations previously discussed, the use of CT scan digital analysis still involved recurrent exposure to radiation.

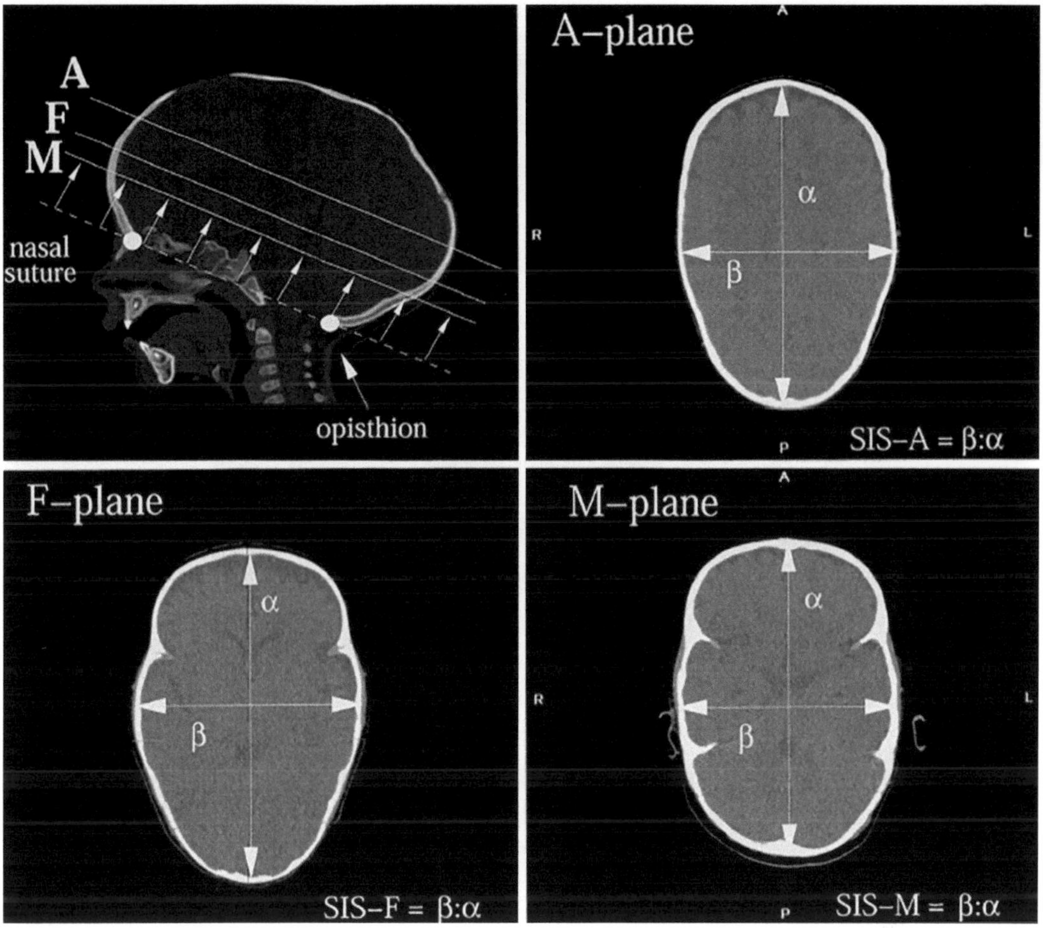

Fig. 51.4 SSI-A, SSI-F, and SSI-M were computed from CT bone slices defined by internal anatomical landmarks based on cerebral ventricles just above the top of the lateral ventricles (A-plane), the Foramina of Munro (F-plane), and at the level of the maximal dimension of the fourth ventricle (M-plane). (Reproduced with permission from Ruiz-Correa S, Sze RW, Starr JR, Lin HT, Speltz ML, Cunningham ML, et al. New scaphocephaly severity indices of sagittal craniosynostosis: a comparative study with cranial index quantifications. Cleft Palate Craniofac J. 2006;43(2):211–21)

51.3.4 Three-Dimensional Vector Analysis

3D vector analysis (3DVA) has been validated as a tool for craniofacial morphologic assessment with the purposes of diagnosis, surgical planning, and outcome assessment in the setting of the shortcomings of cranial anthropometric and 2D techniques [3, 15]. However, 3DVA software is used to generate a 3D matrix of the imported pre- and postoperative CT scan DICOM data, which is presented as a concurrent axial, coronal, and sagittal view. The user must then select the dorsum sella, nasion, and vertex. Vectors are then generated from the dorsum sella to the cranial surface such that a cranial point cloud representation comprised of more than 37,000 points is created (Fig. 51.5, top) [3, 9, 15]. This results in a 3D representation in a graphical form that is programmed to generate a set of clinically meaningful anthropometric values, and a digital "craniofacial fingerprint" is created (Fig. 51.5, bottom) [3]. This allowed for the generation of a color histogram superimposed over the cranial

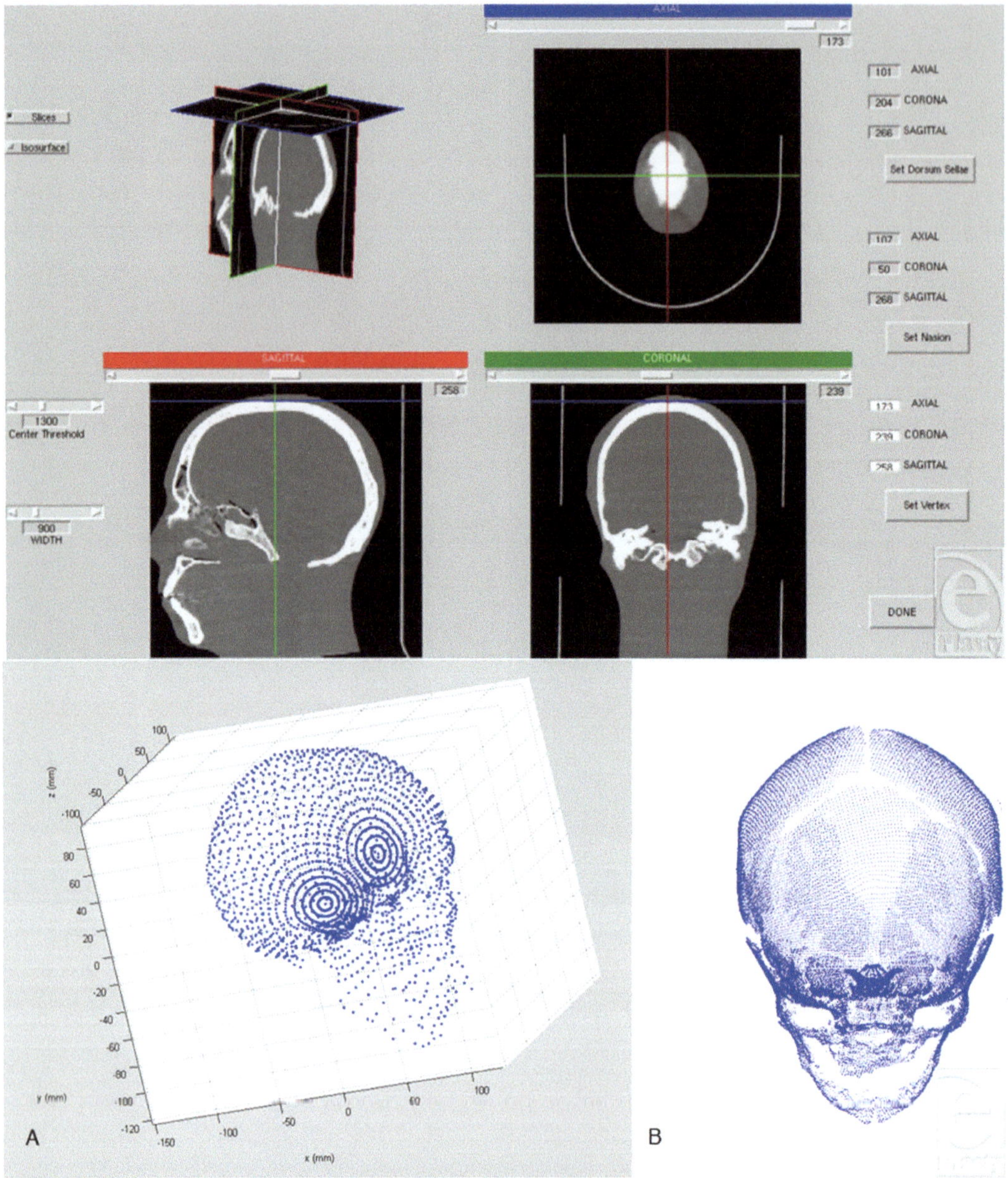

Fig. 51.5 (Top) Orthographic viewer. After DICOM data are imported, the user defines the nasion, vertex, and dorsum sella in three planes viewed concurrently: axial, coronal, and sagittal. In this way, the analysis is corrected for rotation, translation, and alignment. (Bottom) 3DVA-generated cranial surface point clouds. (Bottom left) Automated measurement of vectors from dorsum sella to outer cortex of calvarium using 3DVA at a low-frequency interval of 10°. Subject is an adult human skull embedded in a doped-lucite matrix. (Bottom right) Automated measurement of vectors from dorsum sella to outer cortex of calvarium using 3DVA at a high-frequency interval of 2°. "Craniofacial Fingerprint." Subject is a pediatric patient; open fontanelles are clearly discenable. (Reproduced under the Creative Commons Attribution License from Marcus JR, Domeshek LF, Das R, Marshall S, Nightingale R, Stokes TH, et al. Objective three-dimensional analysis of cranial morphology. Eplasty. 2008;8:e20)

point cloud that demonstrates deviations from normal controls (Fig. 51.6) [3, 9]. The same group went on to use 3DVA to generate a normative database that was accurate and reproducible [3]. Strengths of 3DVA include its ability to distinguish between varying pathologies and its ability to differentiate subtle morphologic differences in patients with the same disease process. Although 3DVA provides a 3D analysis of craniofacial morphology and provides a quantitative and reproducible assessment, long-term studies would necessitate repeat exposure to ionizing radiation [9].

51.3.5 3D Digital Stereophotogrammetry

3D digital stereophotogrammetry has emerged as a useful tool to obtain objective, reproducible, noninvasive information for the assessment of craniosynostosis, with an additional advantage of not requiring exposure to ionizing radiation [9, 25–29]. It has been used to differentiate between patients with and without craniosynostosis, predict what suture is fused, and objectively quantify postsurgical aesthetic outcomes (Fig. 51.7) [26].

Weinberg et al. [29] evaluated 19 standardized, linear facial measurements derived from 17 landmarks on the face favoring the oral–nasal region with digital calipers as well as 3D photographs captured with the Genex 3D system. The 3D imaging system allows each point on the object's surface to have a corresponding pixel in the x, y, and z coordinates. They also assessed the precision and accuracy of the measurements with and without landmarks. They demonstrated that the precision of the 3D photographs was superior to that of the digital calipers, and the highest precision was obtained from measurements taken with 3D photogrammetry with landmarks labeled before the images were captured [29].

Van Veelen et al. [28] used 3D photogrammetry to measure intracranial volume in patients that underwent early extended strip craniectomy or late total cranial remodeling, and volume measurements were related to CI, head circumference, and signs of elevated intracranial pressure. Additionally, the volume measurements derived from the 3D photogrammetry were compared with those obtained from 3D CT. The authors demonstrated that pre- and postoperative volume was increased in all patients that underwent surgery when compared with age-matched controls. Patients who underwent late total cranial remodeling had a slightly larger intracranial volume than patients that underwent early strip craniectomy. Volume measurements obtained on 3D photogrammetry demonstrated a high level of reproducibility and had a strong correlation with measurements obtained on CT [28]. Mertens et al. [25] used 3D photogrammetry to evaluate the effect of early extended strip craniectomy for sagittal synostosis versus a late modified pi procedure on intracranial volume and CI and showed that both techniques are effective at normalizing these variables, but surgical duration and blood loss were significantly lower in patients undergoing early strip craniectomy.

In contrast, Seeberger et al. [27] used 3D photogrammetry to compare the intracranial volume of children with sagittal synostosis to age- and sex-matched controls and demonstrated that male patients with sagittal synostosis had significantly smaller intracranial volumes compared with their unaffected counterparts. Although these results conflict with the previous studies, they illustrate the utility of 3D photogrammetry in the evaluation of craniosynostosis and highlight the benefit of reducing patient exposure to ionizing radiation. Other strengths of this modality include its noninvasive nature, ease of collection in potentially uncooperative pediatric patients, and the ability to generate a 3D archive of a patient's facial morphology [9].

Recent advances have coupled the use of 3D photogrammetry with deep learning for craniosynostosis diagnosis [30]. Preoperative 3D stereophotographs were obtained in patients with scaphocephaly, trigonocephaly, and anterior plagiocephaly and in unaffected infants, and

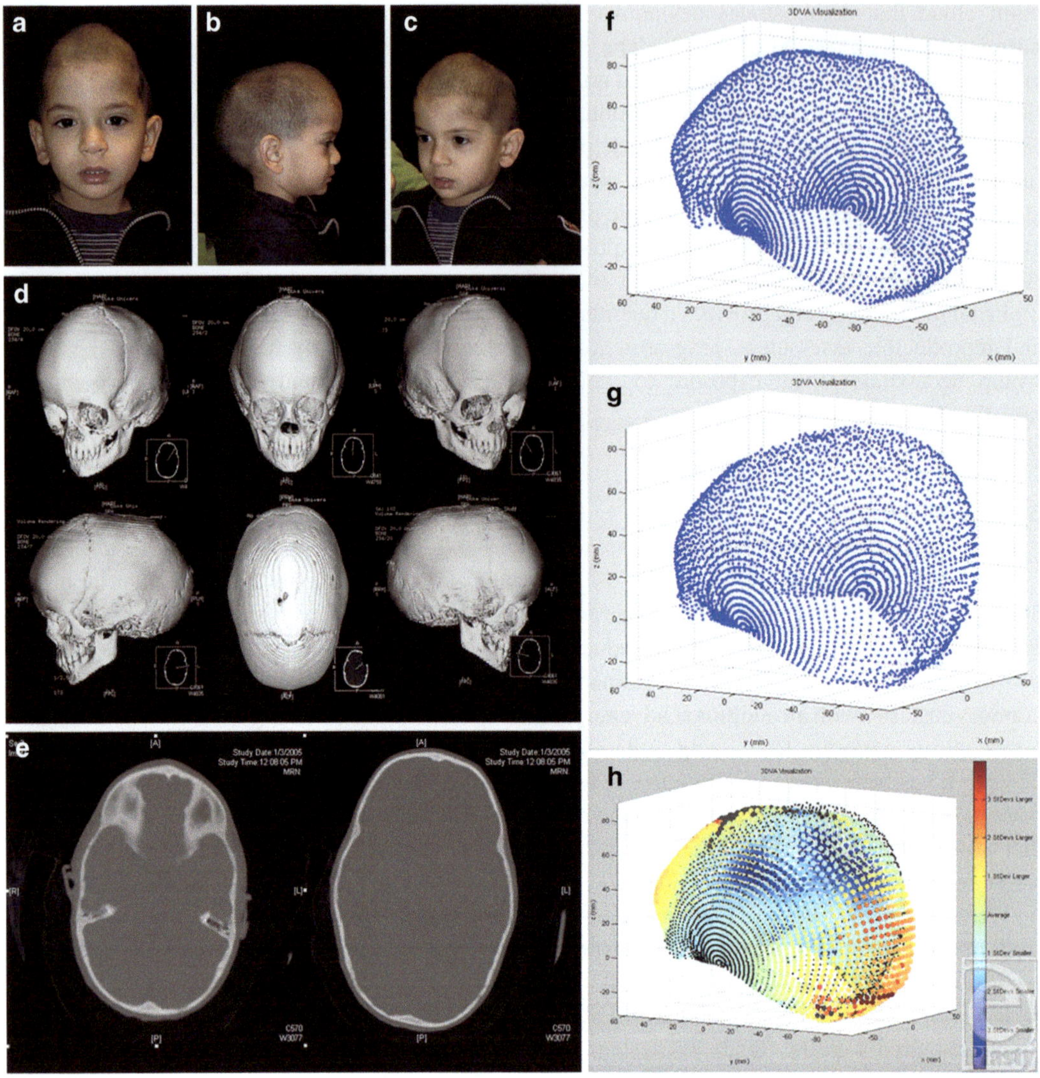

Fig. 51.6 Sagittal synostosis. (**a–c**) Nine-month-old with narrow bitemporal width, AP elongation, high anterior vertex, but no frontal bossing. (**d, e**) 3D CT demonstrating sagittal synostosis. The closed metopic suture perhaps contributed to this particular shape pattern, atypical for scaphocephaly. (**f**) 3DVA-generated point cloud for the patient's DICOM data. (**g**) 3DVA-averaged data for normal 9-month-old males ($N = 4$). (**h**) Subject's data set (colored points) compared with normative data set (black points). The color scale describes each point's distance (in number of standard deviations) from the population mean. Note anterior vertex and low occipital bossing and high occiput recession. (Reproduced under the Creative Commons Attribution License from Marcus JR, Domeshek LF, Das R, Marshall S, Nightingale R, Stokes TH, et al. Objective three-dimensional analysis of cranial morphology. Eplasty. 2008;8:e20)

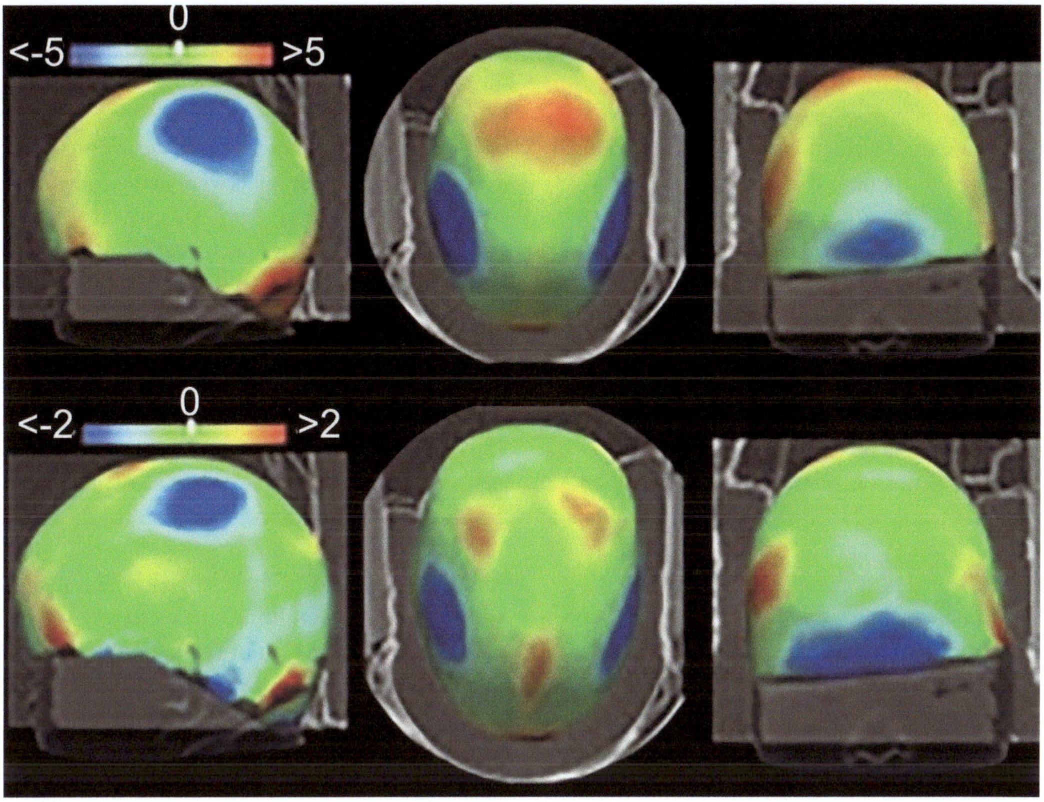

Fig. 51.7 Head shape metrics calculated for one example patient with sagittal craniosynostosis from the preoperative computed tomographic image. (Top) Local malformations (mm) and (bottom) curvature discrepancies (mm^{-1}). Positive malformations represent overdevelopment, and negative values represent underdevelopment. Positive curvature discrepancies represent sharper areas than the normative model, whereas negative values represent flatter areas. (Reproduced with permission from Porras AR, Tu L, Tsering D, Mantilla E, Oh A, Enquobahrie A, et al. Quantification of head shape from three-dimensional photography for presurgical and postsurgical evaluation of craniosynostosis. Plast Reconstr Surg. 2019;144(6):1051e–60e)

a deep learning network was used to classify the shape as control or one of the corresponding craniosynostosis subtypes. To validate the deep learning network, a tenfold cross validation was used, and the 3D stereophotographs were correctly classified in 195 of 196 subjects, illustrating the ability of deep learning algorithms to accurately predict subtypes of craniosynostosis as well as controls [30].

51.4 Metopic Synostosis

Similar challenges in the assessment of metopic synostosis such as a lack of objective and reproducible measurements have been described and further limited by exposure to ionizing radiation with serial imaging assessments [31, 32]. In response to these challenges, several techniques have been devised.

51.4.1 Quantitative Measurements Using CT

Patients with a diagnosis of isolated metopic synostosis were evaluated pre- and postoperatively with high-resolution, thin-section CT scans [33]. A total of 14 measurements were derived from the CT scans from bony landmarks and quantified with a fine-point caliper, a 0.5-mm ruler, and a 1° protractor. Preoperatively, patients had a narrowed intercoronal distance at a value of 92% of the general population, narrowed anteromedial wall interorbital distance at 79% of the general population, narrowed lateral orbital wall distance at 94% of the general population, and elevated medial orbital wall protrusion at 115% of the general population. Operative intervention corrected these abnormalities by 1-year postoperatively [33].

Trigonocephaly severity indices have been derived from CT scans of patients diagnosed with metopic synostosis to stratify the severity of the cranial dysmorphology [34]. CT scans underwent volumetric reformatting to trace 2D planes defined by several landmarks, and severity indices were generated. In concert, the metopic severity index was also derived. The authors demonstrated that the severity indices, which were outcome shape-based and therefore reflect outline information that represents global information, achieved more accuracy than the metopic severity index with is a linear distanced-based measurement [34].

51.4.2 The Metopic Angle

Data from a retrospective review of patients that underwent endoscopic strip craniectomy for metopic synostosis were imported into the STARscanner Laser Data Acquisition System to obtain cranial vault contour data [31, 35]. In the system, reference is defined by the tragus and root of the nose, and all measurements were fashioned with respect to the reference plane. The metopic angle was derived from images of the anterior–posterior diameter of the cranial contour. A line perpendicular to this diameter is laterally extended until it meets the contour of the frontal bone bilaterally. Tangential lines to the contour of the frontal bones are then drawn, and the metopic angle is formed at the tangential intersection (Fig. 51.8) [31, 35]. The authors demonstrated that the metopic angle at 3 months and 1 year postoperatively in patients that underwent endoscopic strip craniectomy for metopic synostosis were comparable with those of age-matched controls [31].

51.4.3 Anterior-Posterior Volume Ratio

The STARscanner imaging acquisition system has been used to create a novel assessment tool, the anterior–posterior volume ratio for the evaluation of metopic synostosis patients that have undergone fronto-orbital advancement [36]. This system uses multiple surface lasers to create a 3D reconstruction of the patient's head. A technician then identifies several soft tissue landmarks on the 3D image including the sellion, left tragus, and right tragus. Using this information, the system creates several axial reference planes that are used to calculate multiple linear measurements, which are ultimately used to create volumetric data (Fig. 51.9) [36]. The volumetric data allow the cranial vault to be divided into four quadrants that are further classified as anterior or posterior. The anterior–posterior volume ratio is defined as the ratio of the sum of the anterior cranial vault volumes to the sum of the posterior vault volumes and was shown to increase postoperatively as expected, although this study was limited by its small sample size [36].

51.4.4 The Metopic Index

The metopic index (MI) represents a simple anthropometric cranial measurement that can be derived from CT scans as well as cranial landmarks that can be palpated on physical examination [32]. In a retrospective analysis of patients with metopic synostosis, CT scans were converted to 3D reconstructions. The MI was calculated from the midfrontozygomatic diameter (the

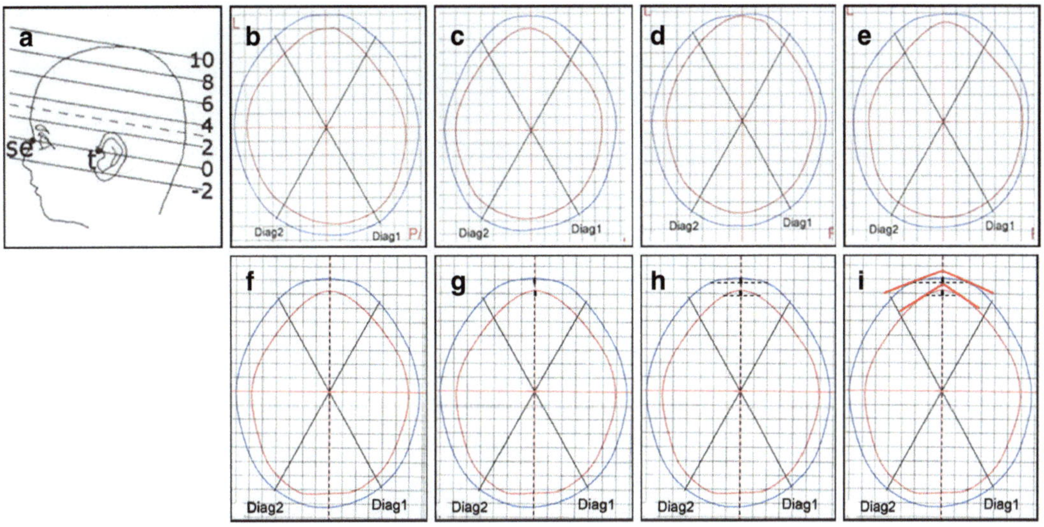

Fig. 51.8 Laser scans. The STARscanner Laser Data Acquisition System allows collection of images of the vault circumference in different planes. Our reference plane is defined by tragion (t) and sellion (Se), as surrogates for porion and nasion, respectively. All the measurements were made in a plane parallel with the reference plane situated at 3/10th of the height of the vault from the reference plane (**a**). To allow for direct comparisons, the cranial contour at each point postoperatively (blue) was plotted on the same diagram with the preoperative vault contour (red). The 1-year postoperative diagrams of 4 different patients are presented (**b**–**e**). (**f**–**i**) The steps used to calculate the metopic angle. Initially, the anteroposterior diameter is drawn and measured (**f**). A distance equal to 1/40th of this diameter is measured from the most anterior point (**g**). A perpendicular line to the anteroposterior diameter is developed at this level and extended laterally until it intersects the frontal bone contour bilaterally (**h**). At those intersection points, tangential lines to the frontal bone contour are drawn bilaterally. The metopic angle is formed at the intersection of these 2 tangents (**i**). (Reproduced with permission from Gociman B, Agko M, Blagg R, Garlick J, Kestle JR, Siddiqi F. Endoscopic-assisted correction of metopic synostosis. J Craniofac Surg. 2013;24(3):763–8)

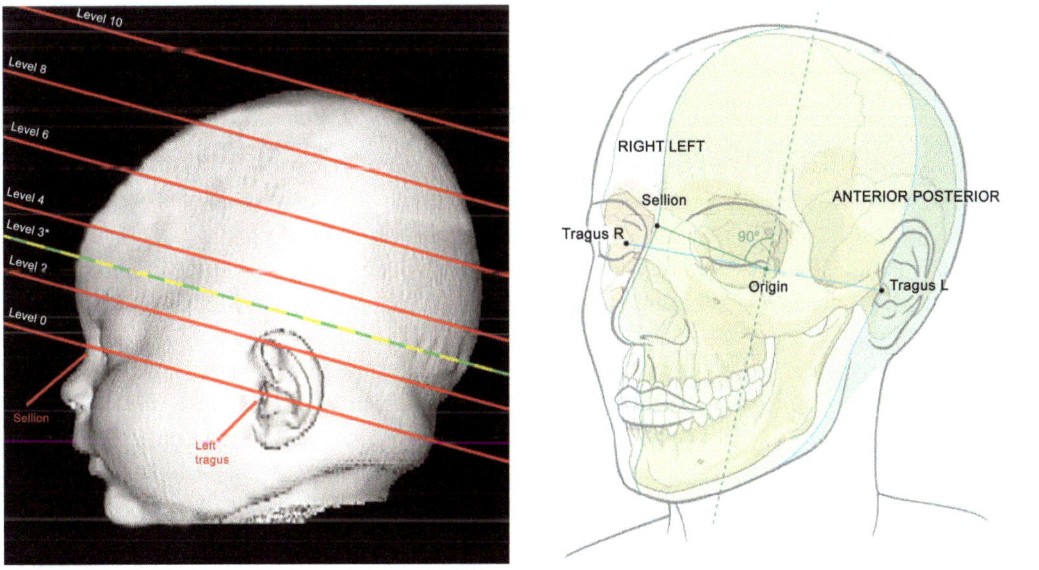

Fig. 51.9 (Left) Schematic representation of the levels for which the STAR scanner produces linear measurements and the landmarks that are used for acquisition. *Level 3 was determined to be the most useful plane for analysis. (Right) Line connecting the tragia delineates the anterior and posterior segments and a line from the selion perpendicular to this line divides the cranium into the left and right segments. (Reproduced with permission from Weathers WM, Khechoyan D, Wolfswinkel EM, Mohan K, Nagy A, Bollo RJ, et al. A novel quantitative method for evaluating surgical outcomes in craniosynostosis: pilot analysis for metopic synostosis. Craniomaxillofac Trauma Reconstr. 2014;7(1):1–8)

minimum width between the midfrontozygomatic points, or the midpoint along the recess above the brow ridge between the anteroinferolateral frontal bone and frontal bone zygomatic process) divided by the euryon–euryon distance (maximal cranial width determined from the lateral extremes of the skull) (Fig. 51.10). The authors showed that the mean preoperative MI in patients with trigonocephaly was significantly lower than that of age-matched controls but normalized after operative intervention [32].

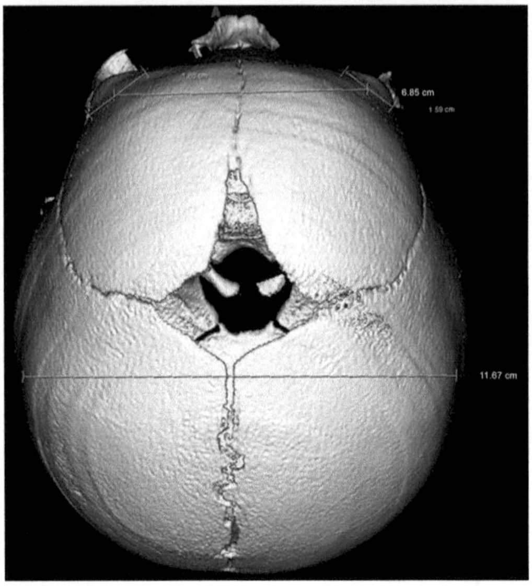

Fig. 51.10 Superior projection of a 3D reconstruction of a CT scan obtained in a child without craniosynostosis. Displayed are the midfrontozygomatic diameter (6.85 cm) and the eurion-eurion diameter (11.67 cm). The metopic index is therefore 0.59, which is within the range of normal based upon measurements obtained in control subjects. (Reproduced with permission from Wang JY, Dorafshar AH, Liu A, Groves ML, Ahn ES. The metopic index: an anthropometric index for the quantitative assessment of trigonocephaly from metopic synostosis. J Neurosurg Pediatr. 2016;18(3):275–80)

51.4.5 3D Stereophotogrammetry

As previously discussed, the use of 3D stereophotogrammetry is particularly advantageous because it provides objective, quantitative, and reproducible data without subjecting the developing brain to radiation exposure [25, 26, 28, 29, 37]. However, 3D photogrammetry has been used to demonstrate that preoperative frontal and total intracranial volumes are smaller in patients with metopic synostosis but that fronto-orbital advancement normalized these values 10 days postoperatively [38]. Similarly, Kuehle et al. [39] used 3D photography to demonstrate that the preoperative intracranial volume in male patients with trigonocephaly is lower than that of age-matched controls, but fronto-orbital remodeling is corrective (Fig. 51.11).

Meulstee et al. [37] analyzed 3D photographs of trigonocephalic patients using principal component analysis to identify the mean cranial shape in this population in comparison with the variation in cranial shape that is observed in the general population. With the principal component analysis, the authors distinguished metopic synostosis patients from age-matched controls [37]. Linden et al. [40] used 3D photogrammetry to evaluate forehead contours pre- and postoperatively in patients that underwent corrective surgery for metopic synostosis. Their results showed that forehead contours differed significantly preoperatively and immediately postoperatively but that the changes immediately postoperatively persisted at the 1-year postoperative time point (Fig. 51.12). de Jong et al. [41] performed a mean head shape and volume evaluation derived from 3D photos in children with trigonocephaly who underwent endoscopic-assisted strip craniectomy combined with helmet therapy. Using a mean shape evolution analysis, they obtained the anterior fossa to total volume ratio and showed that this value increased postoperatively. Thus, 3D photogrammetry is a useful tool to evaluate pre- and postoperative cranial morphology as well as long-term outcomes with the major advantages of ease of use and lack of radiation exposure [9].

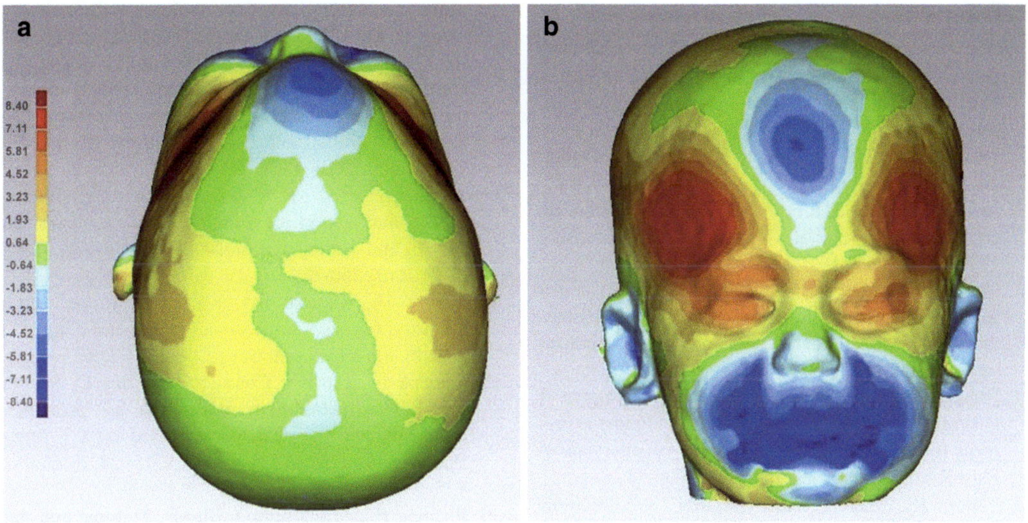

Fig. 51.11 Volumetric heat maps of a patient with trigonocephaly showing changes after fronto-orbital remodeling: (**a**) axial view; (**b**) frontal view. Pre- and postoperative 3D photogrammetric data were merged, and areas of volume changes were indicated in colors: red indicates an increase in intracranial volume in milliliters; blue indicates a decrease in intracranial volume in milliliters. (Reproduced with permission from Kuehle R, Ewerbeck N, Ruckschloss T, Ristow O, El Damaty A, Freudlsperger C, et al. Photogrammetric evaluation of corrective surgery for trigonocephaly. Int J Oral Maxillofac Surg. 2022;51(1):70–7)

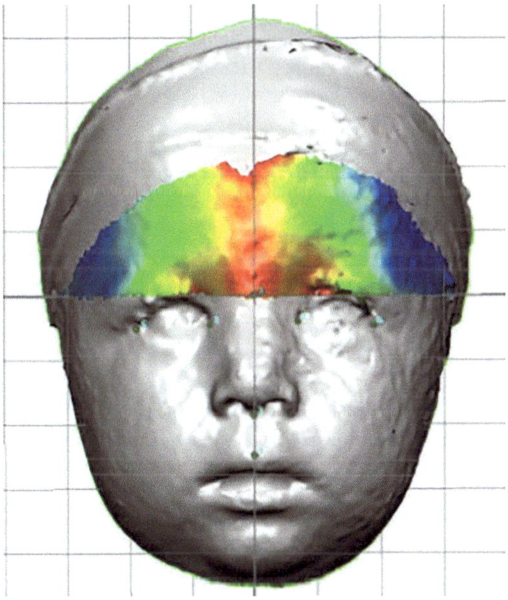

Fig. 51.12 Example of a color map overlaying a preoperative and over 1-year postoperative images "best fit" in 3-D orientation. Color mapping was used to highlight changes in the upper third of the face and further demonstrate the relative volume deficit at the midline, shown in red, and the lateral expansion in blue after surgical correction. (Reproduced with permission from Linden OE, Baratta VM, Gonzalez JA, Byrne ME, Klinge PM, Sullivan SR, et al. Surgical correction of metopic craniosynostosis: a 3D photogrammetric analysis of cranial vault outcomes. Cleft Palate Craniofac J. 2019;56(2):231–5)

51.5 Conclusions

Although predicting the need for operative intervention in craniosynostosis surgery has its roots in subjective assessments such as the Whitaker classification, major advances in the evaluation of cranial morphology have been achieved. Driving these advancements is the development of objective, reproducible, and quantifiable evaluation tools that can be standardized across centers and surgeons. Although the evolution of assessment has involved subjective measures, direct anthropometric measurements from palpable patient landmarks, quantitative analysis of 2D and 3D CT, and most recently 3D photogrammetry coupled with deep learning, the primary goal of improving patient care and patient outcomes has remained at the forefront. Nevertheless, the future of evaluation tools in craniosynostosis harbors much promise for further development.

References

1. Hankinson TC, Fontana EJ, Anderson RC, Feldstein NA. Surgical treatment of single-suture craniosynostosis: an argument for quantitative methods to evaluate cosmetic outcomes. J Neurosurg Pediatr. 2010;6(2):193–7.
2. Jane JA, Edgerton MT, Futrell JW, Park TS. Immediate correction of sagittal synostosis. J Neurosurg. 1978;49(5):705–10.
3. Marcus JR, Domeshek LF, Das R, Marshall S, Nightingale R, Stokes TH, et al. Objective three-dimensional analysis of cranial morphology. Eplasty. 2008;8:e20.
4. Panchal J, Marsh JL, Park TS, Kaufman B, Pilgram T, Huang SH. Sagittal craniosynostosis outcome assessment for two methods and timings of intervention. Plast Reconstr Surg. 1999;103(6):1574–84.
5. Venes JL, Sayers MP. Sagittal synostectomy. Technical note. J Neurosurg. 1976;44(3):390–2.
6. Wes AM, Naran S, Sun J, Mazzaferro D, Xu W, Nguyen P, et al. The Whitaker classification of craniosynostosis outcomes: an assessment of interrater reliability. Plast Reconstr Surg. 2017;140(4):579e–86e.
7. Whitaker LA, Bartlett SP, Schut L, Bruce D. Craniosynostosis: an analysis of the timing, treatment, and complications in 164 consecutive patients. Plast Reconstr Surg. 1987;80(2):195–212.
8. Guo J, Mei X, Tang K. Automatic landmark annotation and dense correspondence registration for 3D human facial images. BMC Bioinformatics. 2013;14:232.
9. Lloyd MS, Buchanan EP, Khechoyan DY. Review of quantitative outcome analysis of cranial morphology in craniosynostosis. J Plast Reconstr Aesthet Surg. 2016;69(11):1464–8.
10. McCarthy JG, Glasberg SB, Cutting CB, Epstein FJ, Grayson BH, Ruff G, et al. Twenty-year experience with early surgery for craniosynostosis: I. Isolated craniofacial synostosis—results and unsolved problems. Plast Reconstr Surg. 1995;96(2):272–83.
11. Seruya M, Oh AK, Boyajian MJ, Posnick JC, Myseros JS, Yaun AL, et al. Long term outcomes of primary craniofacial reconstruction for craniosynostosis: a 12-year experience. Plast Reconstr Surg. 2011;127(6):2397–406.
12. Lajeunie E, Le Merrer M, Bonaiti-Pellie C, Marchac D, Renier D. Genetic study of scaphocephaly. Am J Med Genet. 1996;62(3):282–5.
13. Hunter AG, Rudd NL, Craniosynostosis I. Sagittal synostosis: its genetics and associated clinical findings in 214 patients who lacked involvement of the coronal suture(s). Teratology. 1976;14(2):185–93.
14. Kolar JC, Salter EM. Preoperative anthropometric dysmorphology in metopic synostosis. Am J Phys Anthropol. 1997;103(3):341–51.
15. Marcus JR, Domeshek LF, Loyd AM, Schoenleber JM, Das RR, Nightingale RW, et al. Use of a three-dimensional, normative database of pediatric craniofacial morphology for modern anthropometric analysis. Plast Reconstr Surg. 2009;124(6):2076–84.
16. Ruiz-Correa S, Sze RW, Starr JR, Lin HT, Speltz ML, Cunningham ML, et al. New scaphocephaly severity indices of sagittal craniosynostosis: a comparative study with cranial index quantifications. Cleft Palate Craniofac J. 2006;43(2):211–21.
17. Al-Shaqsi SZ, Rai A, Forrest C, Phillips J. Standardization of cranial index measurement in sagittal craniosynostosis. J Craniofac Surg. 2019;30(2):366–9.
18. Fearon JA, Ruotolo RA, Kolar JC. Single sutural craniosynostoses: surgical outcomes and long-term growth. Plast Reconstr Surg. 2009;123(2):635–42.
19. Posnick JC, Lin KY, Chen P, Armstrong D. Sagittal synostosis: quantitative assessment of presenting deformity and surgical results based on CT scans. Plast Reconstr Surg. 1993;92(6):1015–24; discussion 225–6.
20. Posnick JC, Armstrong D, Bite U. Metopic and sagittal synostosis: intracranial volume measurements prior to and after cranio-orbital reshaping in childhood. Plast Reconstr Surg. 1995;96(2):299–309; discussion 10–5.
21. David LR, Plikaitis CM, Couture D, Glazier SS, Argenta LC. Outcome analysis of our first 75 spring-assisted surgeries for scaphocephaly. J Craniofac Surg. 2010;21(1):3–9.
22. Posnick JC, Bite U, Nakano P, Davis J, Armstrong D. Indirect intracranial volume measurements using CT scans: clinical applications for craniosynostosis. Plast Reconstr Surg. 1992;89(1):34–45.
23. Marcus JR, Stokes TH, Mukundan S, Forrest CR. Quantitative and qualitative assessment of morphology in sagittal synostosis: mid-sagittal vector analysis. J Craniofac Surg. 2006;17(4):680–6.
24. Khechoyan D, Schook C, Birgfeld CB, Khosla RK, Saltzman B, Teng CC, et al. Changes in frontal morphology after single-stage open posterior-middle vault expansion for sagittal craniosynostosis. Plast Reconstr Surg. 2012;129(2):504–16.
25. Mertens C, Wessel E, Berger M, Ristow O, Hoffmann J, Kansy K, et al. The value of three-dimensional photogrammetry in isolated sagittal synostosis: impact of age and surgical technique on intracranial volume and cephalic index horizontal line a retrospective cohort study. J Craniomaxillofac Surg. 2017;45(12):2010–6.
26. Porras AR, Tu L, Tsering D, Mantilla E, Oh A, Enquobahrie A, et al. Quantification of head shape from three-dimensional photography for presurgical and postsurgical evaluation of craniosynostosis. Plast Reconstr Surg. 2019;144(6):1051e–60e.
27. Seeberger R, Hoffmann J, Freudlsperger C, Berger M, Bodem J, Horn D, et al. Intracranial volume (ICV) in isolated sagittal craniosynostosis measured by 3D photocephalometry: a new perspective on a controversial issue. J Craniomaxillofac Surg. 2016;44(5):626–31.

28. van Veelen MC, Jippes M, Carolina JA, de Rooi J, Dirven CMF, van Adrichem LNA, et al. Volume measurements on three-dimensional photogrammetry after extended strip versus total cranial remodeling for sagittal synostosis: a comparative cohort study. J Craniomaxillofac Surg. 2016;44(10):1713–8.
29. Weinberg SM, Scott NM, Neiswanger K, Brandon CA, Marazita ML. Digital three-dimensional photogrammetry: evaluation of anthropometric precision and accuracy using a Genex 3D camera system. Cleft Palate Craniofac J. 2004;41(5):507–18.
30. de Jong G, Bijlsma E, Meulstee J, Wennen M, van Lindert E, Maal T, et al. Combining deep learning with 3D stereophotogrammetry for craniosynostosis diagnosis. Sci Rep. 2020;10(1):15346.
31. Gociman B, Blagg R, Agko M, Goodwin I, Kestle JR, Siddiqi F. The metopic angle: a novel assessment tool of the trigonocephalic frontal deformity and its correction. J Craniofac Surg. 2014;25(6):2101–4.
32. Wang JY, Dorafshar AH, Liu A, Groves ML, Ahn ES. The metopic index: an anthropometric index for the quantitative assessment of trigonocephaly from metopic synostosis. J Neurosurg Pediatr. 2016;18(3):275–80.
33. Posnick JC, Lin KY, Chen P, Armstrong D. Metopic synostosis: quantitative assessment of presenting deformity and surgical results based on CT scans. Plast Reconstr Surg. 1994;93(1):16–24.
34. Ruiz-Correa S, Starr JR, Lin HJ, Kapp-Simon KA, Sze RW, Ellenbogen RG, et al. New severity indices for quantifying single-suture metopic craniosynostosis. Neurosurgery. 2008;63(2):318–24; discussion 24–5.
35. Gociman B, Agko M, Blagg R, Garlick J, Kestle JR, Siddiqi F. Endoscopic-assisted correction of metopic synostosis. J Craniofac Surg. 2013;24(3):763–8.
36. Weathers WM, Khechoyan D, Wolfswinkel EM, Mohan K, Nagy A, Bollo RJ, et al. A novel quantitative method for evaluating surgical outcomes in craniosynostosis: pilot analysis for metopic synostosis. Craniomaxillofac Trauma Reconstr. 2014;7(1):1–8.
37. Meulstee JW, Verhamme LM, Borstlap WA, Van der Heijden F, De Jong GA, Xi T, et al. A new method for three-dimensional evaluation of the cranial shape and the automatic identification of craniosynostosis using 3D stereophotogrammetry. Int J Oral Maxillofac Surg. 2017;46(7):819–26.
38. Freudlsperger C, Steinmacher S, Bachli H, Somlo E, Hoffmann J, Engel M. Metopic synostosis: measuring intracranial volume change following fronto-orbital advancement using three-dimensional photogrammetry. J Craniomaxillofac Surg. 2015;43(5):593–8.
39. Kuehle R, Ewerbeck N, Ruckschloss T, Ristow O, El Damaty A, Freudlsperger C, et al. Photogrammetric evaluation of corrective surgery for trigonocephaly. Int J Oral Maxillofac Surg. 2022;51(1):70–7.
40. Linden OE, Baratta VM, Gonzalez JA, Byrne ME, Klinge PM, Sullivan SR, et al. Surgical correction of metopic craniosynostosis: a 3-D photogrammetric analysis of cranial vault outcomes. Cleft Palate Craniofac J. 2019;56(2):231–5.
41. de Jong G, Tolhuisen M, Meulstee J, van der Heijden F, van Lindert E, Borstlap W, et al. Radiation-free 3D head shape and volume evaluation after endoscopically assisted strip craniectomy followed by helmet therapy for trigonocephaly. J Craniomaxillofac Surg. 2017;45(5):661–71.

Complications and Long-Term Surgical Outcome in Craniosynostoses

52

Matthieu Vinchon, Pierre-Aurélien Beuriat, Alexandru Szathmari, and Federico Di Rocco

52.1 Introduction

The life of a child affected by craniosynostosis is impacted in many and highly variable ways, on account both of his condition and of the surgery it leads to. Craniosynostoses are serious malformations, with often dire consequences, even more so when associated with faciostenosis. On the other hand, despite constant effort to optimize results and decrease morbidity, surgery is always an important undertaking and is associated with a number of unwanted consequences, during operation, in the immediate postoperative course, or later in life. For these reasons, it is important to know the complications of synostoses and of their treatment, in order to inform the decision to operated, taken conjointly by the surgeon and the child's parents, as well as anticipate surgical difficulties. In the present chapter, we shall review chronologically the different complications of craniosynostoses before, during, and after surgery, their management and prevention. We shall conclude on the issues of surgical decision and informed consent and the need for consensual quantitative scales to evaluate morphological results as well as surgical complications.

52.2 Preoperative Complications

52.2.1 Birth Difficulties

The calvarial sutures play an important role in the biomechanics of birth, and their fusion can have dire consequences [1]. In an earlier, unpublished study conducted in Lille during the years 2016–2021, among 233 new cases of craniosynostoses, we found that the overall prevalence of dystocia (difficult or instrumented birth) was 45.5%; among these, 30.5% were delivered by C section (compared with 20% in the general population in France during that period), 24.4% of them because of fetal distress. The prevalence of C-section was highest among boys, and patients with metopic or multisutural synostosis (Fig. 52.1). Dystocia was the cause of birth trauma in four identified cases: one with sagittal synostosis who developed a large subperiosteal hema-

M. Vinchon (✉)
Department of Pediatric Neurosurgery, Hospices Civils de Lyon, Lyon, France

Service de Neurochirurgie Pédiatrique, Hôpital Femme Mère Enfant, Bron, France

P.-A. Beuriat · A. Szathmari · F. Di Rocco
Department of Pediatric Neurosurgery, Hospices Civils de Lyon, Lyon, France
e-mail: pierre-aurelien.beuriat@chu-lyon.fr; alexandru.szathmari@chu-lyon.fr; federico.dirocco@chu-lyon.fr

F. Di Rocco, J. Kestle (eds.), *Neurosurgical Aspects of Craniosynostosis*,
https://doi.org/10.1007/978-3-031-69386-1_52

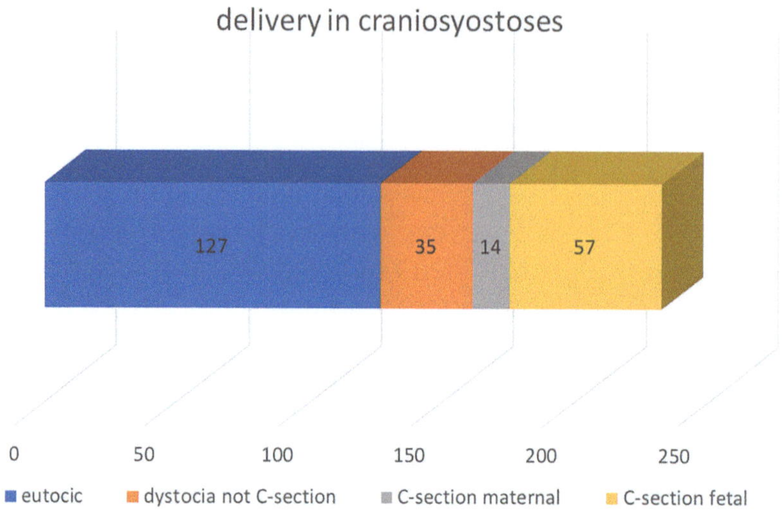

Fig. 52.1 Conditions of birth in 233 cases of craniosynostoses followed during the period 2016–2019 in Lille. Close to half of these children had delivery difficulties, 30.3% born by C-section, 24.4% by C-section for fetal distress. These birth difficulties can be anticipated in case of prenatal diagnosis, and may be a confusion factor regarding the developmental outcome

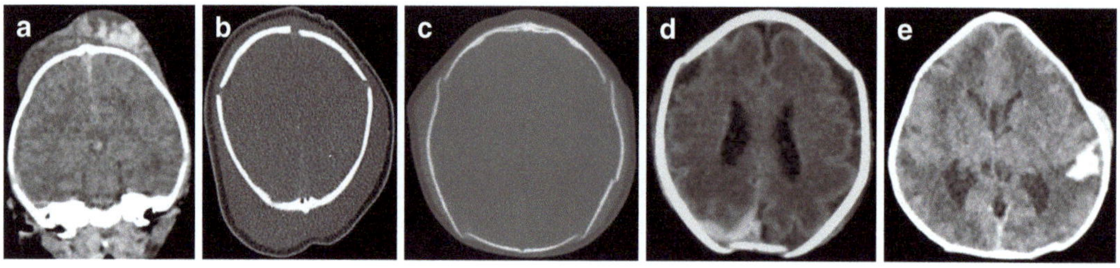

Fig. 52.2 Birth trauma in children with craniosynostosis: (**a**, **b**) sagittal synostosis, with the characteristic bilateral cephalhematoma, because no periosteal midline adherence limits its spread; (**c**, **d**) metopic synostosis, with difficult forceps delivery, scalp laceration, fracture of the petrous bone and subdural bleeding; (**e**) a newborn with complex multisuture synostosis who developed intracerebral hemorrhage

toma (Fig. 52.2a, b); one with metopic synostosis who had petrous bone fracture and subdural bleeding associated with forceps delivery (Fig. 52.2c, d); one with unilambdoid synostosis who developed a subdural hemorrhage; and one with complex multisuture synostosis who developed intracerebral hemorrhage (Fig. 52.2e). Although the mechanical trauma was predominantly mild and had no or few consequences, dystocia could also cause fetal distress during and after birth, with potential impact on the patient's later development. Birth difficulties could thus be a confounding factor when studying the developmental impact of brain compression by the synostosis. Although the majority of children with craniosynostosis are delivered by natural vaginal delivery, a prenatal diagnosis should reinforce the vigilance regarding possible dystocia and lower the threshold for cesarean section.

52.2.2 Brain Compression

Brain decompression by calvarial expansion is the cornerstone of surgery for craniosynostoses. However, the relation between reduced intracranial volume and intracerebral pressure is complex, certainly underpinned by poorly understood hydrodynamic mechanisms [2].

Multiple suture synostoses, mostly syndromic, are associated with raised intracranial pressure (ICP), which increases with the number of fused sutures [3]. Calvarial growth restriction is often the main presenting symptom of multisuture craniosynostoses, sometimes present at birth in case of cloverleaf malformation, or later during progression toward oxycephaly, with progressive closure of the different sutures [4].

By contrast, in unisutural synostoses, the initial presentation in early childhood is mostly related to morphological concerns, and the brain is generally not compressed initially. Typically, the closure of the sagittal suture is compensated by the coronal and metopic sutures, giving the child his typical dolichocephalic appearance with a bulging forehead and an above-normal head circumference. However, in older children, sagittal synostosis can mimic pseudotumor cerebri [5], and is a not uncommon finding in clinically eloquent tonsillar herniation [6]. Similarly, ICP can rise late after correction of unisutural synostosis, because of nonsynchronous multisuture synostosis [7].

Regarding metopic synostosis, the occurrence of brain compression and the benefit of decompressive surgery are controversial. While some authors have documented intracranial hypertension [8], others, using sophisticated imaging techniques, found no evidence of brain compression [9]. Better developmental outcomes have been reported in all types of craniosynostoses when surgery was performed before the age of 1 year [10]; however, in this retrospective study, the reason why some children were operated early, and others later, was not analyzed. A more recent study has found that late surgery was associated with confounding factors susceptible to influence developmental outcome, such as social context, prematurity, and comorbidities [11].

52.2.3 Psychosocial Impact of Morphological Disgrace

Difficulties can arise during childhood because of the morphological disgrace, leading to problems of self-image, taunting, and even harassment by schoolmates (and even occasionally by teachers!). The psychological impact at school age should not be taken lightly. Compounded with the parental stress, which children and infants feel and absorb like sponges, this psychological burden may play a significant role in the future life of these patients. Very rarely, the demand for morphological correction is not expressed until adult age [12]. Moreover, in familial cases, the demand for early morphological correction for their child, coming from affected parents, is revealing.

52.3 Intraoperative Complications

52.3.1 Anesthesia and Installation

Complications of anesthesia and installation are the shared responsibility of the surgeon and the anesthetist. Among these, the risk of complications of venous and arterial catheters, and pression sores on the scalp or eyeballs (Fig. 52.3) must be decreased by scrupulous attention from both teams.

52.3.2 Bleeding

Intraoperative bleeding occurs whatever the technique chosen, is the most threatening complications during surgery, with a potential for fatal consequences, and requires blood transfusion in a number of patients. The importance of bleeding relates to the body proportions in infants, with a larger head and a limited blood volume (estimated around 500 mL at 3 months and 750 mL at 3 months) compared to adults. Diffuse bleeding comes from the scalp, the dura-mater (in particular arachnoid villi, which appear around 9 months) and above all from the bone, especially at the skull base. In craniosynostosis surgery, bleeding is increased by enlarged trans-osseous veins and intracranial hypertension. Clotting problems can result from profuse bleeding and hypothermia, so a high degree of vigilance and close interactions between surgeon and anesthetist are warranted, in order to avoid entering a fatal spiral.

Rigorous anesthesia protocols are followed in order to monitor hemodynamics; near-infrared spectroscopy can help to determine if and when transfusion must be decided (Fig. 52.4). In case of profuse bleeding, supplementation with platelets and clotting factors may also be needed. Transfusion following all the security protocols incurs extremely low additional risk, whereas reluctance or delay to transfuse can have fatal consequences. Although all precautions to diminish the risk of bleeding should be taken, we consider that transfusion should not be regarded as a complication. In consequence, the acceptance

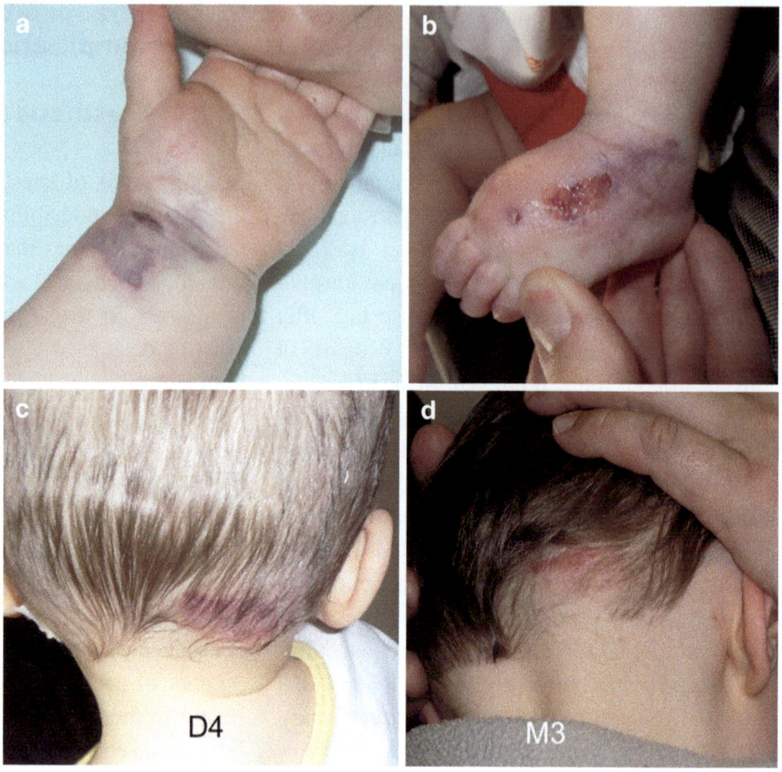

Fig. 52.3 Complications of arterial catheter (**a**), of peripheral venous catheters (**b**), of positioning (**c**, **d**) are a shared responsibility of the surgeon and anesthetist

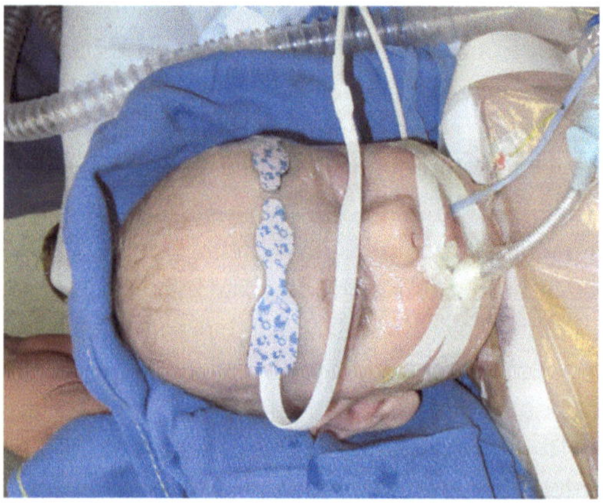

Fig. 52.4 Near-infrared spectroscopy can be used when the forehead is not in the operative field (sagittal synostosis and posterior pole surgeries), and helps to determine if and when transfusion is needed

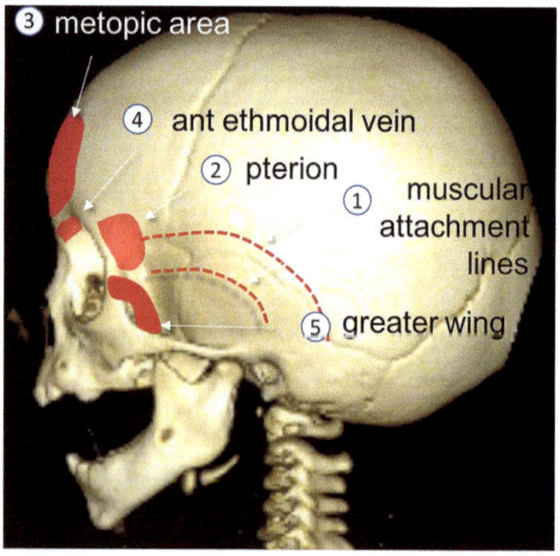

Fig. 52.5 Location of trans-osseous veins in metopic synostosis, numbered according to the timing of their occurrence during fronto-orbital remodeling

from parent that transfusion may be needed is a prerequisite for surgery.

Intraoperative blood loss is anticipated preoperatively by iron supplementation and/or erythropoietin, and mitigated during surgery by hemodilution and volume expansion. Meticulous hemostasis at each stage of the operation requires precise knowledge of where the bleeding comes from, notably the location of trans-osseous veins (Figs. 52.5 and 52.6). Permanent communication

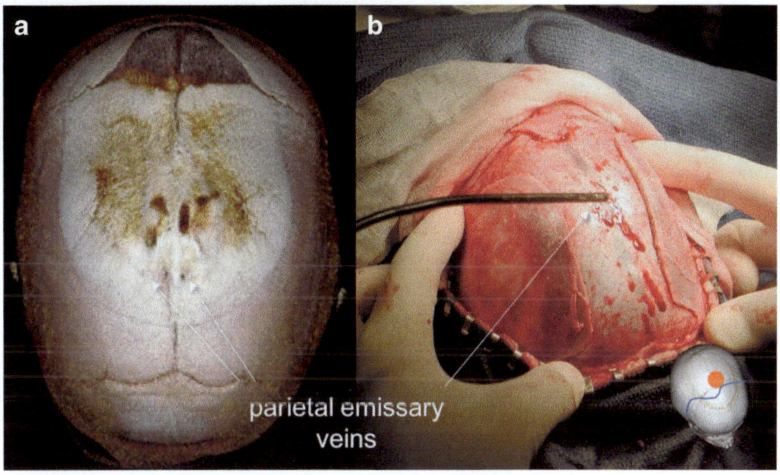

Fig. 52.6 Parietal emissary veins in sagittal synostosis: (**a**) 3D-CT scanner; (**b**) operative view of the exposed sagittal sinus, patient in the prone position

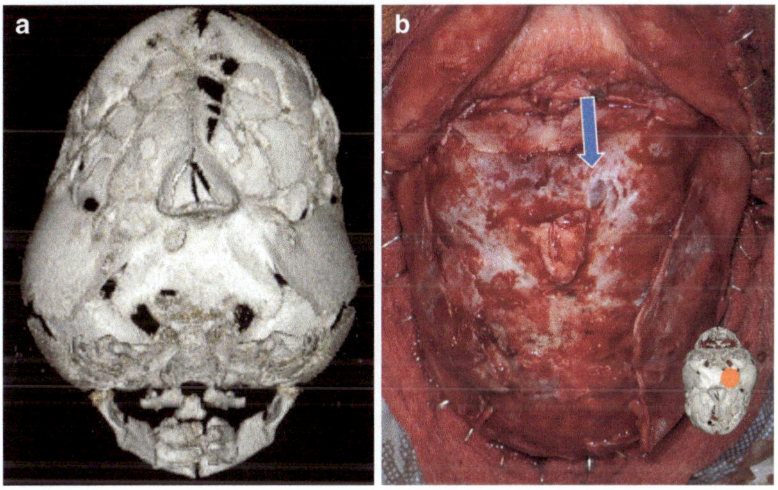

Fig. 52.7 Cloverleaf skull, operated on D5 of life because of life-threatening intracranial hypertension with tonsillar herniation. (**a**) CT-scanner showing the lacunae and complex sutural pattern around the lesser fontanelle. (**b**) Operative view showing limited dural tear close to the posterior fontanel

between surgeon and anesthetist before, during, and after surgery is vital for the successful management of this potentially lethal complication.

52.3.3 Dural Tear

Even though most dural tears occur at a distance from the venous sinuses, dural lesions, even when involving only the outer layer, increase blood loss, and, if left unattended, can initiate a meningocele. Bleeding can become catastrophic if a dural tear involves a venous sinus (Fig. 52.7). The risk of dural tear is diversely evaluated, because not all authors take note of minimal splits of the dural outer layer. Endoscopic techniques may not lead to more dural tears [13], but make these more difficult to cope with. The risk of dural tear is higher in newborns, in children with longstanding intracranial hypertension, in craniofacial advancement [14] and in redo surgery [15], especially after previous dural repair. Dural adherences are intense along the sutures, in particular underneath the fontanels and epactal bones, and on the midline of the skull base. Opening of the sagittal sinus is thus at higher risk when the metopic suture is still patent [1]. The adherence of patent sutures to the dura is especially tricky in unilambdoid synostosis, because the lateral sinus is often lacking on the synostotic side [16], and the sinus on the nonsynostotic, adherent side is compensatorily enlarged.

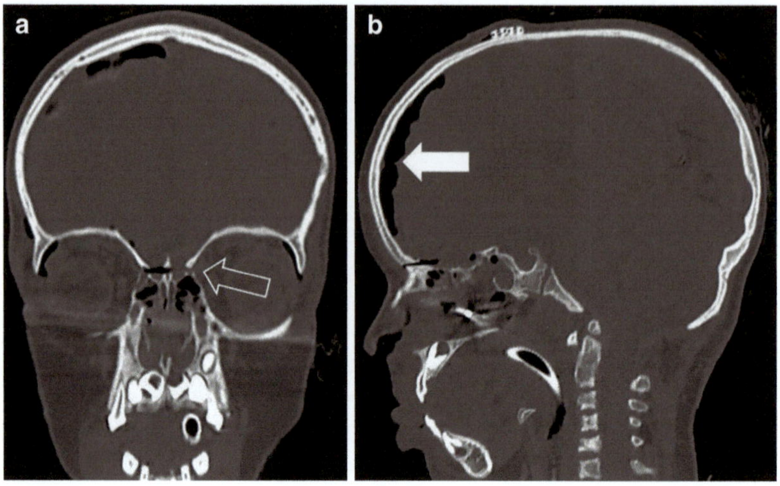

Fig. 52.8 Two-years female operated for Crouzon disease with Le Fort 3 osteotomy because of severe sleep apneas. She developed rhinorrhea because of ethmoidal dural tear (empty arrow); note intradural pneumocephalus (full arrow), which required craniotomy for duraplasty

Dural tear at the skull base is a not uncommon complication of the different techniques of fronto-orbital advancement in craniofaciosynostoses [14, 17], with a high risk of cerebrospinal fluid leakage and meningeal infection. Although these leaks can often dry spontaneously, intracranial dural repair is sometimes necessary (Fig. 52.8).

Partial dural tears, limited to the outer dural layer, should be reapproximated by a few stitches whenever possible, sometimes completed with fibrin glue. Complete dural tears must be repaired with a running suture as watertight as possible, which may require harvesting an epidural graft.

The prevention of dural tears involves careful dissection of bone from permeable fontanels, and of sutures from the underlying sinuses before using the craniotome. Use of the burr over the pterional and asterial fontanels should be especially cautious. Dissection of the dura from the bone can be tedious, on account of adherences and uneven inner surface of the calvaria, as well as frequent bleeding from the middle meningeal artery or dural veins. In very small infants with cloverleaf malformation, patient dissection of the lacunae and epactal bones, followed by piecemeal removal of the bone septa, often extending deep between the sulci, is the most delicate time of suturectomy [18].

52.4 Early Postoperative Period

52.4.1 The Emotional Shock

In the immediate postoperative days, parental distress is almost constant [19]. In addition to the child being in pain, or drowsy and feeding poorly on account of opioid medications, he often presents with facial edema, of variable severity but which can be major and complicated by chemosis, and even subluxation of the tarsal cartilage. The child's ordeal appeals to his parent's feelings of guilt over their decision to have him operated, and echoes with the guilt which is very widespread in parents of a child with inborn diseases, especially if genetically determined. When the edema subsides, the change of facial features, which was the purpose of the operation, can be difficult to cope with. The rare complaint "it's not my child anymore" is only the most radical expression of a widespread parental unease. To make things worse, parental stress is absorbed by the child, so that parental and infantile stress amplify each other in a play of mirrors. This often translates into sleepless nights back home, regressive reactions, with often prolonged cosleeping. This postoperative stress should not be overlooked and must be anticipated. Physical contact, cradling, cuddling should be encouraged immediately after surgery. Before surgery, parents should be informed of the oncoming physical changes and convinced that the child's appearance will be "more normal," and that he will have "the head he should have had." Contacts with patients associations can be a precious resource for these parents, who can thus interact with others who "have been through that" before them.

52.4.2 Infection

Infection is a rare complication but can prolong hospital stay and have dire consequences. A sepsis can result of operative site infection (OSI) or venous or urinary catheter. However, aseptic fever is common, on account of the large subcutaneous exposure, and should not lead to untimely antibiotic treatments. By contrast, the reappearance of fever and scalp edema after initial subsidence should raise alarm of OSI.

OSI occurs in up to 7% [20], and can be epidermal, dermal, or deep. OSI is sometimes elicited by the child's scratching his wound, or initiated by inflammation caused by absorbable sutures, or skin necrosis due to tension closure associated with ambitious calvarial expansion. It can also be a consequence of incidental respiratory or ocular infection present at the time of surgery; in these cases, it is wise to postpone the scheduled operation, provided that the infection is circumstantial and not chronic, in relation with faciostenosis, and also that the child has no menacing intracranial hypertension. Other potential factors associated with postoperative infection are the long duration of surgery [21], the extended incision, opening of the facial sinuses, the creation of an epidural dead space, skin breakdown, the presence of implanted material, especially external distractors [22] or springs, and prolonged use of venous or urinary catheter.

Whereas superficial scalp infection usually requires only local measures (removal of scabs and remaining sutures plus local antiseptics), superficial suppuration may be aggressive, the scab protecting an ecosystem in which staphylococcus aureus thrives; in addition to scab removal, oral antibiotics may be necessary. Deep suppuration is rare but can be associated with septic signs, and require debridement, drainage, and irrigation in addition to antibiotics [23]. The management of these postoperative empyemas should be as conservative as possible, because wide opening and dismantling of the construct would devascularize the bone flaps, and bone necrosis would have catastrophic morphological consequences (Fig. 52.9).

Prevention of local and deep infection implies rigorous asepsis, before, during, and after surgery, and high-quality layered closure without excessive tension. The child must be prevented from scratching his wound, sometimes with the help of antihistamine medications. Prophylactic antibiotics are administered routinely during surgery, justified by the extent of surgery, its duration, and the potential gravity of OSI; however, protocols vary and are mostly tradition-based [24].

52.4.3 Complications of Implants and Fixation Devices

Aseptic subcutaneous granulomas can develop on absorbable sutures and plates, and take months to disappear, but require nothing more than reassuring words. During surgery, simple precautions can decrease these benign but vexing complications, like avoiding to place knots over salient facial features, cutting threads short, and burying the knots in bone perforations. Bone fixation with wires is generally well tolerated but can lead to skin compromise or perforation [23], as well as migrate inward into the dura as the calvaria grows by apposition-resorption, and should be used sparingly (Fig. 52.10). The same happens with much more serious consequences with non-absorbable plates [25], springs, and prosthetic materials [26]. Absorbable plates are generally well tolerated but can also cause aseptic granulomas, and migrate, both inward and outward [27, 28].

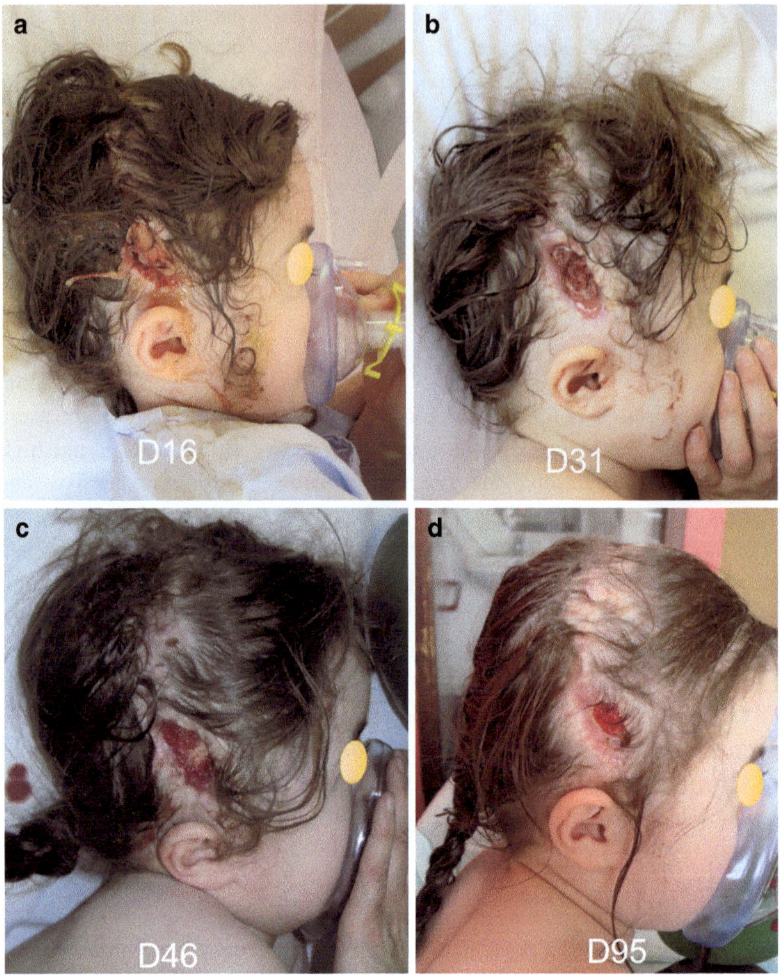

Fig. 52.9 Crouzon syndrome, first operated for posterior pole expansion at 6 months, reoperated at 5 years for fronto-orbital advancement. The child presented with fistulization of an epidural empyema, which was treated with antibiotics, prolonged drainage-irrigation and directed scarring

52.4.4 Scalp and Calvarial Breakdown

Skin or bone disruption generally results of excessive tension of the scalp, after generous volume expansion; it almost never happens after external trauma.

Skin breakdown occurs mostly in children with multisuture synostosis, especially in older children and after redo surgery. Even when the underlying bone is exposed, it rarely causes serious infection, but may require prolonged directed scarring, or sometimes reoperation. Breakdown is prevented by progressive scalp traction, which is one of the important advances brought about by distraction techniques. Alternately, scalp expansion using a balloon expander can be proposed, provided that the child's calvaria is already rigid enough not to cave in, and surgery can be programmed some time in advance.

Bone dislocation is a rare but worrisome complication. Cranioplasties are at best semirigid constructs, especially in young infants, and the mechanical compression by scalp traction can be enough to cause breakdown of construct. The lordosis of the fronto-orbital bandeau is caused by breakage of plates [29] or bone dislocation at the pterion, especially if the coronal suture is incompletely fused (Fig. 52.11). The fronto-malar synfibrosis is also a weak point, where fixation of the

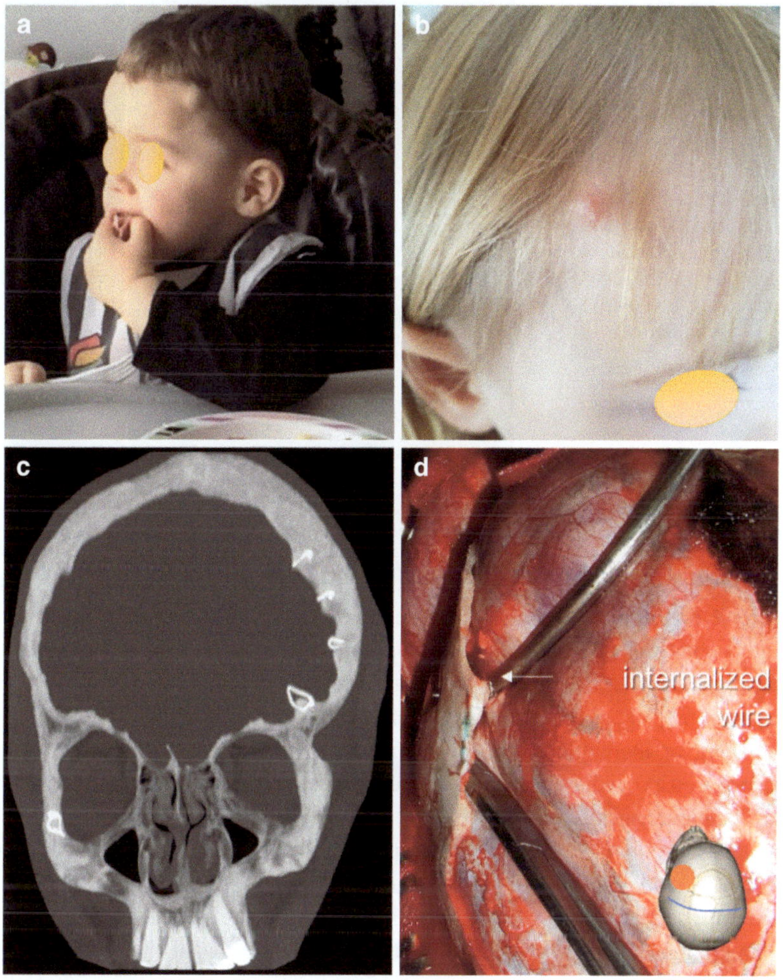

Fig. 52.10 Complications of wires: outward migration of wires (**a**, **b**) can threaten or perforate the scalp (**b**), while their inward migration (**c**, **d**), caused by resorptional calvarial growth, brings these into contact or conflict with the dura (**d**)

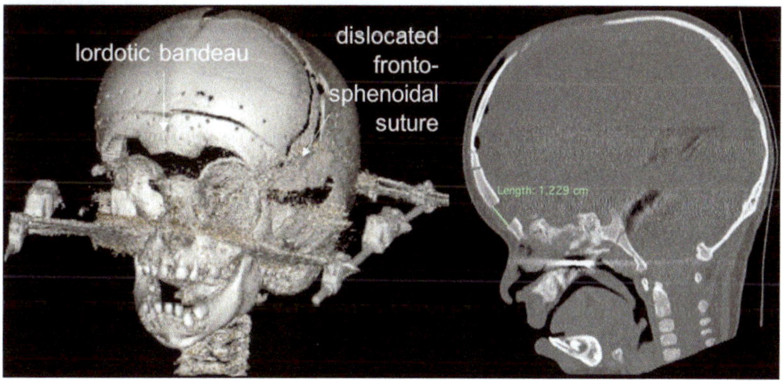

Fig. 52.11 Breakdown of construct caused by dislocation of the fronto-sphenoidal suture under the tension of scalp, resulting in lordosis of the bandeau, lifted 12 mm, with eye exposure and pulsating exophthalmos, and requiring reoperation for refixation of bandeau

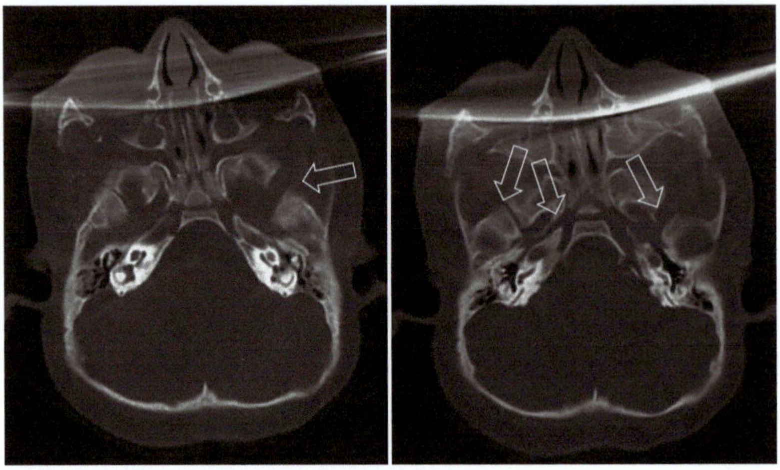

Fig. 52.12 Fifteen-months child with Crouzon disease, operated for fronto-orbital advancement with transfacial pin; axial CT scanner performed on D14 of craniofacial distraction because of abducens palsy, showed spheno-temporal ("Le Fort 6") dislocation (arrows)

lateral orbital pillar can give way. Bone breakdown also occurs in redo surgery, because regenerative bone becomes brittle. The occurrence of "gull-winging" (the uplifting of the parietal bone by disjunction of sutures) happens after posterior distraction [30], as the consequence of distracting a patent or incompletely fused suture. Anterior distraction procedures can also cause skull base dislocation, causing optic neuropathy after monobloc osteotomy [31], or oculomotor paralysis on account of spheno-petrous ("Le Fort 6") dislocation (Fig. 52.12). All these complications impose reoperations and/or reappraisal of the surgical strategy.

52.4.5 Growing Fracture

Postoperative leptomeningeal cysts or growing fractures develop as a result of untended intraoperative dural tear or postoperative dural necrosis, with the brain herniating through the rent and preventing it from healing. It can develop after endoscopic surgery, because dural tear can be unnoticed or because dural repair is most uneasy [32]. The pressure gradient causes focal hydrodynamic disturbance, with enlarged Virchow-Robin spaces [33].

Anatomical repair of the dura and calvaria is necessary (Fig. 52.13). Whenever possible, autologous materials are highly preferable [33, 34]. The management of postoperative leptomeningeal cysts can be challenging because of the tension of the brain (which may require temporary lumbar drainage); of the proximity of the dural defect to the sinuses; of the extent of bone defect requiring a large donor site; of the young age of the child whose thin calvaria is difficult to split. However, modern high-speed motors and piezoelectric saws allow the splitting of calvaria in very young children [35].

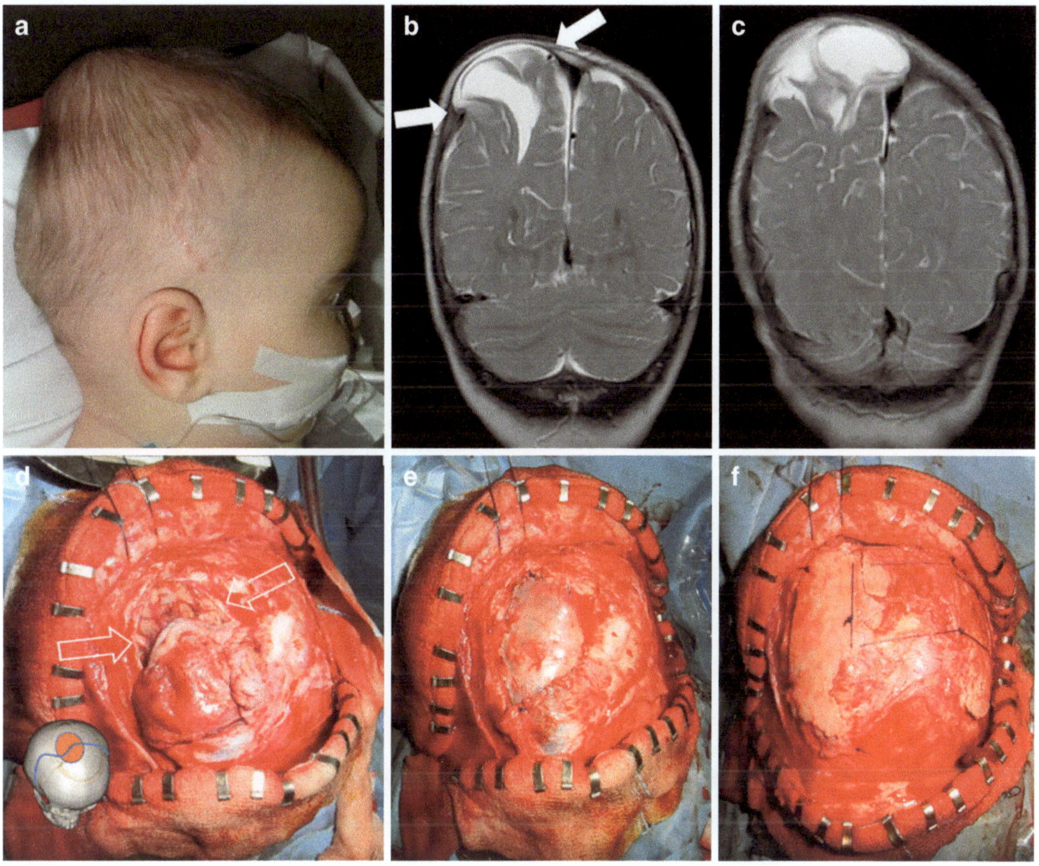

Fig. 52.13 Figure growing fracture. (**a**) Seven-months male operated 2 months earlier for sagittal synostosis (H-craniectomy with linear coagulation of the dura mater and no drainage, causing dural necrosis). (**b**) Note the thickened bone margins (full arrows) due to uplifting of the periosteal tissues. (**b**, **c**) The herniated brain tissue is highly edematous, due to expansion of Virchow-Robin spaces. (**e**) The margins of the dural defect are much retracted (empty arrows), requiring a large pericranial autograft (**f**). (**g**) The bone defect is bridged with split calvarial autograft

52.5 Late Surgical Outcome

52.5.1 The Scar

Whatever the surgery, it leaves a scar. However much, as A. Raimondi quipped, the infant's scalp may be "forgiving," the scar can be a problem for the child's self-image and a source of embarrassment. Its perception is highly variable: while some children shun going to the swimming pool for fear that their scar might show through wet hair, others glorify it with creative hairstyle (Fig. 52.14). Like any bodily imperfection, the scar can be a fixation point for teasing, taunting, and harassment at school age, as well as self-depreciation at adolescence. In order to make the scar as stealthy as possible, its curve should as much as possible keep a 90° orientation relative to the direction of hair. When a father has a receding hairline, his son's incision may need to be more posterior than usual. In complex synostoses, it should be kept in mind that repeated surgeries may be needed in the future, and that the bicoronal incision should be versatile enough to give access to both the posterior and anterior poles. This may be problematic when the initial surgery was endoscopic, with two scars, one very anterior, and the other very posterior.

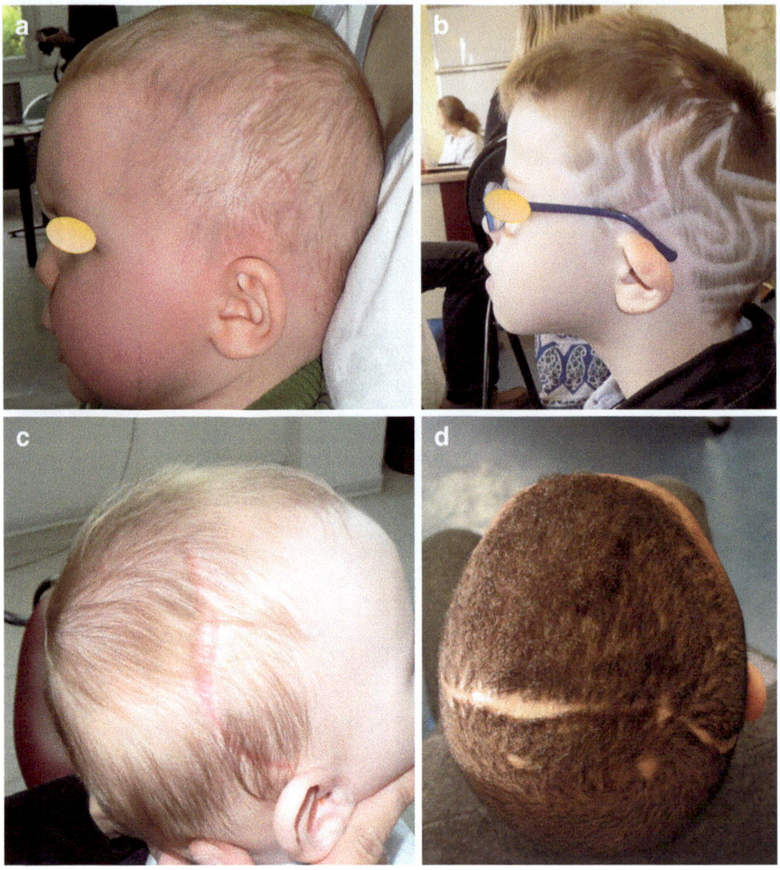

Fig. 52.14 (**a**) Discrete "lazy S" incision, curved in order to stay perpendicular to the natural direction of hair, leaves the most discreet scar. (**b**) "Zig-zag" scar, intended to be easily hidden, but glorified by creative haircut. (**c**) Early, wide and red scar, destined to whiten with time. (**d**) Persistent cheloid scar of the scalp incision and of the drain

52.5.2 Redo Operations

Reoperations can be needed, sometimes many years after the initial surgery. The larger or lesser importance of these reoperations led Whitaker et al. to propose a grading of surgical results as: (1) not requiring reoperation; (2) minor reoperation proposed; (3) reoperation less than initial surgery necessary; and (4) reoperation as large or more than initial surgery [36]. In addition to the operative complications mentioned above, many of which can required additional surgery, other operations may become necessary during follow-up.

Incomplete reossification of the calvaria leaves pulsating lacunae. These occur in about 5% of operated cases, and appear to be more frequent in fronto-orbital advancement [37], and occipital pole remodeling [38]. Lacunae most often sit close to the midline, especially at the vertex, and occur most often after extensive midline bone resection [39], all the more in older children. On account of their location, calvarial lacunae present no risk of traumatic brain injury, and no limitations should be imposed on the child's activities. Lacunae thus present mostly an aesthetic problem, although some children also experience the "syndrome of the trephined," with headaches or learning difficulties, and changes in the cerebral blood flow have been documented in some cases [38]. The surgical management of persistent lacunae can be proposed after the fifth or sixth birthday, and the most desirable technique is autologous graft by split calvaria [35] (Fig. 52.15).

Temporal hollowing is specific problem with metopic synostosis, and can result from atrophy of the temporal muscle compounded with excessive restoration of frontal bosses. The progressive nature of this imperfection, which becomes more

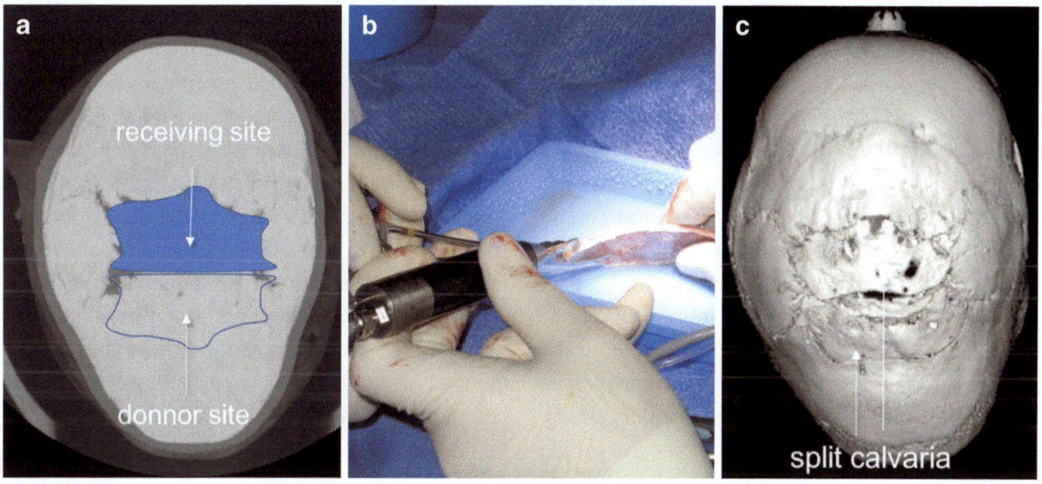

Fig. 52.15 Persisting lacuna at the vertex after craniectomy at 4 months for sagittal synostosis; repair age 4 years, using split calvaria. (**a**) The craniotomy for the donor site is tailored on a template outlined around the limits of the lacuna. (**b**) The flap is then split using the piezoelectric saw. (**c**) Both bone tables are fixed rigidly in place is order to fill the lacuna and the donor site

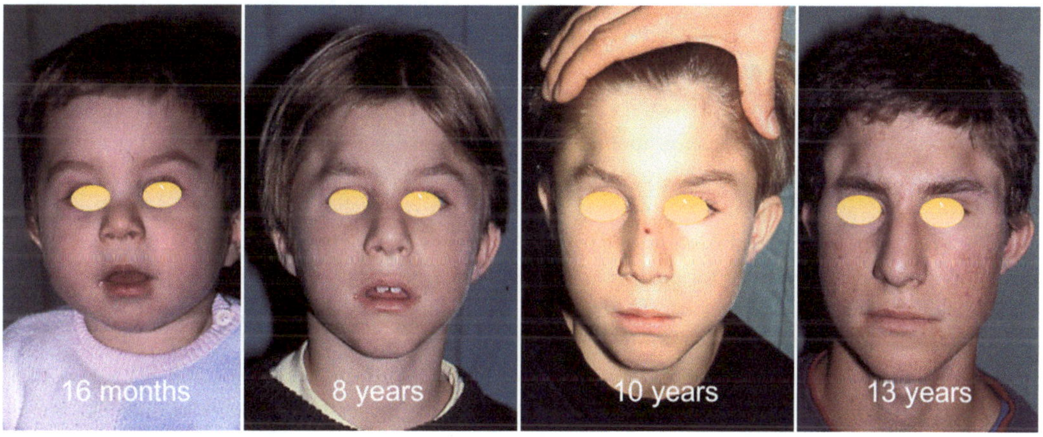

Fig. 52.16 Progressive temporal hollowing after surgery for metopic synostosis

apparent with time (Fig. 52.16), suggests that bone growth is focally disturbed by surgery, possibly because the greater wing of the sphenoid needs the strain of muscles to sustain its growth. Temporal hollowing can be well accepted, or lead to a demand for esthetic correction; this is easily performed by lipofilling, which can be repeated as needed, but should preferably be delayed until adolescence. Different technical refinements have been proposed in order to reduce the prevalence of temporal hollowing, like large temporal "elephant ears" [40], or tongue-and groove bandeau advancement, with mixed results leaving room for improvement.

52.5.3 Other Craniofacial Operations

Other major craniofacial operations are often needed in craniofaciostenoses, in order to correct midface retrusion or hypertelorism. Secondary multisuture synostosis should be expected in syndromic craniofaciostenoses [4] as well as in lambdoid synostosis [16], but are rare in sagittal synostosis, occurring in about 2% of cases [39], and are almost never found in nonsyndromic metopic synostosis. Secondary closure of new sutures attests of the progressive nature of the disease, and these reoperations should not be regarded as complications of surgery. However, this information regarding this evolution should be given to parents as early as the first consultation, in particular in case of prenatal diagnosis.

In addition, other relatively minor operations may be needed, such as onlay grafts, rhinoplasty, removal of facial scars, correction of slant eyes or of strabismus. Ideally, all these operations, which are mostly destined to improve cosmesis, should be performed at the end of growth and on demand from the patient himself.

The large array of different operations, implicating different surgical specialists, at different ages, underlines the importance of prolonged multidisciplinary follow-up.

52.5.4 Morphological Result

Although the Whitaker classification mentioned above [36] is convenient and widely accepted [41], this classification is focused on reinterventions, not on morphology, and does not quantify the preoperative dysmorphism; for these reasons, it does not evaluate accurately morphological results. Obviously, the objective quantification of something as subjective as morphological disgrace has proved difficult.

The evaluation of results by satisfaction questionnaires filled by the parents may be fraught with complacency, or by the fear of another operation. In one study, parents were generally as satisfied as surgeons on all items, except for syndromic cases [42], where doctors appeared ready to accept suboptimal results, possibly because no good surgical solution exists. Similarly, another study found a better acceptance by doctors, compared with parents, of what is inevitable (the scar, alopecia) or for which they have no good surgical remedy (calvarial asymmetry, bony bumps) [41]. This discrepancy shows a mismatch between surgeons' and parents' expectations; whereas parents might have inordinately high hopes of normalization, surgeons might be more centered on what they can expect from their usual technique. Blinded morphological evaluation by independent surgeons avoids the complacency bias, but not the professional one [43]: the criteria by which surgeons judge may be at odds from what the patients expect. In a self-declarative evaluation by adult patients operated in infancy for nonsyndromic craniosynostosis, values regarding self-esteem and depression scores were in the normal range; these patients satisfied themselves with all the imperfections of surgical techniques from a past era, except asymmetry of facial features [44]. A blinded evaluation of "attractiveness" by laypersons confirmed the negative impact of craniofacial asymmetry [45]; the method in this study, enrolling as evaluators independent female professionals of a daycare center, is probably a step in the right direction. All these subjective evaluations would also be more in line with the patients' expectations, with the input of patients associations.

Multiple efforts have been devoted recently to the creation of pre and postoperative quantitative evaluation scales of the deformity, much-needed tools if we want to scale postoperative results, and compare one technique with another. The Rotterdam team has proposed a score for scaphocephaly, summing semi-quantitative subscores in the same spirit as the long-established Glasgow Coma Scale [39, 46]. The evaluation by an independent panel is necessarily based on documents, and 2D pictures are obviously misleading; for this reason, 3D photogrammetry is a promising tool [47]. We hope that in a near future, a consensus will emerge on quantitative morphological scales adapted to each of the different craniosynostoses.

52.6 Clinical Outcome

52.6.1 Mortality

Overall mortality is very low in craniosynostoses, and it affects almost exclusively syndromic cases [48]. Already from birth, some of these patients are beyond surgical resources, and they die because of breathing and feeding difficulties, and also possibly because of associated tonsillar herniation. Intraoperative mortality is poorly documented in literature, and mostly caused by uncontrolled bleeding; this outcome, although hopefully exceptional, cannot be dismissed.

52.6.2 Development

What is the real influence of cerebral compression on development? As mentioned above, the relation between intracranial volume and brain compression is not linear. Furthermore, intracranial hypertension occurs most regularly in multisuture synostoses, which have almost always a genetic background, so that the two factors cannot be separated. The correlation between developmental outcome and the age at surgery might be an indication of the developmental impact of brain compression [10, 49], but other factors, like a syndromic context, or a lack of parental motivation for surgery are confusing factors [11].

The impact of focal cerebral compression on development is also elusive. The Leeds group found a discrepancy between verbal and performance IQ (VIQ > PIQ) in unisutural craniosynostoses [50], which they ascribed to parietal compression, and which could be reversed by early surgery [49]. On the other hand, other researchers found no correlation between the severity of deformity and cerebral compression in metopic synostosis [8]. Shimoji found even paradoxical results, development being more impaired in milder forms of metopic synostosis [51]; this might suggest different referral patterns, and confirms that the importance of trigonocephalic deformation plays a secondary role, if any role at all in the patient's development. Overall, these studies suggest that the developmental impact of each type of synostosis is a specific problem.

52.6.3 Influence of the Syndromic Context

In syndromic craniosynostoses, gene or chromosomal disorders as well as environmental factors causing the synostosis can have a marked impact on development. In a previous, unpublished series of 188 cases of metopic synostosis operated over 20 years, the only significant and independent variable impacting negatively the development was syndromic context, which was identified in 31%. In FGFR3 mutation, experimental models in mice have shown that a developmental impact existed irrespective of the presence or absence of synostosis, and could be salvaged by targeted therapy by high-affinity FGFR tyrosine kinase inhibitor BGJ398 [52]. This suggests that the mutation affects brain function directly, and opens exciting new treatment perspectives.

In addition, comorbidities and complications of many syndromic craniosynostoses are susceptible to impact on psychomotor and cognitive development [11]. Tonsillar herniation can cause sleep apneas, predominantly central [53], which can combine with obstructive apneas caused by midface retrusion, compromising wake periods and hindering learning. Hand and foot malformations in Apert syndrome require early management in order to allow psychomotor development [54]. Optic nerve atrophy caused by raised ICP, found in 12.3% of syndromic craniosynostoses, affects predominantly FGFR-related diseases [55], and deafness associated with Muenke syndrome, or resulting from tubal dysfunction in faciostenoses [56], can also both impair learning. In addition, careful brain imaging can disclose alterations of the cerebellar vermis and corpus callosum, which can be the consequence of deformation as well as associated malformations, and can impact on the child's development [57].

52.7 The Operative Decision and the Informed Consent

The decision to operate is taken jointly by the surgeon and the child's parents, based on the expected positive and adverse effects of surgery. The aims of surgery must therefore be clearly defined, and the potential complications well known by the surgeon and exposed to the parents. As mentioned above, much uncertainty surrounds the natural history of unoperated craniosynostoses, while many unknowns lay in the future after surgery, especially in syndromic cases. Unlike in multisuture synostoses, for which consent for surgery is comparatively straightforward, the aim of surgery for unisutural craniosynostosis is in a large part morphological. In that regard, the treatment can be seen as morphological surgery with a risk of severe morbidity and even mortality; few other fields of cranial surgery have such potential benefit-risk imbalance. The expected improvement of morphological appearance and better conformity with the social norm, as well as the potentially traumatic change of their child's facial features contribute to make the decision to operate an agonizing process for the parents.

Although emotions are the substance of which we are made, and society is the medium in which we live, surgeons are often poorly trained in psychology and sociology, often wrongly dismissed as "soft sciences." In addition, their position as professionals, which requires objectivity, sometimes hinders a more heartfelt approach. In this regard also, patients associations can be a precious resource for these parents, helping them to cope with the mixed feeling and stress associated with decision-making.

52.8 The Future

The invasiveness of classical craniofacial surgery and the potentially high morbidity prompted the development of less invasive techniques and the boom of endoscopic surgery for craniosynostoses. However, the abundant literature published on these techniques appears to focus almost exclusively on easily measured outcome variables, such as transfusion rate and duration of hospital stay, with no indication on the long-term morphological results.

This points to the need for a consensual quantitative morphological rating based on objective criteria, which would allow to compare the patients pre and postoperatively, and one technique with another. A morphological scoring proposed for scaphocephaly allows the comparison of techniques [39, 43], and other scales are in development.

In order to weight the other pan of the scale, we also need a quantitative grading of complications. A classification of complications, sorted by their timing relative to operation, and their consequences for the patient, was proposed by the team in Leeds [58], and should certainly be a source of inspiration.

In order to be meaningful, the two quantitative scales, results and complications, should not be simple lists of items, but require a ponderation of variables. In that regard, direct interview or collaboration of the patients themselves is invaluable to identify what really matters to them [44]; and here again, the input of patients associations would be a precious help.

References

1. Vinchon M. The metopic suture: natural history. Neurochirurgie. 2019;65(5):239–45. https://doi.org/10.1016/j.neuchi.2019.09.006. Epub 2019 Sep 25.
2. Langvatn EA, Frič R, Due-Tønnessen BJ, Eide PK. Intracranial volume versus static and pulsatile intracranial pressure values in children with craniosynostosis. J Neurosurg Pediatr. 2019;24(1):66–74. https://doi.org/10.3171/2019.2.PEDS18767.
3. Tamburrini G, Caldarelli M, Massimi L, Santini P, Di Rocco C. Intracranial pressure monitoring in children with single suture and complex craniosynostosis: a review. Childs Nerv Syst. 2005;21(10):913–21. https://doi.org/10.1007/s00381-004-1117-x. Epub 2005 May 3.
4. Pellerin P, Vinchon M, Dhellemmes P, Guerreschi P. Crouzon syndrome: posterior fossa volume studies in vestibular orientation. Childs Nerv Syst. 2021;37(10):3105–11. https://doi.org/10.1007/s00381-021-05186-9. Epub 2021 Apr 27.
5. Martinez-Lage JF, Alamo L, Poza M. Raised intracranial pressure in minimal forms of craniosynostosis. Childs Nerv Syst. 1999;15(1):11–5; discussion 16. https://doi.org/10.1007/s003810050319.
6. Sgulò FG, Spennato P, Aliberti F, Di Martino G, Cascone D, Cinalli G. Contemporary occurrence of hydrocephalus and Chiari I malformation in sagittal craniosynostosis. Case report and review of the literature. Childs Nerv Syst. 2017;33(1):187–92. https://doi.org/10.1007/s00381-016-3189-9. Epub 2016 Jul 22.
7. Vinchon M, Pellerin P, Guerreschi P, Baroncini M, Dhellemmes P. Atypical scaphocephaly: a review. Childs Nerv Syst. 2012;28(9):1319–25. https://doi.org/10.1007/s00381-012-1807-8. Epub 2012 Aug 8.
8. Blum JD, Beiriger J, Kalmar C, Avery RA, Lang SS, Villavisanis DF, Cheung L, Cho DY, Tao W,

Whitaker R, Bartlett SP, Taylor JA, Goldstein JA, Swanson JW. Relating metopic craniosynostosis severity to intracranial pressure. J Craniofac Surg. 2022;33(8):2372–8. https://doi.org/10.1097/SCS.0000000000008748. Epub 2022 Jul 22.
9. de Planque CA, Florisson JMG, Tasker RC, Rijken BFM, van Veelen MLC, Mathijssen IMJ, Lequin MH, Dremmen MHG. A diffusion tensor imaging analysis of white matter microstructures in non-operated craniosynostosis patients. Neuroradiology. 2022;64(12):2391–8. https://doi.org/10.1007/s00234-022-02997-8. Epub 2022 Jun 27.
10. Renier D, Arnaud E, Marchac D. Craniosténoses: résultats fonctionnels et morphologiques post-opératoires [Craniosynostosis: functional and morphologic postoperative results]. Neurochirurgie. 2006;52(2–3 Pt 2):302–10. French. https://doi.org/10.1016/s0028-3770(06)71223-1.
11. Lynn JV, Buchman LK, Breuler CJ, Buchman SR. Surgical timing and neurocognitive development among patients with craniosynostosis: analysis of confounders. Plast Reconstr Surg. 2023;151(4):821–9. https://doi.org/10.1097/PRS.0000000000010004. Epub 2023 Mar 29.
12. Marchac D, Renier D, Arnaud E. Unoperated craniosynostosis patients: correction in adulthood. Plast Reconstr Surg. 2008;122(6):1827–38. https://doi.org/10.1097/PRS.0b013e31818cc388.
13. Arts S, Delye H, van Lindert EJ. Intraoperative and postoperative complications in the surgical treatment of craniosynostosis: minimally invasive versus open surgical procedures. J Neurosurg Pediatr. 2018;21(2):112–8. https://doi.org/10.3171/2017.7.PEDS17155. Epub 2017 Nov 24.
14. Dunaway DJ, Britto JA, Abela C, Evans RD, Jeelani NU. Complications of frontofacial advancement. Childs Nerv Syst. 2012;28(9):1571–6. https://doi.org/10.1007/s00381-012-1804-y. Epub 2012 Aug 8.
15. Wagner CS, Pontell ME, Hitchner MK, Barrero CE, Salinero LK, Swanson JW, Bartlett SP, Taylor JA. Prior fronto-orbital advancement associated with complications from transcranial midface surgery in patients with syndromic craniosynostosis. Childs Nerv Syst. 2023; https://doi.org/10.1007/s00381-023-05879-3. Epub ahead of print.
16. Vinchon M, Guerreschi P, Karnoub MA, Wolber A. Synostosis of the lambdoid suture: a spectrum. Childs Nerv Syst. 2021;37(6):1991–2000. https://doi.org/10.1007/s00381-020-05003-9. Epub 2021 Jan 6.
17. Hassan AM, Chappell AG, Murthy N, Stoehr JR, Alden T, Gosain AK. Posterior cranial vault distraction (PCVD): common complication rates and strategies of prevention and management. J Craniofac Surg. 2021;32(1):62–6. https://doi.org/10.1097/SCS.0000000000006980.
18. Vinchon M, Guerreschi P, Karnoub MA, Wolber A. Linear craniectomy for early posterior decompression in craniosynostoses: technique and results. Childs Nerv Syst. 2021;37(10):3113–8. https://doi.org/10.1007/s00381-021-05117-8. Epub 2021 Mar 13.
19. Lim J, Davis A, Tang AR, Shannon CN, Bonfield CM. Caregiver stress in children with craniosynostosis: a systematic literature review. Childs Nerv Syst. 2019;35(2):217–25. https://doi.org/10.1007/s00381-018-3959-7. Epub 2018 Aug 29.
20. Hennedige A, Richardson D, Duncan C, Parks C, Sinha A, Ellenbogen J, Robertson B. Part 1: surgical correction in 231 trigonocephaly patients—the Alder Hey experience. J Craniofac Surg. 2021;32(6):2123–8. https://doi.org/10.1097/SCS.0000000000007475.
21. Puthumana JS, Lopez CD, Lake IV, Yang R. Evaluation of complications and outcomes in craniosynostosis by age of operation: analysis of the national surgical quality improvement program-pediatric. J Craniofac Surg. 2023;34(1):29–33. https://doi.org/10.1097/SCS.0000000000008872. Epub 2022 Aug 11.
22. Goldstein JA, Paliga JT, Taylor JA, Bartlett SP. Complications in 54 frontofacial distraction procedures in patients with syndromic craniosynostosis. J Craniofac Surg. 2015;26(1):124–8. https://doi.org/10.1097/SCS.0000000000001320.
23. Natghian H, Song M, Jayamohan J, Johnson D, Magdum S, Richards P, Wall S. Long-term results in isolated metopic synostosis: the Oxford experience over 22 years. Plast Reconstr Surg. 2018;142(4):509e–15e. https://doi.org/10.1097/PRS.0000000000004768.
24. Holle J, Finger T, Lugonja J, Schmidt F, Schaumann A, Gratopp A, Thomale UW, von Bernuth H, Schulz M. The influence of perioperative antibiotic prophylaxis on wound infection and on the colonization of wound drains in patients after correction of craniosynostosis. Front Pediatr. 2021;9:720074. https://doi.org/10.3389/fped.2021.720074.
25. Mullens CL, Grome LJ, Serrano CA, Qaiser R, Mason AC. Titanium hardware extrusion following pediatric cranioplasty. Int Surg. 2018;13:1–5. https://doi.org/10.1016/j.inat.2018.01.002.
26. Ma IT, Symon MR, Bristol RE, Beals SP, Joganic EF, Adelson PD, Shafron DH, Singh DJ. Outcomes of titanium mesh cranioplasty in pediatric patients. J Craniofac Surg. 2018;29(1):99–104. https://doi.org/10.1097/SCS.0000000000004045.
27. Aldana PR, Wieder K, Postlethwait RA, James HE, Steinberg B. Ultrasound-aided fixation of biodegradable implants in pediatric craniofacial surgery. Pediatr Neurosurg. 2011;47(5):349–53. https://doi.org/10.1159/000337874. Epub 2012 May 9.
28. Yang L, Xu M, Jin X, Xu J, Lu J, Zhang C, Tian T, Teng L. Complications of absorbable fixation in maxillofacial surgery: a meta-analysis. PLoS One. 2013;8(6):e67449. https://doi.org/10.1371/journal.pone.0067449.
29. Hayden Gephart MG, Woodard JI, Arrigo RT, Lorenz HP, Schendel SA, Edwards MS, Guzman R. Using bioabsorbable fixation systems in the treatment of pediatric skull deformities leads to good outcomes and low morbidity. Childs Nerv Syst. 2013;29(2):297–301.

https://doi.org/10.1007/s00381-012-1938-y. Epub 2012 Oct 26.
30. Iida C, Sakamoto Y, Miwa T, Yoshida K, Kishi K. Posterior distraction first or fronto-orbital advancement first for severe syndromic craniosynostosis. J Craniofac Surg. 2019;30(1):47–9. https://doi.org/10.1097/SCS.0000000000004897.
31. Alonso N, Goldenberg D, Fonseca AS, Kanashiro E, Matsushita H, da Silva Freitas R, Shin JH. Blindness as a complication of monobloc frontofacial advancement with distraction. J Craniofac Surg. 2008;19(4):1170–3. https://doi.org/10.1097/SCS.0b013e318176ac83.
32. Aryan HE, Meltzer HS, Gerras GG, Jandial R, Levy ML. Leptomeningeal cyst development after endoscopic craniosynostosis repair: case report. Neurosurgery. 2004;55(1):235–7; discussion 237–8. https://doi.org/10.1227/01.neu.0000126951.74653.a6.
33. Zemann W, Metzler P, Jacobsen C, Kruse AL, Lübbers HT, Könü D, Obwegeser JA. Growing skull fractures after craniosynostosis repair: risk factors and treatment algorithm. J Craniofac Surg. 2012;23(5):1292–5. https://doi.org/10.1097/SCS.0b013e31825435d5.
34. Rinehart GC, Pittman T. Growing skull fractures: strategies for repair and reconstruction. J Craniofac Surg. 1998;9(1):65–72.
35. Vercler CJ, Sugg KB, Buchman SR. Split cranial bone grafting in children younger than 3 years old: debunking a surgical myth. Plast Reconstr Surg. 2014;133(6):822e–7e. https://doi.org/10.1097/PRS.0000000000000222.
36. Whitaker LA, Bartlett SP, Schut L, Bruce D. Craniosynostosis: an analysis of the timing, treatment, and complications in 164 consecutive patients. Plast Reconstr Surg. 1987;80(2):195–212.
37. Prevot M, Renier D, Marchac D. Lack of ossification after cranioplasty for craniosynostosis: a review of relevant factors in 592 consecutive patients. J Craniofac Surg. 1993;4(4):247–54; discussion 255–6.
38. Szathmari A, Morgado A, Beuriat PA, Petrescu P, Di Rocco F, Mottolese C. Cranioplasty for bone defects after craniosynostosis surgery. Case series with literature review. Neurochirurgie. 2020;66(2):97–101. https://doi.org/10.1016/j.neuchi.2019.10.015. Epub 2020 Feb 24.
39. Vinchon M, Guerreschi P, Karnoub MA, Wolber A. Morphological and surgical results in sagittal synostosis: early craniectomy versus later cranioplasty. Childs Nerv Syst. 2021;37(7):2335–41. https://doi.org/10.1007/s00381-021-05178-9. Epub 2021 Apr 22.
40. Pellerin P, Vinchon M, Dhellemmes P, Wolber A, Guerreschi P. Trigonocephaly: Lille's surgical technique. Childs Nerv Syst. 2013;29(12):2183–8. https://doi.org/10.1007/s00381-013-2229-y. Epub 2013 Jul 31.
41. Messerer M, Cottier R, Vandenbulcke A, Belouaer A, Daniel RT, Broome M, Cossu G. Aesthetic results in children with single suture craniosynostosis: proposal for a modified Whitaker classification. Childs Nerv Syst. 2023;39(1):221–8. https://doi.org/10.1007/s00381-022-05678-2. Epub 2022 Sep 22.
42. Kluba S, Rohleder S, Wolff M, Haas-Lude K, Schuhmann MU, Will BE, Reinert S, Krimmel M. Parental perception of treatment and medical care in children with craniosynostosis. Int J Oral Maxillofac Surg. 2016;45(11):1341–6. https://doi.org/10.1016/j.ijom.2016.03.017. Epub 2016 Apr 23.
43. van Veelen ML, Mihajlović D, Dammers R, Lingsma H, van Adrichem LN, Mathijssen IM. Frontobiparietal remodeling with or without a widening bridge for sagittal synostosis: comparison of 2 cohorts for aesthetic and functional outcome. J Neurosurg Pediatr. 2015;16(1):86–93. https://doi.org/10.3171/2014.12.PEDS14260. Epub 2015 Apr 24.
44. Svalina A, Heikura E, Savolainen T, Serlo W, Sinikumpu JJ, Silvola AS, Salokorpi N. Appearance or attitude: what matters to craniosynostosis patients? Association of self-esteem, depressive symptoms, and facial aesthetics in patients with sagittal and metopic synostosis. Childs Nerv Syst. 2022;38(10):1929–36. https://doi.org/10.1007/s00381-022-05587-4. Epub 2022 Jun 23.
45. Collett BR, Gray KE, Kapp-Simon KA, Birgfeld C, Cunningham M, Rudo-Stern J, Ung D, Buono L, Speltz ML. Laypersons' ratings of appearance in children with and without single-suture craniosynostosis. J Craniofac Surg. 2013;24(4):1331–5. https://doi.org/10.1097/SCS.0b013e3182997885.
46. Van Veelen MC, Kamst N, Touw C, Mauff K, Versnel S, Dammers R, de Jong THR, Prasad V, Mathijssen IM. Minimally invasive, spring-assisted correction of sagittal suture synostosis: technique, outcome, and complications in 83 cases. Plast Reconstr Surg. 2018;141(2):423–33. https://doi.org/10.1097/PRS.0000000000004037.
47. Abdel-Alim T, Kurniawan M, Mathijssen I, Dremmen M, Dirven C, Niessen W, Roshchupkin G, van Veelen ML. Sagittal craniosynostosis: comparing surgical techniques using 3D photogrammetry. Plast Reconstr Surg. 2023; https://doi.org/10.1097/PRS.0000000000010441. Epub ahead of print.
48. Vinchon M. What remains of non-syndromic bicoronal synostosis? Neurochirurgie. 2019;65(5):252–7. https://doi.org/10.1016/j.neuchi.2019.09.002. Epub 2019 Sep 13.
49. Bellew M, Mandela RJ, Chumas PD. Impact of age at surgery on neurodevelopmental outcomes in sagittal synostosis. J Neurosurg Pediatr. 2019:1–8. https://doi.org/10.3171/2018.8.PEDS18186. Epub ahead of print.
50. Bellew M, Chumas P. Long-term developmental follow-up in children with nonsyndromic craniosynostosis. J Neurosurg Pediatr. 2015;16(4):445–51. https://doi.org/10.3171/2015.3.PEDS14567. Epub 2015 Jul 24.
51. Shimoji T, Shimabukuro S, Sugama S, Ochiai Y. Mild trigonocephaly with clinical symptoms: analysis of surgical results in 65 patients. Childs Nerv Syst.

2002;18(5):215–24. https://doi.org/10.1007/s00381-002-0568-1. Epub 2002 May 7.
52. Cornille M, Moriceau S, Khonsari RH, Heuzé Y, Loisay L, Boitez V, Morice A, Arnaud E, Collet C, Bensidhoum M, Kaci N, Boddaert N, Paternoster G, Rauschendorfer T, Werner S, Mansour SL, Di Rocco F, Oury F, Legeai-Mallet L. FGFR3 overactivation in the brain is responsible for memory impairments in Crouzon syndrome mouse model. J Exp Med. 2022;219(4):e20201879. https://doi.org/10.1084/jem.20201879. Epub 2022 Mar 7.
53. Rijken BF, Lequin MH, van der Lijn F, van Veelen-Vincent ML, de Rooi J, Hoogendam YY, Niessen WJ, Mathijssen IM. The role of the posterior fossa in developing Chiari I malformation in children with craniosynostosis syndromes. J Craniomaxillofac Surg. 2015;43(6):813–9. https://doi.org/10.1016/j.jcms.2015.04.001. Epub 2015 Apr 14.
54. Kim JS, Block LM, Zhu X, Davit AJ. Management of paronychia in patients with Apert syndrome. Tech Hand Up Extrem Surg. 2020;25(1):30–4. https://doi.org/10.1097/BTH.0000000000000295.
55. Fearon JA, Barrientos S, Ditthakasem K, Herbert M. Optic nerve atrophy in syndromic craniosynostosis. Plast Reconstr Surg. 2022;150(2):381e–6e. https://doi.org/10.1097/PRS.0000000000009367. Epub 2022 Jun 8.
56. Couloigner V, Khalfallah SA. Craniosynostosis and ENT. Neurochirurgie. 2019;65(5):318–21. https://doi.org/10.1016/j.neuchi.2019.09.015. Epub 2019 Sep 27.
57. Aldridge K, Collett BR, Wallace ER, Birgfeld C, Austin JR, Yeh R, Feil M, Kapp-Simon KA, Aylward EH, Cunningham ML, Speltz ML. Structural brain differences in school-age children with and without single-suture craniosynostosis. J Neurosurg Pediatr. 2017;19(4):479–89. https://doi.org/10.3171/2016.9.PEDS16107. Epub 2017 Feb 3.
58. Shastin D, Peacock S, Guruswamy V, Kapetanstrataki M, Bonthron DT, Bellew M, Long V, Carter L, Smith I, Goodden J, Russell J, Liddington M, Chumas P. A proposal for a new classification of complications in craniosynostosis surgery. J Neurosurg Pediatr. 2017;19(6):675–83. https://doi.org/10.3171/2017.1.PEDS16343. Epub 2017 Mar 31.

Quality of Life Metrics in Craniosynostosis: A Guide for Surgeons and Healthcare Practitioners

53

Nebras M. Warsi, Johanna N. Riesel, and Abhaya V. Kulkarni

53.1 Introduction

A diagnosis of craniosynostosis can carry profound implications for patients, caregivers, and their families [1]. Commonly, surgeons are not only tasked with operative management, but also with providing guidance throughout the challenging decision-making process associated with these complex craniofacial disorders. Traditionally, outcomes have been indexed by surgical variables such as cephalic index, postoperative appearance, operative time, intraoperative blood loss, and overall complication rates [2, 3]. However, a growing body of evidence suggests that parents, caregivers, and—as they grow older—patients themselves, have significant anxiety regarding and limitations related to a broad range of health metrics including cosmesis, self-image, societal integration, neurocognitive outcomes, and psychosocial health [1, 4–6].

N. M. Warsi · A. V. Kulkarni (✉)
Division of Neurosurgery, Hospital for Sick Children, Toronto, ON, Canada

Division of Neurosurgery, Department of Surgery, University of Toronto, Toronto, ON, Canada
e-mail: nebras.warsi@mail.utoronto.ca; abhaya.kulkarni@sickkids.ca

J. N. Riesel
Division of Plastic and Reconstructive Surgery, Hospital for Sick Children, Toronto, ON, Canada
e-mail: johanna.riesel@sickkids.ca

Quality of life (QoL), defined as the perception of the patient's position in life in the context of their goals and expectations, is an overarching measure that may be used to index these key patient and parental variables [5]. QoL analyses in this population are complex: significant heterogeneity exists between outcomes for syndromic and nonsyndromic diagnoses, and further prognostic challenges arise due to the presence of comorbid deficits, baseline functional status of the child, and operative approaches chosen. Specific to paediatric studies, another question pertains to the relative emphasis of parental reports versus those obtained from children themselves. Given that most patients undergo surgery in infancy, if children are to be interviewed for QoL outcomes, the optimal age(s) to do so are unclear. Across paediatric QoL studies, parental- and child-reported measures have been shown to differ, and children's own reports and priorities may shift as they enter schooling and adolescence [7, 8].

The present chapter serves as a guide for surgeons and other healthcare practitioners to navigate a variety of QoL issues as they relate to craniosynostosis. We begin with an overview of commonly employed QoL metrics in craniosynostosis and then examine specific issues pertaining to syndromic and nonsyndromic forms of this disorder. Through this analysis, readers will be presented with a detailed examination of patient and caregiver-level concerns that may be

F. Di Rocco, J. Kestle (eds.), *Neurosurgical Aspects of Craniosynostosis*,
https://doi.org/10.1007/978-3-031-69386-1_53

employed to better counsel families and develop mutual surgical goals and expected outcomes.

53.1.1 Pearls

- In addition to commonly discussed surgical metrics, QoL outcomes represent key components of preoperative counseling discussions.
- Significant variation exists in expected QoL with and without intervention across the spectrum of craniosynostosis pathology.
- While novel surgical techniques are increasingly employed to treat craniosynostosis, examination of associated QoL benefits has been limited. As such, many open questions remain, and further research is needed in this area.

53.2 Quality of Life Measures in Craniosynostosis

A variety of qualitative, quantitative, and combined measures have been employed to index QoL in craniosynostosis. Among these metrics, the most general form of QoL analysis has been open-ended interview of parents and older patients to discuss self-perceptions of function, psychosocial wellbeing, developmental progress, and overall disease impact [6, 9]. However, purely qualitative assessments provide limited ability to directly compare responses between subjects and across studies. Objective clinical scales utilized include the Short-Form Health Survey 36-Item (SF-36) [10], Glasgow Children's Benefit Inventory (GCBI), World Health Organization Quality of Life Scale (WHOQoL) [11, 12], Who Health Organization Disability Assessment Schedule (WHODAS) [13], Health Utility Index Mark 3 (HUI-3) [14], Infant Toddler Quality of life Questionnaire (ITQoL) [10], Child Health Questionnaire Parental Form 50 and Child Form 87 (CHD-PF50/CF87) [10], TNO-AZL Questionnaire for Children's Quality of Life (TACQoL) [15], and the Child Behaviour Checklist (CBCL) [15, 16]. Given the prevalence of obstructive sleep apnea (OSA) in syndromic patients, the OSA-18 is a targeted assessment of physical, cognitive, and sleep disturbances related to sleep apnea [17]. More recently, the FACE-Q craniofacial module has been developed to capture aesthetic and functional outcomes, adverse events, and health-related QoL items specific to paediatric craniofacial disorders including craniosynostosis [18]. Notably, of all scales examined, the FACE-Q is unique in assessing cosmetic outcomes explicitly. Table 53.1 provides an overview of the different clinical factors encompassed by these QoL assessment tools.

Table 53.1 Overview of QoL domains covered by the most utilized standardized questionnaires in craniosynostosis (adapted from Park et al., 2021 [4])

	Physical	Cognitive	Psychological	Social	Education	Sleep
SF-36	✓	✓	✓	✓		
GCBI	✓				✓	
WHOQoL	✓		✓	✓		
WHODAS	✓	✓				
HUI-3	✓	✓	✓			
ITQoL	✓			✓		✓
CHD-PF50/CF87	✓		✓	✓	✓	
TACQoL	✓		✓	✓		✓
CBCL	✓					
OSA-18	✓		✓			✓
FACE-Q	✓		✓	✓	✓	

53.3 Nonsyndromic Craniosynostosis

Nonsyndromic synostosis commonly affects a single suture and is not associated with significant medical comorbidities or extracranial deformations. In rare instances, multisuture craniosynostosis can be seen without identifiable affiliated syndrome, but for the purposes of this chapter, "single suture craniosynostosis" will be synonymous with "non-syndromic craniosynostosis." In cases of nonsyndromic craniosynostosis, the sagittal suture is most commonly affected [4]. In the absence of elevated intracranial pressure, single suture craniosynostosis has historically been considered purely cosmetic; however, the recent literature suggests that subtle neurocognitive and QoL impairments may also exist within these populations [15, 19, 20]. In comparison with syndromic craniosynostosis, QoL impairments in nonsyndromic cases are more subtle, and there is substantially less agreement between studies as to overall QoL across different metrics.

Subtle neurocognitive impairment has primarily been observed in patients with isolated sagittal synostosis. This is likely due to the relative prevalence of the condition as compared to synostosis of the other cranial sutures. Boltshauser et al. reported on 30 patients with untreated isolated sagittal synostosis at an average age of 9.25 years [15]. Interestingly, the majority of patients and parents were pleased with their current situation and rated the deformity as significantly less evident than in infancy. TACQoL assessments were also within normal range. However, patients reported a higher incidence of bullying and their scores in attention and memory were significantly lower than in healthy controls.

The data regarding the impact of surgical intervention are mixed. In comparison to healthy controls, Cloonan et al. found that, at age 5, parental reports of school functioning and social QoL were lower in children treated for single and multisuture nonsyndromic craniosynostosis as compared to healthy controls [16]. However, in long-term follow-up of patients with a mean age of 23 years, Mazzafero et al. found that treated patients report higher WHOQoL scores than normative populations; however, a risk of bias does exist as this study utilized mail-in questionnaires [11]. Forms were completed by 32/52 contacted patients, suggesting that perhaps those patients who were more satisfied with their QoL and functioning better may have been more likely to participate in the study. One additional study examined patients treated for isolated sagittal synostosis and reported no difference in education, employment, and psychosocial measures as compared to healthy controls [21]. Sader et al. reported a North American comparative study of operative versus conservative management for single-suture disease [22]. When adjusting for disease severity and patient age, no significant differences in the physical, psychosocial, and total QoL domains were found between the treated and untreated groups. While this study raises critical questions with regard to the patient and caregiver-level benefits of craniofacial intervention, the results must be interpreted with caution as the treated group was comprised of much younger patients with a higher severity of their deformity. Furthermore, head shape "severity" was subjectively reported in a retrospective fashion, which makes this value difficult to interpret. Additionally, there are currently no validated methods for accurately rating head shape severity, and as such, there are little data to correlate head shape severity with neurocognitive or operative outcomes. Taken together, the existing literature suggests that careful patient selection and identification of specific patient and caregiver goals as related to QoL should form a core component of presurgical consultation.

A single study examined the influence of surgical timing and technique on outcomes in nonsyndromic synostosis [23]. Shavlokhova et al. reported that earlier surgical intervention is associated with better familial function, higher self-esteem, and school performance. The amount of intraoperative transfusion was also associated with lower familial and school domain scores, perhaps associated with more complex surgery and longer hospital stay, though these data were not directly reported. No difference between the type of surgical technique was reported in terms of QoL outcomes.

Regarding open versus endoscopic strip craniectomy (ESC) across different forms of single suture synostosis, a pair of systematic reviews have demonstrated lower intraoperative blood loss, operative time, and surgical stay in association with endoscopic surgery [2, 3]. However, no studies to date have examined QoL outcomes associated with this technique. Based on Shavlokhova et al.'s results, it is possible that reduced intraoperative transfusion rates and shorter hospital stays associated with endoscopic surgery may correlate with improved QoL; however, this will need to be formally examined and at present remains an open question. Furthermore, the required orthotic helmeting following the ESC may be a burden to families, but this has also not yet been studied. Additional novel treatments, such as distraction and spring-mediated distraction have not yet been assessed in the QoL literature.

53.4 Syndromic Craniosynostosis

Syndromic forms of craniosynostosis generally represent complex multisuture deformities often in combination with developmental, behavioural, and systemic medical disorders [4]. Apert, Crouzon, Pfeiffer, Muenke, and Saethre-Chotzen syndromes represent the most common paediatric craniofacial syndromes associated with craniosynostosis [24]. Worldwide, approximately 12–31% of total cases of craniosynostosis are associated with a syndromic diagnosis [25–28]. Significant contributors to poor QoL in these populations include the need for multistage craniofacial procedures, surgical and nonsurgical management of comorbid conditions, associated physical deformities, and comorbid neuropsychological impairments [4, 6]. It is important to note that there is variability in the comorbidities seen in syndromic cases of craniosynostosis. For example, patients with Crouzon syndrome often have normal intelligence levels, and patients with Pfeiffer syndrome have a broad range of associated comorbidities ranging from mild to severely debilitating. The following QoL data should be read with this variability in mind.

Psychosocial impairments in syndromic craniosynostosis are commonly reported in the literature. Patients show lower self-esteem and suffer from significantly higher rates of abuse, bullying, anxiety, and depression as compared to normative populations [6]. Psychosocial stressors such as these are also shown to worsen with adolescence as patients gradually became more aware of their condition and internalize negative body image perceptions [6, 10]. Overall social integration, familial cohesion, and parental stress as indexed by the SF-36, ITQoL, and CHD-CF87 rate significantly worse for syndromic patients as compared to healthy controls [10, 29]. Subjective interviews of adults living with Apert and Crouzon syndromes also demonstrate higher proportions of patients continuing to live with parents and requiring daily assistance than in the general population [13, 30]. Surgical management, at least for Apert syndrome, is associated with partial improvement in the majority of psychosocial metrics [9].

Amongst these patients, significant impairments are also seen in the domains of physical health and educational/professional attainment. Anomalies most strongly implicated with functional limitations include complex syndactyly, visual and/or speech impairment, cognitive deficits, and behavioural issues [10]. Patients with Apert syndrome in particular report increased incidence of daily pain limiting physical function, mostly in the hands [10]. In comparison to these patients, those with Crouzon syndrome demonstrate significantly higher WHOQoL scores in measures of physical function, though still below those of the general population [31]. In both Apert and Crouzon patients, greater need for daily assistance and higher disability burden were most often cited as reasons for poorer educational and professional attainment [29, 30, 32].

OSA, thought to be secondary to midface hypoplasia and pharyngeal collapse, has been observed in up to 75% of syndromic patients [33]. Midface hypoplasia is due to skull base fusion commonly seen in patients with syndromic craniosynostosis. Bannink et al. found that the presence and severity of OSA serve as independent predictors of QoL in these populations [17]. Specifically, they found that OSA-18 scores for sleep disturbance, physical suffering, and caregiver concerns were significantly higher in craniosynostosis groups as compared to healthy controls, and correlated with OSA severity [17]. Early intervention is critical to mitigate the downstream sequelae that result from unmanaged OSA. A variety of treatment modalities may be appropriate based on the patient's phenotypic expression of midface hypoplasia and airway collapse, including, but not limited to adenoidectomy, continuous positive airway pressure, nasopharyngeal tubes or airways (NPT or NPA), and tracheostomy. One retrospective study by Randhawa et al. found long-term nasopharyngeal airway (NPA) placement was associated with clinically significant improvements in OSA-18 scores as well as learning, vitality, and physicals measures across the GCBI [34]. This treatment was also subjectively preferred to tracheostomy based on parental interviews; however, the NPA may not be sufficient in all patient populations. Given that ongoing OSA is linked with hypoxia-induced cognitive and behavioural deficits, targeted treatments for patients suffering from OSA is critical. Based on Randhawa et al.*'s* results [34], long-term NPA may serve as an effective treatment for certain patients with this condition with demonstrated improvements to QoL, though no direct comparisons between NPA and standard tracheostomy have been performed to date.

53.5 Conclusions

Craniosynostosis is associated with diminished QoL as reported by parents, caregivers, and patients. While QoL impairments in nonsyndromic forms of craniosynostosis are less severe in comparison to syndromic diagnoses, they remain common and relate predominantly to self-esteem, perceived appearance by peers, and mild neurocognitive deficits. In contrast, patients with syndromic synostosis commonly present with associated deformities and comorbidities and demonstrate significant impairment in psychosocial, physical, educational, and professional domains of life, even after surgical intervention (though the latter can improve certain domains of QoL). Surgical treatment for both syndromic and nonsyndromic malformations is associated with improved QoL, as is treatment of comorbid OSA in syndromic synostoses. Surgeons and practitioners should be aware of these salient QoL metrics such that they may guide patients and families through informed decision-making and goal setting regarding the treatment of children with craniosynostosis.

References

1. Kuta V, Curry L, McNeely D, Walling S, Chorney J, Bezuhly M. Understanding families' experiences following a diagnosis of non-syndromic craniosynostosis: a qualitative study. BMJ Open. 2020;10(9):e033403.
2. Yan H, Abel TJ, Alotaibi NM, Anderson M, Niazi TN, Weil AG, et al. A systematic review and meta-analysis of endoscopic versus open treatment of craniosynostosis. Part 1: the sagittal suture. J Neurosurg Pediatr. 2018;22:352.
3. Yan H, Abel TJ, Alotaibi NM, Anderson M, Niazi TN, Weil AG, et al. A systematic review of endoscopic versus open treatment of craniosynostosis. Part 2: the nonsagittal single sutures. J Neurosurg Pediatr. 2018;22:361.
4. Park KM, Tripathi NV, Al-Mufarrej F. Quality of life in patients with craniosynostosis and deformational plagiocephaly: a systematic review. Int J Pediatr Otorhinolaryngol. 2021;149:110873.
5. Skevington SM, Lotfy M, O'Connell KA. The World Health Organization's WHOQOL-BREF quality of life assessment: psychometric properties and results of the international field trial a report from the WHOQOL Group. Qual Life Res. 2004;13:299.
6. Visram SM, Gill D, Shute JT, Cunningham SJ. Qualitative study to identify issues affecting quality of life in adults with craniofacial anomalies. Br J Oral Maxillofac Surg. 2019;57:47.
7. Haverman L, Limperg PF, Young NL, Grootenhuis MA, Klaassen RJ. Paediatric health-related quality of life: what is it and why should we measure it? Arch Dis Child. 2017;102(5):393.
8. McLaughlin JF. The measurement of health-related quality of life (HRQL) in children with cerebral palsy. Eur J Neurol. 2001;8(Suppl 5):183–93. http://ovidsp.ovid.com/ovidweb.cgi?T=JS&PAGE=reference&D=med4&NEWS=N&AN=11851747.
9. Allam KA, Wan DC, Khwanngern K, Kawamoto HK, Tanna N, Perry A, et al. Treatment of Apert syndrome: a long-term follow-up study. Plast Reconstr Surg. 2011;127:1601.

10. Bannink N, Maliepaard M, Raat H, Joosten KFM, Mathijssen IMJ. Health-related quality of life in children and adolescents with syndromic craniosynostosis. J Plast Reconstr Aesthet Surg. 2010;63:1972.
11. Mazzaferro DM, Naran S, Wes AM, Magee L, Taylor JA, Bartlett SP. Quality of life in adults with nonsyndromic craniosynostosis. Plast Reconstr Surg. 2018;141:1474.
12. Lloyd MS, Venugopal A, Horton J, Rodrigues D, Nishikawa H, White N, et al. The quality of life in adult patients with syndromic craniosynostosis from their perspective. J Craniofac Surg. 2016;27:1510.
13. Sakamoto Y, Takenouchi T, Miwa T, Kishi K. Assessment of long-term quality of life in patients with syndromic craniosynostosis. J Plast Reconstr Aesthet Surg. 2021;74:336.
14. De Jong T, Maliepaard M, Bannink N, Raat H, Mathijssen IMJ. Health-related problems and quality of life in patients with syndromic and complex craniosynostosis. Childs Nerv Syst. 2012;28:879.
15. Boltshauser E, Ludwig S, Dietrich F, Landolt MA. Sagittal craniosynostosis: cognitive development, behaviour, and quality of life in unoperated children. Neuropediatrics. 2003;34:293.
16. Cloonan YK, Collett B, Speltz ML, Anderka M, Werler MM. Psychosocial outcomes in children with and without non-syndromic craniosynostosis: findings from two studies. Cleft Palate Craniofac J. 2013;50:406.
17. Bannink N, Maliepaard M, Raat H, Joosten KFM, Mathijssen IMJ. Obstructive sleep apnea-specific quality of life and behavioral problems in children with syndromic craniosynostosis. J Dev Behav Pediatr. 2011;32:233.
18. Klassen AF, Rae C, Riff W, Denadai R, Murray DJ, Bracken S, et al. FACE-Q craniofacial module: part 2 psychometric properties of newly developed scales for children and young adults with facial conditions. J Plast Reconstr Aesthet Surg. 2021;74:2330.
19. Kljajić M, Maltese G, Tarnow P, Sand P, Kölby L. The cognitive profile of children with nonsyndromic craniosynostosis. Plast Reconstr Surg. 2019;143:1037e.
20. Bellew M, Chumas P. Long-term developmental follow-up in children with nonsyndromic craniosynostosis. J Neurosurg Pediatr. 2015;16:445.
21. Salokorpi N, Savolainen T, Sinikumpu JJ, Ylikontiola L, Sándor GK, Pirttiniemi P, et al. Outcomes of 40 nonsyndromic sagittal craniosynostosis patients as adults: a case-control study with 26 years of postoperative follow-up. Oper Neurosurg. 2019;16:1.
22. Sader N, Mehta V, Hart S, Bliss L, Moore H, DaSilva M, et al. Quality of life and satisfaction in surgical versus conservative treatment of nonsyndromic children with craniosynostosis. J Neurosurg Pediatr. 2021;29:1–6.
23. Shavlokhova V, Grüninger S, Hoffmann J, Freudlsperger C, Engel M. Health-related quality of life in children after surgical treatment of nonsyndromal craniosynostosis. J Craniomaxillofac Surg. 2021;49:655.
24. Sawh-Martinez R, Steinbacher DM. Syndromic craniosynostosis. Clin Plast Surg. 2019;46:141.
25. Dempsey RF, Monson LA, Maricevich RS, Truong TA, Olarunnipa S, Lam SK, et al. Nonsyndromic craniosynostosis. Clin Plast Surg. 2019;46:123.
26. Kweldam CF, Van Der Vlugt JJ, Van Der Meulen JJNM. The incidence of craniosynostosis in the Netherlands, 1997-2007. J Plast Reconstr Aesthet Surg. 2011;64:583.
27. Neusel C, Class D, Eckert AW, Firsching R, Göbel P, Götz D, et al. Multicentre approach to epidemiological aspects of craniosynostosis in Germany. Br J Oral Maxillofac Surg. 2018;56:881.
28. Boulet SL, Rasmussen SA, Honein MA. A population-based study of craniosynostosis in metropolitan Atlanta, 1989-2003. Am J Med Genet A. 2008;146A:984.
29. Taghinia AH, Yorlets RR, Doyle M, Labow BI, Upton J. Long-term functional upper-extremity outcomes in adults with Apert syndrome. Plast Reconstr Surg. 2019;143:1136.
30. Tovetjärn R, Tarnow P, Maltese G, Fischer S, Sahlin PE, Kölby L. Children with Apert syndrome as adults: a follow-up study of 28 scandinavian patients. Plast Reconstr Surg. 2012;130:572e.
31. Raposo-Amaral CE, Neto JGJ, Denadai R, Raposo-Amaral CM, Raposo-Amaral CA. Patient-reported quality of life in highest-functioning Apert and Crouzon syndromes: a comparative study. Plast Reconstr Surg. 2014;133:182e.
32. Fischer S, Tovetjärn R, Maltese G, Sahlin PE, Tarnow P, Kölby L. Psychosocial conditions in adults with Crouzon syndrome: a follow-up study of 31 Swedish patients. J Plast Surg Hand Surg. 2014;48:244.
33. Inverso G, Brustowicz KA, Katz E, Padwa BL. The prevalence of obstructive sleep apnea in symptomatic patients with syndromic craniosynostosis. Int J Oral Maxillofac Surg. 2016;45:167.
34. Randhawa PS, Ahmed J, Nouraei SR, Wyatt ME. Impact of long-term nasopharyngeal airway on health-related quality of life of children with obstructive sleep apnea caused by syndromic craniosynostosis. J Craniofac Surg. 2011;22:125.

54 Long Follow-Up Results in Craniosynostoses

Niina Salokorpi and Willy Serlo

The main goal of any health care intervention is to cure the patients, relieve symptoms, prolong survival, and improve well-being along with the quality of life (QoL) of the patient. Quality of life includes aspects such as life satisfaction, wealth, levels of safety and freedom, health perceptions and physical, psychological, social, and cognitive well-being [1, 2].

These aspects should be held in mind when speaking about the results of any treatment, not only the craniosynostosis surgery. As described in previous chapters, the craniosynostosis include a wide spectrum of pathologies, some of which have mainly aesthetical influence while others additionally cause permanent problems in physical health and cognitive performance levels.

Historically, the success of the craniosynostosis surgery has been evaluated by measurable objective outcome parameters such as anatomical measurements including cranial index (CI) and intracranial volume (ICV). Additionally, evaluation of postoperative complications, morbidity, mortality, and the necessity for reoperations were used [3–8]. These, clinically very relevant measurements, reflect well the surgeons' opinions about the outcome. However, this does not reflect what the patients themselves consider important as an assessment of the outcome. This question becomes even more complicated when taking into account that while craniosynostosis is treated in early childhood, the patient's own opinion about the outcome of the treatment could be asked only many years later. The size and shape of the skull and face develops until adulthood. Craniocerebral disproportion and restrictions of the airways may cause delayed morbidity. Thus, conclusions of the long-term outcome should not be made before the growth of the patient is complete.

When evaluating the outcome at a certain age, one should keep in mind that the patient has lived all their life so far with that residual pathology. Nobody can say afterwards, if the patient's life would have been different if a different treatment decision would have been made earlier since the particular patient has experience only of living with this particular appearance. This aspect could be to some extent surpassed by comparing some objective measurements and factors between patients and controls. This could include, for example, comparing self-esteem, depression

N. Salokorpi
Research Unit of Clinical Medicine, Oulu University Hospital and University of Oulu, Oulu, Finland

Medical Research Center Oulu (MRC Oulu), University of Oulu and Oulu University Hospital, Oulu, Finland
e-mail: niina.salokorpi@oulu.fi

W. Serlo (✉)
Department of Neurosurgery, Neurocenter, Oulu University Hospital, Oulu, Finland

Department of Children and Adolescents, Oulu University Hospital, Oulu, Finland
e-mail: willy.serlo@oulu.fi

F. Di Rocco, J. Kestle (eds.), *Neurosurgical Aspects of Craniosynostosis*,
https://doi.org/10.1007/978-3-031-69386-1_54

score, QoL, satisfaction with own appearance, and general physical health issues.

Depending on the type of craniosynostosis, the patients may have only aesthetical problems, but also physical, mental, or developmental disabilities due to the primary condition [9–11].

The primary goals of the surgery can differ and thus can change what is accepted as a good outcome. In some cases, the primary goal is normalization of the patient's craniofacial appearance. Thus, when evaluating the outcome, the main stress is on the aesthetics. In patients who exhibit, for example, an increase in ICP, it could be considered that a poorer aesthetic outcome is acceptable, since the main goal of the treatment is to save the patient's life and allow the brain to grow. In such situations, one must pose the question: "I saved the patient but is this enough?" Does the surgery prevent neurocognitive deficits and improve QoL? What is the impact of the surgery itself on the patient's QoL and cognition?

Any craniosynostosis surgery aims to normalize patients' appearance [12]. Despite the treatment, the facial appearance of craniosynostosis patients can remain different from what we assume to be "normal," resembling what is expected, and preferably aesthetically pleasing. This can negatively influence a person's self-esteem, body image, social relationships, and behavior later in life [6, 13–17]. Having a residual dysmorphic face and head shape can attract unfavorable attention and possibly even cause rejection from strangers and peers. This may have a secondary psychosocial effect by negatively influencing the patients' social behavior and cause difficulties in educational environments and even poor school performance [18]. Thus, patients encounter psychological difficulties and must adapt to the demands of their environment in many aspects including, behavior, psychological well-being, social experiences, and satisfaction with appearance [15].

Thus, evaluation of long-term follow-up should be done from the surgeons and patients' points of view, preferably when patients have reached adulthood. Such evaluation should be broad, covering the earlier mentioned aspects.

Historically, several different simplified classifications for the assessment of the results of craniosynostoses treatment have been proposed. Whitaker in 1987 proposed a IV category scale for assessment according to the need for additional surgery [19]. This classification has been widely used in many studies [6, 8, 20, 21]. Sloan et al. proposed classification of the surgical results into seven classes [22], and Aryan et al. proposed in 2005 a simplified version of Sloan's classification [23]. The latter has four categories, where only one category infers the need for operative corrections, while the other three categories correspond to less severe degrees of deformity. These classifications have their role, since they allow the evaluation of the aesthetical outcome to some extent based on the surgeon's opinion retrospectively from usually rather reticent medical records [24, 25].

Whilst these evaluation scales are easy to use, they are very limited. More sophisticated methods are required.

One of the first attempts to determine a correlation between appearance and QoL after craniosynostosis surgery, thus evaluating the results of the surgery from the patient's point of view, was published by Lloyd et al. in 2016 [21]. However, the facial aesthetics were evaluated using the Whitaker classification, mentioned earlier. Another attempt was made by Kluba and associates, who asked parents how satisfied they were with the results of treatment using a 5-point rating scale. They found that parents were mainly satisfied with the surgical results and were stricter in their evaluation when compared to surgeons [26]. Joly and associates evaluated the results after suturectomy for metopic and coronal synostosis by asking children and parents if the head shape was normal in their opinion. They also used the Whitaker scale to evaluate the results. In this study, the children's mean age at the time of evaluation was 14 years; thus, the follow-up was reasonably long, and children were old enough to express their reliable opinion. Interestingly, while surgeons were satisfied only with three patients' appearances out of 17, the patients themselves found their head and facial shape to be normal in 11 out of 17 cases [6]. In this study, there is a discrepancy between the surgeons' and patients' opinions about appearance, confirming the necessity for paying attention to what matters to patients.

One option to standardize aesthetic evaluations is by using independent third person panels. In orthodontics, there are numerous studies on patients' self-satisfaction with pre- and postoperative aesthesis, as well as third person quantitative evaluation of aesthetic outcome [27, 28]. When studying persons treated for severe malocclusions, it was found that the QoL and self-perceived aesthetic satisfaction improve extensively after treatment [27]. These variables may be determinants of the outcomes among craniosynostoses patients, as well.

The studies by Metzler and Bendon evaluated surgical results from photographs; however, the grading was concentrated on deformity and evaluation of the necessity for reoperations [29, 30].

During the last few years, a few studies were published evaluating the impact of craniosynostosis on health-related quality of life (HRQoL) [21, 31, 32]. The latest study on QoL in craniosynostosis patients was published by Shavlokhova in 2021 and carried out on adolescents operated on due to nonsyndromic craniosynostoses in infancy. They found no QoL limitations in later life when compared to the average population [33].

In previous studies, it was found that the overall quality of life is lower than average in patients with syndromic and complex craniosynostosis [31, 32].

In a study of 28 adults with Apert syndrome, it was found that the patients managed relatively well in terms of education and employment, although the highest level of education was lower than with controls. The social relations (marriage, number of friends) of these patients appeared to require improvement [11]. More optimistic results were reported by Allam and associates who followed up eight Apert syndrome patients for over 15 years and assessed their social and educational progress. It was demonstrated that these patients can function quite well in society, can achieve a high level of education, hold full-time employment, and integrate well socially [10].

From a clinical viewpoint, surgically treated sagittal craniosynostosis patients are expected to have a minimal risk of late sequelae. Clinical follow-up is usually continued no later than school age. There are several studies suggesting single suture craniosynostoses are associated with mild to moderate developmental and educational difficulties which become apparent at school age [34–36]. However, patients with sagittal synostosis have the best performance in neuropsychological tests [35].

The authors shed some light on this topic by carrying out a study evaluating adult patients treated for sagittal synostosis with an average follow-up time of 26.5 years (range 17–37) and comparison with age and gender matched controls [37]. Patients filled in extensive questionnaires and were asked to evaluate their own satisfaction on the Visual Analogue Scale (VAS). Patients and controls standardized photographs were evaluated by panels. The results were very encouraging, since it appeared that patients managed as well in adult life as controls.

The study revealed that the patients were equally satisfied with their appearance as were controls. Lay and dentists panels found the patients' appearance to be slightly less attractive than controls, but the difference was less than 10% on a 100 mm VAS. The socioeconomic situation and general health of patients equaled that of controls. Being operated on for sagittal craniosynostosis did not influence a patient's education level, employment status or finding a life partner [37].

Interestingly there was no significant difference between the patients and controls complaints regarding their facial appearance. In both groups, the most common subjects to complain about were teeth, shape of head, or face. The majority of patients' dissatisfaction with their appearance was not related to the craniosynostosis itself [37, 38].

The authors attempted to find parameters from 3D images that would correlate with subjective satisfaction with their own appearance in adult metopic and sagittal craniosynostosis patients operated on in early childhood. Though some difference was found between patients and controls in 3D parameters, there was no significant correlation between these findings and satisfaction with own appearance [39].

While exhibiting the correct direction, still neither of these studies sufficiently reflects the results of the surgery from the patient-oriented point of view. Different scales and questions are used in each study. The heterogeneity of the deformities, the wide variety of operative techniques and consequently a small number of patients in each series, makes the comparison even more obscure.

To allow cross-study comparisons and to facilitate meta-analyses the outcome measures must be validated and consistent. Core outcome sets should include data meaningful to both patients and physicians [40]. This creates a next challenge, since there is a necessity to ensure accurate reporting of the patients' subjective experience. Thus, there is a requirement for structured validated patient-reported outcome measurement instruments.

Several questions are important for the reliable comparison of surgical results and should be considered.

First, the preoperative degree of pathology should be documented properly including systemic findings. Second, surgical techniques have changed over the decades and perioperative treatment improved significantly. Thus, patients that have attained adulthood have been often operated on with methods now abandoned [37, 38]. Additionally, one should bear in mind that in the pediatric population, the health and well-being of a child are inseparable from their parents' well-being [40, 41]. Findings made by Feragen et al. suggest that many parents of craniosynostosis children experience stressful and potentially traumatic symptoms due to their child's complex treatment, which may in turn affect the family. These adverse experiences could have a negative effect, and they could additionally serve as a trigger towards personal growth and positive change [42]. This could include increased compassion, valuing of close relations, and discovery of new strengths within oneself or changing life's perspective [43].

When evaluating long-term follow-up, social and cultural aspects should be taken into account. Perception of beauty is influenced by the individual's geographic, ethnic, cultural, and demographic background. However, objective measurements remain the foundation for aesthetic evaluations. Differences in aesthetic preferences can lead to dissatisfaction with the results. Increasing global environment, role of social media, cultural differences, and international variability must be considered when reporting outcomes [44].

When speaking of all these challenges, one should remember that there is no means of 100% testing which treatment decision was better after all, since there is no real basis for comparison. The surgery was done in early childhood, and the patient outcome can be compared to other patients or normal cohorts. Nobody really knows what a patients' life would have been if different surgical decision would have been made.

Since the studies on the previously discussed aspects of long-term follow-up are so far scarce, with this chapter we pose more questions than answers. The authors want to initiate discussion on this topic, stimulating further and more profound research. The clinicians treating patients daily should regularly have time for reflecting on their own results and experience and share their thoughts with others.

References

1. Thoma A, Cornacchi SD, Lovrics PJ, Goldsmith CH, Evidence-Based Surgery Working Group. Evidence-based surgery. Users' guide to the surgical literature: how to assess an article on health-related quality of life. Can J Surg. 2008;51:215–24.
2. McDowell I. Measuring health: a guide to rating scales and questionnaires. Oxford University Press; 2009. p. 1–764.
3. Thoma A, Ignacy TA. Health services research: impact of quality of life instruments on craniofacial surgery. J Craniofac Surg. 2012;23:283–7.
4. Tapia VJ, Epstein S, Tolmach OS, Hassan AS, Chung NN, Gosman AA. Health-related quality-of-life instruments for pediatric patients with diverse facial deformities: a systematic literature review. Plast Reconstr Surg. 2016;138:175–87.

5. Breik O, Mahindu A, Moore MH, Molloy CJ, Santoreneos S, David DJ. Apert syndrome: surgical outcomes and perspectives. J Craniomaxillofac Surg. 2016;44:1238–45.
6. Joly A, Pare A, Sallot A, Arsene S, Listrat A, Travers N, Goga D, Laure B. Long-term assessment of suturectomy in trigonocephaly and anterior plagiocephaly. J Craniofac Surg. 2016;27:627–30.
7. Ozlen F. Surgical treatment of trigonocephaly: technique and long-term results in 48 cases. J Neurosurg Pediatr. 2011;7:300.
8. Seruya M, Oh AK, Boyajian MJ, Posnick JC, Keating RF. Treatment for delayed presentation of sagittal synostosis: challenges pertaining to occult intracranial hypertension. J Neurosurg Pediatr. 2011;8:40–8.
9. Kapp-Simon KA, Speltz ML, Cunningham ML, Patel PK, Tomita T. Neurodevelopment of children with single suture craniosynostosis: a review. Childs Nerv Syst. 2007;23:269–81.
10. Allam KA, Wan DC, Khwanngern K, Kawamoto HK, Tanna N, Perry A, Bradley JP. Treatment of apert syndrome: a long-term follow-up study. Plast Reconstr Surg. 2011;127:1601–11.
11. Tovetjarn R, Tarnow P, Maltese G, Fischer S, Sahlin PE, Kolby L. Children with Apert syndrome as adults: a follow-up study of 28 Scandinavian patients. Plast Reconstr Surg. 2012;130:573e–7e.
12. Farkas LG, Deutsch CK. Anthropometric determination of craniofacial morphology. Am J Med Genet. 1996;65:1–4.
13. Feragen KB, Borge AIH. Peer harassment and satisfaction with appearance in children with and without a facial difference. Body Image. 2010;7:97–105.
14. Stock NM, Feragen KB. Psychological adjustment to cleft lip and/or palate: a narrative review of the literature. Psychol Health. 2016;31:777–813.
15. Feragen KB, Stock NM. Psychological adjustment to craniofacial conditions (excluding oral clefts): a review of the literature. Psychol Health. 2017;32:253–88.
16. Kostanski M, Gullone E. Adolescent body image dissatisfaction: relationships with self-esteem, anxiety, and depression controlling for body mass. J Child Psychol Psychiatry. 1998;39:255–62.
17. Bous RM, Hazen RA, Baus I, Palomo JM, Kumar A, Valiathan M. Psychosocial adjustments among adolescents with craniofacial conditions and the influence of social factors: a multi-informant study. Cleft Palate Craniofac J. 2020;57:624–36.
18. Becker DB, Petersen JD, Kane AA, Cradock MM, Pilgram TK, Marsh JL. Speech, cognitive, and behavioral outcomes in nonsyndromic craniosynostosis. Plast Reconstr Surg. 2005;116:400–7.
19. Whitaker LA, Bartlett SP, Schut L, Bruce D. Craniosynostosis: an analysis of the timing, treatment, and complications in 164 consecutive patients. Plast Reconstr Surg. 1987;80:195–212.
20. Mesa JM, Fang F, Muraszko KM, Buchman SR. Reconstruction of unicoronal plagiocephaly with a hypercorrection surgical technique. Neurosurg Focus. 2011;31:E4.
21. Lloyd MS, Venugopal A, Horton J, Rodrigues D, Nishikawa H, White N, Solanki G, Noons P, Evans M, Dover S. The quality of life in adult patients with syndromic craniosynostosis from their perspective. J Craniofac Surg. 2016;27:1510–4.
22. Sloan GM, Wells KC, Raffel C, McComb JG. Surgical treatment of craniosynostosis: outcome analysis of 250 consecutive patients. Pediatrics. 1997;100:E2.
23. Aryan HE, Jandial R, Ozgur BM, Hughes SA, Meltzer HS, Park MS, Levy ML. Surgical correction of metopic synostosis. Childs Nerv Syst. 2005;21:392–8.
24. Salokorpi N, Sinikumpu J-J, Iber T, Zibo HN, Areda T, Ylikontiola L, Sándor GK, Serlo W. Frontal cranial modeling using endocranial resorbable plate fixation in 27 consecutive plagiocephaly and trigonocephaly patients. Childs Nerv Syst. 2015; https://doi.org/10.1007/s00381-015-2657-y.
25. Serlo WS, Ylikontiola LP, Vesala AL, Kaarela OI, Iber T, Sándor GKB, Ashammakhi N. Effective correction of frontal cranial deformities using biodegradable fixation on the inner surface of the cranial bones during infancy. Childs Nerv Syst. 2007;23:1439–45.
26. Kluba S, Rohleder S, Wolff M, Haas-Lude K, Schuhmann MU, Will BE, Reinert S, Krimmel M. Parental perception of treatment and medical care in children with craniosynostosis. Int J Oral Maxillofac Surg. 2016;45:1341–6.
27. Silvola AS, Varimo M, Tolvanen M, Rusanen J, Lahti S, Pirttiniemi P. Dental esthetics and quality of life in adults with severe malocclusion before and after treatment. Angle Orthod. 2014;84:594–9.
28. Claudino D, Traebert J. Malocclusion, dental aesthetic self-perception and quality of life in a 18 to 21 year-old population: a cross section study. BMC Oral Health. 2013;13:3.
29. Metzler P, Zemann W, Jacobsen C, Lubbers HT, Gratz KW, Obwegeser JA. Assessing aesthetic outcomes after trigonocephaly correction. Oral Maxillofac Surg. 2014;18:181–6.
30. Bendon CL, Johnson HP, Judge AD, Wall SA, Johnson D. The aesthetic outcome of surgical correction for sagittal synostosis can be reliably scored by a novel method of preoperative and postoperative visual assessment. Plast Reconstr Surg. 2014;134:775e–86e.
31. Bannink N, Maliepaard M, Raat H, Joosten KF, Mathijssen IM. Health-related quality of life in children and adolescents with syndromic craniosynostosis. J Plast Reconstr Aesthet Surg. 2010;63:1972–81.
32. de Jong T, Maliepaard M, Bannink N, Raat H, Mathijssen IM. Health-related problems and quality of life in patients with syndromic and complex craniosynostosis. Childs Nerv Syst. 2012;28:879–82.
33. Shavlokhova V, Grüninger S, Hoffmann J, Freudlsperger C, Engel M. Health-related quality of life in children after surgical treatment of non-syndromal craniosynostosis. J Craniofac Surg. 2021;49:655–8.

34. Speltz ML, Kapp-Simon KA, Cunningham M, Marsh J, Dawson G. Single-suture craniosynostosis: a review of neurobehavioral research and theory. J Pediatr Psychol. 2004;29:651–68.
35. Bellew M, Chumas P. Long-term developmental follow-up in children with nonsyndromic craniosynostosis. J Neurosurg Pediatr. 2015;16:445–51.
36. Kapp-Simon KA, Collett BR, Barr-Schinzel MA, Cradock MM, Buono LA, Pietila KE, Speltz ML. Behavioral adjustment of toddler and preschool-aged children with single-suture craniosynostosis. Plast Reconstr Surg. 2012;130:635–47.
37. Salokorpi N, Savolainen T, Sinikumpu J-J, Ylikontiola L, Sándor GK, Pirttiniemi P, Serlo W. Outcomes of 40 nonsyndromic sagittal craniosynostosis patients as adults: a case-control study with 26 years of postoperative follow-up. Oper Neurosurg. 2019; https://doi.org/10.1093/ons/opy047.
38. Salokorpi N. Treatment of craniosynostoses. Oulun yliopisto; 2017.
39. Svalina A, Vuollo V, Serlo W, Sinikumpu J-J, Silvola A-S, Salokorpi N. Craniofacial characteristics and cosmetic satisfaction of patients with sagittal and metopic synostosis: a case-control study using 3D photogrammetric imaging. Childs Nerv Syst. 2021; https://doi.org/10.1007/s00381-021-05434-y.
40. Szpalski C, Weichman K, Sagebin F, Warren SM. Need for standard outcome reporting systems in craniosynostosis. Neurosurg Focus. 2011;31:E1.
41. Feragen KJB, Myhre A, Stock NM. "Will you still feel beautiful when you find out you are different?": parents' experiences, reflections, and appearance-focused conversations about their Child's visible difference. Qual Health Res. 2022;32:3–15.
42. Feragen KB, Stock NM, Myhre A, Due-Tønnessen BJ. Medical stress reactions and personal growth in parents of children with a rare craniofacial condition. Cleft Palate Craniofac J. 2020;57:228–37.
43. Joseph S, Linley PA. Growth following adversity: theoretical perspectives and implications for clinical practice. Clin Psychol Rev. 2006;26:1041–53.
44. Heidekrueger PI, Szpalski C, Weichman K, Juran S, Ng R, Claussen C, Ninkovic M, Broer PN. Lip attractiveness: a cross-cultural analysis. Aesthet Surg J. 2017;37:828–36.

MIX
Papier aus verantwortungsvollen Quellen
Paper from responsible sources
FSC® C105338

If you have any concerns about our products,
you can contact us on
ProductSafety@springernature.com

In case Publisher is established outside the EU,
the EU authorized representative is:
Springer Nature Customer Service Center GmbH
Europaplatz 3, 69115 Heidelberg, Germany

Printed by Libri Plureos GmbH
in Hamburg, Germany